# DIAGNOSTIC IMAGING
# PEDIATRIC
# NEURORADIOLOGY

## A. James Barkovich, MD

Professor of Radiology, Neurology, Pediatrics and Neurosurgery
University of California at San Francisco
San Francisco, California

## Kevin R. Moore, MD

Pediatric Neuroradiologist
Primary Children's Medical Center

Adjunct Assistant Professor of Radiology
Section of Neuroradiology
University of Utah, School of Medicine
Salt Lake City, Utah

## Blaise V. Jones, MD

Division Chief, Neuroradiology
Cincinnati Children's Hospital Medical Center

Associate Professor, Radiology and Pediatrics
University of Cincinnati College of Medicine
Cincinnati, Ohio

## Gilbert Vézina, MD

Director, Program in Neuroradiology
Children's National Medical Center

Professor of Radiology and Pediatrics
The George Washington University School of Medicine and
Health Sciences
Washington, DC

## Bernadette L. Koch, MD

Associate Director, Radiology
Cincinnati Children's Hospital Medical Center

Associate Professor, Radiology and Pediatrics
University of Cincinnati College of Medicine
Cincinnati, Ohio

## Charles Raybaud, MD, FRCPC

Head of the Division of Neuroradiology
The Hospital for Sick Children

Professor of Radiology
University of Toronto
Toronto, Ontario

## P. Ellen Grant, MD

Division Chief, Pediatric Radiology
Massachusetts General Hospital
Athinoula A. Martinos Center for Biomedical Imaging

Associate Professor of Radiology
Harvard Medical School
Boston, Massachusetts

## Susan I. Blaser, MD, FRCPC

Pediatric Neuroradiologist
The Hospital for Sick Children

Associate Professor of Neuroradiology
The University of Toronto
Toronto, Ontario

## Gary L. Hedlund, DO

Pediatric Neuroradiologist
Chairman, Department of Medical Imaging
Primary Children's Medical Center
Salt Lake City, Utah

## Anna Illner, MD

Pediatric Neuroradiologist
Texas Children's Hospital

Assistant Professor of Radiology
Baylor College of Medicine
Houston, Texas

AMIRSYS®
Names you know, content you trust®

AMIRSYS®

Names you know, content you trust®

# First Edition

Text - Copyright A. James Barkovich, MD 2007

Drawings - Copyright Amirsys Inc 2007

Compilation - Copyright Amirsys Inc 2007

Composition by Amirsys Inc, Salt Lake City, Utah

Printed in Canada by Friesens, Altona, Manitoba, Canada

ISBN-13: 978-1-4160-4918-0
ISBN-10: 1-4160-4918-5
ISBN-13: 978-0-8089-2395-4 (International English Edition)
ISBN-10: 0-8089-2395-1 (International English Edition)

# Notice and Disclaimer

Library of Congress Cataloging-in-Publication Data

Diagnostic imaging pediatric neuroradiology / A. James Barkovich ... [et al.]. -- 1st ed.
    p. ; cm.
 Includes bibliographical references and index.
 ISBN-13: 978-1-4160-4918-0
 ISBN-10: 1-4160-4918-5
 ISBN-13: 978-0-8089-2395-4 (international English ed.)
 ISBN-10: 0-8089-2395-1 (international English ed.)
 1. Pediatric neurology--Diagnosis. 2. Pediatric diagnostic imaging. 3. Nervous system--Radiography. I. Barkovich, A. James, 1952-
 [DNLM: 1. Central Nervous System Diseases--radiography--Outlines. 2. Child. 3. Head--radiography--Outlines. 4. Neck--radiography--Outlines. 5. Neuroradiography--methods--Outlines. 6. Spine--radiography--Outlines. WS 18.2 D536 2007]

 RJ488.5.R33D43 2007
 618.92'8--dc22

                                    2007009069

To my wife, Karen, and our boys, Matthew, Krister, and Emil.
They keep me focused on what is really important.

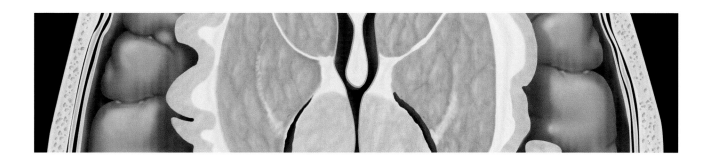

# DIAGNOSTIC IMAGING: PEDIATRIC NEURORADIOLOGY

We at Amirsys and Elsevier are proud to present Diagnostic Imaging: Pediatric Neuroradiology, the eleventh volume in our acclaimed Diagnostic Imaging (DI) series. We began this precedent-setting, image- and graphics-rich series with David Stoller's Diagnostic Imaging: Orthopaedics. The next volumes, DI: Brain, DI: Head and Neck, DI: Abdomen, DI: Spine, DI: Pediatrics, DI: Obstetrics, DI: Chest, DI: Breast and DI: Ultrasound are now joined by James Barkovich's fabulous new textbook, DI: Pediatric Neuroradiology.

Dr. Barkovich and his crack team of acknowledged experts in pediatric neuroimaging have chosen and exquisitely illustrated the most important disorders of the brain, spine, head and neck that occur in children. This extensive diagnostic list includes not only diseases that are predominately or exclusively pediatric. They have also included a number of important "adult" diagnoses that can be found in children. Some of these "adult" disorders may have a somewhat different imaging spectrum when they occur in children.

Again, the unique bulleted format of the DI series allows our authors to present approximately twice the information and four times the images per diagnosis compared to the old-fashioned traditional prose textbook. All the DI books follow the same format, which means that our many readers find the same information in the same place—every time! And in every body part! The innovative visual differential diagnosis "thumbnail" provides you with an at-a-glance look at entities that can mimic the diagnosis in question and has been highly popular (and much copied). "Key Facts" boxes provide a succinct summary for quick, easy review.

In summary, Diagnostic Imaging: Pediatric Neuroradiology is a product designed with you, the reader, in mind. Today's typical practice settings demand efficiency in both image interpretation and learning. You may see a relatively small percentage of pediatric patients. When (not if) you do, you need the right information, right at your fingertips! We think you'll find this new volume a highly efficient and wonderfully rich resource that will significantly enhance your practice—and find a welcome place on your bookshelf. Enjoy!

Anne G. Osborn, MD
Executive Vice President & Editor-in-Chief, Amirsys, Inc.

H. Ric Harnsberger, MD
CEO & Chairman, Amirsys, Inc.

Paula J. Woodward, MD
Senior Vice President & Medical Director, Amirsys, Inc.

# PREFACE

This book presents a new approach to Pediatric Neuroradiology in which a great deal of information is presented in a bulleted format. The information is concise, and the figures are plentiful and of high quality. As someone who grew up reading textbooks, I will admit that it took a while for the concept of a bulleted textbook of Pediatric Neuroradiology to grow on me. I worried that the nuances of this fascinating specialty, which are often woven into the text of a traditional textbook, might get lost. A loss of nuances would be dangerous in a rapidly evolving field where there is little true understanding of the disorders and where the borderlines between disorders blur if examined closely enough. However, such a book is very useful in the daily practice of neuroradiology, where it is often important to find an answer quickly. Indeed, by searching through many images and reading the Key Facts and selected bulleted information in every chapter, an understanding of the most likely diagnosis and the differential diagnoses is quickly achieved. Thus, this is a very useful book for the practicing radiologist.

Although it initially seemed that this book would be a lengthy undertaking, it was proved once again that, when good people are recruited, even the most challenging tasks can be beautifully accomplished in a reasonable time. This book is largely the work of my hard-working, talented and accomplished co-authors; their contributions along with the assistance of Amirsys staff, has allowed this book to very successfully accomplish its task: to present in an easily accessible manner most of the important disorders of the brain, spine, head and neck that are found in children. In this book, these disorders are beautifully illustrated with many representative MRI, CT, proton spectroscopy, and angiographic images. A short and thoughtful differential diagnosis is presented for each diagnosis. The clinical manifestations of each disorder are listed. For those interested in the underlying genetics or pathology, those important details are included, as well. The reader will notice that some of the disorders presented in this book are often seen in adults and might be considered "adult" rather than "pediatric" disorders by some. However, many disorders can present in either children or adults: "pediatric" disorders in adults and vice versa. Therefore, it was decided that, for the convenience of the user, it was better to be inclusive and put a few such diagnoses in this text. We hope the readers will appreciate this feature and find that it saves them time.

The authors hope that the readers will find this book of Pediatric Neuroradiology a useful tool for learning and that it will be both convenient and useful in their practices.

A. James Barkovich, MD
Professor of Radiology, Neurology, Pediatrics and Neurosurgery
University of California at San Francisco
San Francisco, California

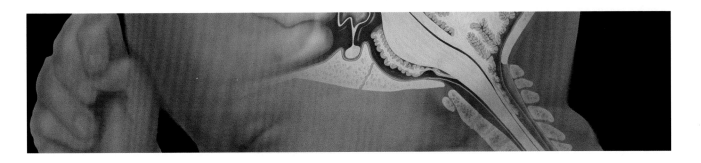

# ACKNOWLEDGMENTS

## Illustrations
Richard Coombs, MS
Lane R. Bennion, MS
James A. Cooper, MD

## Image/Text Editing
Douglas Grant Jackson
Amanda Hurtado
Christopher Odekirk

## Medical Text Editing
Henry J. Baskin, Jr., MD
Jeffrey S. Anderson, MD

## Contributing Authors
H. Ric Harnsberger, MD
H. Christian Davidson, MD

## Associate Editor
Kaerli Main

## Production Lead
Melissa A. Hoopes

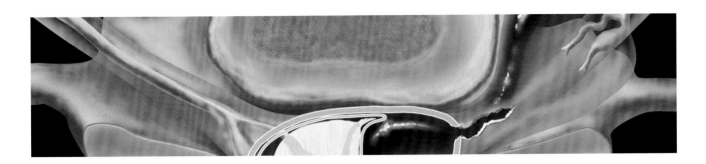

# SECTIONS

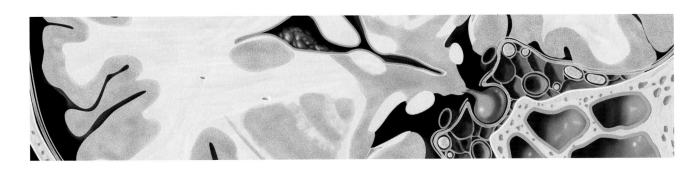

# TABLE OF CONTENTS

# PART II
## Head & Neck

## SECTION 1
## Temporal Bone & Skull Base

## SECTION 2
## Orbit, Nose and Sinuses

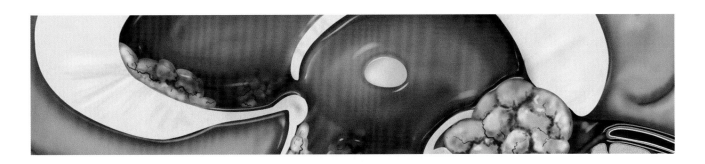

# ABBREVIATIONS

H: Proton

3T (imaging): 3 Tesla

ACA: Anterior cerebral artery

AcoA: Anterior communicating artery

ACTH: Adrenocorticotrophic hormone

ADC: Apparent diffusion coefficient

AICA: Anterior inferior cerebellar artery

ApoE: Apolipoprotein E

BA: Basilar artery

BCKD: Branched-chain Alpha-keto dehydrogenase

BFGF: Basic fibroblast growth factor

CBLL: Cerebellar

Cf: Compare

CHARGE: Coloboma; Heart defects; Atresia of choanae; Retardation of growth; Genitourinary abnormalities; Ear abnormalities

Cho: Choline

CN(s): Cranial nerve(s)

CNS: Central nervous system

COW: Circle of Willis

CPA-IAC: Cerebellopontine angle-internal auditory canal

Cr: Creatine

CSF: Cerebrospinal fluid

CST: Cavernous sinus thrombosis

CVT: Cerebral venous thrombosis

DSA: Digital subtraction angiography

ECA: External carotid artery

F/U: Follow-up

FDG: Fluordeoxygluose

GA1: Glutaric academia type 1

GFAP: Glial fibrillary acidic protein

GM1/2: Gangliosidosis 1/2

HA: Headache

HGBL(s): Hemangioblastoma(s)

HHT: Hereditary hemorrhagic telangiectasia

HMPAO: Hexamethylopropyleneamine oxime

HU: Hounsfield unit

HUS: Hemolytic-uremic syndrome

ICA: Internal carotid artery

ICH: Intracranial hemorrhage

IC-PCoA: Internal carotid-posterior communicating artery junction

INO: Internuclear ophthalmopligia

Ino: Inositol

ION: Inferior olivary nucleus

IVH: Intraventricular hemorrhage

LHX3: LIM homeobox 3 gene

LHX4: LIM homeobox 4 gene

LV: Lateral ventricle

MCA: Middle cerebral artery

MEN1: Multiple endocrine neoplasia 1

MIB-1: Histologic marker of cell proliferation

MIH: Melanotropin release-inhibiting hormone

MIP: Maximum intensity projection

MSH: Melanotropin stimulating hormone

NAT: Nonaccidental trauma

NF: Neurofibromatosis

NSE: Neural-specific enolase

**NTD(s):** Neural tube defect(s)

**OMIM:** Online Mendelian Inheritance in Man

**PAS:** Periodic acid schiff

**PCA:** Posterior cerebral artery

**PCoA:** Posterior communicating artery

**PICA:** Posterior inferior cerebellar artery

**PVSs:** Perivascular space(s)

**rCBF:** Relative cerebral blood flow

**rCBV:** Relative cerebral blood volume

**S/P:** Following (status post)

**SAH:** Subarachnoid hemorrhage

**SPECT:** Single photon emission computed tomography

**SPGR:** Spoiled gradient refocused

**SSAC(s):** Suprasellar arachnoid cyst(s)

**SSS:** Superior sagittal sinus

**TBI:** Traumatic brain injury

**TOF:** Time of flight

**TS:** Transverse sinus

**VA:** Vertebral artery

**VACTERL:** Vertebral Anal Cardiac Tracheal Esophageal Renal Limb

**VEGF:** Vascular endothelial growth factor

**VHL:** von Hippel Lindau

**WM:** White matter

**WWS:** Walker-Warburg syndrome

# DIAGNOSTIC IMAGING
## PEDIATRIC
## NEURORADIOLOGY

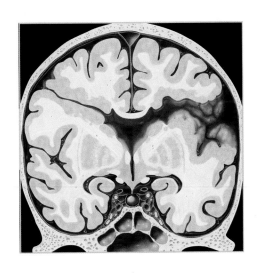

# PART I
**Brain**

---

Cerebral Hemispheres  [1]

Sella/Suprasellar  [2]

Pineal Region  [3]

Cerebellum/Brain Stem  [4]

Ventricular System  [5]

Meninges, Cisterns, Calvarium, Skull Base  [6]

Blood Vessels  [7]

Multiple Regions, Brain  [8]

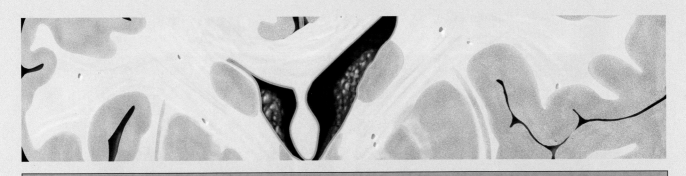

# SECTION 1: Cerebral Hemispheres

# CONCEPTS OF BRAIN MALFORMATION

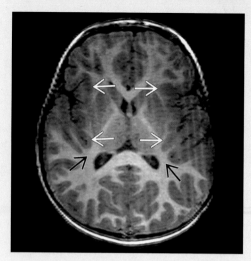

Axial T1WI MR shows normal appearance of Sylvian fissures ➡. Cortex is of normal & uniform thickness. Opercula cover the insulae. A thick band of white matter ➡ lies between parietal operculum & trigone.

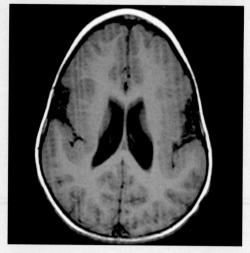

Axial T1WI MR shows bilateral sylvian polymicrogyria. The cortex is thickened, opercular are underdeveloped, and white matter is thinned between posterior operculum and trigone.

## TERMINOLOGY

### Synonyms
- Malformation, dysmorphism, dysgenesis

### Definitions
- Malformation: Result of absence or disruption of normal developmental brain processes
  - May result from abnormal gene expression
    - Many different genes identified, characterized
  - May result from injury to brain at time when gene is expressed
    - Injury may be from ischemia, infection, toxin (maternal ingestion or metabolic disorder)

## IMAGING ANATOMY

### General Anatomic Considerations
- Examine entire brain in three planes
  - Sagittal for midline and lateral structures
  - Coronal for cerebellum, temporal and parietal lobes
  - Axial for sylvian fissures, midbrain, frontal and occipital lobes

### Critical Anatomic Structures
- Cerebral cortex: Proper development and connections critical for normal cognition and neurologic function
  - Initially smooth, agyric
    - Sulci and gyri develop as development proceeds
  - Sylvian fissure: 16 weeks
  - Parieto-occipital sulcus: 23 weeks
  - Calcarine sulcus: 24 weeks
  - Cingulate sulcus: 24 weeks
  - Marginal sulcus: 27 weeks
  - Collateral sulcus: 26 weeks
  - Occipito-temporal sulcus: 33 weeks
  - Central sulcus: 25 weeks
  - Precentral sulcus: 27 weeks
  - Postcentral sulcus: 28 weeks
  - Superior frontal sulcus: 27-28 weeks
  - Inferior frontal sulcus: 29 weeks
  - Interparietal sulcus: 27 weeks

- Superior temporal sulcus (posterior): 27 weeks
- Cerebral commissures important for transfer of information in brain
  - Corpus callosum: Connects neocortical cerebral hemispheric white matter
    - Look for rostrum, genu, body, isthmus, splenium
  - Hippocampal commissure: Connects fornices
    - Cannot separate hippocampal commissure from callosal splenium on sagittal images
    - Sometimes seen better when corpus is hypogenetic or absent
  - Anterior commissure: Connects temporal lobes
    - Lies at junction of callosal rostrum and lamina terminalis (anterior wall of 3rd ventricle)
- Sylvian fissures (central portion of cerebral hemisphere): Many important pathways run around or near sylvian fissures
  - First appear at 16 weeks gestational age
  - Initially flat and uncovered
  - Slowly covered by opercula: Frontal, parietal, and temporal
- Cerebellum: Many important functions, including cognition
  - Connects with cerebrum, brain stem, and spinal cord
  - Forms from the uppermost segment (r1) of the midline dorsal metencephalon
  - Vermis: Forms from the anterior part of r1
  - Hemispheres: Form from the posterior part of r1
  - Brain stem: Strong developmental associations between cerebellum and midbrain tegmentum, ventral pons, inferior olives
- Basal cerebral nuclei: Thalami, caudate nuclei, putamina, globi pallidi, subthalamic nuclei
  - Connected in complex network with each other and with cerebral cortex
  - Nomenclature: Striatum (caudate + putamen); basal ganglia (caudate + putamen + globus pallidus); lentiform nucleus (putamen + globus pallidus)

### Anatomic Relationships
- Cerebral cortex

# CONCEPTS OF BRAIN MALFORMATION

## Key Facts

### Etiology
- Malformations may result from abnormal gene expression or disruption when gene is expressed

### Imaging
- Imaging technique must be optimized for age
  - Thinner sections required in infants
  - Long TR, TE conventional spin echo images optimal for T2 contrast in neonates
- Brain must be visualized in multiple planes
- Acquisition of 3D data set with thin partitions allows reformation in multiple planes

### Evaluation of Images
- Must know normal appearance of brain at patient's age to recognize abnormal

- Evaluate cerebral commissures, cerebral cortex, white matter, interhemispheric fissure, basal ganglia, cerebellum, brain stem
- Lateral convexities, midline structures (commissures, 3rd ventricle, pineal region, brain stem, vermis) best evaluated in sagittal plane
- Superior convexities best evaluated in coronal plane
- Cerebellar hemispheres, basal ganglia best evaluated in coronal, axial planes
- Learn fundamental embryology to best understand imaging appearance of brain malformations

### Diagnostics
- Knowledge of basic genetics, close collaboration with geneticists aid in diagnosis of malformations

---

- Cortex is thin (2-3 mm) with smooth gray-white junction
- Precentral cortex is especially thin
- Formed from cells originating in germinal matrices (ventricular zones)
  - Glutamatergic neurons from zones in dorsal walls of lateral ventricles
  - GABAergic and other inhibitory neurons from more ventral ventricular walls (ganglionic eminences)
- Sylvian fissures
  - Initially open with rounded margins surrounding insula
    - Frontal lobe: Anterior, superior
    - Parietal lobe: Posterior, superior
    - Temporal lobe: Inferior
  - At mid-gestation margins of fissures become squared
  - Frontal, parietal, temporal opercula grow, cover insular cortex by end of first postnatal year
- Commissures: Corpus callosum
  - Superior callosal axons connect medial hemispheres; inferior axons connect lateral hemispheres
  - Genu: Connects anterior frontal lobes
  - Body: Connects posterior frontal lobes and parietal lobes
  - Splenium: Connects occipital lobes
- Other commissures
  - Hippocampal commissure connects cingula
  - Anterior commissure connects anterior temporal lobes
- Cerebellum: Glutamatergic neurons form in rhombic lips; GABAergic neurons form in dorsal ventricular zone
  - Deep cerebellar nuclei: Glutamatergic
  - Granule cortical neurons: Glutamatergic
  - Unipolar brush cells (cortical): Glutamatergic
  - Purkinje cells (cortical): GABAergic
  - Inhibitory interneurons (cortical): GABAergic
- Basal cerebral nuclei
  - Cells derive from ventral ventricular walls (ganglionic eminences)
  - Most are GABAergic or cholinergic

## ANATOMY-BASED IMAGING ISSUES

### Key Concepts or Questions
- Knowledge of normal anatomy is critical in identifying malformations
  - Identification of subtle anomalies otherwise difficult
- Single malformation or malformation syndrome
  - Malformation syndrome composed of multiple anomalies
  - Associated anomalies may be external to CNS
- Genetic vs. acquired malformation
  - Genetic: Mutations result in formation of abnormal proteins ⇒ abnormal brain development
  - Acquired: Injury during period when normal proteins are expressed ⇒ abnormal brain development

### Imaging Approaches
- See in multiple planes with optimal tissue contrast
- Optimal gray matter-white matter contrast varies according to age
  - Best on T2WI prior to age 10 months
    - Spin-echo T2 prior to 8 months, inversion recovery T2 after 8 months
  - Best on T1WI after 10 months
    - Inversion recovery > spoiled gradient echo > spin echo
- Look at cerebral and cerebellar cortex (thickness and gyral pattern), midline structures (proper size and morphology), white matter (proper volume and signal intensity), and interhemispheric fissure (entire cerebrum)
  - Sagittal plane best for lateral cerebral convexities, cerebellar vermis, brain stem
  - Coronal plane best for cerebellar hemispheres, walls of lateral ventricles, temporal lobes
  - Axial plane best for basal ganglia, insular cortex, interhemispheric fissure
- Always evaluate brain stem when cerebellum is small or dysmorphic

# CONCEPTS OF BRAIN MALFORMATION

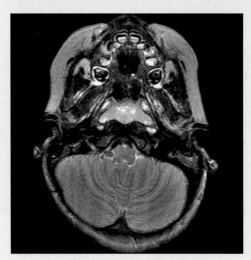

Axial T2WI MR shows normal cerebellar anatomy. Folia and fissures are concentric, running parallel to the inner table of the occipital bone.

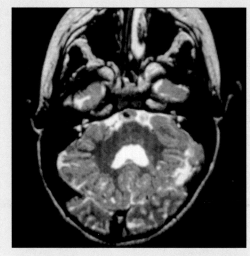

Axial T2WI MR shows a diffusely dysmorphic cerebellar cortex. Folia and fissures have random orientation. 4th ventricle is too large. No discrete vermis is identified.

## Imaging Protocols

- Three dimensional spoiled gradient echo T1WI through entire brain
  - Excellent gray-white contrast
  - Isotropic voxels
  - Reformat in at least two orthogonal planes
- T2WI with optimal gray-white contrast
  - Conventional spin echo has better contrast resolution than turbo spin echo
  - Heavily T2WI (TR = 3000 ms, TE = 120 ms) before 12 months
- Contrast-enhancement rarely useful
- Diffusion tensor tractography (DTT) becoming important to identify white matter abnormalities
  - Best if diffusion gradient is applied in multiple directions

## Imaging Pitfalls

- Isointensity of gray matter and white matter at certain stages of development
  - Must use sequences that have maximal contrast between gray matter and white matter
  - Sequences must vary with age/stage of myelination of patient
- Malformations may not be appreciated if seen in the wrong plane
  - View entire brain in at least 2 (prefer 3) planes
  - May need to reformat 3D data set in oblique planes

## PATHOLOGIC ISSUES

### Classification

- Cerebral commissures
  - Which commissures involved?
    - If corpus callosum: Genu, body, splenium, or rostrum
  - Interhemispheric cyst?
    - Type I or type II
  - Associated malformations?
- Malformations of cortical development classified based on developmental stage that went wrong

- Malformations secondary to abnormalities of stem cell development/apoptosis
  - Focal cortical dysplasias, hemimegalencephaly, microcephalies
  - All ⇒ abnormal signal extending from ventricle to pia
- Malformations secondary to abnormal neuronal migration
  - Heterotopia, lissencephalies, congenital muscular dystrophies
  - Heterotopia ⇒ nodules of gray matter in white matter
  - Lissencephalies ⇒ thick cortex, smooth inner margin ± cell-sparse layer
  - Congenital muscular dystrophies ⇒ delayed myelination, cerebellar dysplasia
- Malformations secondary to abnormal cortical organization
  - Polymicrogyria, schizencephalies
  - Cortex is "festooned" with irregular cortical-white matter junction
- Cerebellar malformations
  - Focal versus diffuse malformation
    - If focal, vermis versus hemisphere
  - Hypoplastic versus dysmorphic structure
  - Brain stem affected?
- Holoprosencephaly
  - Alobar, semilobar, lobar, or middle interhemispheric variant
  - Key features: Deep cerebral nuclei, hemispheres continuous across midline

## RELATED REFERENCES

1. Barkovich AJ et al: A developmental and genetic classification for malformations of cortical development. Neurology. 65(12):1873-87, 2005
2. Patel S et al: Analysis and classification of cerebellar malformations. AJNR Am J Neuroradiol. 23(7):1074-87, 2002
3. Plawner LL et al: Neuroanatomy of holoprosencephaly as predictor of function: beyond the face predicting the brain. Neurology. 59(7):1058-66, 2002

## IMAGE GALLERY

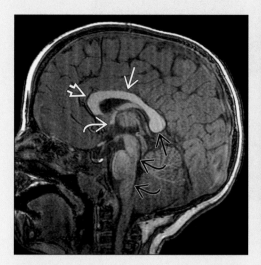 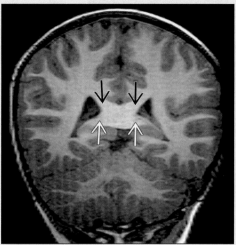

*(Left)* Sagittal T1WI MR shows normal midline structures: Anterior commissure ➡, callosal genu ➡, body ➡, splenium and hippocampal commissure ➡, brain stem ➡, chiasm, pituitary, and vermis. *(Right)* Coronal T1WI MR shows the two components of the splenium. The upper portion ➡ is composed of axons from the occipital lobes, the lower part ➡ connects the hippocampal crura.

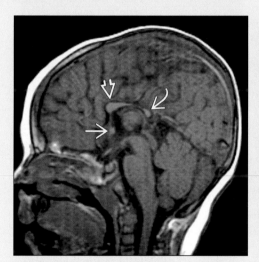 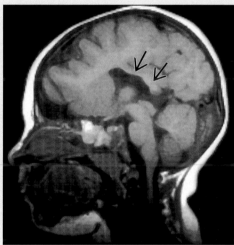

*(Left)* Sagittal T1WI MR shows hypogenesis of the corpus callosum ➡ with normal hippocampal ➡ and anterior ➡ commissures. *(Right)* Sagittal T1WI MR shows presence of the callosal splenium and posterior body ➡ without genu or anterior body. This morphology strongly suggests a diagnosis of semilobar holoprosencephaly.

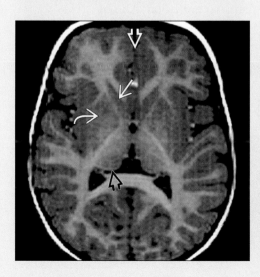 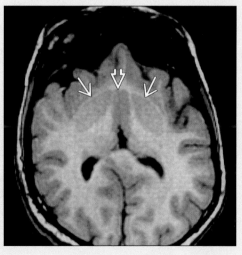

*(Left)* Axial T1WI MR shows normal caudate heads ➡, lentiform nuclei ➡, and thalami ➡, separated in the midline by the interhemispheric fissure ➡ and the third ventricle. *(Right)* Axial T1WI MR shows absence of anterior interhemispheric fissure, lack of separation of caudate nuclei in the midline ➡, and medially deviated basal ganglia ➡ in holoprosencephaly.

# HOLOPROSENCEPHALY

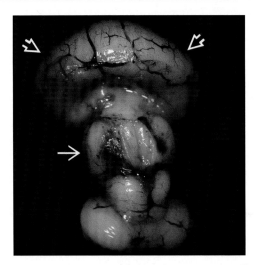

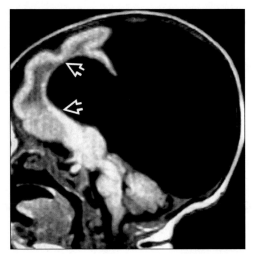

Anteroposterior gross pathology shows a very small cerebrum ⇨ with complete absence of interhemispheric fissure. Basal ganglia ⇨ are small, fused, and not distinct from the midbrain.

Sagittal T1WI MR of alobar holoprosencephaly shows a small focus of brain ⇨ within the anterior calvarium with a large dorsal cyst pushing it forward and pushing the cerebellum and brainstem down.

## TERMINOLOGY

### Abbreviations and Synonyms

- Holoprosencephaly (HPE), interhemispheric fissure (IHF), middle interhemispheric variant (MIH), interhemispheric cyst (IHC)

### Definitions

- Spectrum of congenital forebrain malformations characterized by lack of formation of midline structures
- Traditionally divided into alobar, semilobar, and lobar forms, plus MIH (also called syntelencephaly)

## IMAGING FINDINGS

### General Features

- Best diagnostic clue
  - Alobar HPE (most severe) ⇒ "pancake" of anterior cerebral tissue
  - Semilobar HPE ⇒ caudate heads fused in midline
  - Lobar HPE (least severe)⇒ absent anterior midline falx and fissure, hypoplastic genu

  - MIH ⇒ sylvian fissures connected across midline over vertex (86%)
- Location
  - Most severe involvement is anterior, ventral and medial
  - Least severe is posterior, dorsal and lateral
- Size: Microcephalic unless large dorsal cyst is present

### CT Findings

- NECT
  - Alobar: Monoventricle, often incompletely covered posteriorly by brain ⇒ dorsal "cyst"
    - No interhemispheric fissure or sylvian fissures
    - Dorsal cyst and hydrocephalus cause macrocephaly
  - Semilobar: Absent septum pellucidum, partial occipital and temporal horns
  - Lobar: Absent septum pellucidum; formed lateral ventricles but dysplastic frontal horns
  - Skull base/vault
    - Cleft palate; variable optic canal hypoplasia
    - Absent or hypoplastic ethmoid sinus, anterior falx (and superior sagittal sinus), crista galli

## DDx: Holoprosencephaly Mimics

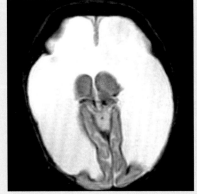

Hydranencephaly

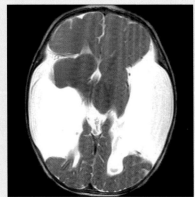

Schizencephaly

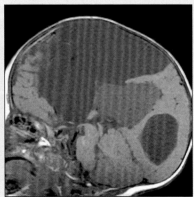

ACC with IHC

# HOLOPROSENCEPHALY

## Key Facts

### Terminology
- Spectrum of congenital forebrain malformations characterized by lack of formation of midline structures

### Imaging Findings
- Alobar ⇒ absent corpus callosum, dorsal cyst, cerebral tissue flattened anteriorly
- Semilobar ⇒ posterior corpus callosum present and titled back
- Lobar ⇒ genu of corpus callosum "fades" away
- Grayscale Ultrasound: Diagnosable on fetal ultrasound (and fetal MR)

### Top Differential Diagnoses
- Severe Hydrocephalus
- Bilateral Open-Lip Schizencephaly

- Callosal Agenesis (ACC) with Interhemispheric Cyst
- Hydranencephaly

### Pathology
- Mutations affecting signaling genes that regulate dorsal-ventral patterning of neural tube
- Result ⇒ more lateral structures are in midline and "fused"

### Clinical Issues
- "Face predicts brain": Severe midline anomaly ⇒ severe HPE
- Over-represented in fetal demise, stillbirths

### Diagnostic Checklist
- Distinguish HPE from mimics (which have better prognosis)

---

○ MIH: Normal IHF anterior frontal and occipital lobes; absent IHF posterior frontal/parietal lobes

## MR Findings
- T1WI
  - Sagittal imaging
    - Alobar ⇒ absent corpus callosum, dorsal cyst, cerebral tissue flattened anteriorly
    - Semilobar ⇒ posterior corpus callosum present and titled back
    - Lobar ⇒ genu of corpus callosum "fades" away
    - MIH ⇒ central body of callosum absent, with dysmorphic gray matter (GM) in defect
  - Axial imaging
    - Amadeus ventricle in alobar HPE
    - Small or absent 3rd ventricle
    - Crossing sulcus/gyrus resembles schizencephalic clefts in MIH
- T2WI
  - Delayed myelin maturation in classical HPE, but normal in middle hemispheric variant (MIH)
  - Following are variable (worst in alobar, mildest in lobar)
    - Degree of frontal lobe hypoplasia, basal nuclei fusion
    - Presence of dorsal cyst (suprapineal recess)
    - Degree of hypoplasia or absence of olfactory nerves (best seen on coronal views)
    - Subcortical heterotopia anterior to interhemispheric fissure and subjacent to shallow frontal sulci
  - Semilobar and lobar HPE are often microcephalic
- MRA: Azygous or absent anterior cerebral artery (ACA)
- MRV
  - Absent superior sagittal, inferior sagittal and straight sinuses
  - Cortical veins and deep veins drain directly to torcular

## Radiographic Findings
- Radiography: Hypotelorism, fused metopic suture or single frontal "plate" of bone, variable degree of microcephaly

## Ultrasonographic Findings
- Grayscale Ultrasound: Diagnosable on fetal ultrasound (and fetal MR)
- Color Doppler: Absent superior sagittal sinus, variable absence of deep and midline venous structures

## Imaging Recommendations
- Best imaging tool: MR
- Protocol advice: Multiplanar MR with special attention to midline structures

## DIFFERENTIAL DIAGNOSIS

### Severe Hydrocephalus
- Macrocephalic (HPE usually microcephalic)
- PD/intermediate best to show residual thin mantle of cortex underneath calvaria
- Preservation of falx

### Bilateral Open-Lip Schizencephaly
- Large and bilateral schizencephaly can mimic semilobar or alobar HPE
- Residual posterior cerebral tissue along falx
- Anterior falx preserved

### Callosal Agenesis (ACC) with Interhemispheric Cyst
- Much better prognosis than alobar HPE
- Thalamic fusion (HPE has nonseparated basal ganglia)
- IHC displaces cerebral tissue to sides of cranium, not to front

### Hydranencephaly
- Obliteration of parenchyma in carotid territory
- Residual cerebral tissue is along top of tentorium (posterior cerebral artery territory)

### Other Holoprosencephaly Spectrum Disorders
- Septo-optic dysplasia
- Central incisor syndrome

# HOLOPROSENCEPHALY

- Nonspecific midline dysplasias & frontonasal dysplasia, agnathia-otocephaly, anencephaly

## PATHOLOGY

### General Features
- General path comments
  - Anomaly of dorsal-ventral induction of neural tube
    - Lack of ventral midline induction ⇒ classical holoprosencephaly
    - Lack of dorsal midline induction ⇒ middle interhemispheric variant
- Genetics
  - Cytogenetic abnormality in 50%: Especially trisomy 13; also 18q-, 18p-, 3p, 7-, trisomy 9, 1q15q, 11q12-q13
  - Familial HPE: 5+ implicated genes
    - HPE1 (21q22.3), HPE2 (SIX3 - 2p21), HPE3 (Sonic hedgehog gene - 7q36), HPE4 (TGIF-18p), HPE5 (ZIC2 - 13q32)
- Etiology
  - Mutations affecting signaling genes that regulate dorsal-ventral patterning of neural tube
  - Most medial aspects of hemispheres fail to form
    - Result ⇒ more lateral structures are in midline and "fused"
- Epidemiology: 1 to 1.4 per 10,000 live births
- Associated abnormalities
  - Maternal risk factors
    - ETOH, diabetes, retinoic acid, hypocholesterolemia
    - Infants of diabetic mothers ⇒ alobar HPE with normal facies
  - Facial anomalies ⇒ central incisor; proboscis; single naris; single nasal bone/absent internasal suture and caudal metopic suture
    - +/- Midline facial clefting; premaxillary agenesis if severe; absent superior lingual frenulum
  - Non-facial/non-CNS anomalies 65%

### Gross Pathologic & Surgical Features
- Extreme hypoplasia of neocortex
- Severe cases ⇒ absence of frontal lobes and basal ganglia
  - Dorsal cyst (especially in association with noncleaved thalamus) felt to represent expansion of partially blocked posterodorsal 3rd ventricle
- Milder cases ⇒ more frontal lobe development, more basal ganglia

### Staging, Grading or Classification Criteria
- Alobar, semilobar, lobar classification of DeMyer
- MIH described as HPE variant by Barkovich in 1993, clinically milder
- Arrhinencephaly ⇒ absence of olfactory bulbs
  - Associated finding with HPE versus variant
- Septo-optic dysplasia ⇒ more severe cases overlap with HPE in etiology and presentation

## CLINICAL ISSUES

### Presentation
- Most common signs/symptoms
  - Mentally retarded, microcephalic, disturbed endocrine function, athetosis, ± facial anomalies
  - Worst (classic alobar HPE) = cyclopia, proboscis, midline facial clefting, microcephaly
  - Most common "brain plus face" malformation
    - "Face predicts brain": Severe midline anomaly ⇒ severe HPE
    - Function predicted by degree of non-separation of brain structures, frontal lobe hypoplasia
- Other signs/symptoms
  - Seizures (50%) and mental retardation: Most severe with cortical malformations
  - Severity of pituitary/hypothalamic malfunction correlates with degree of hypothalamic non-separation

### Demographics
- Age: Presentation in infancy (can be diagnosed with fetal US or MRI)
- Gender: M:F = 1.4:1

### Natural History & Prognosis
- Over-represented in fetal demise, stillbirths
- Clinical severity relates to degree of hemispheric and deep gray nuclei non-separation

### Treatment
- Treat seizures and endocrine dysfunction

## DIAGNOSTIC CHECKLIST

### Consider
- Distinguish HPE from mimics (which have better prognosis)

### Image Interpretation Pearls
- Alobar HPE and mimics all displace residual brain
  - Recognize presence of posterior residual or lateral displacement to spot mimics

## SELECTED REFERENCES

1. Barkovich AJ: Pediatric Neuroimaging. 4th ed. Lippincott Williams & Wilkins. 364-74, 2005
2. Hayashi M et al: Neuropathological evaluation of the diencephalon, basal ganglia and upper brainstem in alobar holoprosencephaly. Acta Neuropathol. 107(3):190-6, 2004
3. Pulitzer SB et al: Prenatal MR findings of the middle interhemispheric variant of holoprosencephaly. AJNR Am J Neuroradiol. 25(6):1034-6, 2004
4. Barkovich AJ et al: Analysis of the cerebral cortex in HPE with attention to the Sylvian fissures. AJNR. 23:143-50, 2002
5. Blaas HG et al: Brains and faces in holoprosencephaly: pre- and postnatal description of 30 cases. Ultrasound Obstet Gynecol. 19(1):24-38, 2002
6. Simon EM et al: The dorsal cyst in holoprosencephaly and the role of the thalamus in its formation. Neuroradiology. 43(9):787-91, 2002
7. Simon EM et al: The middle interhemispheric variant of holoprosencephaly. AJNR. 23(1):151-6, 2002

# HOLOPROSENCEPHALY

## IMAGE GALLERY

### Variant

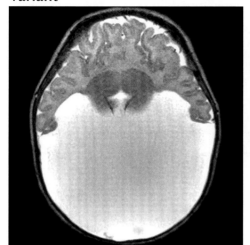
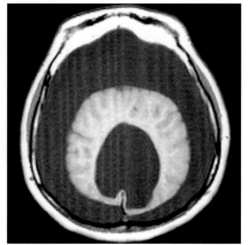

*(Left)* Axial T2WI MR shows alobar HPE with large dorsal cyst. Note the small, unseparated basal ganglia and absent 3rd ventricle. *(Right)* Axial T1WI MR shows a ball of tissue surrounding a round monoventricle. Large bilateral chronic subdural hematomas surround the cerebrum. Note the absence of a falx cerebri.

### Typical

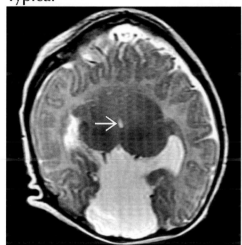
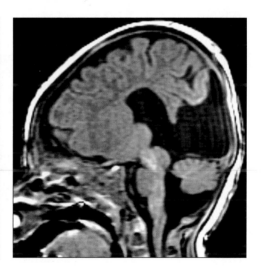

*(Left)* Axial T2WI MR shows typical semilobar HPE. Deep gray nuclei are nearly normal in size but incompletely separated. Small 3rd ventricle ➡ and dorsal cyst are present. Almost no frontal lobe is seen. *(Right)* Sagittal T1WI MR shows typical semilobar HPE with small dorsal cyst and presence of the posterior body/splenium of corpus callosum.

### Typical

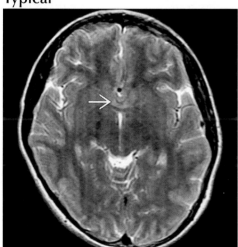
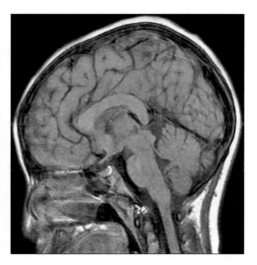

*(Left)* Axial T2WI MR shows very mild lobar HPE. Hemispheres lack separation ➡ only immediately anterior to the anterior commissure. Basal ganglia and frontal lobes are nearly normal. *(Right)* Sagittal T1WI MR of same patient as previous image shows very mild anomaly of corpus callosum with absent genu and rostrum, and dysplastic splenium.

# SYNTELENCEPHALY

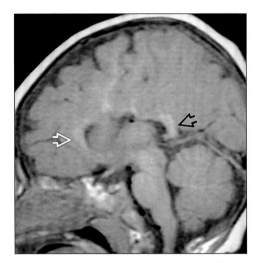

Sagittal T1WI MR shows typical appearance of MIH. Callosal genu ➡ and splenium ▷ are present without intervening body. No cingulum is present, showing abnormal sulcation of the midline.

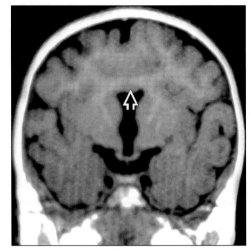

Coronal T1WI MR shows absence of interhemispheric fissure in the posterior frontal lobes. Heterotopic gray matter ➡ lines the roof of the lateral ventricles. Basal ganglia are normal.

## TERMINOLOGY

### Abbreviations and Synonyms
- Middle interhemispheric variant of holoprosencephaly (MIH); syntelencephaly, holoprosencephaly (HPE)

### Definitions
- Variant of HPE characterized by lack of separation of posterior frontal lobes

## IMAGING FINDINGS

### General Features
- Best diagnostic clue: Midline continuity of posterior frontal/parietal lobes + normal separation of frontal/occipital poles
- Size: Typically normocephalic
- Morphology
  - "Fusion" of dorsal aspect of cerebral hemispheres, usually posterior frontal lobes
  - Normal ventral hemispheres, basal ganglia, hypothalamus

### MR Findings
- T1WI
  - Abnormal sylvian fissure (SF) spans both hemispheres
  - Fused posterior frontal or parietal lobes
  - Dysgenetic corpus callosum (CC): Genu and splenium only
  - Dorsal cyst in 25%
  - Hypothalamus, thalami, basal ganglia normal
- T2WI: Similar to T1WI
- MRA: Azygous anterior cerebral artery (ACA)

### Imaging Recommendations
- Best imaging tool: MR thin sections in 3 planes

## DIFFERENTIAL DIAGNOSIS

### Classic Holoprosencephaly
- Failure of cleavage of hypothalamus, basal ganglia, prefrontal cerebrum

### Bilateral Schizencephaly
- Clefts communicate with ventricles

## DDx: Syntelencephaly Mimics

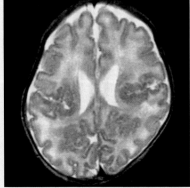

Perisylvian Polymicrogyria

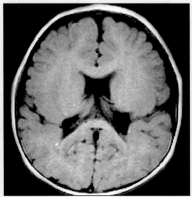

Bilateral Schizencephaly

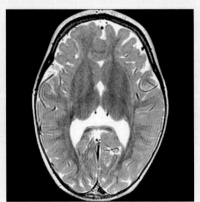

Lobar Holoprosencephaly

# SYNTELENCEPHALY

## Key Facts

### Terminology
- Variant of HPE characterized by lack of separation of posterior frontal lobes

### Top Differential Diagnoses
- Classic Holoprosencephaly
- Bilateral Schizencephaly
- Bilateral Perisylvian Polymicrogyria (PMG)

### Pathology
- Linked to ZIC2 mutation at 13q32, other dorsal induction genes

### Clinical Issues
- Spasticity, hypotonia, seizures, developmental delay (DD): "Cerebral palsy"

## Bilateral Perisylvian Polymicrogyria (PMG)
- Absence of interhemispheric fusion

## PATHOLOGY

### General Features
- General path comments: Mitosis/apoptosis of embryonic roof plate form interhemispheric fissure (IHF) after neural tube closure (fetal weeks 3-4)
- Genetics
  - Linked to ZIC2 mutation at 13q32, other dorsal induction genes
    - In mice, these genes involved in differentiation of embryonic roof plate
    - In contrast to genes linked to classic HPE (i.e., Sonic hedgehog), dorsal > ventral neuraxis ⇒ lack of severe midline facial dysmorphisms in MIH
- Etiology: Impaired expression of roof plate properties alters mitosis and apoptosis leading to faulty dorsal IHF formation, "fusion" of the cerebral hemispheres

### Gross Pathologic & Surgical Features
- IHF present at frontal, occipital poles; hemispheric fusion posterior frontal and parietal lobes; fused SF
- Deep gray nuclei (basal ganglia, hypothalami) normal

### Microscopic Features
- Callosal fibers identified anteriorly, posteriorly

## CLINICAL ISSUES

### Presentation
- Most common signs/symptoms
  - Spasticity, hypotonia, seizures, developmental delay (DD): "Cerebral palsy"
    - Mild facial dysmorphisms frequent: Hypertelorism, cleft lip/palate

### Demographics
- Age: Presents in infancy

### Natural History & Prognosis
- Static course: Mild/moderate psychomotor delay

## SELECTED REFERENCES

1. Lewis AJ et al: Middle interhemispheric variant of holoprosencephaly: a distinct cliniconeuroradiologic subtype. Neurology. 59(12): 1860-5, 2002
2. Marcorelles P et al: Unusual variant of holoprosencephaly in monosomy 13q. Pediatr Dev Pathol. 5(2):170-8, 2002
3. Simon EM et al: The middle interhemispheric variant of holoprosencephaly. AJNR Am J Neuroradiol. 23(1): 151-6, 2002

## IMAGE GALLERY

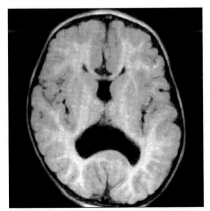 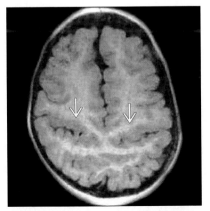 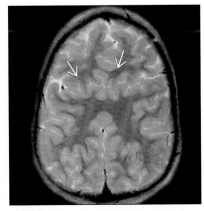

*(Left)* Axial T1WI MR shows absent septum pellucidum and slightly dysplastic ventricular system. Nearly normal callosal genu and splenium, basal ganglia, and frontal interhemispheric fissure are present. *(Center)* Axial T1WI MR in same patient shows the absent interhemispheric fissure and the sylvian fissures ➡ extending upward almost to the midline at that level. *(Right)* Axial T2WI MR in a different patient from previous image shows continuity ➡ of the bilateral interhemispheric fissures over the dorsum of the cerebral hemispheres at the level of the fusion.

# COMMISSURAL ANOMALIES

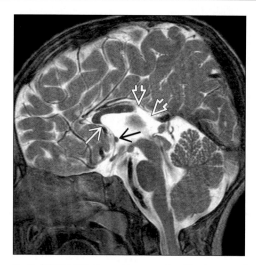
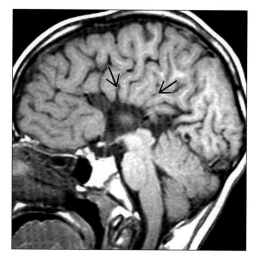

*Sagittal T2WI MR shows hypogenesis with absence of posterior body and splenium ➡. Also absent is the late forming anterior-inferior genu ➡. Normal anterior commissure ➡.*

*Sagittal T1WI MR shows characteristic outward radiation of medial hemispheric sulci ➡, without intervening cingulum, in a child with complete agenesis of the corpus callosum.*

## TERMINOLOGY

### Abbreviations and Synonyms
- Corpus callosum (CC) agenesis, CC hypogenesis, commissural agenesis

### Definitions
- Congenital malformation resulting in hypoplasia or absence of cerebral commissures: Corpus callosum, anterior commissure (AC), hippocampal commissure (HC)

## IMAGING FINDINGS

### General Features
- Best diagnostic clue
  - Axial: Parallel lateral ventricles
  - Coronal: Anterior horns resemble "Viking helmet" or "Texas longhorn"
- Size: CC remnants vary in size, shape
- Morphology
  - Axonal bundles cross midline, connecting cerebral hemispheres
    - CC between centra semiovale
    - AC in superior lamina terminalis
    - HC between fornices, merges with splenium

### CT Findings
- CTA: "Meandering" anterior cerebral arteries (ACAs)
- NECT
  - Lateral ventricles are key to diagnosis
    - Lateral ventricles appear parallel in dysgenesis of CC
    - Colpocephaly (dilated posteriorly)
    - Pointed frontal horns
  - Variable findings
    - Midline cyst or lipoma

### MR Findings
- T1WI
  - Sagittal
    - Gyri radiate out from 3rd ventricle
    - Everted cingulate gyrus, absent cingulate sulcus
  - Coronal
    - Longhorn-shaped anterior horns
    - Elongated foramina of Monro
    - "Keyhole" temporal horns & vertical hippocampi

## DDx: Callosal Deformity/Absence

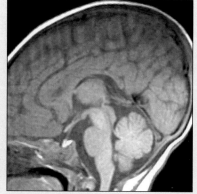
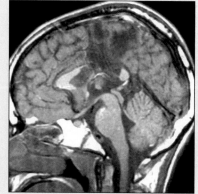
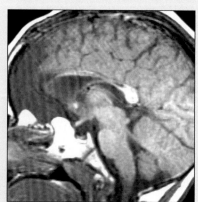

*Normal Neonate*  *Gunshot Trauma*  *Callosotomy*

# COMMISSURAL ANOMALIES

## Key Facts

### Terminology
- Corpus callosum (CC) agenesis, CC hypogenesis, commissural agenesis
- Congenital malformation resulting in hypoplasia or absence of cerebral commissures: Corpus callosum, anterior commissure (AC), hippocampal commissure (HC)

### Imaging Findings
- Axonal bundles cross midline, connecting cerebral hemispheres
- Lateral ventricles appear parallel in dysgenesis of CC
- Gyri radiate out from 3rd ventricle
- Longhorn-shaped anterior horns
- Colpocephaly
- WM tracts more loosely packed with dysgenesis, resulting in relative dilation of trigones

- Probst bundles are densely packed WM tracts running parallel to interhemispheric fissure

### Top Differential Diagnoses
- Destruction of Callosum
- Immature Callosum

### Pathology
- Multiple genes contribute to formation of CC
- 0.5-70 per 10,000 live births
- 4% of CNS malformations
- Associated with multiple named syndromes and malformations (50-80%)
- Agenesis with interhemispheric cyst
- Type 1 ⇒ cyst is diverticulum of lateral ventricle
- Type 2 ⇒ multiple interhemispheric cysts, hyperdense/hyperintense to CSF

---

- o Ventriculomegaly seen in type I interhemispheric cyst variant
  - ▪ Cyst is a diverticulum of lateral ventricle
- T2WI
  - o Colpocephaly
    - ▪ Result of loss of normal white matter (WM) architecture in posterior frontal and parietal lobes
    - ▪ Densely packed WM tracts converging into CC account for concave shape of ventricular trigone
    - ▪ WM tracts more loosely packed with dysgenesis, resulting in relative dilation of trigones
  - o Probst bundles are densely packed WM tracts running parallel to interhemispheric fissure
    - ▪ Axons normally would cross through CC
    - ▪ Run between cingulate gyrus and ventricles, indenting medial wall of ventricles
    - ▪ Hypointense on T2WI, like internal capsule and anterior commissure
- MRA
  - o ACAs "meander", no CC genu to curve around
  - o ± Azygous ACA
- MRV
  - o Occasional midline venous anomalies
    - ▪ Persistent falcine sinus common
- DTI
  - o Fiber tracts from all brain regions converge on remnant of CC
  - o In complete agenesis, may form Probst bundles

## Ultrasonographic Findings
- Grayscale Ultrasound
  - o Coronal
    - ▪ Absent CC
    - ▪ Trident lateral ventricles
    - ▪ Widely spaced lateral ventricles, colpocephaly
  - o Sagittal
    - ▪ Radially arranged gyri "point to" 3rd ventricle
- Color Doppler: ACAs wander between frontal lobes

## Angiographic Findings
- Conventional
  - o ACAs don't conform to normal CC shape
  - o ± Azygous ACA

### Imaging Recommendations
- Best imaging tool: Sagittal and coronal MR
- Protocol advice: Multiplanar MR (look for additional malformations)

# DIFFERENTIAL DIAGNOSIS

## Destruction of Callosum
- Surgery (callosotomy), trauma
- Periventricular pattern of injury in premature/neonates ⇒ periventricular leukomalacia (PVL)
- Metabolic (Marchiafava-Bignami with necrosis, longitudinal splitting of CC)

## Attenuation of Callosum
- Hydrocephalus stretches CC and flattens fiber tracts
- Thinning often remains even after successful treatment

## Immature Callosum
- CC may be difficult to perceive in neonate
  - o Look for cingulate gyrus

## Malformations with Colpocephaly
- Chiari 2, lobar holoprosencephaly
  - o Have some degree of dysgenesis of CC

# PATHOLOGY

## General Features
- General path comments
  - o Associated with midline anomalies ⇒ lipoma, dorsal/interhemispheric cysts, inferior vermian hypoplasia
  - o Cortical maldevelopment ⇒ heterotopia, frontal schizencephaly, ARX-related lissencephaly
  - o Ocular/spinal/facial anomalies/sincipital cephaloceles
  - o Embryology
    - ▪ Axons from cingulum migrate first

# COMMISSURAL ANOMALIES

- Cortical axons migrate towards midline chemical signals
- When reaching midline, growth cone is changed, becomes repulsed by midline signal
- Follows signals in new hemisphere to subplate
- Receives neurotrophin, forms synapse
- Posterior genu and anterior body form first, followed by posterior body, splenium, and finally rostrum
- Genetics
  - Multiple genes contribute to formation of CC
    - Multiple potential sites of disruption
  - Genetics of associated syndromes and malformations better delineated
- Etiology
  - Axons fail to form (rare, seen only in severe cortical malformations like cobblestone lissencephaly)
  - Axons not guided to midline (mutations in adhesion molecules)
  - Axons reach midline but fail to cross
    - Absence or malfunction of midsagittal guiding material
    - Axons turn back, form Probst bundles
  - Miscellaneous
    - Toxic: Fetal alcohol exposure may affect adhesion molecules
    - Infection: In utero cytomegalovirus (CMV)
    - Inborn errors of metabolism: Non-ketotic hyperglycinemia, pyruvate dehydrogenase deficiency, maternal phenylketonuria (PKU), Zellweger
- Epidemiology
  - 0.5-70 per 10,000 live births
  - 4% of CNS malformations
- Associated abnormalities
  - Most common anomaly seen with other central nervous system (CNS) malformations
  - Associated with multiple named syndromes and malformations (50-80%)
    - Aicardi Syndrome: X-linked dominant, CC dysgenesis, interhemispheric cysts (type 2b) infantile spasms, retinal lacunae
    - Dandy Walker, Chiari 2, Rubinstein-Taybi, Smith-Lemli-Opitz, multiple others

## Gross Pathologic & Surgical Features

- Leaves of septum pellucidum laterally displaced to form membranous roof of lateral ventricles
  - Project between fornices, longitudinal callosal bundles (Probst)
- Anterior and hippocampal commissures usually small
  - Occasionally hippocampal commissure enlarges and mimics splenium

## Staging, Grading or Classification Criteria

- Agenesis with interhemispheric cyst
  - Type 1 ⇒ cyst is diverticulum of lateral ventricle
  - Type 2 ⇒ multiple interhemispheric cysts, hyperdense/hyperintense to CSF

## CLINICAL ISSUES

### Presentation

- Most common signs/symptoms
  - Seizures, developmental delay, microcephaly
  - Absence of callosum variably symptomatic
    - Associated syndromes or malformations often account for symptoms
  - Hypopituitarism, hypothalamic malfunction
  - Absent/small AC ⇒ poor cognition
- Other signs/symptoms: Hypertelorism

### Demographics

- Age: Any age, usually identified early childhood
- Gender: If isolated finding M > F

### Natural History & Prognosis

- Sporadic/isolated agenesis/dysgenesis: 75% normal or near normal at 3 years
  - Subtle cognitive defects become apparent with increasing complexity of school tasks

### Treatment

- Treat associated endocrine deficiencies, seizures

## DIAGNOSTIC CHECKLIST

### Consider

- Aicardi syndrome
  - Especially if type II cysts are present with polymicrogyria, heterotopia

### Image Interpretation Pearls

- Look for additional lesions
- Remember order of formation of callosum to differentiate destruction from hypogenesis

## SELECTED REFERENCES

1. Bedeschi MF et al: Agenesis of the corpus callosum: clinical and genetic study in 63 young patients. Pediatr Neurol. 34(3):186-93, 2006
2. Ren T et al: Imaging, anatomical, and molecular analysis of callosal formation in the developing human fetal brain. Anat Rec A Discov Mol Cell Evol Biol. 288(2):191-204, 2006
3. Aicardi J: Aicardi syndrome. Brain Dev. 27(3):164-71, 2005
4. Pavone P et al: Callosal anomalies with interhemispheric cyst: expanding the phenotype. Acta Paediatr. 94(8):1066-72, 2005
5. Lee SK et al: Diffusion tensor MR imaging visualizes the altered hemispheric fiber connection in callosal dysgenesis. AJNR Am J Neuroradiol. 25(1):25-8, 2004
6. Kuker W et al: Malformations of the midline commissures: MRI findings in different forms of callosal dysgenesis. Eur Radiol. 13(3):598-604, 2003
7. Moutard ML et al: Agenesis of corpus callosum: prenatal diagnosis and prognosis. Childs Nerv Syst. 19(7-8):471-6, 2003
8. Barkovich AJ et al: Callosal agenesis with cyst: a better understanding and new classification. Neurology. 56(2):220-7, 2001

## IMAGE GALLERY

### Typical

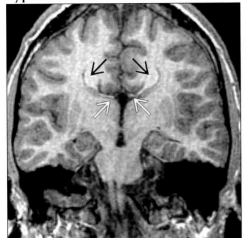
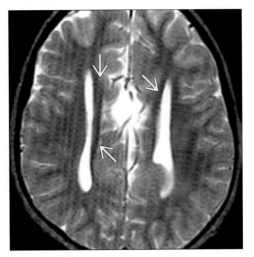

*(Left)* Coronal T1WI MR shows the classic "Texas longhorn" configuration caused by impression of Probst bundles ⇨ on frontal horns; they blend with fornices ➡ inferiorly. Cingula are small. *(Right)* Axial T2WI MR shows the parallel lateral ventricles characteristic of agenesis of the corpus callosum. Probst bundles are seen as bands of white matter medial to the ventricles ➡.

### Typical

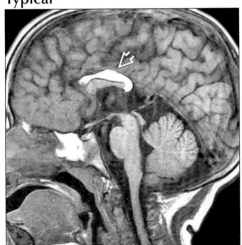
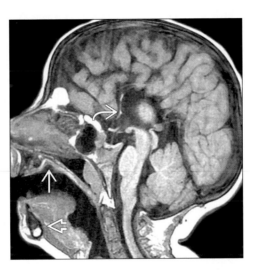

*(Left)* Sagittal T1WI MR shows callosal hypogenesis (absent body, splenium, inferior genu) associated with interhemispheric (sometimes called pericallosal) lipoma ➡. *(Right)* Sagittal T1WI MR in a child with Rubinstein-Taybi syndrome shows agenesis of CC with small AC ➚, absent HC. High palate ➡ and micrognathia ➡ are also characteristic of the syndrome.

### Variant

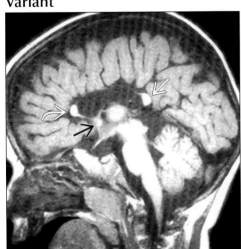
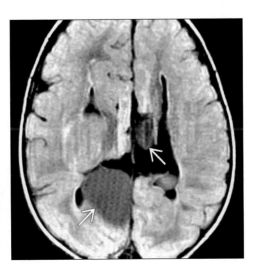

*(Left)* Sagittal T1WI MR shows severe hypogenesis of CC with only genu ➡ present. Posteriorly, the HC ➡, which usually merges with the splenium, is seen. Note slightly enlarged AC ➡. *(Right)* Axial FLAIR MR in a child with Aicardi syndrome shows callosal agenesis with parallel ventricles and Type 2b interhemispheric cysts ➡.

# MICROCEPHALY

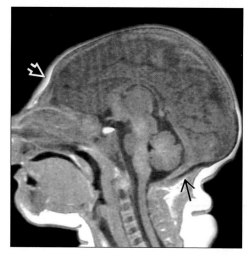

Sagittal T1WI MR shows marked decrease in the cranial-to-facial proportions. Note the slanting forehead ➡ and flat occiput ➡. These features contribute to the conical head shape.

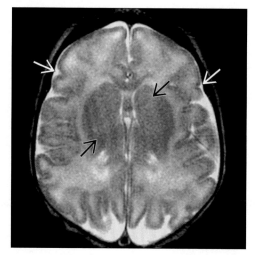

Axial T2WI MR shows a simplified gyral pattern with too few gyri and sulci that are too shallow ➡. Also note lack of internal capsule myelination ➡. MSG, group 2.

## TERMINOLOGY

### Abbreviations and Synonyms

- Micrencephaly, primary (genetic) microcephaly, microcephaly with simplified gyral pattern (MSG), microlissencephaly, secondary (nongenetic) microcephaly

### Definitions

- Microcephaly: Small head size
  - Primary (genetic): Mendelian inheritance OR associated with genetic syndrome
    - MSG: Head circumference (HC) > 3 standard deviations (SDs) below mean, too few gyri, shallow sulci
    - Microlissencephaly: HC > 3 SDs below mean, pachy or agyria
  - Secondary (nongenetic): Results from noxious agent that affects fetal/infant brain growth
- Micrencephaly: Brain reduced in size

## IMAGING FINDINGS

### General Features

- Best diagnostic clue: ↓ Craniofacial proportions, sutural overlap, simplified gyri, shallow sulci
- Imaging findings: Dictated by the cause of microcephaly
  - MSG
    - Group 1: Small, but grossly normal brain, gyral simplification, shallow sulci, normal myelination
    - Group 2: Simplified gyral pattern, shallow sulci, delayed WM myelination
    - Group 3: Fewer gyri and sulci than groups 1 and 2, subependymal heterotopia, arachnoid cysts
    - Group 4: Significant prenatal or neonatal problems, polyhydramnios, imaging similar to group 1
    - Group 5: Microlissencephaly, profoundly microcephalic, expanded subarachnoid spaces (SAS), very small smooth brains
  - Primary microcephaly: ± Pachygyria, lissencephaly, holoprosencephaly
  - Secondary (nongenetic) microcephaly

## DDx: Microcephaly

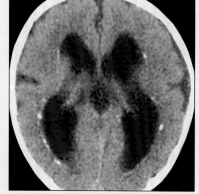

Cytomegalovirus

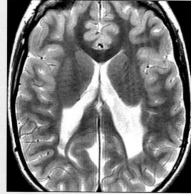

Periventricular Leukomalacia

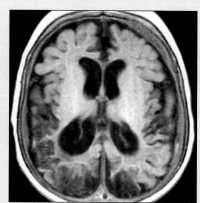

Nonaccidental Head Injury Remote

# MICROCEPHALY

## Key Facts

### Terminology
- Microcephaly: Small head size
- Micrencephaly: Brain reduced in size

### Imaging Findings
- Best diagnostic clue: ↓ Craniofacial proportions, sutural overlap, simplified gyri, shallow sulci
- Imaging findings: Dictated by the cause of microcephaly
- Radiography: ↓ Craniofacial ratio, slanted forehead, overlapping sutures
- Small cranial vault, sutures overlapping
- Primary (genetic) microcephaly, MSG or microlissencephaly
- Small yet normal brain ⇔ simplified gyral pattern (oligogyria) ⇔ lissencephaly
- ± Various telencephalic anomalies: Callosal absence or dysgenesis, holoprosencephaly
- Destructive changes: Encephalomalacia, Ca++ in TORCH infections, ± subdural collections
- Sulci (¼-½ normal depth), cortex simplified ⇔ pachygyric ⇔ heterotopic ⇔ lissencephalic

### Pathology
- Primary microcephaly is associated with many syndromes

### Clinical Issues
- Clinical Profile: Receding forehead, flat occiput, small cranium ⇒ conical shaped head; large face and ears

### Diagnostic Checklist
- MR provides the most sensitive tool for investigating the simplified cortex in microcephaly

---

- Hypoxic ischemic encephalopathy (HIE): ± Cortical, white matter, or basal ganglia volume loss
- TORCH infection: Ca++, abnormal WM, neuronal migration anomalies, ± germinolytic cysts
- Fetal alcohol syndrome (FAS): Callosal abnormalities, ventriculomegaly
- Nonaccidental head injury (NAHI): Encephalomalacia, chronic subdurals, ± parenchymal lacerations
- Lateral radiograph, CT scout, or sagittal MR: ↓ Craniofacial proportions (skull/face ratio)
  - Normal craniofacial ratios: Premature (5:1), term (4:1), 2 years (3:1), 3 years (2.5:1), 12 years (2:1), adult (1.5:1)
- Fetal sonography or fetal MR Findings
  - Difficult to confirm microcephaly until late 2nd or early 3rd trimester

### CT Findings
- NECT
  - Small cranial vault, sutures overlapping
  - Ca++ in TORCH and TORCH look-alikes (Aicardi-Goutieres syndrome)
  - Cortical surface: Normal ⇔ simplified ⇔ migrational abnormalities
  - White matter attenuation: Normal ⇔ diminished (secondary to hypomyelination or demyelination)

### MR Findings
- T1WI
  - Primary (genetic) microcephaly, MSG or microlissencephaly
    - Small yet normal brain ⇔ simplified gyral pattern (oligogyria) ⇔ lissencephaly
    - Normal myelination ⇔ hypomyelination ⇔ demyelination
    - ± Various telencephalic anomalies: Callosal absence or dysgenesis, holoprosencephaly
    - ± Cerebellar hypoplasia (more common in genetic causes of microcephaly)
  - Secondary (nongenetic) microcephaly
    - Destructive changes: Encephalomalacia, Ca++ in TORCH infections, ± subdural collections
- T2WI
  - Primary (genetic) microcephaly, MSG or microlissencephaly
    - Sulci (¼-½ normal depth), cortex simplified ⇔ pachygyric ⇔ heterotopic ⇔ lissencephalic
    - ↓ Commisural fiber tracts, normal basal ganglia volume, ± cerebellar hypoplasia
    - White matter maturation: Normal ⇔ hypomyelinated ⇔ demyelinated
  - Secondary (nongenetic) microcephaly
    - White matter: Hyperintensity ⇒ gliosis, cavitation, demyelination, hypointensity ⇒ (Ca++), ↓ WM volume
    - Cortex: Normal ⇔ simplified ⇔ polymicrogyria (think TORCH)
    - Midline anomalies: Absent corpus callosum, holoprosencephaly
- FLAIR: Periventricular: Cavitation (↓ signal), gliosis (↑ signal), ± chronic subdural collections ⇒ hyperintense
- T2* GRE: Sequelae to nonaccidental trauma: Hypointensity from hemorrhage, ± parenchymal shear injury
- DWI: T2 shine-through when associated with gliosis or demyelination
- MRS: ↓ NAA, MI and CHO may be ↑ in states of ongoing demyelination and neurodegeneration

### Radiographic Findings
- Radiography: ↓ Craniofacial ratio, slanted forehead, overlapping sutures

### Ultrasonographic Findings
- Grayscale Ultrasound
  - Small fontanel due to sutural overlap, sulcal and ventricular expansion
  - ± Basal ganglia or thalamic Ca++ (TORCH or HIE), ± periventricular volume loss (TORCH or HIE)

### Imaging Recommendations
- Best imaging tool

# MICROCEPHALY

- ○ NECT detects: Ca++ (TORCH, pseudo-TORCH), edema, encephalomalacia, and subdural collections
- ○ MR depicts: Gyral pattern, cortical organization, myelination, midline anomalies, gliosis, hemorrhage
- Protocol advice
- ○ Consider NECT for detection of Ca++
- ○ MR brain: GRE T2* (blood and Ca++), 3D SPGR to evaluate brain topography, FLAIR for detecting subdurals

## DIFFERENTIAL DIAGNOSIS

### Secondary (Nongenetic) Microcephaly

- Antenatal causes: Pre-eclampsia, maternal infection (TORCH), maternal diabetes, FAS, hyperphenylalaninemia
- Perinatal causes: HIE infection
- Postnatal: Prolonged status epilepticus, HIE, hypoglycemia, meningo-encephalitis, neurodegenerative, child abuse
- Noxious insult: Radiation, maternal use of anticonvulsants, ETOH, cocaine, hyper-vitamin A

## PATHOLOGY

### General Features

- General path comments
- ○ Whatever the cause, there is reduced growth of the brain, ↓ proliferation of neurons and glia
- ○ Embryology-anatomy
  - Several pathways in which genes affect neuronal progenitor cells & brain size
  - ASPM mutations cause dividing neurons to arrest in metaphase
  - Microcephalin involved in cell cycle regulation
- Genetics
- ○ Primary (genetic) microcephaly is typically autosomal recessive (example: Familial form → 1:40,000 births)
- ○ Primary microcephaly is associated with many syndromes
  - MCPH genetic heterogeneity: Mutations MCPH5 (1q31) most prevalent
  - Down (21-trisomy), Edward (18-trisomy), Cri-du-chat (5p-), Cornelia de Lange, Rubinstein-Taybi
- Etiology: Heterogeneous: Inherited or acquired
- Epidemiology
- ○ Microcephaly in the general population: 0.6-1.6%
- ○ Genetically determined microcephaly: Familial 1:40,000, Down syndrome 1:800
- Associated abnormalities: Frequently seen as a component of other severe malformations

### Gross Pathologic & Surgical Features

- Skull capacity < 1,300 mL, brain weight < 900 grams
- Simplified gyral pattern (oligogyria)
- Short central sulcus, sulci (shallow, narrow or wide)
- Sulcus parieto-occipitalis may be enlarged ~ simian fissure
- Island of Reil remains uncovered (incomplete operculization)

- Acquired microcephaly: ± Cystic degeneration of white matter, infarcts, Ca++, hemorrhagic products

### Microscopic Features

- MCPH5: No evidence of abnormal neuronal migration or architecture
- Some types have abnormalities of cortex layers 2, 3

### Staging, Grading or Classification Criteria

- Grouped by: Myelination, neuronal organization and migration, and associated congenital anomalies

## CLINICAL ISSUES

### Presentation

- Most common signs/symptoms: Severe mental retardation, ± seizures, developmental delay
- Clinical Profile: Receding forehead, flat occiput, small cranium ⇒ conical shaped head; large face and ears
- Criteria for the diagnosis of microcephaly: Head circumference > 3 SD below the mean for age and sex

### Demographics

- Age
- ○ Primary (genetic) microcephaly often reveals itself either in utero or shortly after birth
- ○ Secondary (nongenetic) microcephaly usually results from insults within the first two years of life
- Gender: Variable based upon type
- Ethnicity: Common genetic forms ~ pan-ethnic, certain syndromic causes show ethnicity

### Natural History & Prognosis

- Dictated by the cause of microcephaly

### Treatment

- Supportive, genetic testing available for some microcephalic disorders

## DIAGNOSTIC CHECKLIST

### Consider

- Cerebellar hypoplasia is more common in primary microcephaly
- When midline anomalies accompany microcephaly, consider fetal alcohol syndrome (FAS)

### Image Interpretation Pearls

- MR provides the most sensitive tool for investigating the simplified cortex in microcephaly

## SELECTED REFERENCES

1. Ornoy A et al: Fetal effects of primary and secondary cytomegalovirus infection in pregnancy. Reprod Toxicol. 21(4):399-409, 2006
2. Bond J et al: ASPM is a major determinant of cerebral cortical size. Nat Genet. 32(2):316-20, 2002
3. Custer DA et al: Neurodevelopmental and neuroimaging correlates in nonsyndromal microcephalic children. J Dev Behav Pediatr. 21(1):12-8, 2000
4. Barkovich AJ et al: Microlissencephaly: a heterogeneous malformation of cortical development. Neuropediatrics. 29(3):113-9, 1998

## IMAGE GALLERY

### Typical

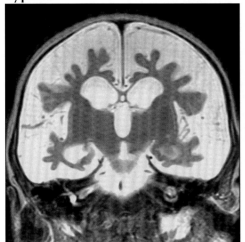
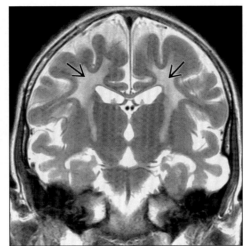

*(Left)* Coronal T2WI MR shows global cerebral atrophy in an infant who suffered a profound hypoxic ischemic insult at birth. The head circumference was 4 SDs below the mean. *(Right)* Coronal T2WI MR shows cerebral hemispheric demyelination →. Diagnosis: Microcephaly secondary to Aicardi-Goutieres syndrome, disorder associated with aberrant interferon function.

### Typical

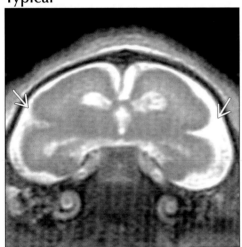
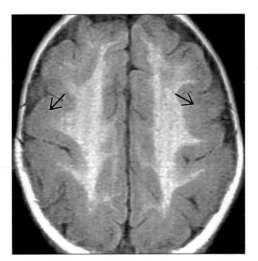

*(Left)* Coronal T2WI MR shows profound microcephaly. Note the enlarged subarachnoid spaces → and the extremely small smooth brain. There is reduction in WM volume. MSG, group 5. *(Right)* Axial T1WI MR shows thickened cerebral cortex → with broad gyri and too few sulci in a developmentally delayed, microcephalic patient. Diagnosis is pachygyria.

### Typical

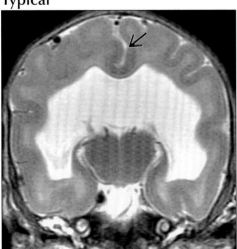
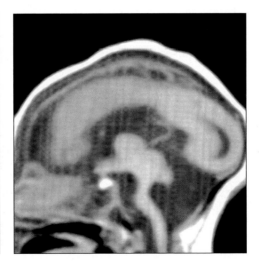

*(Left)* Coronal T2WI MR shows partial formation of interhemispheric fissure → and absent falx in an infant with microcephaly, profound developmental delay. Diagnosis: Semilobar holoprosencephaly. *(Right)* Sagittal T1WI MR shows an example of microlissencephaly with cerebellar hypoplasia. Note the nearly complete absence of sulcation and the very small cerebellum and brain stem.

# HEMIMEGALENCEPHALY

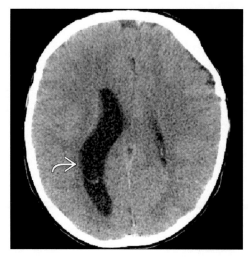
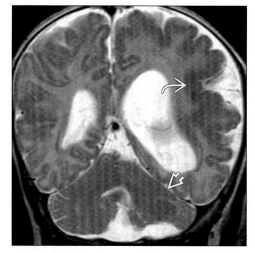

*Axial NECT shows enlargement of the right hemisphere with ipsilateral ventricular enlargement ➔. No other diagnosis will increase parenchymal volume without decreasing ventricle size.*

*Coronal T2WI MR shows irregular thickened cortex ➔, linear abnormal signal in the white matter, and ventriculomegaly in an infant with cerebral and cerebellar ➔ hemimegalencephaly.*

## TERMINOLOGY

### Abbreviations and Synonyms
- Hemimegalencephaly (HME), unilateral megalencephaly, focal megalencephaly

### Definitions
- Hamartomatous overgrowth of part or all of a hemisphere
- Defect of cellular organization and neuronal migration

## IMAGING FINDINGS

### General Features
- Best diagnostic clue
  - Enlarged hemisphere with thickened cortical ribbon
  - Large ipsilateral ventricle with abnormally shaped frontal horn
  - Broad featureless gyri with shallow sulci
  - Abnormal primitive veins overlying shallow sulci
- Size: May affect entire hemisphere, or single lobe
- Morphology: Sulci typically shallow, with enlarged gyri

## CT Findings
- CTA: May show enlarged ipsilateral vessels which are tortuous or bizarre
- NECT
  - Large cerebral hemisphere with deviation of posterior falx and occipital pole to opposite side
  - Ipsilateral ventricle is large with abnormally shaped frontal horn
  - Thickened cortex with increased attenuation, occasional calcification (Ca++)
- CECT: Large vessels, developmental venous anomalies (DVAs)

## MR Findings
- T1WI
  - Thick cortex: Pachygyria, polygyria, fused gyri and shallow sulci
  - Gray matter heterotopia scattered throughout hemisphere
  - Rarely affects ipsilateral cerebellum and brainstem
  - Alteration of white matter (WM) signal
    - ↑ Signal ⇒ accelerated myelination, Ca++
    - ↓ Signal ⇒ dysmyelination, hypomyelination
- T2WI

## DDx: Thickened Cortex in Children

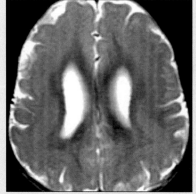
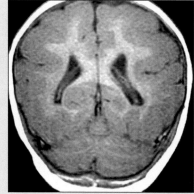
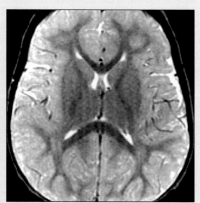

*Band Heterotopia*     *Pachygyria*     *Cortical Edema*

# HEMIMEGALENCEPHALY

## Key Facts

### Terminology
- Hamartomatous overgrowth of part or all of a hemisphere
- Defect of cellular organization and neuronal migration

### Imaging Findings
- Enlarged hemisphere with thickened cortical ribbon
- Large ipsilateral ventricle with abnormally shaped frontal horn
- Some associated with ipsilateral hemihypertrophy
- Size, signal intensity of affected hemisphere can change
- Progression of myelination, development of Ca++
- Volume loss 2° to unremitting seizures
- Gray/white differentiation can be blurred
- Dysplastic cortex often hypointense on T2WI

### Pathology
- Abnormal proliferation, migration and differentiation of neurons
- Associated with neurocutaneous and overgrowth syndromes
- Neurons are decreased in number
- Glial cells are increased in number

### Clinical Issues
- Hemispherectomy removes seizure focus: Halts injury to contralateral hemisphere; early surgery allows brain plasticity to take over function of resected areas
- Contralateral hemisphere must be normal
- Shunting of post-operative cavity often necessary
- Possible increased risk of hemorrhage into surgical cavity with minor trauma

---

- ○ Size, signal intensity of affected hemisphere can change
  - ■ Progression of myelination, development of Ca++
  - ■ Volume loss 2° to unremitting seizures
- ○ Gray/white differentiation can be blurred
- ○ Dysplastic cortex often hypointense on T2WI
  - ■ Especially in neonates and infants
- FLAIR: ↑ Signal in WM, poor gray/white definition, reflecting altered myelination
- T2* GRE: Sensitive for Ca++
- DWI: Diffusion tractography can show increased number/density of fiber tracts
- T1 C+
  - ○ Enhancement of DVAs
  - ○ Occasional parenchymal enhancement
- MRV: Anomalous venous pattern
- MRS: With seizures, progressive ↓ NAA and ↑ creatine, choline, and myoinositol ⇒ reflects glial proliferation
- Magnetoencephalography (MEG)
  - ○ Somatosensory maps may predict severity of cortical lamination defects

### Radiographic Findings
- Radiography
  - ○ Asymmetric calvaria
  - ○ Some associated with ipsilateral hemihypertrophy

### Ultrasonographic Findings
- Grayscale Ultrasound
  - ○ Displaced midline and hemispheric overgrowth
    - ■ Diagnosis can be made in fetus and neonate
- Color Doppler
  - ○ ± Enlarged ipsilateral arteries
  - ○ Frequent dysplastic, primitive venous system

### Nuclear Medicine Findings
- PET: Glucose hypometabolism of affected hemisphere in 50%

### Angiographic Findings
- Conventional
  - ○ ± High flow shunting to involved side

- ○ Modified Wada testing can be used to suppress seizures from abnormal hemisphere to unmask contralateral seizure activity

### Imaging Recommendations
- Best imaging tool: Multiplanar MR
- Protocol advice
  - ○ Image before seizures lead to significant atrophy of involved hemisphere
  - ○ Close analysis of contralateral hemisphere essential
    - ■ Contralateral malformations, seizure foci contraindication to hemispherectomy
    - ■ Thin slice T1WI to identify heterotopia

## DIFFERENTIAL DIAGNOSIS

### Disorders of Neuronal Migration
- Unilateral ⇒ schizencephaly, focal polymicrogyria, focal cortical dysplasia
- Bilateral/diffuse ⇒ agyria/pachygyria, band heterotopia, x-linked subependymal heterotopia

### Tuberous Sclerosis (TS)
- Lobar or hemispheric hamartomatous overgrowth
  - ○ Both are disorders of cellular proliferation
- Superficial resemblance of balloon cells in hemimegalencephaly and TS
  - ○ But immunohistochemistry and electron microscopic profiles different

### Syndromes with Disordered Migration/Organization
- Fukuyama muscular dystrophy
- Muscle-eye-brain disease
- Congenital bilateral perisylvian syndrome

### Hemiatrophy
- Rasmussen syndrome: Chronic focal encephalitis
  - ○ Unilateral frontal-temporal atrophy
  - ○ Progressive atrophy, signal change of caudate & putamen

# HEMIMEGALENCEPHALY

## Gliomatosis Cerebri
- Low grade glioma diffusely infiltrating multiple lobes
- Rare in children
  - Multifocal glioma is more common in children, higher grade

## Cortical Edema
- Cortical injury may result in diffuse or unilateral swelling

## PATHOLOGY

### General Features
- General path comments
  - Abnormal proliferation, migration and differentiation of neurons
  - Embryologic theories
    - Insult to developing brain leads to development of too many synapses, persistence of supernumerary axons and potential for white matter overgrowth
    - Localized epidermal growth factor (EGF) in cortical neurons and glial cells may lead to excessive proliferation
- Genetics: Associated with some proliferation and hemihypertrophy syndromes
- Epidemiology: Account for ~ 3% of cortical dysplasias that are diagnosed by imaging
- Associated abnormalities
  - Associated with neurocutaneous and overgrowth syndromes
    - Neurofibromatosis type 1, tuberous sclerosis, Klippel-Trenaunay-Weber, Proteus syndrome
    - Unilateral hypomelanosis of Ito, epidermal nevus syndrome, congenital infiltrating lipomatosis, incontinentia pigmenti

### Gross Pathologic & Surgical Features
- Large hemisphere, shallow sulci, fused & disorganized gyri
- Regional polymicrogyria, pachygyria and heterotopia

### Microscopic Features
- Giant neurons, loss of horizontal layering of neurons
  - Neurons are decreased in number
- White matter hypertrophy & gliosis
  - Glial cells are increased in number
- Balloon cells ⇒ hypertrophic atypical cells that have variable reactivity for neuronal and glial proteins
  - Contain few lysosomes, microfilaments, microtubules and abundant lipofuscin granules

## CLINICAL ISSUES

### Presentation
- Most common signs/symptoms
  - Seizures
    - Infantile spasms, focal and generalized
  - Macrocrania
- Other signs/symptoms
  - Developmental delay, hemiparesis
  - Systemic overgrowth syndromes

## Demographics
- Age: Usually diagnosed during first year of life

## Natural History & Prognosis
- Intractable seizures ⇒ progressive injury to "good" hemisphere
- Hemispherectomy removes seizure focus: Halts injury to contralateral hemisphere; early surgery allows brain plasticity to take over function of resected areas

## Treatment
- Anticonvulsants often ineffective
- Occasional shunting to control head size and cerebellar displacement
- Surgical hemispherectomy
  - Contralateral hemisphere must be normal
  - Modified hemispherectomy ⇒ resect frontal, temporal, parietal lobes, infarct occipital
  - Reports of endovascular hemispherectomy ⇒ embolization of major arteries to infarct abnormal hemisphere/lobes
  - Shunting of post-operative cavity often necessary
  - Possible increased risk of hemorrhage into surgical cavity with minor trauma

## DIAGNOSTIC CHECKLIST

### Consider
- Hemihypertrophy syndromes: Remember potential airway compromise, sedation risk

### Image Interpretation Pearls
- Myelin maturation ⇒ WM signal change
- Hemisphere may atrophy over time
- One of the only diagnoses to cause ipsilateral parenchymal and ventricular enlargement

## SELECTED REFERENCES

1. Agid R et al: Prenatal MR diffusion-weighted imaging in a fetus with hemimegalencephaly. Pediatr Radiol. 36(2):138-40, 2006
2. Salamon N et al: Contralateral hemimicrencephaly and clinical-pathological correlations in children with hemimegalencephaly. Brain. 129(Pt 2):352-65, 2006
3. Tinkle BT et al: Epidemiology of hemimegalencephaly: a case series and review. Am J Med Genet A. 139(3):204-11, 2005
4. Devlin AM et al: Clinical outcomes of hemispherectomy for epilepsy in childhood and adolescence. Brain. 126(Pt 3):556-66, 2003
5. Flores-Sarnat L et al: Hemimegalencephaly: part 2. Neuropathology suggests a disorder of cellular lineage. J Child Neurol. 18(11):776-85, 2003
6. Flores-Sarnat L: Hemimegalencephaly: part 1. Genetic, clinical, and imaging aspects. J Child Neurol. 17(5):373-84; discussion 384, 2002
7. Galluzzi P et al: Hemimegalencephaly in tuberous sclerosis complex. J Child Neurol. 17(9):677-80, 2002
8. Ishibashi H et al: Somatosensory evoked magnetic fields in hemimegalencephaly. Neurol Res. 24(5):459-62, 2002
9. Hoffmann KT et al: MRI and 18F-fluorodeoxyglucose positron emission tomography in hemimegalencephaly. Neuroradiology. 42(10):749-52, 2000

## IMAGE GALLERY

### Typical

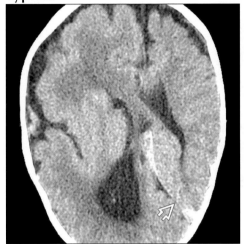 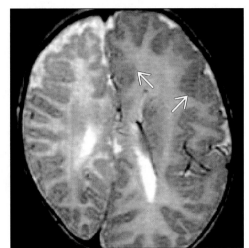

*(Left)* Axial NECT shows marked overgrowth of the right cerebral hemisphere due to HME. Note the marked deviation of the posterior falx cerebri ➡ by the enlarged occipital lobe. *(Right)* Axial T2WI MR shows irregularity of the cortical ribbon ➡ in large hemisphere. Note decreased signal in the left hemisphere white matter due to decreased water content.

### Variant

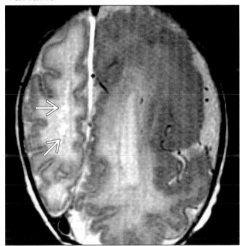 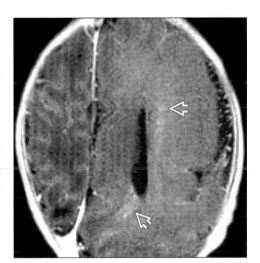

*(Left)* Axial T2WI MR shows morphologic and signal abnormalities of HME in the left hemisphere. Foci of abnormal signal in right hemisphere WM ➡ are due to prenatal injury. *(Right)* Axial T1WI MR shows diffusely increased signal in the left hemisphere white matter, with focal areas of more hyperintense signal ➡ reflecting calcification, myelin clumping, or gliosis.

### Variant

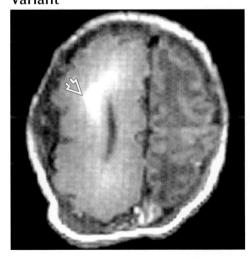 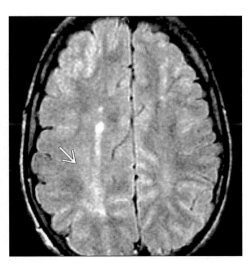

*(Left)* Axial T1WI MR in this 4 month old shows absence of cortical definition in the enlarged right hemisphere, with abnormal hyperintense signal in the white matter ➡. *(Right)* Axial FLAIR MR shows subtle increased signal in the right hemisphere white matter ➡, with enlarged gyri and blurring of gray-white differentiation. Pathology-confirmed hemimegalencephaly.

# LISSENCEPHALY

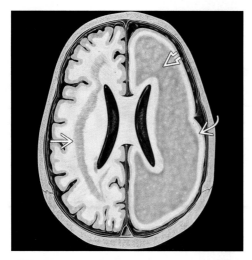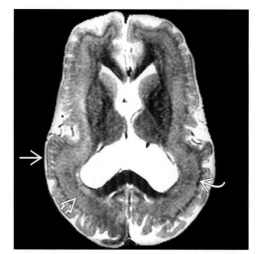

*Axial graphic composite shows thin gray matter band ➡ in right hemisphere. The left hemisphere is lissencephalic with thick subcortical gray matter band ⬧ and thin outer cortex ⬀.*

*Axial T2WI MR shows band heterotopia with a thin wavy cortex ➡, adjacent thin white matter layer ➡ and thick subcortical gray matter band ⬧ paralleling the cortex.*

## TERMINOLOGY

### Abbreviations and Synonyms

- Classical lissencephaly (LIS); type 1 lissencephaly (LIS1); pachygyria-agyria complex; X-linked lissencephaly (XLIS)
- Band heterotopia (BH), double cortex (DCX)

### Definitions

- Classical type 1 lissencephaly is a congenital developmental disorder characterized by arrested neuronal migration, 4-layer cortex, and smooth (or relatively smooth) brain surface
  - Phenotypic spectrum correlates with gene alterations, most commonly LIS1 and DCX (also called XLIS)

## IMAGING FINDINGS

### General Features

- Best diagnostic clue
  - LIS: Hour-glass configuration of brain; often somewhat incomplete (pachygyria-agyria)

- BH: Thinner, symmetric subcortical ribbons of gray matter (GM), paralleling cortex and embedded in white matter (WM)
  - LIS 2° cytomegalovirus: Thin cortex/subcortical calcifications
- Location
  - LIS1: More severe parietal/occipital
  - XLIS (DCX): More severe subfrontal/temporal
- Size
  - Thickness of band of GM predicts configuration/thickness of overlying cortex AND underlying WM
    - Thin band predicts near normal cortical thickness/appearance
    - Thick band predicts thin, abnormally convoluted overlying cortex
- Morphology
  - LIS
    - Thick inner band GM, cell sparse WM zone, thin outer layer GM
    - Shallow Sylvian fissure ⇒ brain with "hour-glass" configuration
    - Usually some gyral formation (pachygyria-agyria complex)

## DDx: Lissencephaly

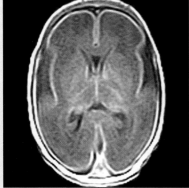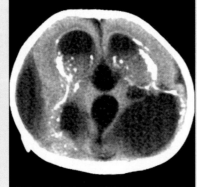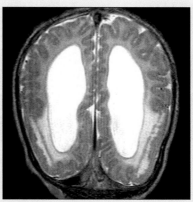

| 25 Week Premie | Cytomegalovirus | Cobblestone |

# LISSENCEPHALY

## Key Facts

### Terminology
- Classical lissencephaly (LIS); type 1 lissencephaly (LIS1); pachygyria-agyria complex; X-linked lissencephaly (XLIS)
- Band heterotopia (BH), double cortex (DCX)
- Classical type 1 lissencephaly is a congenital developmental disorder characterized by arrested neuronal migration, 4-layer cortex, and smooth (or relatively smooth) brain surface

### Imaging Findings
- LIS: Hour-glass configuration of brain; often somewhat incomplete (pachygyria-agyria)
- BH: Thinner, symmetric subcortical ribbons of gray matter (GM), paralleling cortex and embedded in white matter (WM)

- LIS 2° cytomegalovirus: Thin cortex/subcortical calcifications
- LIS1: More severe parietal/occipital
- XLIS (DCX): More severe subfrontal/temporal
- Thickness of band of GM predicts configuration/thickness of overlying cortex AND underlying WM

### Pathology
- Epidemiology: 1-4:100,000 live births
- 4-layer cortex

### Diagnostic Checklist
- Fetal MR, US: Agyric (smooth) cortex is normal up to 26 weeks!
- Specific fetal signs: Presence or absence of parieto-occipital fissure; shallow Sylvian fissure

---

- BH
  - Thick inner GM band + thin, abnormal cortex OR
  - Thin/partial inner band + normal cortex

## CT Findings
- NECT
  - Always isodense with GM
  - +/- Small midline septal Ca++ (Miller-Dieker)
- CECT: No enhancement

## MR Findings
- T1WI: Distinct GM-WM layers; cell-sparse WM layer may have ↓ signal
- T2WI
  - Distinct layering; ↑ signal cell-sparse WM layer
  - CMV related lissencephaly lacks thick cortex
- T2* GRE
  - Midline calcification in Miller-Dieker
  - CMV related lissencephaly: Periventricular and subcortical white matter calcifications
- MRS: ↓ N-acetylaspartate (NAA) in affected cortex

## Ultrasonographic Findings
- Grayscale Ultrasound: Late intrauterine documentation possible

## Nuclear Medicine Findings
- PET: Inner cellular layer has higher glucose utilization than outer layer (fetal pattern)

## Angiographic Findings
- Conventional
  - MCA branches laterally placed due to shallow Sylvian fissures
  - Wavy vessels on surface of brain
  - Lack of formed gyral blush

## Imaging Recommendations
- Best imaging tool: MR
- Protocol advice: MR + thin slice SPGR (surface coil/3D reconstruction) for subtle, focal band heterotopia and adjunctive surface reconstruction (gyral array)

# DIFFERENTIAL DIAGNOSIS

## Lissencephaly Syndromes and Variants
- Miller-Dieker syndrome: LIS1 plus deficiency of 14-3-3epsilon ⇒ Miller-Dieker syndrome (severe LIS plus facial features)
- ARX mutations: XLIS with abnormal genitalia (XLAG)
  - Males have XLAG, females have callosal agenesis
- Lissencephaly with cerebellar hypoplasia (LCH)
  - Can be seen with LIS1 and XLIS mutations
  - Severe cerebellar and hippocampal involvement suggests RELN mutation (7q22)
  - +/- Microcephaly, hydrocephalus, microcalcification, axonal swelling, agenesis of corpus callosum, hypoplastic brainstem, stippled epiphyses, loose skin, lymphedema, arthrogryposis

## Cobblestone or Type 2 Lissencephalies
- "Pebbly" surface of brain, cerebellar and ocular abnormalities, congenital muscular dystrophy

## Bilateral, Diffuse Subependymal Heterotopia
- Mutation filamin-1 gene (required for cell migration to cortex) on Xq28
- Nodular heterotopia lines ventricles, simulates tuberous sclerosis, no enhancement, no Ca++

# PATHOLOGY

## General Features
- General path comments
  - Surface gyral pattern predicts gene mutation
  - Embryology
    - Subependymal germinal zones proliferate, form neuroblasts, glia
    - Neuroblasts leave ventricular surface by "leading edge" extension/growth cone formation (requires "filamen")
    - Neuroblasts attach to radially arranged glial fibers (RGFs)
    - Neuroblasts migrate along RGFs to mantle (via cell-adhesion, ligand-receptor interactions)

# LISSENCEPHALY

- RGFs guide/nourish migrating neuroblasts
- Neuroblasts disengage from RGFs (requires "reelin" secreted by layer 1 pioneer neurons)
- Earliest neuroblasts disengage in cortical subplate
- Later waves pass through initial layer, form 6-layered cortex
- Genetics
  - Deletion of genes that govern specific stages of neuronal migration
    - Large deletion LIS1 gene located on 17p13.3 plus deficiency of 14-3-3epsilon ⇒ Miller-Dieker
    - Smaller deletion LIS1gene (also called PAFAH1B1 gene) ⇒ isolated LIS1/BH
    - DCX (found in the leading edge of migrating neurons and growth cone of migrating neurons) mutated in XLIS
    - XLIS/BH: XLIS gene on Xq22.3-q23, mothers (focal band heterotopia), sons (lissencephaly)
- Etiology
  - Genetic: Mutations alter molecular reactions at any/multiple migration points ⇒ migrational arrest
    - LIS is one of most common neuronal migrational disorders associated with consanguinity
  - Acquired: Toxins/infections ⇒ reactive gliosis/macrophage infiltration disturbs neuronal migration/cortical positioning
    - CMV-infected cells can fail to migrate or arrest
    - Toxins (alcohol/irradiation) ⇒ abnormal migration
- Epidemiology: 1-4:100,000 live births
- Associated abnormalities: +/- Cardiac or facial anomalies

## Gross Pathologic & Surgical Features
- Variable cortical, gyral thickness and maturity
- Variable thickness of subcortical WM

## Microscopic Features
- 4-layer cortex
  - Superficial molecular or marginal layer
  - Thin outer cortical layer of neurons (large, abnormal position)
  - "Cell-sparse" WM zone
  - Thick deep cortical layer of neurons (lack orderly arrangement)
- Sparse underlying WM
- Hypoplastic corticospinal tracts, heterotopia of olives

## Staging, Grading or Classification Criteria
- Graded by location (frontal/posterior), thickness of cortex/inner band GM
  - Agyria with frontotemporal pachygyria most common

# CLINICAL ISSUES

## Presentation
- Most common signs/symptoms
  - LIS: Developmental delay and seizures
  - BH: Seizures may be late onset & cognitive function may be normal if well developed cortex

- Clinical Profile: Cognitive function, age of seizure onset/severity depends on location/amount of abnormally positioned GM

## Demographics
- Age: Severe forms LIS identified in infancy, milder BH forms identified in older child or adult
- Gender
  - LIS1: Full mutations ⇒ severe posterior lissencephaly, mosaic mutations ⇒ posterior BH
  - XLIS/DCX (anterior): Responsible for most familial BH, 80% sporadic female cases, 25% sporadic males
    - Mothers (focal band heterotopia), sons (lissencephaly)
    - Missense mutations ⇒ less severe malformations (BH or pachygyria-BH) in some males

## Natural History & Prognosis
- Variable life span dependent upon extent of malformation
  - Focal subcortical BH often lead normal life
  - LIS, thick complete band/thin cortical ribbon: Significant mental retardation, motor deficits, seizures, early demise

## Treatment
- Treat seizures (corpus callosotomy an option for intractable epilepsy)

# DIAGNOSTIC CHECKLIST

## Consider
- Gyral pattern predicts inheritance pattern

## Image Interpretation Pearls
- Fetal MR, US: Agyric (smooth) cortex is normal up to 26 weeks!
- Specific fetal signs: Presence or absence of parieto-occipital fissure; shallow Sylvian fissure

# SELECTED REFERENCES

1. Ghai S et al: Prenatal US and MR imaging findings of lissencephaly: review of fetal cerebral sulcal development. Radiographics. 26(2):389-405, 2006
2. Barkovich AJ et al: A developmental and genetic classification for malformations of cortical development. Neurology. 65(12):1873-87, 2005
3. Sicca F et al: Mosaic mutations of LIS1 gene cause subcortical band heterotopia. Neurology. 61(8):1042-6, 2003
4. Toyo-oka K et al: 14-3-3 epsilon is important for neuronal migration by binding to NUDEL: a molecular explanation for Miller-Dieker syndrome. Nat Genet. 34(3):274-85, 2003
5. Kaminaga T et al: Proton magnetic resonance spectroscopy in disturbances of cortical development. Neuroradiology. 43(7):575-80, 2001
6. Gressens P: Mechanisms and disturbances of neuronal migration. Pediatr Res. 48:725-30, 2000
7. Pfund Z et al: Lissencephaly: fetal pattern of glucose metabolism on positron emission tomography. Neurology. 55(11):1683-8, 2000
8. Pilz DT et al: LIS1 and XLIS (DCX) mutations cause most classical lissencephaly, but different patterns of malformation. Hum Mol Genet. 7(13):2029-37, 1998

## IMAGE GALLERY

### Typical

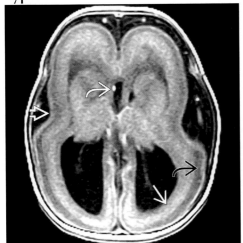
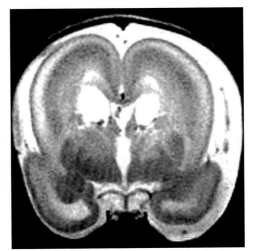

*(Left)* Axial T1WI MR in Miller-Dieker shows typical midline calcification ➔, thin outer gray matter layer ➔, cell-sparse white matter layer ➔ and thick inner gray matter band ➔. *(Right)* Coronal T2WI MR shows similar findings. Note completely smooth cortex and shallow Sylvian fissures.

### Typical

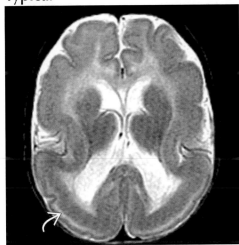
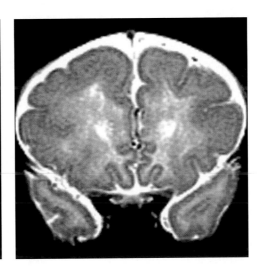

*(Left)* Axial T2WI MR shows more common pattern with more severe parietal/occipital involvement in LIS1. Note the presence of a cell-sparse white matter layer ➔ posteriorly. *(Right)* Coronal T2WI MR shows a nearly normal appearance of inferior frontal lobes and anterior temporal lobes in the same patient. The cortical layers are better blended than posteriorly.

### Typical

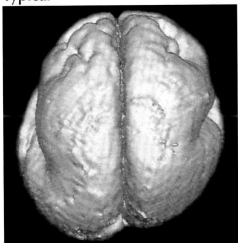
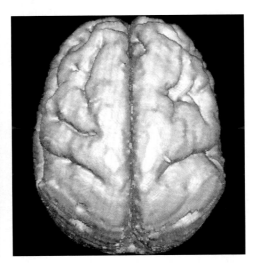

*(Left)* Axial three dimensional reconstruction from MR data set in a severe frontal pachygyria and posterior agyria. *(Right)* Axial 3 dimensional reconstruction from MR data set shows pachygyria with broad, flat gyri separated by shallow sulci.

# HETEROTOPIC GRAY MATTER

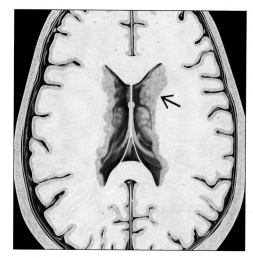

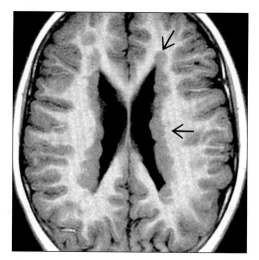

Axial graphic shows extensive bilateral subependymal heterotopia ➡ lining the lateral ventricles. Gray matter cortical ribbon is thin and the sulci are shallow.

Axial T1WI MR shows extensive bilateral subependymal heterotopic gray matter nodules ➡ lining the bodies of both lateral ventricles. Overlying cortex is normal.

## TERMINOLOGY

### Abbreviations and Synonyms
- Heterotopic gray matter (HGM)

### Definitions
- Arrested/disrupted neurons along migration path from periventricular germinal zone to cortex
  - Can be inherited
  - Can be acquired (maternal trauma, infection, or toxin)

## IMAGING FINDINGS

### General Features
- Best diagnostic clue: Nodule or ribbon, isointense with gray matter (GM), located in wrong place (± thin overlying cortex)
- Location: Anywhere from ventricular wall to subpial space
- Size: Diffuse or focal
- Morphology
  - Subependymal heterotopia (most common)
    - GM nodules indent or adjacent to ventricle
  - Band heterotopia ("double cortex")
    - Thick inner GM band deep to thin, abnormal cortex (seizure risk)
    - Thin/partial inner band deep to normal cortex = normal function
  - Classic lissencephaly
    - Part of agyria, agyria/pachygyria spectrum
    - Thick inner band GM, cell sparse WM zone, thin outer layer GM
    - Shallow Sylvian fissure with "hour-glass" cerebral configuration
  - Cobblestone cortex (formerly called lissencephaly type 2)
    - Usually occurs with congenital muscular dystrophies
    - Neurons "overmigrate" through gaps in limiting membrane ⇒ "pebbled" surface of brain
    - Associated ocular, cerebellar anomalies common
  - Subcortical heterotopia: Large foci have thinned and dysplastic overlying cortex, small foci don't
    - Focal HGM nodules
    - Large nodular HGM (can mimic neoplasm!)

## DDx: Periventricular

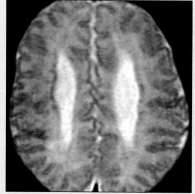

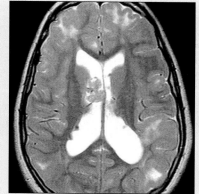

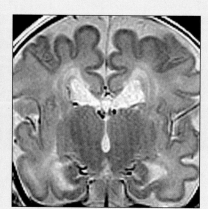

CMV Calcification

SEN in TSC

Migrating Neurons

## Key Facts

### Imaging Findings

- Subependymal heterotopia (most common)
- Band heterotopia ("double cortex")
- Classic lissencephaly
- Cobblestone cortex (formerly called lissencephaly type 2)
- Subcortical heterotopia: Large foci have thinned and dysplastic overlying cortex, small foci don't
- Imaging characteristics match gray matter (GM)
- Margins may be distinct or blurred
- If subcortical, look for continuity with cortex and ventricular surface

### Top Differential Diagnoses

- Tuberous Sclerosis
- Zellweger Syndrome (Peroxisomal Disorder)
- Cytomegalovirus

### Pathology

- Genetic: Mutations alter molecular reactions at multiple migration points ⇒ migrational arrest ⇒ HGM
- Acquired: Toxins/infections ⇒ reactive gliosis/macrophage infiltration ⇒ disturbed neuronal migration/cortical positioning

### Clinical Issues

- Mild cases or simple subcortical nodules can be asymptomatic and only incidental findings on imaging or autopsy

### Diagnostic Checklist

- HGM is common and commonly associated with other anomalies
- HGM doesn't enhance and doesn't calcify

---

  - Swirling, curvilinear GM mass continuous both with cortex, underlying ventricular surface

## CT Findings

- NECT: Always isodense with GM (extremely rare dysplastic Ca++)
- CECT: No enhancement
- Xenon-CT: ↑ Regional cerebral blood flow (rCBF) during functional testing suggests HGM is functional

## MR Findings

- T1WI
  - Imaging characteristics match gray matter (GM)
  - Margins may be distinct or blurred
- T2WI
  - Imaging characteristics of GM
  - If subcortical, look for continuity with cortex and ventricular surface
- FLAIR: No abnormal signal
- DWI: White matter pathways (tractography) pass through band heterotopia; connectivity patterns may explain absence of focal neurologic deficits
- MRS: Choline and NAA are variable

## Ultrasonographic Findings

- Grayscale Ultrasound: Fetal US and fetal MR have documented subependymal heterotopia

## Nuclear Medicine Findings

- PET: Band heterotopia: Glucose uptake similar to or > than normal cortex
- Brain scan (HMPAO-SPECT): Perfusion similar to normal cortex

## Imaging Recommendations

- MR + thin slice SPGR (surface coil/3D reconstruction) for subtle lesions

## DIFFERENTIAL DIAGNOSIS

### Tuberous Sclerosis

- SENs of tuberous sclerosis have signal of mature white matter, not gray matter

- SENs often calcify, may enhance
- Linear white lines of TS: From ventricle to cortex

### Zellweger Syndrome (Peroxisomal Disorder)

- Abnormal neuronal migration, hypomyelination, band heterotopia

### Many Syndromes and Complicated Brain Malformations Include HGM Amongst Findings

- Agenesis CC, Chiari 2 are the most common of these

### Cytomegalovirus

- Periventricular calcifications

## PATHOLOGY

### General Features

- General path comments
  - GM nodules/masses in wrong location
  - Embryology complicated, process dependent upon multiple molecular mechanisms
    - Cell cycle control, cell-cell adhesion, growth factor, neurotransmitter release, interaction with matrix proteins
  - Specific (normal) orderly pattern of development
    - Subependymal germinal zones proliferate, form neuroblasts & glia
    - Neuroblasts leave ventricular surface by "leading edge" extension/growth cone formation (requires filamen)
    - Neuroblasts attach to radially arranged glial fibers (RGFs)
    - Neuroblasts migrate along RGFs to mantle (requires cell-adhesion, ligand-receptor interactions)
    - RGFs guide/nourish migrating neuroblasts
    - Neuroblasts disengage from RGFs (requires reelin secreted by layer 1 pioneer neurons)
    - Earliest neuroblasts disengage in cortical subplate
    - Later waves pass through initial layer, form 6 layered cortex

# HETEROTOPIC GRAY MATTER

- Genetics
  - Transitory "pioneer cells" arrive first in corticogenesis (layer 1)
  - Genetics = complete/partial deletion/mutation of genes that govern specific stages of neuronal migration
    - Migrational failure occurs at multiple stages
  - Type 1 (classic or Miller-Dieker) lissencephaly: Large deletion LIS1 gene located on 17p13.3
  - Isolated lissencephaly/posterior band heterotopia: Smaller deletion LIS1
  - Isolated lissencephaly/anterior band heterotopia: XLIS gene on Xq22.3-q23
  - Microcephaly with periventricular nodular heterotopia: ARGEF2 gene mutation
  - Bilateral, diffuse subependymal heterotopia: Filamin-1 gene FLN-A (required for cell migration to cortex) on Xq28
  - Isolated foci (large masses or single small foci) of HGM occur with many, many other syndromes and malformations: 22q11 microdeletions, Chr 5p mutations
- Etiology
  - Genetic: Mutations alter molecular reactions at multiple migration points ⇒ migrational arrest ⇒ HGM
  - Acquired: Toxins/infections ⇒ reactive gliosis/macrophage infiltration ⇒ disturbed neuronal migration/cortical positioning
    - CMV-infected cells can fail to migrate ⇒ lissencephaly
    - Toxins (alcohol, XRT) ⇒ slow/abnormal migration
- Epidemiology
  - 17% of neonatal CNS anomalies at autopsy
  - Found in up to 40% of patients with intractable epilepsy

## Gross Pathologic & Surgical Features

- Spectrum: Agyria to normal cortex + small ectopic nodules GM
- Persistent fetal leptomeningeal vascularization if severe

## Microscopic Features

- Multiple neuronal cell types, immature/dysplastic neurons
  - Excess of excitatory over inhibitory neuronal circuitry
- Neuronal numbers, positioning abnormal
- Subjacent microstructural white matter abnormalities

## Staging, Grading or Classification Criteria

- Classification by specific location, type, and size of HGM may predict specific gene mutation
  - Nodular/band/curvilinear, anterior/posterior, subcortical, subependymal

# CLINICAL ISSUES

## Presentation

- Most common signs/symptoms: Cognitive function, age of seizure (Sz) onset/severity depend on location/amount of abnormally positioned GM

- Clinical Profile: Young child with developmental delay and Sz

## Demographics

- Age
  - Severe cases present in infancy with Sz & associated malformations
  - Mild cases or simple subcortical nodules can be asymptomatic and only incidental findings on imaging or autopsy
- Gender: Males with X-linked disorders have significantly worse brain malformation and outcome

## Natural History & Prognosis

- Variable life span dependent upon extent of malformation
  - Lissencephaly: Months to few years
  - Focal heterotopia: Can be normal if Szs controlled

## Treatment

- Surgery reserved for intractable Sz
  - Resect small accessible epileptogenic nodules
  - Corpus callosotomy if bilateral or diffuse unresectable lesions

# DIAGNOSTIC CHECKLIST

## Consider

- HGM is common and commonly associated with other anomalies

## Image Interpretation Pearls

- HGM doesn't enhance and doesn't calcify
- Subcortical HGM can appear mass-like, mimic tumor

# SELECTED REFERENCES

1. Bonilha L et al: Microstructural white matter abnormalities in nodular heterotopia with overlying polymicrogyria. Seizure. 2006
2. Hetts SW et al: Anomalies of the corpus callosum: an MR analysis of the phenotypic spectrum of associated malformations. AJR Am J Roentgenol. 187(5):1343-8, 2006
3. Barkovich AJ et al: A developmental and genetic classification for malformations of cortical development. Neurology. 65(12):1873-87, 2005
4. Guerrini R et al: Neuronal migration disorders, genetics, and epileptogenesis. J Child Neurol. 20(4):287-99, 2005
5. Eriksson SH et al: Exploring white matter tracts in band heterotopia using diffusion tractography. Ann Neurol. 52(3):327-34, 2002
6. Barkovich AJ et al: Gray matter heterotopia. Neurology. 55(11):1603-8, 2000
7. Barkovich AJ: Morphologic characteristics of subcortical heterotopia: MR imaging study. AJNR Am J Neuroradiol. 21(2):290-5, 2000
8. Gressens P: Mechanisms and disturbances of neuronal migration. Pediatr Res. 48(6):725-30, 2000
9. Morioka T et al: Functional imaging in periventricular nodular heterotopia with the use of FDG-PET and HMPAO-SPECT. Neurosurg Rev. 22(1):41-4, 1999
10. Marsh L et al: Proton magnetic resonance spectroscopy of a grey matter heterotopia. Neurology 47(6):1571-4, 1996
11. Shimodozono M et al: Functioning heterotopic grey matter? Increased blood flow with voluntary movement & sensory stimulation. Neuroradiology. 37(6):440-2,1995

## IMAGE GALLERY

### Typical

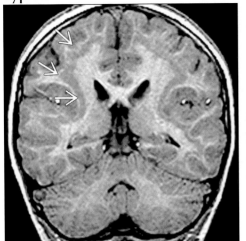
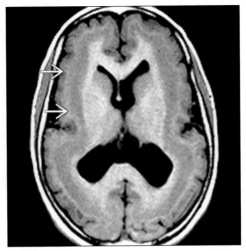

*(Left)* Coronal T1WI MR shows bilateral thin curvilinear bands of subcortical gray matter ➡. The overlying sulci and gyri are near normal. *(Right)* Axial T1WI MR in a different child shows a wider band of heterotopic gray matter ➡. The overlying sulci are too few in number and very shallow; the gyri are abnormally wide.

### Typical

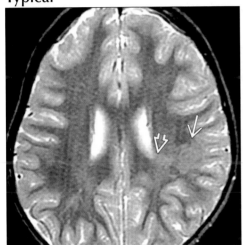
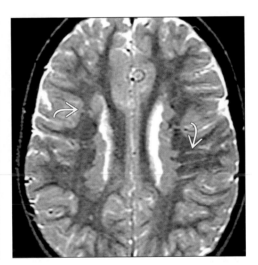

*(Left)* Axial T2WI MR shows a blurred curvilinear streak of gray matter extending from the cortex ➡ to the ventricular surface ➡ in this case of subcortical heterotopia. *(Right)* Axial T2WI MR shows bilateral subependymal nodular heterotopia. Note the thin, sharp strands of gray matter ➡ connecting the subependymal rests to the cortex, an uncommon finding.

### Typical

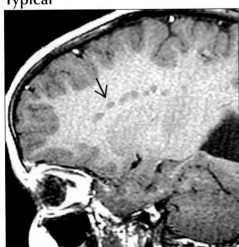
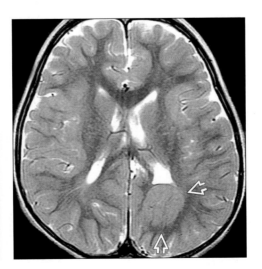

*(Left)* Sagittal T1WI MR in a patient with megalencephaly shows a "string of small pearls" ➡ of periventricular nodular heterotopia; this is a common finding and should be recognized. *(Right)* Axial T2WI MR shows a large mass of subcortical heterotopic gray matter ➡ extending from the left trigone to occipital cortex in a patient presenting with focal seizures.

# POLYMICROGYRIA

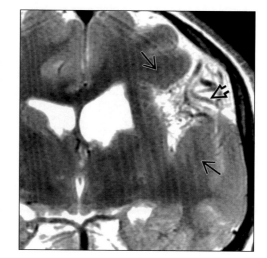

*Coronal graphic shows the cobblestone or pebbly gyri characteristic of polymicrogyria involving the perisylvian cortex ➡. Also note the irregular cortical-white matter interface ➡.*

*Coronal T2WI MR shows left perisylvian polymicrogyria. Note the irregular cortical-white matter junction ➡. Also note the open sylvian fissure and dysplastic leptomeningeal vessels ➡.*

## TERMINOLOGY

### Abbreviations and Synonyms
- Polymicrogyria (PMG) sometimes referred to as cortical dysplasia
- Polymicrogyria/schizencephaly complex

### Definitions
- Polymicrogyria
  - Malformation due to abnormality in late neuronal migration and cortical organization
    - Schizencephaly is also a disorder of late neuronal migration and cortical organization
  - Neurons reach the cortex but distribute abnormally, forming multiple small undulating gyri

## IMAGING FINDINGS

### General Features
- Best diagnostic clue
  - Polymicrogyria ⇒ cortical-white matter junction is always irregular

- Appearance of PMG is influenced by the state of brain maturation and and slice thickness of the imaging study
- Location: Polymicrogyria: Predilection for perisylvian regions, when bilateral often syndromic
- Morphology
  - Variable appearance ⇒ normal or thick cortex, small irregular gyri, indistinct cortical-white matter junction
  - Paradoxically, cortex may range from bumpy and irregular ⇔ smooth

### CT Findings
- NECT
  - Excessive small convolutions or apparent thickening of cortex, shallow or flat sulci
  - ± Periventricular Ca++ if secondary to CMV
  - < 5% of affected patients, PMG cortex will show calcification

### MR Findings
- T1WI
  - Irregular cortical surface, cortex isointense to gray matter, indistinct cortical-white matter interface
  - Sulci always abnormal: Shallow or absent

## DDx: Cortical Malformations

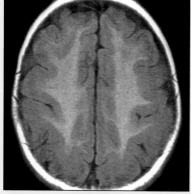

*Pachygyria*

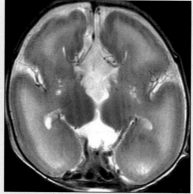

*Lissencephaly (ARX)*

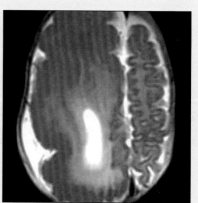

*Hemimegalencephaly*

# POLYMICROGYRIA

## Key Facts

### Terminology
- Polymicrogyria (PMG) sometimes referred to as cortical dysplasia

### Imaging Findings
- Polymicrogyria ⇒ cortical-white matter junction is always irregular
- Radiography: Polymicrogyric newborns, infants often microcephalic
- Polymicrogyria (two imaging patterns) ⇒ influenced by degree of myelination
- < 12 months: Thin appearing, small, fine undulating cortex with normal thickness (2-3 mm)
- > 18 months: Thick, bumpy cortex (5-8 mm), ± hypomyelination, ± cortical infolding

### Top Differential Diagnoses
- Pachygyria: Smooth cortical-white matter interface
- Lissencephaly: Smooth brain lacking gyri and sulci (many genes: LIS1, DCX, ARX)
- Congenital CMV: Association with polymicrogyria, NCCT aides detection of periventricular Ca++

### Clinical Issues
- Most common signs/symptoms: Polymicrogyria ⇒ faciopharyngoglossomasticatory diplegia, developmental delay, seizure, hemiparesis

### Diagnostic Checklist
- Polymicrogyria ⇒ always present near schizencephaly
- Irregular cortical-white matter interface and shallow or absent overlying sulci

---

- T2WI
  - Polymicrogyria (two imaging patterns) ⇒ influenced by degree of myelination
    - < 12 months: Thin appearing, small, fine undulating cortex with normal thickness (2-3 mm)
    - > 18 months: Thick, bumpy cortex (5-8 mm), ± hypomyelination, ± cortical infolding
- FLAIR: Hyperintense signal at sites of dysplastic white matter
- T2* GRE: Hypointense foci at sites of periventricular Ca++ ⇒ CMV
- T1 C+: Amplifies dysplastic leptomeningeal veins overlying regions of polymicrogyria, seen in ~ 51% of PMG cases
- MRV: Demonstrates persistent embryonic veins overlying abnormal cortex
- MRS: ↓ NAA at seizure-precipitating, atrophic and/or hypomyelinated sites, may be normal

### Radiographic Findings
- Radiography: Polymicrogyric newborns, infants often microcephalic

### Nuclear Medicine Findings
- PET
  - Increased metabolism during ictus
  - Hypometabolic interictally

### Other Modality Findings
- Fetal MR and US: Agyric cortex normal up to 26 weeks
- Prenatal MR can defect PMG other anomalies of cortical development as early as 24 weeks

### Imaging Recommendations
- Best imaging tool
  - MR ⇒ volume 3DFT spoiled gradient acquisition (T1) and 3DFT FSE (T2); ≤ 1.5 mm partition size
  - Evaluation in three planes
  - NECT as supplement to detect Ca++ in suspected (TORCH) infection

- Protocol advice: Techniques that accentuate cortical-white matter interface: Volume 3D SPGR (T1WI)

## DIFFERENTIAL DIAGNOSIS

### Cortical Malformations
- Pachygyria: Smooth cortical-white matter interface
- Lissencephaly: Smooth brain lacking gyri and sulci (many genes: LIS1, DCX, ARX)
- Hemimegalencephaly: Disorder of neuronal proliferation, migration, and differentiation
- Congenital CMV: Association with polymicrogyria, NCCT aides detection of periventricular Ca++
- Microlissencephaly: Disorder of stem cell proliferation, HC < 3 SDs below the mean
- Malformations of cortical development not otherwise classified
  - Malformations secondary to inborn errors of metabolism
  - Zellweger syndrome: Deficiency of peroxisomes, severe hypomyelination, cortical malformation
  - Mitochondrial and pyruvate metabolism disorders

## PATHOLOGY

### General Features
- General path comments
  - Polymicrogyria ⇒ disorder of late neuronal migration and cortical organization
  - Location: Unilateral (40%), bilateral (60%), frontal (70%), parietal (63%), temporal (38%), and occipital (7%)
- Genetics
  - Bilateral PMG syndromes ⇒ Most X-linked, some autosomal dominant and recessive
  - Polymicrogyria: Deletions of: 22q11.2 (DiGeorge critical region), Xq28 and 16q12.2-21
  - Familial PMG includes unilateral, bilateral frontoparietal, and bilateral diffuse PMG
- Etiology

# POLYMICROGYRIA

- o Polymicrogyria ⇒ intrauterine infection, ischemia, toxins, vascular problems related to twinning, or gene mutations
- o Molecular mechanisms: Neurite extension, synaptogenesis, and neuronal maturation
- Epidemiology: Malformations of cortical development found in ~ 40% of children with intractable epilepsy
- Associated abnormalities
  - o Syndromes associated with polymicrogyria
    - Congenital bilateral perisylvian syndrome (CBPS) ⇒ faciopharyngoglossomasticatory diplegia, ± esophageal malformations (Foix-Chavany-Marie)
    - Aicardi ⇒ infantile spasms, absent corpus callosum, chorioretinal lacunae, vertebral anomalies
    - Syndrome of congenital hemiplegia and epilepsy
    - Syndrome of megalencephaly with polymicrogyria and hydrocephalus
    - Otosclerosis and bilateral perisylvian PMG
    - Others: Zellweger, Adams-Oliver, Arima, micro, Galloway-Mowat, and Delleman syndrome

## Gross Pathologic & Surgical Features

- Polymicrogyria ⇒ multiple small gyri, gyri lie in haphazard orientation

## Microscopic Features

- Polymicrogyria ⇒ range of histology reflecting derangement of the six layered lamination of the cortex
  - o Cortical layers 4 and 5 most involved
  - o Leptomeningeal embryonic vasculature overlies malformation
  - o Myelination within the subcortical or intracortical fibers changes the cortical appearance on MR imaging
- Epileptogenic focus is typically not within the dysplastic cortex but adjacent to the PMG and is known as the paramicrogyral zone

## Staging, Grading or Classification Criteria

- Polymicrogyria ⇒ unlayered or four layered cytoarchitecture

## CLINICAL ISSUES

### Presentation

- Most common signs/symptoms: Polymicrogyria ⇒ faciopharyngoglossomasticatory diplegia, developmental delay, seizure, hemiparesis
- Other signs/symptoms: Hemiplegia, hydrocephalus
- Clinical Profile: Onset and severity of seizures relates to extent of malformation

### Demographics

- Age: Signs and symptoms vary with severity of gene mutation, and resultant phenotypic expression
- Gender: X-linked inheritance ⇒ boys

### Natural History & Prognosis

- Variable life span based on: Severity of genetic mutation, resultant malformation and associated anomalies

- Bilateral forms of PMG carry worse prognosis

## Treatment

- Options, risks, complications
  - o Medical management of seizures and supportive care
  - o Corpus callosotomy if bilateral or diffuse unresectable lesions and intractable epilepsy

## DIAGNOSTIC CHECKLIST

### Consider

- Polymicrogyria ⇒ always present near schizencephaly
  - o Irregular cortical-white matter interface and shallow or absent overlying sulci

### Image Interpretation Pearls

- Fetal appearance of the newborn brain ⇔ lissencephaly
- Primitive sylvian fissures with thick cortex ⇔ polymicrogyria

## SELECTED REFERENCES

1. Araujo D et al: Language and motor FMRI activation in polymicrogyric cortex. Epilepsia. 47(3):589-92, 2006
2. Chang BS et al: A familial syndrome of unilateral polymicrogyria affecting the right hemisphere. Neurology. 66(1):133-5, 2006
3. Morris EB 3rd et al: Histopathologic findings of malformations of cortical development in an epilepsy surgery cohort. Arch Pathol Lab Med. 130(8):1163-8, 2006
4. Munakata M et al: Morphofunctional organization in three patients with unilateral polymicrogyria: combined use of diffusion tensor imaging and functional magnetic resonance imaging. Brain Dev. 28(6):405-9, 2006
5. Barkovich AJ et al: A developmental and genetic classification for malformations of cortical development. Neurology. 65(12):1873-87, 2005
6. de Wit MC et al: Re: polymicrogyria versus pachygyria in 22q11 microdeletion. Am J Med Genet A. 136(4):419; author reply 420-1, 2005
7. Guerrini R: Genetic malformations of the cerebral cortex and epilepsy. Epilepsia. 46 Suppl 1:32-7, 2005
8. Jansen A et al: Genetics of the polymicrogyria syndromes. J Med Genet. 42(5):369-78, 2005
9. Piao X et al: Genotype-phenotype analysis of human frontoparietal polymicrogyria syndromes. Ann Neurol. 58(5):680-7, 2005
10. Riel-Romero RM et al: Developmental venous anomaly in association with neuromigrational anomalies. Pediatr Neurol. 32(1):53-5, 2005
11. Titomanlio L et al: A new syndrome of congenital generalized osteosclerosis and bilateral polymicrogyria. Am J Med Genet A. 138(1):1-5, 2005
12. Righini A et al: Early prenatal MR imaging diagnosis of polymicrogyria. AJNR Am J Neuroradiol. 25(2):343-6, 2004
13. Takanashi J et al: The changing MR imaging appearance of polymicrogyria: a consequence of myelination. AJNR Am J Neuroradiol. 24(5):788-93, 2003
14. Barkovich AJ et al: Syndromes of bilateral symmetrical polymicrogyria. AJNR Am J Neuroradiol. 20(10):1814-21, 1999
15. Kuzniecky R et al: The congenital bilateral perisylvian syndrome: imaging findings in a multicenter study. CBPS Study Group. AJNR Am J Neuroradiol. 15(1):139-44, 1994

# POLYMICROGYRIA

## IMAGE GALLERY

### Typical

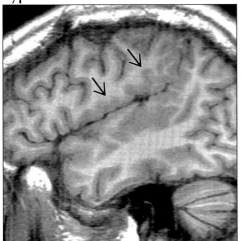
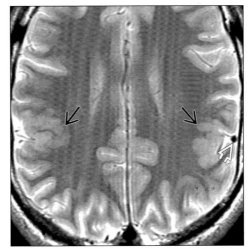

*(Left)* Sagittal T1WI MR shows perisylvian polymicrogyria. The festooned morphology of the perisylvian cortex shows an irregular interface ➡ with the adjacent white matter. *(Right)* Axial T2WI MR shows bilateral perisylvian/suprasylvian polymicrogyria ➡. Note irregularity of the cortical-white matter junction in the involved cortex and enlarged overlying vein ➡.

### Typical

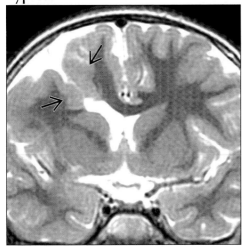
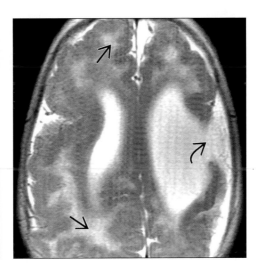

*(Left)* Coronal T2WI MR shows closed-lip schizencephaly lined by polymicrogyric cortex ➡. Polymicrogyria is always seen adjacent to schizencephalic cleft. *(Right)* Axial T2WI MR shows the sequela of congenital CMV infection, with extensive bi-hemispheric polymicrogyria, open-lip schizencephaly ➡ and diffuse, multifocal demyelination ➡.

### Variant

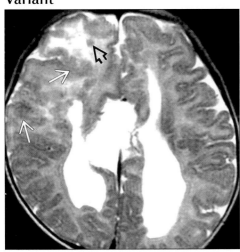
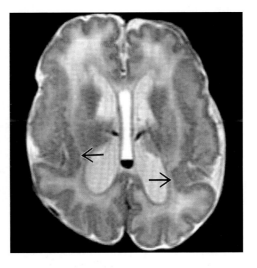

*(Left)* Axial T2WI MR shows polymicrogyria ➡ in Aicardi syndrome. Note the focal subcortical heterotopia ➡ and surrounding demyelination. The corpus callosum is also absent. *(Right)* Axial T2WI MR shows bilateral posterior perisylvian polymicrogyria ➡ in this infant with Zellweger syndrome. Ventricles are enlarged and too many frontal sulci are present.

# SCHIZENCEPHALY

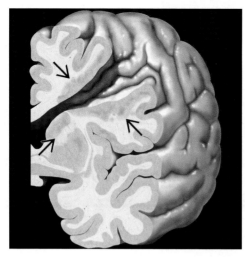

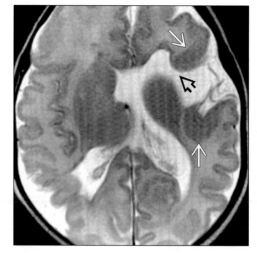

Coronal oblique graphic shows an open-lip schizencephaly in the frontal lobe. Note irregular gray-white interface of the cortex lining the cleft ➡, indicating its dysplastic nature.

Axial T2WI MR shows an open-lip left frontal schizencephalic cleft ➡ that communicates with the anterior portion of the sylvian fissure, with dysplastic cortex lining its margins ➡.

## TERMINOLOGY

### Abbreviations and Synonyms
- Schizencephaly, agenetic porencephaly

### Definitions
- Clefts in the brain parenchyma that extend from the cortical surface to the ventricle (pia to ependyma), lined by dysplastic gray matter (GM)

## IMAGING FINDINGS

### General Features
- Best diagnostic clue
  - Abnormal cleft in hemisphere, connecting ventricle and subarachnoid space, lined by gray matter
    - Look for dimple in wall of ventricle if cleft is narrow/closed
- Location: Frontal and parietal lobes near central sulcus most common
- Size
  - "Closed-lip" lesions are small, with walls apposed to each other
  - "Open-lip" lesions can be very large, mimicking hydranencephaly
- Morphology
  - Up to half of schizencephalies are bilateral
    - When bilateral, 60% open on both sides, 20% open on only one side
    - When unilateral, 2/3 are open

### CT Findings
- NECT
  - Cleft of cerebrospinal fluid (CSF) density
  - GM lining clefts can be slightly hyperdense
  - Dimple on wall of ventricle where cleft intersects it
    - May be best clue for closed-lip lesions
  - Calcifications (Ca++) when associated with cytomegalovirus (CMV)
  - Large open-lip schizencephaly can be associated with expansion/thinning of overlying calvaria
    - Chronic effect of CSF pulsations
    - May require CSF diversion
- CECT: Large, primitive appearing veins near cleft

### MR Findings
- T1WI

## DDx: Clefts in the Brain

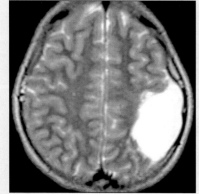

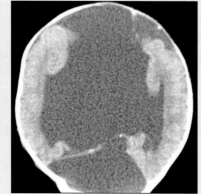

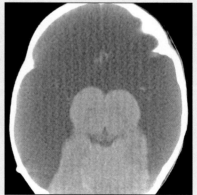

Remote Infarct | ACC/IHC | Hydranencephaly

# SCHIZENCEPHALY

## Key Facts

### Terminology
- Clefts in the brain parenchyma that extend from the cortical surface to the ventricle (pia to ependyma), lined by dysplastic gray matter (GM)

### Imaging Findings
- Look for dimple in wall of ventricle if cleft is narrow/closed
- Location: Frontal and parietal lobes near central sulcus most common
- Up to half of schizencephalies are bilateral
- Distinction of GM lining the cleft can be difficult prior to myelination
- Abnormal GM along cleft typically hypointense on T2WI

### Top Differential Diagnoses
- Encephaloclastic Porencephaly
- Transmantle Heterotopia

### Pathology
- Early prenatal insult affecting germinal zone prior to neuronal migration
- Insult can be genetically determined, or 2° to infection, trauma, vascular insult
- 1/3 of children with schizencephaly will have non-CNS abnormalities

### Clinical Issues
- Seizures are reportedly more common in unilateral schizencephaly
- Magnitude of clefts and associated lesions govern severity of impairment

---

- ○ Distinction of GM lining the cleft can be difficult prior to myelination
- ○ Closed lip ⇒ irregular tract of GM extending from cortical ribbon to ventricle
  - ■ GM lining cleft can appear "cobblestone" ⇒ dysplastic
  - ■ GM/white matter (WM) border may be indistinct or irregular
- ○ Open lip ⇒ "canal" of CSF may be wide and wedge-shaped or have nearly parallel walls
  - ■ GM lining cleft may be harder to discern in open-lip schizencephaly
- T2WI
  - ○ Infolding of gray matter along transmantle clefts
    - ■ In unmyelinated infant, GM/WM distinction more clear on T2WI
    - ■ Abnormal GM along cleft typically hypointense on T2WI
- T2* GRE: May show Ca++ if associated with CMV
- T1 C+: Associated developmental venous anomalies (DVAs) well shown with contrast
- MRA
  - ○ MCA candelabra can "fall" into large clefts
  - ○ Displaced along walls of cleft in subarachnoid space, not free within "canal"
- 3D surface rendered MR
  - ○ Best defines relationship of gyri/sulci to cleft in cerebral mantle
- Functional MR
  - ○ Functional reorganization of the undamaged hemisphere reported

### Ultrasonographic Findings
- Grayscale Ultrasound: Diagnosable by fetal ultrasound and fetal MR; progressive changes have been reported

### Nuclear Medicine Findings
- PET: Normal or ↑ glucose metabolism and perfusion of wall of cleft (normal gray matter activity)

### Imaging Recommendations
- Best imaging tool: MR
- Protocol advice

- ○ Prior to myelination ⇒ T2WI; use multiple planes
- ○ After myelination complete ⇒ T1WI
  - ■ Thin slice "volume" acquisitions that allow multiplanar and surface-rendered reformatting

## DIFFERENTIAL DIAGNOSIS

### Encephaloclastic Porencephaly
- Cleft in brain due to insult after neuronal migration complete
- Lined by gliotic WM, not dysplastic GM!

### Hydranencephaly
- Destruction of tissue in middle and anterior cerebral artery territory
- Residual parenchyma displaced inferiorly and posteriorly

### Holoprosencephaly
- Semilobar can mimic bilateral open-lip schizencephaly
- Midline fusion anomalies
- Residual parenchyma displaced anteriorly

### Agenesis of Corpus Callosum with Interhemispheric Cyst (ACC/IHC)
- Type 1 cyst ⇒ diverticulum of 3rd ventricle
- Residual parenchyma displaced laterally

### Post-Operative Cavities
- History should suffice

### Transmantle Heterotopia
- May actually represent a form of closed-lip schizencephaly

## PATHOLOGY

### General Features
- General path comments
  - ○ Can be due to acquired insult or inherited mutation
    - ■ Intrauterine insults include: Infection (CMV), maternal trauma or toxin exposure

# SCHIZENCEPHALY

- ▪ Reported with alloimmune thrombocytopenia (acquired, but subsequent pregnancies have same risk of intrauterine damage)
  - ○ Experimental schizencephaly induced by mumps virus
    - ▪ Antigen detected in ventricular zone neuroepithelial cells & radial glial fibers ⇒ destruction & disordered migration
- • Genetics
  - ○ EMX2 (gene locus 10q26.1) is a regulatory gene with a role in structural patterning of developing forebrain
    - ▪ EMX2 is expressed in germinal matrix of developing neocortex
    - ▪ Mutations in the homeobox gene EMX2 seen in some cases (controversial)
- • Etiology
  - ○ Early prenatal insult affecting germinal zone prior to neuronal migration
    - ▪ "Spot-weld" effect, preventing normal migration and organization
    - ▪ Insult can be genetically determined, or 2° to infection, trauma, vascular insult
- • Epidemiology
  - ○ Bilateral clefts are more commonly reported by pathology
  - ○ Unilateral slightly more commonly reported by imaging
- • Associated abnormalities
  - ○ Hippocampal and callosal anomalies
  - ○ Septo-optic dysplasia (SOD, de Morsier syndrome)
    - ▪ Absence of the septum pellucidum in 70% of schizencephaly, especially bilateral
    - ▪ Schizencephaly is usually bilateral in SOD
    - ▪ Optic nerve hypoplasia in 1/3 of schizencephaly
    - ▪ Imaging is not sensitive in detection of optic nerve hypoplasia (≈ 50%)
  - ○ 1/3 of children with schizencephaly will have non-CNS abnormalities

## Gross Pathologic & Surgical Features
- • Transmantle clefts with separated or apposed gray matter lining
- • Abnormal cortical array of pachygyria, polymicrogyria, or near normal-sized gyri "dive" into cleft
- • Thalami, corticospinal tracts may be atrophied or not formed

## Microscopic Features
- • Little, if any glial scarring
- • Loss of normal laminar architecture
- • Polymicrogyria, or heterotopic gray matter

## Staging, Grading or Classification Criteria
- • Type I (closed-lip): Fused pial-ependymal seam lined by gray matter forms "furrow" in cortex
- • Type II (open-lip): Large, gray matter lined, fluid-filled cerebrospinal fluid clefts

## CLINICAL ISSUES

### Presentation
- • Most common signs/symptoms

- ○ Unilateral ⇒ seizures and mild motor deficit ("congenital" hemiparesis)
- ○ Bilateral ⇒ severe developmental delay, paresis, spasticity
  - ▪ Seizures are reportedly more common in unilateral schizencephaly
- • Other signs/symptoms: Microcephaly or plagiocephaly

## Natural History & Prognosis
- • Magnitude of clefts and associated lesions govern severity of impairment

## Treatment
- • Treat seizures and hydrocephalus; physiotherapy for motor deficits

## DIAGNOSTIC CHECKLIST

### Consider
- • Image to confirm etiology of "congenital hemiparesis": Perinatal stroke versus unilateral schizencephaly

### Image Interpretation Pearls
- • Multiplanar imaging to avoid "in-plane" oversight of closed-lip schizencephaly
  - ○ If plane of imaging is the same as plane of cleft, abnormality easily overlooked
- • Lateral ventricle walls should be smooth
  - ○ "Dimple" in wall ⇒ look for closed-lip schizencephaly
  - ○ "Angle" of wall ⇒ consequence of periventricular injury (PVL)
  - ○ "Lump" on wall ⇒ GM heterotopion or subependymal nodule of tuberous sclerosis

## SELECTED REFERENCES

1. Curry CJ et al: Schizencephaly: heterogeneous etiologies in a population of 4 million California births. Am J Med Genet A. 137(2):181-9, 2005
2. Granata T et al: Schizencephaly: clinical spectrum, epilepsy, and pathogenesis. J Child Neurol. 20(4):313-8, 2005
3. Guerrini R: Genetic malformations of the cerebral cortex and epilepsy. Epilepsia. 46 Suppl 1:32-7, 2005
4. Cecchi C: Emx2: a gene responsible for cortical development, regionalization and area specification. Gene. 291(1-2):1-9, 2002
5. Dale ST et al: Neonatal alloimmune thrombocytopenia: antenatal and postnatal imaging findings in the pediatric brain. AJNR Am J Neuroradiol. 23(9):1457-65, 2002
6. Raybaud C et al: Schizencephaly: correlation between the lobar topography of the cleft(s) and absence of the septum pellucidum. Childs Nerv Syst. 17(4-5):217-22, 2001
7. Sato N et al: MR evaluation of the hippocampus in patients with congenital malformations of the brain. AJNR Am J Neuroradiol. 22(2):389-93, 2001
8. Takano T et al: Experimental schizencephaly induced by Kilham strain of mumps virus: pathogenesis of cleft formation. Neuroreport. 10(15):3149-54, 1999

# SCHIZENCEPHALY

## IMAGE GALLERY

### Variant

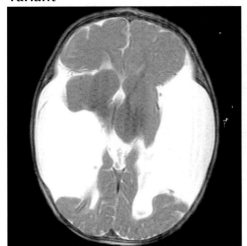
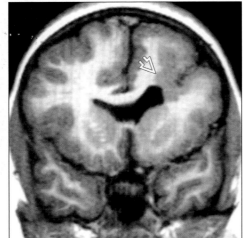

*(Left)* Axial T2WI MR shows bilateral large open lip schizencephaly connecting trigones with sylvian fissures in both hemispheres. These large clefts can closely mimic hydranencephaly. *(Right)* Coronal T1WI MR shows a typical closed-lip schizencephaly ➡ in left hemisphere. Note abnormal sulcation through most of both hemispheres. This portends a guarded prognosis.

### Typical

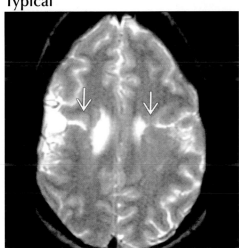
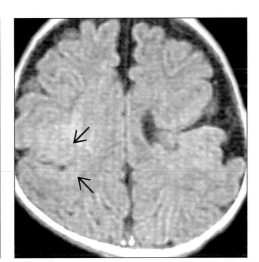

*(Left)* Axial T2WI MR in a child with seizures shows bilateral schizencephalic clefts. Note that the dysplastic gray matter lining the clefts ➡ extends into the lateral ventricles as heterotopia. *(Right)* Axial T1WI MR shows a very subtle right sided lesion ➡ in addition to larger left sided one. T2WI provides the best gray-white differentiation and anatomical detail in the neonate.

### Typical

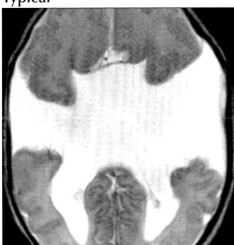
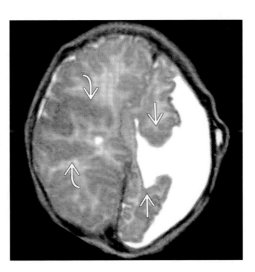

*(Left)* Axial T2WI MR shows large bilateral open-lip schizencephaly causing "bat-wing" appearance of ventricular system. Septum pellucidum absent and optic nerves were small; septo-optic dysplasia. *(Right)* Axial T2WI MR shows a large open lip schizencephaly, lined by dysplastic cortex ➡, in left hemisphere. Deep infoldings of dysplastic cortex ➡ are seen in contralateral hemisphere.

# NORMAL MYELINATION & METABOLIC DISEASE

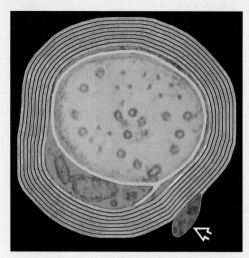

Graphic of myelinated axon shows oligodendroglial cell process ⮞ producing multiple layers of myelin (blue), wrapping around central axon (yellow), increasing speed of action potentials.

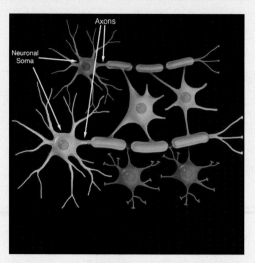

Graphic shows oligodendrocytes (blue) extending processes to coat axons with segments of myelin. Nodes of Ranvier (red) separate myelin segments. Astrocytes (purple) extend processes to the nodes.

## TERMINOLOGY

### Synonyms
- Inborn errors of metabolism, leukodystrophies

### Definitions
- Disorders caused by abnormalities of myelin formation or by the breakdown or normal myelin or other normal brain tissue
  - Tissue breakdown due to either the accumulation of toxic metabolites or the lack of formation of necessary metabolites

## IMAGING ANATOMY

### General Anatomic Considerations
- Myelination progresses generally caudal to rostral
  - Pathways that mature earlier myelinate earlier
    - Posterior fossa: Medial longitudinal fasciculus, lateral lemniscus, medial lemniscus early; corticospinal tract and transverse pontine fibers later
    - Cerebrum: Sensorimotor pathways and visual pathways myelinate early, association pathways myelinate late

### Critical Anatomic Structures
- Myelin sheath
  - Surrounds axon
  - Composed of multiple segments, separated by nodes of Ranvier
    - Each segment is modified plasma membrane, originating as extension of oligodendroglial cell process
    - Nodes of Ranvier are sites of multiple sodium channels where axon depolarization takes place
  - Function: Myelin segments increase resistance to propagation of action potentials in axon
    - Impulse therefore jumps to next node

- Because of low capacitance of sheath, remaining axonal membrane between the nodes depolarizes with little energy requirement & markedly increased speed
- Structure of myelin
  - Multiple layers wound in a spiral around central axon
  - Characteristic protein-lipid-protein-lipid-protein structure
  - Major structural proteins are proteolipid protein and myelin basic proteins
    - Abnormalities in the formation of these proteins cause absent or unstable myelin
  - Major lipids are cholesterol, phospholipids, and galactolipids in 4:3:2 ratio
    - Cerebroside (galactosylceramide) is most characteristic myelin lipid
    - Absent cerebroside in lab animals ⇒ reduced conduction velocity, myelin degeneration

## ANATOMY-BASED IMAGING ISSUES

### Key Concepts or Questions
- Imaging results of myelination
  - Shortened T1 and T2 relaxation times
  - Reduced diffusivity
    - Diffusivity reduced more perpendicular to axon than parallel to axon
  - Increased fractional anisotropy (FA)
  - Increased magnetization transfer (MT)

### Imaging Approaches
- MR is only imaging technique that assesses myelination
  - T1 weighted images show myelination as increasing hyperintensity
  - T2 weighted images show myelination as increasing hypointensity
  - Diffusion imaging shows myelination as decreasing diffusivity

# NORMAL MYELINATION & METABOLIC DISEASE

## Key Facts

### Myelination

- Myelination occurs in orderly predictable patterns
  - Brain stem tracts, auditory tracts, sensorimotor tracts early
  - Association tracts (anterior frontal, anterior temporal, parietal) late
- MR is sensitive to myelination
  - Qualitative (T1 and T2 weighted images)
  - Quantitative (mag transfer, diffusion, T2 relaxometry)
- Knowledge of normal patterns of myelination important for early identification of disease

### Metabolic Disorders

- Knowledge of normal brain myelination is important in making the diagnosis of metabolic disorder

- First imaging finding may be myelination delay
- Suspect metabolic disorder in developmentally delayed child with bilateral symmetric signal abnormality
  - White matter (lobe, subcortical vs. deep vs. periventricular)
  - Gray matter (basal ganglia -- specific nuclei) vs. cortex
  - Both gray and white matter
  - Assess for cerebellar involvement
- Contrast enhancement suggests focal inflammatory process, helps specify diagnosis
- Proton spectroscopy is a valuable adjunct in making the diagnosis in several disorders

---

- On diffusion tensor imaging (DTI), $\lambda 1$ (major eigenvalue) decreases less than $\lambda 2$ (median eigenvalue) and $\lambda 3$ (minor eigenvalue)
  - FA maps show myelination as increasing FA
  - MT imaging shows myelination as increasing MT
- Many ways to assess myelination by MR
  - Qualitative method: Assess milestones when changes of myelination appear on T1, T2 weighted images
    - Middle cerebellar peduncle: T1WI - birth; T2WI - 2 months
    - Posterior limb internal capsule, posterior portion: T1WI - 36 gestational weeks; T2WI - 40 gestational weeks
    - Anterior limb internal capsule: T1WI - 2-3 months; T2WI - 7-11 months
    - Genu of corpus callosum: T1WI - 4-6 months; T2WI - 5-8 months
    - Splenium of corpus callosum: T1WI - 3-4 months; T2WI - 4-6 months
    - Central occipital WM: T1WI - 3-5 months; T2WI - 9-14 months
    - Peripheral occipital WM: T1WI - 4-7 months; T2WI - 11-15 months
    - Central frontal WM: T1WI - 3-6 months; T2WI - 11-16 months
    - Peripheral frontal WM: T1WI - 7-11 months; T2WI - 14-24 months
  - Quantitative methods: Assess changes in diffusivity, FA, MT and compare with values of age-matched patients

### Imaging Protocols

- Protocol for suspected metabolic disease
  - Sagittal T1 weighted images
  - Axial T2WI and FLAIR (if more than 12 months old)
  - Coronal FLAIR (T2WI if 12 months old or less)
  - Diffusion weighted imaging
  - Single voxel short echo (TE < 30 msec) MR spectrum at basal ganglia
  - Intermediate to long echo (135 msec $\leq$ TE $\leq$ 288 msec) MR spectrum in gray and white matter

### Imaging Pitfalls

- Prematurely born infants should have myelination appropriate for their postnatal age minus time of prematurity
  - e.g., If born at 28 weeks and is 3 months old, expect myelination of term neonate (3 months old minus 3 months premature)
- Hypomyelination may be caused by premature birth or metabolic disorder
  - Prematures with white matter injury have delayed myelination due to damage to oligodendrocytes

## PATHOLOGIC ISSUES

### General Pathologic Considerations

- Inborn errors of metabolism: Abnormal myelin or myelin that breaks down due to intrinsic toxins

### Classification

- Metabolic disorders can affect white matter or gray matter (or both)
- Classify as to what structures are involved and in what patterns

## PATHOLOGY-BASED IMAGING ISSUES

### Key Concepts or Questions

- Acute presentation or longstanding problem
  - Acute presentation may suggest toxic exposure
- Family history
  - Strongly suggests metabolic disorder
- Inciting event
  - Acute exacerbations sometimes triggered by foods, infections, or trauma

### Imaging Approaches

- Assess myelination: T1 and T2 weighted images
- Look for areas of acute/chronic injury: T2 weighted, FLAIR, and diffusion weighted (DW) images

# NORMAL MYELINATION & METABOLIC DISEASE

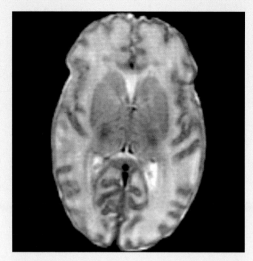

Axial T2WI MR of a prematurely born infant with adjusted age 35 gestational weeks shows completely unmyelinated supratentorial white matter (hyperintense compared with gray matter).

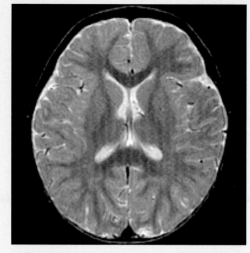

Axial T2WI MR of a normal 2 year old shows myelinated supratentorial white matter. After myelination, the white matter becomes hypointense compared with gray matter.

- ○ Injury may involve gray matter, white matter, or both
- ○ Injury usually bilateral and symmetrical
- ○ Acutely injured areas typically show swelling, reduced diffusivity on DW images
- ○ Chronically injured areas have atrophy, increased diffusivity
- • Best approach to white matter (WM) is that of Van der Knaap and Valk: Assess location and quality of brain abnormalities
  - ○ Lobe involved
  - ○ Periventricular WM vs. deep WM vs. subcortical WM
  - ○ Internal capsule (anterior vs. posterior limb) external capsule
  - ○ Corpus callosum: Rostrum, genu, body, splenium
  - ○ Cerebellum, cerebellar peduncles, hila of dentate nuclei
  - ○ Midbrain, pons, medulla
  - ○ Symmetry, extension (small vs. large, isolated vs. confluent)
  - ○ Appearance (swelling, atrophy, cysts)
  - ○ Signal intensity
  - ○ Demarcation (sharp vs. vague vs. mixed)
  - ○ Myelination (normal vs. absent vs. delayed)
- • Proton MR spectroscopy is diagnostic in some disorders
  - ○ Absent creatine peak (3.03 ppm) in creatine synthesis disorders
  - ○ Markedly elevated NAA peak (2.01 ppm) in Canavan disease
  - ○ Elevated phenylalanine (7.37 ppm) in phenylketonuria
  - ○ Elevated branched chain ketoacids (0.9 ppm) in maple syrup urine disease
  - ○ Elevated glycine (3.55 ppm) in nonketotic hyperglycinemia
- • Contrast-enhancement may be present in acute phase of some disorders
  - ○ X-linked adrenoleukodystrophy
  - ○ Krabbe disease
  - ○ Alexander disease

## CLINICAL IMPLICATIONS

### Clinical Importance
- • Metabolic disorders result from disruption of a metabolic pathway
  - ○ Necessary chemical may not be produced
  - ○ Toxic chemical may not be detoxified or excreted
  - ○ Chemical may be produced but in insufficient quantity
- • Biochemical dysfunction may involve multiple systems (gastrointestinal, genitourinary, musculoskeletal) or be isolated to CNS
  - ○ CNS involvement may have many manifestations
    - ▪ Developmental delay
    - ▪ Acute encephalopathy
    - ▪ Chronic encephalopathy
    - ▪ Seizures
    - ▪ Focal neurological deficits
  - ○ Manifestations depend upon what part of brain is affected

## RELATED REFERENCES

1. Cecil KM: MR spectroscopy of metabolic disorders. Neuroimaging Clin N Am. 16(1):87-116, viii, 2006
2. Vigneron DB: Magnetic resonance spectroscopic imaging of human brain development. Neuroimaging Clin N Am. 16(1):75-85, viii, 2006
3. Barkovich AJ: Pediatric Neuroimaging. 4th Ed. Philadelphia, Lippincott Williams & Wilkins. 2005
4. van der Knaap MS et al: Magnetic Resonance of Myelination and Myelin Disorders. 3rd Ed. Berlin, Springer. 2005
5. van der Knaap MS et al: Pattern recognition in magnetic resonance imaging of white matter disorders in children and young adults. Neuroradiology. 33(6):478-93, 1991
6. van der Knaap MS et al: MR imaging of the various stages of normal myelination during the first year of life. Neuroradiology. 31(6):459-70, 1990

## IMAGE GALLERY

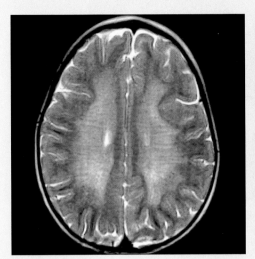 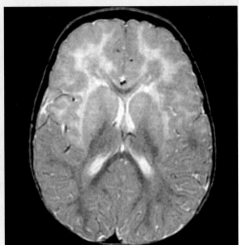

*(Left)* Axial T2WI MR of a 2 year old with metachromatic leukodystrophy shows abnormal hyperintensity, with striations, of deep and periventricular white matter, sparing of subcortical regions. *(Right)* Axial T2WI MR in infant with Alexander disease shows involvement of subcortical, deep, and periventricular white matter in frontal lobes. Basal ganglia are also hyperintense.

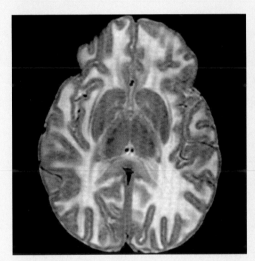 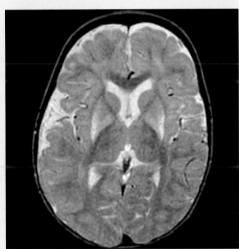

*(Left)* Axial T2WI MR in 18 month old patient with megalencephaly with subcortical cysts shows involvement of all white matter: Subcortical, deep, and periventricular. Internal capsules are involved. *(Right)* Axial T2WI MR in 2 year old with glutaric aciduria I shows abnormal hyperintensity in globi pallidi, putamina, and deep frontal white matter. Subcortical white matter is spared.

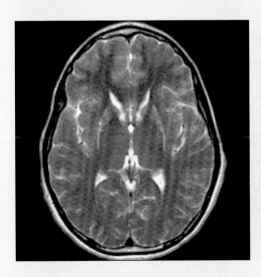 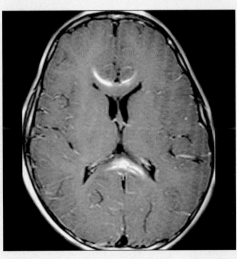

*(Left)* Axial T2WI MR in child with Huntington disease shows shrunken, hyperintense putamina and caudate heads. White matter is normal, as are thalami and globi pallidi. *(Right)* Axial T1 C+ MR in child with X-linked adrenoleukodystrophy shows contrast-enhancement of genu and splenium of corpus callosum. Enhancement results from inflammation/blood-brain barrier injury.

# HYPOMYELINATION

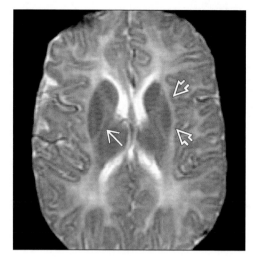

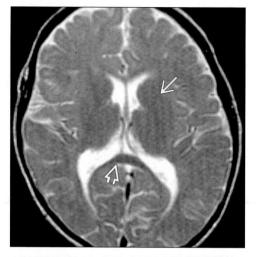

Axial T2WI MR in a 13 year old with Pelizaeus Merzbacher disease shows hyperintense signal throughout the cerebral WM, including the internal ➡ and external ➡ capsules.

Axial T2WI MR in a 3.5 year old with 18q-syndrome shows minimal hypointense signal in the internal capsules ➡ and splenium ➡. On T2WI, myelination should appear complete by this age.

## TERMINOLOGY

### Abbreviations and Synonyms
- Undermyelination, delayed myelin maturation

### Definitions
- Diminished or absent degree of white matter (WM) myelination for age
- Myelin "milestones" not achieved
- May be primary hypomyelination syndrome or secondary to other pathology

## IMAGING FINDINGS

### General Features
- Best diagnostic clue
  - Poor gray-white differentiation on T1WI in children > 1 year
  - Poor gray-white differentiation on T2WI in children > 2 years
- Location: Key areas to assess are internal capsule, pyramidal tracts, optic radiations, and peripheral frontal lobe WM rami

- Size
  - Hypomyelination will result in reduced brain volume
    - Thin corpus callosum evident on sagittal images
- Morphology: Typically normal

### CT Findings
- NECT
  - May appear normal
  - Lack of myelin results in hypodensity on NECT
    - Accentuated gray-white differentiation

### MR Findings
- T1WI
  - Myelinated WM is hyperintense on T1WI
  - WM structures become hyperintense in predictable chronology
  - Myelination on T1WI is complete by 1 year of age
- T2WI
  - Mature WM is hypointense on T2WI
    - Reflects displacement of interstitial water by thickened myelin sheaths
  - Lags hyperintensity on T1WI by 4-8 months
    - T1 signal reflects presence of myelin
    - T2 signal reflects displacement of water

## DDx: Leukodystrophies

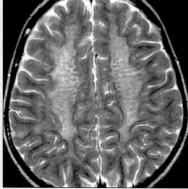

Metachromatic Leukodystrophy

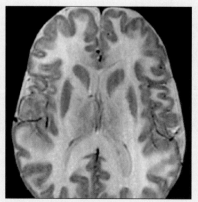

Canavan Disease

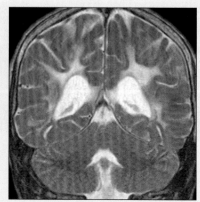

Adrenoleukodystrophy

# HYPOMYELINATION

## Key Facts

### Imaging Findings
- Location: Key areas to assess are internal capsule, pyramidal tracts, optic radiations, and peripheral frontal lobe WM rami
- Myelinated WM is hyperintense on T1WI
- Myelination on T1WI is complete by 1 year of age
- Mature WM is hypointense on T2WI
- T1 signal reflects presence of myelin
- T2 signal reflects displacement of water
- Myelination on T2WI appears complete by 3 years of age, usually by 2 years of age
- T1WI most helpful in children < 10 months
- T2WI most helpful in children > 10 months
- DTI and FA can provide data on WM prior to myelin deposition

### Top Differential Diagnoses
- Pelizaeus-Merzbacher disease (PMD)
- Spastic paraplegia type 2 (SPG2)
- Hypomyelination with atrophy of basal ganglia and cerebellum (H-ABC)
- 18q-syndrome
- Jacobsen syndrome (11q-)
- Hypomyelination with trichothiodystrophy
- Leukodystrophies

### Diagnostic Checklist
- Remember to adjust chronologic age for degree of prematurity
- Assess myelination prior to learning chronologic age of patient

---

- ○ Myelination on T2WI appears complete by 3 years of age, usually by 2 years of age
- ○ "Terminal zones"
  - Regions of persistent hyperintense signal on T2WI in otherwise normal brains
  - Typically around trigones of lateral ventricles
  - Likely due to concentration of interstitial water migrating to ventricles in these areas
  - Must be distinguished from periventricular leukomalacia or perivascular spaces
- PD/Intermediate: Helpful for distinguishing gliosis from undermyelination from terminal zones
- FLAIR
  - ○ Typically "bland" in children < 2 years
    - May be confusing in infants
    - Best used as an adjunct to T2WI
- DWI
  - ○ ADC values predate T1 and T2 weighted signal changes
    - ADC drops as WM diffusivity decreases
  - ○ Fractional anisotropy globally increases with brain maturation
  - ○ Fractional anisotropy (FA) maps delineate unmyelinated tracts throughout the brain
  - ○ FA and spectroscopy can separate hypomyelination from demyelination
- T1 C+: Hypomyelination associated with leukodystrophies can show abnormal enhancement
- MRS
  - ○ Normal NAA peaks in hypomyelination
  - ○ Relative increases in myo-inositol, choline, and lipid resonances with hypomyelination
  - ○ Significant increases in choline may indicate demyelination

### Imaging Recommendations
- Best imaging tool: MR
- Protocol advice
  - ○ T1WI most helpful in children < 10 months
  - ○ T2WI most helpful in children > 10 months
  - ○ DTI and FA can provide data on WM prior to myelin deposition

## DIFFERENTIAL DIAGNOSIS

### Primary Hypomyelination Syndromes
- Chromosome deletions and mutations
  - ○ Pelizaeus-Merzbacher disease (PMD)
  - ○ Spastic paraplegia type 2 (SPG2)
  - ○ Hypomyelination with atrophy of basal ganglia and cerebellum (H-ABC)
  - ○ 18q-syndrome
  - ○ Jacobsen syndrome (11q-)
  - ○ Hypomyelination with congenital cataracts (DRCTNNB1A)
  - ○ Hypomyelination with trichothiodystrophy

### Prematurity
- Use of normal milestones assumes full-term gestation
- Adjust chronologic age for degree of prematurity
- Even after adjustment, white matter injury results in myelin delay

### External Stresses
- Chronic debilitating conditions in infancy
  - ○ Congenital vascular malformations (AVF)
  - ○ Malnutrition
- Treatments for diseases in neonate
  - ○ Organ transplantation
  - ○ Chemotherapy
- Myelination typically rebounds with treatment of primary illness

### Syndromes with Demyelination or Myelin Vacuolation
- Mucopolysaccharidoses
  - ○ Hunter, Hurler
- Mitochondrial encephalopathies
  - ○ Electron transport chain (ETC) defects
  - ○ Mitochondrial membrane abnormalities
- Leukodystrophies
  - ○ Metachromatic leukodystrophy (MLD)
  - ○ Globoid leukodystrophy (Krabbe)
  - ○ Adrenoleukodystrophy (ALD)
  - ○ Canavan disease

# HYPOMYELINATION

## PATHOLOGY

### General Features
- General path comments: PMD and 18q-syndrome are prototypes of primary hypomyelination
- Genetics
  - 10-30% of PMD and SPG2 caused by defects in proteolipid protein (PLP) gene (Xq21-q22)
  - 18q-syndrome can cause hemizygous deletion (one copy of gene missing) of myelin basic protein gene
    - MBP gene on deleted segment of long arm of chromosome 18
- Etiology
  - Defects in PLP prevent normal myelin compaction
    - Compaction displaces water and accounts for T2 hypointensity
    - Myelin becomes unstable and breaks down without PLP
  - MBP is thought to stabilize myelin spiral at major dense line
- Epidemiology: True primary hypomyelination syndromes (PMD, SPG2, 18q-, H-ABC, 11q-) are rare
- Associated abnormalities: Craniofacial malformations associated with 18q-syndrome

### Gross Pathologic & Surgical Features
- Smaller brain volume

### Microscopic Features
- Pelizaeus-Merzbacher disease
  - Patchy myelin deficiency; no sparing of subcortical U-fibers
  - Islands of persistent perivascular myelin result in classic "tigroid" appearance
  - Absent or deficient compact myelin sheaths, "redundant myelin balls"

### Staging, Grading or Classification Criteria
- Define degree of myelination by age at which it would be appropriate → "degree of myelination appropriate for x months of age"

## CLINICAL ISSUES

### Presentation
- Most common signs/symptoms: Developmental delay, hypotonia
- Other signs/symptoms
  - Classic PMD: Head titubation, hypotonia, only 50% able to sit
  - 18q-syndrome: Developmental delay, short stature, delayed bone age, limb anomalies
  - Jacobsen syndrome: Developmental delay, short stature, thrombocytopenia, trigonocephaly, pyloric stenosis
  - H-ABC: Dystonia, choreoathetosis, rigidity, learning difficulties

### Demographics
- Age: Primary hypomyelination syndromes typically present in infancy
- Gender

  - Classic PMD is X-linked recessive and thus exclusive to males
  - Jacobsen syndrome: M < F (1:3)
- Ethnicity
  - No single group identified as at risk
  - PMD may represent a group of phenotypically similar but genetically distinct entities

### Natural History & Prognosis
- Late progression of symptoms may occur in some

### Treatment
- No treatment yet for heritable disorders of hypomyelination

## DIAGNOSTIC CHECKLIST

### Consider
- Possible to distinguish hypomyelination, demyelination, myelin vacuolization using diffusion, spectroscopy
- Remember to adjust chronologic age for degree of prematurity

### Image Interpretation Pearls
- Assess myelination prior to learning chronologic age of patient
  - Avoid predetermination bias
- Correlate imaging findings with clinical history and neurological exam to narrow scope of differential

## SELECTED REFERENCES

1. van der Voorn JP et al: Childhood white matter disorders: quantitative MR imaging and spectroscopy. Radiology. 241(2):510-7, 2006
2. Grossfeld PD et al: The 11q terminal deletion disorder: a prospective study of 110 cases. Am J Med Genet A. 129(1):51-61, 2004
3. Battini R et al: Unusual clinical and magnetic resonance imaging findings in a family with proteolipid protein gene mutation. Arch Neurol. 60(2):268-72, 2003
4. Hudson LD: Pelizaeus-Merzbacher disease and spastic paraplegia type 2: two faces of myelin loss from mutations in the same gene. J Child Neurol. 18(9):616-24, 2003
5. Linnankivi TT et al: 18q-syndrome: brain MRI shows poor differentiation of gray and white matter on T2-weighted images. J Magn Reson Imaging. 18(4):414-9, 2003
6. Pizzini F et al: Proton MR spectroscopic imaging in Pelizaeus-Merzbacher disease. AJNR Am J Neuroradiol. 24(8):1683-9, 2003
7. Plecko B et al: Degree of hypomyelination and magnetic resonance spectroscopy findings in patients with Pelizaeus Merzbacher phenotype. Neuropediatrics. 34(3):127-36, 2003
8. Takanashi J et al: Brain N-acetylaspartate is elevated in Pelizaeus-Merzbacher disease with PLP1 duplication. Neurology. 58(2):237-41, 2002
9. van der Knaap MS et al: New syndrome characterized by hypomyelination with atrophy of the basal ganglia and cerebellum. AJNR Am J Neuroradiol. 23(9):1466-74, 2002
10. Woodward K et al: CNS myelination and PLP gene dosage. Pharmacogenomics. 2(3):263-72, 2001
11. Barkovich AJ: Concepts of myelin and myelination in neuroradiology. AJNR Am J Neuroradiol. 21(6):1099-109, 2000

## IMAGE GALLERY

### Typical

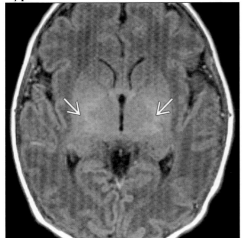
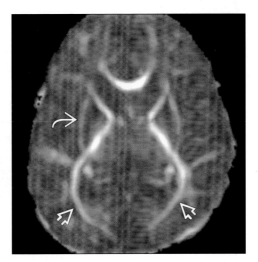

*(Left)* Axial T1WI MR in a normal 9 day old shows minimal bright signal from myelin in the posterior limbs of the internal capsules ➡. *(Right)* In contrast, the fractional anisotropy map generated from DTI acquisition (same neonate as previous image) shows anisotropy throughout the brain, including the external capsules ➡ and optic radiations ➡.

### Typical

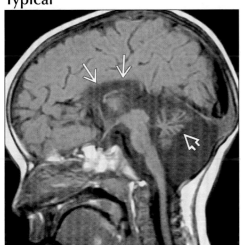
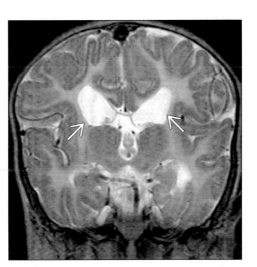

*(Left)* Sagittal T2WI MR in this 2 year old with H-ABC shows marked cerebellar atrophy ➡ and diminished cerebral and cerebellar myelination. Corpus callosum ➡ is very thin. *(Right)* Coronal T2WI MR (same child as previous image) shows absence of dark myelin signal in the peripheral WM, as well as severe atrophy of the caudate heads causing enlargement of frontal horns ➡.

### Variant

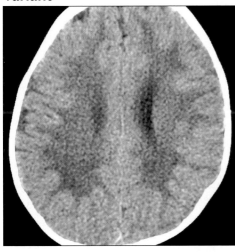
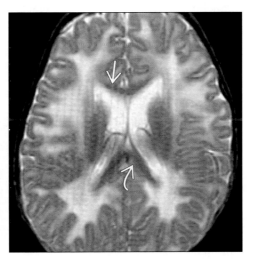

*(Left)* Axial NECT shows accentuation of gray-white differentiation caused by abnormally hypodense WM in this 12 month old with Jacobsen syndrome (11q deletion). *(Right)* Axial T2WI MR (same child as previous image) shows extensive hyperintense signal in the cerebral WM, with some myelination visible in the genu ➡ and splenium ➡ of the corpus callosum.

# LEUKODYSTROPHIES

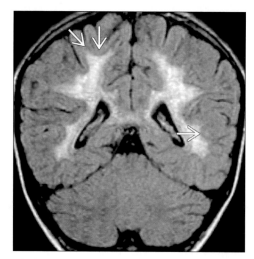

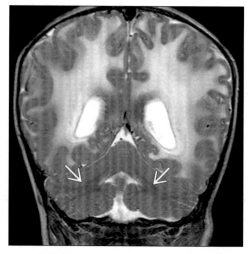

*Coronal FLAIR MR shows bilateral and symmetric periventricular and deep white matter signal abnormality but sparing of sub-cortical U-fibers ➡ in child with metachromatic leukodystrophy.*

*Coronal T2WI MR in another case of MLC shows characteristic diffuse deep and periventricular hemispheric white matter involvement, with sparing of the cerebellar white matter ➡.*

## TERMINOLOGY

### Definitions

- Inborn errors of metabolism (IEMs) that cause a defect in the production or maintenance of myelin as their primary manifestation
- Syndromes in which destruction or demyelination of white matter (WM) is the primary manifestation
  - X-linked adrenoleukodystrophies (ALD) ⇒ deficiency of the peroxisomal enzyme acyl-CoA synthetase
  - Metachromatic leukodystrophy (MLD) ⇒ deficiency of the lysosomal enzyme arylsulfatase-A (ARSA)
  - Krabbe disease [globoid cell leukodystrophy (GLD)] ⇒ deficiency of the lysosomal enzyme galactosylceramidase I
  - Megaloencephalic leukoencephalopathy with cysts (MLC) ⇒ mutations in the MLC1 gene
  - Alexander disease ⇒ mutations in gene for glial fibrillary acidic protein (GFAP)
  - Canavan disease ⇒ absence/deficiency of aspartoacyclase
  - Giant axonal neuropathy (GAN) ⇒ mutation in gene for cytoplasmic protein gigaxonin

- Leukoencephalopathy with brain stem and spinal cord involvement and raised lactate (LBSL) ⇒ cause unknown
- Leukoencephalopathy with vanishing white matter (VWM) ⇒ caused by mutations in eukaryotic initiation factor (eIF2B)
- Hypomyelination syndromes ⇒ primary manifestation is a delay or deficiency in the production of myelin
  - Pelizaeus-Merzbacher disease (PMD)
  - 18q- syndrome
  - Spastic paraplegia type 2 (SPG2)
  - Hypomyelination with atrophy of the basal ganglia and cerebellum (H-ABC)
  - Jacobsen syndrome: 11q-
- Syndromes that affect other organs in addition to WM
  - Mucopolysaccharidoses ⇒ caused by deficiencies of lysosomal enzymes that degrade glycosaminoglycans
  - Oculocerebrorenal syndrome (Lowe syndrome) ⇒ golgi complex enzyme deficiency
  - Merosin-deficient congenital muscular dystrophies (CMD)
  - Trichothiodystrophies: Cockayne syndrome, galactosemia

## DDx: Acquired White Matter Injury

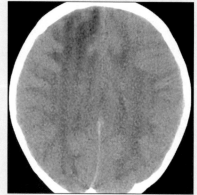

*ADEM*

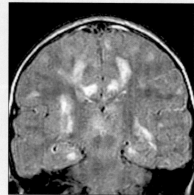

*Viral Encephalitis*

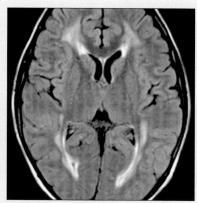

*Radiation Injury*

# LEUKODYSTROPHIES

## Key Facts

### Terminology
- Inborn errors of metabolism (IEMs) that cause a defect in the production or maintenance of myelin as their primary manifestation
- Syndromes in which destruction or demyelination of white matter (WM) is the primary manifestation
- Hypomyelination syndromes ⇒ primary manifestation is a delay or deficiency in the production of myelin
- Syndromes that affect other organs in addition to WM
- Syndromes associated with cortical malformation
- Syndromes caused by enzyme deficiencies that produce high serum levels of metabolites that are neurotoxic

### Imaging Findings
- Abnormal signal in WM, usually symmetric; periventricular, deep or subcortical
- Failure to achieve myelination milestones
- LBSL
- Myelin destruction may increase diffusion by increasing extracellular space
- Myelin sheath swelling (myelin vacuolization) may reduce diffusion
- Some have characteristic enhancement patterns
- Findings on MRS generally reflect neuronal loss and increased cellular turnover

### Diagnostic Checklist
- Contrast-enhanced MR and MRS are key tools in diagnosis

---

- Syndromes associated with cortical malformation
  - Zellweger syndrome ⇒ caused by near complete absence of peroxisomes
  - Neonatal ALD ⇒ caused by deficiency of peroxisomal biogenesis
- Syndromes caused by enzyme deficiencies that produce high serum levels of metabolites that are neurotoxic
  - Maple syrup urine disease (MSUD) ⇒ defect in catabolism of leucine, isoleucine, and valine (BCKD complex)
  - Phenylketonuria (PKU) ⇒ accumulation of phenylalanine
  - Hyperhomocystinemia (homocystinuria) ⇒ accumulation of homocystine
  - Nonketotic hyperglycinemia ⇒ accumulation of glycine
  - Urea cycle disorders ⇒ accumulation of ammonia

## IMAGING FINDINGS

### General Features
- Best diagnostic clue
  - Abnormal signal in WM, usually symmetric; periventricular, deep or subcortical
  - Failure to achieve myelination milestones
- Location
  - Some initially affect periventricular ± deep WM
    - MLD
    - GLD
    - X-linked ALD
    - GAN
    - LBSL
  - Some initially affect subcortical WM
    - MLC
    - Canavan disease
    - VWM
  - Alexander disease ⇒ subcortical, deep and periventricular frontal WM
  - GLD ⇒ increased attenuation in thalami early

  - Canavan ⇒ T2/FLAIR signal abnormalities in globi pallidi, thalami early
- Size
  - Some leukodystrophies cause macrocephaly
    - Alexander disease, Canavan disease, MLC

### CT Findings
- NECT
  - Decreased WM attenuation
  - Increased density in basal ganglia early in GLD
  - Most progress to atrophy in later stages of disease

### MR Findings
- T1WI
  - Best sequence for hypomyelination in children < 1 year
  - Periventricular rim of ↑ signal in Alexander disease
  - Optic nerve enlargement in Krabbe disease
- T2WI
  - Hyperintense signal of affected WM
  - 3-zone involvement of periventricular WM in X-linked ALD
  - Periventricular rim of ↓ signal in Alexander disease
- FLAIR
  - Best sequence for demyelination in children > 2 years old
  - Distinguishes cysts from abnormal WM in MLC
  - Distinguishes abnormal from "vanished" WM in VWM
- DWI
  - Myelin destruction may increase diffusion by increasing extracellular space
  - Some processes increase diffusion after destruction of myelin/axons
    - ALD ⇒ increased diffusion and ↑ ADC
    - GLD ⇒ increased diffusion and ↑ ADC
    - Alexander disease ⇒ increased diffusion and loss of anisotropy
  - Myelin sheath swelling (myelin vacuolization) may reduce diffusion
    - Canavan disease ⇒ reduced diffusivity
  - Some reduce diffusion during active demyelination
    - MLD ⇒ reduced diffusion in early phase

# LEUKODYSTROPHIES

○ Fractional anisotropy (FA) can show some preservation of myelin sheath integrity in less severely affected WM in MLC
- T1 C+
  ○ Some have characteristic enhancement patterns
    - ALD ⇒ zone of active inflammation
    - GLD ⇒ lumbar nerve roots
    - Alexander disease ⇒ ventricular lining, periventricular rim, frontal WM, optic chiasm, fornix, basal ganglia, thalamus, dentate nucleus, brainstem structures
- MRS
  ○ Findings on MRS generally reflect neuronal loss and increased cellular turnover
  ○ Alexander disease ⇒ ↑ ↑ myo-inositol (mI), ± ↑ choline (Cho), ± ↓ N-acetylaspartic acid (NAA)
  ○ MLD ⇒ ↑ Cho, ↑ mI
  ○ ALD ⇒ ↑ Cho, ↑ mI; ↓ ↓ NAA indicates irreversible neuronal loss
  ○ GLD ⇒ ↑ Cho, ↑ mI, ↓ NAA
  ○ Canavan has ↑ NAA, one of the only conditions where this is found
  ○ MSUD can show a peak at 0.9 ppm, representing branched chain alpha ketoacids

## Imaging Recommendations
- Best imaging tool: Contrast-enhanced MR with MRS
- Protocol advice: MRS: Sample both abnormal and normal-appearing WM

## DIFFERENTIAL DIAGNOSIS

### Radiation and Chemotherapy Injury
- Late delayed injury due to vascular compromise
- Loss of myelin with edema

### Viral Encephalitis
- Bilateral, symmetrical gray and white matter injury
- Often affects thalami, basal ganglia, hippocampi, cingulum

### Acute Disseminated Encephalomyelitis (ADEM)
- Acute autoimmune demyelinating disease common in children

### Multiple Sclerosis
- Typically teenagers
- Characteristic morphology

### Neonatal Hypoxic Ischemic Encephalopathy
- Periventricular pattern of injury

## PATHOLOGY

### General Features
- General path comments
  ○ MLD ⇒ accumulation of sulfatide
  ○ ALD ⇒ accumulation of long-chain fatty acids
  ○ GLD ⇒ accumulation of psychosine and cerebroside
  ○ Canavan disease ⇒ accumulation of NAA
  ○ Alexander disease ⇒ excess Rosenthal fibers

○ MLC ⇒ vacuolating myelinopathy without axonal damage
○ VWM ⇒ vacuolating leukodystrophy with foamy cytoplasm in oligodendroglia
- Genetics
  ○ MLD ⇒ ARSA gene located at 22q13.31
  ○ X-linked ALD ⇒ ABCD1 gene at Xq28
  ○ GLD ⇒ gene for galactosylceramidase mapped to chromosome 14q24.3-14q32.1
  ○ Alexander disease ⇒ gene for GFAP mapped to chromosome 17q21
  ○ Canavan disease ⇒ aspartoacyclase gene is on chromosome 17
  ○ MLC ⇒ MLC1 gene is at chromosome 22q13
  ○ GAN ⇒ gene mapped to chromosome 16q24
  ○ VWM ⇒ gene mapped to chromosome 20pter-q12
- Epidemiology
  ○ Rare diseases that can be increased in incidence in closed communities
  ○ Improved detection of milder manifestations with genetic screening has resulted in apparent increases in incidence

## CLINICAL ISSUES

### Natural History & Prognosis
- Severely affected children typically have progressive neurologic deterioration and death in childhood
- With more sophisticated genetic testing, milder forms with prolonged lifespan are being diagnosed

## DIAGNOSTIC CHECKLIST

### Image Interpretation Pearls
- Contrast-enhanced MR and MRS are key tools in diagnosis

## SELECTED REFERENCES

1. van der Knaap MS et al: Alexander disease: ventricular garlands and abnormalities of the medulla and spinal cord. Neurology. 66(4):494-8, 2006
2. van der Knaap MS et al: Vanishing white matter disease. Lancet Neurol. 5(5):413-23, 2006
3. van der Voorn JP et al: Childhood white matter disorders: quantitative MR imaging and spectroscopy. Radiology. 241(2):510-7, 2006
4. Patay Z: Diffusion-weighted MR imaging in leukodystrophies. Eur Radiol. 15(11):2284-303, 2005
5. Schiffmann R et al: The latest on leukodystrophies. Curr Opin Neurol. 17(2):187-92, 2004
6. Serkov SV et al: Five patients with a recently described novel leukoencephalopathy with brainstem and spinal cord involvement and elevated lactate. Neuropediatrics. 35(1):1-5, 2004
7. Brockmann K et al: Cerebral proton magnetic resonance spectroscopy in infantile Alexander disease. J Neurol. 250(3):300-6, 2003
8. Brockmann K et al: Proton MRS profile of cerebral metabolic abnormalities in Krabbe disease. Neurology. 60(5):819-25, 2003
9. Engelbrecht V et al: Diffusion-weighted MR imaging in the brain in children: findings in the normal brain and in the brain with WM diseases. Radiology. 222(2):410-8, 2002

## IMAGE GALLERY

### Variant

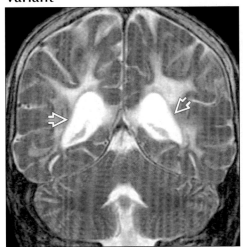 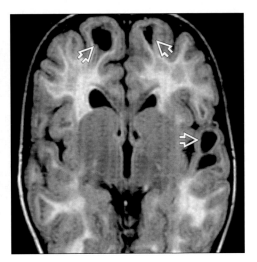

*(Left)* Coronal T2WI MR shows bilateral posterior periventricular and deep WM hyperintensity and volume loss in a child with X-linked adrenoleukodystrophy. Note ex vacuo ventriculomegaly ➦. *(Right)* Axial FLAIR MR in megaloencephalic leukoencephalopathy with subcortical cysts shows diffuse abnormal WM signal with sparing of the internal capsules and characteristic subcortical cysts ➦.

### Variant

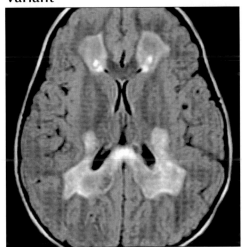 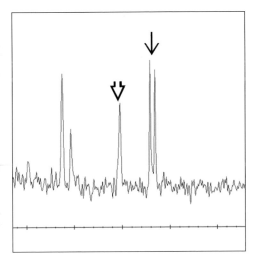

*(Left)* Axial FLAIR MR in LBSL patient shows sharply-defined, symmetric periventricular and deep white matter signal abnormality with sparing of both the internal capsules and subcortical U-fibers. *(Right)* MRS with TE = 288 msec in LBSL shows reduced NAA at 2.01 ppm ➦ and a prominent lipid/lactate doublet at 1.3 ppm ➡.

### Typical

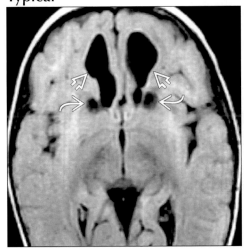 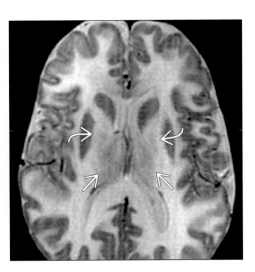

*(Left)* Axial FLAIR MR shows large foci of cystic destruction in the frontal WM ➦ and caudate heads ➥ of a child with Alexander disease. These cysts occur at a late stage of the illness. *(Right)* Axial T2WI MR in a child with Canavan disease shows periventricular, deep, and subcortical WM involvement, plus thalami ➡ and globi pallidi ➡ involvement; very characteristic.

# MITOCHONDRIAL ENCEPHALOPATHIES

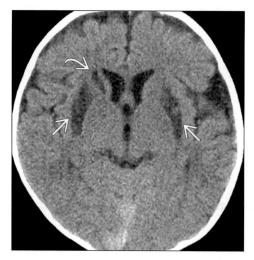

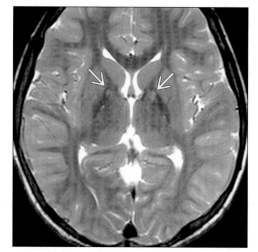

*Axial NECT shows well-defined hypodense lesions in the caudate ⟶ and putamina ⟶ in this infant with Leigh syndrome. Bilateral basal ganglia lesions are common in MEMs.*

*Axial T2WI MR shows the classic "eye of the tiger" pattern ⟶ in a teenager diagnosed with pantothenate kinase-associated neurodegeneration, formerly called Hallervorden-Spatz syndrome.*

## TERMINOLOGY

### Abbreviations and Synonyms

- Mitochondrial encephalomyelopathies (MEMs)
  - Subacute necrotizing encephalomyelopathy or Leigh syndrome (LS)
    - Pyruvate dehydrogenase complex defects
    - Cytochrome oxidase (COX, complex IV) deficiency
    - Adenosine triphosphatase (ATPase) 6 gene mutations (complex V)
    - Other electron transport chain (ETC) enzyme deficiencies (complex I, II, III)
  - Pantothenate kinase-associated neurodegeneration (PKAN), or Hallervorden-Spatz syndrome
  - Glutaric acidurias, type I (GA1) and type 2 (GA2)
  - Myopathy, encephalopathy, lactic acidosis, and stroke-like episodes (MELAS)
  - Myoclonic epilepsy with ragged-red fibers (MERRF)
    - Seen primarily in adults
  - Kearns-Sayre syndrome (KSS), progressive external ophthalmoplegia
  - Menkes disease (trichopoliodystrophy), Alpers disease, Friedreich ataxia
  - Fatal infantile myopathy, benign infantile myopathy
  - Familial mitochondrial encephalopathy with macrocephaly, cardiomyopathy, and complex I deficiency

### Definitions

- Genetically based disorders of mitochondrial function resulting in progressive or intermittent brain injury
- Characteristically due to deficiencies/defects of enzymes affecting the respiratory (electron-transport) chain, Krebs cycle, and/or other components of energy production by mitochondria

## IMAGING FINDINGS

### General Features

- Best diagnostic clue
  - MEMs have a broad range of imaging appearances, characterized by regions of brain destruction, volume loss, and/or mineralization
  - They typically affect both gray and white matter
  - Most disorders of mitochondrial function will cause lesions in the basal ganglia

## DDx: Symmetric Basal Ganglia Lesions

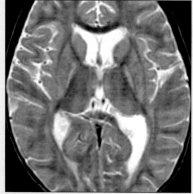

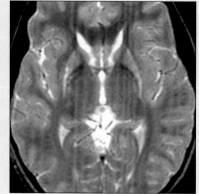

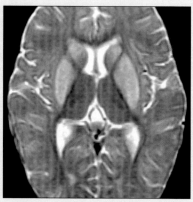

*Near Drowning*

*Huntington Chorea*

*EBV Encephalitis*

# MITOCHONDRIAL ENCEPHALOPATHIES

## Key Facts

### Terminology
- Genetically based disorders of mitochondrial function resulting in progressive or intermittent brain injury
- Characteristically due to deficiencies/defects of enzymes affecting the respiratory (electron-transport) chain, Krebs cycle, and/or other components of energy production by mitochondria

### Imaging Findings
- MEMs have a broad range of imaging appearances, characterized by regions of brain destruction, volume loss, and/or mineralization
- Most disorders of mitochondrial function will cause lesions in the basal ganglia
- Collections mimic subdural hematomas from child abuse

- PKAN causes characteristic T2 hypointensity in globus pallidus (GP)
- LS typically causes a speckled pattern in deep nuclei
- Detection of lactate characteristic of MEMs
- Absence of lactate does not exclude diagnosis, however

### Pathology
- Epidemiology: As a group, MEMs are relatively common ~ 1:8,500

### Diagnostic Checklist
- Think of MEMs when encountering an atypical presentation of stroke, severe encephalitis, or seizure
- Don't forget to consider MEMs when an infant presents with subdurals
- Can also have retinal hemorrhages!

---

- Typically bilateral and symmetric
  - MELAS causes peripheral stroke-like lesions
- Location
  - Variable
    - Most common in basal ganglia (BG), brainstem, thalami, dentate nuclei
    - Less commonly diffuse white matter (WM), peripheral cortex, cerebellum
- Size: Focal/diffuse atrophy is characteristic of GA1, Menkes
- Morphology
  - BG lesions often conform to original shape of nuclei
  - Edema/swelling characteristic of acute lesions; volume loss characteristic of late disease

### CT Findings
- NECT
  - Focal hypodensities
  - Increased density can be seen in BG in PKAN, KSS
    - May reflect dystrophic calcification (Ca++)
  - Diffuse decreased density of WM
  - GA1, Menkes ⇒ volume loss with subdural collections
    - Collections mimic subdural hematomas from child abuse
    - Typically hyperattenuating relative to CSF

### MR Findings
- T1WI
  - Hypointense lesions
    - Foci of hyperintensity may reflect Ca++, blood products, myelin breakdown (rare)
  - Friedreich ataxia ⇒ cerebellar, spinal atrophy
- T2WI
  - MEMs typically cause hyperintense lesions on T2WI and FLAIR
  - PKAN causes characteristic T2 hypointensity in globus pallidus (GP)
    - Due to excess and premature iron deposition
    - Central area of hyperintensity reflects gliosis
    - Combination of hypo- and hyper-intensity lesions ⇒ "eye of the tiger" sign
  - LS typically causes a speckled pattern in deep nuclei

- Sparing (islands of preserved signal) around vessels?
- DWI
  - MEMs may or may not cause foci of restricted diffusion
    - DWI is not reliable for detection or exclusion of MEMs
- MRS
  - Detection of lactate characteristic of MEMs
    - Absence of lactate does not exclude diagnosis, however
    - May only be elevated during acute crises
  - Chronic lesions typically have ↓ NAA

### Nuclear Medicine Findings
- PET: GA1: ↓ Glucose uptake in BG, thalami, insula, and temporal opercular cortex

### Imaging Recommendations
- Best imaging tool: MR is modality of choice in investigation of suspected metabolic disease of any sort
- Protocol advice
  - MRS can be helpful, although often nonspecific
  - ↑ Lactate and restricted diffusion can be clue to true etiology

## DIFFERENTIAL DIAGNOSIS

### Perinatal Asphyxia
- Central pattern of injury affects ventrolateral thalamus and basal ganglia
  - T1 hyperintensity seen acutely ⇒ myelin breakdown/clumping?

### Kernicterus
- T2 prolongation in GP, subthalamic nuclei, hippocampi

### Near Drowning
- History generally definitive
- High lactate implies poorer prognosis

# MITOCHONDRIAL ENCEPHALOPATHIES

## Juvenile Huntington Disease
- Symmetric T2 prolongation in putamina
- Caudate atrophy presents later

## Neurofibromatosis Type 1
- Signal abnormalities in basal ganglia most common brain manifestation

## Encephalitis
- Viral encephalitides can cause symmetric basal ganglia T2 prolongation
- Acute disseminated encephalomyelitis can affect basal ganglia, mimic MELAS/MERRF

## Wilson Disease
- Signal changes in basal ganglia most often secondary to hepatic failure
  - T2 changes evident in older children, teens

## PATHOLOGY

### General Features
- General path comments
  - Main role of mitochondria ⇒ production of ATP for cell energy
    - Mitochondria contain their own DNA, inherited from mother
  - Most MEMs can be caused by variable number of mutations affecting structure/function of mitochondrial-based enzymes
  - Broad phenotypic presentation due to varied distribution of mitochondria throughout various cell types
- Genetics
  - LS ⇒ group of disorders caused by defective terminal oxidative metabolism
    - Defects in pyruvate dehydrogenase complex ⇒ X-linked
    - Cytochrome oxidase (COX) deficiency (respiratory chain complex IV) ⇒ SURF1 gene on chromosome 9
    - Several others genes and enzyme complexes affected
  - PKAN ("classic" form) ⇒ defects on chromosome 22p12.3-13 (PKAN2 gene)
  - MELAS ⇒ mitochondrial DNA defects (tRNA gene)
  - GA1 ⇒ deficiency of glutaryl-coenzyme A dehydrogenase; gene on chromosome 19p13.2
  - Friedreich ataxia ⇒ chromosome 9q13
    - Mutations of frataxin ⇒ causes deficiency of respiratory chain complexes I-III
  - Menkes ⇒ X-linked, Xq12-q13.3
  - Alpers ⇒ mutations of mitochondrial DNA polymerase gamma subunits
- Etiology: Most pronounced effects are on striated muscle and deep cerebral nuclei ⇒ presumed highest ATP demand
- Epidemiology: As a group, MEMs are relatively common ~ 1:8,500
- Associated abnormalities
  - KSS ⇒ ophthalmoplegia, heart block, retinitis pigmentosa
  - Alpers ⇒ micronodular cirrhosis
  - Menkes ⇒ brittle sparse hair ("kinky" hair disease), osteoporosis
  - Friedreich ataxia ⇒ hypertrophic cardiomyopathy, diabetes

## CLINICAL ISSUES

### Presentation
- Most common signs/symptoms
  - Psychomotor delay/regression, hypotonia
  - Stroke-like episodes, episodic paresis
- Other signs/symptoms
  - Ataxia, ophthalmoplegia, ptosis, vomiting, swallowing and respiratory difficulties, dystonia
  - Seizure, peripheral neuropathy

### Demographics
- Age
  - Majority have clinical symptoms in infancy
  - MELAS usually presents in teens

### Natural History & Prognosis
- Age at onset and severity correlates with degree of enzyme deficit
- Metabolic stressors (e.g., infection) may unmask disease or cause deterioration
- LS ⇒ progressive neurodegeneration leading to respiratory failure and death in childhood
- PKAN ⇒ non-uniform progression, 11 year life expectancy after diagnosis
- GA1 ⇒ progressive atrophy with severe dystonia
- MELAS ⇒ progressive course with episodic insults
- KSS, Friedreich ataxia ⇒ significant morbidity from cardiac effects

### Treatment
- In general, MEMs are treated supportively and symptomatically

## DIAGNOSTIC CHECKLIST

### Image Interpretation Pearls
- Think of MEMs when encountering an atypical presentation of stroke, severe encephalitis, or seizure
- Don't forget to consider MEMs when an infant presents with subdurals
  - Can also have retinal hemorrhages!

## SELECTED REFERENCES
1. Mizrachi IB et al: Pitfalls in the diagnosis of mitochondrial encephalopathy with lactic acidosis and stroke-like episodes. J Neuroophthalmol. 26(1):38-43, 2006
2. Gago LC et al: Intraretinal hemorrhages and chronic subdural effusions: glutaric aciduria type 1 can be mistaken for shaken baby syndrome. Retina. 23(5):724-6, 2003
3. Rossi A et al: Leigh Syndrome with COX deficiency and SURF1 gene mutations: MR imaging findings. AJNR Am J Neuroradiol. 24(6):1188-91, 2003

## IMAGE GALLERY

### Typical

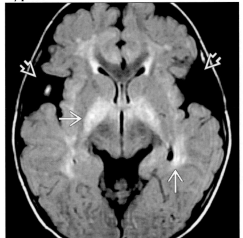
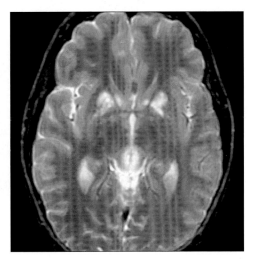

*(Left)* Axial FLAIR MR shows striking sylvian fissure enlargement ⇨ in association with abnormal signal in the periventricular WM and globi pallidi ⇨ of a child with glutaric aciduria type I. *(Right)* Axial T2WI MR shows T2 hyperintensity in putamina, caudate heads, medial thalami in patient with neuropathy, ataxia, and retinitis pigmentosa (NARP), caused by MTATP6 mutation.

### Typical

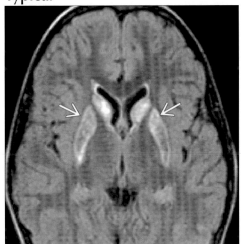
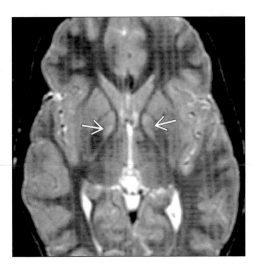

*(Left)* Axial FLAIR MR shows symmetric signal ⇨ abnormalities in the putamina and caudate heads in a child with complex III deficiency. *(Right)* Axial T2WI MR in a child with Kearns Sayre syndrome also shows symmetric signal abnormalities ⇨ in the globus pallidus. MR imaging 2 years later revealed diffuse WM injury.

### Variant

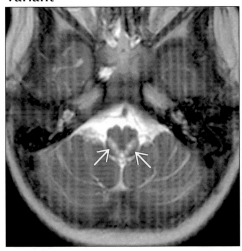
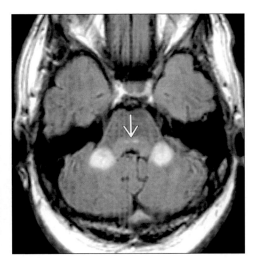

*(Left)* Axial T2WI MR shows symmetric lesions ⇨ in the dorsal medulla oblongata of a child with Leigh syndrome. Brain stem lesions are common, particularly with cytochrome oxidase defects. *(Right)* Axial FLAIR shows lesions in dorsal pons ⇨ and middle cerebellar peduncles in a child with Leigh syndrome. Symmetric brainstem and cerebellar lesions should prompt investigation for MEMs.

# MELAS

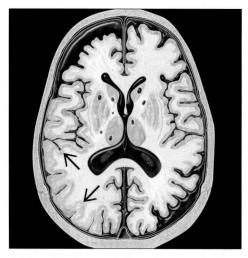

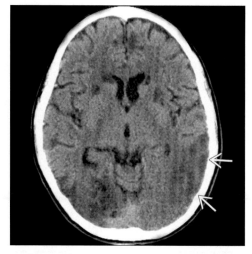

*Axial graphic shows pathology of MELAS. The acute onset of gyral swelling that crosses vascular territories is depicted ➡. Note old lacunar infarcts, and generalized/focal atrophy.*

*Axial NECT shows subtle low density in left temporo and occipital cortex ➡. Prior strokes in multiple areas: right occipital, medial frontal lobes, basal ganglia lacunar infarctions.*

## TERMINOLOGY

### Abbreviations and Synonyms

- Mitochondrial myopathy, encephalopathy, lactic acidosis, and stroke-like episodes (MELAS)

### Definitions

- Inherited disorder of intracellular energy production caused by mitochondrial dysfunction

## IMAGING FINDINGS

### General Features

- Best diagnostic clue
  - Acute: Stroke-like cortical lesions
    - "Shifting spread" (appearance, disappearance, reappearance elsewhere) is classic
    - Lesions cross typical vascular territories
  - Elevated lactate in CSF, normal-appearing brain on MRS
    - Correlates well with other mitochondrial encephalopathy (ME) markers
- Location
  - Parieto-occipital > temporo-parietal region
  - Basal ganglia (BG)
- Size
  - Variable
  - Multiple lesions common
- Morphology
  - Acute: Cortical edema that often spares underlying white matter (WM)
  - Chronic: Atrophy, deep WM and BG lacunar infarcts

### CT Findings

- CTA: Usually normal
- NECT
  - Acute: Edematous cortex
  - Chronic: Atrophy, lacunar infarcts, BG Ca++
- CECT: Variable gyral enhancement

### MR Findings

- T1WI
  - Acute: Edematous cortex
  - Subacute: Band of cortical hyperintensity consistent with cortical necrosis
  - Chronic: Progressive atrophy of BG, temporal-parietal-occipital cortex with preservation of hippocampal, entorhinal structures

## DDx: MELAS Mimics

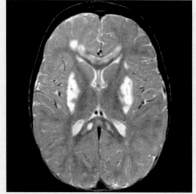

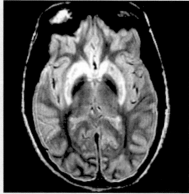

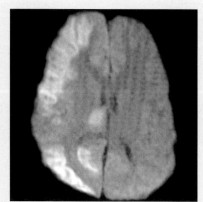

*Leigh Syndrome*

*Wilson Disease*

*Embolic Stroke*

# MELAS

## Key Facts

### Terminology
- Mitochondrial myopathy, encephalopathy, lactic acidosis, and stroke-like episodes (MELAS)
- Inherited disorder of intracellular energy production caused by mitochondrial dysfunction

### Imaging Findings
- Acute: Stroke-like cortical lesions
- Elevated lactate in CSF, normal-appearing brain on MRS
- Lactate (Lac) doublet peak at 1.3 ppm in 60-65%
- Presence/amount of Lac at MRS varies with type of ME; regional and temporal variation
- Xenon CT shows focal hyperperfusion during acute strokelike episode, hypoperfusion later
- Best imaging tool: MR with multivoxel MRS

### Top Differential Diagnoses
- Hyperhomocysteinemia
- Leigh Disease
- Embolic/Thrombotic/Watershed Strokes

### Pathology
- A-to-G translation at nucleotide 3243 of mtDNA

### Clinical Issues
- Acute onset: Headache, followed by hemianopsia, psychosis, aphasia
- Progressive course with periodic acute exacerbation

### Diagnostic Checklist
- Think of MEs in patient with an acute stroke-like cortical lesion that crosses usual vascular territories

---

- T2WI
  - Acute: Hyperintense cortex/subcortical WM
  - Chronic: Multifocal hyperintensities in basal ganglia, deep WM
- FLAIR: Acute: Cortical edema, hyperintensity
- T2* GRE: No hemorrhage
- DWI
  - Acute: Reduced diffusion
    - ADC variable; often normal or only slightly decreased (may help distinguish from acute ischemic stroke)
- T1 C+: Acute: Cortical enhancement
- MRA: Normal without major vessel occlusion
- MRS
  - Lactate (Lac) doublet peak at 1.3 ppm in 60-65%
    - Lac peak inverts with intermediate TE (135-144 msec) due to J-coupling
    - Changes may precede DWI abnormalities
  - Cautions
    - Presence/amount of Lac at MRS varies with type of ME; regional and temporal variation
    - Lac not always elevated, especially in chronic lesions
    - Lac may be elevated in CSF but not brain (measure ventricular lac)
    - Multivoxel more sensitive than single voxel techniques
    - Failure to interrogate proper region of interest (ROI) reduces sensitivity
    - Other causes of elevated CNS Lac (e.g., hypoxia, ischemia, neoplasm, infection) must be excluded
    - If child is sedated with phenobarbital, doublet at 1.15 ppm may be present and mimic elevated Lac (however doesn't invert)

### Angiographic Findings
- Conventional
  - Acute
    - Dilated cortical arteries, prominent capillary blush without arterial occlusion

### Other Modality Findings
- Xenon CT shows focal hyperperfusion during acute strokelike episode, hypoperfusion later
- Electromyographic findings consistent with myopathy found in majority of cases
- EEG may show focal periodic epileptiform discharges

### Imaging Recommendations
- Best imaging tool: MR with multivoxel MRS
- Protocol advice: Acquire spectra with TE of both 35, 144 msec

## DIFFERENTIAL DIAGNOSIS

### Hyperhomocysteinemia
- Predisposes to vasculopathy, infarctions
- Watershed ischemia/infarcts common

### Leigh Disease
- COX defect +/- SURF1 gene mutation
  - Causes subacute necrotizing encephalomyopathy
  - Progressive impairment of cognitive, motor function
- Imaging shows bilateral symmetric putaminal lesions > globi pallidi
- Other lesions in caudate nuclei, subthalamic nuclei, periaqueductal GM, brainstem

### Other Toxic/Metabolic Basal Ganglia Lesions
- Pattern may give clue to etiology (e.g., "eye of panda" in Wilson disease)
- Cyanide, carbon monoxide poisoning

### Kearns-Sayre Syndrome (KSS)
- Ataxia, ophthalmoplegia, retinitis pigmentosa
- Diffuse symmetric Ca++ in basal ganglia, caudate nuclei, subcortical WM
- Hyperintense basal ganglia on T1-, T2WI; cerebellar WM, posterior columns of medulla often involved

### Embolic/Thrombotic/Watershed Strokes
- Ischemic areas are in arterial or inter-arterial distributions

# MELAS

- No Lac elevation in normal unaffected brain, CSF

## PATHOLOGY

### General Features
- General path comments
  - MEs divided into somewhat ill-defined categories based on clinical, histopathologic, biochemical, genetic features
    - Many overlapping syndromes exist (e.g., Leigh-MELAS)
- Genetics
  - Maternally-transmitted
  - A-to-G translation at nucleotide 3243 of mtDNA
- Etiology
  - Respiratory chain is under dual genetic control
    - At least 13 proteins are encoded by mitochondrial DNA
    - Over 80 proteins encoded by nuclear DNA
  - Defects in respiratory chain metabolism
    - Defective mitochondrial protein synthesis
    - NAD+ and NADP+ depletion occurs
    - Catabolic metabolism shifts from Krebs cycle to anaerobic glycolysis
    - Pyruvate, lactate accumulate
    - Result ⇒ cellular energy failure
  - May also cause hyperperfusion, vasogenic edema, enhancement during acute strokelike episodes
  - Caution: Relationship of phenotype to genotype complex, variable in most MEs
- Epidemiology
  - Overall prevalence of mitochondrial disorders = 5.7 per 100,000 in population > 14 y
  - Uncommon but important cause of pediatric stroke
- Associated abnormalities: Some cortical malformations associated with A3243G mutations

### Gross Pathologic & Surgical Features
- Diffuse generalized atrophy
- Multiple focal cortical, deep WM/BG infarcts
- Prominent mineralization of BG
- Perivascular Ca++ in both GM, WM may occur

### Microscopic Features
- Trichrome stain may show increased numbers of ragged-red fibers in skeletal muscle
- Immunohistochemistry: COX-positive ragged-red fibers (may help distinguish from MERRF)
- Electron Microscopy: Swelling, increase in number of dysfunctional mitochondria in smooth muscle, endothelial cells of small arteries and pial arterioles

## CLINICAL ISSUES

### Presentation
- Most common signs/symptoms
  - Acute onset: Headache, followed by hemianopsia, psychosis, aphasia
  - Other signs/symptoms
    - Seizures
    - Muscle weakness (myopathy)
    - Sensorineural hearing loss
    - Chronic: Cognitive deficits, dementia, small stature
- Clinical Profile: Older child or young adult with muscle weakness and epilepsy or acute stroke-like syndrome

### Demographics
- Age
  - Onset of stroke-like episodes usually occurs in childhood/early adulthood
    - Mean age onset = 15 y
    - 90%+ symptomatic by 40 y
- Gender: M:F ≈ 2:1

### Natural History & Prognosis
- Recurrent strokelike events with either permanent or reversible neurologic deficits
- Progressive course with periodic acute exacerbation

## DIAGNOSTIC CHECKLIST

### Consider
- Think of MEs in patient with an acute stroke-like cortical lesion that crosses usual vascular territories

### Image Interpretation Pearls
- Obtain MRS in CSF, uninvolved (normal-appearing) brain

## SELECTED REFERENCES

1. Mizrachi IB et al: Pitfalls in the diagnosis of mitochondrial encephalopathy with lactic acidosis and stroke-like episodes. J Neuroophthalmol. 26(1):38-43, 2006
2. Matsumoto J et al: Mitochondrial encephalomyopathy with lactic acidosis and stroke (MELAS). Rev Neurol Dis. 2(1):30-4, 2005
3. Abe K et al: Comparison of conventional and diffusion weighted MRI and proton MR spectroscopy in patients with mitochondrial encephalomyopathy, lactic acidosis, and stroke-like events. Neuroradiology. 46(2):113-7, 2004
4. Chol M et al: The mitochondrial DNA G13513A MELAS mutation in the NADH dehydrogenase 5 gene is a frequent cause of Leigh-like syndrome with isolated complex I deficiency. J Med Genet. 40(3):188-91, 2003
5. Iizuka T et al: Slowly progressive spread of the stroke-like lesions in MELAS. Neurology. 61(9):1238-44, 2003
6. Jeppesen TD et al: Late onset of stroke-like episode associated with a 3256C-->T point mutation of mitochondrial DNA. J Neurol Sci. 214(1-2):17-20, 2003
7. Sparaco M et al: MELAS: clinical phenotype and morphological brain abnormalities. Acta Neuropathol (Berl). 106(3):202-12, 2003
8. Wang XY et al: Serial diffusion-weighted imaging in a patient with MELAS and presumed cytotoxic oedema. Neuroradiology. 45(9):640-3, 2003
9. Carvalho KS et al: Arterial strokes in children. Neurol Clin. 20(4):1079-100, vii, 2002
10. Sartor H et al: MELAS: a neuropsychological and radiological follow-up study. Mitochondrial encephalomyopathy, lactic acidosis and stroke. Acta Neurol Scand. 106(5):309-13, 2002

## IMAGE GALLERY

### Typical

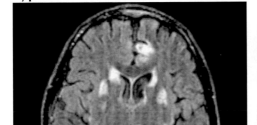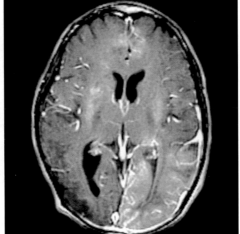

*(Left) Axial FLAIR MR shows differing degree of hyperintensity of the left occipital infarct ➡ compared to the other regions. Note also how the left posterior stroke crosses vascular boundaries. (Right) Axial T1 C+ MR shows pial/cortical enhancement of only some of the regions of injury, suggesting injuries of differing ages.*

### Typical

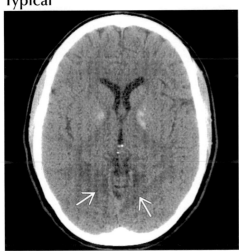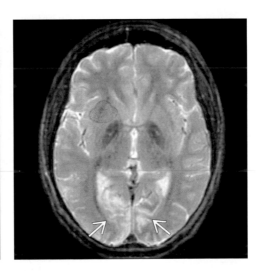

*(Left) Axial NECT shows bilateral globus pallidus calcification and low density in the medial occipital lobes ➡. Such calcification is abnormal in children and young adults. (Right) Axial T2WI MR in same patient as previous image shows bilateral medial occipital brain injuries ➡. Foci of hyperintensity in the globi pallidi correspond to the calcifications on CT.*

### Typical

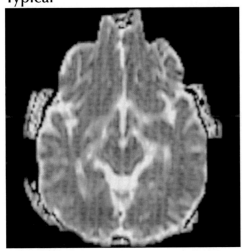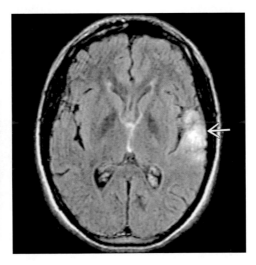

*(Left) Axial ADC in same patient as previous image shows reduced diffusivity in the occipital lobes at the site of the abnormal T2 changes, suggesting acute infarct. Diffusion abnormality is characteristically mild. (Right) Axial FLAIR MR two years later in the same patient shows new lesion ➡ in the left anterior temporal lobe. Occipital lobes look nearly normal.*

# GANGLIOSIDOSIS (GM2)

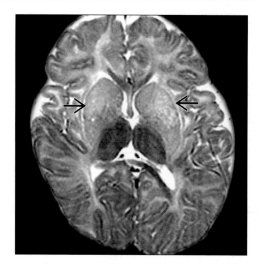

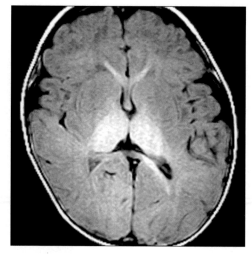

Axial T2WI MR shows characteristic findings of Sandhoff disease (SD). There is delayed myelination, diffuse, symmetric thalamic hypointensity with hyperintensity of the corpus striatum ➡.

Axial T1WI MR (same patient as previous image) shows corresponding thalamic hyperintensity. Note hypomyelination of hemispheric white matter with sparing of corpus callosum in this 1 year old.

## TERMINOLOGY

### Abbreviations and Synonyms
- GM2 Gangliosidosis (GM2)
- Tay-Sachs disease, Sandhoff disease

### Definitions
- Inherited lysosomal storage disorder characterized by GM2 ganglioside accumulation in brain
- Three major biochemically distinct, but clinically indistinguishable, types
  - Tay-Sachs disease (TS)
  - Sandhoff disease (SD)
  - GM2 variant AB (rare)
- TS and SD exist in infantile, juvenile, and adult forms
- GM2 variant AB exists in infantile form only

## IMAGING FINDINGS

### General Features
- Best diagnostic clue
  - Infantile GM2: Symmetric T1, T2 shortening thalami (hyperdense on CT) with mild T2 hyperintensity corpus striatum, white matter
  - Juvenile, adult GM2: Cerebellar atrophy
- Location
  - Infantile GM2: Thalami, corpus striatum (CS), cerebral >> cerebellar white matter (WM)
  - Juvenile, adult GM2: Cerebellum
- Morphology: Infantile GM2: Corpus callosum spared
- Juvenile, adult GM2: T2 hyperintense cerebral WM + atrophy may accompany cerebellar atrophy
- Infantile GM2, late: Thalamic, cerebral, cerebellar atrophy

### CT Findings
- NECT
  - Infantile GM2
    - Hyperdense thalami (classic but variable)
    - Hypodense CS, WM
  - Juvenile, adult GM2
    - Cerebellar atrophy
    - ± Cerebral WM hypodensity, atrophy
- CECT: No abnormal enhancement

## DDx: T2 Hypointense Thalami

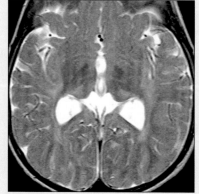

Status Marmoratus

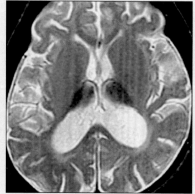

Neuronal Ceroid Lipofuscinosis

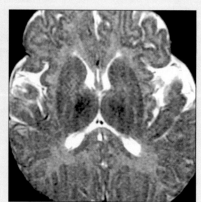

Krabbe Disease

# GANGLIOSIDOSIS (GM2)

## Key Facts

### Terminology
- Inherited lysosomal storage disorder characterized by GM2 ganglioside accumulation in brain

### Imaging Findings
- Infantile GM2: Symmetric T1, T2 shortening thalami (hyperdense on CT) with mild T2 hyperintensity corpus striatum, white matter
- Juvenile, adult GM2: Cerebellar atrophy

### Top Differential Diagnoses
- Status Marmoratus
- Neuronal Ceroid Lipofuscinosis (NCL)
- Krabbe Disease
- Juvenile GM1 Gangliosidosis

### Pathology
- Autosomal recessive inheritance
- Accumulation GM2 ganglioside in neuronal lysosomes causes neuronal degeneration, apoptosis with secondary hypo- or demyelination

### Clinical Issues
- TS more common in Ashkenazi Jews, French Canadians, Cajuns, and Druze
- Infantile GM2: Rapidly progressive psychomotor regression culminating in paralysis, blindness, deafness; death typically by 4 yrs of age
- Juvenile GM2: More slowly progressive with death between 5 and 15 years of age
- Supportive therapy, seizure control

## MR Findings
- T1WI
  - Infantile GM2
    - Hyperintense thalami
    - Hypointense WM
- T2WI
  - Infantile GM2
    - TS: Hypointense ventral thalamus, ± hyperintense posterior thalamus
    - SD: Mild diffuse thalamic hypointensity
    - Both: Hyperintense CS (mild), cerebral WM
  - Juvenile, adult GM2
    - Cerebellar atrophy
    - ± Hyperintense cerebral WM, atrophy
    - Rare, hyperintense "mass-like" brainstem involvement
- DWI: Variably reduced diffusivity ventral thalamus in TS
- T1 C+: No abnormal enhancement
- MRS
  - Infantile GM2: ↓ NAA, ↑ choline, myo-inositol
  - Juvenile, adult GM2: ↓ NAA in normal-appearing thalami, cerebral WM reported

## Ultrasonographic Findings
- Infantile GM2: Echogenic thalami

## Imaging Recommendations
- MR (CT may confirm thalamic abnormality)

## DIFFERENTIAL DIAGNOSIS

### Status Marmoratus
- Hyperdense (variable T2 hypo-, T1 hyperintense) thalami, ± basal ganglia on background of atrophy, WM hypodensity
- History of profound perinatal ischemia

### Neuronal Ceroid Lipofuscinosis (NCL)
- Thalami, globi pallidi are hyperdense (CT), hypointense (T2WI)
- Cerebral, cerebellar atrophy

### Krabbe Disease
- Hyperdense thalami, caudate and dentate nuclei
- T2 hyperintense cerebral + cerebellar WM with involvement of corpus callosum

### Juvenile GM1 Gangliosidosis
- Imaging findings identical to SD
- GM1 ganglioside accumulates in brain & abdominal viscera

## PATHOLOGY

### General Features
- General path comments
  - Neuronal accumulation GM2 ganglioside caused by deficient lysosomal enzyme, β-hexosaminidase A
  - Embryology-anatomy
    - GM2 ganglioside resides in neuronal membranes; plays role cell-cell recognition, synaptogenesis
    - β-hexosaminidase A (Hex A) & GM2 activator protein (GMAP) required for lysosomal GM2 ganglioside catabolism
    - Hex A is 1 of 3 isoenzymes of β-hexosaminidase formed by dimerization of α and β subunits
    - Hex A = αβ dimer; Hex B = ββ dimer; Hex S = αα dimer
    - Hex A and Hex B are major forms; Hex S is minor form with unclear physiologic function
- Genetics
  - Autosomal recessive inheritance
    - TS: > 100 different mutations α subunit, Chr 15q23-q24
    - SD: > 30 different mutations β subunit, Chr 5q13
    - GM2 variant AB: ~ 4 different mutations GMAP, Chr 5q31.3-q33.1
    - GM2 variant B1 (rare): α Subunit mutation → normal α subunit production but catalytically inactive Hex A for GM2 ganglioside hydrolysis
    - Mutations allowing residual Hex A activity (0.5-4% of normal activity) account for milder juvenile/adult phenotypes

# GANGLIOSIDOSIS (GM2)

- Etiology
  - Accumulation GM2 ganglioside in neuronal lysosomes causes neuronal degeneration, apoptosis with secondary hypo- or demyelination
    - GM2 ganglioside accumulation in myelin membrane may also contribute to demyelination
  - Exact mechanism by which GM2 ganglioside accumulation causes neuronal apoptosis is unknown
    - Activated microglia, macrophages, and astrocytes suggest an inflammatory component
    - Identification of autoantibodies in mouse models SD suggest autoimmune component
- Epidemiology
  - TS: 1:30 carrier frequency Ashkenazi Jews, French Canadians
    - ↑ Incidence Cajuns, Druze
    - 1:300 Sephardic Jews and non-Jewish
  - SD, GM2 variant AB: Pan-ethnic, but increased in small gene pools
    - 1:1,000 Jewish, 1:600 non-Jewish, 1:16-29 Creole population of Cordoba, Argentina, 1:7 Maronite Christian Cypriots
  - Incidence TS US and Canada ↓ by > than 90% since 1970 2° to carrier screening and prenatal diagnosis

## Gross Pathologic & Surgical Features
- Infantile GM2: Early megalencephaly; late atrophy
  - Gelatinous, hemispheric white matter, ± cavitation
- Juvenile/adult: Cerebellar atrophy

## Microscopic Features
- GM2 ganglioside accumulation in cerebral neurons
- Less severe GM2 ganglioside accumulation in glial, Purkinje, anterior horn, and retinal ganglion cells
- EM: GM2 ganglioside contained in "membranous cytoplasmic bodies" (MCBs) in neuronal cytoplasm, proximal nerve processes, axons
  - MCBs in cytoplasm cause distortion and ballooning
  - MCBs proximal nerve processes form meganeurites
- Hypomyelination, demyelination and Wallerian degeneration
- Juvenile/adult GM2: Ganglioside accumulation in anterior horn cells, cerebellar neurons, basal ganglia, brainstem
  - MCBs occasionally absent
- SD: Additional storage GM2 (and globoside) in viscera

## CLINICAL ISSUES

### Presentation
- Most common signs/symptoms
  - Infantile GM2: Psychomotor retardation/regression
  - Juvenile/adult GM2: Atypical spinocerebellar ataxia
  - Other signs/symptoms
    - Infantile: Macrocranium, hypotonia, seizures, blindness (90% with cherry-red spot macula), exaggerated startle response to noise
    - Juvenile/adult: Dysarthria, extrapyramidal dysfunction; psychosis/depression (30%) late
- Clinical Profile
  - Diagnosis: Documentation Hex A deficiency in serum leukocytes, cultured skin fibroblasts, amniotic fluid, or chorionic villus sample

- Abnormal results should be followed by DNA analysis to detect mutation and/or exclude a pseudodeficiency allele

## Demographics
- Age
  - Infantile GM2: Symptom onset first year of life
  - Juvenile GM2: Symptom onset by 2-6 yrs of age
  - Adult GM2: Symptom onset 1st-3rd decades
- Gender: No gender predilection
- Ethnicity
  - TS more common in Ashkenazi Jews, French Canadians, Cajuns, and Druze
  - SD, GM2 variant AB: Pan-ethnic but increased in small gene pools

## Natural History & Prognosis
- Infantile GM2: Rapidly progressive psychomotor regression culminating in paralysis, blindness, deafness; death typically by 4 yrs of age
- Juvenile GM2: More slowly progressive with death between 5 and 15 years of age
  - Death usually 2° to respiratory infection preceded by several years decerebrate rigidity in a vegetative state
- Adult: Prolonged survival to age 60-80 can occur

## Treatment
- Supportive therapy, seizure control
- Future therapies: Enzyme replacement, bone marrow & CNS stem cell transplantation, substrate deprivation, retroviral-vector-mediated gene therapy

## SELECTED REFERENCES

1. Maegawa GH et al: The natural history of juvenile or subacute GM2 gangliosidosis: 21 new cases and literature review of 134 previously reported. Pediatrics. 118(5):e1550-62, 2006
2. Aydin K et al: Proton MR spectroscopy in three children with Tay Sachs disease. Pediatr Radiol. 35(11):1081-5, 2005
3. Inglese M et al: MR imaging and proton spectroscopy of neuronal injury in late-onset GM2 gangliosidosis. AJNR Am J Neuroradiol. 26(8):2037-42, 2005
4. Yamaguchi A et al: Possible role of autoantibodies in the pathophysiology of GM2 gangliosidoses. J Clin Invest. 113 (2):200-8, 2004
5. Jeyakumar M et al: Central nervous system inflammation is a hallmark of pathogenesis in mouse models of GM1 and GM2 gangliosidosis. Brain. 126(Pt 4):974-87, 2003
6. Nassogne MC et al: Unusual presentation of GM2 gangliosidosis mimicking a brain stem tumor in a 3-year-old girl. AJNR Am J Neuroradiol. 24(5):840-2, 2003
7. Pelled D et al: Reduced rates of axonal and dendritic growth in embryonic hippocampal neurones cultured from a mouse model of Sandhoff disease. Neuropathol Appl Neurobiol. 29(4):341-9, 2003
8. Yuksel A et al: Neuroimaging findings of four patients with Sandhoff disease. Pediatr Neurol. 21(2):562-5, 1999
9. Chavany C et al: Biology and potential strategies for the treatment of GM2 gangliosidoses. Mol Med Today. 4(4):158-65, 1998
10. Myerowitz R: Tay-Sachs disease-causing mutations and neutral polymorphisms in the Hex A gene. Hum Mutat. 9(3):195-208, 1997
11. Brismar J et al: Increased density of the thalamus on CT scans in patients with GM2 gangliosidoses. AJNR Am J Neuroradiol. 11(1):125-30, 1990

# GANGLIOSIDOSIS (GM2)

## IMAGE GALLERY

### Typical

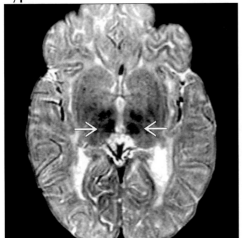
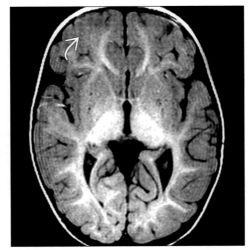

*(Left)* Axial T2WI MR shows typical hypointensity of the ventral thalamus ➜ in Tay-Sachs disease. Signal in the posterior thalamus is normal in this case but often is hyperintense. *(Right)* Axial T1WI MR in same patient as previous image shows diffuse thalamic hyperintensity, identical to that seen in SD. Note hypomyelination of the frontal white matter ➔ in this 1-year old patient.

### Typical

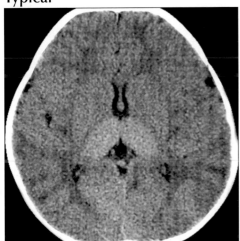
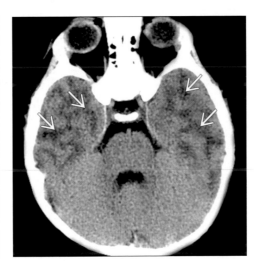

*(Left)* NECT shows classic appearance of the thalami in infantile GM2. There is symmetric, diffuse thalamic hyperdensity and white matter hypointensity. *(Right)* NECT in same patient as previous image again shows diffuse cerebral white matter hypodensity ➔. Note that the posterior fossa has a normal appearance.

### Typical

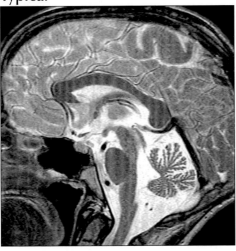
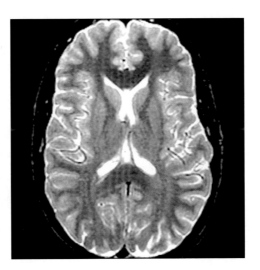

*(Left)* Sagittal T2WI MR shows diffuse cerebellar vermian atrophy seen in this patient with juvenile GM2. Cerebellar atrophy is a typical finding in this form of the disease. *(Right)* Axial T2WI MR in same patient as previous image shows normal appearing supratentorial structures. Occasionally, cerebral white matter hyperintensity and atrophy are also present in juvenile GM2.

# METACHROMATIC LEUKODYSTROPHY (MLD)

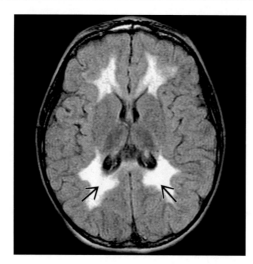

Axial FLAIR MR shows confluent hyperintensity of the periventricular white matter. Posterior periventricular and peritrigonal WM ➡ is involved early in the disease.

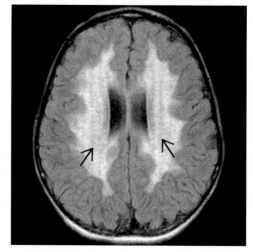

Axial FLAIR MR shows linear areas of hypointensity ➡ extending from ventricular wall to cerebral cortex. These "spared" areas of myelin, called radial stripes, are best seen on T2 images.

## TERMINOLOGY

### Abbreviations and Synonyms
- Sulfatide lipoidosis

### Definitions
- Lysosomal storage disorder due to ↓ arylsulfatase A (ARSA)
  - Defect in catabolism of sphingolipid, sulfatide (a normal constituent of myelin)

## IMAGING FINDINGS

### General Features
- Best diagnostic clue: Confluent "butterfly-shaped" central cerebral hemispheric WM T2 signal ↑
- Location
  - Central cerebral hemispheric WM
    - Early: Spares subcortical U-fibers
    - Late: Involvement of subcortical U-fibers
- Morphology: Symmetric, confluent periventricular high T2 signal

### CT Findings
- NECT: Symmetric ↓ central cerebral WM attenuation, atrophy
- CECT: No WM enhancement (lacks inflammation)
- CT perfusion: ↓ Perfusion to hemispheric WM

### MR Findings
- T1WI
  - Early: ↓ T1 signal within periventricular WM
  - Late: Cerebral atrophy
- T2WI
  - Early in disease
    - Confluent periventricular hyperintensity ("butterfly pattern")
    - Radial stripes (relative sparing of myelin in perivenular regions)
    - Early sparing of subcortical U-fibers
  - Later in disease progression
    - Progressive peripheral extension of T2 hyperintensity (demyelination)
    - Involvement of U-fibers, corpus callosum, descending pyramidal tracts, internal capsules
    - Progressive cerebral atrophy
- PD/Intermediate: ↑ Signal within periventricular WM

## DDx: Metachromatic Leukodystrophy Look-Alikes

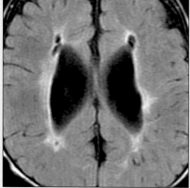

Periventricular Leukomalacia

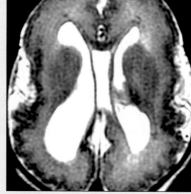

Cytomegalovirus

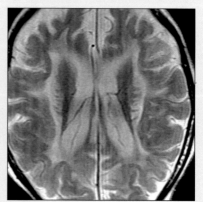

Pseudo-TORCH

# METACHROMATIC LEUKODYSTROPHY (MLD)

## Key Facts

### Terminology
- Lysosomal storage disorder due to ↓ arylsulfatase A (ARSA)

### Imaging Findings
- Best diagnostic clue: Confluent "butterfly-shaped" central cerebral hemispheric WM T2 signal ↑
- Radial stripes (relative sparing of myelin in perivenular regions)
- Early sparing of subcortical U-fibers
- Progressive peripheral extension of T2 hyperintensity (demyelination)
- Involvement of U-fibers, corpus callosum, descending pyramidal tracts, internal capsules
- Progressive cerebral atrophy
- DWI: ↓ ADC values in affected areas
- MRS: ↑ Choline

- MRI: Include FLAIR
- MRS: Sample central hemispheric WM

### Top Differential Diagnoses
- Pelizaeus-Merzbacher Disease
- TORCH
- Pseudo-TORCH
- Periventricular Leukomalacia (PVL)

### Pathology
- Associated abnormalities: Symptomatic gallbladder disease

### Clinical Issues
- Late infantile form (most common)
- Begins insidiously in the second year of life
- Strabismus, gait disturbance, ataxia, weakness, hypotonia

---

- FLAIR: "Butterfly pattern" of periventricular hyperintensity
- T2* GRE: No petechial hemorrhage
- DWI: ↓ ADC values in affected areas
- T1 C+: No WM enhancement
- MRS: ↑ Choline

## Ultrasonographic Findings
- Thick gallbladder wall, ± sludge or polypoid ingrowths

## Nuclear Medicine Findings
- PET: 123I-IMP shows cerebral hypoperfusion

## Imaging Recommendations
- Best imaging tool: Early MRI & MRS in pre-symptomatic enzyme deficient siblings
- Protocol advice
  - MRI: Include FLAIR
  - MRS: Sample central hemispheric WM

## DIFFERENTIAL DIAGNOSIS

### Pelizaeus-Merzbacher Disease
- Usually manifests in the neonate and infant
- Lack of myelination without myelin destruction
- Cerebellum may be markedly atrophic

### TORCH
- Variable WM hyperintensity (demyelination & gliosis)
- Non-progressive
- Varied patterns of Ca++ depending on etiology

### Pseudo-TORCH
- Progressive cerebral and cerebellar demyelination
- Brainstem, basal ganglia and periventricular Ca++
- Elevated CSF neurotransmitters

### Periventricular Leukomalacia (PVL)
- Usually symmetric periventricular bright T2 signal
- Periventricular volume loss (non-progressive)
- Static spastic diplegia or quadriplegia

### Sneddon Syndrome (Arylsulfatase A Pseudodeficiency)
- Demyelination may be precipitated by hypoxic event
- Periventricular WM bright T2 signal
- ARSA pseudodeficiency
- Confirmed by skin biopsy

### Krabbe Disease
- Early involvement of cerebellar WM
- CT shows ↑ attenuation of thalami

### Megaloencephalic Leukoencephaly with Subcortical Cysts (MLC)
- Slowly progressive, sparing of cognition

## PATHOLOGY

### General Features
- General path comments
  - Systemic storage of sulfatide due to deficient ARSA
    - Symptomatic storage: CNS, peripheral nerves and gallbladder
    - Asymptomatic storage: Kidneys, pancreas, adrenals, and liver
  - Diagnosis confirmed by
    - Detecting excessive urine sulfatide
    - Absent or deficient ARSA activity in fibroblasts and/or leukocytes
- Genetics
  - Autosomal recessive
    - ARSA gene located at 22q13.31qter
    - Considerable genotype-phenotype variability
    - > 40 different mutations documented (459+1G>A; P426L)
  - Compound heterozygosity with missense mutations associated with very late onset
- Etiology
  - Absent or deficient activity of ARSA ⇒ sulfatide accumulation
    - Sulfatide not able to be degraded ∴ ↑ storage in lysosomes ⇒ lethal demyelination

# METACHROMATIC LEUKODYSTROPHY (MLD)

- Epidemiology
  - In the United States incidence of all forms of MLD 1:100,000
    - ↑ In Habbanite Jewish (1:75 live births)
    - ↑ In Navajo Indians (1:2,500 live births)
- Associated abnormalities: Symptomatic gallbladder disease

## Gross Pathologic & Surgical Features
- Early
  - Megalencephaly & demyelination
  - Lack of inflammatory component to WM
- Late
  - Progressive cerebral hemispheric demyelination ⇒ atrophy

## Microscopic Features
- CNS
  - PAS-positive metachromatic material accumulates within glial cells and neurons
  - Sulfatide deposition within plasma membranes
  - Sulfatide membrane-bound inclusions at the inner layer of myelin sheaths
  - Demyelination may be extensive yet inflammatory component is lacking
- Biochemistry
  - Three isoenzymes of ARSA (A, B, & C)
    - Markedly ↓ ARSA activity in late infantile, juvenile, and adult forms of MLD
    - Sulfatide content in WM is considerably higher in the late infantile form

# CLINICAL ISSUES

## Presentation
- Most common signs/symptoms
  - Late infantile form (most common)
    - Begins insidiously in the second year of life
    - Strabismus, gait disturbance, ataxia, weakness, hypotonia
    - ± Cherry-red macular spot
    - Bulbar signs ⇒ progressive hypotonia ⇒ decerebrate posturing ⇒ optic atrophy
    - Children frequently die within 4 years of diagnosis
  - Juvenile form
    - Appears between 5 and 10 years
    - Impaired school performance (nonverbal learning disability)
    - Spastic gait, ataxia, intellectual impairment
    - Brisk deep tendon reflexes
    - Progressive spasticity ⇒ progressive dementia ⇒ decerebrate posturing ⇒ seizures
    - Rare to survive longer than 20 years
  - Adult form
    - May present as MS
    - Dementia between third and fourth decades
    - Some adults present with schizophrenia
    - Progressive: Corticobulbar, corticospinal, and cerebellar changes
- Clinical Profile: Toddler with visuomotor impairment and abdominal pain

## Demographics
- Age
  - Variable depending on form
    - Late infantile form presents between 1 & 2 yrs
- Gender: Males and females affected equally
- Ethnicity: ↑ Incidence in Habbanite Jews and Navajo Indians

## Natural History & Prognosis
- Variable depending on clinical form

## Treatment
- Bone marrow transplant
  - May arrest motor and intellectual deterioration
- Attempts to promote ARSA enzymatic activity have shown poor results
- Future role of retroviral-vector-mediated ARSA gene transfer

# DIAGNOSTIC CHECKLIST

## Consider
- If WM involvement appears as "worst case MLD", involving internal capsule and brainstem ⇒ MLD look-alike, consider
  - Pseudo-TORCH
  - Vacuolating megaloencephalic leukoencephaly with subcortical cysts

## Image Interpretation Pearls
- "Butterfly pattern" of cerebral hemispheric WM
- Radial periventricular stripes on T2WI
- Early sparing of subcortical U-fibers
- Lack of WM enhancement (no inflammatory component)

# SELECTED REFERENCES

1. Patay Z: Diffusion-weighted MR imaging in leukodystrophies. Eur Radiol. 15(11):2284-303, 2005
2. Toldo I et al: Spinal cord and cauda equina MRI findings in metachromatic leukodystrophy: case report. Neuroradiology. 47(8):572-5, 2005
3. van der Voorn JP et al: Histopathologic correlates of radial stripes on MR images in lysosomal storage disorders. AJNR Am J Neuroradiol. 26(3):442-6, 2005
4. Oguz KK et al: Diffusion-weighted imaging findings in juvenile metachromatic leukodystrophy. Neuropediatrics. 35(5):279-82, 2004
5. Sener RN: Metachromatic leukodystrophy. Diffusion MR imaging and proton MR spectroscopy. Acta Radiol. 44(4):440-3, 2003
6. Sener RN: Metachromatic leukodystrophy: diffusion MRI findings. AJNR Am J Neuroradiol. 23(8):1424-6, 2002
7. Parmeggiani A et al: Sneddon syndrome, arylsulfatase A pseudodeficiency and impairment of cerebral white matter. Brain Dev. 22(6):390-3, 2000
8. Faerber EN et al: MRI appearances of metachromatic leukodystrophy. Pediatr Radiol 29(9):669-72, 1999
9. Stillman AE et al: Serial MR after bone marrow transplantation in two patients with metachromatic leukodystrophy. AJNR Am J Neuroradiol. 15(10):1929-32, 1994

# METACHROMATIC LEUKODYSTROPHY (MLD)

## IMAGE GALLERY

### Typical

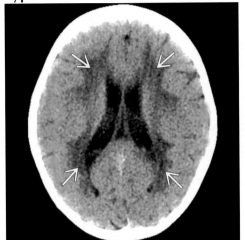
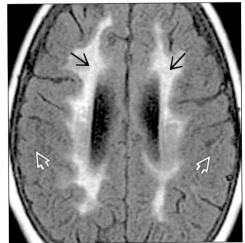

*(Left)* Axial NECT shows symmetric periventricular WM hypoattenuation ➡. The presence of periventricular Ca++ would suggest an alternative diagnosis such as CMV or pseudo-TORCH. *(Right)* Axial T2WI MR shows a characteristic "butterfly" pattern ➡ of central periventricular demyelination. Note the sparing of peripheral, subcortical WM ➡.

### Typical

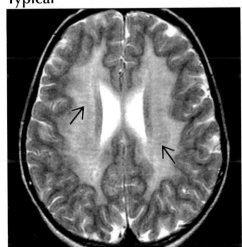
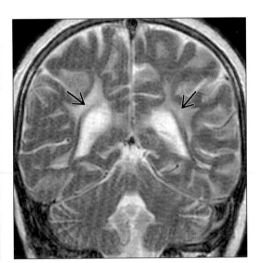

*(Left)* Axial T2WI MR shows symmetric cerebral hemispheric WM hyperintensity secondary to demyelination. Note the hypointense radial stripes ➡ that are seen best on this T2 weighted image. *(Right)* Coronal T2WI MR shows the presence of prolonged T2 relaxation within the peritrigonal WM ➡, a region that is involved early in patients with metachromatic leukodystrophy.

### Typical

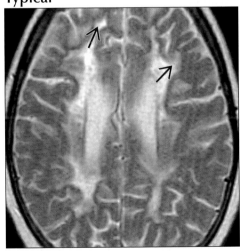
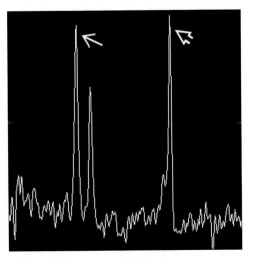

*(Left)* Axial T2WI MR shows the findings of progressive MLD. Prolonged T2 relaxation extends outward to the subcortical WM ➡. Note the loss of volume (atrophy) of white matter. *(Right)* MRS using the PRESS technique and a TE of 288, demonstrates a non-specific elevation in choline ➡ with normal to slightly reduced NAA ➡ in this white matter voxel.

# KRABBE

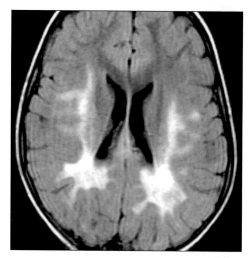 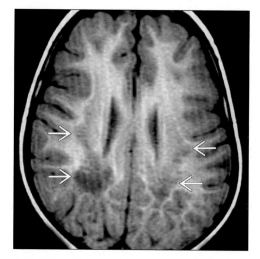

*Axial FLAIR MR shows abnormal hyperintense signal in the periventricular and deep white matter with a posterior predominance. Note that there is sparing of subcortical WM at this stage.*

*Axial T1WI MR (same child as previous image) shows irregular hypointense signal ➡ in the same distribution. Lesions are due to a combination of demyelination and oligodendrocyte loss.*

## TERMINOLOGY

### Abbreviations and Synonyms
• Globoid cell leukodystrophy (GLD)

### Definitions
• Leukodystrophy caused by a deficiency of the lysosomal enzyme galactocerebroside β-galactosidase (galatosylceramidase I)

## IMAGING FINDINGS

### General Features
• Best diagnostic clue: Faint hyperdensity in thalami on CT in an infant (3-6 months) that is extremely irritable and has depressed deep tendon reflexes
• Location: Thalami, basal ganglia, cerebellar nuclei, white matter (WM), corticospinal & pyramidal tracts

### CT Findings
• NECT
  ○ Symmetric hyperdensities in thalami

■ May also be seen in basal ganglia (BG), corona radiata, cerebellar nuclei
■ Disappear over time
○ Deep, periventricular WM hypodensity
○ Volume loss late in disease course
○ Juvenile and adult onset less likely to show hyperdensities

### MR Findings
• T1WI
  ○ Thalami may show some hyperintensity early in disease
  ○ Optic nerve enlargement
  ○ Volume loss late in disease course
• T2WI
  ○ Patchy T2 hyperintensity in deep, periventricular WM
    ■ Coalesces over time to become confluent and diffuse
    ■ Spares subcortical WM early on
    ■ Posteriorly > anteriorly early in disease
  ○ Hyperintense T2 signal in cerebellar nuclei and WM
  ○ May see hypointensity in thalamus early in disease
  ○ May see hyperintensity along corticospinal tracts

### DDx: Leukodystrophies

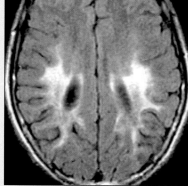 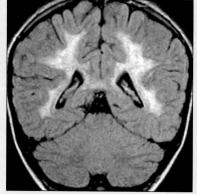 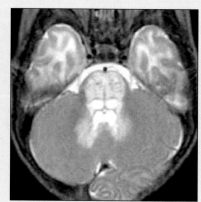

*Adrenoleukodystrophy*     *Metachromatic Leukodystrophy*     *Maple Syrup Urine Disease*

# KRABBE

## Key Facts

### Terminology
- Leukodystrophy caused by a deficiency of the lysosomal enzyme galactocerebroside β-galactosidase (galatosylceramidase I)

### Imaging Findings
- Best diagnostic clue: Faint hyperdensity in thalami on CT in an infant (3-6 months) that is extremely irritable and has depressed deep tendon reflexes
- Optic nerve enlargement
- Volume loss late in disease course
- Patchy T2 hyperintensity in deep, periventricular WM
- Hyperintense T2 signal in cerebellar nuclei and WM
- Effects of hemapoietic stem cell transplantation can be tracked with diffusion tensor imaging (DTI)

### Top Differential Diagnoses
- X-Linked Adrenoleukodystrophy (ALD)
- Metachromatic Leukodystrophy (MLD)
- Maple Syrup Urine Disease (MSUD)
- GM2 Gangliosidoses (e.g., Tay-Sachs)

### Pathology
- WM injury due to accumulation of cerebroside and psychosine (galactosylsphingosine)
- Perivascular large multinucleated "globoid" and mononuclear epithelioid cells in demyelinated zones
- Severe oligodendrocyte loss

### Clinical Issues
- Neonatal: Most common symptom is extreme irritability
- Seizures result in medical attention

---

- FLAIR: Better delineates WM signal abnormalities
- DWI
  - Reduced diffusion early in disease course
    - May reflect decrease in extracellular space due to axonal swelling
  - Diffusivity of WM increases with disease progression
    - Likely reflects increase in extracellular space due to neuronal/axonal loss
  - Effects of hemapoietic stem cell transplantation can be tracked with diffusion tensor imaging (DTI)
- T1 C+
  - May see enhancement at junction of normal and abnormal WM
  - May see enhancement of cranial nerves
- MRS
  - Reduction in NAA
  - Elevated choline
  - ± Lactate elevation
  - ± Macromolecule elevation (0.8-1.4 ppm)

## Imaging Recommendations
- Best imaging tool: MR with DWI or DTI
- Protocol advice: Consider Krabbe when encountering bilateral thalamic or BG hyperdensity on CT in an infant

## DIFFERENTIAL DIAGNOSIS

### X-Linked Adrenoleukodystrophy (ALD)
- Stereotypical advancing demyelination splenium → parietal periventricular WM
- Typically presenting in older children (boys) than GLD

### Metachromatic Leukodystrophy (MLD)
- Dysmyelination/demyelination of periventricular WM
- Typically presents in 2nd year of life

### Maple Syrup Urine Disease (MSUD)
- Edema in deep cerebellar and perirolandic WM, dorsal brain stem
- Presents in first few days of life

### Neuronal Ceroid Lipofuscinosis (NCL)
- Inherited neurodegenerative disorders associated with accumulation of abnormal pigment lipofuscin
- Hypointense/hyperdense thalami & putamina; hyperintense periventricular WM

### GM2 Gangliosidoses (e.g., Tay-Sachs)
- Presents in infancy
- Hypointense (MR)/hyperdense (DT) thalami; patchy hyperintense WM

### Status Marmoratus
- End result of acute near-total asphyxia

## PATHOLOGY

### General Features
- General path comments
  - WM injury due to accumulation of cerebroside and psychosine (galactosylsphingosine)
  - Canine variant affects West Highland and Cairn terriers
    - Important research substrate
- Genetics
  - Autosomal recessive lysosomal disorder
  - Gene mapped to chromosome 14 ⇒ 14q24.3 to 14q32.1
    - Different mutations associated with differing severity for both age of onset & progression
    - Solitary mutation in 40–50% of infantile cases with European, Mexican ancestry
    - 65 mutations & polymorphisms described
    - Majority of adult form mutations occur at 5' end of the gene; infantile cases cluster at 3' end
- Etiology
  - Gene defects result in deficiency of lysosomal galactosylceramidase I (a.k.a., galactocerebroside β-galactosidase)
    - Galactosylceramidase I metabolizes psychosine & galactosylceramide to sphingosine & ceramide

# KRABBE

- Galactosylceramidase II & III can catalyze galactosylceramide but not psychosine
- Causes marked accumulation of psychosine
- Psychosine is toxic to oligodendrocytes
  - Sulfotransferase may also be deficient → suggests galactosylceramide degradation may be complex
- Epidemiology
  - 1:25-50,000 in Sweden
  - 1:100,000 US

## Gross Pathologic & Surgical Features
- Small, atrophic brain
- Enlarged optic nerves/chiasm
  - Described by Krabbe in 1 of original 5 cases
  - Due to accumulation of globoid cells

## Microscopic Features
- Perivascular large multinucleated "globoid" and mononuclear epithelioid cells in demyelinated zones
  - "Globoid" cells = macrophages containing PAS-positive galactocerebrosides
- Myelin loss with astrogliosis & dysmyelination
- Severe oligodendrocyte loss
- Demyelination is marked within cerebrum, cerebellum, brainstem, spinal cord with segmental involvement of peripheral nerves
- Globoid cell inclusions in sweat gland epithelial cells

## Staging, Grading or Classification Criteria
- Infantile: Before age 2
  - Most common & most severe
  - Variants: Irritative-hypertonic, neonatal feeding abnormality, hemiplegic, prolonged floppy
- Late infantile-juvenile: After age 2
  - Considerable biochemical, clinical variations
  - Variants: Visual failure, cerebellar ataxia, spastic-onset, acute polyneuropathy, dementia-psychosis
- Adult: After age 10
  - Corticospinal, pyramidal tract symptoms
  - Mimics a peripheral neuropathy
  - May go undiagnosed for many years

## CLINICAL ISSUES

### Presentation
- Most common signs/symptoms
  - Neonatal: Most common symptom is extreme irritability
    - Seizures result in medical attention
    - Hypersensitivity to sensory stimuli (e.g., hyperacusis), fevers, feeding problems, failure to thrive, optic atrophy, cortical blindness
  - Infantile-juvenile
    - Visual failure, cerebellar ataxia, spasticity, polyneuropathy, dementia, psychosis
  - Adult
    - Hemiparesis, spastic paraparesis, cerebellar ataxia, intellectual impairment, visual failure, peripheral polyneuropathy, talipes cavus
- Clinical Profile
  - Diagnosis made with leukocyte or skin fibroblast β-galactosidase assay

- Molecular assay available for genetic counseling, prenatal testing

## Demographics
- Age: Most commonly infantile
- Gender: M = F
- Ethnicity: 6:1,000 in the Druze community in Israel

## Natural History & Prognosis
- Neonatal: Rapidly progressive, few live > 2 years
  - Hypertonicity → flaccidity as PNS involved
- Infantile-juvenile: More protracted course, slower rate of progression
- Adult: Heterogeneous, progresses more slowly
  - MR may remain normal for many years, even in presence of symptoms

## Treatment
- Hematopoietic stem cell transplantation (bone marrow or umbilical cord blood)
  - Halts disease progression in mild forms of Krabbe
  - Both clinical & radiologic manifestations may reverse or retard
    - Improvement of peripheral nerve conduction
- Gene therapy for Krabbe (as well as all lysosomal storage disorders) holds promise

## SELECTED REFERENCES
1. Siddiqi ZA et al: Peripheral neuropathy in Krabbe disease: effect of hematopoietic stem cell transplantation. Neurology. 67(2):268-72, 2006
2. Escolar ML et al: Transplantation of umbilical-cord blood in babies with infantile Krabbe's disease. N Engl J Med. 352(20):2069-81, 2005
3. McGraw P et al: Krabbe disease treated with hematopoietic stem cell transplantation: serial assessment of anisotropy measurements--initial experience. Radiology. 236(1):221-30, 2005
4. van der Voorn JP et al: Histopathologic correlates of radial stripes on MR images in lysosomal storage disorders. AJNR Am J Neuroradiol. 26(3):442-6, 2005
5. Brockmann K et al: Proton MRS profile of cerebral metabolic abnormalities in Krabbe disease. Neurology. 60(5):819-25, 2003
6. Haq E et al: Molecular mechanism of psychosine-induced cell death in human oligodendrocyte cell line. J Neurochem. 86(6):1428-40, 2003
7. Suzuki K: Globoid cell leukodystrophy (Krabbe's disease): update. J Child Neurol. 18(9):595-603, 2003
8. Bajaj NP et al: Adult onset of Krabbe's disease resembling hereditary spastic paraplegia with normal neuroimaging. J Neurol Neurosurg Psychiatry. 72(5):635-8, 2002
9. Jatana M et al: Apoptotic positive cells in Krabbe brain and induction of apoptosis in rat C6 glial cells by psychosine. Neurosci Lett. 330(2):183-7, 2002
10. Guo AC et al: Evaluation of white matter anisotropy in Krabbe disease with diffusion tensor MR imaging: initial experience. Radiology. 218(3):809-15, 2001
11. Farina L et al: MR imaging and proton MR spectroscopy in adult Krabbe disease. AJNR Am J Neuroradiol. 21(8):1478-82, 2000
12. Jones BV et al: Optic nerve enlargement in Krabbe's disease. AJNR Am J Neuroradiol. 20(7):1228-31, 1999

## IMAGE GALLERY

### Typical

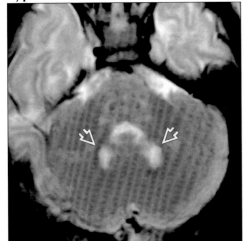

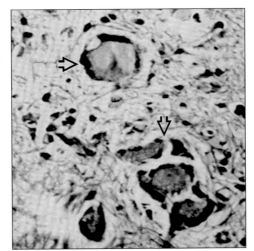

*(Left)* Axial T2WI MR in an infant with Krabbe disease shows hyperintensity ⊟ in the deep cerebellar nuclei, with rims of surrounding hypointensity. *(Right)* Micropathology, high power shows characteristic multinucleated globoid cells ⊟, with abundant cytoplasm and peripherally displaced nuclear material.

### Typical

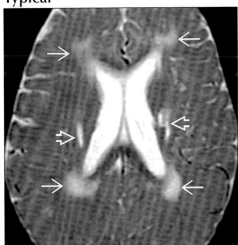

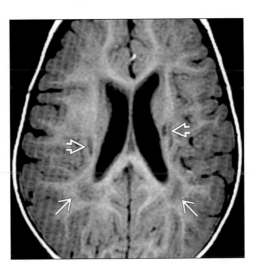

*(Left)* Axial T2WI MR shows patchy signal abnormalities ⊟ in the periventricular white matter and frank cystic necrosis ⊟ in the descending pyramidal tracts. *(Right)* Axial T1WI MR in the same child as previous image shows the necrotic foci as well-defined hypointense lesions ⊟. Regions of demyelination ⊟ are considerably more subtle.

### Typical

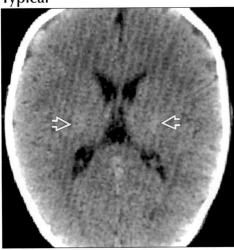

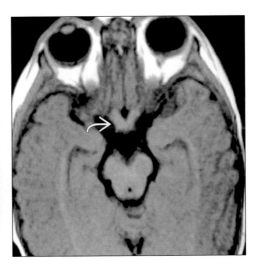

*(Left)* Axial NECT shows faint hyperintensities ⊟ in the thalami of an infant with Krabbe disease. These are thought to represent microcalcifications that resolve with disease progression. *(Right)* Axial T1WI MR shows symmetric enlargement of the optic nerves ⊟ in a child with Krabbe disease. Enlargement is due to focal accumulation of globoid cells.

# X-LINKED ADRENOLEUKODYSTROPHY

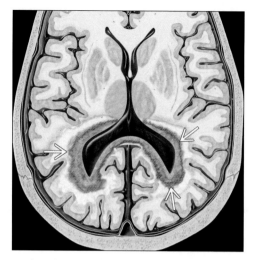

Axial graphic illustrates typical layers of involvement in classic childhood cerebral X-ALD. Intermediate zone of inflammation ➡ enhances, moves peripherally with progression.

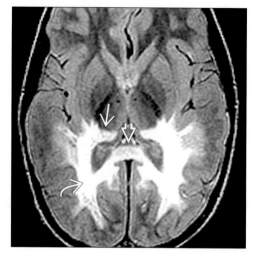

Axial FLAIR MR shows a similar pattern of intense, symmetrical demyelination of splenium ⬌, peritrigonal white matter, forceps major ⬈ and pulvinar areas ➡ with "U-fiber" sparing.

## TERMINOLOGY

### Abbreviations and Synonyms

- X-linked adrenoleukodystrophy (X-ALD): Severe progressive form usually affecting pre-teen males
- Adrenomyeloneuropathy (AMN): Mild adult or spino-cerebellar form, half have some cerebral involvement

### Definitions

- Inherited disorder of peroxisome metabolism ⇒ impaired β-oxidation of very long chain fatty acids (VLCFA)
  - X-ALD and AMN account for 80% of cases
  - At least 6 variants other than classic childhood cerebral X-ALD (CCALD) exist: Pre-symptomatic X-ALD; adolescent (AdolCALD); adult (ACALD); AMN; Addison only; symptomatic female carriers

## IMAGING FINDINGS

### General Features

- Best diagnostic clue: Enhancing (CT or MR) peritrigonal demyelination in CCALD
- Location
  - Classic CCALD: Splenium/peritrigonal white matter (WM)
    - Pattern: Splenium ⇒ peritrigonal WM ⇒ corticospinal tracts/fornix/commisural fibers/visual and auditory pathways
    - Typically spares subcortical U-fibers
- Morphology
  - Usually symmetrical, confluent, posterior involvement; frontal pattern occurs in 15%
  - Central (splenium) to peripheral gradient is usual

### CT Findings

- NECT
  - ↓ Density splenium/posterior WM
  - ± Ca++ of involved WM
- CECT: CCALD: Linear enhancement of intermediate zone typical

---

## DDx: Posterior Increased Signal

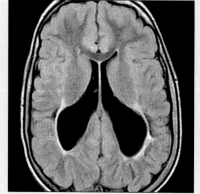

Periventricular Leukomalacia

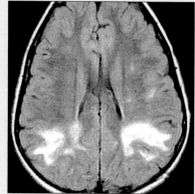

PRES

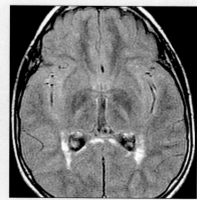

Infantile Refsum

# X-LINKED ADRENOLEUKODYSTROPHY

## Key Facts

### Terminology
- X-linked adrenoleukodystrophy (X-ALD): Severe progressive form usually affecting pre-teen males
- Inherited disorder of peroxisome metabolism ⇒ impaired β-oxidation of very long chain fatty acids (VLCFA)
- X-ALD and AMN account for 80% of cases
- At least 6 variants other than classic childhood cerebral X-ALD (CCALD) exist: Pre-symptomatic X-ALD; adolescent (AdolCALD); adult (ACALD); AMN; Addison only; symptomatic female carriers

### Imaging Findings
- Best diagnostic clue: Enhancing (CT or MR) peritrigonal demyelination in CCALD
- Classic CCALD: Splenium/peritrigonal white matter (WM)
- Pattern: Splenium ⇒ peritrigonal WM ⇒ corticospinal tracts/fornix/commisural fibers/visual and auditory pathways
- Typically spares subcortical U-fibers
- Usually symmetrical, confluent, posterior involvement; frontal pattern occurs in 15%
- X-ALD: ↓ NAA even in normal-appearing WM predicts progression; ↑ Cho, myo-inositol, lactate
- Best imaging tool: MR + contrast

### Pathology
- Complete myelin loss (U-fibers preserved), astrogliosis

### Diagnostic Checklist
- X-ALD presenting at atypical ages may have atypical appearances (lack of enhancement, asymmetry, and frontal rather than posterior predominance)

## MR Findings
- T1WI: ↓ T1 signal of involved WM; leading edge may be slightly ↑
- T2WI
  - ↑ T2 signal of involved WM
    - CCALD: Splenium ⇒ peritrigonal WM ⇒ corticospinal tracts/fornix/commisural fibers/visual and auditory pathways
    - AMN: Cerebellum, spinal cord, most common intracranial feature is corticospinal involvement, but may resemble CCALD
- FLAIR: Same as T2WI
- DWI
  - Need ADC map to overcome "T2 shine through"
  - DTI: Reduced brain "connectivity", ↑ isotropic diffusion and reduced fractional anisotropy in obvious WM change and in pre-symptomatic WM
- T1 C+
  - Leading edge (intermediate zone) enhances
    - Enhancement strongly linked to progression
- MRS
  - X-ALD: ↓ NAA even in normal-appearing WM predicts progression; ↑ Cho, myo-inositol, lactate
    - Peaks between 0.9 and 2.4 ppm probably represent VLCFA macromolecules
  - AMN: ↓ NAA in internal capsule, corticospinal tracts, parieto-occipital WM
- Spinal MR: Spinal atrophy in AMN

## Nuclear Medicine Findings
- PET: Hypometabolism of occipital lobes
- SPECT: Tc-99m HMPAO shows ↑ in regional cerebral blood flow in enhancing zone, but decrease elsewhere

## Imaging Recommendations
- Best imaging tool: MR + contrast
- Protocol advice
  - Enhanced MR shows posterior involvement of WM with rim enhancement
  - DWI/DTI and MRS may predict onset of pre-symptomatic disease

## DIFFERENTIAL DIAGNOSIS

### Periventricular Leukomalacia (PVL)
- Periventricular gliosis and volume loss following injury of prematurity; doesn't enhance

### Neonatal Hypoglycemia (Acute and Follow-up)
- May involve splenium, calcar avis, and posterior peritrigonal WM, but doesn't enhance

### Inborn Errors of Metabolism with Posterior Predominance
- White matter disease with lactate (WML): Doesn't enhance
- Infantile Refsum (peroxisomal disorder)

### Metachromatic Leukodystrophy
- Frontal and posterior white matter, doesn't enhance

### Alexander Disease
- Enhances, but frontal predominance
- Subcortical white matter involved

## PATHOLOGY

### General Features
- General path comments
  - VLCFA accumulate in all tissues of body
  - Symptomatic accumulation: CNS myelin, adrenal cortex, Leydig cell testes
    - Adrenal failure: Skin bronzing
    - Testes: Early androgenetic alopecia in adults
- Genetics: X-ALD: X-linked recessive, Xq28; mutations ABCD1 gene (> 300 described!)
- Etiology
  - Peroxisomes ubiquitous organelles involved in catabolic pathways
    - Involved with myelin formation/stabilization
    - Defect in VLCFA importer ⇒ impaired β-oxidation VLCFA

# X-LINKED ADRENOLEUKODYSTROPHY

- VLCFA accumulate in WM ⇒ brittle myelin
  - ABCD1 is ATPase transporter protein: "Traffic" ATPase, required for transport hydrophilic molecules across peroxisomal membrane
  - Modifying/exacerbating factors affect phenotype
    - Down-regulation of gene
    - Inflammatory/traumatic triggers
- Epidemiology: X-ALD and variants: 1 per 16,800 births in North America

## Gross Pathologic & Surgical Features
- Atrophy, WM softened

## Microscopic Features
- Complete myelin loss (U-fibers preserved), astrogliosis
- Ca++ (late), prominent inflammatory changes
- 3 zones with specific features
  - Innermost zone of necrosis, gliosis and ± Ca++
  - Intermediate zone of active demyelination and inflammation
  - Peripheral zone of demyelination without inflammation

## Staging, Grading or Classification Criteria
- Loes MR scoring system: Severity score based upon location and extent of disease and atrophy
  - Pattern 1: Parieto-occipital WM (rapid progression if contrast-enhancement present and very young)
  - Pattern 2: Frontal WM (same as pattern 1)
  - Pattern 3: Corticospinal tract (adults, slower progression)
  - Pattern 4: Corticospinal tract and cerebellar WM (adolescents, slower progression)
  - Pattern 5: Concomitant parieto-occipital and frontal WM (mainly childhood, extremely rapid)

# CLINICAL ISSUES

## Presentation
- Most common signs/symptoms: Skin bronzing, behavioral difficulties, hearing problems
- Classic childhood cerebral X-ALD (CCALD): 35-50%, but percentage ↓ as new forms diagnosed
  - Pre-teen male (3-10 years): Behavioral, learning, gait, hearing, vision difficulties
  - "Addison/adrenal insufficiency" (skin bronzing, nausea & vomiting, fatigue) may predate X-ADL diagnosis
- Adrenomyeloneuropathy (AMN) (25%)
  - 14-60 years
  - Spinal involvement > > brain involvement; peripheral nerve involvement
  - Brain inflammatory reaction eventually in 50%
  - Brain MR: Variable pattern demyelination, enhancement (especially corticospinal tracts)
- Presymptomatic ALD (12%)
  - Abnormal genetic testing (due to known symptomatic brother or maternal uncle), but normal imaging, symptom free
- 20-50% female carriers show AMN-like symptoms
  - Symptomatic due to skewed X-inactivation, but milder, late onset
- Other presentations less common

- AdolCALD: 10-20 years, symptoms and course similar to CCALD
- ACALD: May be misdiagnosed as psychiatric disorder; very rapid progression; diffuse rather than posterior pattern

## Demographics
- Age: CCALD: Pre-teen males
- Gender
  - Males in classic X-ALD
  - Female carries may show AMN-like symptoms
- Ethnicity
  - CCALD predominates in North America and France
  - AMN predominates in Netherlands

## Natural History & Prognosis
- CCALD: Progresses to spastic quadriparesis, blindness, deafness, vegetative state
- AMN: Spasticity, weak legs and sphincter, sexual dysfunction

## Treatment
- CCALD: Vegetative state, death in 2-5 years without BMT
  - Lorenzo oil may prolong time before symptoms if MR still normal
  - Variable results: Cholesterol-lowering drugs, dietary VLCFA restriction, glycerol trioleate/trierucate intake, plasmapheresis, interferon, immuno-ablation
  - Early bone marrow transplantation (BMT) stabilizes demyelination: **Rare** reversal demyelination

# DIAGNOSTIC CHECKLIST

## Consider
- X-ALD presenting at atypical ages may have atypical appearances (lack of enhancement, asymmetry, and frontal rather than posterior predominance)

## Image Interpretation Pearls
- Always give contrast to unknown leukodystrophy/leukoencephalopathy

# SELECTED REFERENCES

1. Hudspeth MP et al: Immunopathogenesis of adrenoleukodystrophy: Current understanding. J Neuroimmunol. 2006
2. Moser HW. Related Articles et al: Therapy of X-linked adrenoleukodystrophy. NeuroRx. 3(2):246-53, 2006
3. Fatemi A et al: MRI and proton MRSI in women heterozygous for X-linked adrenoleukodystrophy. Neurology. 60(8):1301-7, 2003
4. Loes DJ et al: Analysis of MRI patterns aids prediction of progression in X-linked adrenoleukodystrophy. Neurology. 61(3):369-74, 2003
5. Eichler FS et al: Proton MR spectroscopic & diffusion tensor brain MR imaging in X-linked adrenoleukodystrophy: initial experience. Radiology. 225(1):245-52, 2002
6. Melhem ER et al: X-linked adrenoleukodystrophy: the role of contrast-enhanced MR imaging in predicting disease progression. AJNR Am J Neuroradiol. 21(5):839-44, 2000
7. van Geel BM et al: X linked adrenoleukodystrophy: clinical presentation, diagnosis, and therapy. J Neurol Neurosurg Psychiatry. 63(1):4-14, 1997

## IMAGE GALLERY

### Typical

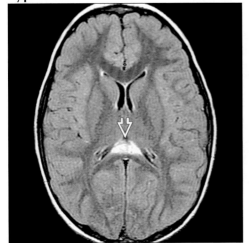
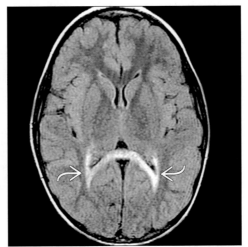

*(Left) Axial FLAIR MR shows focal intense central hyperintensity (demyelination) in the splenium ➡ of the corpus callosum. This is usually the first site involved by the disease. (Right) Axial FLAIR MR on follow-up imaging in the same child as previous image shows progressive extension of inflammation/demyelination into callosal radiations and the peritrigonal white matter ➡.*

### Typical

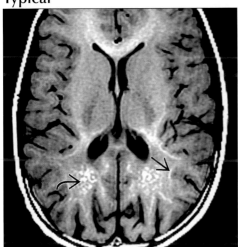
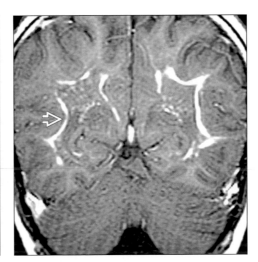

*(Left) Axial T1WI MR shows posterior demyelination with speckled calcifications/spared myelin ➡ and lack of involvement of the subcortical U-fibers ➡. (Right) Coronal T1 C+ MR in the same patient as previous image shows linear enhancement ➡ at the leading edge of demyelination, subjacent to the spared subcortical U-fibers.*

### Typical

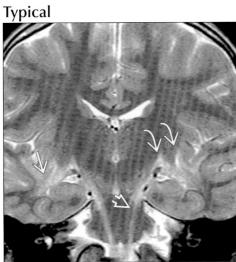
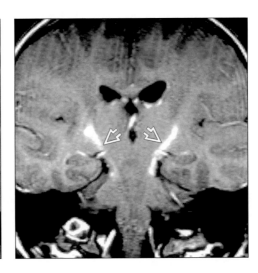

*(Left) Coronal T2WI MR shows demyelination of the corticospinal tracts ➡ and the temporal stem white matter ➡. Involvement of the geniculate bodies ➡ is also seen. (Right) Coronal T1 C+ MR in another patient shows symmetrical enhancement ➡ of the corticospinal tracts, a very common finding in adrenoleukodystrophy.*

# ZELLWEGER SYNDROME

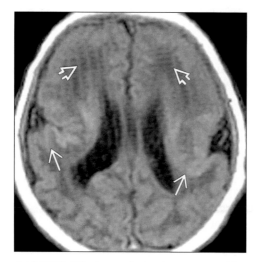

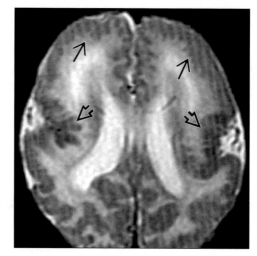

*Axial T1WI MR shows abnormal cortex resembling polymicrogyria: Note irregular inner surface ➡. Note the marked hypomyelination for a child of 22 months ➡. (Courtesy C. Glasier, MD).*

*Axial T2WI MR shows microgyria in the frontal lobes ➡. Thickened perisylvian cortex vaguely mimics pachygyria ➡. Note the hyperintense hypomyelinated white matter at 22 months of age.*

## TERMINOLOGY

### Abbreviations and Synonyms
- Cerebrohepatorenal syndrome of Zellweger

### Definitions
- Near complete absence of peroxisomes

## IMAGING FINDINGS

### General Features
- Best diagnostic clue: Hypomyelination, microgyria, germinolytic cysts
- Location: Microgyria involving anterior frontal and temporal regions

### CT Findings
- NECT: Flat supraorbital ridge, subependymal cysts, simplified gyral pattern

### MR Findings
- T1WI: Hypomyelination, caudothalamic subependymal cysts
- T2WI: Microgyria

- MRS: ↓ NAA, ↑ lipids and lactate

### Imaging Recommendations
- Best imaging tool: MRI & MRS
- Protocol advice: 3D SPGR for cortical malformations, FLAIR for germinolytic cysts

## DIFFERENTIAL DIAGNOSIS

### Congenital CMV
- Periventricular Ca++, Subependymal cysts, ± cortical malformation

### Pseudo-TORCH
- Basal ganglia, thalamic and periventricular Ca++

### Congenital Bilateral Perisylvian Syndrome
- Absent germinolytic cysts, normal white matter

### Pseudo-Zellweger
- Cerebellar malformations more common

### Infantile Refsum Disease
- Heralds with hepatomegaly and jaundice

### DDx: Zellweger Mimics

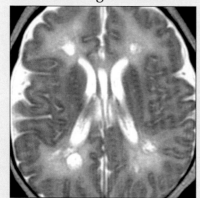

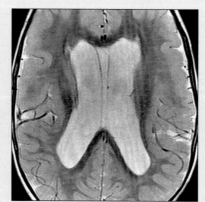

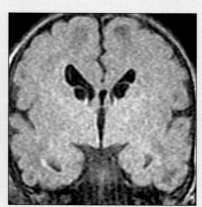

*Congenital CMV*

*Perisylvian Syndrome*

*Infantile Refsum*

# ZELLWEGER SYNDROME

## Key Facts

### Terminology
- Near complete absence of peroxisomes

### Imaging Findings
- Best diagnostic clue: Hypomyelination, microgyria, germinolytic cysts
- T1WI: Hypomyelination, caudothalamic subependymal cysts
- MRS: ↓ NAA, ↑ lipids and lactate

- Protocol advice: 3D SPGR for cortical malformations, FLAIR for germinolytic cysts

### Top Differential Diagnoses
- Congenital CMV
- Congenital Bilateral Perisylvian Syndrome
- Infantile Refsum Disease

### Diagnostic Checklist
- Dysmorphic newborn with hypotonia and seizures

---

### Neonatal Adrenoleukodystrophy
- Lacks facial dysmorphism

## PATHOLOGY

### General Features
- General path comments: Absence of peroxisomes→ multiple metabolic disturbances
- Genetics: Autosomal-recessive, Locus 7q11, 7q21 (PEX1), 8q (PEX2), 6q (PEX3)
- Etiology: Lack of peroxisome formation
- Associated abnormalities
  ○ Glaucoma, cataracts, retinal pigment degeneration
  ○ Hepatomegaly (78%), renal cortical cysts (97%)
  ○ Skeletal: Stippled chondral calcification (patellar)

### Gross Pathologic & Surgical Features
- Hypomyelination, cortical & cerebellar malformations

### Microscopic Features
- Microgyria, subependymal germinolytic cysts
- Sudanophilic leukodystrophy

## CLINICAL ISSUES

### Presentation
- Most common signs/symptoms
  ○ Broad forehead, hypoplastic supraorbital ridge and nasal bridge

  ○ Severe hypotonia, seizures, optic atrophy
- Clinical Profile: Hypotonic from birth, dysmorphic facies

### Demographics
- Age: Onset shortly after birth
- Gender: More common in males

### Natural History & Prognosis
- Most die in first 3 months

### Treatment
- No proven definitive treatment
- Oral plasmalogen, bile acid therapy, co-enzyme Q10

## DIAGNOSTIC CHECKLIST

### Consider
- Dysmorphic newborn with hypotonia and seizures

### Image Interpretation Pearls
- Germinolytic cysts, hypomyelination and microgyria

## SELECTED REFERENCES
1. Mochel F et al: Contribution of fetal MR imaging in the prenatal diagnosis of Zellweger syndrome. AJNR Am J Neuroradiol. 27(2):333-6, 2006
2. Barkovich AJ et al: MR of Zellweger syndrome. AJNR 18(6):1163-70, 1997

## IMAGE GALLERY

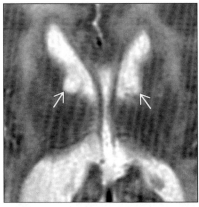 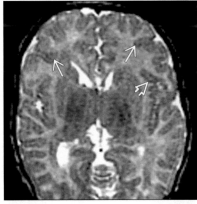 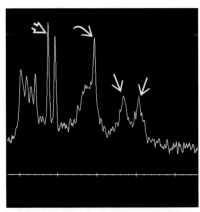

*(Left)* Axial T2WI MR shows characteristic germinolytic cysts, extending into the posterior caudate heads at the bilateral caudothalamic notch ➡. Right lateral ventricle is enlarged. *(Center)* Axial T2WI FS MR shows microgyria involving the frontal lobes ➡ and insular cortex ➡. Microgyria in the perirolandic and sylvian regions is a hallmark of Zellweger syndrome. *(Right)* MRS in a 2 year old, using single voxel PRESS technique and short TE (35 msec), shows prominent macromolecular peaks ➡. Note the mild decline of NAA ➡ and elevated choline ➡.

# OTHER PEROXISOMAL DISORDERS

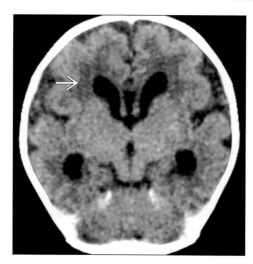

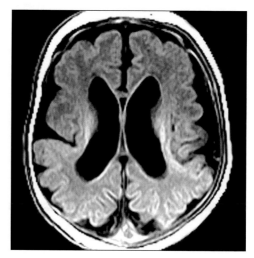

*Axial NECT in neonate with peroxisome assembly disorder, but no patellar stippling, subependymal or renal cysts, shows microcephaly, hypodense white matter ⇒ and simplified gyral pattern.*

*Axial T1WI MR in same infant as previous image at 1 month of age shows simplified gyri, volume loss and ventriculomegaly. Findings are similar to, but less severe than classic Zellweger syndrome patients.*

## TERMINOLOGY

### Abbreviations and Synonyms

- Peroxisomal disorders; peroxisomal biogenesis or assembly disorders (PBD); single peroxisomal enzyme (transporter) deficiencies (PED)
- PBD: Zellweger syndrome (ZS), neonatal adrenoleukodystrophy (NALD), infantile Refsum disease (IRD), rhizomelic chondrodysplasia punctata (RCDP) type 1
  - Zellweger spectrum disorders (ZSD): Triad of ZS, NALD, IRD (but not RCDP)
  - RCDP type 1: Normal β-oxidation of very long chain fatty acids (VLCFA), therefore different profile
- PED comprised of ≥ 10 disorders with gene mutation affecting a single protein in a peroxisomal function
  - Peroxisomal fatty acid β-oxidation
    - X-ALD; deficiencies of alkyl-DHAP-synthase (RCDP type 3); Acyl-CoA oxidase, D-bifunctional protein (D-BP), sterol carrier protein X (SCPx) & 2-methylacylCoA racemase (AMACR)
  - Ether phospholipid biosynthesis (esp. plasmalogens)
    - DHAP-alkyl transferase (DHAPAT; RCDP type 2)

  - Phytanic acid α-oxidation: Adult Refsum disease (ARD)
  - Glyoxylate detox: Primary hyperoxaluria type 1 (PH1)
  - Hydrogen peroxide metabolism: Acatalasemia

### Definitions

- Peroxisomes: Membrane-bound subcellular organelles involved in catabolic and anabolic pathways
- PEX genes encode peroxins (proteins required for peroxisome biosynthesis)

## IMAGING FINDINGS

### General Features

- Best diagnostic clue: ZSD and look-alikes: Neocortical dysplasia, peri-Sylvian polymicrogyria (PMG), hypomyelination
- Location
  - Supra- and infratentorial involvement
    - Early, severe: Gray (GM) & white matter (WM)
    - Late, mild: Often limited to WM

## DDx: Common Peroxisomal Disorders

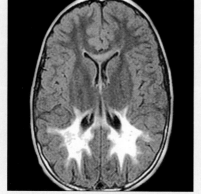

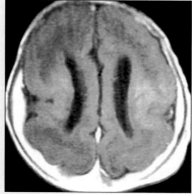

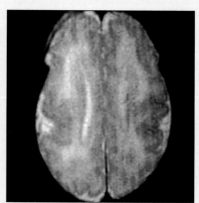

*X-Linked ALD*   *Zellweger Bleed*   *Zellweger PMG*

# OTHER PEROXISOMAL DISORDERS

## Key Facts

### Terminology
- Peroxisomal disorders; peroxisomal biogenesis or assembly disorders (PBD); single peroxisomal enzyme (transporter) deficiencies (PED)
- PBD: Zellweger syndrome (ZS), neonatal adrenoleukodystrophy (NALD), infantile Refsum disease (IRD), rhizomelic chondrodysplasia punctata (RCDP) type 1
- PED comprised of ≥ 10 disorders with gene mutation affecting a single protein in a peroxisomal function
- Peroxisomes: Membrane-bound subcellular organelles involved in catabolic and anabolic pathways
- PEX genes encode peroxins (proteins required for peroxisome biosynthesis)

### Imaging Findings
- Best diagnostic clue: ZSD and look-alikes: Neocortical dysplasia, peri-Sylvian polymicrogyria (PMG), hypomyelination
- Early, severe: Gray (GM) & white matter (WM)

### Pathology
- Epidemiology: Peroxisomal disorders 1:5,000 births
- Intact peroxisomal function required for normal brain formation, deficiency ⇒ neocortical dysgenesis
- Peroxisomes normally located near developing myelin sheaths in oligodendroglial cells at peak of myelin formation
- Deficiency leads to:
- Defect in formation or maintenance of central WM
- Nonspecific myelin reduction

## CT Findings
- NECT: X-ALD: Occasional punctate WM calcifications

## MR Findings
- T2WI
  - ZSD continuum: ZS most severe, NALD intermediate, IRD least severe
    - ZS: ↑ Intensity WM/myelin delay, neocortical dysplasia/PMG, atrophy, late cerebral and cerebellar demyelination
    - NALD: PMG, progressive WM disease
    - IRD: No neuronal migration anomalies, WM non-progressive ± improves
  - D-BP & Acyl-CoA oxidase deficiencies: ZS-like
    - D-BP: Occasional thalami & globus pallidus involvement (unlike PBD)
  - RCDP: ↑ Intensity periventricular WM, centrum semiovale, delayed occipital myelination
  - SCPx: Thalamic, pons, occipital ↑ intensity
  - AMACR: Deep WM ↑ intensity
- FLAIR: ZSD: Subependymal cysts
- DWI
  - X-ALD: Intermediate zone ↓ ADC
  - PBD: ↑ ADC values
- T1 C+
  - X-ALD: Leading edge enhancement
  - Acyl-CoA oxidase deficiency: Enhancing centrum semiovale lesions

## Radiographic Findings
- Radiography
  - ZS & RCDP: Rhizomelia, stippled epiphyses
  - RCDP & DHAP deficiencies: Coronal vertebral clefts
  - ARD: Short metacarpals/metatarsals (30%)

## Ultrasonographic Findings
- ZS: Renal cysts
- ZSD & D-BP: Hepatomegaly

## Imaging Recommendations
- Best imaging tool: MR
- Protocol advice: MR, DWI, MRS, C+

## DIFFERENTIAL DIAGNOSIS

### ZSD Mimics
- Bilateral peri-Sylvian PMG
- Congenital cytomegalovirus infections

### RCDP 1 Mimics
- X-linked dominant chondrodysplasia punctata: Conradi–Hünermann–Happle syndrome (CDPX2)
- Warfarin embryopathy

## PATHOLOGY

### General Features
- General path comments
  - PBD: Organelle fails to form, multiple peroxisomal functions defective
  - PBD have PEX gene mutations
    - PEX 1,6,12,26: ZS, NALD, IRD
    - PEX 2: ZS, IRD
    - PEX 5,10,13: ZS, NALD
    - PEX 3, 14, 16,19: ZS
    - PEX 7: RCDP 1
  - PED: Single peroxisomal enzyme deficiency
    - ARD: Phytanoyl-CoA hydroxylase
    - X-ALD: ABCD1 gene mutation
    - Acyl-CoA oxidase: ZS-like phenotype (less severe)
    - D-BP: ZS-like phenotype (severe)
    - SCPx: Sterol carrier protein X, single family
    - PH1: AGXT gene mutation, glyoxylate aminotransferase 1 (AGT) deficient (catalyzes transamination of glyoxylate to glycine) ⇒ ↑ glyoxylate oxidation to oxalate ⇒ renal stones ± systemic hyperoxaluria
    - Acatalasemia: Impaired hydrogen peroxide detoxification ⇒ ↑ risk of diabetes
- Genetics
  - Phenotype severity varies with nature of mutation
    - PEX1: G843D does not abolish peroxisomal protein import completely = milder phenotype (NALD, IRD)

# OTHER PEROXISOMAL DISORDERS

- PEX1: c.2097-2098insT mutation abolishes import completely = severe phenotype (ZS)
- PEX7: L292X = classical, severe RCDP phenotype
- PEX7: A218V = milder RCDP phenotype
  - PED may clinically resemble PBD
    - D-BP & Acyl-CoA oxidase deficiencies: ZS-like
    - Defects involving first 2 steps of plasmalogens (DHAP-alkyl transferase, DHAP-synthase deficiencies): RCDP/PEX7-like
- Etiology: VLCFA and phytanic acid incorporated into cell membranes ⇒ cell dysfunction, atrophy and death
- Epidemiology: Peroxisomal disorders 1:5,000 births

## Gross Pathologic & Surgical Features

- Intact peroxisomal function required for normal brain formation, deficiency ⇒ neocortical dysgenesis
- Peroxisomes normally located near developing myelin sheaths in oligodendroglial cells at peak of myelin formation
  - Deficiency leads to:
    - Defect in formation or maintenance of central WM
    - Nonspecific myelin reduction

## Microscopic Features

- Neuropathologic lesions
  - Abnormalities in neuronal differentiation/migration
  - Inflammatory dysmyelination or non-inflammatory demyelination of WM
- Postdevelopmental neuronal degeneration
  - Adrenomyeloneuropathy (AMN): Spinal cord axonopathy
  - IRD, RCDP: Cerebellar atrophy
- PH1: Rare reports of oxalate crystals in brain
- ZS: Additional olivary dysplasia

# CLINICAL ISSUES

## Presentation

- Most common signs/symptoms: CNS involvement manifests during development and/or later in life
- Other signs/symptoms
  - BPD
    - ZSD: Frontal bossing, marked hypotonia, hepatomegaly, perinatal apnea, seizures, jaundice, cataracts, retinopathy, deaf
    - RCDP: Rhizomelia, dwarfism/short-stature, broad nasal bridge (koala bear face), epicanthus, microcephaly, mental retardation, cataracts
  - PED
    - D-BP & Acyl-CoA oxidase deficiencies: ZS-like
    - ARD: Classic tetrad of peripheral polyneuropathy, cerebellar ataxia, ↑ CSF protein, retinitis pigmentosa; also ichthyosis, psychiatric disorders, cardiac arrhythmias, anosmia, deaf
    - X-ALD: Behavioral, learning, hearing difficulties, skin-bronzing
    - SCPx: Dystonia, azoospermia/hypogonadism, hyposmia
    - AMACR: Rare, variable findings (tremor, pyramidal signs, seizures, sensory motor neuropathy)

- PH1: Renal stones or renal failure with systemic oxalosis (bone pain, fractures, myocarditis, embolic stroke, retinopathy)

## Demographics

- Age
  - Most: Neonatal
  - X-ALD, classic Refsum: Childhood or adult onset

## Natural History & Prognosis

- PBD: Variable neurodevelopmental delays, retinopathy, deafness, liver disease
  - ZSD & look-alikes share imaging and clinical phenotype; most fail to gain milestones, severe phenotypes die within first year of life
  - RCDP & look-alikes: Severe and mild phenotypes
- PED: Variable
  - X-ALD: Progression to vegetative state if untreated
  - PH1: Progression to systemic oxalosis (myocardium, bone marrow, eyes, peripheral nerves); rapidly progressive (death in first year) and mild phenotypes

## Treatment

- PBD: Limited by multiple malformations and metabolic defects originating in-utero
- PED: X-ALD (cholesterol lowering drugs, VLCFA restriction, bone marrow transplant); ARD (phytanic acid restriction); PH1 (pyridoxin ⇒ ↓ production oxalate; alkalinize urine to ↑ oxalate solubility)

# DIAGNOSTIC CHECKLIST

## Consider

- Plasma biochemical abnormalities may be absent!
- Analysis of cultured skin fibroblasts indicated if strong imaging and clinical suspicion

# SELECTED REFERENCES

1. Ferdinandusse S et al: Clinical and biochemical spectrum of D-bifunctional protein deficiency. Ann Neurol. 59(1):92-104, 2006
2. Ferdinandusse S et al: Mutations in the gene encoding peroxisomal sterol carrier protein X (SCPx) cause leukencephalopathy with dystonia and motor neuropathy. Am J Hum Genet. 78(6):1046-52, 2006
3. Funato M et al: Aberrant peroxisome morphology in peroxisomal beta-oxidation enzyme deficiencies. Brain Dev. 28(5):287-92, 2006
4. van den Brink DM et al: Phytanic acid: production from phytol, its breakdown and role in human disease. Cell Mol Life Sci. 63(15):1752-65, 2006
5. van Woerden CS et al: High incidence of hyperoxaluria in generalized peroxisomal disorders. Mol Genet Metab. 88(4):346-50, 2006
6. Wanders RJ et al: Peroxisomal disorders: The single peroxisomal enzyme deficiencies. Biochim Biophys Acta. 1763(12):1707-20, 2006
7. Barth PG et al: Neuroimaging of peroxisome biogenesis disorders (Zellweger spectrum) with prolonged survival. Neurology. 62(3):439-44, 2004
8. Clarke CE et al: Tremor and deep white matter changes in alpha-methylacyl-CoA racemase deficiency. Neurology. 63(1):188-9, 2004

## IMAGE GALLERY

### Typical

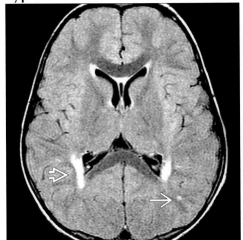 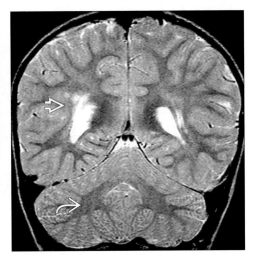

*(Left) Axial FLAIR MR in a 3 year old with mild-phenotype chondrodysplasia punctata shows increased signal in peritrigonal white matter ⮞. A focus of white matter bright signal is present ➡. (Right) Coronal T2WI MR in the same patient as previous image, shows peritrigonal signal increase ⮞ and normal dentate nuclei and cerebellar white matter ➡.*

### Typical

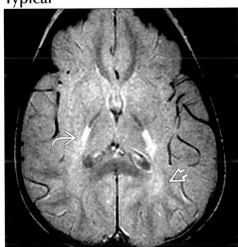 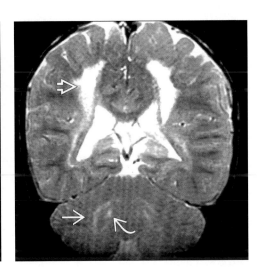

*(Left) Axial PD/Intermediate MR in a 4 year old with infantile Refsum shows posterior limb demyelination ➡, mild peritrigonal WM hyperintensity ⮞, and delayed peripheral WM arborization. (Right) Coronal T2WI MR in the same patient as previous image shows hyperintensity ⮞ in parietal white matter. Milder hyperintensity is present in the cerebellar white matter ➡ and dentate nuclei ➡.*

### Typical

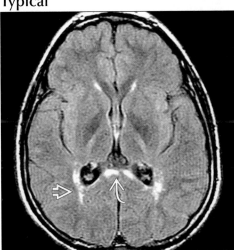 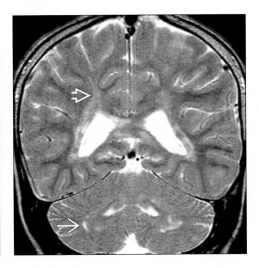

*(Left) Axial FLAIR MR in a 14 year old with infantile Refsum shows resolution of internal capsule hyperintensity. The corpus callosum is now involved ⮞. Mild peritrigonal changes remain ➡. (Right) Coronal T2WI MR in a 14 year old with infantile Refsum shows marked improvement in parietal white matter signal ⮞, but persistent cerebellar white matter involvement ➡.*

# MAPLE SYRUP URINE DISEASE

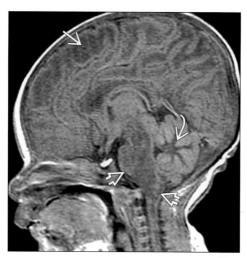

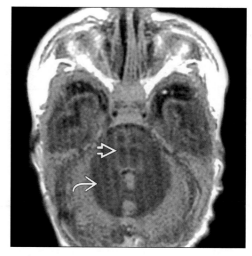

Sagittal T1WI MR shows marked brainstem swelling ➡ and low signal. There is edema of fastigial white matter ➡ and to a lesser degree, the supratentorial white matter ➡.

Axial T1WI MR shows the typical pattern of MSUD edema: Swelling and low intensity involving the cerebellar white matter ➡ and brainstem ➡.

## TERMINOLOGY

### Abbreviations and Synonyms
- Maple syrup urine disease (MSUD)
- Leucine encephalopathy

### Definitions
- MSUD is an inherited disorder of branched chain amino acid metabolism presenting in newborns with neurologic deterioration, ketoacidosis and hyperammonemia

## IMAGING FINDINGS

### General Features
- Best diagnostic clue
  - Radiologist may be first to suggest diagnosis based on classic appearing MSUD edema
    - Cerebellar white matter, brain stem, globi pallidi (GP)
    - Thalamus, cerebral peduncles, corticospinal tracts (to cortex)
- Location
  - Cerebellar and brainstem edema > supratentorial
  - Edema of corticospinal tracts

### CT Findings
- NECT
  - Early: Diffuse edema not sparing brainstem and cerebellum
    - Recognize here for best neurocognitive outcome
  - Subacute: Rapid formation of typical (classic) MSUD edema pattern
    - Subacute: Cerebral peduncles, dorsal brainstem and cerebellar edema > supratentorial hemispheres
    - Margins become sharp during subacute phase

### MR Findings
- T1WI: ↓ Signal intensity, margins may be sharp
- T2WI
  - Late: Generalized and MSUD edema disappear
    - Resolve to "pallor" and volume loss
- FLAIR: Insensitive to fluid shifts in the newborn
- DWI
  - Markedly reduced diffusivity (↑ intensity on DWI, ↓ intensity on ADC map)
  - DTI: ↓ Anisotropy
- MRS: Broad peak at 0.9 ppm

## DDx: Not Maple Syrup Urine Disease

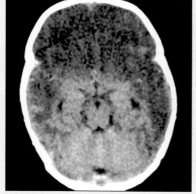

HIE Cerebellum NL

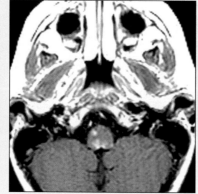

Alexander Gad T1WI

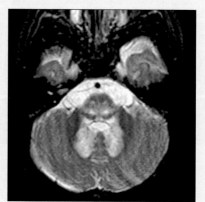

SURF1 Mitochondrial

# MAPLE SYRUP URINE DISEASE

## Key Facts

### Terminology
- MSUD is an inherited disorder of branched chain amino acid metabolism presenting in newborns with neurologic deterioration, ketoacidosis and hyperammonemia

### Imaging Findings
- Radiologist may be first to suggest diagnosis based on classic appearing MSUD edema
- Cerebellar white matter, brain stem, globi pallidi (GP)

### Pathology
- Heterogeneous clinical & molecular phenotypes: > 50 different mutations in genes governing enzyme components of branched-chain α-ketoacid dehydrogenase complex (BCKD)

### Clinical Issues
- Initial symptoms of classic MSUD: Poor feeding, vomiting, poor weight gain, increasing lethargy
- Patients in crisis often (but not always) smell like maple syrup (or burnt sugar)
- MSUD has potentially favorable outcome with strict dietary control & aggressively treated metabolic crises
- Metabolic "intoxication" (at any age) provoked by infection, injury, stress, fasting, or even pregnancy

### Diagnostic Checklist
- Neonatal testing for MSUD is not universal
- Not all MSUD occurs in population isolates
- Neonatal brain edema which includes the posterior fossa and brainstem is highly suggestive of MSUD

## Ultrasonographic Findings
- Grayscale Ultrasound: ↑ Echogenicity of GP, periventricular white matter, and areas typically involved by MSUD edema

## Imaging Recommendations
- Best imaging tool: Diffusion-weighted imaging during the hyperacute phase
- Protocol advice: MR with diffusion-weighted imaging best, but CT can make diagnosis in critically ill infant

## DIFFERENTIAL DIAGNOSIS

### Disorders Causing Brainstem and Cerebellar Swelling
- Mitochondrial SURF1 mutations: Lactate may be seen in this and in MSUD during crisis
- Late onset Alexander disease: Abnormal signal and enhancement of brainstem and aqueduct

### Hypoxic-Ischemic Encephalopathy
- No symptom free interval, usually positive history
- Cerebellum, brainstem relatively spared (MSUD involves these areas)

### Hexachlorophene Toxicity
- Myelin splitting disorder described in premature babies washed in hexachlorophene in 1960s & 70s

### Marchiafava-Bignami
- Myelin splitting disorder (corpus callosum) of adult red-wine drinkers

## PATHOLOGY

### General Features
- General path comments
  ○ Maternal ingestion of fenugreek during labor gives false impression of MSUD as urine shares a component and smell with MSUD urine
  ○ Embryology-anatomy

- Involves early myelinated areas (myelin splitting disease, spares areas where myelin isn't present)
- Genetics
  ○ Heterogeneous clinical & molecular phenotypes: > 50 different mutations in genes governing enzyme components of branched-chain α-ketoacid dehydrogenase complex (BCKD)
    ■ For example, E1α (33%), E1β (38%), E2 (19%)
  ○ Autosomal recessive
- Etiology
  ○ Branched chain organic aciduria result from abnormalities of enzyme catabolism of branched chain amino acids (leucine, isoleucine, valine)
  ○ MSUD: ↓ Activity BCKD ⇒ accumulation of branched-chain L-amino (BCAA) and metabolites (neurotoxic)
  ○ Leucine accumulation, in particular neurotoxic
  ○ ↑ Plasma isoleucine associated with maple odor
- Epidemiology: 1:850,000 general population; but as frequent as 1:170 in population isolates
- Associated abnormalities: ↑ Leucine impairs cell volume regulation ⇒ edema: Brain, muscle, liver, pancreas

### Gross Pathologic & Surgical Features
- Brainstem edema
- Spongy degeneration: White matter, basal ganglia

### Microscopic Features
- ↓ Oligodendrocytes and astrocytes
- Alterations in neuronal migration, maturation
  ○ Aberrant orientation of neurons
  ○ Abnormal dendrites/dendritic spines

### Staging, Grading or Classification Criteria
- Classical (80%), intermediate, and intermittent forms of MSUD; thiamine responsive MSUD

## CLINICAL ISSUES

### Presentation
- Most common signs/symptoms

# MAPLE SYRUP URINE DISEASE

○ Initial symptoms of classic MSUD: Poor feeding, vomiting, poor weight gain, increasing lethargy
  ▪ In neonates, develop within 4-7 days
○ Patients in crisis often (but not always) smell like maple syrup (or burnt sugar)
  ▪ Resuscitation with non-protein containing oral or IV hydrating fluids may "clear" the odor
  ▪ Maple syrup odor may be difficult to identify in first days of life unless urine soaked diaper is allowed to dry
  ▪ Maple syrup odor of cerumen "more predictable"
○ Neonates in communities with known ↑ risk of MSUD may be diagnosed within hours of blood sampling
  ▪ If tested and receive immediate results and therapy is instituted ⇒ excellent outcome
  ▪ Tandem mass spectrometry of whole blood filter paper shortens diagnosis time
  ▪ Guthrie test insensitive before 24 hours, requires incubation period and has high false positive rate
• Clinical Profile
  ○ Normal at birth
  ○ Presents after disease free interval, usually within the first 48 hours to 2 weeks of life
  ○ Mimic of sepsis: Acute encephalopathy, vomiting, seizures, neurological distress, lethargy, coma, leukopenia/thrombopenia
    ▪ Additionally free water retention, renal salt wasting and hyponatremia, dehydration
  ○ Plasma detection of alloisoleucine diagnostic for MSUD
    ▪ May not appear until 6th day of life
  ○ Ketosis or ketoacidosis
  ○ Hyperammonemia
  ○ Typical EEG: "Comb-like-rhythms"
  ○ Prenatal diagnosis can be performed on cultured amniocytes or chorion villus cells

## Demographics
• Age: May be diagnosed on day 1 if suspected
• Ethnicity
  ○ 1/170 live births in certain population isolates
    ▪ Founder effect in old order Mennonites
  ○ High carrier rate in Middle East and Ashkenazi Jewish decendents

## Natural History & Prognosis
• Breast feeding may delay onset of symptoms to second week of life
• MSUD has potentially favorable outcome with strict dietary control & aggressively treated metabolic crises
  ○ Response to therapy can be variable
  ○ Exposure to high levels branched chain amino acids (BCAA) and their metabolites neurotoxic
  ○ Uncontrolled BCAA levels lead to profound cognitive impairment/death
  ○ Pretreatment plasma leucine > 40 mg/100 mL OR encephalopathy > days associated with poor cognitive outcome
• May survive to adulthood if well controlled
  ○ Metabolic "intoxication" (at any age) provoked by infection, injury, stress, fasting, or even pregnancy
• Late (adulthood): ± Peripheral neuropathy

• Exfoliative skin and corneal lesions from inadequate amino-acid intake

## Treatment
• Acute "metabolic rescue" to reverse cerebral edema, control oxidative stress
• May require hemodialysis during acute crisis to limit neurotoxicity/damage
• Metabolically appropriate diet (protein-modified) minimizes severity
  ○ Inhibit endogenous protein catabolism while sustaining protein synthesis
  ○ Prevent deficiencies of essential amino acids
  ○ Maintain normal serum osmolarity
  ○ Dietary therapy must be lifelong
  ○ Commercially available formulas, foods are available without branched-chain amino acids or with reduced levels of branched-chain amino acids
  ○ Creatine and antioxidant therapy
• Orthotopic liver transplantation increases availability of BCKD (rarely used)
• Gene therapy experimental

## DIAGNOSTIC CHECKLIST

### Consider
• Neonatal testing for MSUD is not universal
• Not all MSUD occurs in population isolates
• Even if testing performed, results may be available only after 1 to 2 weeks in non-endemic areas

### Image Interpretation Pearls
• Neonatal brain edema which includes the posterior fossa and brainstem is highly suggestive of MSUD

## SELECTED REFERENCES

1. Funchal C et al: Creatine and antioxidant treatment prevent the inhibition of creatine kinase activity and the morphological alterations of C6 glioma cells induced by the branched-chain alpha-keto acids accumulating in MSUD. Cell Mol Neurobiol. 26(1):67-79, 2006
2. Funchal C et al: Morphological alterations and induction of oxidative stress in glial cells caused by the branched-chain alpha-keto acids accumulating in maple syrup urine disease. Neurochem Int. 49(7):640-50, 2006
3. Simon E et al: Variant maple syrup urine disease (MSUD)--the entire spectrum. J Inherit Metab Dis. 29(6):716-24, 2006
4. Van der Knaap MS et al: Maple syrup urine disease. In: Magnetic Resonance of Myelin, Myelination, & Myelin Disorders. Berlin, Springer-Verlag. 311-20, 2005
5. Parmar H et al: MSUD: Diffusion-weighted and diffusion-tensor magnetic resonance imaging findings. J Comput Assist Tomogr. 28(1):93-7, 2004
6. Henneke M et al: Identification of twelve novel mutations in patients with classic and variant forms of maple syrup urine disease. Hum Mutat. 22(5):417, 2003
7. Morton DH et al: Diagnosis and treatment of MSUD: a study of 36 patients. Pediatrics. 109:999-1008, 2002
8. Fariello G et al: Cranial ultrasonography in maple syrup urine disease. AJNR Am J Neuroradiol. 17(2):311-5, 1996
9. Brismar J et al: Maple syrup urine disease: findings on CT and MR scans of the brain in 10 infants. AJNR Am J Neuroradiol. 11(6):1219-28, 1990

# MAPLE SYRUP URINE DISEASE

## IMAGE GALLERY

### Typical

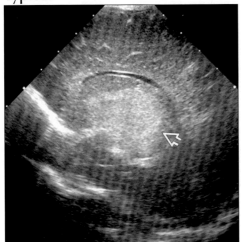
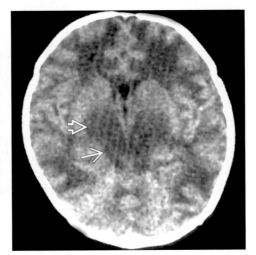

*(Left)* Sagittal ultrasound shows extensive thalamic swelling and hyperechogenicity ➡ secondary to MSUD edema. *(Right)* Axial NECT shows typical extension of edema from the brainstem into the cerebral peduncles ➡ and thalami ➡. Frontal white matter is also edematous.

### Typical

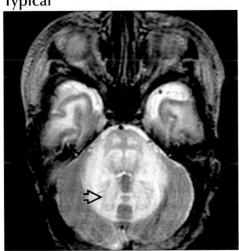
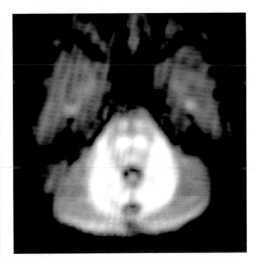

*(Left)* Axial T2WI MR shows classic MSUD edema, with swelling and hyperintensity involving the brainstem and cerebellar white matter. The dentate nuclei ➡ are outlined by the cerebellar edema. *(Right)* Axial DWI MR shows marked hyperintensity due to reduced diffusion from intramyelinic edema in typical MSUD pattern.

### Typical

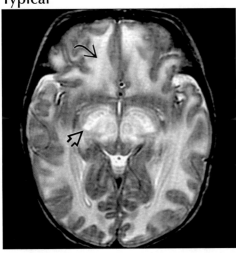
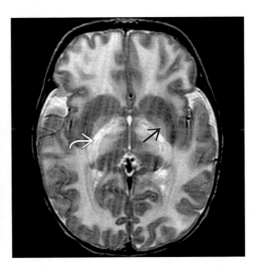

*(Left)* Axial T2WI MR shows marked edema of the cerebral peduncles and thalami ➡. There is extensive, but milder supratentorial white matter edema ➡ and sparing of the cortical ribbon. *(Right)* Axial T2WI MR in same patient as previous image shows abnormally increased signal intensity in posterior limbs of internal capsules ➡ and more subtle increase in globi pallidi ➡ during the acute phase.

# UREA CYCLE DISORDERS

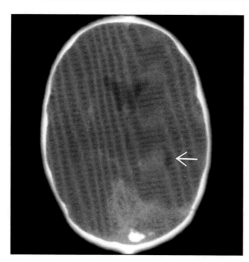

Axial NECT shows diffuse severe cerebral edema due to hyperammonemia in infant with citrullinemia. Enlarged frontal horns and temporal horn ➡ are due to edema restricting CSF resorption.

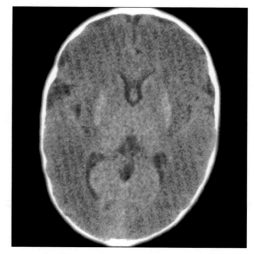

Axial NECT in a more subacute phase of citrullinemia shows persistent edema, but the thalami and lentiform nuclei are now somewhat hyperdense.

## TERMINOLOGY

### Abbreviations and Synonyms

- N-Acetylglutamate synthase deficiency (NAGS)
- Carbamyl phosphate synthetase 1 deficiency (CPS1)
- Ornithine transcarbamylase deficiency (OTC)
- Argininosuccinate synthetase deficiency (ASS, classic citrullinemia)
- Argininosuccinate ligase deficiencies (ASL)
- Arginase deficiency (AD)
- Arginase deficiency (hyperargininemia, ARG)
- Hyperornithinemia-hyperammonemia-homocitrullinuria syndrome (HHH)
- Lysinuric protein intolerance (LPI)

### Definitions

- Urea cycle incorporates nitrogen → urea (water soluble → excreted in urine) preventing accumulation of toxic nitrogen products
- Each disorder represents an enzyme deficiency

## IMAGING FINDINGS

### General Features

- Best diagnostic clue: Neonatal encephalopathy with brain swelling, ↑ urine ammonia, respiratory alkalosis, ↑ plasma glutamine/alanine
- Location
  ○ Neonates and infants ⇒ deep gray nuclei, particularly globi pallidi; frontal lobes; insular cortex
  ○ Adult forms of disease ⇒ cortex (especially insulae) more prominently than basal ganglia
- Size: Swelling (edema) in acute phase

### CT Findings

- NECT
  ○ Acute: Severe edema involving cortex, subcortical white matter, basal ganglia
  ○ Subacute: Subcortical hypodensities (basal ganglia, cortex resume normal signal)
  ○ Chronic: Atrophy of affected regions
- CECT: No enhancement

### MR Findings

- T1WI

### DDx: Urea Cycle Disorders

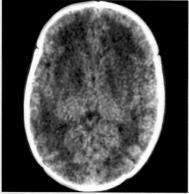

Mitochondrial

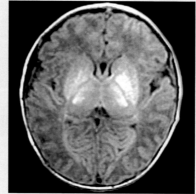

Hypoxia-Ischemia

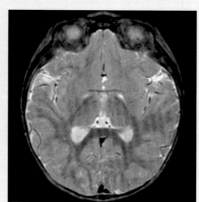

Methylmalonic Acidemia

# UREA CYCLE DISORDERS

## Key Facts

### Terminology
- N-Acetylglutamate synthase deficiency (NAGS)
- Carbamyl phosphate synthetase 1 deficiency (CPS1)
- Ornithine transcarbamylase deficiency (OTC)
- Argininosuccinate synthetase deficiency (ASS, classic citrullinemia)
- Argininosuccinate ligase deficiencies (ASL)
- Arginase deficiency (AD)
- Arginase deficiency (hyperargininemia, ARG)
- Hyperornithinemia-hyperammonemia-homocitrullinuria syndrome (HHH)
- Lysinuric protein intolerance (LPI)

### Imaging Findings
- Best diagnostic clue: Neonatal encephalopathy with brain swelling, ↑ urine ammonia, respiratory alkalosis, ↑ plasma glutamine/alanine

- Neonates and infants ⇒ deep gray nuclei, particularly globi pallidi; frontal lobes; insular cortex
- Adult forms of disease ⇒ cortex (especially insulae) more prominently than basal ganglia

### Top Differential Diagnoses
- Nonketotic Hyperglycinemia
- Organic Acidemias
- Non-Inherited Disorders Associated with Transient Hyperammonemia
- Mitochondrial Disorders
- Hypoxic-Ischemic Encephalopathy

### Clinical Issues
- Progressive neurologic deterioration
- 100% death if untreated (↓ mortality in older patients)

---

- Acute and subacute phases
  - ↑ Signal in deep gray nuclei, particularly globi pallidi and insular/perirolandic cortex
  - ↑ Signal in insular/perirolandic cortex
  - ↑ Signal in depths of frontal sulci
- Chronic phases
  - Shrunken basal ganglia
  - Ulegyria
- Preservation of posterior fossa structures
- T2WI
  - Acute and subacute phases
    - ↑ Signal in deep gray nuclei
    - ↑ Signal in insular and frontal cortex
    - Diffuse brain edema, infarctions
  - Chronic: Symmetric subcortical cysts
- FLAIR
  - Acute and subacute phases
    - Hyperintensity in deep gray nuclei and cortical sulci
  - Chronic phase
    - Prominent ventricles and sulci
    - Symmetric subcortical cysts
- MRS
  - ↑ Glutamine/glutamate
  - ↓ Myoinositol on short TE
  - Presence of lipids/lactate

### Imaging Recommendations
- Best imaging tool
  - Emergent: Noncontrast CT
  - Nonemergent: MR
- Protocol advice
  - Noncontrast brain MR
    - Include T1, T2, MR spectroscopy

## DIFFERENTIAL DIAGNOSIS

### Nonketotic Hyperglycinemia
- Also presents with neonatal encephalopathy, stupor
- Absence of basal ganglia injuries
- MR spectroscopy shows elevated glycine at 3.6 ppm
- May have callosal, cortical anomalies

### Organic Acidemias
- Bilateral symmetrical basal ganglia involvement
- Some present in neonatal period
- Associated with metabolic acidosis and ketosis

### Non-Inherited Disorders Associated with Transient Hyperammonemia
- Sepsis
- Prematurity
- Respiratory distress

### Mitochondrial Disorders
- Can present in neonates, infants with encephalopathy
- Often involve basal ganglia, cerebral white matter, cortex
- MR spectroscopy shows lactate elevation in parenchyma, CSF

### Hypoxic-Ischemic Encephalopathy
- Thalami and putamina more than globi pallidi
- Perirolandic cortex, dorsal brain stem
- MR spectroscopy shows elevated lactate in parenchyma during first week

## PATHOLOGY

### General Features
- General path comments
  - Cerebral edema, neuronal loss, astrocyte swelling
    - Severity depends on duration of hyperammonemia
    - Survivors ⇒ ventriculomegaly, symmetric white matter injuries, bilateral lentiform nuclear injuries, insular cortical injury
    - Sparing of cerebellum
  - Assay for deficient enzyme from liver cells/erythrocytes
- Genetics
  - All are autosomal recessive except OTC (X-linked)
    - CPS1: 2q35
    - ASS: 9q34

# UREA CYCLE DISORDERS

- ASL: 7cen-q11.2
- ARG: 6q23
- LPI: 14q11.2
- OTC: Xp21.1
  - Heterozygous OTC female → may have no symptoms
- Etiology
  - Symptoms due to high levels of ammonia resulting in conversion of glutamate → glutamine in astrocytes
  - High osmolality ⇒ swelling, intracranial hypertension, cerebral hypoperfusion
- Epidemiology
  - Onset: Neonatal (most common), infancy, child, adult
    - Manifest in periods of diet with ↑ protein content or ↑ catabolism
    - Age of onset determined largely by type of mutation
  - OTC is most common (1:14,000 population), followed by citrullinemia, CPS1, ASL
- Associated abnormalities
  - Propensity for
    - Hypertension
    - Electrolyte abnormalities (hypokalemia and hypomagnesemia)
    - Gastrointestinal disorders (anorexia, microcytic anemia)

## Gross Pathologic & Surgical Features

- Diffuse cerebral edema
- Generalized neuronal cell loss
- Chronic phase
  - Ventriculomegaly
  - Cystic degeneration of white matter
  - Atrophy of bilateral lentiform nuclei
  - Ulegyria

## Microscopic Features

- Alzheimer type II astrocytes
- Splitting/vacuolation of myelin
- Spongiform changes in deep layers of cerebral cortex, basal ganglia

# CLINICAL ISSUES

## Presentation

- Most common signs/symptoms
  - Complete defect in urea cycle: Neonatal presentation
    - May be normal at birth
    - Develop encephalopathy after 24-48 hours
    - Progressive lethargy, poor suck, hypothermia, hypotonia, vomiting, hyperventilation ⇒ apnea
    - Coarse/friable hair
    - All develop hepatic insufficiency
  - Partial defect in urea cycle: Presentation in infancy, childhood, adulthood
    - Childhood: Anorexia, ataxia, behavioral abnormalities (biting, self-injury, hyperactivity)
    - Adulthood: Headache, nausea, dysarthria, ataxia, hallucinations, visual impairment
- Clinical Profile

- ↑ Ammonium blood levels
- Neonatal screening with tandem mass spectrometry
- Segregate patients based on citrulline levels in plasma
  - Absent/trace ⇒ CPS1, NAGS, or OTC deficiency
  - Normal/reduced ⇒ LPI, HHH, ARG
  - Moderate elevation ⇒ ASL
  - Marked elevation ⇒ citrullinemia

## Demographics

- Age
  - Any age
  - Most commonly presents in neonates

## Natural History & Prognosis

- Progressive neurologic deterioration
  - 100% death if untreated (↓ mortality in older patients)
- High morbidity (severe neurological deficits) in survivors

## Treatment

- Liver transplant
  - Typically performed between 6 and 12 months of age
- Alternative pathway therapy: Sodium benzoate/sodium phenylbutyrate
- Protein restriction, replace with essential amino acids
- Hemodialysis in infants diagnosed during hyperammonemic coma

# DIAGNOSTIC CHECKLIST

## Image Interpretation Pearls

- Consider urea cycle disorder in infant with extensive temporo-parietal and basal ganglia injuries
- Consider urea cycle disorder in child with bilateral insular edema

# SELECTED REFERENCES

1. Choi JH et al: Two cases of citrullinaemia presenting with stroke. J Inherit Metab Dis. 29(1):182-3, 2006
2. Kojic J et al: Brain glutamine by MRS in a patient with urea cycle disorder and coma. Pediatr Neurol. 32(2):143-6, 2005
3. Nassogne MC et al: Urea cycle defects: management and outcome. J Inherit Metab Dis. 28(3):407-14, 2005
4. Smith W et al: Urea cycle disorders: clinical presentation outside the newborn period. Crit Care Clin. 21(4 Suppl):S9-17, 2005
5. Leonard JV et al: The role of liver transplantation in urea cycle disorders. Mol Genet Metab. 81 Suppl 1:S74-8, 2004
6. Kleppe S et al: Urea cycle disorders. Curr Treat Options Neurol. 5:309-19, 2003
7. Takanashi J et al: Brain MR imaging in neonatal hyperammonemic encephalopathy resulting from proximal urea cycle disorders. AJNR Am J Neuroradiol. 24(6):1184-7, 2003
8. Leonard JV et al: Urea cycle disorders. Semin Neonatal. 7:27-35, 2002
9. Mian A et al: Urea-cycle disorders as a paradigm for inborn errors of hepatocyte metabolism. Trends Mol Med. 8(12):583-9, 2002
10. Choi CG et al: Localized proton MR spectroscopy in infants with urea cycle defect. AJNR. 22:834-37, 2001

## IMAGE GALLERY

### Typical

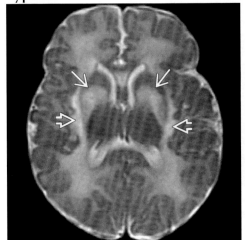

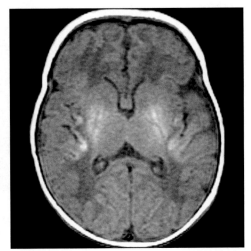

*(Left)* Axial T2WI MR in neonate with OTC shows edema of subinsular white matter ⇨ and globi pallidi ➡. *(Right)* Axial T1WI MR of same patient shows hyperintensity of posterior insular cortex and of globi pallidi and posterior putamina bilaterally.

### Typical

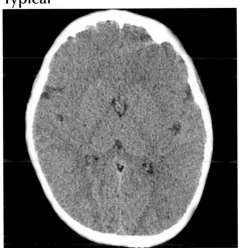

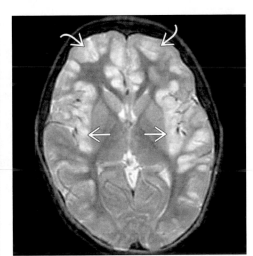

*(Left)* Axial NECT in an older child with OTC shows effacement of sulci and compression of ventricles due to edema from hyperammonemia. Basal ganglia and thalami are normal. *(Right)* Axial T2WI MR in the same patient shows edema of the bilateral insulae ➡ and frontal cortex ➡, with sparing of the basal ganglia and thalami.

### Typical

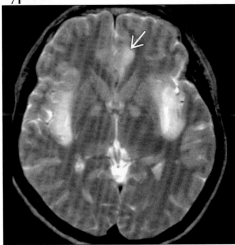

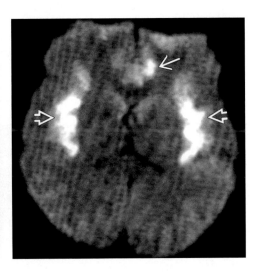

*(Left)* Axial T2WI MR in a young adult with citrullinemia shows edema of the bilateral insulae and underlying extreme capsules, bilateral globi pallidi, and left cingulum ➡. *(Right)* Axial DWI MR of the same patient shows reduced diffusivity in the bilateral insulae ⇨ and in the left cingulum ➡.

# GLUTARIC ACIDURIA TYPE 1

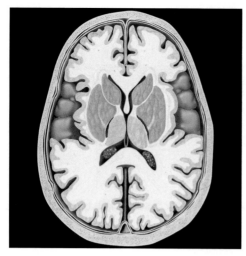

Axial graphic shows glutaric aciduria type I in crisis. There is enlargement of the Sylvian fissures and there is acute striatal necrosis.

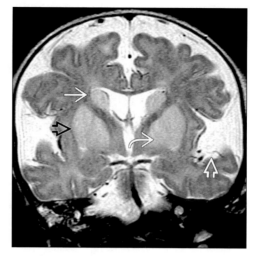

Coronal T2WI MR shows typical large pericerebral and Sylvian fissure ⊞, CSF spaces, with increased signal intensity of the caudate heads ⊞, globi pallidi ⊞ and putamina ⊞.

## TERMINOLOGY

### Abbreviations and Synonyms
- GA1; glutaric acidemia type 1; mitochondrial glutaryl-coenzyme A dehydrogenase (GCDH) deficiency

### Definitions
- Inborn error of metabolism characterized by encephalopathic crises, acute striatal injury and resultant severe dystonia

## IMAGING FINDINGS

### General Features
- Best diagnostic clue: Wide operculae & bright basal ganglia (BG)
- Morphology
  - Wide opercula (frontotemporal atrophy) = "bat wing" dilatation of Sylvian fissures
  - Child abuse mimic: Easily torn bridging veins within enlarged cerebrospinal fluid (CSF) spaces ⇒ subdural hematomas (SDH)

### CT Findings
- NECT
  - Wide Sylvian fissures (93%) & mesencephalic cistern (86%)
  - Early macrocephaly, late atrophy (mostly ventricular enlargement)
  - SDH with minimal trauma
  - BG hypodensity
- CECT: No enhancement

### MR Findings
- T1WI
  - Sylvian fissure "cyst-like" spaces isointense to CSF
  - Fronto-temporal atrophy
  - Subependymal pseudocysts (disappear by 6 months)
- T2WI
  - ↑ Signal caudate/putamina > globus pallidus; BG atrophy over time
  - If severe: ± White matter (WM), thalami, dentate nuclei, medial lemniscus, substantia involvement
  - Myelin maturation delay (± periventricular WM and U-fiber involvement)
- FLAIR: Same as T2WI

## DDx: Glutaric Aciduria Type 1 Mimics

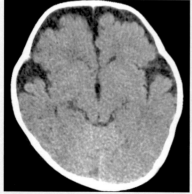

*Physiologic EVOH*

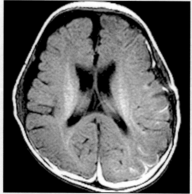

*Non-Accidental Trauma*

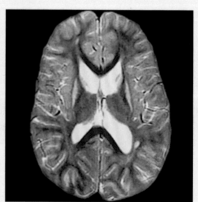

*Huntington Dz*

# GLUTARIC ACIDURIA TYPE 1

## Key Facts

### Terminology

- GA1; glutaric acidemia type 1; mitochondrial glutaryl-coenzyme A dehydrogenase (GCDH) deficiency
- Inborn error of metabolism characterized by encephalopathic crises, acute striatal injury and resultant severe dystonia

### Imaging Findings

- Wide opercula (frontotemporal atrophy) = "bat wing" dilatation of Sylvian fissures
- Child abuse mimic: Easily torn bridging veins within enlarged cerebrospinal fluid (CSF) spaces ⇒ subdural hematomas (SDH)

### Top Differential Diagnoses

- Non-Accidental Injury (a.k.a., Child Abuse)

### Pathology

- Autosomal recessive
- Genetically and clinically heterogeneous
- Amish variant, riboflavin sensitive, less WM involvement: Ala421-to-val
- Epidemiology: 1:30,000 newborns

### Clinical Issues

- Symptomatic: Most severely handicapped, 20% die before 5 yrs
- Prognosis poor if has already presented with encephalopathic crisis
- Intrauterine diagnosis available
- Early treatment may prevent or ameliorate crises and imaging features

---

- DWI: Acute: Reduced diffusion in BG and selected WM tracts
- T1 C+: No enhancement
- MRS
  - ↑ Chol/Cr ratio, ↓ NAA
  - During crisis: ± ↑ Lactate

### Nuclear Medicine Findings

- PET: Fluoro-2-deoxyglucose (FDG-18): Silent thalamic and cortical involvement manifests as ↓ uptake with normal MR

### Imaging Recommendations

- Best imaging tool: MR
- Protocol advice: MRS, DWI

## DIFFERENTIAL DIAGNOSIS

### Non-Accidental Injury (a.k.a., Child Abuse)

- GA1 does not cause fractures
- SDH in GA1 from torn-bridging veins in presence of large CSF, atrophy
- SDH in GA1 do not occur without enlarged CSF spaces

### Other Disorders with Bilateral Middle Cranial Fossa "Cyst-Like" Spaces

- Mucopolysaccharidoses (and other lysosomal storage disorders)
  - Pachymeningeal storage leads to CSF pathway obstruction, loculations
- "Idiopathic" middle cranial fossae arachnoid cysts
  - 5% may be bilateral, usually asymptomatic, lack DWI restriction
  - CSF intensity; may be slightly different on FLAIR (protein, blood products)
- Physiologic subarachnoid space enlargement
  - Transient extraventricular obstructive hydrocephalus (EVOH)
  - 3-8 months of age; macrocrania, large subarachnoid space; self-limiting

### Striate Atrophy or Gliosis

- Leigh disease (mitochondrial); H-ABC (hypomyelination, atrophy of basal ganglia & cerebellum; Huntington disease

## PATHOLOGY

### General Features

- General path comments
  - Embryology: Toxic effects in utero impede operculization during 3rd trimester
  - Mild hepatocellular dysfunction during crisis
- Genetics
  - Autosomal recessive
  - GCDH gene mutations (Chr 19p13.2) result in amino acid substitutions
  - Genetically and clinically heterogeneous
    - European variant (most common): Arg402-to-trp
    - Amish variant, riboflavin sensitive, less WM involvement: Ala421-to-val
    - Many Palestinian mutations
    - Severe, 1% residual enzyme, symptoms despite treatment (Tx): Glu365 to lys
  - Rare adult-onset: Compound heterozygosity with a deletion and novel missense mutation
  - Fetal testing available if familial mutation known
- Etiology
  - GCDH required for metabolism of lysine, hydroxylysine & tryptophan
  - ↓ GCDH ⇒ accumulation glutaric, glutaconic, glutylarylcarnitine & 3-OH-glutaric acid
  - Accumulated substances likely toxic to striate cells and white matter
- Epidemiology: 1:30,000 newborns

### Gross Pathologic & Surgical Features

- Macrocrania, frontotemporal atrophy/hypoplasia; ↑ CSF spaces, ± SDH
- Hypo- and de-myelination

# GLUTARIC ACIDURIA TYPE 1

## Microscopic Features
- Myelin vacuolation and splitting
- Excess intramyelinic fluid
- Spongiform changes, neuronal loss BG

## Staging, Grading or Classification Criteria
- Symptomatic: Fronto-temporal atrophy, BG swelling
- Presymptomatic: Symptom-free; BG normal; but CSF spaces still enlarged

## CLINICAL ISSUES

### Presentation
- Most common signs/symptoms
  - Macrocrania presents early (even in-utero); initially normal development
  - Acute encephalopathy, seizures, dystonia, choreoathetosis, mental retardation
- Clinical Profile: Macrocrania and dystonia
- Acute onset group: Majority
  - Episodic crises follow trigger (infection, immunization, surgery)
    - Acute Reye-like encephalopathy, ketoacidosis, ↑ NH3, vomiting
    - Dystonia, opisthotonus, seizures, excessive sweating
    - Follow-up: Alert child (intellect preserved > > motor); rapid infantile head growth ⇒ frontal bossing; severe dystonia
- Insidious onset: 25%
  - No precipitating crisis, still ⇒ dystonia
- Presymptomatic may remain asymptomatic
  - Diagnose, treat, avoid catabolic stress
- Rare asymptomatic without treatment
  - Still frontotemporal atrophy, but normal BG
- Diagnosis: Frequent long interval between presentation and diagnosis
  - Tandem mass spectrometry of newborn filter-paper blood specimens
    - May miss mild biochemical phenotype
  - Chromatography-mass spectroscopy of urine
  - Deficient or absent GCDH activity in fibroblasts
  - Laboratory (may be relatively normal between crises)
    - Metabolic acidosis/ketosis, hypoglycemia, ↓ carnitine
    - Urinary organic acids: ↑ Glutaric, glutaconic and 3-OH-glutaric acid

### Demographics
- Age: Generally manifests during 1st year of life
- Gender: No predilection
- Ethnicity: 10% carrier rate in old order Amish

### Natural History & Prognosis
- Symptomatic: Most severely handicapped, 20% die before 5 yrs
- Presymptomatic: Many (not all) remain asymptomatic with diagnosis and therapy
- Treat before first encephalopathic crisis; avoid catabolic crises
- Prognosis poor if has already presented with encephalopathic crisis

## Treatment
- Intrauterine diagnosis available
  - DNA analysis: Cultured amniotic fluid cells & chorionic villi biopsy
  - Fetal sonography: Dilated peri-Sylvian CSF in 3rd trimester
- Early treatment may prevent or ameliorate crises and imaging features
  - Low-protein diet (reduced tryptophan & lysine), synthetic protein drink
  - Riboflavin (Vit B2) to ensure cofactor supply for GCDH
  - Oral carnitine replacement; gamma aminobutyric acid (GABA) analog (baclofen)
- Anti-cholinergic drugs, botulin toxin type A, pallidotomy have been used to treat dystonia

## DIAGNOSTIC CHECKLIST

### Image Interpretation Pearls
- Consider GA in young children with macrocrania, "cysts" in Sylvian fissures and abnormal basal ganglia

## SELECTED REFERENCES

1. Kolker S et al: Guideline for the diagnosis and management of glutaryl-CoA dehydrogenase deficiency (glutaric aciduria type I). J Inherit Metab Dis. 2007
2. Korman SH et al: Glutaric aciduria type 1: Clinical, biochemical and molecular findings in patients from Israel. Eur J Paediatr Neurol. 2006
3. Lindner M et al: Neonatal screening for glutaric aciduria type I: strategies to proceed. J Inherit Metab Dis. 29(2-3):378-82, 2006
4. Oguz KK et al: Diffusion-weighted MR imaging and MR spectroscopy in glutaric aciduria type 1. Neuroradiology. 47(3):229-34, 2005
5. Elster AW: Glutaric aciduria type I: value of diffusion-weighted magnetic resonance imaging for diagnosing acute striatal necrosis. J Comput Assist Tomogr. 28(1):98-100, 2004
6. Kurul S et al: Glutaric aciduria type 1: proton magnetic resonance spectroscopy findings. Pediatr Neurol. 31(3):228-31, 2004
7. Kolker S et al: Adult onset glutaric aciduria type I presenting with a leukoencephalopathy. Neurology. 60(8):1399, 2003
8. Strauss KA et al: Type I glutaric aciduria, part 1: natural history of 77 patients. Am J Med Genet. 121C(1):38-52, 2003
9. Strauss KA et al: Type I glutaric aciduria, part 2: a model of acute striatal necrosis. Am J Med Genet. 121C(1):53-70, 2003
10. Twomey EL et al: Neuroimaging findings in glutaric aciduria type 1. Pediatr Radiol. 33(12):823-30, 2003
11. Al-Essa M et al: Fluoro-2-deoxyglucose (18FDG) PET scan of the brain in glutaric aciduria type 1: clinical and MRI correlations. Brain Dev. 20(5):295-301, 1998
12. Hoffman GF et al: Clinical course, early diagnosis, treatment, and prevention of disease in glutaryl-Co A dehydrogenase deficiency. Neuropediatrics 27:115-23, 1996
13. Brismar J et al: CT and MR of the brain in glutaric acidemia type I: a review of 59 published cases and a report of 5 new patients. AJNR Am J Neuroradiol. 16(4):675-83, 1995

## IMAGE GALLERY

### Typical

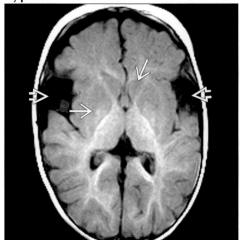 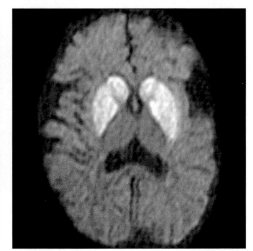

*(Left)* Axial T1WI MR shows large Sylvian fissures ⇒ and mildly decreased signal intensity of the lentiform nuclei ⇒. *(Right)* Axial DWI MR in the same patient as previous image, shows hyperintensity (reduced diffusion) of the caudate heads, globi pallidi and putamina bilaterally, indicating an acute process.

### Typical

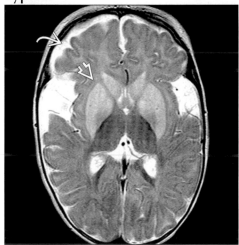 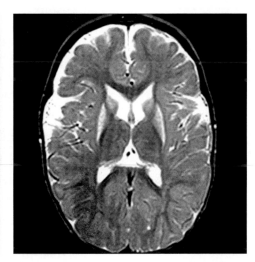

*(Left)* Axial T2WI MR shows prominent Sylvian fissures, asymmetric pericerebral fluid ⇒ and striatal edema/hyperintensity ⇒, during an episode of acute crisis. *(Right)* Axial follow-up T2WI obtained in the same patient as previous image, shows atrophy and probably astrogliosis of the caudate heads, putamina and globi pallidi. Note compensatory enlargement of frontal horns.

### Typical

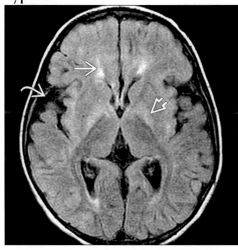 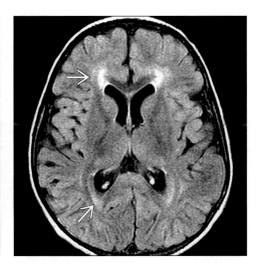

*(Left)* Axial FLAIR MR shows subtle increased signal intensity ⇒ in the globi pallidi and frontal white matter ⇒ in a child with mild phenotype. There is mild Sylvian fissure prominence ⇒. *(Right)* Axial FLAIR MR shows moderate periventricular white matter involvement ⇒ in the same child as previous image, with mild phenotype.

# CANAVAN DISEASE

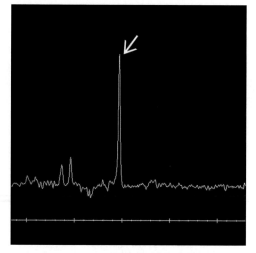

Axial T2WI MR shows diffuse hyperintensity of the hemispheric white matter reflecting spongy degeneration and demyelination. Note the early involvement of subcortical U-fibers ⇨.

MRS using single voxel, PRESS with a long TE (288) shows marked elevation in NAA ⇨.

## TERMINOLOGY

### Abbreviations and Synonyms
• Canavan-Van Bogaert-Bertrand disease

### Definitions
• Spongiform leukodystrophy

## IMAGING FINDINGS

### General Features
• Best diagnostic clue: Megalencephaly and diffuse demyelination
• Location: Subcortical U-fibers, thalami and globi pallidi

### CT Findings
• NECT: Putaminal hypoattenuation may precede subcortical leukodystrophy

### MR Findings
• T1WI: Hypointense WM and striatum
• T2WI: Subcortical U-fiber WM involvement, symmetric involvement of striatum

• DWI: ± Reduced diffusion (depends on stage)
• T1 C+: Lack of enhancement
• MRS: Marked ↑ NAA (also seen with Salla disease)

### Imaging Recommendations
• Best imaging tool: MRI & MRS
• Protocol advice: MRI brain, MRS

## DIFFERENTIAL DIAGNOSIS

### Alexander Disease (Fibrinoid Leukodystrophy)
• Predilection for frontal WM

### Megalencephaly with Leukoencephalopathy and Cysts (MLC)
• Subcortical cysts, normal basal ganglia

### Glutaric Aciduria Type 1
• Large sylvian fissures, basal ganglia T2 hyperintensity

### Pelizaeus-Merzbacher Disease
• Profound deficient myelin development

## DDx: Canavan Disease Look-Alikes

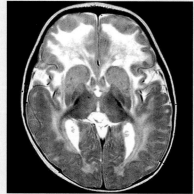
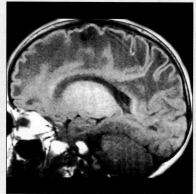
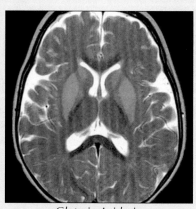

Alexander Disease        MLC        Glutaric Aciduria

# CANAVAN DISEASE

## Key Facts

### Terminology
- Spongiform leukodystrophy

### Imaging Findings
- T2WI: Subcortical U-fiber WM involvement, symmetric involvement of striatum
- MRS: Marked ↑ NAA (also seen with Salla disease)
- Best imaging tool: MRI & MRS

### Top Differential Diagnoses
- Alexander Disease (Fibrinoid Leukodystrophy)
- Megalencephaly with Leukoencephalopathy and Cysts (MLC)
- Glutaric Aciduria Type 1
- Pelizaeus-Merzbacher Disease

### Diagnostic Checklist
- Perform MRS in all suspected leukodystrophies
- MRS shows marked ↑ NAA

## PATHOLOGY

### General Features
- General path comments: Spongy degeneration of white matter
- Genetics: Autosomal recessive, mapped to short arm of Ch 17
- Etiology: Deficiency of aspartoacyclase (an enzyme with role in myelin synthesis)

### Gross Pathologic & Surgical Features
- Extra fluid in astrocytes

### Microscopic Features
- Spongiform degeneration of white matter

### Staging, Grading or Classification Criteria
- Age of onset predicts course

## CLINICAL ISSUES

### Presentation
- Most common signs/symptoms
  - Three clinical variants: Infantile variant most common
    - Congenital (first few days of life): Early encephalopathy, rapid death
    - Infantile (3-6 months): Hypotonia, macrocephaly, seizures, peripheral spasticity, optic atrophy
    - Juvenile: Onset at 4-5 years; slower progression
- Clinical Profile: Megalencephaly, axial hypotonia, optic atrophy

### Demographics
- Age: Typically evident by 2 to 4 months
- Gender: No sex predilection
- Ethnicity: ↑ Risk for Ashkenazi Jewish
- Epidemiology of lesion
  - High carrier state (1:37-58) among screened Ashkenazi Jewish

### Natural History & Prognosis
- Relentless, death by end of first decade

### Treatment
- No treatment currently available, ± gene therapy and acetate supplementation

## DIAGNOSTIC CHECKLIST

### Consider
- Perform MRS in all suspected leukodystrophies

### Image Interpretation Pearls
- MRS shows marked ↑ NAA

## SELECTED REFERENCES

1. Patay Z: Diffusion-weighted MR imaging in leukodystrophies. Eur Radiol. 15(11):2284-303, 2005

## IMAGE GALLERY

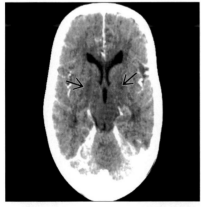 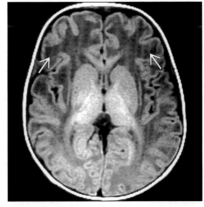 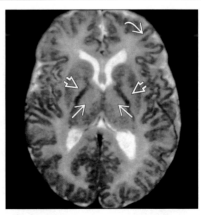

*(Left) Axial CECT shows decreased attenuation within the globi pallidi ⇒. On CT, these basal ganglia changes may appear prior to the detection of peripheral WM hypoattenuation. (Center) Axial T1WI MR shows profoundly hypointense hemispheric white matter. Note the extensive symmetric early involvement of the subcortical U-fibers ⇒. (Right) Axial T2WI MR shows symmetric thalamic ⇒ and globi pallidi ⇒ hyperintensity. Note the symmetric and extensive WM demyelination with subcortical U-fiber involvement ⇒.*

# ALEXANDER DISEASE

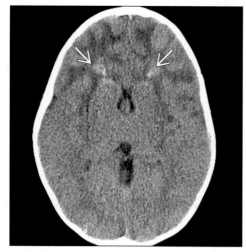
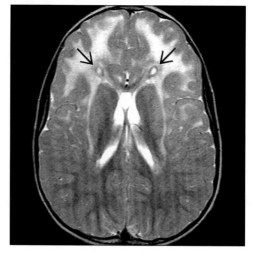

*NECT shows typical appearance of infantile AD. There is focal hyperdensity in the frontal periventricular rim and caudate heads ➡ surrounded by diffuse frontal white matter hypodensity.*

*Axial T2WI MR shows hypointensity in periventricular rim ➡ at frontal horns. There is diffuse symmetric frontal WM hyperintensity, subtle hyperintensity in the caudate heads & putamina.*

## TERMINOLOGY

### Abbreviations and Synonyms
- Alexander disease (AD)
- Fibrinoid leukodystrophy

### Definitions
- Rare leukoencephalopathy characterized by accumulation of cytoplasmic inclusions, Rosenthal fibers (RFs), in astrocytes
- Infantile form most common; characterized by macrocephaly, seizures, psychomotor regression
- Milder juvenile and adult forms; characterized by brainstem and cerebellar dysfunction

## IMAGING FINDINGS

### General Features
- Best diagnostic clue
  - Infantile form: Enhancing, bifrontal, white matter (WM) signal abnormality in macrocephalic infant
  - Other common findings
    - T1 hyperintense, T2 hypointense enhancing periventricular rim
    - Symmetric, T2 hyperintense caudate heads > putamina, thalami
  - Variably involved
    - Periaqueductal midbrain, dorsal medulla, dentate nuclei, optic chiasm, fornix
  - Juvenile and adult forms
    - Lesions of the cerebellum (especially dentate nuclei), medulla and spinal cord predominate
    - Frontal WM, basal ganglia (BG) changes less pronounced
- Location
  - WM
    - Frontal predominance (periventricular & subcortical)
    - External, extreme capsules
  - Periventricular rim
  - Basal ganglia, thalami, brain stem (BS), dentate nuclei, fornix, optic chiasm, spinal cord
- Morphology
  - Spared red nuclei, claustrum "stand out on T2"
  - ± Ventricular "garlands" in juvenile, adult cases
    - Probable blood vessels in areas of high density RFs

## DDx: Leukodystrophies with Macrocephaly

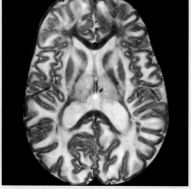
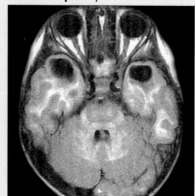
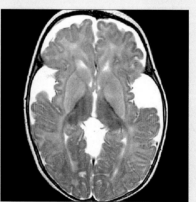

| *Canavan Disease* | *MLC* | *Glutaric Aciduria Type 1* |

# ALEXANDER DISEASE

## Key Facts

### Terminology
- Rare leukoencephalopathy characterized by accumulation of cytoplasmic inclusions, Rosenthal fibers (RFs), in astrocytes

### Imaging Findings
- Infantile form: Enhancing, bifrontal, white matter (WM) signal abnormality in macrocephalic infant
- Best imaging tool: MR C+ with MRS

### Top Differential Diagnoses
- Canavan Disease
- Megaloencephalic Leukoencephalopathy with Subcortical Cysts (MLC)
- Glutaric Aciduria Type 1 (GA-1)
- Mucopolysaccharidoses (MPS)

### Pathology
- AD characterized by RF accumulation in astrocytes & hypo-/demyelination
- Heterozygous (dominant) mutations GFAP (17q21) identified in > 95% cases AD

### Clinical Issues
- Variable rate of progression ultimately leading to death in all subtypes

### Diagnostic Checklist
- Enhancing, symmetric bifrontal WM disease in macrocephalic infant highly characteristic of AD
- Juvenile, adult cases may mimic posterior fossa tumors

---

- ± Obstructive hydrocephalus (especially infantile form) 2° to periaqueductal disease
- Swelling early; atrophy & cystic encephalomalacia late

## CT Findings
- NECT
  - Hypodense frontal white matter
  - Dense periventricular rim, ± BG
- CECT: Intense enhancement typical of early disease

## MR Findings
- T1WI
  - Hypointense WM (mainly frontal), deep gray structures
  - Hyperintense periventricular rim
- T2WI
  - Hyperintense WM (mainly frontal, involves subcortical WM), deep gray structures
  - Frequently hypointense periventricular rim
  - ↓ Signal BG described in late disease
- FLAIR: Cystic degeneration frontal WM (late disease)
- DWI: Normal to increased diffusivity
- T1 C+
  - Intense enhancement typical of early disease
    - Esp frontal WM, periventricular rim infantile AD
    - Cerebellar and medullary enhancement in juvenile, adult cases may resemble tumor
- MRS: ↓ NAA/Cr, ± ↑ myo-inositol/Cr, ± lactate

## Nuclear Medicine Findings
- F-18 fluorodeoxyglucose (FDG) PET
  - Hypometabolism in affected frontal white matter
  - Preserved overlying cortical glucose metabolism

## Imaging Recommendations
- Best imaging tool: MR C+ with MRS
- Protocol advice: Enhance all "unknown" cases hydrocephalus and abnormal WM
- Proposed MR criteria for diagnosis of typical infantile AD (4 out of 5 required)
  - 1) Extensive cerebral WM changes with frontal predominance
  - 2) ↑ T1, ↓ T2 periventricular rim

- 3) Abnormal signal BG, thalami
- 4) BS lesions
- 5) Contrast-enhancement of any of the following: Frontal WM, periventricular rim, BG, thalami, BS, dentate nuclei, cerebellar cortex, optic chiasm, fornix

## DIFFERENTIAL DIAGNOSIS

### Canavan Disease
- WM: Diffuse; subcortical U-fibers involved early
- Deep gray: Globi pallidi, thalami
- No enhancement
- Characteristic ↑↑ NAA peak MRS

### Megaloencephalic Leukoencephalopathy with Subcortical Cysts (MLC)
- WM: Diffuse with involvement of subcortical U-fibers
- Deep gray: Not involved
- No enhancement
- Characteristic anterior temporal subcortical cysts

### Glutaric Aciduria Type 1 (GA-1)
- WM: Periventricular WM involved in severe disease
- Deep gray: Symmetric BG
- No enhancement
- Characteristic widened opercula 2° to extension of middle cranial fossa cysts into the opercula

### Mucopolysaccharidoses (MPS)
- WM: Mild periventricular
- Deep gray: Not involved
- No enhancement
- Characteristic cribriform appearance WM, corpus callosum 2° glycosaminoglycan-filled Virchow-Robin spaces

## PATHOLOGY

### General Features
- General path comments

# ALEXANDER DISEASE

- o AD characterized by RF accumulation in astrocytes & hypo-/demyelination
- o Embryology-anatomy
  - Astrocytes play role in formation of myelin by oligodendrocytes
  - Astrocytic end-feet form part of blood-brain barrier (BBB)
  - Glial fibrillary acidic protein (GFAP) = major intermediate filament protein of astrocytes
- Genetics
  - o Heterozygous (dominant) mutations GFAP (17q21) identified in > 95% cases AD
    - ≥ 45 different mutations identified
    - Same mutation may cause all three clinical forms of AD ⇒ other genetic or environmental factors influence AD phenotype
    - Mutations cause gain in function
    - Majority mutations arise de novo
- Etiology
  - o RFs: Abnormal intracellular protein aggregates containing GFAP, and small stress proteins: αβ-crystalline, hsp27, and ubiquitin
  - o Mechanism by which GFAP mutation induces RF formation in AD is uncertain
    - Theory: Accumulation RFs in astrocytes causes astrocyte dysfunction, including BBB disruption, and loss of normal interaction with other cells, especially oligodendrocytes, leading to hypo-/demyelination
  - o RFs also identified in astrocytomas, hamartomas, and glial scars
- Epidemiology: Rare; unknown incidence

## Gross Pathologic & Surgical Features

- Megaloencephalic, heavy brain with large ventricles
- Swollen, transparent, gelatinous white matter with cortical thinning; cavitation late
- BG swelling early; atrophy and cystic change late

## Microscopic Features

- RFs: Eosinophilic, electron-dense, cytoplasmic inclusions in fibrous astrocytes
  - o Highest concentration RFs in end-feet subependymal, subpial, perivascular astrocytes ⇒ accounts for intense enhancement in these locations
- Hypomyelination/myelin loss frontal lobes > caudal brain, ± cerebellar white matter, dentate nuclei, BS
- Generalized astrocytosis ± neuraxonal degeneration

# CLINICAL ISSUES

## Presentation

- Most common signs/symptoms
  - o Infantile: Macrocephaly, seizures, developmental delay/arrest, spasticity
  - o Juvenile: Developmental regression, bulbar/ pseudobulbar signs, ataxia, spasticity
  - o Adult: Bulbar/pseudobulbar signs, ataxia
- Other signs/symptoms: Bladder/bowel dysfunction juvenile, adult forms
- Clinical Profile: Infant with macrocephaly, seizures
- Cerebrospinal fluid (CSF) analysis: Variable ↑ protein, and presence of αβ-crystalline, hsp27, lactate

- Diagnosis: MR and GFAP gene analysis from peripheral blood sample

## Demographics

- Age
  - o Infantile: Birth to 2 years
  - o Juvenile: 2-12 years
  - o Adult: > 12 years old
- Gender: M = F infantile form; M > F juvenile form
- Ethnicity: No known racial predilection

## Natural History & Prognosis

- Natural History
  - o Variable rate of progression ultimately leading to death in all subtypes
    - Neonatal variant of infantile subtype is most rapidly fatal; infantile form is next most severe
    - Juvenile form is more slowly progressive
    - Adult form is mildest
- Prognosis: Related to age at onset of disease
  - o Infantile: Average survival = 3 yrs after disease onset
  - o Juvenile: Average survival = 8 yrs after disease onset
  - o Adult: Average survival = 15 yrs after disease onset

## Treatment

- Supportive; hydrocephalus in infantile form may respond to shunting
- Potential future therapeutic role for agents causing down-regulation of GFAP expression

# DIAGNOSTIC CHECKLIST

## Image Interpretation Pearls

- Enhancing, symmetric bifrontal WM disease in macrocephalic infant highly characteristic of AD
- Juvenile, adult cases may mimic posterior fossa tumors
  - o Careful scrutinization BG, WM will aid in diagnosis

# SELECTED REFERENCES

1. van der Knaap MS et al: Alexander disease: ventricular garlands and abnormalities of the medulla and spinal cord. Neurology. 66(4):494-8, 2006
2. Li R et al: Glial fibrillary acidic protein mutations in infantile, juvenile, and adult forms of Alexander disease. Ann Neurol. 57(3):310-26, 2005
3. van der Knaap MS et al: Unusual variants of Alexander's disease. Ann Neurol. 57(3):327-38, 2005
4. Mignot C et al: Alexander disease: putative mechanisms of an astrocytic encephalopathy. Cell Mol Life Sci. 61(3):369-85, 2004
5. Brockmann K et al: Cerebral proton magnetic resonance spectroscopy in infantile Alexander disease. J Neurol. 250(3):300-6, 2003
6. Gordon N: Alexander disease. Eur J Paediatr Neurol. 7(6):395-9, 2003
7. Johnson AB et al: Alexander's disease: clinical, pathologic, and genetic features. J Child Neurol. 18(9):625-32, 2003
8. Messing A et al: Alexander disease: new insights from genetics. J Neuropathol Exp Neurol. 60(6):563-73, 2001
9. Rodriguez D et al: Infantile Alexander disease: spectrum of GFAP mutations and genotype-phenotype correlation. Am J Hum Genet. 69(5):1134-40, 2001
10. van der Knaap MS et al: Alexander disease: diagnosis with MR imaging. AJNR Am J Neuroradiol. 22(3):541-52, 2001

# ALEXANDER DISEASE

## IMAGE GALLERY

### Typical

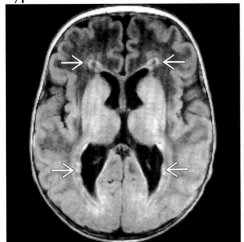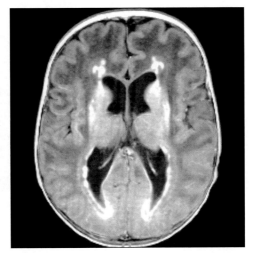

*(Left)* Axial T1WI MR shows extensive hypointensity in the frontal WM extending into the external capsule, hyperintense basal ganglia, hyperintense garlands ➡ in/around walls of ventricles. *(Right)* Axial T1 C+ MR in same patient as previous image shows enhancement of the periventricular rim, caudate heads and putamina. In AD, enhancement occurs in areas of greatest Rosenthal fiber deposition.

### Typical

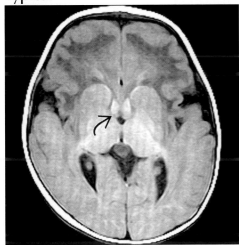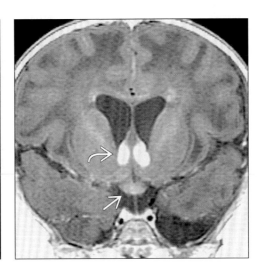

*(Left)* Axial T1WI MR shows swelling and hyperintensity in the columns of the fornices ➢ in addition to hyperintensity of the frontal periventricular rim and anterior margin of the caudate heads. *(Right)* Coronal T1 C+ MR in same patient as previous image shows intense enhancement ➡ of the forniceal columns. Subtle thickening and enhancement of the optic chiasm ➡ is also noted.

### Typical

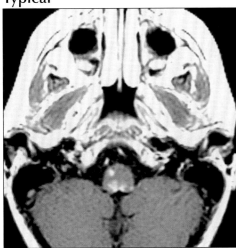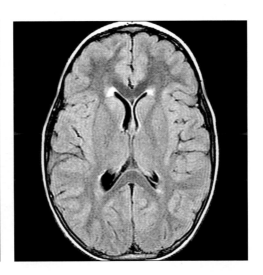

*(Left)* Axial T1 C+ MR shows typical findings of juvenile AD, with predominance of posterior fossa abnormalities. Several small regions of enhancement are present in the peripheral medulla. *(Right)* Axial FLAIR MR in same patient as previous image shows largely normal white matter with minimal periventricular hyperintensity. The clue to diagnosis of AD is in the hyperintense caudate heads.

# MLC

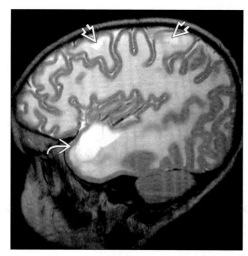

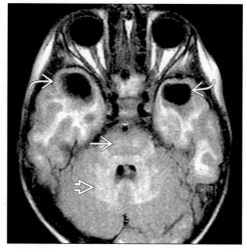

*Sagittal T2WI MR shows typical temporal pole ⇨ and subcortical fronto-parietal ⇨ cysts in a 2 year old with macrencephaly. Note the complete absence of myelination.*

*Axial FLAIR MR shows bilateral temporal pole cysts ⇨ and diffusely increased signal intensity of supratentorial, pontine ⇨, and cerebellar ⇨ white matter.*

## TERMINOLOGY

### Abbreviations and Synonyms
- Megaloencephalic leukoencephalopathy (MLC) with subcortical cysts
- Formerly known as van der Knaap disease; vacuolating megaloencephalic leukoencephalopathy with benign, slowly progressive course; leukoencephalopathy with swelling and cysts

### Definitions
- Neurodegenerative leukoencephalopathy with genetic mutation affecting astrocyte dysfunction

## IMAGING FINDINGS

### General Features
- Best diagnostic clue
  - Swollen white matter
  - Subcortical white matter involved early in course of disease
  - Subcortical cysts especially temporal poles, frontoparietal lobes

- Cysts can be several cm in size
  - Eventually volume loss and ↑ number cysts
- Location
  - MLC: White matter diffusely affected; includes subcortical U-fibers
    - Subcortical cysts (especially anterior temporal and frontoparietal)
    - Pontine and cerebellar WM involvement more subtle
- Size: Macrocephaly
- Morphology
  - Gyri appear somewhat swollen; sulci normal
  - Some cerebellar atrophy may develop late in disease

### CT Findings
- NECT: Involved WM shows ↓ attenuation
- CECT: No contrast-enhancement

### MR Findings
- T1WI
  - Involved WM ↓ signal on T1WI
  - Cysts are isointense to CSF
- T2WI
  - Diffuse WM swelling & ↑ signal on T2WI
    - Diffuse supratentorial white matter

## DDx: MLC1 Look-Alikes

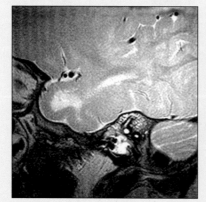

*Cytomegalovirus*

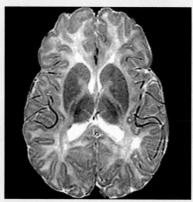

*Hypomyelination*

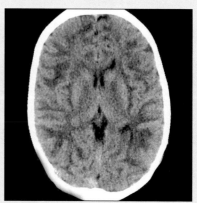

*Canavan*

# MLC

## Key Facts

### Terminology
- Megaloencephalic leukoencephalopathy (MLC) with subcortical cysts
- Neurodegenerative leukoencephalopathy with genetic mutation affecting astrocyte dysfunction

### Imaging Findings
- Swollen white matter
- Subcortical white matter involved early in course of disease
- Subcortical cysts especially temporal poles, frontoparietal lobes
- Cysts can be several cm in size
- Eventually volume loss and ↑ number cysts

### Top Differential Diagnoses
- Other Nonenhancing Leukodystrophies

- Congenital Cytomegalovirus Infection

### Pathology
- Autosomal recessive; gene localized on chr 22q(tel)
- Currently 50 mutations of MLC1 gene known
- Etiology: Inborn genetic error involving astrocytic end processes
- Rare spongiform leukoencephalopathy

### Clinical Issues
- Other signs/symptoms: Symptoms milder than very abnormal MR suggests
- Normal development during first year of life
- Loss of milestones begins during second year
- Slow deterioration in childhood
- Phenotype-genotype variability

---

- Subcortical U-fibers, posterior limbs internal capsule not spared
- Less pronounced corpus callosum, pontine tracts, cerebellar white matter involvement
  - Anterotemporal and frontoparietal cysts
    - May be "lost" in diffuse WM swelling
    - Best seen on FLAIR and T1 weighted images
- FLAIR
  - Involved WM ↑ signal on FLAIR
  - Anterotemporal and frontoparietal subcortical cysts
    - Approximate CSF signal
    - Well seen on FLAIR
- DWI: MLC: DTI shows ↓ anisotropy, ↑ ADC values
- T1 C+: No contrast-enhancement
- MRS: All metabolites ↓ in cystic regions; ↓ NAA in WM, ± lactate doublet, ± ↑ Cho, myo-I

### Imaging Recommendations
- Best imaging tool: MR
- Protocol advice: MR, MRS, DWI, contrast administration (to exclude the enhancing leukodystrophies)

## DIFFERENTIAL DIAGNOSIS

### Other Nonenhancing Leukodystrophies
- Metachromatic leukodystrophy
  - ARSA gene mutation
  - Look for WM "stripes" on T2WI
  - Spares internal capsule and subcortical U-fibers
- Canavan disease (Acetoaspartyluria)
  - Mutation in gene encoding ASPA
  - Elevated NAA, not decreased as in MLC
- Leukoencephalopathy with vanishing white matter (VWM)
  - Mutations in genes that encode eIF2B subunits: EIF2B1-5
  - Progressive replacement of all WM with CSF-intensity
    - Subcortical cysts with CSF-intensity in MLC
  - Alternatively called CACH: Childhood ataxia central hypomyelination

- Pelizaeus-Merzbacher disease
  - PLP1 gene mutation
  - Hypomyelination without cysts

### Congenital Cytomegalovirus Infection
- Temporal pole cysts
- Micro- not macrocephaly

## PATHOLOGY

### General Features
- General path comments
  - MLC1 expressed in brain and leukocytes
    - Distal astroglial processes affected most
  - No systemic or other organ involvement
- Genetics
  - Autosomal recessive; gene localized on chr 22q(tel)
    - Currently 50 mutations of MLC1 gene known
    - MLC1 (KIAAOO27) encodes putative CNS membrane transporter
    - MLC1 mutation in 80% patients with typical clinical and MR features
  - MLC2 gene remains hypothetical
- Etiology: Inborn genetic error involving astrocytic end processes
- Epidemiology
  - Rare spongiform leukoencephalopathy
    - In some communities with high levels consanguinity carrier rate as high as 1/40

### Gross Pathologic & Surgical Features
- Spongiform leukoencephalopathy
- Primarily affects myelin initially
- Eventually axons, cortex involved

### Microscopic Features
- Neuropathologic reports are rare
  - Myelin splitting and vacuolization of outermost lamellae of myelin sheaths
  - ↑ Extracellular spaces, ↓ numbers of fibers
  - Cortex: ↓ Neuronal density with neuronal degenerative changes

# MLC

## CLINICAL ISSUES

### Presentation

- Most common signs/symptoms
  - Macrocephaly
  - Slow gross motor development & deterioration
  - Early onset progressive ataxia
  - Slow motor deterioration & spasticity
  - Very slow cognitive decline
- Other signs/symptoms: Symptoms milder than very abnormal MR suggests
- Clinical Profile
  - Normal development during first year of life
    - Early macrocephaly
  - Loss of milestones begins during second year
    - Ataxia and pyramidal tract involvement
    - Slow motor deterioration
    - Seizures
  - Slow deterioration in childhood
    - Very slow cognitive decline, although learning problems in 50%
    - Ability to walk lost in first decade in 50%
  - Phenotype-genotype variability

### Demographics

- Age
  - Macrocephaly before the age of 1 year
  - Neurodevelopmental deterioration begins during second year
  - Adolescent and adult presentations very rare
- Gender: M = F
- Ethnicity
  - Common MLC mutations in population isolates due to founder effect
    - Specific Indian community (Agarwal): Insertion (c.135_136insC)
    - Libyan Jewish (c.176G>A) mutation
    - Japanese (p.Ser93Leu) mutation
    - Turkish (several)
    - Many "private" mutations

### Natural History & Prognosis

- Imaging and clinical features progress very slowly
  - Milder phenotype
    - Attend college
    - Live independently
    - Retain walking ability to 4th decade
    - Life expectancy to 40s or later
  - More severe phenotype
    - Delayed talking
    - Early loss of walking
    - Severe cognitive impairment
    - Life expectancy to teens

### Treatment

- Treat symptoms (seizures, spasticity)

## DIAGNOSTIC CHECKLIST

### Consider

- Not all symmetrical leukodystrophies are metachromatic leukodystrophy
  - If U-fibers or cysts involved, consider MLC

### Image Interpretation Pearls

- Describe specific tract and location involvement (e.g., internal capsules)
- Always enhance the unknown leukoencephalopathy

## SELECTED REFERENCES

1. Gorospe JR et al: Alexander disease and megalencephalic leukoencephalopathy with subcortical cysts: leukodystrophies arising from astrocyte dysfunction. Ment Retard Dev Disabil Res Rev. 12(2):113-22, 2006
2. Ilja Boor PK et al: Megalencephalic leukoencephalopathy with subcortical cysts: an update and extended mutation analysis of MLC1. Hum Mutat. 27(6):505-12, 2006
3. Itoh N et al: An Adult Case of Megalencephalic Leukoencephalopathy with Subcortical Cysts with S93L Mutation in MLC1 Gene: A Case Report and Diffusion MRI. Eur Neurol. 56(4):243-5, 2006
4. Montagna G et al: Vacuolating megalencephalic leukoencephalopathy with subcortical cysts: functional studies of novel variants in MLC1. Hum Mutat. 27(3):292, 2006
5. Morita H et al: MR imaging and 1H-MR spectroscopy of a case of van der Knaap disease. Brain Dev. 28(7):466-9, 2006
6. Boor PK et al: MLC1: a novel protein in distal astroglial processes. J Neuropathol Exp Neurol. 64(5):412-9, 2005
7. Boor PK et al: MLC1: a novel protein in distal astroglial processes. J Neuropathol Exp Neurol. 64(5):412-9, 2005
8. Juneja M et al: Megalencephalic leukoencephalopathy with subcortical cysts. Indian J Pediatr. 72(2):179-80, 2005
9. Pascual-Castroviejo I et al: Vacuolating megalencephalic leukoencephalopathy: 24 year follow-up of two siblings. Neurologia. 20(1):33-40, 2005
10. Riel-Romero RM et al: Megalencephalic leukoencephalopathy with subcortical cysts in two siblings owing to two novel mutations: case reports and review of the literature. J Child Neurol. 20(3):230-4, 2005
11. Schiffmann R et al: The latest on leukodystrophies. Curr Opin Neurol. 17(2):187-92, 2004
12. Teijido O et al: Localization and functional analyses of the MLC1 protein involved in megalencephalic leukoencephalopathy with subcortical cysts. Hum Mol Genet. 13(21):2581-94, 2004
13. Brockmann K et al: Megalencephalic leukoencephalopathy with subcortical cysts in an adult: quantitative proton MR spectroscopy and diffusion tensor MRI. Neuroradiology. 45(3):137-42, 2003
14. Patrono C et al: Genetic heterogeneity of megalencephalic leukoencephalopathy and subcortical cysts. Neurology. 61(4):534-7, 2003
15. Tsujino S et al: A common mutation and a novel mutation in Japanese patients with van der Knaap disease. J Hum Genet. 48(12):605-8, 2003
16. Leegwater PA et al: Identification of novel mutations in MLC1 responsible for megalencephalic leukoencephalopathy with subcortical cysts. Hum Genet. 110(3):279-83, 2002
17. Leegwater PA et al: Mutations of MLC1 (KIAA0027), encoding a putative membrane protein, cause megalencephalic leukoencephalopathy with subcortical cysts. Am J Hum Genet. 68(4):831-8, 2001
18. van der Knaap MS et al: Defining and categorizing leukoencephalopathies of unknown origin: MR imaging approach. Radiology. 213(1):121-33, 1999
19. van der Knaap MS et al: Histopathology of an infantile-onset spongiform leukoencephalopathy with a discrepantly mild clinical course. Acta Neuropathol (Berl). 92(2):206-12, 1996

## IMAGE GALLERY

### Typical

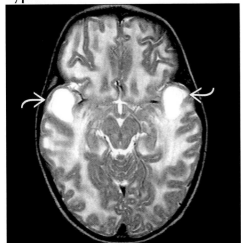
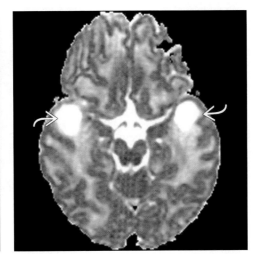

*(Left)* Axial T2WI MR shows bilateral temporal pole cysts ➔. Signal intensity is diffusely increased throughout supratentorial white matter. Subcortical U-fibers are involved. *(Right)* Axial ADC shows high diffusivity in the temporal pole cysts ➔ and, to a lesser extent, in the cerebral white matter of the same child as previous image.

### Typical

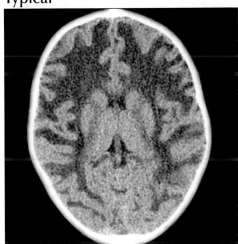
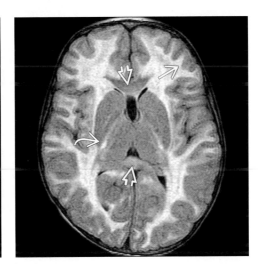

*(Left)* Axial NECT shows diffuse low attenuation and swelling of supratentorial white matter. Note the normal ventricular size and absence of sulcal enlargement. *(Right)* Axial FLAIR MR shows diffusely increased signal intensity of white matter. Subcortical U-fibers ➔, internal capsules ➔, and, to a lesser extent, corpus callosum ➔ are involved.

### Typical

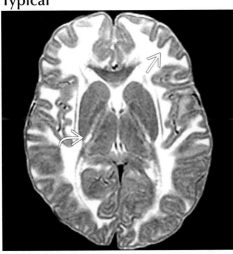
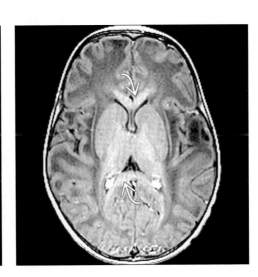

*(Left)* Axial T2WI MR shows similar findings with involvement of internal capsules ➔, subcortical U-fibers ➔ and diffuse white matter swelling. *(Right)* Axial T1 C+ MR shows lack of contrast-enhancement of the involved white matter. Note that some myelination is present in corpus callosum ➔.

# PKAN

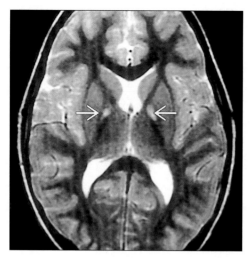 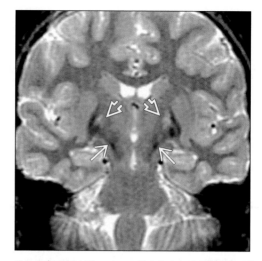

*Axial T2WI MR shows classic "eye-of-the-tiger" appearance of PKAN. The globus pallidi are abnormally hypointense with central foci of hyperintensity ➡, resembling a tiger's eyes.*

*Coronal T2WI MR captures all main imaging features of PKAN: "Eye-of-the-tiger" sign in the GP ⇒ with symmetric hypointensity in the surrounding GP & substantia nigra ➡.*

## TERMINOLOGY

### Abbreviations and Synonyms
- Pantothenate kinase-associated neurodegeneration (PKAN)
- Neurodegeneration with brain iron accumulation (NBIA)
- Hallervorden-Spatz syndrome
- NBIA = new umbrella term for neurodegenerative disorders characterized by brain iron accumulation
  - NBIA includes PKAN, aceruloplasminemia, neuroferritinopathy, and others
- PKAN and NBIA preferred terms due to 3rd Reich association of Julius Hallervorden

### Definitions
- PKAN: Form of NBIA caused by mutation pantothenate kinase 2 (PANK2) gene chromosome 20
- Classic form causes extrapyramidal motor impairment in young children

## IMAGING FINDINGS

### General Features
- Best diagnostic clue: "Eye-of-the-tiger" sign: Bilateral, symmetric foci T2 hyperintensity globus pallidus (GP) surrounded by pallidal T2 hypointensity
- Location
  - GP, substantia nigra (SN)
    - "Eye" in "eye-of-the-tiger" medial GP
- Morphology: Focal GP hyperintensity surrounded by GP hypointensity has appearance of tiger eyes
- Variable atrophy
- Iron deposition (ferritin-bound) responsible for T2 hypointense imaging appearance

### CT Findings
- NECT: Variable: Hypodense, hyperdense or normal GP
- CECT: No abnormal enhancement

### MR Findings
- T1WI
  - Variable: Hyperintense or normal
    - Ferritin-bound iron has greater T1 shortening than hemosiderin-bound

### DDx: Disorders with ↑ T2 GP

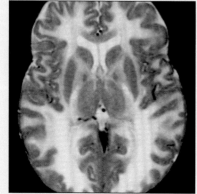 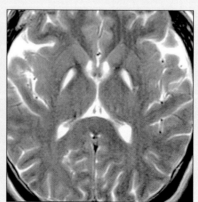 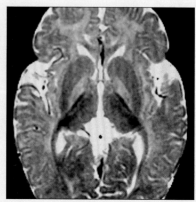

*Canavan*     *Carbon Monoxide*     *Kernicterus*

# PKAN

## Key Facts

### Terminology
- NBIA = new umbrella term for neurodegenerative disorders characterized by brain iron accumulation
- NBIA includes PKAN, aceruloplasminemia, neuroferritinopathy, and others
- PKAN: Form of NBIA caused by mutation pantothenate kinase 2 (PANK2) gene chromosome 20
- Classic form causes extrapyramidal motor impairment in young children

### Imaging Findings
- Best diagnostic clue: "Eye-of-the-tiger" sign: Bilateral, symmetric foci T2 hyperintensity globus pallidus (GP) surrounded by pallidal T2 hypointensity

### Top Differential Diagnoses
- Metabolic Disorders with ↓ T2 Signal GP

- Ischemic/Toxic/Metabolic Disorders with ↑ T2 Signal in GP

### Pathology
- 1:1 correlation between PANK2 mutation and "eye-of-the-tiger" sign MR

### Clinical Issues
- Classic PKAN: Young child with gait, postural deficits
- Atypical PKAN: Teenager with speech, psychiatric disturbance
- Classic PKAN: Fatal; mean duration disease after symptom onset = 11 years
- Atypical PKAN: Eventual severe impairment, ± death, adulthood

---

- T2WI
  - GP: "Eye-of-the-tiger"
    - Hyperintense "eye" predates surrounding T2 hypointensity
  - Variable hypointensity substantia nigra
    - More common older patients
- FLAIR: "Eye" in "eye-of-the-tiger" persists
- T2* GRE: T2 hypointensities "bloom" due to paramagnetic effect iron
- T1 C+: No abnormal enhancement
- MRS: ↓ NAA in GP (neuronal loss)

### Nuclear Medicine Findings
- PET: Hemispheric hypometabolism described in adult patients with dementia
- Tc-99m SPECT: ↑ Activity medial GP
  - Possible chelation Tc-99m by pallidal cysteine

### Imaging Recommendations
- Best imaging tool: MR
- Protocol advice
  - Include GRE sequence
  - T2 hypointensity more conspicuous on spin echo (vs. fast spin echo) and high field strength magnets

## DIFFERENTIAL DIAGNOSIS

### Metabolic Disorders with ↓ T2 Signal GP
- Neuronal ceroid lipofuscinosis: ↓ T2 GP/thalami; cerebral and cerebellar atrophy
- Fucosidosis: ↓ T2 GP; ↑ T2, atrophy white matter; cutaneous lesions; hepatosplenomegaly

### Ischemic/Toxic/Metabolic Disorders with ↑ T2 Signal in GP
- Metabolic
  - Methylmalonic acidemia (MMA): ↑ T2 GP, ± periventricular white matter (WM)
  - Kearns-Sayre/L-2-Hydroxyglutaric aciduria: ↑ T2 GP (> than other deep gray) and peripheral WM
  - Canavan: ↑ T2 GP (> than other deep gray) and subcortical WM; macrocephaly; ↑↑ NAA

- Ischemic/toxic
  - Anoxic encephalopathy: ↑ T2 GP (and other deep gray) and cortex
  - Carbon monoxide poisoning: ↑ T2 GP (± other deep gray, cortex, WM)
  - Cyanide poisoning: ↑ T2 BG followed by hemorrhagic necrosis
  - Kernicterus: ↑ T2/T1 GP neonate

## PATHOLOGY

### General Features
- General path comments
  - Iron accumulation likely 2° phenomenon in PKAN
    - Serial MRs in PKAN patients show hypertense foci GP predating surrounding hypointensity
  - Embryology-anatomy
    - Normal progressive, physiologic brain iron accumulation GP, SN > red & dentate nuclei
    - ↓ T2 signal GP identified in majority of normals by age ≥ 25, but never before age 10
- Genetics
  - Autosomal recessive (50% sporadic)
  - PANK2 mutation on chromosome 20p12.3-p13
    - 1:1 correlation between PANK2 mutation and "eye-of-the-tiger" sign MR
    - PANK2 gene encodes mitochondrial-targeted pantothenate kinase 2, key enzyme in biosynthesis of coenzyme A (CoA)
    - CoA essential to energy metabolism, fatty acid synthesis and degradation, among other functions
    - Null mutations more common in early-onset, rapidly progressive disease
    - Missense mutations more common in late-onset, more slowly progressive disease ⇒ suggests residual pantothenate kinase 2 activity in late-onset (less severe) disease
  - HARP: Hypoprebetalipoproteinemia, acanthocytosis, retinitis pigmentosa and pallidal degeneration
    - Allelic with PKAN

# PKAN

- Prominent orofacial dystonia; early onset parkinsonism
- Etiology
  - Leading theory
    - PANK2 mutation ⇒ CoA deficiency ⇒ energy and lipid dyshomeostasis ⇒ production oxygen free radicals ⇒ phospholipid membrane destruction
    - Basal ganglia and retina prone to oxidative damage 2° to high metabolic demand
  - Contributing factors
    - Cysteine accumulation GP 2° to ↓ phosphopantothenate causes iron chelation and peroxidative cell membrane damage
    - Lewy bodies, glial inclusions, and axonal spheroids further compromise glial and neuronal cell function
- Epidemiology: Rare; incidence unknown

## Gross Pathologic & Surgical Features
- Symmetric rust-brown pigmentation GP (interna > externa) and pars reticulata SN
  - In addition to iron, intra- and extraneuronal ceroid lipofuscin and melanin contribute to pigmentation
- Variable atrophy

## Microscopic Features
- Classic features
  - Abnormal iron accumulation GP interna and pars reticulata SN
    - Iron located in astrocytes, microglial cells, neurons and around vessels
  - Neuronal loss, gliosis and glial inclusions primarily involving GP interna and pars reticulata SN
  - Round or oval, non-nucleated, axonal swellings ("spheroids") in GP, SN, cortex, and brainstem
- "Loose" tissue consisting of reactive astrocytes, dystrophic axons and vacuoles in anteromedial GP corresponds to "eye-of-the-tiger" on MR
- Variably present neurofibrillary tangles, Lewy bodies, and acanthocytes (on blood smear)

## Staging, Grading or Classification Criteria
- Clinical Classification
  - PKAN divided into classic and atypical disease
    - Classic PKAN: Early onset; more rapidly progressive disease; uniform phenotype
    - Atypical PKAN: Late onset; more slowly progressive disease; heterogeneous phenotype

# CLINICAL ISSUES

## Presentation
- Most common signs/symptoms
  - Classic PKAN: Dystonia
    - Other extrapyramidal signs/symptoms: Dysarthria, rigidity, choreoathetosis
    - Upper motor neuron signs/symptoms and cognitive decline frequent
    - Pigmentary retinopathy 66%
  - Atypical PKAN: Psychiatric and speech disturbances
    - Other signs/symptoms: Pyramidal, extrapyramidal disturbances (including freezing), dementia
- Clinical Profile
  - Classic PKAN: Young child with gait, postural deficits
  - Atypical PKAN: Teenager with speech, psychiatric disturbance
- Normal serum and CSF iron levels
- Confirmatory PANK2 mutation analysis should be performed in all suspected cases of PKAN

## Demographics
- Age
  - Classic PKAN: Majority present before 6 years of age
  - Atypical PKAN: Mean age at presentation = 13 years

## Natural History & Prognosis
- Natural History
  - Classic PKAN: Rapid, non-uniform progression with periods of deterioration interspersed with stability ultimately leading to death early adulthood
  - Atypical PKAN: More slowly progressive with loss of ambulation 15-40 years after disease onset
- Prognosis
  - Classic PKAN: Fatal; mean duration disease after symptom onset = 11 years
  - Atypical PKAN: Eventual severe impairment, ± death, adulthood
- MR imaging findings may precede symptoms

## Treatment
- No curative treatment; iron chelation ineffective
- Palliation of symptoms: Stereotactic pallidotomy, baclofen, trihexyphenidyl
- Potential for pantothenate replacement therapy

# DIAGNOSTIC CHECKLIST

## Consider
- Patients with hypointense GP without "eye-of-the-tiger" lack PANK2 mutation and therefore are not designated PKAN but rather other form NBIA
- Physiologic GP hypointensity difficult to distinguish from pathologic hypointensity in teenager/adult

# SELECTED REFERENCES

1. Hayflick SJ et al: Brain MRI in neurodegeneration with brain iron accumulation with and without PANK2 mutations. AJNR Am J Neuroradiol. 27(6):1230-3, 2006
2. Koyama M et al: Pantothenate kinase-associated neurodegeneration with increased lentiform nuclei cerebral blood flow. AJNR Am J Neuroradiol. 27(1):212-3, 2006
3. Nicholas AP et al: Atypical Hallervorden-Spatz disease with preserved cognition and obtrusive obsessions and compulsions. Mov Disord. 20(7):880-6, 2005
4. Thomas M et al: Clinical heterogeneity of neurodegeneration with brain iron accumulation (Hallervorden-Spatz syndrome) and pantothenate kinase-associated neurodegeneration. Mov Disord. 19(1):36-42, 2004
5. Hayflick SJ et al: Genetic, clinical, and radiographic delineation of Hallervorden-Spatz syndrome. N Engl J Med. 348(1):33-40, 2003
6. Hayflick SJ. Related Articles et al: Unraveling the Hallervorden-Spatz syndrome: pantothenate kinase-associated neurodegeneration is the name. Curr Opin Pediatr. 15(6):572-7, 2003

## IMAGE GALLERY

### Typical

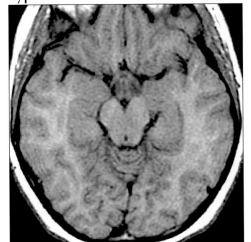 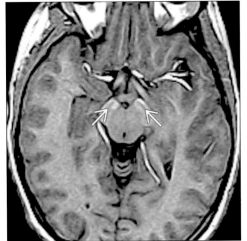

*(Left)* Axial T1WI MR shows no apparent abnormal signal intensity in the substantia nigra in a patient with PKAN. *(Right)* Axial T1WI MR in a patient with PKAN shows hyperintensity of the substantia nigra ➡. The T1 appearance of the GP and SN in PKAN is variable.

### Typical

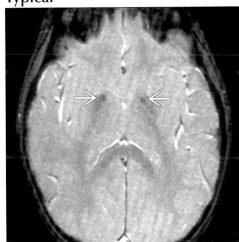 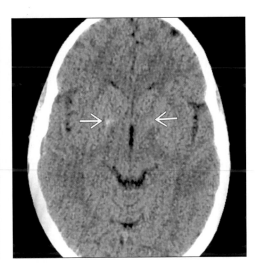

*(Left)* Axial T2* GRE MR shows focal hypointense signal ("blooming") in the bilateral GP ➡ secondary to the paramagnetic effect of iron. *(Right)* Axial NECT shows focal GP calcification ➡ bilaterally. The CT appearance of PKAN is variable. GP may be hypodense or hyperdense secondary to dystrophic calcification as seen in this case.

### Typical

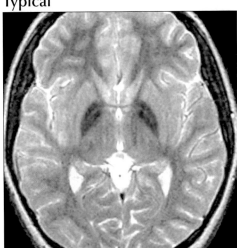 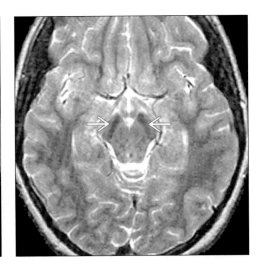

*(Left)* Axial T2WI MR shows diffusely hypointense GP in a 15 year old with spastic gait. Lack of "eye-of-the-tiger" indicates lack of PANK2 mutation. These patients have other forms of NBIA, not PKAN. *(Right)* Axial T2WI MR in same patient as previous image shows hypointense substantia nigra ➡. Nigral hypointensity is usually greater in patients with NBIA other than PKAN.

# HUNTINGTON DISEASE

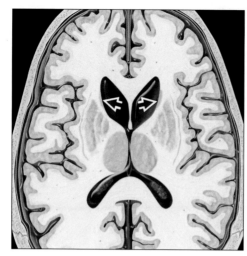

*Axial graphic shows bilateral caudate atrophy, causing convex lateral margins of frontal horns ⇨.*

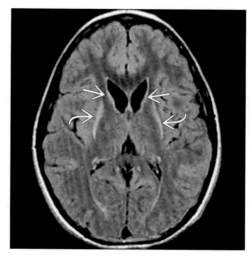

*Axial FLAIR MR shows straightening of the lateral margins of the frontal horns; the caudate heads ⇨ and putamina ⇗ are atrophic and abnormally hyperintense.*

## TERMINOLOGY

### Abbreviations and Synonyms

- Juvenile Huntington disease (HD), Huntington chorea

### Definitions

- Autosomal dominant neurodegenerative disease with loss of GABAergic neurons of basal ganglia (BG)

## IMAGING FINDINGS

### General Features

- Best diagnostic clue: Atrophy of caudate nucleus (CN) ⇒ enlargement of frontal horns of lateral ventricles
- Location
  - Primarily striatum (especially CN, putamen)
  - Cerebral cortex, globus pallidus (GP), thalamus
  - Substantia nigra (SN), brainstem
- Size: Decreased (atrophy)
- Morphology: Loss of convex surface of caudate head

### CT Findings

- NECT
  - Atrophy of CN and putamen, also GP (less severe)
  - Enlargement of frontal horns of lateral ventricles
  - Diffuse cerebral atrophy (reported to be predominantly frontal in some studies)
  - CN atrophy is measured on axial images at level of 3rd ventricle
    - Intercaudate distance (CC) between most medial aspects of CN
    - CC compared with distance between most lateral aspects of frontal horns (FH)
    - CC compared with distance between inner tables (IT) of skull at level of CC measurement
    - ↑ CC relative to FH or IT
    - ↓ FH/CC ratio
    - ↑ CC/IT ratio (bicaudate ratio): Most specific and sensitive measure for HD
- CECT: No contrast-enhancement of affected structures

### MR Findings

- T1WI
  - Shrinkage of CN and ↑ CC
  - MR measurements: ↓ Volume in all BG structures
    - Also reported in presymptomatic stage of HD
  - Diffuse cerebral atrophy

## DDx: Juvenile Huntington Disease

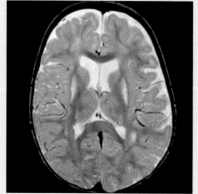

*Glutaric Aciduria*

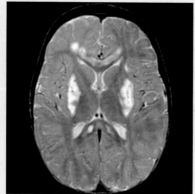

*Leigh Syndrome*

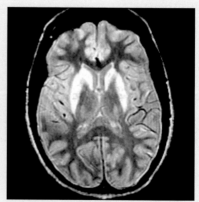

*Wilson Disease*

# HUNTINGTON DISEASE

## Key Facts

### Imaging Findings

- Best diagnostic clue: Atrophy of caudate nucleus (CN) ⇒ enlargement of frontal horns of lateral ventricles
- ↑ CC/IT ratio (bicaudate ratio): Most specific and sensitive measure for HD
- Hyperechogenic lesions primarily in SN and CN
- ↓ FDG uptake in BG before any detectable atrophy

### Top Differential Diagnoses

- Leigh Syndrome
- Wilson Disease
- Hallervorden-Spatz
- Organic Acidemias

### Pathology

- Gross atrophy of CN and putamen

- CAG trinucleotide repeat disease affecting HD gene on chromosome 4p16.3
- Polyglutamine expansion ⇒ huntingtin accumulates in nucleus and cytoplasm ⇒ cytoplasmic huntingtin aggregates in axonal terminals
- Juvenile HD: Involvement of GP and cerebellum
- Severity grades (0-4) based on gross striatal pathology, neuronal loss and gliosis

### Clinical Issues

- Typical childhood presentation: Dystonia, rigidity

### Diagnostic Checklist

- Caudate/putamen atrophy is main radiologic feature of HD
- ↑ Signal intensity in CN and putamina on PD- and T2WI in children suggests HD

---

- T2WI
  - Hyperintense signal in CN, putamina in juvenile HD
    - Gliosis-related
  - Shrinkage of CN and putamina; ↑ CC
  - Striatum may have ↓ signal due to iron deposition
- MRS
  - ↑ Lactate concentration in occipital cortex of symptomatic HD, also in BG in some patients
    - Lactate level correlates with duration of illness
  - ↓ N-acetylaspartate/creatine in BG (neuronal loss)
  - ↑↑ Choline/creatine ratio in BG (gliosis)
  - Findings consistent with energy metabolism defect

### Ultrasonographic Findings

- Transcranial real time sonography (TCS)
  - Hyperechogenic lesions primarily in SN and CN
    - Hyperechogenic lesions in SN correlate with disease severity
    - CN hyperechogenicity correlates with CN hyperintensity on T2WI
  - Ventricular enlargement depicted by TCS correlates with CT findings
- Functional transcranial Doppler ultrasonography
  - ↓ Vasoreactivity in anterior cerebral artery during motor activation in early stage HD
    - Possibly due to brain peroxynitrite deposition

### Nuclear Medicine Findings

- PET
  - ↓ FDG uptake in BG before any detectable atrophy
  - ± Frontal lobe hypometabolism
- SPECT: Perfusion defects in motor cortex, prefrontal cortex, and BG correlate with clinical disease

### Imaging Recommendations

- Best imaging tool: MR
- Protocol advice: T2WI

## DIFFERENTIAL DIAGNOSIS

### Leigh Syndrome

- Onset usually < 2 years, but many causes ⇒ many patterns
- Injury in putamen, CN, and tegmentum
  - Less commonly white matter, thalamus, brain stem, cerebellum
  - No atrophy of CN or putamina

### Wilson Disease

- Rigidity, tremor, dystonia, gait difficulty, dysarthria
- CT: Low densities in BG, cerebellar nuclei, brainstem, and white matter
- T2WI: Symmetrical signal hyperintensity in CN, putamen, thalamus, midbrain, and pons (gliosis and edema)
  - Characteristic irregular areas of hypointensity in CN and putamen
- Atrophy of CN and brainstem on CT, MR

### Hallervorden-Spatz

- Involuntary movements (choreoathetosis), spasticity
- Progressive dementia in young adults
- Characteristic iron deposition in GP, red nuclei, SN
  - "Eye of the tiger" sign: Central spot of high signal in hypointense GP on T2WI

### Organic Acidemias

- Many have abnormal T2 prolongation in corpus striatum
- Consider glutaric aciduria type 1, propionic acidemia

## PATHOLOGY

### General Features

- General path comments
  - Gross atrophy of CN and putamen
    - Selective neuronal loss and astrogliosis
  - Neuronal loss in deep layers of cerebral cortex
  - Varying degrees of atrophy (GP, thalamus, subthalamic nucleus, SN, cerebellum)

# HUNTINGTON DISEASE

- Genetics
  - Autosomal dominant with complete penetrance
  - CAG trinucleotide repeat disease affecting HD gene on chromosome 4p16.3
    - Toxic gain of function for mutant protein (huntingtin)
    - Extra copies of glutamine in huntingtin
    - Larger number of repeats associated with pediatric presentation
  - Genetic anticipation: ↑ Severity or ↓ age of onset in successive generations
    - More commonly in paternal transmission of mutated allele
  - Homozygosity for HD mutation (very rare)
    - Associated with more severe clinical course
- Etiology
  - Polyglutamine expansion ⇒ huntingtin accumulates in nucleus and cytoplasm ⇒ cytoplasmic huntingtin aggregates in axonal terminals
  - Mutant huntingtin abnormally associates with synaptic vesicles and impairs synaptic function
- Epidemiology
  - Worldwide prevalence: 5-10:100,000 people
  - Less common in African, Asian populations

## Gross Pathologic & Surgical Features

- Diffuse cerebral atrophy, marked in CN & putamen
  - Loss of convex bulge of CN facing lateral ventricle
- Juvenile HD: Involvement of GP and cerebellum
  - Not typically involved in adults

## Microscopic Features

- Neuropathological hallmarks of HD
  - Intranuclear inclusions of mutant huntingtin
  - Perinuclear aggregates in cortex, striatum

## Staging, Grading or Classification Criteria

- Severity grades (0-4) based on gross striatal pathology, neuronal loss and gliosis
- Grade 0: No gross striatal atrophy
  - No detectable histologic neuropathology
  - Typical clinical picture and (+) family history of HD
- Grade 1: No gross striatal atrophy
  - Microscopic neuropathologic changes
- Grade 2: Striatal atrophy, convex CN
- Grade 3: More severe striatal atrophy, flat CN
- Grade 4: Most severe striatal atrophy
  - Concave medial surface of CN

## CLINICAL ISSUES

### Presentation

- Most common signs/symptoms
  - Typical childhood presentation: Dystonia, rigidity
    - Known as Westphal variant of HD
  - Teenage presentation: Psychiatric disease (depression)
    - Dystonia, chorea supervenes later
  - Adult triad: Movement disorder (choreoathetosis), dementia of subcortical type, behavioral changes/psychosis
- Clinical Profile
  - Juvenile HD: Rigidity > chorea

- Rigidity and dystonia may occur as initial symptoms
- Cerebellar signs, dyslalia, rapid cognitive decline
- Seizures, parkinsonism, dystonia, long-tract signs
- Severe depression is often presentation in teens
  - Adult HD: Movement disorder
    - Chorea: Often facial twitching or twitching and writhing of distal extremities; ballism later on
    - Progressive ⇒ impaired gait ("dancing gait")

### Demographics

- Age
  - Juvenile HD (5-10% of cases): Onset < 20 years
  - Mean age of onset: 35-44 y in adult-onset HD
- Gender
  - M = F; gender-related factor affecting disease onset
    - Earlier onset and faster progression of HD in offspring of male patients
    - 70% of juvenile cases have affected father

### Natural History & Prognosis

- Invariable progression
  - Juvenile HD: Rapid progression; survival 7-8 years
  - Adult HD: Progressive; death 15-20 years after onset

### Treatment

- Neuroleptic agents
- Clonazepam can suppress chorea
- Ubiquinone (coenzyme Q10) ⇒ normalization of lactate levels in cortex and striatum
- No current treatment modifies progression of disease

## DIAGNOSTIC CHECKLIST

### Image Interpretation Pearls

- Caudate/putamen atrophy is main radiologic feature of HD
  - Bicaudate diameter: Sensitive for CN atrophy
- Decline in size of GP and putamen correlates with disease progression
- ↑ Signal intensity in CN and putamina on PD- and T2WI in children suggests HD

## SELECTED REFERENCES

1. Rosenblatt A et al: The association of CAG repeat length with clinical progression in Huntington disease. Neurology. 66(7):1016-20, 2006
2. Ruocco HH et al: Clinical presentation of juvenile Huntington disease. Arq Neuropsiquiatr. 64(1):5-9, 2006
3. Alberch J et al: Neurotrophic factors in Huntington's disease. Prog Brain Res. 146:195-229, 2004
4. Postert T et al: Basal ganglia alterations and brain atrophy in Huntington's disease depicted by transcranial real time sonography. J Neurol Neurosurg Psychiatry. 67:457-62, 1999
5. Ho VB et al: Juvenile Huntington Disease: CT and MR features. Am J Neuroradiol. 16:1405-12, 1995
6. Jenkins BG et al: Evidence for impairment of energy metabolism in vivo in Huntington's disease using localized 1H NMR spectroscopy. Neurol. 43:2689-95, 1993

## IMAGE GALLERY

### Typical

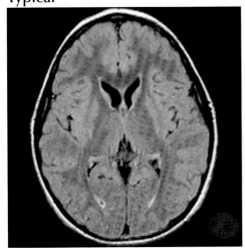
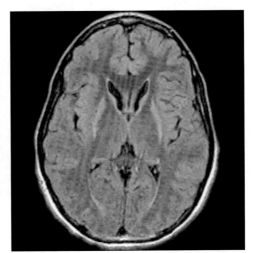

*(Left)* Axial FLAIR MR shows early (grade 1) disease with mild atrophy and hyperintensity of the striatum (caudate and putamen). No cortical atrophy is present, typical of juvenile Huntington disease. *(Right)* Axial FLAIR MR of same patient shows increased (grade 2) degree of caudate head atrophy, resulting in an intermediate degree of enlargement of frontal horns. No cortical atrophy is present.

### Typical

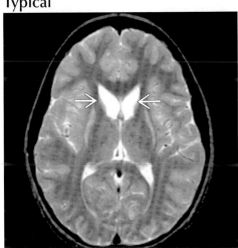
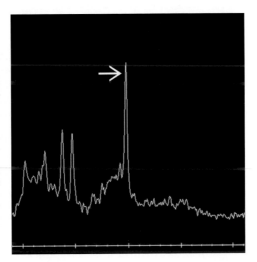

*(Left)* Axial T2WI MR shows severe (grade 3) caudate and putaminal atrophy; the frontal horns have a nearly flat lateral border ➡. *(Right)* MRS shows reduced NAA peak ➡ at 2.01 ppm due to striatal atrophy. Absence of a lactate peak at 1.33 ppm suggests that this is not a mitochondrial disorder.

### Typical

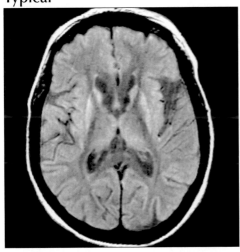
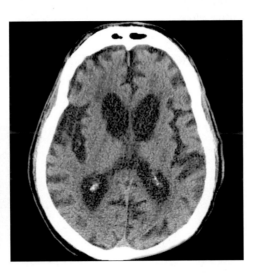

*(Left)* Axial FLAIR MR in an adult patient shows considerable cortical atrophy in addition to the atrophy and hyperintensity of the corpus striatum. Cortical atrophy is common in adult patients. *(Right)* Axial NECT in another adult patient shows severe atrophy of the corpora striata and cerebral cortex.

# WILSON DISEASE

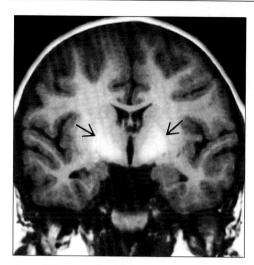

Coronal T1WI MR shows typical initial finding of WD in a child, with bilateral globus pallidus hyperintensity ➡ secondary to liver disease.

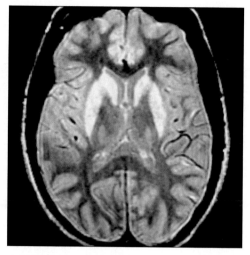

Axial PD/Intermediate MR shows more advanced WD of the CNS, with bilateral hyperintensity of the caudate heads, putamina, globi pallidi, and ventrolateral thalami.

## TERMINOLOGY

### Abbreviations and Synonyms

- Wilson disease (WD), hepatolenticular degeneration, ATP7B disease

### Definitions

- Inborn error of copper metabolism characterized by
  - Liver cirrhosis, Kayser-Fleischer ring of cornea
  - Softening and degeneration of basal ganglia (BG)

## IMAGING FINDINGS

### General Features

- Best diagnostic clue
  - Children: T1 shortening of globi pallidi (GP) 2° to hepatic injury
  - Children and adults: Symmetrical T2 hyperintensity or mixed intensity in putamina, globi pallidi (GP), caudate nuclei, thalami
- Location
  - Children: Hepatic fibrosis ⇒ T1 shortening in GP

- Adults: Putamen (predilection for outer rim), dorsal/central pons, caudate nuclei, GP, thalami (ventrolateral nuclei)
  - Infratentorial: Midbrain, cerebellar nuclei, dentatorubrothalamic, pontocerebellar and corticospinal tracts
- Size: Initially ↑ (swelling of BG), then ↓ (atrophy)
- Morphology: No change in shape of affected structures

### CT Findings

- NECT
  - Widening of frontal horns of lateral ventricles
  - Diffuse cerebral and cerebellar atrophy
  - ± Hypodensity in lenticular nuclei and thalami

### MR Findings

- T1WI
  - T1 signal generally reduced in BG
  - Signal intensity may be ↑ in affected GP, cerebral peduncles in childhood disease due to hepatic component of WD (portal-systemic shunt)
- T2WI
  - Generalized cerebral and cerebellar atrophy
  - Hyperintensity/mixed intensity in putamen, GP, caudate, thalamus

## DDx: Wilson Disease

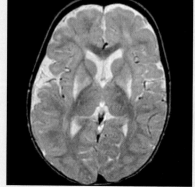

Organic Acidemia

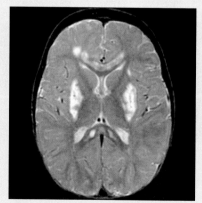

Leigh Syndrome

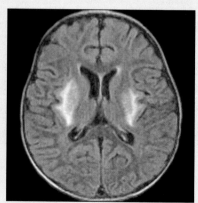

Viral Encephalitis

# WILSON DISEASE

## Key Facts

### Imaging Findings
- Children: T1 shortening of globi pallidi (GP) 2° to hepatic injury
- Children and adults: Symmetrical T2 hyperintensity or mixed intensity in putamina, globi pallidi (GP), caudate nuclei, thalami
- Characteristic "face of the giant panda" sign on axial sections at midbrain level
- Abnormally hyperintense white matter (WM) tracts
- ↓ N-acetyl aspartate/creatine (neuronal loss) in GP
- In adults, BG lesions may differ from those in children
- ↓↓ Glucose metabolism in cerebellum, striatum, and, to lesser extent, in cortex and thalamus

### Top Differential Diagnoses
- Leigh Disease

- Carbon Monoxide Poisoning
- Viral Encephalitides
- Striatonigral Degeneration
- Organic Aciduria

### Pathology
- Edema, necrosis and spongiform degeneration of BG
- Involvement of supra- and infratentorial WM

### Clinical Issues
- Onset of liver disease usually at age 8-16 yrs
- Neurological symptoms rare < 12 yrs

### Diagnostic Checklist
- Less severe changes in signal intensity with longer duration of disease

---

- Concentric-laminar T2 putaminal hyperintensity
- May show hypointensity due to ↑ iron content in BG or cavitations in aggressive WD
- Characteristic "face of the giant panda" sign on axial sections at midbrain level
  - Hyperintensity in tegmentum (except for red nucleus)
  - Hypointensity of superior colliculus
  - Preserved signal intensity of lateral portion of pars reticulata of substantia nigra
- ± Hyperintensity in periaqueductal gray matter, pontine tegmentum, cerebellar dentate nuclei
- Abnormally hyperintense white matter (WM) tracts
  - Dentatorubral if abnormal superior cerebellar peduncle (SCP) and dorsal mesencephalon
  - Dentatothalamic if abnormal SCP, dorsal mesencephalon, and thalamus
  - Pontocerebellar if abnormal base of pons, cerebellar hemispheres, and/or middle cerebellar peduncle
  - Corticospinal if abnormal posterior portion of posterior limb of internal capsule, middle division of cerebral peduncle and/or base of pons
  - ↑ Signal intensity in cerebral, cerebellar white matter
- DWI
  - ↓ Diffusion immediately after onset of neurologic symptoms
  - ↑ Diffusion in subacute and chronic stages
- T1 C+: No contrast-enhancement
- MRS
  - ↓ N-acetyl aspartate/creatine (neuronal loss) in GP
  - ↓ Choline/creatine ratio in GP
  - ↓ Myoinositol/creatine ratio in WD with portosystemic shunting vs WD without shunting
- In adults, BG lesions may differ from those in children
  - Putaminal lesions may not be present
  - GP and substantia nigra may show T2 hypointensity
  - ± Cortical, subcortical lesions (mainly frontal lobe)

### Nuclear Medicine Findings
- PET
  - ↓↓ Glucose metabolism in cerebellum, striatum, and, to lesser extent, in cortex and thalamus

- ↓↓ Dopa-decarboxylase activity (impaired nigrostriatal dopaminergic pathway)
- SPECT
  - (123I)2β-carbomethoxy-3β-(4(123I)iodophenyl)tropane
    - Binds to presynaptic striatal dopamine carriers
  - (123I)iodobenzamide
    - Binds to postsynaptic striatal dopamine D2R
  - In WD patients without neurologic symptoms
    - Normal striatal binding ratios of both tracers
  - In symptomatic WD patients
    - ↓↓ Striatal binding ratios of both tracers
  - In all patients with WD
    - Highly correlated binding ratios of both tracers
    - SPECT parameters significantly correlate with severity of neurologic symptoms
  - Neurologic WD = secondary Parkinsonian syndrome
    - Altered pre- and post-synaptic dopaminergic tracts

### Imaging Recommendations
- Best imaging tool: MRI better than CT for early lesions
- Protocol advice: T2WI, DWI

## DIFFERENTIAL DIAGNOSIS

### Leigh Disease
- Symmetrical spongiform brain lesions with onset in infancy/early childhood
- Lesions predominantly in brainstem, BG (particularly putamen) and cerebral white matter (WM)
- Focal, bilateral and symmetric T2 hyperintense lesions

### Carbon Monoxide Poisoning
- Bilateral GP hypodensity on CT, hyperintensity on T2

### Viral Encephalitides
- Enteroviruses, herpesviruses most common
- Homogeneous T2 hyperintensities in BG and thalami
  - Symmetric or bilateral asymmetric
- White matter tracts, hippocampus often involved
- Posteromedial part of thalamus
  - Spared in WD, always involved in viral encephalitis
- Bilateral thalamic hyperintensities ± hemorrhage

# WILSON DISEASE

## Striatonigral Degeneration

- Hypo- and hyperintense T2 changes in putamen
  - T2 hypointensity of dorsolateral putamen
  - T2 slit-like hyperintensity of putaminal outer rim
  - Highly specific of multiple system atrophy (parkinsonism)

## Organic Aciduria

- Symmetrical diffuse WM changes, wide CSF spaces
- BG changes (↑ T2 signal ± volume loss in caudate and/or lentiform nuclei)

## PATHOLOGY

### General Features

- General path comments
  - Excess copper throughout brain, with unexplained tendency for extensive BG damage
  - Brain lesions usually bilateral, often symmetrical
  - Abnormal WM in extrapyramidal, pyramidal tracts
    - WD considered an extrapyramidal disease
- Genetics
  - Autosomal recessive
  - Responsible gene: ATP7B, chromosome 13q14.3-q21.1
- Etiology
  - Defective incorporation of copper into ceruloplasmin and impaired biliary copper excretion
  - Brain lesions caused by accumulation of copper, chronic ischemia, vasculopathy, or demyelination
- Epidemiology
  - Prevalence: 1 in 30,000 people
  - US carrier frequency: 1 per 90 individuals

### Gross Pathologic & Surgical Features

- Softening and degeneration of basal ganglia
- Widening of cerebral and cerebellar sulci

### Microscopic Features

- Edema, necrosis and spongiform degeneration of BG
- Opalski cells = PAS–positive altered glial cells
- Involvement of supra- and infratentorial WM
  - Capillary endothelial swelling, gliosis
  - Spongiform degeneration, demyelination
- Deep pyramidal cell layers of cerebral cortex involved

### Staging, Grading or Classification Criteria

- Stage 1: Initial period of accumulation of copper by hepatic binding sites
- Stage 2: Acute redistribution of copper within liver and release into circulation
- Stage 3: Chronic accumulation of copper in brain and other extrahepatic tissues

## CLINICAL ISSUES

### Presentation

- Most common signs/symptoms
  - Neurologic: Asymmetric tremor, ataxia, dyskinesia, dysarthria, dystonia (mainly face), incoordination
    - Parkinsonian symptoms: Rigidity, bradykinesia
  - Psychiatric: Hyperkinetic behavior, irritability, emotional lability, difficulty in concentration, depression, psychosis, mania, personality change
  - Acute hepatitis, Kayser-Fleischer ring in cornea
  - Subtle pyramidal signs in up to 20%
- Clinical Profile
  - 40-50% of patients present with liver disease
  - 35-50% with neurological or psychiatric symptoms
  - Corneal rings always present in neurologic WD

### Demographics

- Age
  - Onset of liver disease usually at age 8-16 yrs
  - Neurological symptoms rare < 12 yrs
  - WD often recognized in 2nd-3rd decade
- Gender: M = F; M:F = 1:4 for fulminant WD presentation
- Ethnicity: Higher prevalence in Japan (consanguinity)

### Natural History & Prognosis

- Children: Liver disease most common presentation
- Older individuals: Neuropsychiatric symptoms
  - ↑ Symptom severity with ↑ brain copper deposition
- Once symptomatic, WD is fatal if untreated
- Good prognosis with early chelation treatment
- Best prognosis: Treated asymptomatic siblings

### Treatment

- Penicillamine, trientine, zinc, $NH_4$ tetrathiomolybdate
- Liver transplant (for severe hepatic decompensation)

## DIAGNOSTIC CHECKLIST

### Image Interpretation Pearls

- Less severe changes in signal intensity with longer duration of disease

## SELECTED REFERENCES

1. Favrole P et al: Clinical correlates of cerebral water diffusion in Wilson disease. Neurology. 66(3):384-9, 2006
2. Juan CJ et al: Acute putaminal necrosis and white matter demyelination in a child with subnormal copper metabolism in Wilson disease: MR imaging and spectroscopic findings. Neuroradiology. 47(6):401-5, 2005
3. Kitzberger R et al: Wilson disease. Metab Brain Dis. 20(4):295-302, 2005
4. Semnic R et al: Magnetic resonance imaging morphometry of the midbrain in patients with Wilson disease. J Comput Assist Tomogr. 29(6):880-3, 2005
5. Page RA et al: Clinical correlation of brain MRI and MRS abnormalities in patients with Wilson disease. Neurology. 63(4):638-43, 2004
6. Barthel H et al: Concordant Pre- and Postsynaptic Deficits of Dopaminergic Neurotransmission in Neurologic Wilson Disease. Am J Neuroradiol 24:234-238, 2003
7. Sener RN: Diffusion MR Imaging Changes Associated with Wilson Disease. Am J Neuroradiol 24:965-967, 2003
8. Van Wassenaer-van Hall HN et al: Cranial MR in Wilson Disease: Abnormal White Matter in Extrapyramidal and Pyramidal Tracts. Am J Neuroradiol 16:2021-2027, 1995
9. Hitoshi S et al: Midbrain pathology of Wilson's disease: MRI analysis of three cases. J Neurol Neurosurg Psych 54:624-626, 1991

# WILSON DISEASE

## IMAGE GALLERY

### Typical

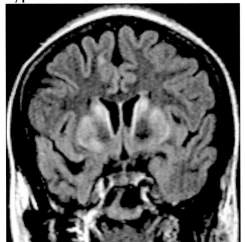
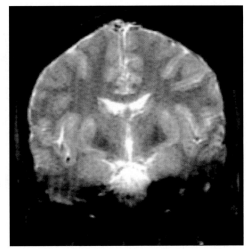

*(Left)* Coronal FLAIR MR shows hyperintensity of the caudate heads and the putamina. The globi pallidi are also affected. Note the characteristic rim of hyperintensity around the putamina. *(Right)* Coronal T2* GRE MR shows hypointensity of globi pallidi due to iron deposition. Subtle hyperintensity of the putamina and caudate heads is present.

### Typical

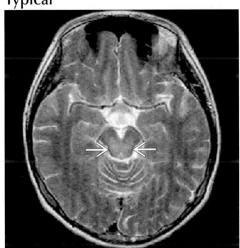
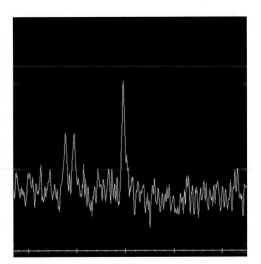

*(Left)* Axial T2WI MR shows subtle hyperintensity ➡ of the midbrain tegmentum. The normal hypointensity of the red nuclei is not visible. *(Right)* MRS with intermediate TE (144 msec) shows ↓ N-acetyl aspartate/creatine in the basal ganglia. Lactate is absent.

### Typical

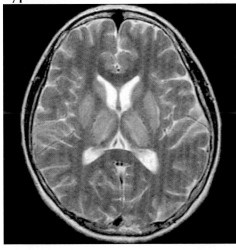
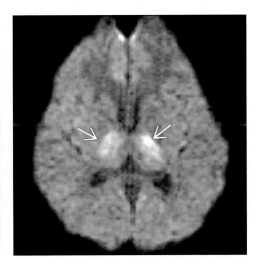

*(Left)* Axial T2WI MR shows mild cortical atrophy and hyperintensity of the basal ganglia and thalami. Note peripheral hyperintensity of the thalami and left lateral putamen. *(Right)* Axial DWI MR shows hyperintensity ➡ in the ventrolateral thalami, indicating reduced diffusivity and active disease in that location.

# HYPOGLYCEMIA

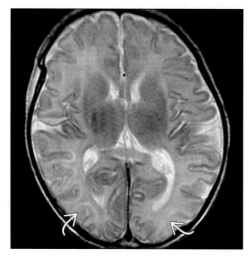

Axial T2WI MR shows hyperintensity of the cortical gray matter ➔ in the occipital lobes causing blurring of the gray-white matter junction ("missing cortex sign").

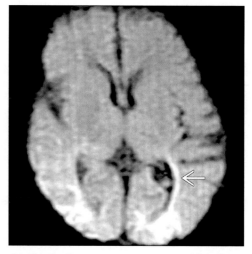

Axial DWI MR shows reduced diffusion in the occipital lobes involving both cortex & white matter. Reduced diffusivity is also present in the optic radiations ➔.

## TERMINOLOGY

### Abbreviations and Synonyms
- Neonatal hypoglycemic brain injury

### Definitions
- Neonatal hypoglycemia → imbalance between supply and utilization of glucose (Gluc) → brain injury

## IMAGING FINDINGS

### General Features
- Best diagnostic clue: Bilateral occipito-parietal edema or infarcts in newborn with seizures
- Location: Parietal, occipital > temporal, basal ganglia

### CT Findings
- NECT: ↓ Bilateral occipito-parietal density

### MR Findings
- Early: ↓ T1, ↑ T2 → infarct > edema
- Subacute: ↑ T1, ↓ T2 cortex → laminar necrosis, Ca++
- Late: Encephalomalacia, gliosis, atrophy
- DWI: Reduced diffusion in acute phase of injury

- MRS: ↓ NAA, (+) lactate

### Imaging Recommendations
- Best imaging tool: MR + DWI

## DIFFERENTIAL DIAGNOSIS

### Venous Thrombosis
- May occur in neonates ± neonatal hypoglycemia

### PRES
- Older children; immunosuppression; diffusion (-)

### Metabolic Stroke
- Lobar edema in urea cycle disorders

## PATHOLOGY

### General Features
- General path comments
  - Newborns with ↓ capacity for mobilizing glucose from glycogenolysis/gluconeogenesis (GNG) OR for utilizing alternative substrates → hypoglycemia

## DDx: Causes of Bilateral Posterior T2 Hyperintensity

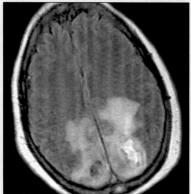

Venous Thrombosis

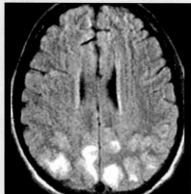

PRES

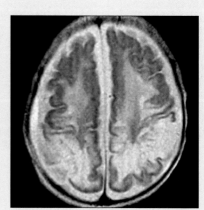

Metabolic Stroke

# HYPOGLYCEMIA

## Key Facts

### Terminology
- Neonatal hypoglycemic brain injury

### Imaging Findings
- Best diagnostic clue: Bilateral occipito-parietal edema or infarcts in newborn with seizures

### Top Differential Diagnoses
- Venous Thrombosis
- PRES

- Metabolic Stroke

### Pathology
- Newborns with ↓ capacity for mobilizing glucose from glycogenolysis/gluconeogenesis (GNG) OR for utilizing alternative substrates → hypoglycemia

### Clinical Issues
- Clinical Profile: Risk factors: Small OR large babies, newborns with metabolic stress

---

- ○ Embryology-anatomy
  - ▪ Gluc crosses placenta, stored as hepatic glycogen
  - ▪ Transition to extrauterine life requires ↑ substrate
  - ▪ GNG: Formation of Gluc from amino acids & fat
- Genetics
  - ○ Persistent hyperinsulinemic hypoglycemia infancy (PHHI): Recessive > dominant, gene 11p15 region
  - ○ Beckwith-Wiedemann (BWS): Gene 11p15 region
- Etiology
  - ○ Inadequate substrate reserve (liver), muscle stores of amino acids (GNG substrates), or lipid stores
    - ▪ Seen with IUGR, preeclampsia, maternal hypoglycemia, bleed
  - ○ ↑ Gluc use: Hypoxia, sepsis, heart disease, ↑ bilirubin
  - ○ Hyperinsulinism: Uncontrolled maternal diabetes, PHHI, BWS
  - ○ Metabolic disorders, midline anomalies + endocrine deficiencies
- Epidemiology
  - ○ 1.3-3 per 1,000 live births
  - ○ PHHI: 1:40,000 Caucasians; ↑ in population isolates

## Gross Pathologic & Surgical Features
- Pale & edematous brain, blurred gray/white boundary

## Staging, Grading or Classification Criteria
- Transitional-adaptive (adaptation to extrauterine life) → mild, brief hypoglycemia, responds to Gluc
- Secondary-associated (additional stresses of HIE, bleed, sepsis) → mild hypoglycemia, responds to Gluc
- Classic-transient (IUGR & ↓ substrate/impaired GNG) → persistent late hypoglycemia, requires ↑ Gluc

- Severe recurrent hypoglycemia → variable onset, severe despite Gluc

## CLINICAL ISSUES

### Presentation
- Most common signs/symptoms: Seizures/jitteriness, hypotonia, tachypnea, tachycardia, temperature instability, diaphoresis
- Clinical Profile: Risk factors: Small OR large babies, newborns with metabolic stress

### Natural History & Prognosis
- Uncontrolled hypoglycemia may cause irreversible brain injury → seizures, ↓ vision, mental retardation

### Treatment
- Maternal diabetic control to ↓ neonatal macrosomia
- Screen at-risk newborns or symptomatic newborns
- Intravenous Gluc to restore normal blood Gluc level
- PHHI → diazoxide, octreotide, frequent feeding, subtotal pancreatectomy, raw cornstarch at night

## SELECTED REFERENCES

1. Filan PM et al: Neonatal hypoglycemia and occipital cerebral injury. J Pediatr. 148(4):552-5, 2006
2. Alkalay AL et al: Neurologic aspects of neonatal hypoglycemia. Isr Med Assoc J. 7(3):188-92, 2005
3. Barkovich AJ et al: Imaging patterns of neonatal hypoglycemia. AJNR Am J Neuroradiol. 19(3):523-8, 1998

## IMAGE GALLERY

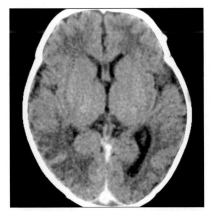 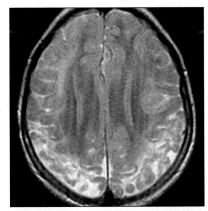 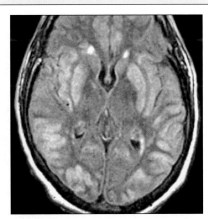

*(Left)* Axial CECT shows conspicuous occipital white matter hypodensity in infant 1 week post event. Early CT findings include blurring of gray-white junction secondary to cortical edema/ischemia. *(Center)* Axial T2WI MR shows typical late findings of neonatal hypoglycemia. There is encephalomalacia and gliosis in the occipital and parietal lobes. *(Right)* Axial FLAIR MR shows hyperintensity and swelling in temporal, occipital, parietal lobe cortices & basal ganglia. Involvement of temporal lobes & basal ganglia is the pattern in older children.

# KERNICTERUS

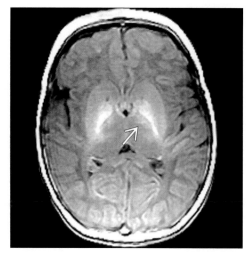
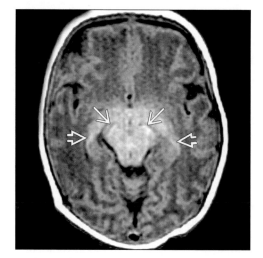

*Axial T1WI MR in a term neonate shows there is increased signal intensity* ➡ *in the entire globus pallidus bilaterally, especially in the medial/posterior nuclei.*

*Axial T1WI MR (same patient as previous image) at the level of midbrain shows thin bands of increased signal* ➡ *in the reticular zone of the substantia nigra and in the hippocampi* ➡.

## TERMINOLOGY

### Abbreviations and Synonyms
- Bilirubin encephalopathy

### Definitions
- Encephalopathy due to deposition of toxic unconjugated bilirubin

## IMAGING FINDINGS

### General Features
- Best diagnostic clue
  - Acute: ↑ T1 signal in globus pallidus (GP), subthalamic nuclei, hippocampi, substantia nigra (SN); ± ↑ T2 signal
  - Chronic: ↑ T2 signal posteromedial border GP and dentate nucleus (DN); T1 normal

### MR Findings
- T1WI
  - Acute: ↑ T1 signal in GP, hippocampi, SN, DN

  - Note: T1 shortening in neonatal GP can be normal; look for other locations
- T2WI: Chronic: ↑ T2 signal/volume loss in posteromedial GP, hippocampi; occasionally DN

### Imaging Recommendations
- Best imaging tool: MR
- Protocol advice: Noncontrast MR (acute or chronic)

## DIFFERENTIAL DIAGNOSIS

### Selective ↑ T2 Globus Pallidus
- Methylmalonic acidemia, succinic semialdehyde dehydrogenase deficiency, L2-hydroxyglutaric aciduria, creatine deficiency, CO exposure

### ↑ T1 Globus Pallidus
- Hyperalimentation (manganese), hepatic failure

## PATHOLOGY

### General Features
- General path comments

## DDx: Increased T2 Signal in the Globus Pallidus

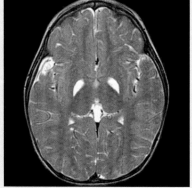
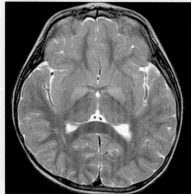
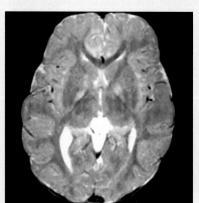

*Methylmalonic Acidemia*

*Creatine Deficiency*

*Neurofibromatosis 1*

# KERNICTERUS

## Key Facts

### Terminology
• Bilirubin encephalopathy

### Imaging Findings
• Acute: ↑ T1 signal in globus pallidus (GP), subthalamic nuclei, hippocampi, substantia nigra (SN); ± ↑ T2 signal
• Chronic: ↑ T2 signal posteromedial border GP and dentate nucleus (DN); T1 normal

### Top Differential Diagnoses
• Methylmalonic acidemia, succinic semialdehyde dehydrogenase deficiency, L2-hydroxyglutaric aciduria, creatine deficiency, CO exposure

### Pathology
• Genetics: Glucose-6-phosphate dehydrogenase (G6PD) deficiency; infants with primary liver disease (Crigler-Najjar, Gilbert disease)
• Most common cause: Erythroblastosis fetalis

○ Heme catabolism by-product ⇒ bilirubin
○ Liver glucuronyl-transferase conjugates bilirubin → excreted by kidneys
○ ↑ Unconjugated bilirubin ⇒ immature/injured blood-brain barrier ⇒ target neurons
○ Free bilirubin ≥ 20 mg/100 dL can be neurotoxic in full term; no tight correlation between total serum bilirubin and kernicterus
• Genetics: Glucose-6-phosphate dehydrogenase (G6PD) deficiency; infants with primary liver disease (Crigler-Najjar, Gilbert disease)
• Etiology
  ○ Most common cause: Erythroblastosis fetalis
  ○ Risk factors for ↑ bilirubin
    ▪ Breast feeding, > 10% loss birth weight, polycythemia, dehydration, hemolytic disorders
  ○ Risk factors that ↑ susceptibility to brain damage
    ▪ Drugs that compete for albumin binding
    ▪ Renal hypoalbuminemia, hepatic failure, prematurity, sepsis
    ▪ ↑ Cerebral blood flow (respiratory acidosis); abnormal blood brain barrier
• Epidemiology: ↑ Incidence with early discharge, breast feeding; poor infant feeding

### Gross Pathologic & Surgical Features
• Yellow staining > than seen on imaging
  ○ GP, "red-zone" of SN, subthalamic nuclei, mamillary bodies, lateral nuclei thalamus, hippocampi
  ○ Cranial nerve nuclei (3, 8)
  ○ Dentate nuclei, cerebellar flocculi, inferior olive

## CLINICAL ISSUES

### Presentation
• Acute, 2-5 days of life: Severe jaundice, somnolence, hypotonia, opisthotonus; rigidity, high-pitched cry

### Natural History & Prognosis
• Chronic: Choreoathetoid cerebral palsy, ataxia, cognitive delay, gaze paresis, deafness

### Treatment
• Early determination of hemolytic disease: Umbilical cord blood for blood type, Rh, Coombs and G6PD
• Anti-D immunoglobulin prophylaxis
• Hydration, phototherapy and exchange transfusion: Can result in resolution of neurologic and radiographic abnormalities

## DIAGNOSTIC CHECKLIST

### Consider
• MRS to exclude mitochondrial, metabolic disorder

## SELECTED REFERENCES

1. Govaert P et al: Changes in globus pallidus with (pre)term kernicterus. Pediatrics. 112(6 Pt 1):1256-63, 2003
2. Rorke LB: Neuropathologic findings in bilirubin encephalopathy (kernicterus). IJNR 4(3):165-70, 1998

## IMAGE GALLERY

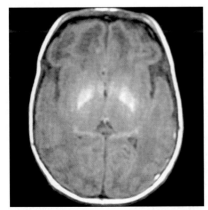 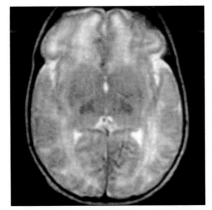 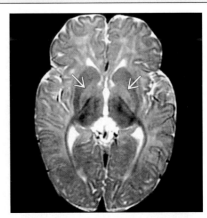

*(Left) Axial T1WI MR in a term neonate, now 11 days old, shows symmetric increased signal in entire globus pallidus bilaterally. (Center) Axial T2WI MR (same patient as previous image) does not show T2 signal abnormality in acute, neonatal phase of kernicterus. Basal ganglia & thalami are normal in appearance. (Right) Axial T2WI MR (same patient as previous image) 9 months later shows bilateral symmetric increased T2 signal in globus pallidus ➡. T2 signal of the pallidum is greater than expected for this age.*

# MESIAL TEMPORAL SCLEROSIS

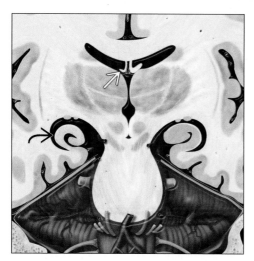

Coronal graphic demonstrates atrophy & loss of internal architecture of right hippocampus →, related to neuronal loss & gliosis characteristic of MTS. Note atrophy of fornix →.

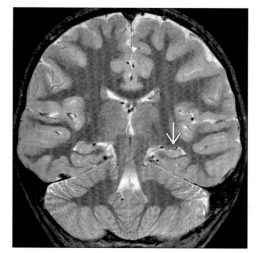

Coronal STIR MR shows asymmetric volume loss & abnormal T2 hyperintensity of left hippocampal formation → compared to normal right mesial temporal lobe.

## TERMINOLOGY

### Abbreviations and Synonyms
- Mesial temporal sclerosis (MTS), hippocampal sclerosis (HS), Ammon horn sclerosis

### Definitions
- Seizure-associated neuronal loss & gliosis in hippocampus, adjacent structures

## IMAGING FINDINGS

### General Features
- Best diagnostic clue: 1° criteria include T2 hyperintensity, hippocampal volume loss, obscuration of internal architecture
- Location
  - Mesial temporal lobe
  - Unilateral > bilateral (20%)

### CT Findings
- NECT: Insensitive to MTS; normal unless marked volume loss

### MR Findings
- T1WI
  - ↓ Hippocampal volume
  - Loss of hippocampal gray-white differentiation
- T2WI
  - Hippocampal ↓ volume, hyperintensity
  - Distortion of internal hippocampal architecture
  - ± Fornix/mamillary body atrophy, temporal horn enlargement, ↓ hippocampal head digitations, parahippocampal gyrus atrophy, ↑ signal in anterior temporal white matter
- FLAIR
  - ↑ Hippocampal signal
  - Pitfall: Hippocampus normally slightly hyperintense to neocortex
- DWI
  - Acute hippocampal injury ⇒ reduced diffusivity
  - Chronic MTS ↑ ADC ⇒ normalized DWI
- T1 C+: No enhancement
- MRS
  - ↓ NAA in hippocampus, ipsilateral temporal lobe
  - NAA/Cho ≤ 0.8 & NAA/Cr ≤ 1.0 suggest MTS

## DDx: Mesial Temporal Lobe Hyperintense Lesions

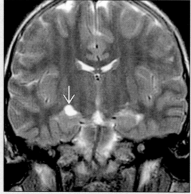

Choroidal Fissure Cyst

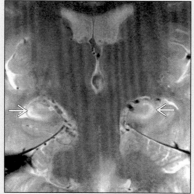

Status Epilepticus

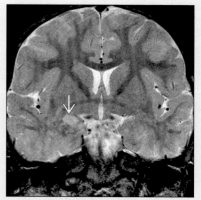

Ganglioglioma

# MESIAL TEMPORAL SCLEROSIS

## Key Facts

### Terminology
- Mesial temporal sclerosis (MTS), hippocampal sclerosis (HS), Ammon horn sclerosis

### Imaging Findings
- Best diagnostic clue: 1° criteria include T2 hyperintensity, hippocampal volume loss, obscuration of internal architecture
- Unilateral > bilateral (20%)

### Top Differential Diagnoses
- Choroidal Fissure Cyst
- Hippocampal Sulcus Remnant
- Status Epilepticus
- Low Grade Neoplasm
- Dysembryoplastic Neuroepithelial Tumor (DNET)

### Pathology
- Mesial temporal lobe atrophy without hemorrhage or necrosis
- Associated abnormalities: Dual pathology in 15+%, cortical dysplasia most common; pediatric >> adult

### Clinical Issues
- Complex partial seizures (CPS) ± 2° generalization
- Clinical features, EEG, & seizure outcome in adolescents with MTS similar to adults

### Diagnostic Checklist
- Coronal high-resolution T2WI best modality to diagnose MTS
- Quantitative volumetric (3D SPGR) imaging increases sensitivity for MTS detection (particularly bilateral)
- Search for dual pathology

## Nuclear Medicine Findings
- FDG PET: Hypometabolism (interictal) in affected mesial temporal lobe (sensitivity 65-75%)
- HMPAO SPECT
  - Interictal: Hypoperfusion in epileptogenic zone (sensitivity 65-75%)
  - Ictal: Focal ↑ uptake in affected temporal lobe
  - Note: Ictal SPECT more sensitive than interictal SPECT

## Imaging Recommendations
- Best imaging tool
  - High-resolution temporal lobe MR
    - Sensitivity 80 → 97%, specificity 83%
  - MRS may help lateralize MTS in discordant cases
- Protocol advice
  - Thin-section coronal T2WI (3-4 mm) & 3D T1 SPGR (1-2 mm) angled perpendicular to hippocampus long axis
  - Coronal FLAIR through temporal lobes
  - Phased-array surface coil or multichannel phased array head coil ↑↑ improves spatial resolution

## DIFFERENTIAL DIAGNOSIS

### Choroidal Fissure Cyst
- Asymptomatic cyst in choroidal fissure; may distort normal hippocampus
- Follows CSF signal, no T2 hyperintensity of mesial temporal lobe

### Hippocampal Sulcus Remnant
- Failure of normal hippocampal sulcus involution ⇒ bilateral hippocampal cysts between dentate gyrus, cornu ammonis
- Asymptomatic normal variant (10-15%)

### Status Epilepticus
- T2 hyperintensity in affected brain ± gyriform enhancement, diffusion restriction
- Clinical history of status epilepticus

### Low Grade Neoplasm
- Focal or diffuse T2 hyperintense temporal lobe mass ± enhancement
- Typically young adult
- Ganglioneuroma, astrocytoma most common

### Dysembryoplastic Neuroepithelial Tumor (DNET)
- Demarcated "bubbly" cortical mass with variable enhancement
- Often associated cortical dysplasia

## PATHOLOGY

### General Features
- General path comments
  - Mesial temporal lobe atrophy without hemorrhage or necrosis
  - Hippocampal formation includes cornu ammonis (CA), dentate gyrus, hippocampal sulcus, fimbria, alveus, fornix, subiculum, parahippocampal gyrus, collateral sulcus
  - Hippocampus has 3 longitudinal portions (head/pes, body, tail) and 4 subfields (CA1-CA4)
    - CA1 (Sommer sector) = most sensitive to ischemia
    - CA2 = most resistant to ischemia
    - CA3 = mildly vulnerable to ischemia
    - CA4 (endfolium) = intermediate vulnerability to ischemia
  - Three hippocampal cell loss patterns described
    - Classic Ammon horn sclerosis ⇒ primary neuronal loss in CA1, CA4; less often dentate, CA2
    - Total Ammon horn sclerosis ⇒ severe neuronal loss of all hippocampal zones
    - Endfolium sclerosis ⇒ cell loss restricted to CA4
- Genetics
  - Familial temporal lobe epilepsy reported
  - Genetic component may predispose some to MTS
- Etiology
  - Etiology controversial whether acquired or developmental

# MESIAL TEMPORAL SCLEROSIS

○ Most likely MTS represents common outcome of both acquired & developmental processes
○ Acquired
  ▪ "Two-hit hypothesis": Initial precipitating injury (IPI) & second factor that ↑ vulnerability to neuronal injury
  ▪ Putative causative factors: Prolonged or complex febrile seizures, multiple seizures in early childhood, status epilepticus, complicated delivery, ischemia
○ Developmental
  ▪ 2nd lesion (usually cortical dysplasia) in ≥ 15% pediatric MTS patients
  ▪ Hippocampal dysgenesis may account for febrile seizures & MTS in small subpopulation of epilepsy patients
• Epidemiology
  ○ Epilepsy affects 0.5-1% of US population
  ○ Complex partial seizures ~ 35% of epilepsy cases
  ○ 15-30% epilepsy patients medically refractory → surgical consultation
• Associated abnormalities: Dual pathology in 15+%, cortical dysplasia most common; pediatric >> adult

## Gross Pathologic & Surgical Features
• Hippocampal body (88%) > tail (61%) > head (51%) > amygdala (12%)

## Microscopic Features
• Chronic fibrillary astrogliosis & neuronal loss

# CLINICAL ISSUES

## Presentation
• Most common signs/symptoms
  ○ Complex partial seizures (CPS) ± 2° generalization
    ▪ ~ 50% of MTS patients have a history of childhood prolonged febrile convulsion (PFC)
• Other signs/symptoms: May progress to tonic-clonic seizures
• Clinical Profile
  ○ Clinical features, EEG, & seizure outcome in adolescents with MTS similar to adults
  ○ Young children (≤ 5 years) have distinct semiology & outcome compared to adults

## Demographics
• Age: May occur at any age; ↑ incidence in young adulthood, adolescence
• Gender: No gender predominance

## Natural History & Prognosis
• Majority of patients have good clinical outcome following febrile seizure
  ○ MTS development uncommon even after prolonged febrile seizures
  ○ Lag period of several years between PFC → MTS, epilepsy onset
  ○ Unfavorable outcome more likely with bitemporal or multifocal epileptiform discharges
• Medical control successful in majority of CPS patients with MTS

## Treatment
• Initial medical management
• Up to 30% MTS patients medically refractory epilepsy → surgical candidates
• Surgical management → anterior temporal lobectomy (ATL) with partial hippocampectomy/amygdalectomy
• 78-90% children seizure-free following surgery
  ○ + MTS (MR): ATL successful ~ 70-95%
  ○ Normal MR: ATL success ~ 40-55%
  ○ Abnormal amygdala: ATL success ~ 50%

# DIAGNOSTIC CHECKLIST

## Consider
• MTS uncommon in children but always associated with epilepsy
• Acute hippocampal injury may demonstrate ↑ T2 signal & volume ± reduced diffusion

## Image Interpretation Pearls
• Coronal high-resolution T2WI best modality to diagnose MTS
  ○ Hippocampal T2 hyperintensity & atrophy most sensitive MTS signs
  ○ Routine axial MR & CT insensitive to MTS
• Quantitative volumetric (3D SPGR) imaging increases sensitivity for MTS detection (particularly bilateral)
• Search for dual pathology

# SELECTED REFERENCES

1. Araujo D et al: Volumetric evidence of bilateral damage in unilateral mesial temporal lobe epilepsy. Epilepsia. 47(8):1354-9, 2006
2. Ng YT et al: Childhood mesial temporal sclerosis. J Child Neurol. 21(6):512-7, 2006
3. Lewis DV: Losing neurons: selective vulnerability and mesial temporal sclerosis. Epilepsia. 46 Suppl 7:39-44, 2005
4. Mittal S et al: Long-term outcome after surgical treatment of temporal lobe epilepsy in children. J Neurosurg. 103(5 Suppl):401-12, 2005
5. Mulani SJ et al: Magnetic resonance volumetric analysis of hippocampi in children in the age group of 6-to-12 years: a pilot study. Neuroradiology. 47(7):552-7, 2005
6. Cendes F: Febrile seizures and mesial temporal sclerosis. Curr Opin Neurol. 17(2):161-4, 2004
7. Farina L et al: Acute diffusion abnormalities in the hippocampus of children with new-onset seizures: the development of mesial temporal sclerosis. Neuroradiology. 46(4):251-7, 2004
8. Ng YT et al: Magnetic resonance imaging detection of mesial temporal sclerosis in children. Pediatr Neurol. 30(2):81-5, 2004
9. Scott RC et al: Hippocampal abnormalities after prolonged febrile convulsion: a longitudinal MRI study. Brain. 126(Pt 11):2551-7, 2003
10. Sinclair DB et al: Pediatric temporal lobectomy for epilepsy. Pediatr Neurosurg. 38(4):195-205, 2003
11. Tarkka R et al: Febrile seizures and mesial temporal sclerosis: No association in a long-term follow-up study. Neurology. 60(2):215-8, 2003
12. Capizzano AA et al: Multisection proton MR spectroscopy for mesial temporal lobe epilepsy. AJNR Am J Neuroradiol. 23(8):1359-68, 2002

# MESIAL TEMPORAL SCLEROSIS

## IMAGE GALLERY

### Typical

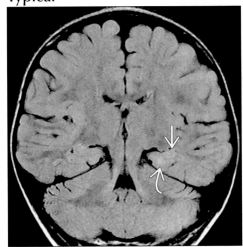 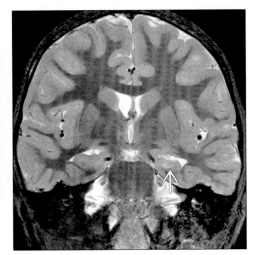

*(Left)* Coronal FLAIR MR demonstrates asymmetric left hippocampal volume loss with abnormal T2 prolongation in hippocampus ➡ and parahippocampal gyrus ➡. The right hippocampus appears normal. *(Right)* Coronal STIR MR shows asymmetric left hippocampal head ("pes") volume loss & flattened undulations ➡ compared to normal right hippocampus. Note ipsilateral temporal horn dilatation.

### Typical

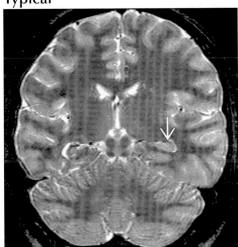 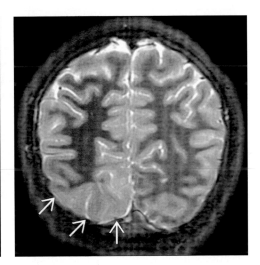

*(Left)* Coronal STIR MR reveals left MTS ➡. Findings meet all three primary diagnostic criteria (T2 hyperintensity, volume loss, obscuration of internal architecture). *(Right)* Coronal STIR MR in an MTS patient shows concurrent right occipital cortical dysplasia ➡. Dual pathology is identified in up to 15% of MTS patients.

### Typical

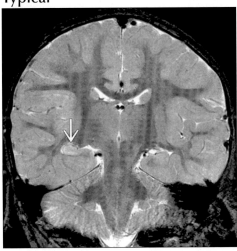 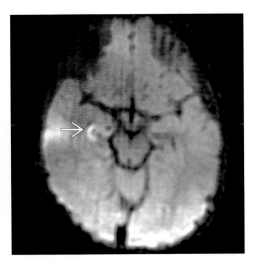

*(Left)* Coronal STIR MR in patient with acute febrile seizure shows abnormal T2 prolongation within right hippocampus without associated volume loss ➡. This is an important differentiating point. *(Right)* Axial DWI MR in patient with acute febrile seizure reveals reduced diffusion ➡ within right hippocampus. ADC map confirmed abnormal diffusivity (not T2 "shine through").

# ACUTE DISSEMINATED ENCEPHALOMYELITIS

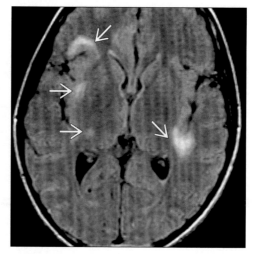

Axial NECT in a child who presented with seizures shows focal decreased attenuation in the white matter of the posterior left temporal lobe ➽ with acute disseminated encephalomyelitis.

Axial FLAIR MR (same child as previous image) shows multiple lesions ➥. There should be a low threshold for performing MR imaging in the appropriate clinical setting for ADEM, even with a normal CT.

## TERMINOLOGY

### Abbreviations and Synonyms
- Acute disseminated encephalomyelitis (ADEM)

### Definitions
- Autoimmune-mediated demyelination
  - Affects both brain and spinal cord
  - Rarely can involve peripheral nerves
    - Overlap with Guillain-Barre syndrome
- Acute hemorrhagic leukoencephalitis (AHEM)
  - Can be regarded as the most severe subtype of ADEM
  - Larger lesions with more mass effect and hemorrhage
- Typically monophasic
  - Multiphasic disseminated encephalomyelitis (MDEM) may actually be variant multiple sclerosis (MS)
  - 15% of patients initially diagnosed with ADEM eventually diagnosed as MS

## IMAGING FINDINGS

### General Features
- Best diagnostic clue: Multifocal hyperintense lesions on T2WI and FLAIR 10-14 days after viral infection or vaccination
- Location
  - Brain ⇒ white matter (WM), basal ganglia, some gray matter (GM)
    - Cerebrum > cerebellum
  - Deep nuclei involvement in 50%
    - May present in delayed fashion, after initial diagnosis
- Size
  - Typically multifocal, small to moderate in size
    - Tumefactive lesions may be large (several cm), with less-than-expected mass effect
- Morphology
  - Amorphous, sometimes spherical or ovoid
    - Less regular in shape than lesions of multiple sclerosis

### CT Findings
- NECT

## DDx: White Matter Lesions in Children

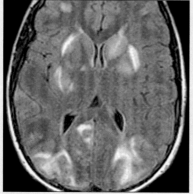

PRES

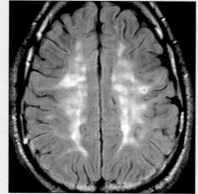

Multiple Sclerosis

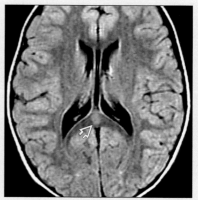

Influenza

# ACUTE DISSEMINATED ENCEPHALOMYELITIS

## Key Facts

### Terminology

- Acute disseminated encephalomyelitis (ADEM)
- Autoimmune-mediated demyelination
- Typically monophasic

### Imaging Findings

- Best diagnostic clue: Multifocal hyperintense lesions on T2WI and FLAIR 10-14 days after viral infection or vaccination
- Brain ⇒ white matter (WM), basal ganglia, some gray matter (GM)
- Initial CT normal in 40%
- Predilection for subcortical white matter
- May involve brainstem, posterior fossa, spinal cord
- Variably reduced diffusivity in acute lesions
- May appear identical to MS

### Top Differential Diagnoses

- Multiple Sclerosis (MS)
- Histiocytosis Syndromes
- Posterior Reversible Encephalopathy Syndrome (PRES)

### Clinical Issues

- Multifocal neurological symptoms; 5-14 days after viral illness/immunization
- Cerebrospinal fluid often abnormal (↑ leukocytes, ↑ protein)
- Usually monophasic, self-limited
- Complete recovery within one month: 50-60%
- Neurologic sequelae (most commonly seizures): 20-30%
- Mortality: 10-30%

---

- Initial CT normal in 40%
- Low density asymmetric WM lesions
- CECT
  - Typically shows more lesions
  - Multifocal subcortical lesions with mild-to-moderate enhancement

## MR Findings

- T1WI: Low signal lesions with minimal mass effect
- T2WI
  - T2 may show hyperintense pontine and brainstem lesions more clearly than FLAIR
    - WM lesions easiest to see on FLAIR
- FLAIR
  - Multifocal FLAIR hyperintensities
    - Range from punctate to mass-like
  - Bilateral but asymmetric
  - Predilection for subcortical white matter
  - May involve brainstem, posterior fossa, spinal cord
- DWI
  - Variably reduced diffusivity in acute lesions
  - Reduced diffusion may portend worse outcome
    - May indicate permanent tissue injury
- T1 C+
  - Punctate enhancement, complete/incomplete ring-enhancement, peripheral enhancement
  - Cranial nerve enhancement
- MRS
  - NAA ↓ within lesions
    - Can normalize with resolution of symptoms
  - May see elevation of lactate and choline in acute lesions
- Other sequences
  - Magnetization transfer ratios (MTRs) in normal-appearing areas of ADEM patients remain normal
    - MTRs are decreased in normal-appearing areas of patients with MS
  - Mean diffusivity on diffusion tensor imaging (DTI) in normal-appearing areas of ADEM patients remains normal
    - Mean diffusivity is increased in MS

## Imaging Recommendations

- Best imaging tool
  - Contrast-enhanced MR
    - May appear identical to MS
- Protocol advice
  - MRS, DTI, and MTR may provide some insight
  - Most helpful data is history of viral prodrome or vaccination

# DIFFERENTIAL DIAGNOSIS

## Multiple Sclerosis (MS)

- MS is defined by multiple lesions separated by space and time
  - Relapsing-remitting course
- Lesions can be identical to ADEM
- MS lesions often more symmetric than ADEM
- "Multiphasic" or "relapsing" ADEM is likely same entity as MS

## Acute Necrotizing Encephalopathy of Childhood (ANEC)

- Primarily reported in Japan, Taiwan, and Korea
- Bilateral symmetric thalamic lesions with edema, necrosis and petechial hemorrhage
- Absence of inflammatory cells at pathology

## Histiocytosis Syndromes

- Langerhans cell histiocytosis (LCH)
  - Cerebellar white matter lesions
  - Bright on T2WI and FLAIR, variably enhancing
- Hemophagocytic lymphohistiocytosis (HLH)
  - Supra- and infratentorial lesions, variably enhancing
  - Associated with parenchymal volume loss

## Posterior Reversible Encephalopathy Syndrome (PRES)

- Reversible WM edema induced by hypertension, seizures, immunosuppressants
- Resolves with treatment of hypertension or reduction of offending medication

# ACUTE DISSEMINATED ENCEPHALOMYELITIS

## Autoimmune-Mediated Vasculitis
- Multifocal GM/WM lesions

## PATHOLOGY

### General Features
- General path comments: Autoimmune-mediated demyelination
- Etiology
  ○ Classically occurs after viral infection or vaccination
    ▪ Specific viral illness: Epstein-Barr, influenza A, mumps, coronavirus
    ▪ After exanthematous diseases of childhood (chickenpox, measles)
    ▪ Vaccines: Diphtheria, influenza, rabies, smallpox, tetanus, typhoid
  ○ Can occur spontaneously
    ▪ Subclinical viral prodrome?
- Epidemiology: Most common para/post-infectious disorder
- Associated abnormalities: Acute hemorrhagic leukoencephalopathy variant associated with ulcerative colitis and asthma

### Microscopic Features
- Acute myelin breakdown
- Perivenous inflammation; lymphocytic infiltrates
- Relative axonal preservation
- Atypical astrogliosis
- Virus generally not found, unlike viral encephalitides
- Similar to experimental allergic encephalomyelitis

### Staging, Grading or Classification Criteria
- 4 patterns of disease classified by Tenembaum et al
  ○ Group A ⇒ lesions < 5 mm
  ○ Group B ⇒ 1 or more lesions > 5 mm
  ○ Group C ⇒ bilateral symmetric thalamic disease
    ▪ Some overlap with ANEC?
  ○ Group D ⇒ AHEM

## CLINICAL ISSUES

### Presentation
- Most common signs/symptoms
  ○ Usually preceded by prodromal phase: Fever, malaise, myalgia
  ○ Multifocal neurological symptoms; 5-14 days after viral illness/immunization
    ▪ Initial symptoms: Headache, fever, drowsiness
    ▪ Cranial nerve palsies, seizures, hemiparesis
    ▪ Decreased consciousness (from lethargy to coma)
- Other signs/symptoms
  ○ Behavioral changes
  ○ Cerebrospinal fluid often abnormal (↑ leukocytes, ↑ protein)
    ▪ Usually lacks oligoclonal bands

### Demographics
- Age: Peak age 3-5 years

### Natural History & Prognosis
- Usually monophasic, self-limited

- Variable prognosis
  ○ Complete recovery within one month: 50-60%
  ○ Neurologic sequelae (most commonly seizures): 20-30%
  ○ Mortality: 10-30%
  ○ Relapses are rare
    ▪ "Relapsing/multiphasic" ADEM
    ▪ May not be a separate entity from relapsing-remitting MS
- Varicella and rubella associated ADEM have preferential patterns
  ○ Rubella-associated ADEM characterized by acute explosive onset, seizures, coma and moderate pyramidal signs
  ○ Varicella-associated ADEM characterized by cerebellar ataxia and mild pyramidal dysfunction

### Treatment
- Immunomodulatory therapy
  ○ Steroids
  ○ Intravenous immunoglobulin
  ○ Plasmapheresis
- MR may show prompt regression in response to treatment

## DIAGNOSTIC CHECKLIST

### Image Interpretation Pearls
- Imaging findings often lag behind symptom onset, resolution
- Distinction from MS dependent upon lack of remittance
- DWI may have some predictive value

## SELECTED REFERENCES

1. Ishizu T et al: CSF cytokine and chemokine profiles in acute disseminated encephalomyelitis. J Neuroimmunol. 175(1-2):52-8, 2006
2. Axer H et al: Initial DWI and ADC imaging may predict outcome in acute disseminated encephalomyelitis: report of two cases of brain stem encephalitis. J Neurol Neurosurg Psychiatry. 76(7):996-8, 2005
3. Mader I et al: MRI and proton MR spectroscopy in acute disseminated encephalomyelitis. Childs Nerv Syst. 21(7):566-72, 2005
4. Richer LP et al: Neuroimaging features of acute disseminated encephalomyelitis in childhood. Pediatr Neurol. 32(1):30-6, 2005
5. Leake JA et al: Acute disseminated encephalomyelitis in childhood: epidemiologic, clinical and laboratory features. Pediatr Infect Dis J. 23(8):756-64, 2004
6. Holtmannspotter M et al: A diffusion tensor MRI study of basal ganglia from patients with ADEM. J Neurol Sci. 206(1):27-30, 2003
7. Inglese M et al: Magnetization transfer and diffusion tensor MR imaging of acute disseminated encephalomyelitis. AJNR Am J Neuroradiol. 23(2):267-72, 2002
8. Tenembaum S et al: Acute disseminated encephalomyelitis: a long-term follow-up study of 84 pediatric patients. Neurology. 59(8):1224-31, 2002
9. Dale RC et al: Acute disseminated encephalomyelitis, multiphasic disseminated encephalomyelitis and multiple sclerosis in children. Brain. 123 Pt 12:2407-22, 2000

## IMAGE GALLERY

### Typical

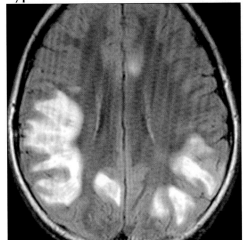
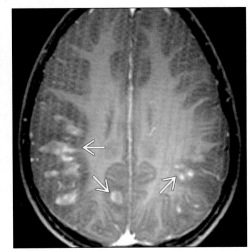

*(Left)* Axial FLAIR MR shows multiple large and confluent lesions of ADEM in both hemispheres. FLAIR sequences are the most sensitive in the detection of ADEM lesions. *(Right)* Axial T1 C+ MR (same child as previous image) shows irregular enhancement in nearly all of the lesions ➡. Lesion size and enhancement may worsen in the subacute phase, despite clinical improvement.

### Typical

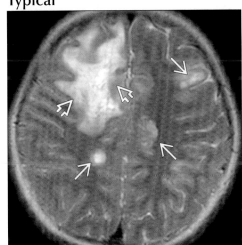
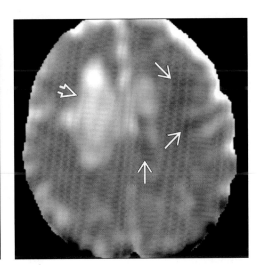

*(Left)* Axial T2WI MR shows a dominant lesion in the right frontal lobe ➡, with several smaller lesions posteriorly and on the left ➡. *(Right)* Axial ADC shows increased diffusivity in the large lesion ➡, but some areas of reduced diffusivity in the smaller lesions ➡ within the left hemisphere.

### Typical

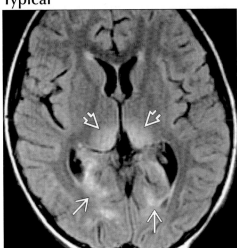
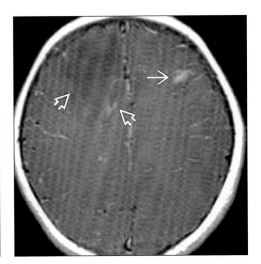

*(Left)* Axial FLAIR MR shows demyelinating lesions in the occipital white matter ➡ and in the posterior thalamus ➡. About 50% of children will have deep nuclei involvement on MR imaging. *(Right)* Axial T1WI MR shows minimal enhancement in a large ADEM lesion in the right frontal lobe ➡, with moderate enhancement of a smaller lesion in the left frontal lobe ➡.

# ACUTE HYPERTENSIVE ENCEPHALOPATHY, PRES

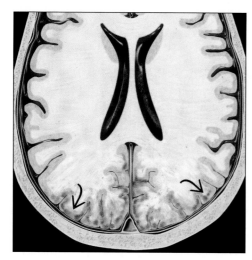

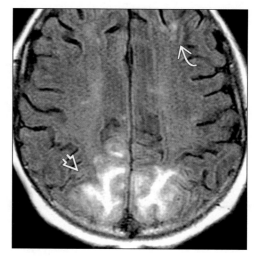

Axial graphic shows classic posterior circulation cortical/subcortical vasogenic edema. Additional petechial hemorrhages ➔ occur less frequently.

Axial FLAIR MR shows bilateral, nearly symmetrical cortical/subcortical involvement ➔ of the parieto-occipital lobes. Faint foci ➔ of frontal PRES lesions are present.

## TERMINOLOGY

### Abbreviations and Synonyms

- Hypertensive encephalopathy; posterior reversible encephalopathy syndrome (PRES); reversible posterior leukoencephalopathy syndrome (RPLS); reversible posterior cerebral edema syndrome

### Definitions

- Disorder of cerebrovascular autoregulation with multiple etiologies, most of which cause acute hypertension (HTN)

## IMAGING FINDINGS

### General Features

- Best diagnostic clue: Patchy cortical/subcortical (PCA) territory lesions in a patient with severe acute/subacute HTN
- Location
  - Most common: Cortex, subcortical white matter
    - Predilection for posterior circulation (parietal, occipital lobes, cerebellum)
    - At junctions of vascular watershed zones
    - Usually bilateral, often somewhat asymmetric
  - Less common: Basal ganglia
  - Rare: Predominate/exclusive brainstem involvement or deep white matter involvement
    - Both have lower "reversibility"
- Size: Extent of abnormalities highly variable
- Morphology: Patchy > confluent

### CT Findings

- CTA
  - Usually normal
  - Rare: Vasospasm with multifocal areas of arterial narrowing
- NECT
  - Patchy bilateral nonconfluent hypodense foci
    - Posterior parietal, occipital lobes > basal ganglia, brainstem
  - Less common: Petechial cortical/subcortical or basal ganglionic hemorrhage

### MR Findings

- T1WI: Hypointense cortical/subcortical lesions
- T2WI
  - Hyperintense cortical/subcortical lesions

## DDx: Posterior Lesions

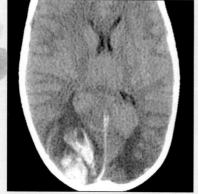

PCA Infarction

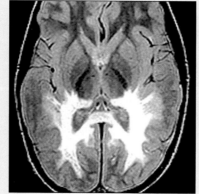

X-Linked ALD

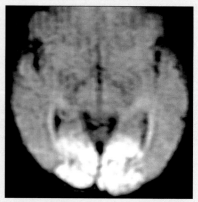

NICU Hypoglycemia

## Key Facts

### Terminology
- Hypertensive encephalopathy; posterior reversible encephalopathy syndrome (PRES); reversible posterior leukoencephalopathy syndrome (RPLS); reversible posterior cerebral edema syndrome
- Disorder of cerebrovascular autoregulation with multiple etiologies, most of which cause acute hypertension (HTN)

### Imaging Findings
- Best diagnostic clue: Patchy cortical/subcortical (PCA) territory lesions in a patient with severe acute/subacute HTN
- Parieto-occipital hyperintense cortical lesions in 95%
- Increased (interstitial) or reduced diffusivity or pseudonormalization

### Pathology
- Breakthrough of autoregulation causes blood brain barrier disruption

### Clinical Issues
- Headache, confusion, seizure, visual disturbance
- Caution: Some patients, especially children, are normotensive or have minimally elevated BP!
- Most cases resolve completely with blood pressure normalization
- Most reversible: Eclampsia
- Favorable outcome with prompt recognition, treatment of HTN

### Diagnostic Checklist
- In some cases (especially children), systemic BP may be only minimally elevated

---

- ○ Less common
  - Extensive brain stem hyperintensity
  - Generalized white matter edema
- PD/Intermediate: Multifocal hyperintensities
- FLAIR
  - ○ Parieto-occipital hyperintense cortical lesions in 95%
  - ○ ± Symmetric lesions in basal ganglia
  - ○ Does not discriminate between vasogenic, cytotoxic edema (both have increased signal intensity)
- T2* GRE: Blooms if hemorrhage present
- DWI
  - ○ Most common: Normal 58%
  - ○ Less common: High signal on DWI with reduced ADC (may indicate irreversible infarction)
  - ○ ADC map: Limitations in predicting course
    - Increased (interstitial) or reduced diffusivity or pseudonormalization
  - ○ DTI (diffusion tensor imaging): Anisotropy loss
  - ○ Perfusion: Increased microvascular CBF
- T1 C+: Variable patchy enhancement
- MRS
  - ○ May show widespread transient metabolic abnormalities
    - ↑ Cho, Cr, mildly ↓ NAA

### Nuclear Medicine Findings
- SPECT
  - ○ Variable: Hyper- or hypoperfusion in affected areas

### Imaging Recommendations
- Best imaging tool: Contrast-enhanced MR + DWI
- Protocol advice: Repeat scan after BP normalized

## DIFFERENTIAL DIAGNOSIS

### Acute Cerebral Ischemia
- Clinical history (HTN, time of symptom onset) important
- DWI usually shows restriction (high signal)

### Acute Cerebral Hyperemia
- Ictal/postictal
  - ○ May cause transient gyral edema, enhancement
- Rapid decompression of chronic SDH
  - ○ Generally localized to cortex under the SDH
- Postcarotid endarterectomy, angioplasty or stenting
  - ○ Hyperperfusion syndrome occurs in 5-9% of cases
  - ○ Perfusion MR or CT scans show elevated rCBF

### Inborn Error of Metabolism
- Posterior involvement usual in X-ALD, infantile Refsum, MELAS

### Other Metabolic Derangement
- Hypoglycemia of newborn, age best clue
- Osmotic demyelination
  - ○ Pons, basal ganglia, white matter involvement typical

### Progressive Multifocal Leukoencephalopathy (PML)
- Usually spares cortex, basal ganglia
- Immunocompromised patients

### Acute Demyelinating Disease
- "Horseshoe" > patchy enhancement
- No predilection for posterior circulation

## PATHOLOGY

### General Features
- General path comments: Typically reversible with blood pressure normalization
- Etiology
  - ○ Diverse causes, clinical entities with HTN as common component
  - ○ Acute HTN OR drug toxicity damages vascular endothelium
  - ○ Breakthrough of autoregulation causes blood brain barrier disruption

# ACUTE HYPERTENSIVE ENCEPHALOPATHY, PRES

- Primarily at arteriolar level with HTN, diabetic vasculopathy, etc.
  - Result = vasogenic (not cytotoxic) edema
    - Arteriolar dilatation with cerebral hyperperfusion
    - Hydrostatic leakage (extravasation, transudation of fluid and macromolecules through arteriolar walls)
    - Interstitial fluid accumulates in cortex, subcortical white matter
    - Posterior circulation sparsely innervated by sympathetic nerves (predilection for parietal, occipital lobes)
  - Progression to frank infarction with cytotoxic edema rare in PRES
- Epidemiology
  - Pre-eclampsia in 5% of pregnancies
  - Eclampsia lower (< 1%)
- Associated abnormalities
  - Acute/subacute systemic or malignant HTN
  - Preeclampsia, eclampsia, toxemia
    - Typically occurs after 20 weeks gestation
    - Rare: Headache, seizures up to several weeks postpartum
    - Maternal endothelial dysfunction due to secretion trophoblastic cytotoxic factors
  - Uremic encephalopathies
    - Acute glomerulonephritis
    - Hemolytic uremic syndrome (HUS)
  - Drug toxicity: Chemotherapeutic; immunosuppressive
    - Cyclosporin or FK-506
    - Tacrolimus
    - Cisplatin
    - Interferon-alpha
    - Erythropoietin
  - Other
    - Thrombotic thrombocytopenic purpura (TTP)
    - Vasculitides (SLE, polyarteritis nodosa)

## Gross Pathologic & Surgical Features
- Common
  - Cortical/subcortical edema
  - ± Petechial hemorrhage in parietal, occipital lobes
- Less common: Lesions in basal ganglia, cerebellum, brain stem, anterior frontal lobes

## Microscopic Features
- Usually no residual abnormalities after HTN corrected
- Autopsy in severe cases shows microvascular fibrinoid necrosis, ischemic microinfarcts, variable hemorrhage
- Chronic HTN associated with mural thickening, deposition of collagen, laminin, fibronectin in cerebral arterioles

# CLINICAL ISSUES

## Presentation
- Most common signs/symptoms
  - Headache, confusion, seizure, visual disturbance
  - Caution: Some patients, especially children, are normotensive or have minimally elevated BP!
- Clinical Profile: Young female with acute/subacute systemic HTN, headache ± seizure

## Demographics
- Age: Any age but young > old
- Gender: M < F

## Natural History & Prognosis
- Most cases resolve completely with blood pressure normalization
  - Most reversible: Eclampsia
  - Least reversible
    - HTN or drug related
    - Pre-existing microangiopathy
    - Thalamic, deep white matter, brainstem involvement
- May be life-threatening

## Treatment
- Favorable outcome with prompt recognition, treatment of HTN

# DIAGNOSTIC CHECKLIST

## Consider
- Patchy bilateral low density foci in occipital lobes may be earliest manifestation of PRES
- In some cases (especially children), systemic BP may be only minimally elevated

## Image Interpretation Pearls
- Major ddx of PRES is cerebral ischemia; diffusion is reduced in the latter, usually increased in the former

# SELECTED REFERENCES

1. Pande AR et al: Clinicoradiological factors influencing the reversibility of posterior reversible encephalopathy syndrome: a multicenter study. Radiat Med. 24:659-68, 2006
2. Neuwelt EA: Mechanisms of disease: the blood-brain barrier. Neurosurgery. 54(1):131-40; discussion 141-2, 2004
3. Coutts SB et al: Hyperperfusion syndrome: toward a stricter definition. Neurosurgery. 53(5):1053-58; discussion 1058-60, 2003
4. Kinoshita T et al: Diffusion-weighted MR imaging of posterior reversible leukoencephalopathy syndrome: a pictorial essay. Clin Imaging. 27(5): 307-15, 2003
5. Thambisetty M et al: Hypertensive brainstem encephalopathy: clinical and radiographic features. J Neurol Sci. 208(1-2): 93-9, 2003
6. Covarrubias DJ et al: Posterior reversible encephalopathy syndrome: prognostic utility of quantitative diffusion-weighted MR images. AJNR Am J Neuroradiol. 23(6): 1038-48, 2002
7. Kumai Y et al: Hypertensive encephalopathy extending into the whole brainstem and deep structures. Hypertens Res. 25(5): 797-800, 2002
8. Singhi P et al: Reversible brain lesions in childhood hypertension. Acta Paediatr. 91(9):1005-7, 2002
9. Mukherjee P et al: Reversible posterior leukoencephalopathy syndrome: evaluation with diffusion-tensor MR imaging. Radiology. 219:756-65, 2001
10. Provenzale JM et al: Quantitative assessment of diffusion abnormalities in posterior reversible encephalopathy syndrome. AJNR Am J Neuroradiol. 22(8):1455-61, 2001

## IMAGE GALLERY

### Variant

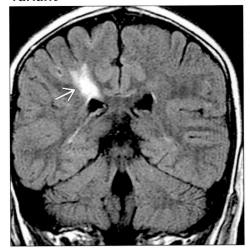
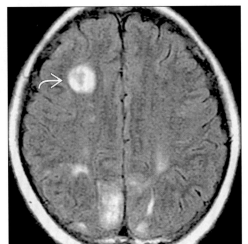

*(Left) Coronal FLAIR MR shows a large white matter lesion ➔ with relative cortical sparing. This lesion had already resolved on follow-up imaging 14 days later. (Right) Axial FLAIR MR shows a rounded frontal lesion ➔ in association with typical posterior PRES lesions. All cleared on follow-up imaging.*

### Typical

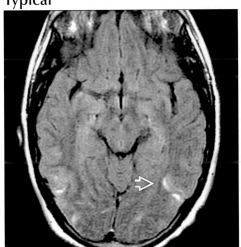
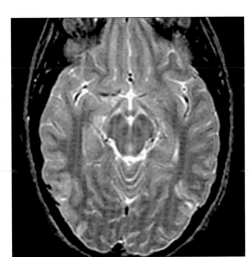

*(Left) Axial FLAIR MR shows extensive bilateral cortical lesions involving the posterior temporal and occipital poles. A few extend into the subcortical white matter ➔. (Right) Axial T2WI MR in the same patient as previous image, shows the lesions less well than does FLAIR imaging.*

### Typical

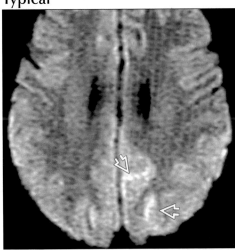
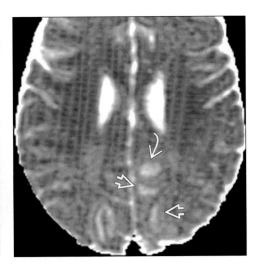

*(Left) Axial DWI MR shows multifocal lesions in the parietal and occipital lobes ➔ in a child with PRES. These are not very bright, suggesting T2 "shine through" rather than reduced diffusion. (Right) Axial ADC from the same study shows these ➔ and additional ➔ lesions are hyperintense, confirming vasogenic edema. All lesions cleared on followup imaging.*

# GERMINAL MATRIX HEMORRHAGE

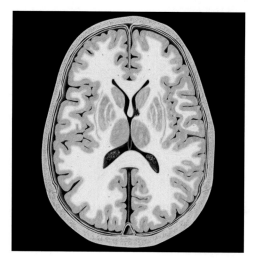

Graphic shows blood in highly vascular germinal matrix, between caudate nucleus and thalamus, extending into occipital horns.

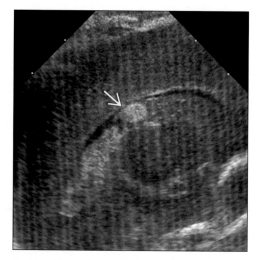

Sagittal oblique ultrasound shows an ovoid echogenic focus ➜ in the right caudothalamic notch, classic location for GMH. Absence of intraventricular hemorrhage makes this grade 1.

## TERMINOLOGY

### Abbreviations and Synonyms
- Germinal matrix hemorrhage (GMH), germinal matrix bleed, preterm caudothalamic hemorrhage, intracranial bleed, germinal matrix-intraventricular hemorrhage (GMH-IVH)

### Definitions
- Hemorrhage which occurs in the germinal zone, a specialized, highly vascular region in the ventricular walls where the neurons and glia are generated

## IMAGING FINDINGS

### General Features
- Best diagnostic clue: Echogenic area in the ventricular wall (usually caudothalamic notch) which may extend into the lateral ventricle(s) or periventricular brain parenchyma
- Location
  - Anywhere in ventricular wall, most often between the caudate nucleus and thalamus

  - Look for extension into ventricular system
  - Cerebellar hemorrhages in 10%, usually small
- Size: Variable
- Morphology: Echogenic when acute, changing to iso- and hypo- echoic with time

### CT Findings
- CT scan preferred over ultrasound for large bleeds
- Excellent at detecting intracranial hemorrhage: Parenchymal, subdural, subarachnoid, intraventricular

### MR Findings
- Usually reserved for infants with complex pathology who are stable enough to travel to the MR suite
- Normal germinal matrix highly cellular, has low signal intensity on T2WIs
  - Usually largely involuted by 26 weeks
- Acute hemorrhage has low signal intensity on T2WIs
- MR is more sensitive, specific, and reproducible than ultrasound, but is not always practical in critically ill premies without the use of MR-compatible incubator

### Ultrasonographic Findings
- Grayscale Ultrasound

## DDx: Germinal Matrix Hemorrhage

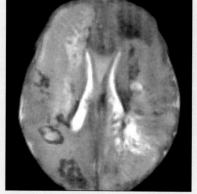

Hemorrhagic Necrosis

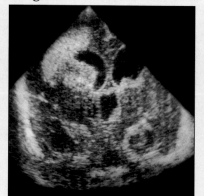

PVHI

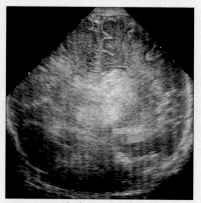

Thalamic Stroke

# GERMINAL MATRIX HEMORRHAGE

## Key Facts

### Terminology
- Hemorrhage which occurs in the germinal zone, a specialized, highly vascular region in the ventricular walls where the neurons and glia are generated

### Imaging Findings
- Best diagnostic clue: Echogenic area in the ventricular wall (usually caudothalamic notch) which may extend into the lateral ventricle(s) or periventricular brain parenchyma

### Top Differential Diagnoses
- Porencephaly or Cystic Periventricular Leukomalacia
- Choroid Plexus Cysts or Hematoma
- Ventriculitis
- Ischemia or Infarction
- Intraventricular Hemorrhage

### Pathology
- Most GMHs occur in the first week of life
- Related to perinatal stresses: Labile blood pressure, hypoxia, hypercarbia, etc.
- Most common in infants < 32 weeks gestation and < 1000 grams
- Higher risk in premies who have congenital heart disease, surgical procedures, severe respiratory distress
- Grade I: Confined to the caudothalamic groove
- Grade II: Extends into the ventricle but does not expand it
- Grade III: Fills and distends the adjacent ventricle
- Grade IV: Parenchymal hemorrhagic venous infarction (PVHI)

---

- ○ Carefully assess the caudothalamic groove for evidence of blood on both sagittal and coronal images
- ○ Acute blood is echogenic, later clot retracts and becomes iso- to hypoechoic
- ○ Fluid-debris levels may be visible in the ventricles
- ○ Secondary hydrocephalus (communicating) is common
- ○ If hemorrhage extends into the ventricles, chemical ventriculitis ensues in 2-3 days
  - Ependymal lining becomes thick and echogenic
- ○ Examine the rest of the brain for
  - Congenital anomalies
  - Extra-axial fluid collections
  - Ventricular size & symmetry
- ○ Cerebellar hemorrhages best seen via posterolateral fontanelle
- Color Doppler
  - ○ Useful to differentiate avascular hematoma from vascular choroid plexus
  - ○ Attempts to use Doppler to predict premies at risk for GMH have not been successful

### Imaging Recommendations
- Best imaging tool
  - ○ Cranial ultrasound via anterior and posterolateral fontanelles
    - High sensitivity and specificity for medium to large hemorrhages
- Protocol advice: Small footprint, high frequency transducer, using multiple focal zones

## DIFFERENTIAL DIAGNOSIS

### Porencephaly or Cystic Periventricular Leukomalacia
- Hypo or anechoic spaces reflecting brain parenchymal loss
- Often follows a hypoxic, ischemic event or high grade germinal matrix bleed

- Most common in watershed zone between deep and superficial vessels
- Can occur in utero or perinatally
- Often bilateral but asymmetric

### Choroid Plexus Cysts or Hematoma
- Cysts and hematoma may both occur in the choroid plexus, sparing the germinal matrix area

### Ventriculitis
- Thickening and increased echoes in the ependyma lining the ventricles
- Often associated with intraventricular hemorrhage or GMH
- Hemorrhagic necrosis in periventricular white matter
- Re-image to determine if communicating hydrocephalus develops after ventriculitis

### Ischemia or Infarction
- Ischemic areas show increased echogenicity
- Lack mass effect of hematoma
- Tend to occur in different areas of the brain, periventricular white matter

### White Matter Injury of Prematurity
- Typically in white matter around ventricle
- Echogenic on US; bright/dark on T1/T2 MR

### Intraventricular Hemorrhage
- Hematoma may be confined to the ventricle without involvement of germinal matrix
- Consider this diagnosis in patients who are older than 34 weeks gestation

## PATHOLOGY

### General Features
- General path comments
  - ○ Germinal matrix is highly cellular region where neurons, glia are generated
  - ○ Blood supply from thin-walled vascular channels

# GERMINAL MATRIX HEMORRHAGE

○ It has matured or "involuted" by 34 weeks gestation, such that hemorrhage becomes very unlikely after this age
○ Most GMHs occur in the first week of life
• Etiology
  ○ Related to perinatal stresses: Labile blood pressure, hypoxia, hypercarbia, etc.
  ○ Probably potentiated by poor or underdeveloped cerebral perfusion autoregulation
• Epidemiology
  ○ Most common in infants < 32 weeks gestation and < 1000 grams
  ○ Higher risk in premies who have congenital heart disease, surgical procedures, severe respiratory distress
  ○ Rate of severe grade III or IV GMH decreased from 70% in 1986 to 23% in 1995 & mortality rate decreased by 30% in the same period

## Gross Pathologic & Surgical Features
• Germinal matrix is gelatinous, friable structure deficient in supporting mesenchyme
  ○ Lack of supporting mesenchyme related to leaking/rupture of capillaries
• Areas of hemorrhagic necrosis, liquefaction, and gliosis

## Microscopic Features
• Minimal astrocytic development before 28 weeks
• Deficiency of astrocytes may reduce stability of capillaries

## Staging, Grading or Classification Criteria
• Germinal matrix grading system created by Papile et al in 1978
• Grade I: Confined to the caudothalamic groove
• Grade II: Extends into the ventricle but does not expand it
• Grade III: Fills and distends the adjacent ventricle
• Grade IV: Parenchymal hemorrhagic venous infarction (PVHI)
  ○ Results from occlusion of ependymal veins, consequent venous infarction
  ○ No longer considered a form of GMH

# CLINICAL ISSUES

## Presentation
• Most common signs/symptoms
  ○ Small bleeds often asymptomatic
  ○ Larger bleeds ⇒ variable: Acute vs. stuttering presentation
    ■ Altered consciousness, motility, tone can progress to stupor, coma, apnea, seizures, decerebrate posturing
• Other signs/symptoms: GMH may occur in utero and follow the same pathway of evolution & complications

## Demographics
• Age: Premature infants in the first week of life (50% on first day)
• Gender: M = F
• Ethnicity: No predisposition

## Natural History & Prognosis
• GMHs may regress or re-bleed and increase in severity of grade
• Secondary hydrocephalus occurring several days after a grade II bleed should not be mislabeled as grade III hemorrhage
• Clot retracts, lyses, and is resorbed; may develop into cyst or area of porencephaly
• Prognosis
  ○ Grade I & II bleeds generally have a good prognosis
  ○ Grade III bleeds have variable long-term deficits
    ■ Spastic diplegia, seizures, developmental delay
    ■ Variability likely related to severity of hemorrhage and degree of associated white matter injury
    ■ May require treatment (ventriculoperitoneal shunting or third ventriculostomy) for communicating hydrocephalus

## Treatment
• Supportive in the acute phase
• Ventricular drainage may be needed in higher grade bleeds

# SELECTED REFERENCES

1. Ballabh P et al: Anatomic analysis of blood vessels in germinal matrix, cerebral cortex, and white matter in developing infants. Pediatr Res. 56(1):117-24, 2004
2. Vasileiadis GT et al: Uncomplicated intraventricular hemorrhage is followed by reduced cortical volume at near-term age. Pediatrics. 114(3):e367-72, 2004
3. Roland EH et al: Germinal matrix-intraventricular hemorrhage in the premature newborn: management and outcome. Neurol Clin. 21(4):833-51, vi-vii, 2003
4. Smyth MD et al: Endoscopic third ventriculostomy for hydrocephalus secondary to central nervous system infection or intraventricular hemorrhage in children. Pediatr Neurosurg. 39(5):258-63, 2003
5. Vollmer B et al: Predictors of long-term outcome in very preterm infants: gestational age versus neonatal cranial ultrasound. Pediatrics. 112(5):1108-14, 2003
6. Fukui K et al: Fetal germinal matrix and intraventricular haemorrhage diagnosed by MRI. Neuroradiology. 43(1):68-72, 2001
7. Blankenberg FG et al: Sonography, CT, and MR imaging: a prospective comparison of neonates with suspected intracranial ischemia and hemorrhage. AJNR Am J Neuroradiol. 21(1):213-8, 2000
8. Tsuji M et al: Cerebral intravascular oxygenation correlates with mean arterial pressure in critically ill premature infants. Pediatrics. 106(4):625-32, 2000
9. Felderhoff-Mueser U et al: Relationship between MR imaging and histopathologic findings of the brain in extremely sick preterm infants. AJNR Am J Neuroradiol. 20(7):1349-57, 1999
10. Ghazi-Birry HS et al: Human germinal matrix: venous origin of hemorrhage and vascular characteristics. AJNR Am J Neuroradiol. 18(2):219-29, 1997
11. Levy ML et al: Outcome for preterm infants with germinal matrix hemorrhage and progressive hydrocephalus. Neurosurgery. 41(5):1111-7; discussion 1117-8, 1997
12. Taylor GA: Effect of germinal matrix hemorrhage on terminal vein position and patency. Pediatr Radiol. 25 Suppl 1:S37-40, 1995
13. Papile et al: Incidence and evolution of subependymal and intraventricular hemorrhage: a study of infants with birth weights less than 1,500 gm. J Pediatr. 92:529-34, 1978

## IMAGE GALLERY

### Typical

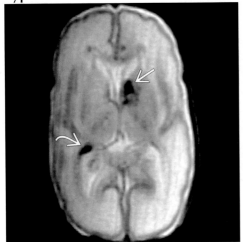
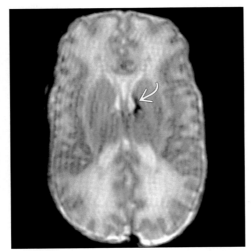

*(Left)* Axial T2WI MR shows grade 1 GMH in the caudothalamic notch ➡. A second GMH ➡ is seen in the anterior right trigone. Germinal matrix lines the ventricles, can bleed anywhere. *(Right)* Axial T2WI MR in the same patient at 6 week follow-up shows evolution of the hemorrhage, with only a small amount of hemosiderin ➡ and minimal ventricular enlargement.

### Typical

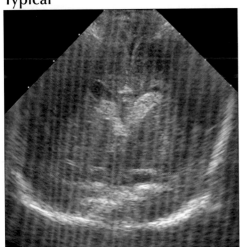
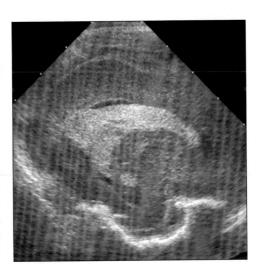

*(Left)* Coronal ultrasound shows grade II GMH. The hemorrhage has broken into the ventricular system but no hydrocephalus has developed. *(Right)* Sagittal ultrasound shows echogenic material filling the ventricle anterior to the foramen of Monro. As no choroid plexus extends anterior to the foramen, this likely is hemorrhage.

### Typical

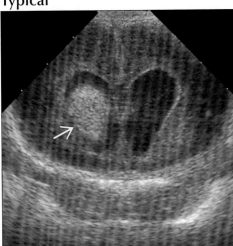
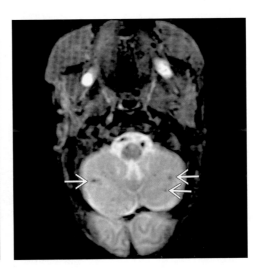

*(Left)* Coronal ultrasound shows large echogenic hematoma ➡ in right frontal horn. The ventricles are significantly enlarged, making this a grade III GMH. *(Right)* Axial T2WI MR shows multiple cerebellar germinal matrix hemorrhages as small areas of low T2 signal intensity ➡.

# WHITE MATTER INJURY OF PREMATURITY

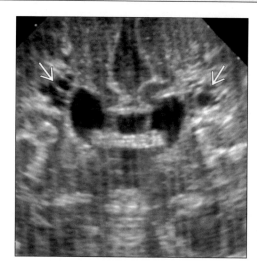

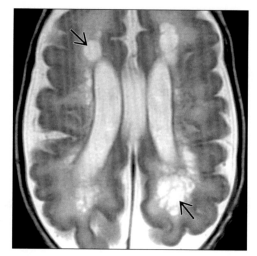

*Coronal ultrasound shows bilateral periventricular white matter cavities ➡ adjacent to the frontal horns. Note mild frontal horn dilatation secondary to early white matter volume loss.*

*Axial T2WI MR shows extensive periventricular cystic white matter injury ➡. Lateral ventricular dilatation and expansion of the subarachnoid spaces reflect parenchymal volume loss.*

## TERMINOLOGY

### Abbreviations and Synonyms
- Periventricular leukomalacia (PVL), perinatal white matter damage, hypoxic-ischemic encephalopathy (HIE)

### Definitions
- Brain injury of prematurity (< 33 weeks)
  - White matter injury (WMI) ⇒ focal or diffuse, noncavitary or cavitary
  - Periventricular hemorrhagic infarction (PVHI) ⇒ associated with large ipsilateral IVH
  - Germinal matrix hemorrhage
  - Intraventricular hemorrhage
  - Cerebellar ⇒ hemorrhage, infarction, and atrophy

## IMAGING FINDINGS

### General Features
- Best diagnostic clue
  - White matter injury of prematurity

- US: Hyperechoic periventricular "flare", loss of normal echotexture, periventricular cysts
- Early MR: Reduced diffusion, foci of T1 shortening, mild T2 shortening
- Late MR: Periventricular liquefaction, ventriculomegaly, and gliosis
- Location
  - WM injury may be focal (adjacent to frontal horns and trigones) or diffuse
  - WM injury due to PVHI shows parenchymal abnormality adjacent to IVH
- Size: Foci of WMI typically in the 2-3 mm range; larger areas may cavitate, carry poorer prognosis
- Morphology: Late findings: Undulating ventricular borders, ventriculomegaly, and volume loss

### CT Findings
- NECT
  - Poor test for the identification of nonhemorrhagic WM injury
  - Late: Ventriculomegaly, undulating lateral ventricular borders, WM volume loss

### MR Findings
- T1WI

## DDx: Mimics of PVL

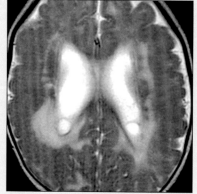

*Congenital CMV*

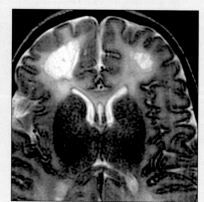

*Citrobacter*

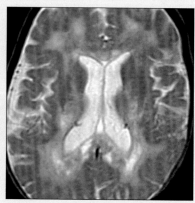

*Zellweger*

## Key Facts

### Terminology

- Periventricular leukomalacia (PVL), perinatal white matter damage, hypoxic-ischemic encephalopathy (HIE)
- Brain injury of prematurity (< 33 weeks)

### Imaging Findings

- US: Hyperechoic periventricular "flare", loss of normal echotexture, periventricular cysts
- Early MR: Reduced diffusion, foci of T1 shortening, mild T2 shortening
- Late MR: Periventricular liquefaction, ventriculomegaly, and gliosis
- Poor test for the identification of nonhemorrhagic WM injury
- Early: ↑ T1 signal in PV WM ⇒ astrogliosis, ± coagulation necrosis, ± hemorrhage

- Late: Ventriculomegaly, volume loss, and ± demyelination
- Reduced diffusion can precede US and MR abnormalities, ADC values may "normalize" as early as 5 days
- Ultrasound: Does not detect noncavitary lesions

### Top Differential Diagnoses

- Normal Periventricular Halo
- Infection

### Diagnostic Checklist

- In the VLBW preterm newborn, US will significantly underestimate white matter injury
- MR is the examination of choice for defining white matter injury in the preterm newborn

---

- ○ Early: ↑ T1 signal in PV WM ⇒ astrogliosis, ± coagulation necrosis, ± hemorrhage
- ○ Late: ⇒ Ventricular enlargement, volume loss, ± cavitation (↓ T1 signal), thin callosum
- T2WI
  - ○ Early: ↓ T2 signal (astrogliosis, coagulation necrosis), blood has much shorter T2 relaxation
  - ○ Late: Ventriculomegaly, volume loss, and ± demyelination
- FLAIR
  - ○ ↑ Periventricular signal (gliosis or coagulation necrosis), ± liquefaction
  - ○ Look also for bright FLAIR signal in brainstem, thalamus, striatum, amygdala
- T2* GRE: ↓ Signal at sites of hemorrhage
- DWI
  - ○ Reduced diffusion can precede US and MR abnormalities, ADC values may "normalize" as early as 5 days
  - ○ May miss or underestimate WM injury if DWI is performed within first 24 hours
  - ○ Always review ADC maps as DWIs may be falsely negative due to the long T2 values of the neonatal brain
  - ○ DTI: Patients with WMI have decreased anisotropy
- MRS: Lactate peak, ↓ NAA, ↑ excitatory neurotransmitters; alterations may antedate MR abnormalities

### Ultrasonographic Findings

- Grayscale Ultrasound
  - ○ Early
    - ▪ Focal WMI hyperechogenicity (flare) adjacent to trigones and frontal horns
    - ▪ Diffuse WMI: More generalized deep white matter hyperechogenicity
  - ○ Late: ± Cavitation, unexplained ventriculomegaly, WM volume loss
  - ○ Beware: US is insensitive to nonhemorrhagic, noncavitary WM injury

### Imaging Recommendations

- Best imaging tool

- ○ Ultrasound: Does not detect noncavitary lesions
- ○ MR (including (DWI, DTI, & MRS)
  - ▪ Clarifies abnormal US exams
  - ▪ Sensitive for defining scope of injury in very low birth weight (VLBW) neonates with "normal" cranial ultrasounds
- Protocol advice
  - ○ Ultrasound screening: In first few days, repeat before discharge
  - ○ MR
    - ▪ Within first 5 days when clinically indicated
    - ▪ When US is abnormal: To define scope of injury and prognosticate
    - ▪ At discharge (near term) whether US was "normal" or "abnormal"

## DIFFERENTIAL DIAGNOSIS

### Normal Periventricular Halo

- Specular reflections from normal WM tracts, peritrigonal, less echogenic than choroid plexus

### Infection

- CMV: Microcephaly, periventricular calcifications, + periventricular demyelination and gliosis, +/- polymicrogyria
- Citrobacter: "Squared-off" abscesses
- Neonatal herpes simplex encephalitis: Early diffusion restriction, neuronal necrosis, ± hemorrhage

### Peroxisomal Disorders (e.g., Zellweger Syndrome)

- Subependymal germinolytic cysts, microgyria, profound hypomyelination

## PATHOLOGY

### General Features

- General path comments
  - ○ Embryology-anatomy

# WHITE MATTER INJURY OF PREMATURITY

- WMI may be due to ⇒ perfusion autoregulation disturbance, infection, metabolic disorders, hydrocephalus
- Genetics: ↑ Spontaneous preterm delivery with the fetal carriage of IL1B+3953*1 (African) and IL1RN*2 (Hispanic) alleles
- Etiology
  - Contributors to white matter injury of prematurity
    - Damage initiators: Low gestational age, chorioamnionitis (⇒ preterm labor)
    - Damage promoters: Vasculitis involving chorionic plate, ↑ inflammatory cytokines, ↑ microglia
    - Maturation-dependent vulnerability: Vulnerability of oligodendrocyte lineage, tenuous BBB, paucity of protectors (proteins), ↓ blood thyroxine, hypocarbia, hypoxia
  - Prenatal hypoxia ⇒ WM damage via inflammatory response, oxidative stress linked to re-oxygenation during perinatal period
- Epidemiology
  - Birth weight < 1500 g ⇒ 45% incidence of WM injury, 15-20% neuromotor disability, 50% cognitive disorder
  - > 50% of patients with cystic WM injury develop cerebral palsy
- Associated abnormalities: Intraventricular hemorrhage, cerebellar hemorrhage and infarction

## Gross Pathologic & Surgical Features
- Autopsy: Pontosubicular necrosis (59%), germinal matrix hemorrhage (50%), WMI (24-50%)

## Microscopic Features
- Focal WMI: Reactive gliosis, coagulative necrosis, ± infarction, ± hemorrhage ⇒ tissue dissolution, ± cavitation
- Diffuse WMI: HIE affects differentiating oligodendroglia, causing more diffuse infarction of periventricular white matter

## Staging, Grading or Classification Criteria
- Sonographic grading of white matter injury (this system does not account for the more common noncavitary WMI)
  - Grade 1: ↑ Periventricular echoes for ≥ 7 days
  - Grade 2: Periventricular echoes that evolve into small fronto-parietal cysts
  - Grade 3: Extensive periventricular cystic lesions

# CLINICAL ISSUES

## Presentation
- Most common signs/symptoms: Spastic diplegia; visual impairment; cognitive impairment
- Other signs/symptoms: ± Hydrocephalus (essential to know head size before making diagnosis)
- Clinical Profile
  - Risk factors for preterm HIE related brain injury
    - Pregnancy: ↓ Gestational age/weight, previous preterm birth, spontaneous preterm labor
    - Intrapartum: Abruption, pre-eclampsia, premature rupture of membranes, chorioamnionitis, group B strep infection
    - Perinatal factors: Respiratory distress, patent ductus arteriosus, ↓ PaCO2, sepsis, anemia, apnea, bradycardia, cardiac arrest

## Demographics
- Age: VLBW (< 1500 g) ~ autopsies and MR studies suggest ~ 50% incidence of WM injury
- Gender: Caucasian males ↑ risk for WM injury of prematurity, African-American females somewhat "immune"
- Ethnicity: Poor antepartum care ↑ the fetal risk for WM injury

## Natural History & Prognosis
- Neonates born ≤ 25 weeks ⇒ 90% are stillborn or die before discharge
  - 50% of survivors ⇒ severely affected (mental retardation, learning disability, attention deficit disorder, spastic diplegia/quadriplegia, seizures, microcephaly, blindness, deafness)
- Motor and visual impairment most common neurologic sequelae of WM injury

## Treatment
- Prenatal care significantly reduces preterm birth
- Supportive, cerebral cooling, possible future for free radical scavengers

# DIAGNOSTIC CHECKLIST

## Consider
- Prior WM injury when US, CT or MR shows unexplained ventricular dilation, look for gliosis and volume loss

## Image Interpretation Pearls
- In the VLBW preterm newborn, US will significantly underestimate white matter injury
- MR is the examination of choice for defining white matter injury in the preterm newborn

# SELECTED REFERENCES

1. Dammann O et al: Neuroimaging and the prediction of outcomes in preterm infants. N Engl J Med. 355(7):727-9, 2006
2. Miller SP et al: Prolonged indomethacin exposure is associated with decreased white matter injury detected with magnetic resonance imaging in premature newborns at 24 to 28 weeks' gestation at birth. Pediatrics. 117(5):1626-31, 2006
3. Hagberg H et al: Effect of inflammation on central nervous system development and vulnerability. Curr Opin Neurol. 18(2):117-23, 2005
4. O'Shea TM et al: Magnetic resonance and ultrasound brain imaging in preterm infants. Early Hum Dev. 81(3):263-71, 2005
5. Partridge SC et al: Diffusion tensor imaging: serial quantitation of white matter tract maturity in premature newborns. Neuroimage. 22(3):1302-14, 2004
6. Ment LR et al: Practice parameter: neuroimaging of the neonate: report of the Quality Standards Subcommittee of the American Academy of Neurology and the Practice Committee of the Child Neurology Society. Neurology. 58(12):1726-38, 2002

# WHITE MATTER INJURY OF PREMATURITY

## IMAGE GALLERY

### Typical

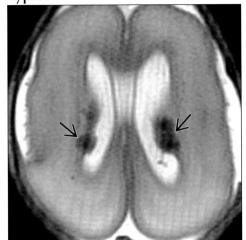
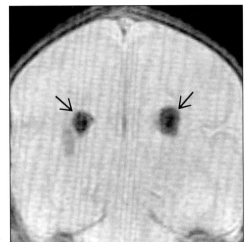

*(Left) Axial T2WI MR shows the smooth appearance of the normal brain at 24 weeks. Note the hypointense periventricular hemorrhages ➡ in the germinal zones. (Right) Coronal T2\* GRE MR in a premature neonate shows blooming ➡ of subependymal germinal matrix hemorrhages secondary to susceptibility effects from the blood.*

### Typical

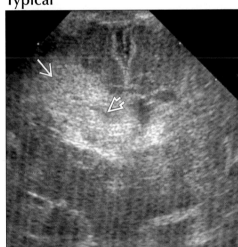
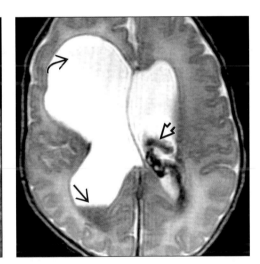

*(Left) Coronal ultrasound shows the features of periventricular hemorrhagic infarction. Note the region of parenchymal echogenicity ➡ and the associated large intraventricular hemorrhage ➡. (Right) Axial T2WI MR shows the late findings of periventricular hemorrhagic infarction. Note the right frontal porencephaly ➡, blood-CSF ➡ level, and choroid plexus hemorrhage ➡.*

### Variant

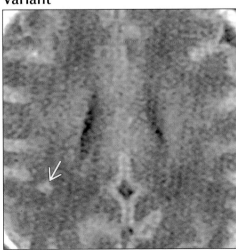
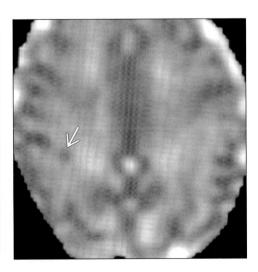

*(Left) Axial T1WI MR shows focal white matter injury. Note the T1 shortening ➡ reflecting astrogliosis and/or early coagulation necrosis. This showed mild decreased T2 signal. GRE was normal. (Right) Axial ADC shows reduced diffusion ➡, suggesting acuity, at the site of focal white matter injury that showed T1 and T2 shortening. GRE imaging showed no evidence of hemorrhage.*

# HIE, TERM

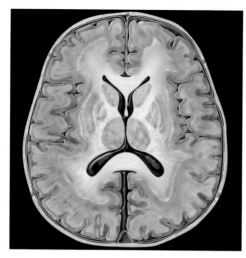

*Axial graphic shows edema of the cortex and subcortical white matter. There is sparing of the deep structures in prolonged partial hypoxic ischemia of the newborn.*

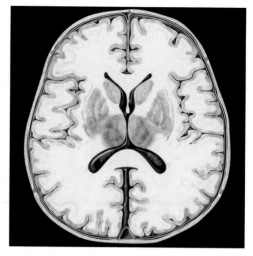

*Axial graphic shows sparing of the cortex and edema of the lateral thalami and of the posterior putamina in profound, acute hypoxic ischemia of the newborn.*

## TERMINOLOGY

### Abbreviations and Synonyms

- Hypoxic ischemic encephalopathy (HIE); hypoxic ischemic insult (HII); formerly perinatal or birth asphyxia, asphyxia neonatorium

### Definitions

- Cerebral hypoperfusion injury
- Acquired condition in term neonates who
  - Show signs of fetal distress prior to delivery
  - Have low Apgars; require resuscitation at birth
  - Have metabolic acidosis (cord pH < 7)
  - Have neurological abnormalities in first 24 hours
- Prolonged partial (PP) injury: As in nuchal cord
  - Chronic repetitive stress, intermittent recovery ⇒ CBF redistribution, preserved deep structures
- Profound acute (PA) injury: As in uterine rupture, uterine abruption or cord prolapse
  - No cerebral blood flow (CBF) redistribution ⇒ areas with high metabolic demand damaged
- Mixed injury: Shock brain

## IMAGING FINDINGS

### General Features

- Best diagnostic clue
  - PP: White matter (WM)/cortex damaged, deep gray nuclei/basal ganglia (BG) spared
  - PA: BG damaged, WM/cortex other than corticospinal tracts (CST) spared
  - Mixed: "Super-scan" on DWI
- Location
  - PP: Parasagittal "border zone" injury
  - PA: Deep gray matter (GM), dorsal brain stem, hippocampi and CST
  - Mixed: Border zone and deep GM

### CT Findings

- NECT
  - PP acute: Loss of cortical "ribbon"; WM edema
  - PP chronic: Ulegyria, border zone & diffuse atrophy
  - PA acute: Subtle ↓ density BG, blurred GM/WM interface; ± petechial bleed
  - PA chronic: Atrophy or slit-like lacunes BG, thalami; ± hazy Ca++ (status marmoratus)

## DDx: Bright Basal Ganglia

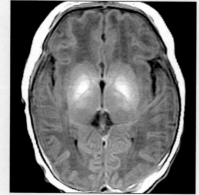

*Acute Kernicterus*

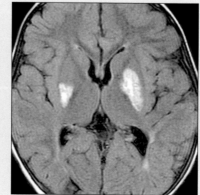

*Leigh Disease*

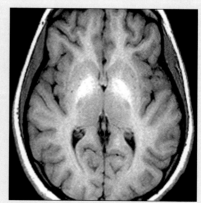

*Manganese TPN*

# HIE, TERM

## Key Facts

### Terminology
- Hypoxic ischemic encephalopathy (HIE); hypoxic ischemic insult (HII); formerly perinatal or birth asphyxia, asphyxia neonatorium
- Cerebral hypoperfusion injury
- Prolonged partial (PP) injury: As in nuchal cord
- Profound acute (PA) injury: As in uterine rupture, uterine abruption or cord prolapse

### Imaging Findings
- PP: Parasagittal "border zone" injury
- PA: Deep gray matter (GM), dorsal brain stem, hippocampi and CST
- PA acute: Subtle ↓ density BG, blurred GM/WM interface; ± petechial bleed
- Reduced diffusivity, ↓ ADC values in acute phase
- Limited window of opportunity to document injury

### Pathology
- Seek inborn errors of metabolism if normal Apgar or > 1 HIE child in family
- Seizure related cell injury
- Epidemiology: HIE: Up to 2/1,000 (0.2%) live births

### Clinical Issues
- Varies from normal outcome (Sarnat I) to spastic quadriparesis, developmental delay, microcephaly, and Sz (Sarnat III)

### Diagnostic Checklist
- DWI crucial, but limited window of opportunity
- Typical periventricular leukomalacia (PVL) pattern may occur in full-terms with HIE AND sepsis

## MR Findings
- T1WI
  - PP acute: Laminar necrosis
  - PA acute: ↓ T1 signal of normally myelinated posterior limb internal capsule (PLIC) if term ≥ 37 wks GA; spuriously normal ≤ 72 hrs!
  - PA acute: ↑ T1 signal in ventrolateral thalamus, BG (especially posterior putamina), peri-Rolandic cortex
  - Mixed acute: ↓ T1 in normally myelinated posterior limb IC & bright cortex
- T2WI
  - PP acute: Blurring of gray-white junction
  - PP chronic: Border zone gliosis, ± cystic encephalomalacia
  - PA chronic: Atrophy/↑ signal posterior putamina/lateral thalami and Rolandic cortex
  - Mixed chronic: Border zone & posterior putamina/lateral thalamic atrophy and gliosis
- FLAIR
  - Acute: Documents cysts, edema poorly shown
  - Chronic: Useful to document extent of gliosis
- T2* GRE: Hemosiderin if subarachnoid hemorrhage or petechial hemorrhagic conversion of ischemia
- DWI
  - Reduced diffusivity, ↓ ADC values in acute phase
  - Limited window of opportunity to document injury
    - Underestimates injury during first 24-48 hours
    - Normalizes around 6 days, even in damaged areas
- T1 C+: Subacute enhancement ⇒ poor outcome
- MRV: More than coincidental ↑ sinovenous occlusion
- MRS
  - Lactate normal < 37 wks gestational age (GA)
  - Lactate in full-term (> 37 wks GA) may be only abnormal finding in first 24 hours!
  - NAA ↓ for age correlates with poor prognosis
  - ↑ α-glutamate/glutamine peaks in BG correlate with ↑ severity of injury

## Radiographic Findings
- Radiography: Late microcephaly, secondary craniostenosis

## Ultrasonographic Findings
- Grayscale Ultrasound
  - More useful in pre-term than full-term: Flare & cysts
  - Useful full-term US signs: ↑ Echogenicity of gyral white matter, cortex, sulci
- Color Doppler: Variable resistive indices & anterior cerebral artery blood flow waveform

## Nuclear Medicine Findings
- PET: Selective damage in BG and areas of primary myelination: ↑ Rates of oxygen-glucose utilization
- Brain scan
  - I-123 iodobenzamide SPECT: Striatum/cerebellum ratio ↓ as ↑ severity of perinatal HIE event
  - Tc-99m annexin V: Animal studies show neuronal apoptosis after HIE even with normal DWI/ADC

## Imaging Recommendations
- Best imaging tool
  - MRS: Lactate may be first or only abnormal finding
  - DWI: Extremely sensitive for early, acute ischemia
  - T1 axial: Loss of PLIC in HIE (infants ≥ 37 wks GA)
- Protocol advice
  - MRS crucial in first 24 hours
  - DWI crucial, but may take > 48 hours to become "positive" ("pseudonormalizes" in 1 wk)
  - Standard MR imaging limited by hypomyelination & ↑ water content of neonatal brain

# DIFFERENTIAL DIAGNOSIS

## Kernicterus (Accentuated by Sepsis, Hypoxia)
- Mimics profound injury on acute T1WI; has confirmed hyperbilirubinemia
- Globus pallidus, (not putamen or thalamus) abnormal

## Metabolic Disorder
- Inherited: Mitochondrial encephalopathy, methylmalonic acidemia
- Manganese (TPN) mimics T1 BG changes of HIE

# HIE, TERM

## PATHOLOGY

### General Features
- General path comments: Multi-organ ischemia common
- Genetics
  - Seek inborn errors of metabolism if normal Apgar or > 1 HIE child in family
  - Inherited prothrombotic disorders ⇒ arterial or venous occlusions
- Etiology
  - PP (as in nuchal cord): Mild or moderate hypoperfusion
    - "Diving reflex" redistribution cerebral blood flow (CBF) to basal ganglia/brainstem/cerebellum
  - PA (as in uterine rupture): Profound hypoperfusion
    - No time to shift CBF, areas of highest metabolic demand damaged
  - Mixed pattern of injury: Mild or moderate hypoperfusion converts to profound near delivery
    - Early compensatory adjustment to ↓ CBF fails ⇒ "pressure-passive" CBF (dependent on systemic BP)
    - BP falls, CBF falls, brain hypoxia/intracellular energy failure follow
  - Asphyxia triggers cascade of cellular biochemical events leading to abnormal function, edema or death of cell
    - Extracellular glutamate accumulates, activates postsynaptic excitatory amino-acid receptors
    - Postsynaptic receptor distribution changes with development ⇒ different damage patterns at different gestational ages
  - Many chances for cell loss
    - Primary neuronal (death at time of insult)
    - Reactive cell death (reperfusion injury)
    - Seizure related cell injury
- Epidemiology: HIE: Up to 2/1,000 (0.2%) live births
- Associated abnormalities
  - Maternal: Infection, pre-eclampsia, diabetes, cocaine
  - Infant: ↓ Gestational age, growth retardation, ↓ Ca++/glucose, sepsis, hyperthermia, seizures, congenital heart disease; ↑ urine S100B protein

### Gross Pathologic & Surgical Features
- PP: Chronic parasagittal ulegyria, gliosis and atrophy
- PA: Chronic hippocampal, BG, thalamic, CST atrophy

### Microscopic Features
- < 30 gestational weeks: Liquefaction, resorption of parenchyma
- > 30 weeks: Reactive astrogliosis, macrophages

### Staging, Grading or Classification Criteria
- Sarnat stages of HIE encephalopathy

## CLINICAL ISSUES

### Presentation
- Most common signs/symptoms
  - Sarnat I (mild): Hyperalert/irritable, mydriasis, EEG normal
  - Sarnat II (moderate): Lethargy, hypotonia, ↓ HR, Sz
  - Sarnat III (severe): Stupor, flaccid, reflexes absent; Sz

- Clinical Profile
  - Periventricular leukomalacia (PVL): Lower extremity spasticity
  - Unilateral/focal lesions: Hemiplegia
  - Parasagittal cystic encephalomalacia: Spastic tetraparesis
  - Bilateral BG damage: Extrapyramidal cerebral palsy

### Demographics
- Age: Full-term perinatal, = ≥ 37 wks GA; immediate prenatal, intrapartum, and postnatal period

### Natural History & Prognosis
- Varies from normal outcome (Sarnat I) to spastic quadriparesis, developmental delay, microcephaly, and Sz (Sarnat III)
- Severe HIE: 50% mortality, significant morbidity in 80% of survivors
- Choreoathetosis after 1 year common in PA survivors

### Treatment
- Correct hypoxia, metabolic disturbances
- Treat seizures and hyperthermia

## DIAGNOSTIC CHECKLIST

### Consider
- Prenatal HIE with recovery or inborn errors of metabolism if imaging doesn't fit history

### Image Interpretation Pearls
- DWI crucial, but limited window of opportunity
- Typical periventricular leukomalacia (PVL) pattern may occur in full-terms with HIE AND sepsis

## SELECTED REFERENCES

1. Barkovich AJ et al: MR imaging, MR spectroscopy, and diffusion tensor imaging of sequential studies in neonates with encephalopathy. AJNR 27(3):533-47, 2006
2. Boichot C et al: Term neonate prognoses after perinatal asphyxia: contributions of MR imaging, MR spectroscopy, relaxation times, and apparent diffusion coefficients. Radiology. 239(3):839-48, 2006
3. Cheong JL et al: Proton MR spectroscopy in neonates with perinatal cerebral hypoxic-ischemic injury: metabolite peak-area ratios, relaxation times, & absolute concentrations. AJNR Am J Neuroradiol. 27:1546-54, 2006
4. Jensen FE. Related Articles et al: Developmental factors regulating susceptibility to perinatal brain injury and seizures. Curr Opin Pediatr. 18(6):628-633, 2006
5. Gazzolo D et al: Urinary S100B protein measurements: A tool for the early identification of hypoxic-ischemic encephalopathy in asphyxiated full-term infants. Crit Care Med. 32(1):131-6, 2004
6. Barkovich AJ et al: Proton spectroscopy and diffusion imaging on the first day of life after perinatal asphyxia: preliminary report. AJNR 22(9):1786-94, 2001
7. Groenendaal F et al: Glutamate in cerebral tissue of asphyxiated neonates during the first week of life demonstrated in vivo using proton magnetic resonance spectroscopy. Biol Neonate. 79(3-4):254-7, 2001
8. Tranquart F et al: D2 receptor imaging in neonates using I-123 iodobenzamide brain SPECT. Clin Nucl Med. 26(1):36-40, 2001

## IMAGE GALLERY

### Typical

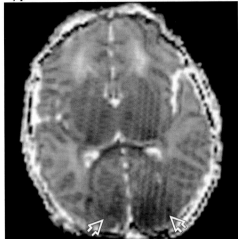

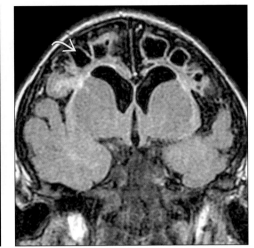

*(Left) Axial ADC shows cortical and subcortical reduced diffusion ➡ in bilateral posterior watershed regions. Peripheral involvement is present with sparing of the deep gray structures. (Right) Coronal FLAIR MR in a different child shows sparing of the deep gray structures at 2 years of age. Extensive cystic encephalomalacia ➡ and gliosis is present in the border zones.*

### Typical

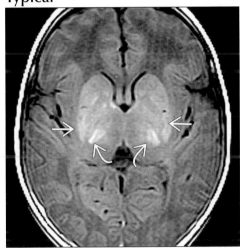

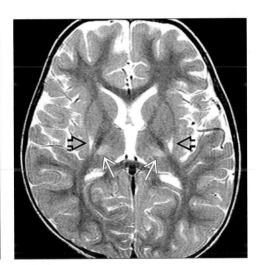

*(Left) Axial T1WI MR shows increased striate and lateral thalamic signal. The posterior limb of the internal capsule is less bright than the adjacent posterior putamina ➡ and thalami ➡. (Right) Axial T2WI MR in another patient follow-up shows typical posterior putamina ➡ and lateral thalamic ➡ atrophy/gliosis. The periphery is spared in this patient who survived uterine rupture.*

### Typical

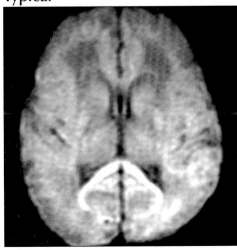

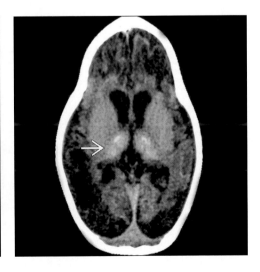

*(Left) Axial DWI MR in a newborn with extensive injury shows reduced diffusivity in both peripheral and deep gray and white matter structures. This "super scan" appearance denotes severe damage. (Right) Axial NECT in a different patient who suffered a severe injury shows microcephaly, premature sutural fusion, cystic encephalomalacia of peripheral structures and thalamic calcification ➡.*

# SICKLE CELL DISEASE, BRAIN

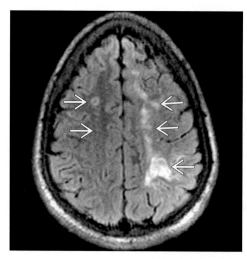

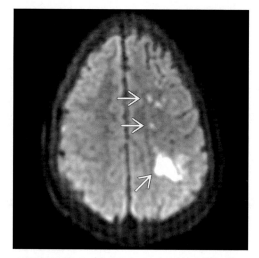

*Axial FLAIR MR shows bilateral subcortical watershed infarction. Hyperintense abnormalities ➡ are seen in the left greater than right border zone between the ACA and MCA.*

*Axial DWI MR (same patient as previous image) shows foci of acute infarction ➡. The FLAIR abnormalities that are not bright on DWI represent foci of subacute/chronic infarction.*

## TERMINOLOGY

### Abbreviations and Synonyms
- Sickle cell disease (SCD)

### Definitions
- Abnormality in hemoglobin (Hgb) → change in shape ("sickling") → increased "stickiness" of erythrocytes (RBCs) → capillary occlusions, ischemia, infarctions, premature RBC destruction (hemolytic anemia)

## IMAGING FINDINGS

### General Features
- Best diagnostic clue
  - Focal narrowing of the distal ICA, MCA, ACA
    - Moyamoya (lenticulostriate collaterals)
- Location: ICA, ACA, MCA; deep white matter, cortex; bone marrow
- Use MR to document previous ischemic events
- Caveat: Cognitive impairment does not correlate with imaging findings

### CT Findings
- CTA: Stenosis of distal ICA, proximal circle of Willis (COW)
- NECT
  - Focal encephalomalacia due to cortical infarction ⇒ diffuse atrophy
  - Calvarial thickening
  - Older moyamoya: Intraventricular bleed may be initial presentation
- CECT: Punctate enhancement in basal ganglia due to moyamoya collaterals

### MR Findings
- T1WI
  - Hemorrhagic infarcts may be seen
  - Punctate flow voids in basal ganglia correspond to moyamoya collaterals
  - Abnormal signal intensity in bone marrow which may be expanded
- T2WI
  - Cortical, deep white matter infarcts
  - Infarction commonly in the cerebral watershed (ACA-MCA) distribution, WM > GM

## DDx: Arteriopathy in Children

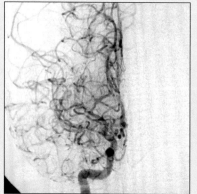

*NF-1, MCA Occlusion*

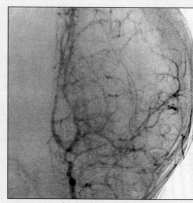

*Idiopathic Arteritis*

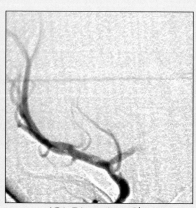

*ICA Dissection, Clot*

# SICKLE CELL DISEASE, BRAIN

## Key Facts

### Terminology
- Abnormality in hemoglobin (Hgb) → change in shape ("sickling") → increased "stickiness" of erythrocytes (RBCs) → capillary occlusions, ischemia, infarctions, premature RBC destruction (hemolytic anemia)

### Imaging Findings
- Moyamoya (lenticulostriate collaterals)
- Hemorrhagic infarcts may be seen
- Cortical, deep white matter infarcts
- Stenosis of distal ICA, proximal COW
- Transcranial Doppler (TCD): Hyperdynamic flow in distal ICA/MCA secondary to proximal stenosis

### Top Differential Diagnoses
- Vasculitis
- Arteriopathy, Moyamoya

- Connective Tissue Disorders
- Thick Skull with Expanded Diploe

### Pathology
- Hgb S becomes "stiff" (hence, erythrocytes are sickle-shaped) when deoxygenated
- Primary cause of stroke in African-American children
- Stroke incidence decreased if Hgb S kept to less than 30% by transfusion (but need initial ischemic event to initiate therapy)

### Clinical Issues
- 11% suffer acute cerebral infarction by age 20 years; risk highest in first decade
- Hgb S found in 10% of African-Americans

---

- ○ Posterior cerebral swelling in hypertensive encephalopathy; can mimic watershed infarction
- FLAIR: Multifocal hyperintensities ± ivy sign of moyamoya
- DWI: Focal hyperintensities due to acute infarctions
- PWI: ↓ rCBF, ↓ rCBV, ↑ TTP, ↑ MTT
- T1 C+: Vascular stasis and leptomeningeal collaterals in MCA territory with proximal MCA stenosis
- MRA
  - ○ Stenosis of distal ICA, proximal COW
    - ▪ Caveat: Turbulent dephasing due to anemia, rapid flow can mimic stenosis on "bright blood" MRA
    - ▪ Suggestion: Use lowest possible TE for bright blood MRA or use black blood MRA if stenosis suspected
  - ○ MRA source images: Multiple dots in basal ganglia due to moyamoya
  - ○ Aneurysms in atypical locations
- MRS: ↑ Lactate, ↓ NAA, ↓ Cho, ↓ Cr in areas of infarction (lactate seen only in acute infarctions)

### Radiographic Findings
- Radiography
  - ○ Thick skull with expanded diploic space
  - ○ Opacified paranasal sinuses

### Ultrasonographic Findings
- Transcranial Doppler (TCD): Hyperdynamic flow in distal ICA/MCA secondary to proximal stenosis
  - ○ Time-averaged mean velocities > 200 cm/s → high risk for ischemic stroke
  - ○ Velocities between 170 and 200 cm/s: Conditional

### Angiographic Findings
- Conventional
  - ○ Stenosis of distal ICA, proximal COW; fusiform aneurysms; moyamoya EC-IC and collaterals
    - ▪ Risk of stroke higher than in other populations
    - ▪ Hydrate, transfuse before catheter study
  - ○ Moyamoya may be associated to persistent primitive carotid-basilar arterial communications

## Imaging Recommendations
- Best imaging tool: MR with DWI, MRA ± DSA
- Protocol advice
  - ○ Diffusion imaging to differentiate acute from subacute/chronic infarction, and from hypertensive encephalopathy
  - ○ MRA to exclude distal ICA, ACA or MCA stenosis, moyamoya collaterals

## DIFFERENTIAL DIAGNOSIS

### Vasculitis
- Idiopathic vs. infectious, autoimmune, or substance abuse etiologies
- Classic imaging findings: Cortical and deep white matter infarcts and parenchymal hemorrhage

### Arteriopathy, Moyamoya
- Prior radiation, neurofibromatosis, Down syndrome: Common risk factors

### Connective Tissue Disorders
- Marfan, Ehlers-Danlos, homocystinuria
- Progressive arterial narrowing and occlusion

### Thick Skull with Expanded Diploe
- Other chronic anemias (thalassemia)

## PATHOLOGY

### General Features
- General path comments
  - ○ Initial endothelial injury from abnormal adherence of sickled RBCs
  - ○ Subsequently internal elastic lamina fragmentation and degeneration of muscularis result in large vessel vasculopathy and aneurysm formation
    - ▪ May be reversed with transfusion (except moyamoya: Not reversible)
- Genetics

# SICKLE CELL DISEASE, BRAIN

- Affected patients can be homozygous or heterozygous for Hgb S
- Mutation in β-globin: Glutamic acid ⇒ valine
- Etiology
  - Heterozygous Hgb S affords increased resistance to malaria (hence prevalence)
  - Hgb S becomes "stiff" (hence, erythrocytes are sickle-shaped) when deoxygenated
    - RBCs lose pliability required to traverse capillaries
    - Result: Microvascular occlusion, cell destruction (hemolysis)
  - Moyamoya collaterals reported in 20-40% of patients with SCD and stroke
- Epidemiology
  - Primary cause of stroke in African-American children
    - Stroke incidence decreased if Hgb S kept to less than 30% by transfusion (but need initial ischemic event to initiate therapy)
- Associated abnormalities
  - Anemia, reticulocytosis, granulocytosis
  - Susceptibility to pneumococci (due to malfunctioning spleen)
  - Occasionally causes pseudotumor cerebri (idiopathic intracranial hypertension without evidence for venous sinus occlusion, etc.)

## Gross Pathologic & Surgical Features
- Bone, brain, renal and splenic infarcts; hepatomegaly

## Microscopic Features
- Severe anemia with sickled cells on smear
- Vascular occlusions due to masses of sickled RBCs

# CLINICAL ISSUES

## Presentation
- Most common signs/symptoms
  - Vasoocclusive crisis with infarctions involving
    - Spleen, brain, bone marrow, kidney, lung, bone, formation of gallstones, priapism, neuropathy, skin ulcers
  - Hypertensive encephalopathy common, clinically can present with acute neurologic deterioration → mimic acute cerebral infarction
- Bone infarcts, avascular necrosis during crisis
- Osteomyelitis, especially Salmonella
- Gross hematuria from renal papillary necrosis and ulceration
- Splenic infarction from exposure to high altitude, e.g., flying
- Infections common, especially pneumococcus after splenic infarction

## Demographics
- Age
  - 11% suffer acute cerebral infarction by age 20 years; risk highest in first decade
    - 24% by age 45 years
  - 1% annual risk for stroke in children with SCD
    - 10% annual risk for stroke if abnormal velocities in the distal ICA or the MCA identified with TCD

- MR detects silent infarction in 22% of children with SCD
- Ethnicity
  - Hgb S found in 10% of African-Americans
  - SCD found primarily in African-Americans and their descendents

## Natural History & Prognosis
- Unrelenting, severe hemolytic anemia beginning at a few months of age after Hgb S replaces Hgb F (fetal)
  - Cognitive dysfunction occurs even in absence of cerebral infarctions
- Poor for homozygous SCD without transfusions
  - Repeated ischemic events leading to strokes with worsening motor and intellectual deficits
- Usually live to adulthood albeit with complications

## Treatment
- Repeated transfusions to keep Hgb S less than 30% decreases both incidence of stroke and intimal hyperplasia in COW vessels
- Hydroxyurea improves hematologic parameters, may be an alternative to chronic transfusions
- Hydration and oxygenation during crises

# DIAGNOSTIC CHECKLIST

## Image Interpretation Pearls
- African-American child with cerebral infarction: Always consider SCD!

# SELECTED REFERENCES

1. Kratovil T et al: Hydroxyurea therapy lowers TCD velocities in children with sickle cell disease. Pediatr Blood Cancer. 2006
2. Switzer JA et al: Pathophysiology and treatment of stroke in sickle-cell disease: present and future. Lancet Neurol. 5(6):501-12, 2006
3. Henry M et al: Pseudotumor cerebri in children with sickle cell disease: a case series. Pediatrics. 113(3 Pt 1):e265-9, 2004
4. Kral MC et al: Transcranial Doppler ultrasonography and neurocognitive functioning in children with sickle cell disease. Pediatrics. 112(2):324-31, 2003
5. Kwiatkowski JL et al: Transcranial Doppler ultrasonography in siblings with sickle cell disease. Br J Haematol. 121(6):932-7, 2003
6. Oguz KK et al: Sickle cell disease: continuous arterial spin-labeling perfusion MR imaging in children. Radiology. 227(2):567-74, 2003
7. Riebel T et al: Transcranial Doppler ultrasonography in neurologically asymptomatic children and young adults with sickle cell disease. Eur Radiol. 13(3):563-70, 2003
8. Steen RG et al: Brain imaging findings in pediatric patients with sickle cell disease. Radiology. 228(1):216-25, 2003
9. Steen RG et al: Cognitive impairment in children with hemoglobin SS sickle cell disease: relationship to MR imaging findings and hematocrit. AJNR Am J Neuroradiol. 24(3):382-9, 2003
10. Carvalho KS et al: Arterial strokes in children. Neurol Clin. 20(4):1079-100, vii, 2002
11. Oyesiku NM et al: Intracranial aneurysms in sickle-cell anemia: clinical features and pathogenesis. J Neurosurg. 75(3):356-63, 1991

## IMAGE GALLERY

### Typical

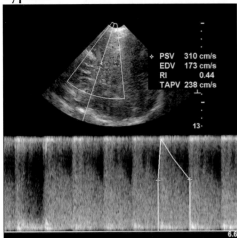

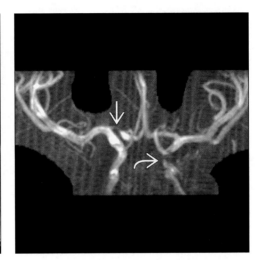

*(Left)* Ultrasound of the left ICA bifurcation reveals abnormally elevated velocities (TAPV = 238). Velocities > 200 cm/s put this patient in a high risk group for stroke. *(Right)* Coronal MRA (same patient as previous image) performed as a follow-up to the abnormal TCD. Severe stenoses of the right A1 ➡ and left distal ICA ➡ are readily apparent.

### Typical

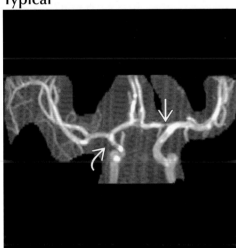

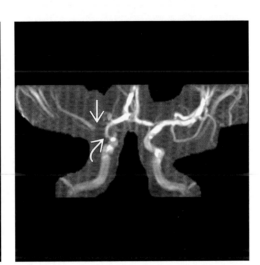

*(Left)* Coronal MRA in a 4 year old shows a stenosis at the origin of the left A1 ➡ and narrowing of the right distal ICA ➡. *(Right)* Coronal MRA (same patient as previous image) 16 months later shows marked evolution of the arteriopathy. There is further narrowing of the right ICA ➡ and new severe compromise of the right MCA ➡.

### Typical

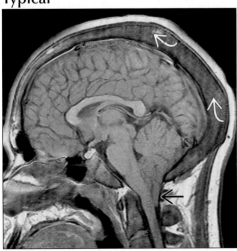

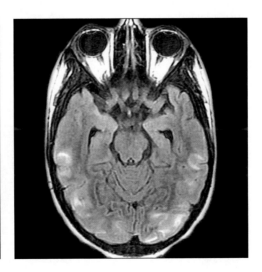

*(Left)* Sagittal T1WI MR shows diffuse thickening of the diploe of the skull ➡ and a Chiari 1 malformation ➡. The diploe has low T1 signal secondary to hyperplasia of red marrow elements. *(Right)* Axial FLAIR MR shows bilateral posterior temporo-occipital edema typical of hypertensive encephalopathy. The edema is primarily subcortical in location, with relative sparing of the cortex.

# CHILDHOOD STROKE

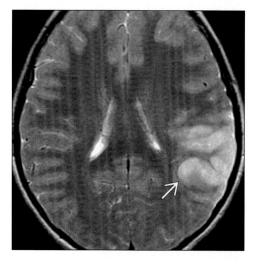

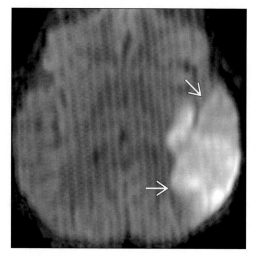

*Axial T2WI MR shows swelling and abnormal signal ➡ typical of a subacute left MCA territory infarct. Approximately 1/3 of childhood strokes will not have an underlying etiology diagnosed.*

*Axial DWI MR in the same child as previous image shows reduced diffusion ➡. Because most childhood strokes present in a delayed fashion, the sensitivity of DWI is less crucial than its specificity.*

## TERMINOLOGY

### Abbreviations and Synonyms
- Cerebrovascular accident (CVA), cerebral infarct, cerebral ischemia

### Definitions
- Acute alteration of neurologic function due to loss of vascular integrity
- This discussion addresses insults occurring outside of the perinatal period

## IMAGING FINDINGS

### General Features
- Best diagnostic clue: Edema, reduced diffusion (acutely) in affected territory
- Location: Proximal and distal middle cerebral artery (MCA) territory most commonly affected
- Morphology
  - Stroke caused by arterial occlusion often conforms to arterial territory
  - Venous territories often less well recognized

### CT Findings
- CTA
  - Invaluable for demonstrating focal vascular abnormalities in acute setting
  - May identify intimal flap in acutely dissected vessel
- NECT
  - Decreased attenuation of affected gray matter (GM)
    - Often wedge-shaped and corresponding to arterial territory
    - Diffuse ischemic injury can result in "reversal sign", with GM diffusely decreased in attenuation relative to white matter (WM)
  - Insular ribbon sign ⇒ loss of distinction of insular cortex
  - Hyperdense MCA sign (HMCAS) ⇒ increased density of thrombosed MCA
  - Hemorrhagic conversion of stroke
    - Cortical hemorrhage often petechial
    - WM or deep nuclear hemorrhage often mass-like ⇒ hematoma within infarcted tissue
  - Hyperdense dural sinus ⇒ "delta" sign
- CECT

## DDx: Focal Cortical Swelling

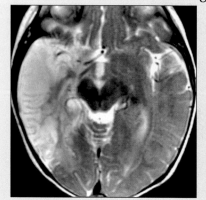

*Herpes Encephalitis*

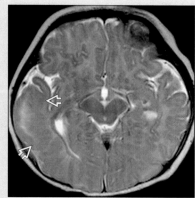

*Tuberous Sclerosis*

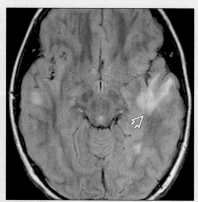

*ADEM*

# CHILDHOOD STROKE

## Key Facts

### Terminology
- Acute alteration of neurologic function due to loss of vascular integrity

### Imaging Findings
- Location: Proximal and distal middle cerebral artery (MCA) territory most commonly affected
- Hyperdense MCA sign (HMCAS) ⇒ increased density of thrombosed MCA
- Enhancement of infarcted territory typically occurs after 5-7 days
- "Climbing ivy" ⇒ bright vessels in sulci distal to arterial occlusion
- Reduced diffusion seen within 45 minutes of arterial occlusion
- Catheter angiography rarely necessary in acute evaluation of childhood stroke

### Pathology
- Anterior circulation > posterior
- Left > right
- Etiology: No underlying cause is discovered in > 33% of cases
- Incidence 2-3/100,000 per year in US

### Clinical Issues
- Under-recognized as significant source of morbidity in pediatric population
- Children with stroke typically present in delayed fashion (> 24 hours)
- Capacity for recovery much greater than in adults

### Diagnostic Checklist
- Have low threshold for use of CTA

---

- ○ Enhancement of infarcted territory typically occurs after 5-7 days
- ○ Enhancement of sagittal sinus wall around non-enhancing clot ⇒ "empty delta" sign

## MR Findings
- T1WI
  - ○ Gyral swelling and hypointensity in affected territory
  - ○ Loss of normal vascular flow void
    - ■ Entry slice artifact can cause false positive!
    - ■ Irregular signal can be seen in normal veins due to slow flow ⇒ acutely thrombosed veins are typically enlarged
- T1WI FS
  - ○ Use of fat-saturation may allow identification of crescent of mural hematoma in dissected vessel
    - ■ Use in combination with MRA (2D or 3D)
- T2WI: Edema evident in affected territory after 4-6 hours of arterial occlusion
- FLAIR
  - ○ More sensitive than T2WI for ischemia-induced cytotoxic edema
  - ○ Also shows loss of normal arterial flow voids
    - ■ "Climbing ivy" ⇒ bright vessels in sulci distal to arterial occlusion
    - ■ Same effect is seen with T1 C+, classically seen in moyamoya
  - ○ Excellent for detection of venous thrombosis
    - ■ Iso/hyperintense thrombus compared to hypointense flowing blood in sinus
- DWI
  - ○ Most sensitive imaging sequence for ischemic injury
  - ○ Reduced diffusion seen within 45 minutes of arterial occlusion
  - ○ Apparent diffusion coefficient (ADC) mapping essential to avoid false positive from "T2 shine through"
- T1 C+
  - ○ Can provide earliest sign of proximal arterial occlusion ⇒ enhancement of arteries in territory distal to occlusion
    - ■ Collateral flow to distal vascular bed is slower

- ■ Normal flow void caused by rapid arterial flow is out-weighed by T1 shortening effect of contrast
- ○ Beware! Contrast effect increased on 3T and gradient echo acquisitions ⇒ normal arteries/veins may show enhancement
- MRA
  - ○ Sensitive in detection of arterial occlusion and stenosis in large and medium sized cerebral vessels
  - ○ Can demonstrate arterial narrowing and dilation in arteritides
- MRV: Can demonstrate focal occlusion, response to treatment
- MRS: ↑ Lactate hallmark of ischemia/infarct
- MR perfusion
  - ○ Can provide valuable information regarding region at risk in setting of acute stroke
    - ■ Ischemic penumbra ⇒ region with diminished perfusion not yet infarcted (perfusion-diffusion mismatch)
    - ■ May define brain salvageable with acute stroke therapy
  - ○ Arterial spin-labeling techniques hold promise for standardized perfusion imaging without contrast administration

## Ultrasonographic Findings
- Grayscale Ultrasound: Affected territory hyperechoic in acute/subacute stage
- Color Doppler
  - ○ Direct Doppler evaluation ideal for surveillance of vascular occlusion in neonate with open sutures
  - ○ Transcranial Doppler evaluation of circle of Willis through temporal squamosa
    - ■ Increased velocities can predict stenoses detectable by MRA
    - ■ Used as screening tool in children with sickle cell anemia

## Nuclear Medicine Findings
- PET and SPECT techniques can be used to investigate normal development, effects of therapy, and subclinical pathology

# CHILDHOOD STROKE

○ Can identify salvageable regions at risk (ischemic penumbra)
○ Can demonstrate effects of synangiosis surgery in moyamoya

## Angiographic Findings
• Catheter angiography rarely necessary in acute evaluation of childhood stroke
  ○ Only justified if contemplating endovascular therapy
• Best modality for detailed evaluation of primary arteriopathies

## Imaging Recommendations
• Best imaging tool: MR with diffusion, MRA, and MRV
• Protocol advice: Contrast can help in assessing timing of injury and in performing perfusion imaging

# DIFFERENTIAL DIAGNOSIS

## Arterial Etiologies
• Arteriopathies
  ○ Moyamoya, vasculitis (radiation, infectious, or autoimmune)
• Emboli ⇒ cardiac (congenital heart disease)
• Aneurysms, vascular malformations
• Cervical dissections ⇒ vertebral > carotid

## Hypoperfusion
• Cardiopulmonary collapse

## Metabolic Encephalopathies
• Mitochondrial encephalopathies, organic acidurias

## Venous Occlusion
• High association with sepsis or adjacent infection (mastoiditis)

## Coagulopathies
• Factor deficiencies, lupus anticoagulant, protein C, protein S

## Non-Ischemic Causes of Cortical Swelling
• Tuberous sclerosis (TSC)
• Encephalitis
  ○ Viral ⇒ herpetic encephalitis
  ○ Autoimmune ⇒ acute disseminated encephalomyelitis (ADEM)

# PATHOLOGY

## General Features
• General path comments
  ○ Anterior circulation > posterior
  ○ Left > right
• Etiology: No underlying cause is discovered in > 33% of cases
• Epidemiology
  ○ Incidence 2-3/100,000 per year in US
    ■ Mortality 0.6/100,000
• Associated abnormalities: Cardiac disease (25-50%), sickle cell (200-400x increased risk), trauma

# CLINICAL ISSUES

## Presentation
• Most common signs/symptoms
  ○ Under-recognized as significant source of morbidity in pediatric population
  ○ Children with stroke typically present in delayed fashion (> 24 hours)
    ■ Poor recognition/understanding of symptoms by child, caregiver, physician
• Other signs/symptoms
  ○ Seizure ⇒ deficit often attributed to post-ictal state (Jacksonian paralysis)
  ○ Speech difficulties, gait abnormality
  ○ Focal deficit often masked by lethargy, coma, irritability
  ○ Preceding transient events occur in 25%

## Demographics
• Age: Incidence/mortality greatest < 1 year

## Natural History & Prognosis
• Capacity for recovery much greater than in adults
  ○ Fewer concomitant risk factors
  ○ Greater capacity for compensatory mechanisms, collateral recruitment

## Treatment
• No randomized trials of therapies
  ○ Clinical window of opportunity/benefit much narrower than in adults
    ■ Acute aggressive therapy may not improve on outcome in large population based on experience in adults
• Aspirin is mainstay of chronic therapy for fixed vascular lesions and vasculopathies
• Transfusion therapy for at-risk children with sickle cell disease

# DIAGNOSTIC CHECKLIST

## Image Interpretation Pearls
• Use same imaging signs as in adults
• Have low threshold for use of CTA

# SELECTED REFERENCES
1. Danchaivijitr N et al: Evolution of cerebral arteriopathies in childhood arterial ischemic stroke. Ann Neurol. 59(4):620-6, 2006
2. Shellhaas RA et al: Mimics of childhood stroke: characteristics of a prospective cohort. Pediatrics. 118(2):704-9, 2006
3. Boardman JP et al: Magnetic resonance image correlates of hemiparesis after neonatal and childhood middle cerebral artery stroke. Pediatrics. 115(2):321-6, 2005
4. Wraige E et al: A proposed classification for subtypes of arterial ischaemic stroke in children. Dev Med Child Neurol. 47(4):252-6, 2005
5. Carvalho KS et al: Arterial strokes in children. Neurol Clin. 20(4):1079-100, vii, 2002
6. Lynch JK et al: Report of the National Institute of Neurological Disorders and Stroke workshop on perinatal and childhood stroke. Pediatrics. 109(1):116-23, 2002

## IMAGE GALLERY

### Variant

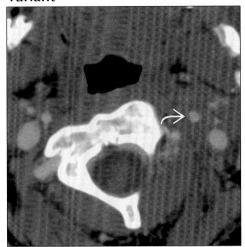 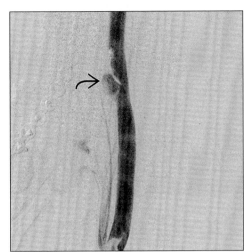

*(Left)* Axial CECT shows a subtle linear defect ➔ representing an arterial dissection in the internal carotid artery of a child presenting with a left hemisphere infarct after mandibular surgery. *(Right)* Lateral catheter angiography (same patient as previous image) obtained several days later shows that the intimal flap seen on the CT has progressed to form a pseudoaneurysm ➔.

### Variant

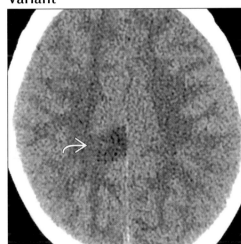 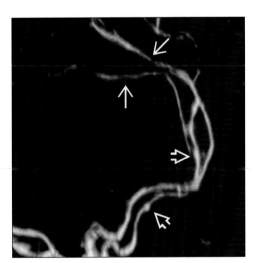

*(Left)* Axial NECT shows a focal region of decreased cortical attenuation ➔ in a child presenting with seizure. Subsequent MR showed reduced diffusion consistent with acute infarct. *(Right)* Sagittal oblique volume rendered MRA in the same child as previous image shows multiple foci of arterial narrowing ➔ and dilation ➔ due to primary arteritis of the CNS (PACNS).

### Variant

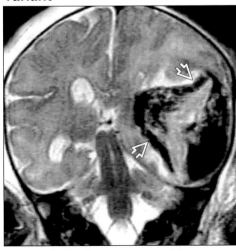 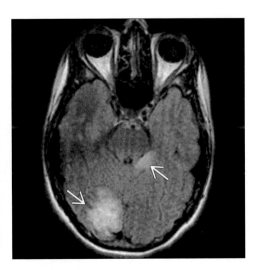

*(Left)* Coronal T2WI MR in a neonate with seizure shows a large hemorrhagic infarct ➔ in the left temporal lobe; this pattern is essentially pathognomonic for thrombosis of the vein of Labbé. *(Right)* Axial FLAIR MR in a 13 year old girl with seizures after using ephedra shows increased cortical and subcortical white matter signal in the right PCA and left superior cerebellar artery distributions ➔.

# HYDRANENCEPHALY

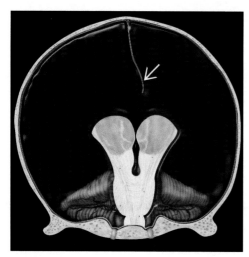

*Coronal graphic shows hydranencephaly. Absent cerebral hemispheres with intact thalami, brainstem, cerebellum. Falx cerebri ➡ appears to "float" in CSF-filled rostral cranial vault.*

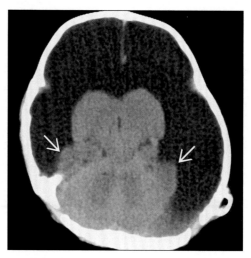

*Axial NECT shows classic hydranencephaly. The cerebral hemispheres are nearly replaced by CSF. The thalami, brainstem, cerebellum and falx are intact. Note temporal lobe remnants ➡.*

## TERMINOLOGY

### Definitions
- In-utero cerebral hemispheric destruction

## IMAGING FINDINGS

### General Features
- Best diagnostic clue
  - Absent cerebrum with CSF-filled cranial vault
  - Falx cerebri and posterior fossa structures intact
- Location: Cerebral hemispheres
- Morphology: "Water bag brain"
- Thalamus, brainstem, cerebellum, choroid plexus intact (Wallerian degeneration brainstem)
- Lobar remnants common along inferior falx

### CT Findings
- CSF attenuation fills cranial vault

### MR Findings
- Cranial vault contains mostly CSF
- Remaining brain has normal signal (no gliosis)

### Ultrasonographic Findings
- Anechoic cranial vault

### Other Modality Findings
- CTA, MRA: Atretic, stenotic, occluded, malformed, or normal supraclinoid ICAs and branch vessels
- Prenatal MR/US: Severe hydrocephalus or hemorrhage may precede hydranencephaly

### Imaging Recommendations
- Best imaging tool
  - Prenatal ultrasound: Allows therapeutic intervention
  - Postnatal MR best delineates extent of destruction

## DIFFERENTIAL DIAGNOSIS

### Severe Hydrocephalus
- Thin mantle of cortex compressed against inner table

### Alobar Holoprosencephaly (HPE)
- Fused midline structures; absent falx

### Severe Bilateral Open-Lip Schizencephaly
- MCA distribution trans-mantle gray matter lined cleft

### DDx: "Water Bag Brain"

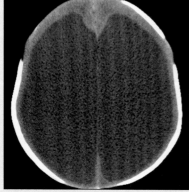

*Hydrocephalus*

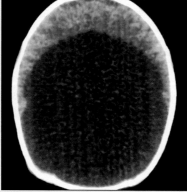

*Alobar Holoprosencephaly*

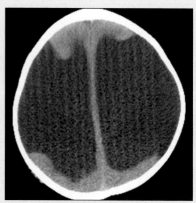

*Schizencephaly*

# HYDRANENCEPHALY

## Key Facts

### Terminology
- In-utero cerebral hemispheric destruction

### Imaging Findings
- Absent cerebrum with CSF-filled cranial vault
- Falx cerebri and posterior fossa structures intact

### Top Differential Diagnoses
- Severe Hydrocephalus
- Alobar Holoprosencephaly (HPE)

- Severe Bilateral Open-Lip Schizencephaly

### Pathology
- Intrauterine compromise of supraclinoid ICAs with intact posterior circulation

### Clinical Issues
- Clinical Profile: Newborn with macrocranium, developmental failure, calvarial transillumination

## PATHOLOGY

### General Features
- General path comments
  - Liquefactive necrosis brain 20-27 weeks gestation
  - Hemihydranencephaly: Very rare unilateral form
- Genetics
  - Sporadic
  - Rare autosomal recessive syndromes
    - Fowler, microhydranencephaly
- Etiology
  - Intrauterine compromise of supraclinoid ICAs with intact posterior circulation
  - Implicated: Hereditary thrombophilic states, intrauterine infection, maternal irradiation/toxin exposure, twin-twin transfusion, intrauterine anoxia
- Epidemiology: < 1:10,000 births; 10x ↑ teenage moms

### Gross Pathologic & Surgical Features
- Leptomeningeal-lined CSF "sacs" in lieu of hemispheres

### Microscopic Features
- Hemosiderin-laden macrophages over remnant brain

## CLINICAL ISSUES

### Presentation
- Most common signs/symptoms: Macrocranium (intact choroid plexus secretes CSF)

- Clinical Profile: Newborn with macrocranium, developmental failure, calvarial transillumination
- Other signs/symptoms
  - Hyperirritability, hyperreflexia, seizures

### Demographics
- Age: Diagnosis usually made first few weeks of life

### Natural History & Prognosis
- Neurological function limited to brainstem
- Prognosis: Death in infancy; prolonged survival rare

### Treatment
- CSF shunt treats macrocephaly; no cognitive change

## DIAGNOSTIC CHECKLIST

### Image Interpretation Pearls
- Intact falx distinguishes hydranencephaly from HPE
- Rim of brain along inner table distinguishes severe hydrocephalus from hydranencephaly

## SELECTED REFERENCES

1. Mittelbronn M et al: Multiple thromboembolic events in fetofetal transfusion syndrome in triplets contributing to the understanding of pathogenesis of hydranencephaly in combination with polymicrogyria. Hum Pathol. 37(11):1503-7, 2006
2. Sutton LN et al: Hydranencephaly versus maximal hydrocephalus: an important clinical distinction. Neurosurgery. 6(1):34-8, 1980

## IMAGE GALLERY

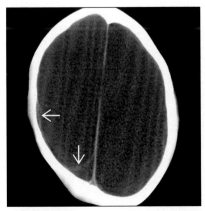 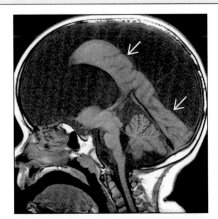 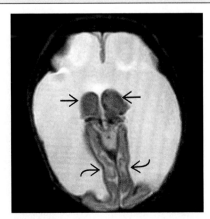

*(Left)* Axial NECT shows absent cerebrum in superior cranial vault. Curved band ➡ probably represents leptomeninges. Absence of brain along inner table distinguishes this from hydrocephalus. *(Center)* Sagittal T1WI MR shows macrocephaly & CSF-filled cranial vault w/parafalcine lobar remnants ➡. Although intact, brainstem is atrophic secondary to Wallerian degeneration. *(Right)* Axial T2WI MR shows partial preservation of thalami ➡ & posteromedial hemispheres ➡, normal findings in hydranencephaly. This preservation & intact falx help differentiation from HPE.

# CEREBRAL CONTUSION

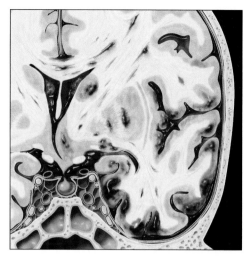

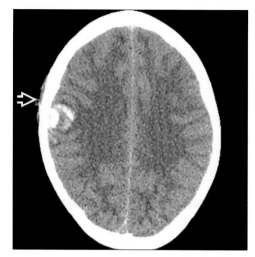

Coronal graphic illustrates hemorrhagic foci involving gray matter of several temporal/frontal gyri as well as deeper white matter & gray nuclei. Mass effect is causing left to right shift.

Axial NECT shows a superficial posterior right frontal hemorrhagic contusion in a 12 year old hit by a golf ball. Overlying scalp tissue ➡ is swollen.

## TERMINOLOGY

### Abbreviations and Synonyms
- Cerebral contusion (CC)

### Definitions
- Injury to brain surfaces involving superficial gray matter

## IMAGING FINDINGS

### General Features
- Best diagnostic clue: Patchy superficial hemorrhages within edematous background
- Location
  - Occur in characteristic locations where brain is adjacent to bony protuberance or dural fold
    - Nearly 50% involve temporal lobes: Temporal pole, inferior surface, perisylvian cortex
    - 33% involve frontal lobe surfaces: Frontal pole, inferior surface (inferior frontal & rectus gyri)
    - 25% parasagittal = "gliding" contusions
  - Less common locations
    - Inferior cerebellar surfaces, parietal/occipital lobes, vermis, cerebellar tonsils
  - Focal contusions may also occur at site of depressed skull fracture
- Size: Barely discernible to large
- Morphology
  - CC evolve with time
    - Early: Patchy, ill-defined superficial foci of punctate or linear hemorrhages along gyral crests
    - 24-48 hours: New lesions appear; size/shape of existing lesions may enlarge
    - Chronic: Encephalomalacia with parenchymal volume loss
  - Multiple, bilateral lesions in 90%

### CT Findings
- NECT
  - Early: May be normal
    - Poorly defined hypodensity & swelling
    - Patchy, ill-defined low-density lesion with small hyperdense foci of petechial hemorrhage
  - 24-48 hours
    - Multiple new hypodense lesions appear

## DDx: Mimics of Cerebral Contusions

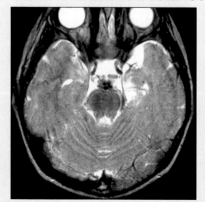

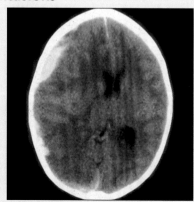

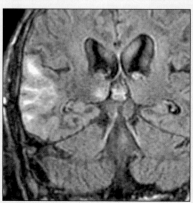

Ganglioglioma

PCA Infarct (+SDH)

MELAS

# CEREBRAL CONTUSION

## Key Facts

### Terminology
- Injury to brain surfaces involving superficial gray matter

### Imaging Findings
- Best diagnostic clue: Patchy superficial hemorrhages within edematous background
- Occur in characteristic locations where brain is adjacent to bony protuberance or dural fold
- Focal contusions may also occur at site of depressed skull fracture
- Petechial hemorrhage may become hematomas
- FLAIR best demonstrates hyperintense cortical edema
- FLAIR may show hyperintense SAH
- Acute: Hypointense hemorrhagic foci "bloom" on GRE (often not seen on other sequences)
- Best imaging tool: MR > CT in detecting presence, delineating extent of lesions

### Top Differential Diagnoses
- Cerebritis
- Infarct
- Low-Grade Neoplasm
- Transient Post-Ictal Changes
- Mitochondrial Disorders
- Other Causes of Cerebral Hemorrhage

### Pathology
- "Coup" lesion(s): Ipsilateral to impact site, from main force blow, associated with calvarial fractures
- "Contrecoup" lesion(s): Opposite impact site, induced by gyral crests striking fixed surface

---

- Lesions often ↑ edema & size → worsening mass effect
- Delayed hyperdense hemorrhages develop in 20%
- Petechial hemorrhage may become hematomas
  - Chronic
    - Become isodense → hypodense
    - Brain parenchymal volume loss
  - Secondary lesions common
    - Herniations/mass effect, hyperdense subarachnoid hemorrhage (SAH), intracerebral hematoma
    - ↑ Ventricles of hydrocephalus
- Xenon-CT
  - ↓ CBF around contusions compared to global CBF
  - ↓ CBF in first 24 hours associated with poor outcome

### MR Findings
- T1WI
  - Acute: Inhomogeneous due to admixture of edema & hemorrhage
  - Chronic: Focal or diffuse atrophy
- FLAIR
  - Acute
    - FLAIR best demonstrates hyperintense cortical edema
    - FLAIR may show hyperintense SAH
  - Chronic
    - Best to follow edema resolution
    - Hypointense hemosiderin, ferritin deposit "stain" in scarred residual parenchyma
    - Hyperintense Wallerian-type axonal degeneration, demyelination, & microglial scaring
    - Hypointense cavitation (cystic encephalomalacia)
- T2* GRE
  - Acute: Hypointense hemorrhagic foci "bloom" on GRE (often not seen on other sequences)
  - Chronic: Hemosiderin, ferritin deposits "bloom" as hypointense "stain" in scarred residual parenchyma
- DWI
  - Acute: Foci of reduced diffusion possible
    - Matches ↓ ADC
    - Extends beyond visible edema
- MRS

- ↓ NAA, ↑ lactate, glutamate/glutamine within first 2 to 4 days if significant neuronal injury has occurred
- Chronically in normal appearing occipitoparietal white & occipital gray matter
  - ↓ NAA in white matter from neuronal injury
  - ↑ Choline in gray matter, suggestive of inflammation
  - NAA & creatine in white & gray matter significantly associated with composite neuropsychological function & neuropsychological tests
  - Gray matter choline abnormality not related to neuropsychological function

### Radiographic Findings
- Radiography: Scalp hematomas or skull fractures

### Nuclear Medicine Findings
- SPECT: Blood-flow imaging with Tc-99m HMPAO
  - Depict focal more extensive changes in children with mild head injury & few findings on MR/CT
  - Negative SPECT in first month predicts good outcome
  - Positive SPECT can predict poor outcome of clinical deterioration & post traumatic headaches

### Imaging Recommendations
- Best imaging tool: MR > CT in detecting presence, delineating extent of lesions
- Protocol advice
  - FLAIR to evaluate edema & SAH
  - GRE for hemorrhagic foci

## DIFFERENTIAL DIAGNOSIS

### Cerebritis
- History of trauma absent
- Herpes typically involves medial temporal lobe & hippocampus

### Infarct
- History of trauma absent

# CEREBRAL CONTUSION

- Characteristic acute stroke-like symptoms (e.g., hemiplegia)

## Low-Grade Neoplasm
- History of trauma absent
- Often asymptomatic
- Solitary lesion, often non-traumatic locations

## Transient Post-Ictal Changes
- History of trauma absent
- Preceding or on-going seizure activity
- Can enhance acutely

## Mitochondrial Disorders
- Cortical swelling in MELAS

## Other Causes of Cerebral Hemorrhage
- AVM/aneurysm, hemorrhagic tumor, coagulopathy, sickle-cell disease, HIV, vasculitis, venous infarct

# PATHOLOGY

## General Features
- Etiology
  - Direct & indirect trauma
    - Direct injury ("coup" lesion) occurs at site of initial impact
    - Indirect injury ("contrecoup" lesion) induced by gyral crests striking fixed surface → bone & dural fold
    - Contrecoup injuries common in frontal, temporal lobes, less often observed in occipital lobes
  - Mechanism = linear differential acceleration (e.g., boxing) or deceleration (e.g., MVA) forces
- Epidemiology
  - Traumatic brain injury: Most common cause of death and acquired brain insult in children
  - Incidence of 0.2% to 0.3% per year
  - Contusions: 45% primary intra-axial traumatic lesions
- Associated abnormalities
  - Soft tissue (scalp, subgaleal) contusions 70%
  - SDH, traumatic SAH, IVH common
  - Skull fracture, possibly depressed 35%

## Gross Pathologic & Surgical Features
- Contusions
  - "Coup" lesion(s): Ipsilateral to impact site, from main force blow, associated with calvarial fractures
  - "Contrecoup" lesion(s): Opposite impact site, induced by gyral crests striking fixed surface
  - Often evolve
    - Petechial hemorrhages (often more evident in 24-48 hours), edema form along gyral crests
    - Small hemorrhages may coalesce
    - Large hematomas may occur in 30-60 minutes
    - Delayed hematomas may develop 24-48 hours later
- Lacerations
  - Intracerebral hematoma with "burst" lobe
  - SDH common; communicates with hematoma via lacerated brain, torn pia-arachnoid
  - SAH common

- May ultimately undergo encephalomalacia change/atrophy
  - Focal encephalomalacia at site of contusion
  - Whole-brain atrophy after mild/moderate injury

## Microscopic Features
- Capillary disruption
- Whole blood extravasation into tissue
  - Plasma content leads to edema
  - Red blood cells account for visible hemorrhage
- Liquefaction & encephalomalacia may occur

# CLINICAL ISSUES

## Presentation
- Most common signs/symptoms
  - Initial symptom: Confusion
  - Focal neurologic deficits vary: Focal cerebral dysfunction, seizures, personality changes
  - Loss of consciousness less common than with diffuse axonal injury (DAI)
- Clinical Profile
  - 2nd most common primary traumatic neuronal injury; DAI = 1st
  - Present in nearly half of moderate/severe closed head injury cases

## Treatment
- Evacuate focal hematoma if symptoms require
- Mitigate secondary effects of closed head injury
  - Raised intracranial pressure
  - Perfusion disturbances

# DIAGNOSTIC CHECKLIST

## Consider
- If negative initial exam, 24-48 hours repeat recommended

## Image Interpretation Pearls
- Look for subtle signs of frontal contrecoup injury on CT: Abnormal thickening and brightness (from blood) along the anterior inferior sagittal falx

# SELECTED REFERENCES

1. Munson S et al: The role of functional neuroimaging in pediatric brain injury. Pediatrics. 117(4):1372-81, 2006
2. MacKenzie JD et al: Brain atrophy in mild or moderate traumatic brain injury: a longitudinal quantitative analysis. AJNR Am J Neuroradiol. 23(9):1509-15, 2002
3. Poussaint TY et al: Imaging of pediatric head trauma. Neuroimaging Clin N Am. 12(2):271-94, ix, 2002
4. Hofman PA et al: MR imaging, single-photon emission CT, and neurocognitive performance after mild traumatic brain injury. AJNR Am J Neuroradiol. 22(3):441-9, 2001
5. Adams JH et al: The neuropathology of the vegetative state after an acute brain insult. Brain. 123 ( Pt 7):1327-38, 2000
6. Liu AY et al: Traumatic brain injury: diffusion-weighted MR imaging findings. AJNR Am J Neuroradiol. 20(9):1636-41, 1999
7. Friedman SD et al: Proton MR spectroscopic findings correspond to neuropsychological function in traumatic brain injury. AJNR Am J Neuroradiol. 19(10):1879-85, 1998

## IMAGE GALLERY

### Typical

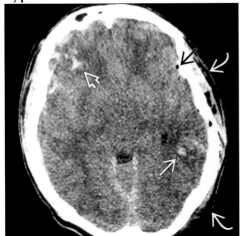
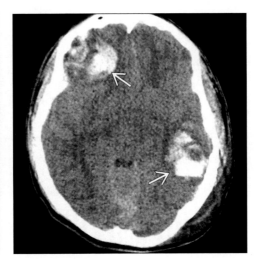

*(Left)* Axial NECT in a 12 year old shows coup ➡ and contrecoup ⟹ contusions with mild amount of hemorrhage and early edema. Pneumocephalus ➡ and extensive left scalp injury ⟹ are evident. *(Right)* Axial NECT (same patient as previous image) 16 hours later shows delayed hemorrhagic transformation of the contusions ➡ and worsening mass effect.

### Typical

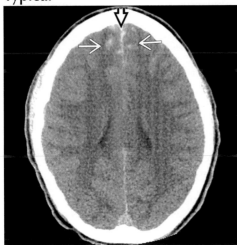
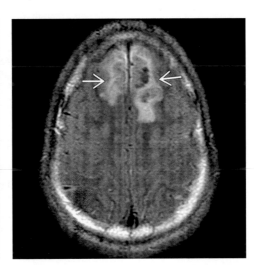

*(Left)* Axial NECT in a 14 year old shows bifrontal parasagittal contrecoup contusions ➡. Subarachnoid hemorrhage ⟹ is evident along the anterior falx. *(Right)* Axial FLAIR MR (same patient as previous image) shows extensive edema/swelling ➡ not well characterized on the CT. In such a case, a non-displaced occipital fracture (coup injury) is often present.

### Typical

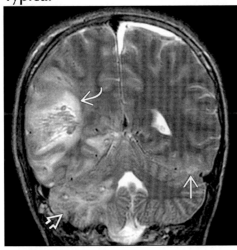
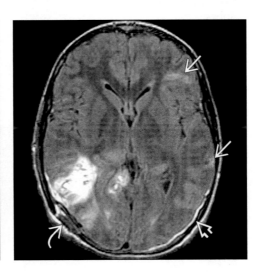

*(Left)* Coronal T2WI MR in an 11 year old shows extensive contusions in the right parieto-occipital junction ➡ and the right cerebellum ⟹, and a small contusion along the left tentorium ➡. *(Right)* Axial FLAIR MR shows a depressed fracture ⟹ & extensive swelling/hemorrhage in the right temporo/occipital lobes, thalamus. Note left sided contrecoup injuries ➡, subdural hematoma ⟹.

# DIFFUSE AXONAL INJURY (DAI)

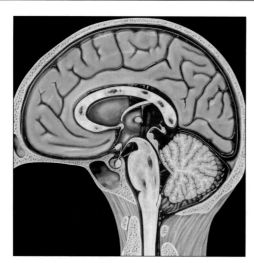

Sagittal graphic illustrates multiple hemorrhagic foci of diffuse axonal injury within the corpus callosum and the brainstem with associated subarachnoid and intraventricular hemorrhage.

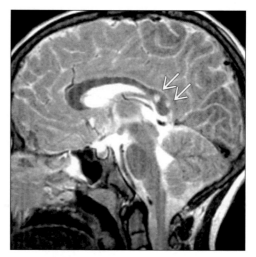

Sagittal T2WI MR shows T2 bright lesions ➡ in the splenium of the CC. The close proximity of the falx cerebri to the posterior CC makes the splenium more vulnerable to injury.

## TERMINOLOGY

### Abbreviations and Synonyms

- Diffuse axonal injury (DAI)
- Traumatic brain injury (TBI)

### Definitions

- Traumatic axonal stretch injury

## IMAGING FINDINGS

### General Features

- Best diagnostic clue: Multifocal punctate hemorrhages at corticomedullary junction, deep cerebral WM, corpus callosum, deep gray matter & upper brainstem
- Location
  - Common
    - Gray/white matter (GM/WM) interface (67%), especially frontotemporal lobes
    - Corpus callosum (20%) → 3/4 of which involve splenium/undersurface of posterior body
    - Brainstem → dorsolateral midbrain & upper pons
  - Less common
    - Caudate, thalamus, internal/external capsule, tegmentum, fornix, corona radiata, cerebellar peduncles
- Size: Punctate to 15 mm
- Morphology
  - Multifocal punctate, round, ovoid, elliptical hemorrhagic foci at characteristic locations
  - Multiple, bilateral lesions in nearly all cases

### CT Findings

- NECT
  - Initially often normal (50-80%)
    - 30% with negative CT are positive on MR
  - Small hypodense foci corresponding to edema at site of shearing injury
  - Hyperdense foci of petechial hemorrhage(s) (20-50%)
  - 10-20% evolve to focal mass lesion with hemorrhagic/edema admixture
  - Delayed scans often reveal "new" lesions

### MR Findings

- T1WI
  - Often unremarkable

## DDx: Multiple Superficial and Deep Cerebral Lesions

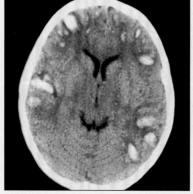

DIC, Hemorrhages

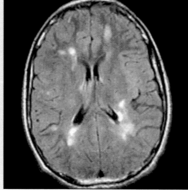

MS, Demyelination

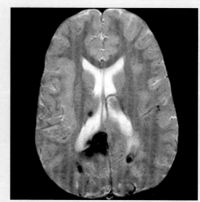

Cavernous Angiomas

# DIFFUSE AXONAL INJURY (DAI)

## Key Facts

### Terminology
- Traumatic axonal stretch injury

### Imaging Findings
- Best diagnostic clue: Multifocal punctate hemorrhages at corticomedullary junction, deep cerebral WM, corpus callosum, deep gray matter & upper brainstem
- 30% with negative CT are positive on MR
- FLAIR: Multiple high signal foci at characteristic locations
- Multifocal hypointense foci on T2* GRE secondary to susceptibility from blood products at characteristic locations
- GRE may be only technique identifying DAI
- SWI detects 5-10 times more lesions than conventional GRE images

### Pathology
- Epidemiology: Seen in up to 40% of children after TBI
- Stage 1: Frontal & temporal lobe gray/white interface
- Stage 2: Lesions in lobar WM & corpus callosum
- Stage 3: Lesions of dorsolateral midbrain & upper pons

### Clinical Issues
- Loss of consciousness (LOC) at moment of impact
- Common consequence of rotational injury in infants/young children
- ↑ Susceptibility from unbalanced head-to-body ratio, weak neck musculature, lack of myelination, larger SAS
- Suggested in patient with clinical symptoms disproportionate to imaging findings

---

- ○ If hemorrhagic, may demonstrate hemoglobin products (signal dependent on age)
- T2WI
  - ○ Multifocal hyperintense foci at characteristic locations
  - ○ If hemorrhagic, may demonstrate hemoglobin products (signal dependent on age)
  - ○ Multifocal hypointense residua may remain for years
- FLAIR: Multiple high signal foci at characteristic locations
- T2* GRE
  - ○ Multifocal hypointense foci on T2* GRE secondary to susceptibility from blood products at characteristic locations
  - ○ Multifocal hypointense foci may remain for years
  - ○ GRE may be only technique identifying DAI
  - ○ Susceptibility-weighted imaging (SWI)
    - High-spatial-resolution 3D fast low-angle shot
    - Extremely sensitive to susceptibility; paramagnetic properties of deoxyhemoglobin and methemoglobin
    - Can be performed with conventional MR imagers
    - SWI detects 5-10 times more lesions than conventional GRE images
- DWI
  - ○ Hyperintense foci of restricted diffusion
  - ○ Decreased ADC & diffusion anisotropy
  - ○ DTI may show severity of WM injury
- MRS
  - ○ In normal-appearing occipitoparietal WM & occipital GM
    - ↓ NAA in WM from neuronal injury
    - ↑ Choline in GM suggestive of inflammation
    - NAA & creatine in WM & GM significantly associated with composite neuropsychological function & neuropsychological tests
    - GM choline abnormality not related to neuropsychological function
  - ○ Decreased NAA/Cr correlates with poor outcome

### Nuclear Medicine Findings
- SPECT: Blood-flow imaging with Tc-99m HMPAO
  - ○ May show focal perfusion abnormalities

### Imaging Recommendations
- Best imaging tool: MR > > CT for detection
- Protocol advice
  - ○ SWI best sequence, although GRE more available
  - ○ Follow-up at 24 hours as 1/6 evolve

## DIFFERENTIAL DIAGNOSIS

### Multifocal Nonhemorrhagic Lesions
- Enlarged Virchow-Robin spaces
- Demyelinating disease → ovoid, may enhance
- Tuberous sclerosis → subcortical tubers
- Non-hemorrhagic metastases → enhancing masses
- Radiation therapy → may cause focal lesions of the splenium

### Multifocal Hemorrhagic Lesions
- Multiple cavernous malformations → often mixed age hemorrhages
- Radiation induced vasculopathy
- Hemorrhagic metastases → enhancing masses
- Disseminated intravascular coagulopathy (DIC)

## PATHOLOGY

### General Features
- General path comments
  - ○ Overlying cortex moves at different speed in relation to underlying deep brain structures resulting in axonal stretching
  - ○ Injury is frequently not diffuse but multifocal → term "traumatic axonal injury" may be more appropriate
- Etiology
  - ○ Trauma induced forces of inertia
    - Differential acceleration/deceleration & rotational/angular forces
    - Head impact not required
  - ○ Axons stretched, rarely disconnected or "sheared" (only in most severe injury)

# DIFFUSE AXONAL INJURY (DAI)

- Non-disruptively injured axons undergo
  - Traumatic depolarization, massive ion fluxes, spreading depression & excitatory amino acid release
  - Metabolic alterations with accelerated glycolysis, lactate accumulation
  - Cellular swelling & cytotoxic edema
- Corpus callosum injury
  - Believed caused by rotational shear-strain forces
  - Falx likely indirectly contributes posteriorly by preventing transient tissue displacement thus allowing greater tensile stresses locally
- Epidemiology: Seen in up to 40% of children after TBI
- Associated abnormalities: Corpus callosal injury associated with intraventricular hemorrhage

## Gross Pathologic & Surgical Features
- Multiple small round/ovoid/linear WM lesions
- Widely distributed: Parasagittal WM, corpus callosum, brain stem tracts (e.g., medial lemnisci, corticospinal tracts)

## Microscopic Features
- 80% DAI lesions are microscopic, nonhemorrhagic
  - Visible lesions are "tip of the iceberg"
- Impaired axoplasmic transport, axonal swelling
- Axonal swelling, 2° "axotomy", "retraction" balls
- Microglial clusters
- Macro-, microhemorrhages (torn penetrating vessels)
- Wallerian degeneration

## Staging, Grading or Classification Criteria
- Adams & Gennarelli staging
  - Stage 1: Frontal & temporal lobe gray/white interface
    - Mild head trauma
  - Stage 2: Lesions in lobar WM & corpus callosum
    - More severe rotational force injury
  - Stage 3: Lesions of dorsolateral midbrain & upper pons
    - Trauma of even greater severity than stage 2
- Correlates with deeper brain involvement from increasing severity of traumatic forces

# CLINICAL ISSUES

## Presentation
- Most common signs/symptoms
  - Loss of consciousness (LOC) at moment of impact
  - Immediate coma typical
    - Persistent vegetative state possible
    - Mild DAI can occur without coma
  - Disconnection & diffuse deafferentation
  - Greater impairment than with cerebral contusions, intracerebral hematoma, extra-axial hematomas
- Clinical Profile
  - Most common 1° traumatic neuronal injury
  - Common consequence of rotational injury in infants/young children
    - ↑ Susceptibility from unbalanced head-to-body ratio, weak neck musculature, lack of myelination, larger SAS

- Suggested in patient with clinical symptoms disproportionate to imaging findings

## Demographics
- Age: Any, may occur in-utero if pregnant woman subjected to sufficient force
- Gender: No predilection

## Natural History & Prognosis
- Specific neuropsychologic outcomes vary
  - Problems with memory, attention, executive skills, speed of motor processing, academic skills, pragmatic language
- Number and volume of lesions detected with SWI negatively correlates with long-term intellectual and neuropsychological functioning
- Severe DAI rarely causes death
  - > 90% remain in a persistent vegetative state (brainstem spared)
  - Prognosis worsens as number of lesions increases
- Brainstem damage (pontomedullary rent) associated with immediate or early death

## Treatment
- No real treatment for diffuse axonal injury
- Supportive therapy
- Treatment of associated abnormalities: Herniation, hematoma, hydrocephalus, seizures, etc.

# DIAGNOSTIC CHECKLIST

## Consider
- Consider DAI if patient symptoms disproportionate to imaging findings

## Image Interpretation Pearls
- Lesions best detected by susceptibility weighted MR

# SELECTED REFERENCES
1. Babikian T et al: Susceptibility weighted imaging: neuropsychologic outcome and pediatric head injury. Pediatr Neurol. 33(3):184-94, 2005
2. Huisman TA et al: Diffusion tensor imaging as potential biomarker of white matter injury in diffuse axonal injury. AJNR Am J Neuroradiol. 25(3):370-6, 2004
3. Tong KA et al: Diffuse axonal injury in children: clinical correlation with hemorrhagic lesions. Ann Neurol. 56(1):36-50, 2004
4. Tong KA et al: Hemorrhagic shearing lesions in children and adolescents with posttraumatic diffuse axonal injury: improved detection and initial results. Radiology. 227(2):332-9, 2003
5. Arfanakis K et al: Diffusion tensor MR imaging in diffuse axonal injury. AJNR Am J Neuroradiol. 23(5):794-802, 2002
6. Hofman PA et al: MR imaging, single-photon emission CT, and neurocognitive performance after mild traumatic brain injury. AJNR Am J Neuroradiol. 22(3):441-9, 2001
7. Sinson G et al: Magnetization transfer imaging and proton MR spectroscopy in the evaluation of axonal injury: correlation with clinical outcome after traumatic brain injury. AJNR Am J Neuroradiol. 22(1):143-51, 2001

## IMAGE GALLERY

### Typical

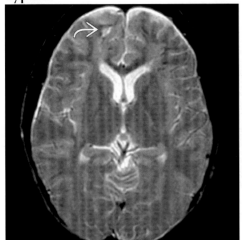 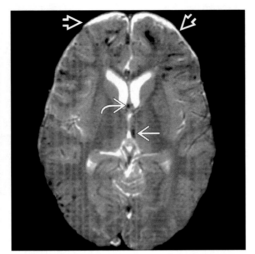

*(Left)* Axial T2WI MR shows diffuse ↑ T2 signal in frontal WM, T2 bright lesion in subcortical WM of the right frontal lobe ➜ and scattered poorly defined T2 dark acute hemorrhages from axonal injury. *(Right)* Axial T2* GRE MR (same patient as previous image) shows better the diffuse DAI in frontal lobes, along right cerebral convexity, and in left thalamus ➜, fornix ➜. Small subdural hygromas are evident ➜.

### Typical

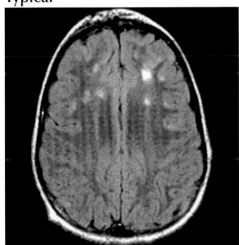 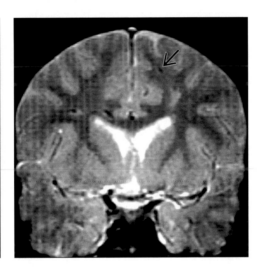

*(Left)* Axial FLAIR MR in a 5 year old shows multiple foci of increased signal in the frontal lobes after head trauma. The injuries are primarily subcortical in location. *(Right)* Coronal T2* GRE MR (same patient as previous image) shows small linear hemorrhages within many of the sites of abnormal ↑ FLAIR signal, and a focus of susceptibility ➜ in the left frontal WM.

### Typical

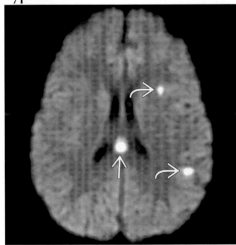 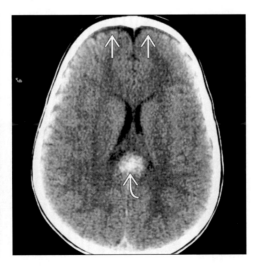

*(Left)* Axial DWI MR obtained days following a MVA shows foci of reduced diffusion in the splenium ➜ and the left corticomedullary junction ➜. Their distribution is classic for DAI. *(Right)* Axial CECT in a different patient shows acute hemorrhage ➜ within the splenium of the corpus callosum. Small hygromas ➜ are seen anterior to the frontal lobes.

# SUBCORTICAL INJURY

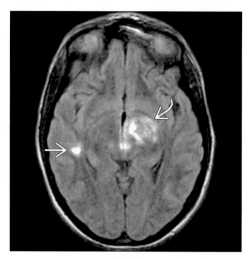

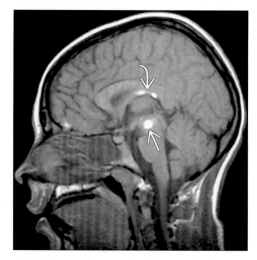

Axial FLAIR MR shows deep, subcortical post traumatic lesion ➡ in the left midbrain/cerebral peduncle. A more superficial injury is seen in the right temporal lobe ➡.

Sagittal T1WI MR (same patient as previous image) shows a hemorrhagic focus ➡ within the midbrain injury. Curvilinear hemorrhage is also evident along the fornix ➡.

## TERMINOLOGY

### Abbreviations and Synonyms
- Subcortical injury (SCI)
- Intraventricular hemorrhage (IVH)
- Choroid hemorrhage (CH)

### Definitions
- SCI: Traumatic lesions of brain stem (BS), basal ganglia, thalamus, & regions around 3rd ventricle
- IVH: Hemorrhage within ventricular system
- CH: Hemorrhage within choroidal tissues

## IMAGING FINDINGS

### General Features
- Best diagnostic clue
  - SCI: Deep gray matter (GM), BS ↑ FLAIR signal
  - IVH: Hyperdense intraventricular cerebrospinal fluid (CSF) on NECT, fluid-heme level common
  - CH: Hyperdense, enlarged choroid on NECT
- Location

- SCI: BS, basal ganglia, thalamus, & regions around 3rd ventricle
  - Most within thalamus & putamen
- IVH: Intraventricular spaces
- CH: Localized within choroid tissue
- Size
  - SCI: Limited to size of BS
  - IVH: Can fill/expand ventricles
  - CH: Limited to size of choroid involved
- Morphology
  - SCI: Petechial, linear
  - IVH: Can cast ventricle
  - CH: Shape of choroid involved

### CT Findings
- NECT
  - SCI: Often normal; petechial hyperdense foci
    - Deep GM nuclei, dorsolateral BS, periaqueductal region
    - Rarely overt hemorrhage
  - IVH
    - Hyperdense intraventricular blood
    - May fill, even expand, ventricle
    - Fluid-heme level common

## DDx: Deep/Thalamic Lesions

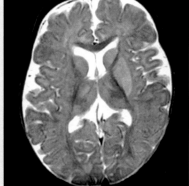

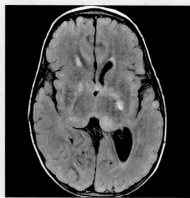

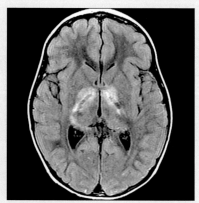

Glutaric Aciduria Type 1

Neurofibromatosis-1

Acute Disseminated Encephalitis

# SUBCORTICAL INJURY

## Key Facts

### Terminology
- SCI: Traumatic lesions of brain stem (BS), basal ganglia, thalamus, & regions around 3rd ventricle
- IVH: Hemorrhage within ventricular system
- CH: Hemorrhage within choroidal tissues

### Imaging Findings
- SCI: Deep gray matter (GM), BS ↑ FLAIR signal
- IVH: Hyperdense intraventricular cerebrospinal fluid (CSF) on NECT, fluid-heme level common
- CH: Hyperdense, enlarged choroid on NECT

### Pathology
- SCI: Petechial hemorrhages of BS, basal ganglia, thalamus, & regions around 3rd ventricle
- IVH: Expected evolutionary hemoglobin changes different than described for intracerebral hematoma

- CH: Blood extravasated into choroid tissue from traumatic rent/tear/laceration

### Clinical Issues
- SCI: Profound neurologic deficits
- IVH: Obtundation, seizures
- SCI: Severely injured patients
- IVH: Hydrocephalus rare manifestation
- CH: Can lead to IVH
- In infants, incompletely myelinated cerebrum more susceptible to hydrocephalus from IVH, SAH; more so with traumatic/ischemic parenchymal injury

### Diagnostic Checklist
- SCI: MR is superior to CT
- IVH/CH: CT is superior to MR

---

- ○ CH: Isolated dense choroidal hemorrhage without associated IVH

### MR Findings
- T1WI
  - ○ SCI: Acutely isointense
  - ○ IVH: Fluid-heme level common
- T2WI
  - ○ SCI: Acutely hyperintense
  - ○ IVH: Fluid-heme
- FLAIR
  - ○ SCI: Most sensitive sequence → foci of hyperintense signal
  - ○ IVH: Detection comparable to CT in acute stage
- T2* GRE: SCI: Susceptibility of petechial hemorrhage
- DWI: SCI: Foci of restricted diffusion in the first hours after injury

### Imaging Recommendations
- Best imaging tool
  - ○ SCI: MR > > > CT
    - Protocol analogous to diffuse axonal injury (DAI)
  - ○ IVH/CH: NECT > > > MR
    - Protocol analogous to subarachnoid hemorrhage
- Protocol advice
  - ○ SCI: FLAIR & GRE
  - ○ IVH/CH: CT = NECT; MR = FLAIR & GRE

## DIFFERENTIAL DIAGNOSIS

### Subcortical Injury
- NF-1 vacuolation
- Metabolic disorders
- Acute disseminated encephalitis (ADEM)/encephalitis
- Cavernous malformation: Symptoms without trauma
- Small vessel ischemia

### Intraventricular Hemorrhage
- Other causes: AVM, moyamoya, aneurysm

### Choroid Hemorrhage
- Normal calcification may mask small hemorrhages

## PATHOLOGY

### General Features
- General path comments
  - ○ SCI
    - Some classify as stage 3 DAI
    - Less common than diffuse axonal injury or cerebral contusion
  - ○ IVH: Blood filling ventricular CSF space
  - ○ CH: Hemorrhage within choroid tissue
- Etiology
  - ○ SCI: Most commonly induced by shear-strain forces that disrupt penetrating and/or choroidal vessels
    - Usually small, typically nonhemorrhagic
    - Larger hemorrhages resulting from shear of penetrating artery
  - ○ SCI: Less commonly
    - Dorsolateral BS impacts tentorial incisura with violent brain motion
    - Anterorostral BS damaged with sudden craniocaudal brain displacement
  - ○ IVH
    - Disruption of subependymal veins (most common)
    - Bleeding from choroid plexus
    - Shearing injuries
    - Basal ganglia/intracerebral hemorrhage with rupture into ventricles
    - Isolated IVH in absence of parenchymal hematoma is unusual
  - ○ CH: Traumatic shear forces damage choroid tissue
- Epidemiology
  - ○ SCI: 5-10% primary traumatic brain injuries
  - ○ IVH: Uncommon in closed head injury
    - 60% patients with corpus callosal DAI
    - 12% patients without corpus callosal DAI
- Associated abnormalities
  - ○ SCI: All stages of DAI (without exception), cerebral contusion, extra-axial hemorrhage
  - ○ IVH: DAI, deep GM/BS/intracerebral hemorrhage, SAH, cerebral contusion
  - ○ CH: DAI, SAH, cerebral contusion

# SUBCORTICAL INJURY

## Gross Pathologic & Surgical Features
- SCI
  - Usually nonhemorrhagic, yet more often hemorrhagic than other forms of primary intra-axial injury
  - Secondary to rich network of perforating vessels within basal ganglia & thalamus
- IVH
  - Gross blood collected within ventricular system
  - Blood-CSF level common
    - High rate of layering, rather than clot formation, most likely relates to intrinsic antithrombotic properties of CSF because of high concentrations of fibrinolytic activators
  - May cast/expand involved ventricle
- CH: Hemorrhagic choroid tissue

## Microscopic Features
- SCI: Petechial hemorrhages of BS, basal ganglia, thalamus, & regions around 3rd ventricle
- IVH: Expected evolutionary hemoglobin changes different than described for intracerebral hematoma
  - Progression occurs much slower
  - Most likely because high ambient oxygen tension of CSF delays degradation
- CH: Blood extravasated into choroid tissue from traumatic rent/tear/laceration

## Staging, Grading or Classification Criteria
- SCI: BS injury (BSI)
  - Primary injury: Direct result of trauma; 4 categories
    - 1: Direct laceration/contusion; rare
    - 2: Diffuse axonal injury (DAI); associated with more superficial DAI; most common primary BSI
    - 3: Multiple primary petechial hemorrhages; not associated with more superficial DAI
    - 4: Pontomedullary rent or separation; may occur without widespread brain injury
  - Secondary injury: Indirect result of trauma, most common cause of BSI, usually herniation
- SCI: When BSI → BS hemorrhage
  - Group 1: Midline rostral anterior BS, posterior to the interpeduncular cistern (69%)
    - Associated with anterior head and/or face impact; 71% survival
  - Group 2: Misc foci of acute BS hemorrhage (18%)
    - Associated with transtentorial herniation & BS compression; 88% survival
  - Group 3: Any BS hemorrhage
    - Associated with transtentorial herniation & BS compression, 100% mortality

## CLINICAL ISSUES

### Presentation
- Most common signs/symptoms
  - SCI: Profound neurologic deficits
    - Low initial Glasgow coma scale scores; coma
  - IVH: Obtundation, seizures

### Natural History & Prognosis
- SCI: Severely injured patients

- Poor prognosis, often die soon after trauma
- Regain consciousness very slowly, incompletely over time, & retain permanent neurological impairment/disability
- SCI: May proceed to brain stem hemorrhage
  - Associated with high mortality
- IVH: Gradually clears as resorbed, although patients > 20 cc of blood do poorly
- IVH: Hydrocephalus rare manifestation
  - Early: CSF outlet obstruction
    - Obstructive, non-communicating hydrocephalus
    - Asymmetric ventricular dilatation
  - Late: Arachnoid dysfunction of CSF resorption
    - Obstructive, communicating hydrocephalus
    - Symmetric ventricular dilatation
- IVH: Hemorrhagic dilation of 4th ventricle is an ominous predictor with 100% reported mortality
- CH: Can lead to IVH
- In infants, incompletely myelinated cerebrum more susceptible to hydrocephalus from IVH, SAH; more so with traumatic/ischemic parenchymal injury

## Treatment
- SCI
  - Supportive therapy
  - Treatment considerations of indirect/associated abnormalities: Herniation, hematoma, hydrocephalus, seizures, etc.
- IVH
  - Ventriculostomy
  - Repeat NECT to evaluate for hydrocephalus, treatment complications

## DIAGNOSTIC CHECKLIST

### Image Interpretation Pearls
- SCI: MR is superior to CT
- IVH/CH: CT is superior to MR

## SELECTED REFERENCES

1. Atzema C et al: Prevalence and prognosis of traumatic intraventricular hemorrhage in patients with blunt head trauma. J Trauma. 60(5):1010-7; discussion 1017, 2006
2. Carpentier A et al: Early morphologic and spectroscopic magnetic resonance in severe traumatic brain injuries can detect "invisible brain stem damage" and predict "vegetative states". J Neurotrauma. 23(5):674-85, 2006
3. Kinoshita T et al: Conspicuity of diffuse axonal injury lesions on diffusion-weighted MR imaging. Eur J Radiol. 56(1):5-11, 2005
4. Bakshi R et al: MRI in cerebral intraventricular hemorrhage: analysis of 50 consecutive cases. Neuroradiology. 41(6):401-9, 1999
5. Shapiro SA et al: Hemorrhagic dilation of the fourth ventricle: an ominous predictor. J Neurosurg. 80(5):805-9, 1994
6. Meyer CA et al: Acute traumatic midbrain hemorrhage: experimental and clinical observations with CT. Radiology. 179(3):813-8, 1991
7. Young WB et al: Prognostic significance of ventricular blood in supratentorial hemorrhage: a volumetric study. Neurology. 40(4):616-9, 1990
8. Gentry LR et al: Traumatic brain stem injury: MR imaging. Radiology. 171(1):177-87, 1989

# SUBCORTICAL INJURY

## IMAGE GALLERY

### Typical

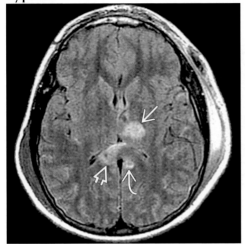
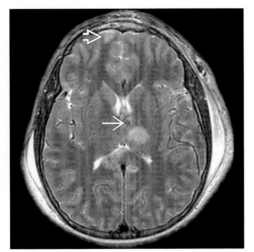

*(Left) Axial FLAIR MR shows deep injuries in the left thalamus ➡, the splenium of the corpus callosum ➡, and the deep left occipital lobe ➡. Marked scalp swelling/hemorrhage is evident. (Right) Axial T2WI MR shows a similar distribution of subcortical injuries and a right frontal superficial contusion ➡. A ventricular drain courses through the anterior third ventricle ➡.*

### Typical

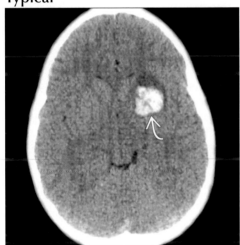
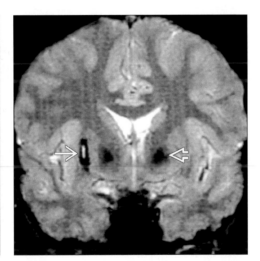

*(Left) Axial NECT in a 6 year old status post MVA with loss of consciousness shows hemorrhage ➡ in the left lentiform nucleus, with surrounding edema, the result of shearing of lenticulostriate artery. (Right) Coronal T2* GRE MR in a different patient status post trauma. A rim of hemosiderin ➡ with T2 bright center persists in right putamen. Hemosiderin deposition is evident in both globi pallidi ➡.*

### Typical

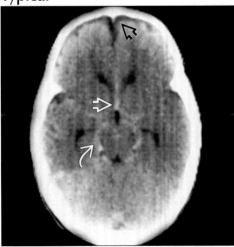
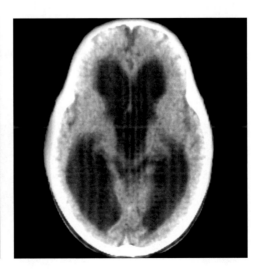

*(Left) Axial CECT in a 6 month old shows post-traumatic SAH around the midbrain ➡ and anterior to the lamina terminalis ➡. Mild diffuse edema, mild hydrocephalus, ↑ anterior SAS ➡ are evident. (Right) Axial NECT (same patient as previous image) 3 months later reveals development of marked atrophy and severe ventriculomegaly; combination of diffuse parenchymal injury and post hemorrhagic hydrocephalus.*

# ASTROBLASTOMA

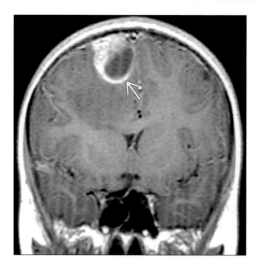

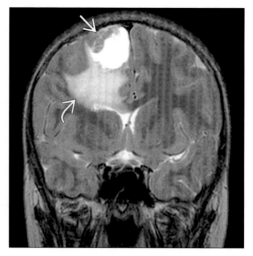

*Coronal T1 C+ MR in a 6 year old shows a mixed solid/cystic lobular mass ➡ in the left frontal lobe with heterogeneous enhancement of the solid aspect & rim-enhancement of the cystic portion.*

*Coronal T2WI MR (same patient as previous image) shows T2 signal of the solid component ➡ to be isointense to grey matter. Marked surrounding vasogenic edema ➤ is evident.*

## TERMINOLOGY

### Definitions
- Rare glial neoplasm with perivascular pseudorosettes and variable biological behavior

## IMAGING FINDINGS

### General Features
- Best diagnostic clue: Large hemispheric circumscribed solid and cystic mass with a "bubbly" appearance
- Location
  ○ Cerebral hemispheres typical, often superficial
  ○ Other locations: Corpus callosum, cerebellum, optic nerves, brainstem, cauda equina
- Size: Variable, typically large at presentation
- Morphology: Circumscribed, lobular solid and cystic mass with dominant solid component

### CT Findings
- NECT
  ○ Solid and cystic lobular mass, solid portion may be mildly hyperdense

  ○ Occasional punctate Ca++, surrounding edema
- CECT: Solid component enhances

### MR Findings
- T1WI: Solid/cystic mass; solid portion hypointense
- T2WI
  ○ Solid and cystic mass with heterogeneous "bubbly" appearance of solid portion
  ○ Solid portion isointense to gray matter
  ○ Relative lack of peritumoral hyperintensity
- T1 C+: Heterogeneous enhancement of solid portion, rim-enhancement of cystic portion
- MRS
  ○ Rare reports show decreased NAA, increased Cho
    ▪ Additional peaks: Lipids, myo-inositol, glycine

## DIFFERENTIAL DIAGNOSIS

### Ependymoma
- Heterogeneous parenchymal/periventricular enhancing mass
- Hemorrhage, necrosis, Ca++, and edema common

## DDx: Hemispheric Cerebral Neoplasms in Children

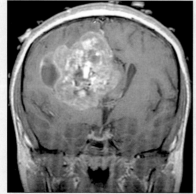

*Ependymoma*

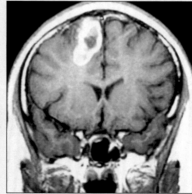

*Oligodendroglioma*

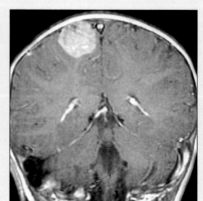

*Ependymoblastoma*

# ASTROBLASTOMA

## Key Facts

### Imaging Findings
- Best diagnostic clue: Large hemispheric circumscribed solid and cystic mass with a "bubbly" appearance
- Cerebral hemispheres typical, often superficial
- T1 C+: Heterogeneous enhancement of solid portion, rim-enhancement of cystic portion

### Top Differential Diagnoses
- Ependymoma
- Primitive Neuroectodermal Tumor (PNET)
- Atypical Teratoid-Rhabdoid Tumor (AT/RhT)
- Oligodendroglioma
- Astrocytoma
- Pleomorphic Xanthoastrocytoma

### Pathology
- General path comments: Cell of origin debated as they share features of astrocytomas and ependymomas

---

### Primitive Neuroectodermal Tumor (PNET)
- Peripheral, heterogeneous parenchymal mass
- Hemorrhage, cysts, and Ca++ common

### Atypical Teratoid-Rhabdoid Tumor (AT/RhT)
- Heterogeneous solid mass with hemorrhage, necrosis, Ca++, cyst formation

### Oligodendroglioma
- Peripheral, cortically-based mass ± enhancement
- Remodeling of inner table of skull common

### Astrocytoma
- JPA: Enhancing solid component, ± cyst
- Fibrillary/malignant: ↑ Mass effect, amount of enhancement with ↑ histologic grade

### Pleomorphic Xanthoastrocytoma
- Mixed cystic and solid with superficial enhancing solid component, meningeal involvement

## PATHOLOGY

### General Features
- General path comments: Cell of origin debated as they share features of astrocytomas and ependymomas
- Epidemiology: Rare, 0.5-2.8% of primary gliomas

### Gross Pathologic & Surgical Features
- Circumscribed solid mass, homogeneous cut surface
- Cysts are common; necrosis may be seen

### Microscopic Features
- Astroblastic pseudorosettes and prominent perivascular hyalinization

### Staging, Grading or Classification Criteria
- Low grade or high grade based on histologic features

## CLINICAL ISSUES

### Presentation
- Most common signs/symptoms: Seizures, focal deficit

### Demographics
- Age: Rare in infants; congenital cases reported

### Treatment
- Surgical resection is treatment of choice
- Adjuvant radiation therapy and chemotherapy for high grade lesions

## SELECTED REFERENCES

1. Burger PC et al: Surgical pathology of the nervous system and its coverings: the Brain: tumors. 4th ed. Philadelphia, Churchill Livingstone. 254-6, 2002
2. Port JD et al: Astroblastoma: radiologic-pathologic correlation and distinction from ependymoma. AJNR Am J Neuroradiol. 23(2):243-7, 2002
3. Brat DJ et al: Astroblastoma: clinicopathologic features and chromosomal abnormalities defined by comparative genomic hybridization. Brain Pathol. 10(3):342-52, 2000

## IMAGE GALLERY

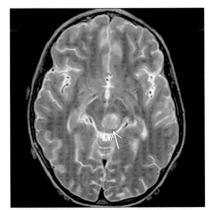 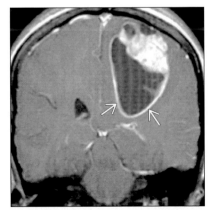 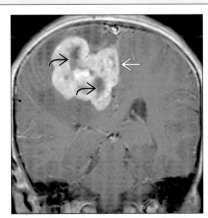

*(Left)* Axial T2WI MR shows a well defined mass ➡ in the left midbrain. Location is unusual for an astroblastoma, but signal intensity is less than usually seen in JPA or fibrillary astrocytoma. *(Center)* Coronal T1 C+ MR shows a hemispheric solid & cystic circumscribed mass with a heterogeneous, "bubbly" appearance of the solid portion & rim-enhancement ➡ of the cystic portion. *(Right)* Coronal T1 C+ MR reveals large, heterogeneous solid mass extending superficially to falx ➡. Central low signal foci ➢ likely represent necrosis, or possibly microcystic change.

# GANGLIOGLIOMA

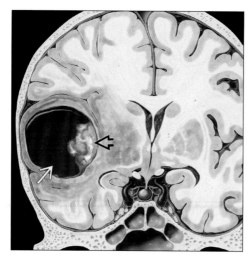

*Coronal graphic shows a discrete cystic ➡ and solid ⊡ temporal lobe mass involving expanded overlying cortex. Calvarial remodeling is seen, typical of superficially located tumors.*

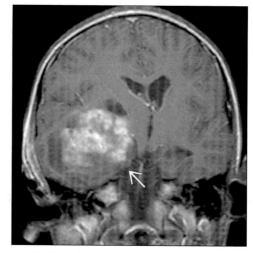

*Coronal T1 C+ MR shows large, heterogeneous right temporal mass with cystic and enhancing solid components, likely originating from mesial cortex ➡. No significant surrounding edema.*

## TERMINOLOGY

### Abbreviations and Synonyms

- Ganglioglioma (GG)

### Definitions

- Epilepsy-associated developmental tumor made of admixture of atypical ganglion cells and neoplastic glial cells

## IMAGING FINDINGS

### General Features

- Best diagnostic clue: Partially cystic enhancing mass involving the cortex in patient with refractory epilepsy
- Location
  - Most common: Supratentorial
    - Cortex: Temporal mostly (40%), then parietal (30%), frontal (18%), or occipital
    - May involve basal ganglia/thalamus, or hypothalamus/optic pathways
  - Other locations uncommon
    - Cerebellum: May be epileptogenic; cerebellar GG and hypothalamic hamartoma only causes for extrahemispheric epilepsy
    - Spinal cord, brainstem/cranial nerves
- Size: Variable, sometimes huge, larger than in adults
- Morphology
  - Three patterns
    - Most common: Circumscribed cyst + solid portion (not all cyst-like lesions are true cysts)
    - Purely solid
    - Uncommon: Infiltrating, poorly-delineated mass
  - GG are larger and more cystic in younger patients (< 10 years)
  - Desmoplastic infantile ganglioglioma (DIG)
    - Before 24 months, mostly temporal, typically huge
    - Cortex-based solid component, cystic component deeper, meninges involved

### CT Findings

- NECT
  - Variable density
    - 38% hypodense
    - 32% mixed hypodense (cyst), isodense (nodule)

## DDx: Other Highly Epileptogenic Lesions

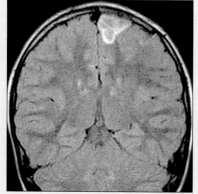

*DNET*

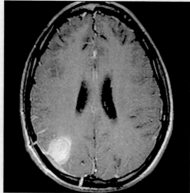

*Pleomorphic Xanthoastrocytoma*

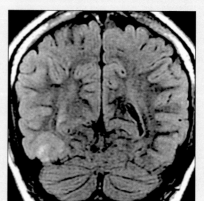

*Focal Cortical Dysplasia*

# GANGLIOGLIOMA

## Key Facts

### Terminology
- Epilepsy-associated developmental tumor made of admixture of atypical ganglion cells and neoplastic glial cells

### Imaging Findings
- Best diagnostic clue: Partially cystic enhancing mass involving the cortex in patient with refractory epilepsy
- Cortex: Temporal mostly (40%), then parietal (30%), frontal (18%), or occipital
- May involve basal ganglia/thalamus, or hypothalamus/optic pathways

### Top Differential Diagnoses
- Other Epilepsy-Associated Glioneuronal Tumors

- Other "Conventional" Gliomas: May Be Indistinguishable

### Pathology
- Associated focal cortical dysplasia (FCD) in surrounding cortex

### Clinical Issues
- Excellent prognosis if benign and resection complete, 80% seizure-free

### Diagnostic Checklist
- Gliomatous component of GG indistinguishable from "conventional" glioma
- Cortical tumor in young patient with refractory epilepsy, think GG!

---

- 15% isodense or hyperdense
  - Ca++ 35-50%
  - No surrounding edema, variable mass effect
  - Bone remodeling common over peripheral tumors
- CECT
  - Enhancement reported in 16-80% of patients
    - Faint or intense, uniform or heterogeneous
    - Can be solid, rim or nodular

### MR Findings
- T1WI: Hypo- to isointense, sometimes hyperintense to gray matter (Ca++)
- T2WI
  - Solid portion hyperintense at least in part, heterogeneous
  - Cystic fluid hyperintense
  - No surrounding edema
- T1 C+
  - Variable enhancement, usually moderate but heterogeneous
    - May be minimal, ring-like, homogeneous
  - Marked meningeal enhancement in desmoplastic infantile ganglioglioma
- MRS: Typical for glial, mostly grade I/JPA tumor: High choline/lactate

### Nuclear Medicine Findings
- PET: Typically decreased activity with FDG PET: Hypometabolism
- 201Tl-SPECT
  - Decreased or normal SPECT activity, increased in high grade GG

### Imaging Recommendations
- Best imaging tool: Multiplanar MR
- Protocol advice: Check for temporal mesial sclerosis (dual pathology)

## DIFFERENTIAL DIAGNOSIS

### Other Epilepsy-Associated Glioneuronal Tumors
- All are superficial, involve the cortex
- Dysembryoplastic neuroepithelial tumor (DNET)
  - Same cortical location, less mass effect, less global enhancement
  - Multicystic "bubbly" appearance
  - Often tapering to the ventricle
- Pleomorphic xanthoastrocytoma (PXA)
  - Supratentorial cortical mass, meningeal involvement common

### Other "Conventional" Gliomas: May Be Indistinguishable
- Juvenile pilocytic astrocytoma (JPA, grade I)
  - Other than hypothalamus/chiasm, supratentorial location rare
  - Doesn't involve cortex, typically
- Low grade astrocytoma (grade II)
  - Circumscribed but infiltrative white matter mass
  - No enhancement
- Malignant gliomas (grade III & IV)
  - Significant surrounding edema
- Supratentorial ependymoma
  - Often epileptogenic, but short history
  - Mostly in white matter
  - Solid, cystic, enhancing, Ca++ common, surrounding edema

### Other Cystic/Necrotic Enhancing Masses
- Abscesses, etc.

### Other Epileptogenic Lesions
- Focal cortical dysplasia (FCD): Thick blurry cortex with no mass effect or enhancement

# GANGLIOGLIOMA

## PATHOLOGY

### General Features
- General path comments
  - Mixed, developmental glioneuronal tumor
  - Associated focal cortical dysplasia (FCD) in surrounding cortex
  - Somehow related to other epilepsy-associated glioneuronal tumors: DNET, PXA
- Genetics
  - Sporadic
    - Tp53 mutations found in malignant degeneration
  - Syndromic
    - GG has been reported in Turcot syndrome
- Etiology
  - Two theories
    - Neoplastic change in FCD or of subpial granule cells
    - Differentiated remnants of embryonal neuroblastoma
- Epidemiology
  - 1-4% of pediatric CNS neoplasms
  - Most common mixed neuronal-glial tumor
  - Most common epilepsy-associated tumor

### Gross Pathologic & Surgical Features
- Firm, well circumscribed, solid or solid/cystic mass
- Involves gray matter, usually cortical

### Microscopic Features
- Mix of mature but neoplastic ganglion cells + neoplastic glial cells (usually astrocytes)
- Dysmorphic, occasionally binucleate neurons
  - Immunohistochemistry of neuronal cells
    - Synaptophysin and neurofilament protein +
    - EM shows dense core granules, variable synapses
    - Neoplastic glial cells are GFAP +
    - Mitoses rare (75% have Ki-67 < 1%, low MIB)
  - Majority exhibit CD34 immunoreactivity (points to dysplastic/neoplastic precursor cells)
- Variants
  - Desmoplastic infantile ganglioglioma (DIG): Large epilepsy-associated, cortex based brain tumor of infancy with meningeal involvement
  - Papillary glioneuronal tumor

### Staging, Grading or Classification Criteria
- Grade I: 80%
- Grade II: Occasional
- Malignant forms: Uncommon (6%), sometimes late secondary degeneration; anaplastic GG (WHO grade III), GBM-like (grade IV)
- GGs take the appearance of their gliomatous component

## CLINICAL ISSUES

### Presentation
- Most common signs/symptoms
  - Resistant epilepsy (about 90%), features dependent on location
  - Other signs/symptoms: Headache, focal deficits
- Clinical Profile: Longstanding refractory epilepsy

### Demographics
- Age: Children, young adults: 80% < 30 y, peak 10-20 y
- Gender: Slight male predominance

### Natural History & Prognosis
- Slow growth, malignant form/degeneration of glial component rare (6%), sometimes years after surgery
- Excellent prognosis if benign and resection complete, 80% seizure-free

### Treatment
- Surgical resection is treatment of choice
- Radiation therapy and/or chemotherapy for aggressive or unresectable tumors

## DIAGNOSTIC CHECKLIST

### Consider
- Gliomatous component of GG indistinguishable from "conventional" glioma

### Image Interpretation Pearls
- Cortical tumor in young patient with refractory epilepsy, think GG!

## SELECTED REFERENCES

1. Giulioni M et al: Lesionectomy in epileptogenic gangliogliomas: seizure outcome and surgical results. J Clin Neurosci. 13(5):529-35, 2006
2. Luyken C et al: Supratentorial gangliogliomas: histopathologic grading and tumor recurrence in 184 patients with a median follow-up of 8 years. Cancer. 101(1):146-55, 2004
3. Trehan G et al: MR imaging in the diagnosis of desmoplastic infantile tumor: retrospective study of six cases. AJNR Am J Neuroradiol. 25(6):1028-33, 2004
4. Im SH et al: Supratentorial ganglioglioma and epilepsy: postoperative seizure outcome. J Neurooncol. 57(1):59-66, 2002
5. Shin JH et al: Neuronal tumors of the central nervous system: radiologic findings and pathologic correlation. Radiographics. 22(5):1177-89, 2002
6. Hayashi Y et al: Malignant transformation of a gangliocytoma/ganglioglioma into a glioblastoma multiforme: a molecular genetic analysis. Case report. J Neurosurg. 95(1):138-42, 2001
7. Koeller KK et al: From the archives of the AFIP: superficial gliomas: radiologic-pathologic correlation. Armed Forces Institute of Pathology. Radiographics. 21(6):1533-56, 2001
8. Nelson JS et al: Pathology and Genetics of Tumours of the Nervous System: Ganglioglioma and Gangliocytoma. Lyon, IARC Press. 96-8, 2000
9. Provenzale JM et al: Comparison of patient age with MR imaging features of gangliogliomas. AJR Am J Roentgenol. 174(3):859-62, 2000
10. Tamiya T et al: Ganglioglioma in a patient with Turcot syndrome. Case report. J Neurosurg. 92(1):170-5, 2000
11. Blumcke I et al: Evidence for developmental precursor lesions in epilepsy-associated glioneuronal tumors. Microsc Res Tech. 46(1):53-8, 1999
12. Komori T et al: Papillary glioneuronal tumor: a new variant of mixed neuronal-glial neoplasm. Am J Surg Pathol. 22(10):1171-83, 1998
13. Kurian NI et al: Anaplastic ganglioglioma: case report and review of the literature. Br J Neurosurg. 12(3):277-80, 1998

# GANGLIOGLIOMA

## IMAGE GALLERY

### Typical

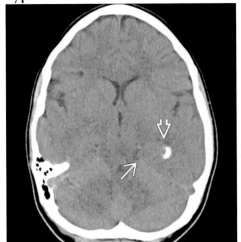
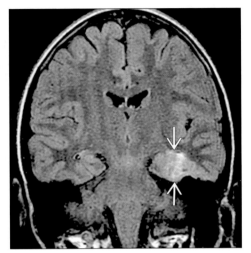

*(Left) Axial NECT in child with longstanding refractory temporal epilepsy, shows calcification ⇨ close to left mesial temporal cortex ➡ with no mass effect or hypoattenuation. (Right) Coronal FLAIR MR (same child as previous image) shows mass ➡ with irregular high signal affecting mesial temporal structures. Hippocampus cannot be identified and temporal horn is effaced.*

### Typical

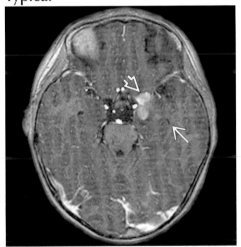
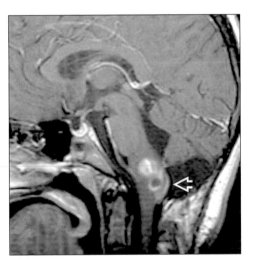

*(Left) Axial T1 C+ MR shows well demarcated, contrast-enhancing cortical nodules ⇨ in left anterior mesial temporal lobe. Note significant mass effect on temporal horn ➡. (Right) Sagittal T1 C+ MR shows ill-defined mass in central and dorsal medulla, with enhancing cysts and nodules ⇨, extending to cervicomedullary junction. Pathology disclosed typical grade I GG.*

### Variant

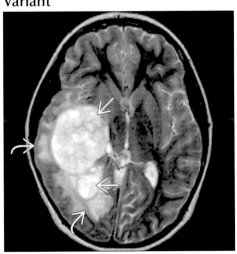
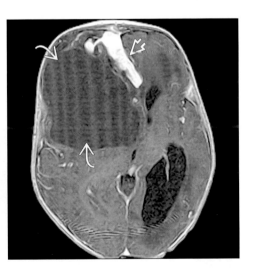

*(Left) Axial T2WI MR shows well demarcated mass lesion ➡ with surrounding white matter edema ➡, atypical for GG. High grade GG with postsurgical dissemination in 4th ventricle. (Right) Axial T1 C+ MR in macrocephalic infant with seizures shows huge cystic mass ➡ and major meningeal involvement associated with solid cortical component ➡: Desmoplastic infantile GG.*

# DESMOPLASTIC INFANTILE GANGLIOGLIOMA

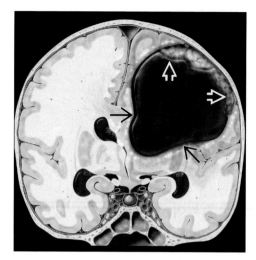

*Coronal graphic shows a young child with enlarged head caused by DIG/DIA. Note dominant cystic component ⇨ with dural-based desmoplastic stroma ⇨. Some edema is seen.*

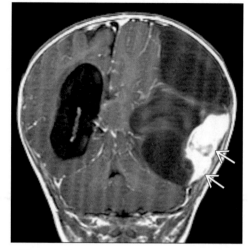

*Coronal T1 C+ MR shows two large left hemispheric cysts and a peripheral plaque of enhancing tumor ⇨ in the left hemisphere. Mass effect from the cysts compresses aqueduct, causing hydrocephalus.*

## TERMINOLOGY

### Abbreviations and Synonyms
- Desmoplastic infantile ganglioglioma (DIG, DIGG) or desmoplastic infantile astrocytoma (DIA)

### Definitions
- DIG: Prominent desmoplastic stroma + neoplastic astrocytes, variable neuronal component
- DIA: Desmoplastic stroma + neoplastic astrocytes

## IMAGING FINDINGS

### General Features
- Best diagnostic clue
  - Large cyst + cortical-based enhancing tumor nodule/plaque
  - Enhancement of adjacent pia PLUS reactive dural thickening
  - Solid portion is hypointense on T2WI
- Location: Frontal > parietal > temporal
- Size: Cysts may be very large, cause macrocephaly, bulging fontanelles in infants

- Morphology: Typically large cyst with nodular/plaque-like solid portion adjacent to, sometimes invading, meninges

### CT Findings
- CTA
  - Hypovascular; supply from intra- and extraparenchymal vessels
  - Vessels markedly stretched around large cyst
- NECT
  - Large heterogeneous solid and cystic mass
  - Well-demarcated hypodense cyst (isodense to CSF)
  - Solid tumor nodule(s) is isodense/slightly hyperdense to GM, no Ca++
- CECT
  - Cyst ⇒ no enhancement
  - Nodule ⇒ marked enhancement

### MR Findings
- T1WI
  - Cyst hypointense, often multilobulated
    - May contain septae
  - Solid portion ⇒ irregular, plaque-like and nodular areas

## DDx: Cysts with Enhancing Nodules

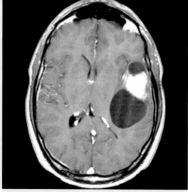

*Pilocytic Astrocytoma*

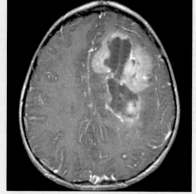

*Primitive Neuroectodermal Tumor*

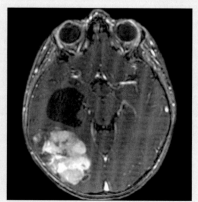

*Pleomorphic Xanthoastrocytoma*

## Key Facts

### Terminology
- Desmoplastic infantile ganglioglioma (DIG, DIGG) or desmoplastic infantile astrocytoma (DIA)

### Imaging Findings
- Large cyst + cortical-based enhancing tumor nodule/plaque
- Location: Frontal > parietal > temporal
- Solid tumor nodule(s) enhance markedly
- Enhancement of leptomeninges, dura adjacent to solid tumor is typical

### Top Differential Diagnoses
- Primitive Neuroectodermal Tumor (PNET)
- Supratentorial Ependymoma
- Pleomorphic Xanthoastrocytoma (PXA)
- Hemangioblastoma

- Ganglioglioma
- Juvenile Pilocytic Astrocytoma (JPA)

### Pathology
- Two distinct components
- Cortical-based solid tumor nodule/plaque with adjacent dural thickening
- Large associated cyst compresses adjacent ventricular system

### Diagnostic Checklist
- Large cystic mass in an infant with T2 hypointense plaque-like solid component adjacent to meninges, think of desmoplastic infantile ganglioglioma
- Important to mention this in differential diagnosis; on first look, pathologists will call this highly malignant tumor

---

- Heterogeneous, slightly hyperintense to surrounding brain
- T2WI
  - Hyperintense, often lobulated, septated cyst
  - Lobular, solid tumor nodule(s) usually low signal, +/- heterogeneous
  - Surrounding interstitial edema in some patients
    - May be related to local ventricular obstruction
- PD/Intermediate: Solid portion hypointense to surrounding brain
- FLAIR
  - Cysts are isointense to CSF
  - Solid portions usually isointense to gray matter
- T2* GRE: No hemorrhage or calcification
- DWI: Reduced diffusivity in solid portion
- T1 C+
  - Solid tumor nodule(s) enhance markedly
  - Enhancement of leptomeninges, dura adjacent to solid tumor is typical

### Radiographic Findings
- Radiography: In infants, macrocephaly with split sutures

### Ultrasonographic Findings
- Grayscale Ultrasound
  - Large, multicystic mass
  - Peripheral solid portion often not identified

### Imaging Recommendations
- Best imaging tool: MR with and without contrast
- Protocol advice
  - MR in three planes
    - T1WI pre-contrast
    - T2WI pre-contrast
    - T1WI post-contrast

## DIFFERENTIAL DIAGNOSIS

### Primitive Neuroectodermal Tumor (PNET)
- Solid tumor is hyperdense on CT, iso to gray matter on T2WI, contains cysts, Ca++, edema

- Large heterogeneously enhancing hemispheric mass
- Large cyst less common than in DIG/DIA

### Supratentorial Ependymoma
- Nonspecific imaging findings but commonly contains Ca++
- Solid portion usually less peripherally located than DIG/DIA
- Cysts are usually less complex

### Pleomorphic Xanthoastrocytoma (PXA)
- Imaging appearance may be identical to DIG
- Occurs in older children, adults
- Temporal lobe most common location

### Hemangioblastoma
- Older patients, usually adults
- Rare above tentorium
- May be solid or cyst with nodule; nodule is T2 hyperintense
- Solid nodule usually vascular, curvilinear flow voids

### Ganglioglioma
- Older children
- Generally smaller in size than DIG
- Ca++ is common
- If present, cysts are small
- Most common in temporal lobe

### Juvenile Pilocytic Astrocytoma (JPA)
- Uncommon in infancy
- Uncommon in cerebral hemispheres
- Cyst is usually smaller; nodule is hyperintense on T2WI

## PATHOLOGY

### General Features
- General path comments
  - May arise from subpial astrocytes
  - Solid portion originates peripherally in cortex
    - Often invades pia
    - Induces meningeal thickening

# DESMOPLASTIC INFANTILE GANGLIOGLIOMA

- Genetics: Not currently known
- Etiology: Probably arise from neural progenitor cells in subcortical zone along with mature subpial astrocytes
- Epidemiology: Seen in all races

## Gross Pathologic & Surgical Features
- Two distinct components
  - Cortical-based solid tumor nodule/plaque with adjacent dural thickening
  - Large associated cyst compresses adjacent ventricular system
- Large cyst(s) containing xanthochromic fluid
- Tumor firmly attached to dura and brain tissue
- Often significant vasogenic edema ⇒ subfalcine, transtentorial herniations
- No necrosis within solid component of tumor, no hemorrhage

## Microscopic Features
- Desmoplasia with mixture of astroglial & neuronal cells
- Cortical portion
  - Abnormal neurons, tumoral astrocytes and small foci of poorly differentiated cells with rare mitoses
- Meningeal portion
  - Neoplastic astrocytes enmeshed in a dense network of connective tissue
  - Prominent reticulin-rich desmoplastic stroma
- Aggregates of poorly differentiated cells in both portions
- Immature neuronal component & neoplastic astrocytes
- Tumor lacks p53 protein expression
- Mitoses are rare, MIB-1 labeling rare

## Staging, Grading or Classification Criteria
- WHO grade 1

# CLINICAL ISSUES

## Presentation
- Most common signs/symptoms
  - Infants
    - ↑ Head size, bulging fontanelles, paresis & seizures (20%)
  - Older children
    - Seizures and focal neurological signs/symptoms
- Clinical Profile: Infant with rapidly progressive macrocephaly

## Demographics
- Age
  - Most are found at 1-24 months (peak: 3-6 months)
  - Children < 24 months, usually ≤ 12 months
    - Occasionally diagnosed in older patients (5-17 yrs)
- Gender: Slightly more common in males (1.7:1.0)

## Natural History & Prognosis
- Median survival rate is > 75% at 15 yrs after diagnosis
- Spontaneous disappearance (rare), anaplasia (very rare)

## Treatment
- Surgical resection curative, no recurrence with complete resection
- Chemotherapy if brain invasion or recurrence

# DIAGNOSTIC CHECKLIST

## Consider
- Large cystic mass in an infant with T2 hypointense plaque-like solid component adjacent to meninges, think of desmoplastic infantile ganglioglioma
- Important to mention this in differential diagnosis; on first look, pathologists will call this highly malignant tumor

## Image Interpretation Pearls
- Solid portion is peripheral in cortex, invades meninges
- Solid portion very hypointense on T2WI

# SELECTED REFERENCES

1. Ganesan K et al: Non-infantile variant of desmoplastic ganglioglioma: a report of 2 cases. Pediatr Radiol. 2006
2. Pommepuy I et al: A Report of a Desmoplastic Ganglioglioma in a 12-year-old Girl with Review of the Literature. J Neurooncol. 76(3):271-5, 2006
3. Nikas I et al: Desmoplastic infantile ganglioglioma: MRI and histological findings case report. Neuroradiology. 46(12):1039-43, 2004
4. Trehan G et al: MR imaging in the diagnosis of desmoplastic infantile tumor: retrospective study of six cases. AJNR Am J Neuroradiol. 25(6):1028-33, 2004
5. Tamburrini G et al: Desmoplastic infantile ganglioglioma. Childs Nerv Syst. 19:292-97, 2003
6. Shin JH et al: Neuronal tumors of the central nervous system: Radiology findings and pathologic correlation. RadioGraphics. 22:1177-89, 2002
7. Tseng JH et al: Chronological changes on magnetic resonance images in a case of desmoplastic infantile ganglioglioma. Pediatr Neurosurg. 36(1):29-32, 2002
8. Lababede O et al: Desmoplastic infantile ganglioglioma (DIG): cranial ultrasound findings. Pediatr Radiol. 31(6):403-5, 2001
9. Mallucci C et al: The management of desmoplastic neuroepithelial tumours in childhood. Childs Nerv Syst. 16(1):8-14, 2000
10. Setty SN et al: Desmoplastic infantile astrocytoma with metastases at presentation. Mod Pathol. 10(9):945-51, 1997
11. Sperner J et al: Clinical, radiological and histological findings in desmoplastic infantile ganglioglioma. Childs Nerv Syst. 10(7):458-62; discussion 462-3, 1994
12. VandenBerg SR: Desmoplastic infantile ganglioglioma and desmoplastic cerebral astrocytoma of infancy. Brain Pathol. 3(3):275-81, 1993
13. VandenBerg SR et al: Desmoplastic supratentorial neuroepithelial tumors of infancy with divergent differentiation potential ("desmoplastic infantile gangliogliomas"). Report on 11 cases of a distinctive embryonal tumor with favorable prognosis. J Neurosurg. 66(1):58-71, 1987

# DESMOPLASTIC INFANTILE GANGLIOGLIOMA

## IMAGE GALLERY

### Typical

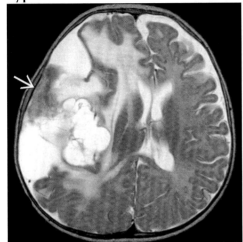
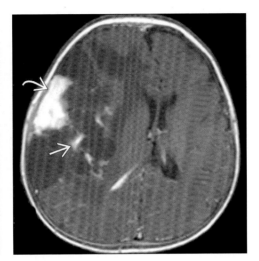

*(Left)* Axial T2WI MR shows typical DIG with multiple cysts in the right hemisphere, along with a hypointense solid peripheral, plaque-like mass ➡. *(Right)* Axial T1 C+ MR in the same patient as previous image shows marked, slightly heterogeneous enhancement of the plaque ➡ of solid tumor. Note other areas of enhancing tumor ➡ within the cyst walls.

### Typical

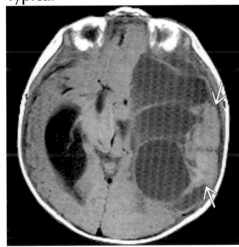
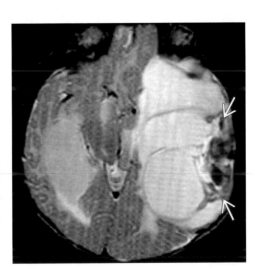

*(Left)* Axial T1WI MR shows a hyperintense plaque-like mass ➡ in the peripheral aspect of the left hemisphere, surrounded by multiple large cysts. Note the distorted midbrain, resulting from mass effect. *(Right)* Axial T2WI MR shows the marked hypointensity of the solid portion of the tumor ➡. The 3rd ventricle and contralateral temporal horn are hydrocephalic due to compression of the aqueduct.

### Typical

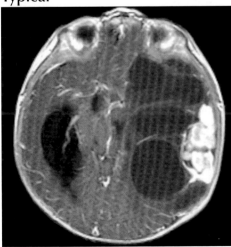
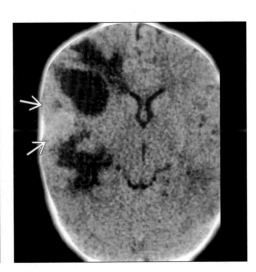

*(Left)* Axial T1 C+ MR shows diffuse heterogeneous enhancement of the solid, plaque-like portion of the tumor. The cyst walls minimally enhance. *(Right)* Axial NECT in a different infant shows that the solid, plaque-like portion of the tumor ➡ is hyperdense compared to both cortex and white matter.

# DNET

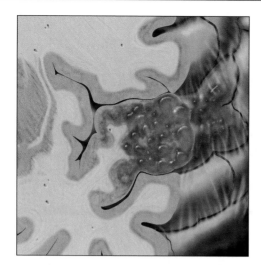

Coronal oblique graphic shows intracortical DNET. The gyrus is expanded by the multiple small cysts in the cerebral cortex and underlying white matter that are characteristic of the tumor.

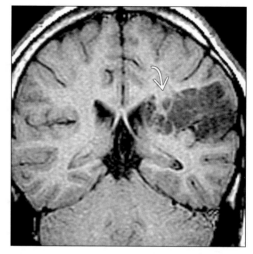

Coronal T1WI MR shows wedge-shaped, multilobular (bubbly) lesion extending from parietal cortex to ventricle. Several small hypointense foci ➔ appear discrete.

## TERMINOLOGY

### Abbreviations and Synonyms

- Dysembryoplastic neuroepithelial tumor (DNET)
  - Occasionally called DNT
  - Formerly called mixed glioma

### Definitions

- Benign, focal, intracortical mass superimposed on background of cortical dysplasia

## IMAGING FINDINGS

### General Features

- Best diagnostic clue: Well-demarcated, wedge shaped, micro- or macrolobular intracortical mass in young patient with longstanding partial seizures
- Location
  - Temporal lobe (often amygdala/hippocampus) most common site
    - Parietal cortex, caudate nucleus, septum pellucidum also frequent sites
  - Intracortical mass scallops inner table of skull and "points" towards ventricle
- Size
  - Variable: Small → involving part of a gyrus
  - Large → up to 7 cm, involving lobule or large portion of lobe
- Morphology
  - Well-circumscribed
  - Wedge-shaped cortical mass with multiple small cyst-like components
  - Minimal or no mass effect
  - Lacks surrounding edema
  - Very slow growth over many years ⇒ may remodel overlying bone

### CT Findings

- CTA: Avascular
- NECT
  - Wedge-shaped low density area
    - Cortical/subcortical lesion
    - Extends towards ventricle in 30%
    - Scalloped inner table in 44-60+%
    - Calcification in 20-36%
  - May resemble stroke on initial CT

## DDx: Cysts & Cystic Tumors

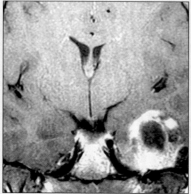

Xanthoastrocytoma

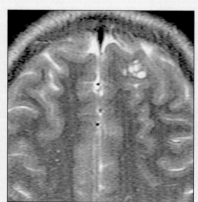

Neuroepithelial Cysts

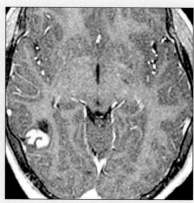

Ganglioglioma

# DNET

## Key Facts

### Terminology
- Dysembryoplastic neuroepithelial tumor (DNET)
- Benign, focal, intracortical mass superimposed on background of cortical dysplasia

### Imaging Findings
- Best diagnostic clue: Well-demarcated, wedge-shaped, micro- or macrolobular intracortical mass in young patient with longstanding partial seizures
- Temporal lobe (often amygdala/hippocampus) most common site
- Intracortical mass scallops inner table of skull and "points" towards ventricle
- Minimal or no mass effect
- Multinodular or septated appearance well seen on T2WI

- Mixed (hypo/isointense) signal with "bright rim" on FLAIR

### Pathology
- Approximately 1-2% of primary brain tumors in patients < 20 years
- Reported in 5-80% of epilepsy specimens
- Several histological types

### Clinical Issues
- Clinical Profile: Longstanding (difficult to control) partial complex seizures in child or young adult
- Gender: M = F
- No or very slow increase in size over time
- Rare recurrence
- Beware of atypical features (enhancement) on pre-op imaging

---

- **But** no temporal evolution to atrophy
- CECT
  - Usually nonenhancing
  - Faint nodular or patchy enhancement in 20%
    - Slightly higher risk of recurrence if enhancement

### MR Findings
- T1WI
  - Pseudocystic mass
  - Hypointense, sharply marginated
  - May have micro- or macronodular appearance
- T2WI
  - Very hyperintense mass
  - Multinodular or septated appearance well seen on T2WI
  - Sharply marginated from surrounding tissues
    - Absence of peritumoral edema
- PD/Intermediate: Hyperintense rim
- FLAIR
  - Mixed (hypo/isointense) signal with "bright rim" on FLAIR
  - No peritumoral edema
- T2* GRE
  - Bleeding into DNET uncommon but does occur
    - Possibly in association with microvascular abnormalities
    - May simulate cavernoma
- DWI
  - Increased diffusivity
  - Similar, but slightly less than CSF
- T1 C+
  - Usually doesn't enhance
  - Faint focal punctate or ring-enhancement in 20%
- MRA: Avascular mass
- MRS: Nonspecific, but lactate present in some

### Nuclear Medicine Findings
- PET
  - F-18 FDG PET demonstrates glucose hypometabolism
  - Lower [C-11] methionine (MET) uptake in DNET than in ganglioglioma or gliomas
- Tc-99m HMPAO SPECT

- Ictal may show hyperperfusion
- Interictal hypoperfusion typical

### Imaging Recommendations
- Best imaging tool: MR
- Protocol advice
  - MR with contrast material
  - FLAIR increases specificity with "bright ring"

## DIFFERENTIAL DIAGNOSIS

### Taylor Type Cortical Dysplasia
- Looks like single tuberous sclerosis lesion
  - Expands single gyrus
  - T2 hyperintensity in subcortical white matter
  - Nonenhancing
  - Blurring of cortical-white matter junction

### Angiocentric Neuroepithelial Tumor (ANET)
- Bright "ring" on T1WI rather than FLAIR
- Perivascular cuffing with tumoral astrocytes on pathology

### Neuroepithelial Cyst
- Nonenhancing single or complex cystic structure
- No bright "ring" on FLAIR

### Ganglioglioma
- Cyst & Ca++ common
- Less hyperintense than DNET
- ± Enhancement

### Pleomorphic Xanthoastrocytoma (PXA)
- Enhancing nodule abuts pia
- Solid portion similar to gray matter intensity on T2
- Look for dural "tail"

## PATHOLOGY

### General Features
- General path comments: Intracortical mass with scalloping of overlying inner table

# DNET

- Genetics
  - Sporadic
  - Nonneoplastic focal cortical dysplasias may be syndrome related
  - Reported cases with NF1
- Etiology
  - Embryology: Dysplastic cells in germinal matrix
  - Extend along migratory path of neurons towards cortex
  - Associated cortical dysplasia common
- Epidemiology
  - < 1% of all primary brain tumors
  - Approximately 1-2% of primary brain tumors in patients < 20 years
  - Reported in 5-80% of epilepsy specimens

## Gross Pathologic & Surgical Features
- Neocortical lesion
- Thick gyrus
- Gelatinous/mucoid consistency of tumor

## Microscopic Features
- Hallmark = "specific glioneuronal element" (SGNE)
  - Columns of heterogeneous cells oriented perpendicular to cortex
  - Oligodendrocyte-like cells arranged around capillaries
  - Other cells show astrocytic, neuronal differentiation
- Several histological types
  - Complex form
    - Multinodular architecture
    - Mixed cellular composition
    - Foci of cortical disorganization
    - SGNE
  - Simple form with SGNE only
  - A third "nonspecific" form has no SGNE
    - But has same neuroimaging characteristics as complex form
- Microcystic degeneration
  - Neurons "float" in pale, eosinophilic mucoid matrix
- Calcification and leptomeningeal involvement common
- Adjacent cortical dysplasia common
- Low proliferative potential with variable MIB-1 index

## Staging, Grading or Classification Criteria
- WHO grade I

# CLINICAL ISSUES

## Presentation
- Most common signs/symptoms: Epilepsy
- Other signs/symptoms: Focal EEG findings common
- Clinical Profile: Longstanding (difficult to control) partial complex seizures in child or young adult

## Demographics
- Age
  - Children and young adults
  - Typically identified before age 20
- Gender: M = F
- Ethnicity: None known

## Natural History & Prognosis
- Benign lesions
- No or very slow increase in size over time
- Rare recurrence
  - Beware of atypical features (enhancement) on pre-op imaging

## Treatment
- Seizures may become intractable
  - Glutamate receptors shown within tumor and margins may explain typical difficult to control seizures
- Surgical resection of epileptogenic foci (may include cortical dysplasia)

# DIAGNOSTIC CHECKLIST

## Consider
- Imaging appearance important in making diagnosis

## Image Interpretation Pearls
- Beware enhancing lesions, they may represent a more ominous lesion than DNET

# SELECTED REFERENCES

1. Parmar H et al: FLAIR ring sign as a marker of dysembryoplastic neuroepithelial tumors (DNET). JCAT In Press, 2007
2. Lellouch-Tubiana A et al: Angiocentric neuroepithelial tumor (ANET): a new epilepsy-related clinicopathological entity with distinctive MRI. Brain Pathol. 15(4):281-6, 2005
3. Takahashi A et al: Frequent association of cortical dysplasia in dysembryoplastic neuroepithelial tumor treated by epilepsy surgery. Surg Neurol. 64(5):419-27, 2005
4. Maehara T et al: Usefulness of [11C]methionine PET in the diagnosis of dysembryoplastic neuroepithelial tumor with temporal lobe epilepsy. Epilepsia. 45(1):41-5, 2004
5. Vuori K et al: Low-grade gliomas and focal cortical developmental malformations: differentiation with proton MR spectroscopy. Radiology. 230(3):703-8, 2004
6. Fernandez C et al: The usefulness of MR imaging in the diagnosis of dysembryoplastic neuroepithelial tumor in children: a study of 14 cases. AJNR Am J Neuroradiol. 24(5):829-34, 2003
7. Stanescu Cosson R et al: Dysembryoplastic neuroepithelial tumors: CT, MR findings and imaging follow-up: a study of 53 cases. J Neuroradiol. 28(4):230-40, 2001
8. Daumas-Duport C et al: Dysembryoplastic neuroepithelial tumors: In: Tumors of the Nervous System. Lyon, France, IARC Press. 6:103-6, 2000
9. Lee DY et al: Dysembryoplastic neuroepithelial tumor: radiological findings (including PET, SPECT, and MRS) and surgical strategy. J Neurooncol. 47(2):167-74, 2000
10. Honavar M et al: Histological heterogeneity of dysembryoplastic neuroepithelial tumour: identification and differential diagnosis in a series of 74 cases. Histopathology. 34(4):342-56, 1999
11. Thom M et al: Spontaneous intralesional haemorrhage in dysembryoplastic neuroepithelial tumours: a series of five cases. J Neurol Neurosurg Psychiatry. 67(1):97-101, 1999
12. Ostertun B et al: Dysembryoplastic neuroepithelial tumors: MR and CT evaluation. AJNR Am J Neuroradiol. 17(3):419-30, 1996

# DNET

I
1

179

## IMAGE GALLERY

### Typical

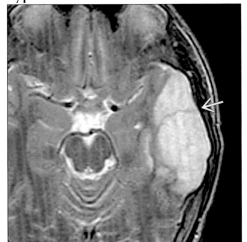 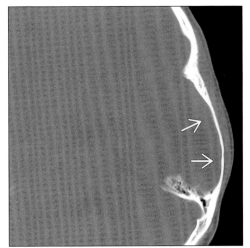

*(Left)* Axial T2WI MR shows large expansile cortical and subcortical hyperintense lesion in left lateral temporal lobe. Note the multinodular, septated ➡ appearance with inner table scalloping. *(Right)* Axial NECT in the same child as previous image shows thinning ➡ and remodeling of the inner table of the pars squamosa of the left temporal bone.

### Typical

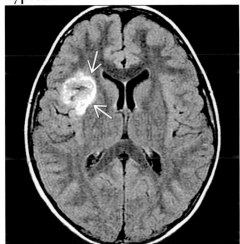 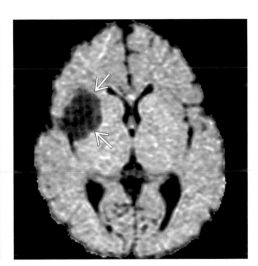

*(Left)* Axial FLAIR MR shows hyperintense mass with a rim of increased signal intensity ➡ in the anterior right frontal operculum and insula; this is the "FLAIR bright ring" sign. *(Right)* Axial DWI MR in the same child as previous image shows marked hypointensity of the mass ➡ on DWI, consistent with a high degree of diffusivity, suggesting its cystic nature.

### Variant

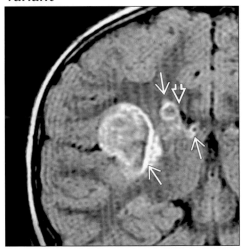 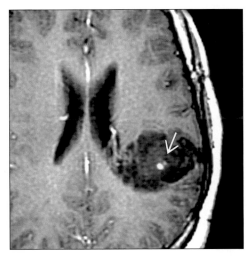

*(Left)* Coronal FLAIR MR shows multiple tumor nodules with the FLAIR bright rim sign ➡. Note the extension of the mass to the lateral ventricle ➡, typical in DNET. *(Right)* Axial T1 C+ MR shows a central focus of enhancement ➡ in this recurrent DNET. When enhancement is present, the tumor has a slightly higher risk of recurrence.

# SUPRATENTORIAL PNET

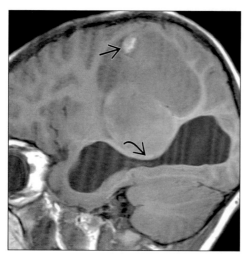

*Sagittal T1WI MR shows a large deep left hemispheric mass with focal early subacute hemorrhage ➡. Note the tumor compressing ➡ the enlarged temporal horn of the lateral ventricle.*

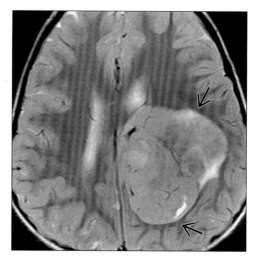

*Axial T2WI MR shows a large lobulated deep hemispheric highly cellular intra-axial tumor with ventricular compression. Tumor is isointense to cortex. Note the lack of peritumoral edema ➡.*

## TERMINOLOGY

### Abbreviations and Synonyms
- Supratentorial primitive neuroectodermal tumor (sPNET)
- Supratentorial primitive neuroepithelial tumor
- Primary cerebral neuroblastoma

### Definitions
- Cerebral embryonal tumor composed of undifferentiated neuroepithelial cells
  - Tumor cells have capacity for differentiation → astrocytic, ependymal, neuronal, muscular, melanotic

## IMAGING FINDINGS

### General Features
- Best diagnostic clue: Complex hemispheric mass with minimal peritumoral edema
- Location: Hemispheric (cortical, subcortical, thalamic) > pineal > suprasellar
- Size

- Variable, based on location and presenting symptoms
  - Hemispheric sPNET larger at diagnosis, mean diameter ~ 5 cm, often huge in newborns
  - Suprasellar PNETs tend to be smaller due to neuroendocrine and visual disturbances
  - Pineal PNETs cause ventricular obstruction and gaze/convergence difficulties
- Morphology: Vary between sharply delimited to diffusely infiltrative

### CT Findings
- NECT
  - Homogeneous to heterogeneous
  - Iso- to hyperattenuating
  - Calcification (50-70%)
  - Hemorrhage and necrosis common
- CECT: Heterogeneous enhancement, prone to cerebrospinal fluid (CSF) spread

### MR Findings
- T1WI
  - Hypo- to isointense to gray matter
  - Homogeneous to heterogeneous
- T2WI

## DDx: Pediatric Cerebral Hemispheric Masses

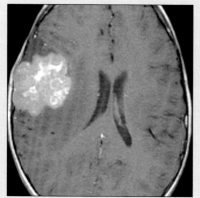

*Oligodendroglioma*

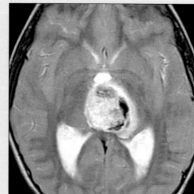

*Thalamic Glioblastoma Multiforme*

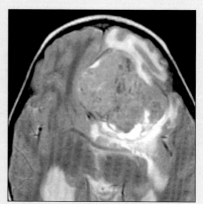

*Atypical Teratoid/Rhabdoid Tumor*

# SUPRATENTORIAL PNET

## Key Facts

### Terminology
- Supratentorial primitive neuroectodermal tumor (sPNET)
- Cerebral embryonal tumor composed of undifferentiated neuroepithelial cells

### Imaging Findings
- Best diagnostic clue: Complex hemispheric mass with minimal peritumoral edema
- Calcification (50-70%)
- Hemorrhage and necrosis common
- CECT: Heterogeneous enhancement, prone to cerebrospinal fluid (CSF) spread
- Solid elements iso- to slightly hyperintense to gray matter (highly cellular)
- Sparse peritumoral edema
- DWI: Restricted diffusion
- Elevated rCBV
- ↓ NAA/Cho, ↓ NAA/Cr, ↓ Cr, ↑ Cho/Cr, + Lac/lipid, + taurine (Tau)
- Best imaging tool: Enhanced MR of brain and spine
- MRS (↑ Tau), perfusion MR (↑ rCBV), enhanced FLAIR (for CSF seeding)

### Top Differential Diagnoses
- Astrocytoma
- Ependymoma
- Oligodendroglioma
- Atypical Teratoid/Rhabdoid Tumor (ATRT)

### Clinical Issues
- Clinical Profile: Infant presenting with macrocephaly, seizures and large hemispheric mass

---

- Solid elements iso- to slightly hyperintense to gray matter (highly cellular)
  - Heterogeneity common
  - Sparse peritumoral edema
  - Ca++ → hypointense foci
  - Blood products → mixed signal intensity
- PD/Intermediate: Slightly hyperintense
- FLAIR
  - Solid components hyperintense
  - Paucity of peritumoral edema
  - Post-enhanced FLAIR improves detection of leptomeningeal metastases
- T2* GRE: Dephasing from blood products
- DWI: Restricted diffusion
- T1 C+
  - Heterogeneous enhancement
  - CSF pathway seeding common
  - Elevated rCBV
  - Subtraction imaging helpful with hemorrhagic masses
- MRS
  - ↓ NAA/Cho, ↓ NAA/Cr, ↓ Cr, ↑ Cho/Cr, + Lac/lipid, + taurine (Tau)
  - ↑ Phosphoethanolamine/glycerophosphoethanolamine, ↑ phosphocholine/glycerophosphocholine

### Ultrasonographic Findings
- Congenital sPNET
  - Large heterogeneous hyperechoic hemispheric mass, + hydrocephalus
- Antenatal sonography
  - Hydrocephalus and hyperechoic hemispheric mass

### Imaging Recommendations
- Best imaging tool: Enhanced MR of brain and spine
- Protocol advice
  - Enhanced MR of entire neuraxis before surgery
  - MRS (↑ Tau), perfusion MR (↑ rCBV), enhanced FLAIR (for CSF seeding)

## DIFFERENTIAL DIAGNOSIS

### Astrocytoma
- Grade I → glioblastoma multiforme (GBM)
- Variable enhancement
- More anaplastic tumors characterized by extensive vasogenic edema
- Calcification uncommon

### Ependymoma
- When supratentorial (30%), usually intra-axial
  - Only 15-25% arise within third or lateral ventricle
- Large at presentation, Ca++ in 50%
- Necrosis and hemorrhage not uncommon

### Oligodendroglioma
- Strong predilection for frontotemporal region
- Peripheral location
- Coarse Ca++ common

### Atypical Teratoid/Rhabdoid Tumor (ATRT)
- Posterior fossa location > 50%, supratentorial 39%
- Necrosis, cysts, and vasogenic edema common
- Early subarachnoid seeding common

### Choroid Plexus Carcinoma
- Parenchymal invasion can be dramatic
- Extensive vasogenic edema
- Strong heterogeneous enhancement

### Tumefactive Multiple Sclerosis (MS)
- For "tumor" size, less mass effect than expected
- Outer enhancing border & inner T2 hypointense border

## PATHOLOGY

### General Features
- General path comments: Embryonal tumor of cerebrum, suprasellar or pineal regions
- Genetics

# SUPRATENTORIAL PNET

- Unlike medulloblastoma (PNET-MB), chromosome 17 aberrations rare
- Somatic mutations in tumor suppressor genes
  - HASH1, hSNF5 on chromosome 22
- Other chromosome anomalies with sPNET
  - Aberrations of short arm of chromosome 11
  - Trisomies of chromosomes 9, 13, 1q, and 18p
- Etiology: Aberrations in tumor suppressor genes may play a role
- Epidemiology
  - Supratentorial PNETs constitute ~ 1% of pediatric brain tumors
  - Of all CNS PNETs, ~ 6% are supratentorial (sPNET)
  - An important hemispheric mass to consider in newborn and infant
- Associated abnormalities
  - Hereditary syndromes
    - Gorlin syndrome
    - Turcot syndrome
    - Hereditary retinoblastoma and risk for secondary malignancies
    - Rubinstein-Taybi syndrome

## Gross Pathologic & Surgical Features
- Variable consistency
  - Solid and homogeneous → cystic, necrotic, hemorrhagic and partially calcified
  - Solid portions soft pink-red coloration, unless prominent desmoplasia
  - Necrosis and hemorrhage common
  - Demarcation between tumor and brain may range from indistinct to sharp

## Microscopic Features
- Similar to medulloblastoma (PNET-MB)
- Composition
  - Undifferentiated or poorly differentiated neuroepithelial cells
  - Pleomorphic nuclei
  - Field necrosis, hemorrhage, Ca++
  - Homer-Wright rosettes & Flexner-Wintersteiner rosettes

## Staging, Grading or Classification Criteria
- WHO grade IV

# CLINICAL ISSUES

## Presentation
- Most common signs/symptoms
  - Vary with site of origin and size of tumor
    - Hemispheric → seizures, disturbed consciousness, motor deficit, elevated ICP
    - Suprasellar → visual disturbance, endocrine problems
    - Pineal → hydrocephalus, Parinaud syndrome
  - Other signs/symptoms
    - Cranial neuropathies due to herniation or diffuse CSF metastases
- Clinical Profile: Infant presenting with macrocephaly, seizures and large hemispheric mass

## Demographics
- Age
  - More common in younger children
    - Median age at diagnosis 35 months
- Gender: M:F = 2:1
- Ethnicity: No ethnic predilection

## Natural History & Prognosis
- Compared to posterior fossa PNET (PNET-MB), sPNETs have poorer survival
  - Supratentorial PNET → 30-35% 5 year survival
  - PNET-MB → 80-85% 5 year survival
- Critical survival factors include
  - Completeness of surgical resection
  - Absence of metastases
  - Patient age > 2 years
  - Smaller, solid tumor (tumor necrosis is unfavorable)
  - Immunohistochemical labeling indices (Ki index > 10%, unfavorable)
  - M stage of tumor
- Heavily calcified sPNETs have slightly better prognosis
- No survival advantage for specific supratentorial location

## Treatment
- Aggressive surgical resection, chemotherapy, craniospinal radiation

# DIAGNOSTIC CHECKLIST

## Consider
- Supratentorial PNET in newborn, infant, or young child presenting with
  - Hemispheric tumor lacking edema, solid portion isointense to gray matter
  - Suprasellar or pineal mass

## Image Interpretation Pearls
- Large hemispheric mass with sparse peritumoral edema
- Taurine elevation on MRS

# SELECTED REFERENCES
1. Astrakas L et al: The clinical perspective of large scale projects: a case study of multiparametric MR imaging of pediatric brain tumors. Oncol Rep. 15 Spec no, 2006
2. Burger PC: Supratentorial primitive neuroectodermal tumor (sPNET). Brain Pathol. 16(1):86, 2006
3. Cha S: Dynamic susceptibility-weighted contrast-enhanced perfusion MR imaging in pediatric patients. Neuroimaging Clin N Am. 16(1):137-47, ix, 2006
4. Poussaint TY et al: Advanced neuroimaging of pediatric brain tumors: MR diffusion, MR perfusion, and MR spectroscopy. Neuroimaging Clin N Am. 16(1):169-92, ix, 2006
5. Kovanlikaya A et al: Untreated pediatric primitive neuroectodermal tumor in vivo: quantitation of taurine with MR spectroscopy. Radiology. 236(3):1020-5, 2005
6. Dai AI et al: Supratentorial primitive neuroectodermal tumors of infancy: clinical and radiologic findings. Pediatr Neurol. 29(5):430-4, 2003

## IMAGE GALLERY

### Typical

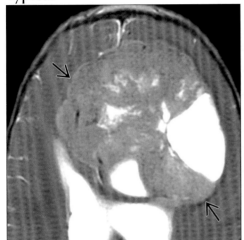

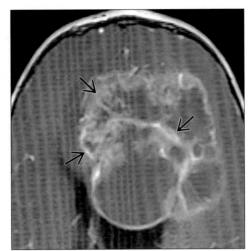

*(Left)* Axial T2WI MR shows a predominantly solid, partially cystic, partially necrotic left frontal lobe mass. The solid portion is isointense with cortex; note the lack of peritumoral edema →. *(Right)* Axial T1 C+ MR shows heterogeneous curvilinear tumor enhancement → following the administration of MR contrast →.

### Variant

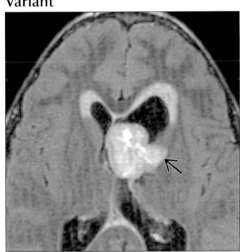

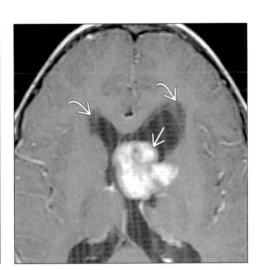

*(Left)* Axial FLAIR MR shows a lobulated exophytic tumor → arising from the left caudate nucleus. The mass grows into the ventricle and obstructs CSF flow at the foramina of Monro. *(Right)* Axial T1 C+ MR shows robust, slightly heterogeneous enhancement of the tumor →. Interstitial edema is demonstrated as bilateral perifrontal T1 hypointensity →.

### Typical

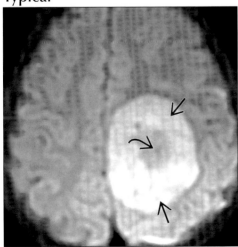

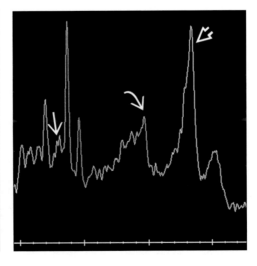

*(Left)* Axial DWI MR shows a predominantly hyperintense hemispheric →. ADC map confirmed reduced diffusion compared to white matter. The necrotic core → demonstrated increased diffusivity. *(Right)* MRS using PRESS technique and a short TE demonstrates: Diminished NAA →, a large lipid peak →, and a small taurine → peak seen just to the left of the elevated choline peak.

# EPENDYMOMA, SUPRATENTORIAL

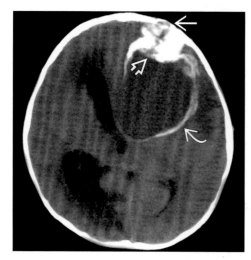

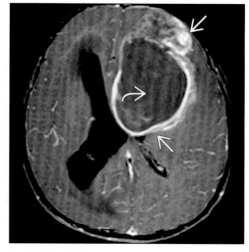

*Axial NECT shows large cystic/solid mass with gross Ca++ of cyst wall ➜ and solid portion of tumor ➜. Note erosion of overlying calvarium ➜, significant mass effect and hydrocephalus.*

*Axial T1 C+ FS MR in same patient as previous image shows well demarcated tumor bulging in ventricle & reaching calvarium. Note high signal of cyst ➜, enhancement of cyst wall & solid portion of tumor ➜.*

## TERMINOLOGY

### Abbreviations and Synonyms
- Supratentorial ependymoma (STE)
  - WHO grade II: Common type; cellular, clear cell, papillary, tanycytic subtypes
  - WHO grade III: Anaplastic ependymoma
- Excludes: Ependymoblastoma which is an embryonal PNET with ependymal rosettes

### Definitions
- Supratentorial tumor made of ependymal cells

## IMAGING FINDINGS

### General Features
- Best diagnostic clue: Heterogeneous signal with solid & cystic components, hemorrhage & Ca++
- Location
  - Typically in parenchyma (~ 80%) not necessarily related to ventricular wall
    - Uncommonly ventricular or cortical ("ectopic")

- Classically frontal, but temporo-parietal location common
- Size: 90% > 4 mm
- Morphology: Well-demarcated, spherical or multilocular heterogeneous tumor

### CT Findings
- NECT
  - Large heterogeneous parenchymal mass
  - Ca++ common (50%); ± cysts, hemorrhage
  - Mass effect
  - Surrounding edema suggests grade III
- CECT: Variable heterogeneous enhancement of solid portion & cyst wall

### MR Findings
- T1WI
  - Heterogeneous, usually iso- to hypointense
    - Cystic foci slightly hyperintense to cerebrospinal fluid (CSF)
    - Hyperintense Ca++, blood products
- T2WI
  - Heterogeneous, usually iso- to hyperintense
    - Strikingly hyperintense cystic foci

## DDx: Heterogeneous Hemispheric Tumors

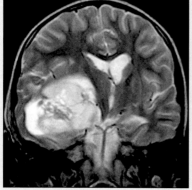

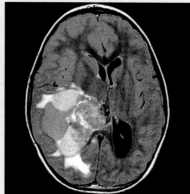

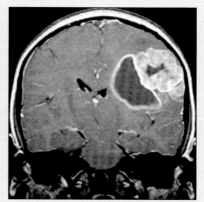

*Ganglioglioma*

*Choroid Plexus Carcinoma*

*Neuroepithelial Tumor*

# EPENDYMOMA, SUPRATENTORIAL

## Key Facts

### Terminology
- Excludes: Ependymoblastoma which is an embryonal PNET with ependymal rosettes

### Imaging Findings
- Best diagnostic clue: Heterogeneous signal with solid & cystic components, hemorrhage & Ca++
- Protocol advice: Early post-surgical MR assessment for prognosis & for second look surgery

### Top Differential Diagnoses
- Juvenile Pilocytic Astrocytoma (JPA)
- Poorly Differentiated Neuroepithelial Tumors
- Choroid Plexus Papilloma (CPP) or Carcinoma (CPC)
- Ganglioglioma, Pleomorphic Xanthoastrocytoma (PXA)

### Pathology
- Radial glia may form stem cells for ependymomas
- Ependymoma 3rd most frequent brain tumor in children, after JPA and medulloblastoma
- 10-50% of them are anaplastic ependymomas (grade III)

### Clinical Issues
- Surgical resection is key element of treatment

### Diagnostic Checklist
- Purely superficial hemispheric tumor may be an ependymoma
- Hugely calcified cystic/solid hemispheric tumor in young child ⇒ think of ependymoma first
- Do not ignore unenhanced CT when available

---

- Hypointense Ca++, variable signal of blood products
- FLAIR
  - Sharp interface between tumor and surroundings
  - Tumor cysts very hyperintense to CSF
  - Mild peritumoral edema
- DWI: Typically similar to surrounding parenchyma
- T1 C+: Mild to moderate, heterogeneous enhancement
- MRS
  - Neoplastic pattern
    - Lactate ↑, NAA ↓, Cho ↑, low NAA/Cho ratio
  - MR spectroscopy alone does not reliably differentiate ependymoma from other tumors

## Radiographic Findings
- Radiography: Ca++ common, skull may be eroded

## Nuclear Medicine Findings
- PET
  - Increased F-18 fluorodeoxyglucose (FDG) uptake
  - May help differentiate recurrent tumor from radiation necrosis

## Imaging Recommendations
- Best imaging tool
  - Brain MR with contrast
    - Spinal mets very uncommon at presentation
    - CT remains useful when available
- Protocol advice: Early post-surgical MR assessment for prognosis & for second look surgery

## DIFFERENTIAL DIAGNOSIS

### Juvenile Pilocytic Astrocytoma (JPA)
- Cyst with mural nodule, Ca++ usually not prominent
- Solid portion enhances vigorously

### Poorly Differentiated Neuroepithelial Tumors
- PNET, atypical teratoid/rhabdoid tumor (AT/RT)

### Choroid Plexus Papilloma (CPP) or Carcinoma (CPC)
- Mimics intraventricular ependymoma
- Ependymoma originates from ventricular wall, CPP and CPC from choroid plexus

### Ganglioglioma, Pleomorphic Xanthoastrocytoma (PXA)
- Mimics cortical, "ectopic" ependymoma

### Oligodendroglioma
- Heterogeneous supratentorial mass with Ca++ in young adults

## PATHOLOGY

### General Features
- General path comments
  - Grade II: Four subtypes encountered in brain
    - Cellular: Most common, densely packed cells with few rosettes & pseudorosettes
    - Papillary: Rare, extensive epithelial surface mimicking CPP
    - Clear-cell: Clear cytoplasm, resembling oligodendroglioma or neurocytoma; predilection for supratentorial location, local recurrence, extraneural metastases
    - Tanycytic: Bundles of elongated cells resembling pilocytic astrocytoma (mostly ventricular)
  - Grade III: Loss of typical features with increased cellularity, pleomorphism, vascular proliferation & necrosis
- Genetics: Associated with aberrations on chromosomes 1q, 6q, 9, 13, 16, 17, 19, 20, 22
- Etiology
  - Classically thought to arise from ependymal cells or ependymal rests at the angle of lateral ventricles
    - But tumor does not necessarily relate to ventricles
  - Radial glia may form stem cells for ependymomas
    - Normal adult ependymal cells are derived from radial glia

# EPENDYMOMA, SUPRATENTORIAL

- Radial glia serves as a scaffold for cellular migration in developing brain
- Could explain why ependymomas may be found anywhere between ventricle and brain surface
- Epidemiology
  - Ependymoma 3rd most frequent brain tumor in children, after JPA and medulloblastoma
    - 40% of ependymomas in children are supratentorial
    - 10-50% of them are anaplastic ependymomas (grade III)

## Gross Pathologic & Surgical Features

- Well-demarcated soft, lobulated, grayish-red mass
  - ± Cysts, necrosis, hemorrhage
  - CSF drop metastases very uncommon

## Microscopic Features

- Common grade II ependymoma
  - Perivascular pseudorosettes
  - Moderately cellular with low mitotic activity and occasional nuclear atypia
  - Immunohistochemistry: S-100, glial fibrillary acidic protein (GFAP), vimentin +
- Grade III anaplastic ependymoma
  - High cellularity, nuclear atypia, hyperchromatism
  - Occasional pseudopalisading or necrosis in most malignant lesions

## Staging, Grading or Classification Criteria

- WHO grade I ependymomas
  - Myxopapillary ependymoma mostly in filum terminale/conus medullaris, exceptional in brain
  - Subependymoma uncommon in children
- WHO grade II: Standard cellular type
  - Usual in supratentorial space
  - Four subtypes: Cellular, papillary, clear cell, tanycytic
- WHO grade III: Anaplastic ependymoma

## CLINICAL ISSUES

### Presentation

- Most common signs/symptoms: Headache, nausea, vomiting; neurological deficits; seizures

### Demographics

- Age
  - Supratentorial ependymoma develops in young children
    - Older than posterior fossa ependymomas however
    - Spinal cord ependymoma develop mostly in adults
  - Age strongly correlates with prognosis, poorer in young children
- Gender: Slight male predominance

### Natural History & Prognosis

- Survival at 5 years is about 50%
- Prognostic predictors
  - Age: Prognosis poorer in young children/infants
  - Location: Affects quality of removal, hence prognosis

- Quality of removal good predictor
  - Need for immediate post-surgical assessment
  - Second surgery may be indicated
- Correlation between grade and prognosis unclear
- Supratentorial ependymoma not typically associated with drop metastases in CSF

### Treatment

- Surgical resection is key element of treatment
  - Gross total resection + XRT correlates with improved survival
  - Chemotherapy not clearly efficient to this day

## DIAGNOSTIC CHECKLIST

### Consider

- Purely superficial hemispheric tumor may be an ependymoma

### Image Interpretation Pearls

- Hugely calcified cystic/solid hemispheric tumor in young child ⇒ think of ependymoma first
- Do not ignore unenhanced CT when available

## SELECTED REFERENCES

1. Agaoglu FY et al: Ependymal tumors in childhood. Pediatr Blood Cancer. 45(3):298-303, 2005
2. Roncaroli F et al: Supratentorial cortical ependymoma: report of three cases. Neurosurgery. 57(1):E192, 2005
3. Shuangshoti S et al: Supratentorial extraventricular ependymal neoplasms: a clinicopathologic study of 32 patients. Cancer. 103(12):2598-605, 2005
4. Spassky N et al: Adult ependymal cells are postmitotic and are derived from radial glial cells during embryogenesis. J Neurosci. 25(1):10-8, 2005
5. Taylor MD et al: Radial glia cells are candidate stem cells of ependymoma. Cancer Cell. 8(4):323-35, 2005
6. Jaing TH et al: Multivariate analysis of clinical prognostic factors in children with intracranial ependymomas. J Neurooncol. 68(3):255-61, 2004
7. Ono S et al: Large supratentorial ectopic ependymoma with massive calcification and cyst formation--case report. Neurol Med Chir (Tokyo). 44(8):424-8, 2004
8. Fouladi M et al: Clear cell ependymoma: a clinicopathologic and radiographic analysis of 10 patients. Cancer. 98(10):2232-44, 2003
9. Korshunov A et al: Gene expression patterns in ependymomas correlate with tumor location, grade, and patient age. Am J Pathol. 163(5):1721-7, 2003
10. Lieberman KA et al: Tanycytomas: a newly characterized hypothalamic-suprasellar and ventricular tumor. AJNR Am J Neuroradiol. 24(10):1999-2004, 2003
11. Choi JY et al: Intracranial & spinal ependymomas: review of MR images in 61 patients. Korean J Radiol. 3(4):219-28, 2002
12. Good CD et al: Surveillance neuroimaging in childhood intracranial ependymoma: how effective, how often, and for how long? J Neurosurg. 94(1):27-32, 2001
13. Akyuz C et al: Intracranial ependymomas in childhood--a retrospective review of sixty-two children. Acta Oncol. 39(1):97-100, 2000
14. Palma L et al: The importance of surgery in supratentorial ependymomas. Long-term survival in a series of 23 cases. Childs Nerv Syst. 16(3):170-5, 2000
15. Armington WG et al: Supratentorial ependymoma: CT appearance. Radiology. 157(2):367-72, 1985

# EPENDYMOMA, SUPRATENTORIAL

## IMAGE GALLERY

### Typical

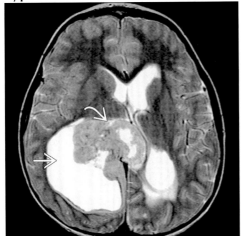
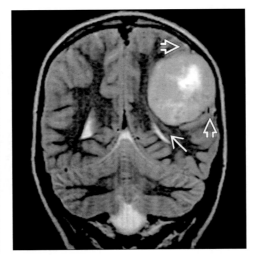

*(Left) Axial T2WI MR shows large cystic ➡ and solid ➡ heterogeneous, well-demarcated ependymoma extending into ventricle & herniating across midline. Note significant hydrocephalus. (Right) Coronal T2WI MR shows well-demarcated gray matter intensity mass with central necrosis, clearly separate from lateral ventricle ➡ but involving parietal cortex ➡.*

### Typical

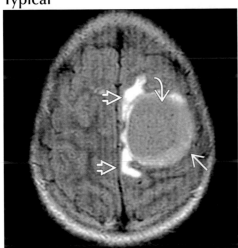
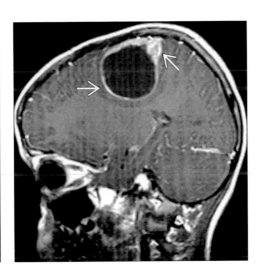

*(Left) Axial FLAIR MR shows predominantly cystic, well-demarcated tumor with thick solid rim ➡. The cyst has high signal intensity ➡. Note significant associated peritumoral edema ➡. (Right) Sagittal T1 C+ MR shows enhancement of the cyst wall and solid portion ➡ of tumor with involvement of the cerebral cortex (tumor abuts calvarium). Histology showed anaplastic ependymoma.*

### Typical

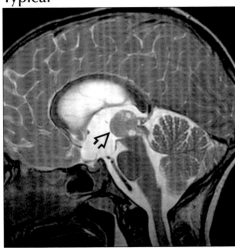
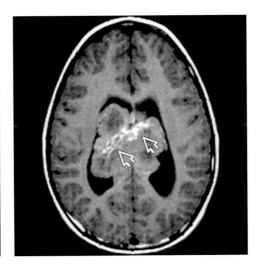

*(Left) Sagittal T2WI MR shows rather small, hypointense tumor ➡ that originated from lateral wall of posterior 3rd ventricle. Note the small intratumoral cysts. (Right) Axial T1WI MR shows heterogeneous intraventricular mass. CT scan showed the mass to be heavily calcified. Hyperintense intratumoral signal ➡ is related to blood products and calcium.*

# ENLARGED PERIVASCULAR SPACES

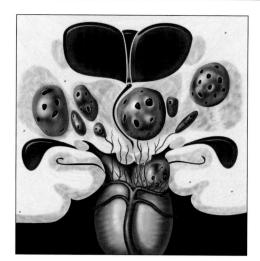

*Coronal graphic shows giant tumefactive perivascular spaces in the midbrain, thalami causing mass effect on the third ventricle and aqueduct with resulting hydrocephalus.*

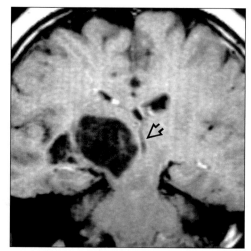

*Coronal T1 C+ MR shows giant tumefactive PVS. The cysts, in the mesencephalothalamic region, cause mass effect on the third ventricle and cerebral aqueduct ⯮ and do not enhance.*

## TERMINOLOGY

### Abbreviations and Synonyms
- Perivascular spaces (PVSs); Virchow-Robin spaces

### Definitions
- Pial-lined interstitial fluid (CSF)-filled structures that accompany penetrating arteries and veins but do not communicate directly with subarachnoid space

## IMAGING FINDINGS

### General Features
- Best diagnostic clue: Fluid-filled spaces that are isointense to CSF, surround/accompany penetrating arteries
- Location
  - Most common site for normal PVSs = basal ganglia (cluster around anterior commissure)
  - Other common locations
    - Subcortical white matter
    - Deep white matter
    - Midbrain
    - Subinsular cortex, extreme capsule
  - Less common sites
    - Thalami
    - Dentate nuclei
    - Corpus callosum, cingulate gyrus
  - Most common location for expanded ("giant" or "tumefactive") PVSs = mesencephalothalamic region
    - Can be found almost anywhere
    - BUT almost never involve cortex (PVSs expand within subcortical white matter)
- Size
  - PVSs usually 5 mm or less
  - Widespread dilatation of PVSs may look very bizarre
  - Giant tumefactive PVSs
    - PVS occasionally expand, attain large size (up to several cm)
    - Multilocular clusters more common than unilocular
    - May cause focal mass effect, hydrocephalus
- Morphology
  - Clusters of well-demarcated, variably-sized parenchymal cysts
  - Multiple > solitary cysts

## DDx: Cystic Lesions

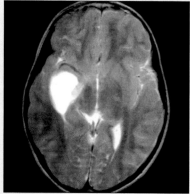

*Ganglioglioma*

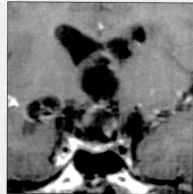

*Racemose Neurocysticercosis*

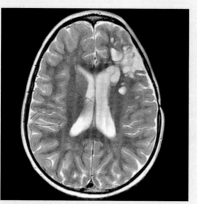

*Radiation Necrosis*

# ENLARGED PERIVASCULAR SPACES

## Key Facts

### Terminology
- Pial-lined interstitial fluid (CSF)-filled structures that accompany penetrating arteries and veins but do not communicate directly with subarachnoid space

### Imaging Findings
- Most common site for normal PVSs = basal ganglia (cluster around anterior commissure)
- Most common location for expanded ("giant" or "tumefactive") PVSs = mesencephalothalamic region
- PVSs usually 5 mm or less
- Clusters of round/ovoid/linear/punctate cyst-like lesions
- Multiple well-delineated cysts isointense with CSF
- Focal mass effect common
- Suppress completely
- DWI: No restricted diffusion
- No enhancement
- Best imaging tool: Routine MR + FLAIR, DWI

### Top Differential Diagnoses
- Cystic Neoplasm
- Infectious/Inflammatory Cysts
- Lacunar Infarcts

### Pathology
- Actually contain interstitial fluid, not CSF

### Clinical Issues
- PVSs occur in all locations, at all ages and are easily seen in most patients on high resolution imaging (3T or multichannel 1.5T)
- "Leave me alone" lesion that should not be mistaken for serious disease

## CT Findings
- NECT
  - Clusters of round/ovoid/linear/punctate cyst-like lesions
    - Low density (attenuation = CSF)
    - No Ca++
- CECT: Do not enhance

## MR Findings
- T1WI
  - Multiple well-delineated cysts isointense with CSF
  - Focal mass effect common
    - Expand overlying gyri
    - Enlarged PVSs in thalami or midbrain may compress aqueduct/3rd ventricle, cause hydrocephalus
- T2WI
  - Appear isointense with CSF
    - Signal intensity within PVSs actually measures slightly < CSF
  - No edema in adjacent brain, may have ↑ SI
  - May see penetrating artery as low signal focus within PVS
- PD/Intermediate: Isointense with CSF
- FLAIR
  - Suppress completely
  - 25% have minimal increased signal in brain surrounding enlarged PVSs
- T2* GRE: No blooming
- DWI: No restricted diffusion
- T1 C+
  - No enhancement
  - ± Visualization of penetrating arteries with contrast
- MRS: Spectra in adjacent brain typically normal

## Angiographic Findings
- Conventional: High-resolution DSA may depict penetrating arteries in area of enlarged PVSs

## Imaging Recommendations
- Best imaging tool: Routine MR + FLAIR, DWI
- Protocol advice: Contrast optional

# DIFFERENTIAL DIAGNOSIS

## Cystic Neoplasm
- Usually in pons, cerebellum, thalamus/hypothalamus
- Single > multiple cysts
- Signal not quite like CSF
- Parenchymal signal abnormalities common
- May enhance

## Infectious/Inflammatory Cysts
- Neurocysticercosis
  - Cysts often have scolex
  - Most are < 1 cm
  - Can be multiple but don't typically occur in clusters
  - Cyst walls often enhance
  - Surrounding edema often present
- Other parasites
  - Hydatid cysts often unilocular
  - Multilocular parasitic cysts typically enhance, mimic neoplasm more than PVSs

## Lacunar Infarcts
- Older patients (adults), children with vasculopathy (e.g., sickle cell disease)
- Common in basal ganglia, white matter
- Adjacent parenchymal hyperintensity

# PATHOLOGY

## General Features
- General path comments
  - Enlarged cystic-appearing spaces
  - Actually contain interstitial fluid, not CSF
- Genetics
  - Usually normal unless PVSs expanded by undegraded mucopolysaccharides (Hurler, Hunter disease)
  - PVSs also expand in
    - Some congenital muscular dystrophies
    - Some chromosomal abnormalities
    - Some malformations of cortical development (especially polymicrogyria)

# ENLARGED PERIVASCULAR SPACES

- Etiology
  - Theory: Interstitial fluid (ISF) accumulates between penetrating vessel, pia
  - Egress of ISF becomes blocked, causing cystic enlargement of PVS
  - Some may result from trauma, local atrophy
- Epidemiology
  - Common nonneoplastic brain "cyst"
  - Common cause of multifocal hyperintensities on T2WI
- Associated abnormalities
  - Hydrocephalus (midbrain expanding PVSs can obstruct aqueduct)
    - Expanding PVSs in midbrain can obstruct aqueduct
    - Expanding PVSs in thalamus can obstruct 3rd ventricle
  - "Cysts" caused by enlarged/obstructed PVSs reported with pituitary adenomas, large aneurysms
  - With progressive cerebral atrophy, can see progressive enlargement of PVSs in the subcortical white matter

## Gross Pathologic & Surgical Features
- Smoothly demarcated, fluid-filled cyst(s)

## Microscopic Features
- Single or double layer of invaginated pia
- Pia becomes fenestrated, disappears at capillary level
- PVSs in cortex usually very small
  - In white matter usually bigger; can be very large
- Surrounding brain usually lacks gliosis, amyloid deposition

## CLINICAL ISSUES

## Presentation
- Most common signs/symptoms
  - Usually normal, discovered incidentally at imaging/autopsy unless part of syndrome, metabolic disorder, cerebral dysplasia
  - Small PVSs seen in many young children in the subcortical white matter at the vertex, usually of no significance
  - Nonspecific symptoms (e.g., headache)
- Clinical Profile: Patient with nonspecific, nonlocalizing symptoms who has bizarre, alarming multicystic-appearing brain mass initially diagnosed as "cystic neoplasm"

## Demographics
- Age
  - PVSs occur in all locations, at all ages and are easily seen in most patients on high resolution imaging (3T or multichannel 1.5T)
  - Present in 25-30% of children (benign normal variant)
- Gender: Giant PVSs: M:F = 1.8:1

## Natural History & Prognosis
- Usually remain stable in size
- Occasionally continue to expand

## Treatment
- "Leave me alone" lesion that should not be mistaken for serious disease
- Shunt ventricles if midbrain lesions cause obstructive hydrocephalus

## DIAGNOSTIC CHECKLIST

## Consider
- Could a multi-cystic nonenhancing mass on MR or CT be a cluster of enlarged PVSs?

## Image Interpretation Pearls
- Prominent but normal PVSs are identified in nearly all children and in virtually every location at high resolution imaging

## SELECTED REFERENCES

1. Groeschel S et al: Virchow-Robin spaces on magnetic resonance images: normative data, their dilatation, and a review of the literature. Neuroradiology. 2006
2. Chaljub G: "Dilated perivascular spaces: a hallmark of mild traumatic brain injury"--a new paradigm? AJNR Am J Neuroradiol. 26(4):692-3, 2005
3. Rohlfs J et al: Enlarged perivascular spaces mimicking multicystic brain tumors. Report of two cases and review of the literature. J Neurosurg. 102(6):1142-6, 2005
4. Salzman KL et al: Giant tumefactive perivascular spaces. AJNR Am J Neuroradiol. 26(2):298-305, 2005
5. Matheus MG et al: Brain MRI findings in patients with mucopolysaccharidosis types I and II and mild clinical presentation. Neuroradiology. 46(8):666-72, 2004
6. Nishi K et al: Histochemical characteristic of perivascular space in the brain with an advanced edema. Leg Med (Tokyo). 5 Suppl 1:S280-4, 2003
7. Papayannis CE et al: Expanding Virchow Robin spaces in the midbrain causing hydrocephalus. AJNR Am J Neuroradiol. 24(7):1399-403, 2003
8. DiFazio MP et al: Ectodermal dysplasia and brain cystic changes: confirmation of a novel neurocutaneous syndrome. J Child Neurol. 17(7):475-8, 2002
9. Hayashi N et al: Polymicrogyria without porencephaly/schizencephaly. MRI analysis of the spectrum and the prevalence of macroscopic findings in the clinical population. Neuroradiology. 44(8):647-55, 2002
10. Ozturk MH et al: Comparison of MR signal intensities of cerebral perivascular (Virchow-Robin) and subarachnoid spaces. J Comput Assist Tomogr. 26(6):902-4, 2002
11. Seto T et al: Brain magnetic resonance imaging in 23 patients with mucopolysaccharidoses and the effect of bone marrow transplantation. Ann Neurol. 50(1):79-92, 2001
12. Song CJ et al: MR imaging and histologic features of subinsular bright spots on T2-weighted MR images: Virchow-Robin spaces of the extreme capsule and insular cortex. Radiology. 214(3):671-7, 2000
13. Mascalchi M et al: Expanding lacunae causing triventricular hydrocephalus. Report of two cases. J Neurosurg. 91(4):669-74, 1999
14. Adachi M et al: Dilated Virchow-Robin spaces: MRI pathological study. Neuroradiology. 40(1):27-31, 1998

## IMAGE GALLERY

Typical

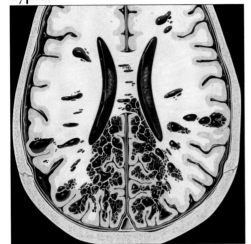
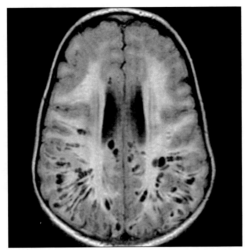

*(Left)* Axial graphic shows multiple dilated PVSs in the subcortical white matter, the centrum semiovale, and the corpus callosum. Most are < 5 mm in size, however widespread extent looks bizarre. *(Right)* Axial FLAIR MR shows multiple enlarged PVSs in a 2 year old with Hunter disease. Extensive dysmyelination of the cerebral white matter is evident, with abnormal T2 hyperintensity.

Typical

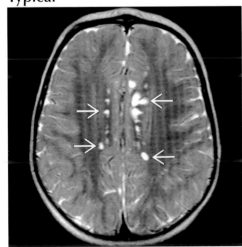
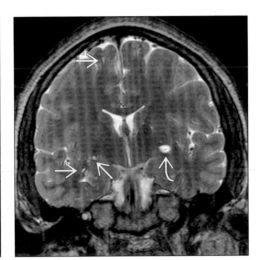

*(Left)* Axial T2WI MR in a 2 year old shows multiple enlarged PVSs ➡ in and around the corpus callosum. Child was asymptomatic for these (normal neurological exam). *(Right)* Coronal T2WI MR shows an enlarged PVS at the base of the left putamen ➡. A penetrating artery (dark signal focus) can be identified within the PVS. Other smaller PVSs are also seen ➡.

Typical

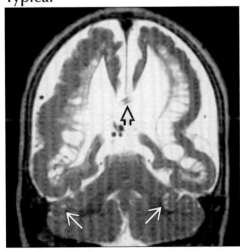
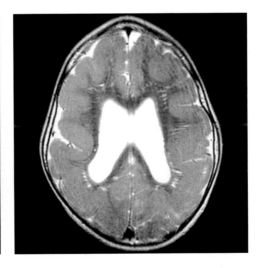

*(Left)* Coronal T2WI MR shows diffusely enlarged PVSs in a 2 year old with cobblestone lissencephaly (Walker Warburg syndrome). A shunt catheter ➡ and cerebellar dysplasia ➡ are also evident. *(Right)* Axial T2WI MR in a 2 year old with pachygyria/agyria shows multiple small PVSs. Moderate ventricular enlargement is noted. ↑ PVS are commonly encountered in malformations of cortical development.

# PORENCEPHALIC CYST

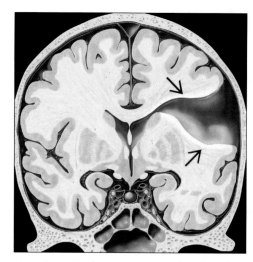

Coronal graphic shows an intraparenchymal CSF-filled cavity that communicates with the lateral ventricle and subarachnoid space, lined with minimally gliotic white matter ➡.

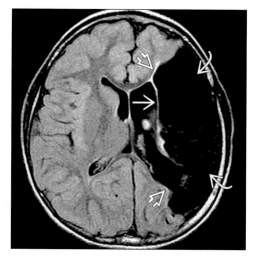

Axial FLAIR MR shows large cavity ➡ that matches territory of left MCA; it is separated from ventricle by thin membrane ➡ and lined by minimally gliotic white matter ➡.

## TERMINOLOGY

### Abbreviations and Synonyms
- Porencephaly

### Definitions
- Definitions/terminology in literature are contradictory, confusing
- Basic definition: Intracerebral cavitation due to late fetal or perinatal injury, sometimes communicating with ventricles/subarachnoid spaces

## IMAGING FINDINGS

### General Features
- Best diagnostic clue: Cystic space in brain parenchyma, enlarged adjacent ventricle on CT, MR, with little or no gliosis
- Location
  - Anywhere in fore & hindbrain; may fit arterial territories (transcerebral), subependymal venous drainage (periventricular white matter sparing the cortex), or isolated deep white matter
  - Unilateral/bilateral
  - Usually connected with one lateral ventricle; covering membrane at the periphery
- Size: Variable, sometimes near complete brain destruction: Hydranencephaly
- Morphology: Rounded or more rectangular, ventricular expansion; but parenchyma decreased in size, usually

### CT Findings
- CTA: No, or tiny vessels over porencephaly
- NECT
  - Intraparenchymal smooth-walled cavity, CSF-isointense, lined with white matter
  - Communication with ventricle or separating membrane
- CECT: No contrast-enhancement

### MR Findings
- T1WI: Smooth-walled cavity within brain parenchyma, isointense to CSF, lined with white matter, sometimes containing residual vascular tracts
- T2WI: Minimal gliosis; loss of brain substance (loss of connecting fibers)
- PD/Intermediate

## DDx: Other Hemispheric Cavities

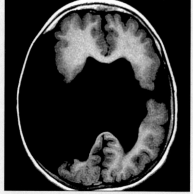

Schizencephaly

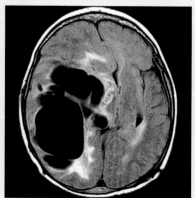

Post-Abscess Cavitation

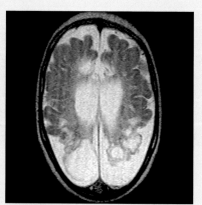

Multicystic Encephalomalacia

# PORENCEPHALIC CYST

## Key Facts

### Terminology
- Basic definition: Intracerebral cavitation due to late fetal or perinatal injury, sometimes communicating with ventricles/subarachnoid spaces

### Imaging Findings
- Best diagnostic clue: Cystic space in brain parenchyma, enlarged adjacent ventricle on CT, MR, with little or no gliosis

### Top Differential Diagnoses
- Arachnoid/Neuroepithelial Cysts
- Early Developmental Cysts: Schizencephaly
- Late Parenchymal Injuries: Scars
- Other Developmental Cysts
- Acquired Disease with Cyst

### Pathology
- Hippocampal sclerosis often coexists with porencephaly, may be bilateral despite unilateral cysts
- Familial porencephaly may be associated with inherited thrombophilia
- CSF-filled cavity with smooth walls, lined by white matter of cerebral hemisphere, sometimes crossed by vascular strand

### Diagnostic Checklist
- Assess hippocampal structures in patients with porencephaly-related seizures
- Brain imaging is unreliable to identify asymptomatic carriers of familial porencephaly, but it may point to the familial disorder

---

- Reliable prediction of cyst contents
  - CSF-isointense content of maldevelopmental/porencephalic cyst
  - Non-CSF-isointense appearance in neoplastic/inflammatory lesion
- FLAIR
  - Accurately depicts CSF content of cyst
  - More accurate than PD in differentiating neoplastic/inflammatory from porencephalic cysts
- T1 C+: Nonenhancing cyst
- MRA: No, or tiny vessels over porencephaly
- MRS: CSF-like

### Ultrasonographic Findings
- Anechoic brain cavity in neonate
- Prenatal ultrasound, MR for congenital porencephaly: Same as post-natal

### Angiographic Findings
- Conventional: Vessels over pial covering membrane are thin; rarely supply cortex beyond porencephaly

### Imaging Recommendations
- Best imaging tool: MR better but CT usually diagnostic
- Protocol advice: Multiple sequences in multiple planes

## DIFFERENTIAL DIAGNOSIS

### Arachnoid/Neuroepithelial Cysts
- CSF-isointense extra-axial cyst that displaces brain tissue away from adjacent skull, with intact cortical ribbon/vessels
- Along the midline, often associated with callosal agenesis/dysgenesis (cortex may not be preserved)

### Early Developmental Cysts: Schizencephaly
- Cystic or closed cleft lined with cortex to ependyma ("pial-ependymal seam"), septum pellucidum typically absent or dehiscent, surrounding cortex polymicrogyric

### Late Parenchymal Injuries: Scars
- Multicystic encephalomalacia

- Posthemorrhagic, postinfectious, postsurgical cavities

### Other Developmental Cysts
- Intraventricular: Choroid or ependymal cysts
- Parenchymal: Neuroglial cysts

### Acquired Disease with Cyst
- Neoplastic: Cyst content different from CSF
- Parasitic

## PATHOLOGY

### General Features
- General path comments: Focal cavity within brain parenchyma with smooth walls, little gliosis
- Genetics
  - Most cases are sporadic
  - Familial porencephaly is a rare condition
    - Autosomal dominant trait with variable expression and incomplete penetrance
    - Involved genes not yet mapped → search for mutations leading to hypercoagulable state
- Etiology
  - Congenital or perinatal: Little or no astrocytic scarring ability, destructive cavity remains
  - Vascular (arterial, venous), hemorrhagic, infectious (CMV, toxoplasmosis)
- Epidemiology: 2.5% incidence of porencephalic cysts among 1,000 congenital and acquired brain lesions
- Associated abnormalities
  - Hippocampal sclerosis often coexists with porencephaly, may be bilateral despite unilateral cysts
  - Familial porencephaly may be associated with inherited thrombophilia

### Gross Pathologic & Surgical Features
- CSF-filled cavity with smooth walls, lined by white matter of cerebral hemisphere, sometimes crossed by vascular strand
- Depending on cause, cortex and periventricular white matter may be lost or somewhat preserved

# PORENCEPHALIC CYST

- Overlying skull may be
  - Remodeled due to long-term direct transmission of non-elastic CSF pulsations through mantle defect
  - Progressively expanded
  - Rarely thickened (Dyke-Davidoff-Masson), if pressure waves are not transmitted (post ventricular drainage)

## Microscopic Features

- Typical porencephalic cyst
  - Fluid-filled, focal cavity with smooth walls and minimal surrounding glial reaction
  - Necrotic tissue completely reabsorbed (liquefaction necrosis), vessels may leave fibrous strands
- May reveal etiology
  - Blood residues
  - Viral particles (CMV), parasites (toxoplasmosis)

## Staging, Grading or Classification Criteria

- Early developmental: Schizencephaly
  - Idiopathic, familial, acquired (e.g., CMV) malformation of cortical development (MCD) with associated polymicrogyria
  - Uni- or bilateral, cortex-lined porus, dehiscent septum pellucidum
  - Spasticity, epilepsy, normo- or micrencephaly
- Late fetal/perinatal: Common porencephaly
  - Destructive, white matter lined cavity, preserved cortex looks normal
  - Typically unilateral, macrocephaly, epilepsy
- Extensive bilateral porencephaly: Hydranencephaly
  - Bilateral destruction of most of hemispheres, may correlate territory of both ICA, both MCA
  - Basal forebrain, central gray matter, hindbrain usually preserved
  - Microcephaly usual
- Post-natal: Multicystic encephalomalacia
  - Incomplete but significant astrocytic scarring

# CLINICAL ISSUES

## Presentation

- Most common signs/symptoms
  - Nothing, or hand preference, or mild hemiparesis, or severe hemiparesis/dystonia
    - Depends on location, amount of tissue destroyed
  - Developmental delay depends on size
  - Epilepsy, sometimes severe: May be due to abnormal neuronal loops from axons rerouted and connecting around the scar
- Clinical Profile
  - No medical history; paresis discovered late in infancy, macrocephaly, epilepsy
  - Severe perinatal disorders less common

## Demographics

- Age: Usually discovered in pediatric age
- Gender: Equal

## Natural History & Prognosis

- Transcerebral cysts tend to expand and compress surrounding brain

## Treatment

- Often no treatment required
- Shunting: Expanding cyst, significant macrocephaly
- Fenestration in selected cases
- Removal of epileptogenic cortex: Severe epilepsy

# DIAGNOSTIC CHECKLIST

## Consider

- Typically prenatal injury in infants born at term
- Assess hippocampal structures in patients with porencephaly-related seizures

## Image Interpretation Pearls

- Brain imaging is unreliable to identify asymptomatic carriers of familial porencephaly, but it may point to the familial disorder

# SELECTED REFERENCES

1. Breedveld G et al: Novel mutations in three families confirm a major role of COL4A1 in hereditary porencephaly. J Med Genet. 43(6):490-5, 2006
2. Guzzetta F et al: Symptomatic epilepsy in children with poroencephalic cysts secondary to perinatal middle cerebral artery occlusion. Childs Nerv Syst. 22(8):922-30, 2006
3. Iida K et al: Cortical resection with electrocorticography for intractable porencephaly-related partial epilepsy. Epilepsia. 46(1):76-83, 2005
4. Lynch JK et al: Prothrombotic factors in children with stroke or porencephaly. Pediatrics. 116(2):447-53, 2005
5. Tonni G et al: Neonatal porencephaly in very low birth weight infants: ultrasound timing of asphyxial injury and neurodevelopmental outcome at two years of age. J Matern Fetal Neonatal Med. 18(6):361-5, 2005
6. Kwong KL et al: Magnetic resonance imaging in 122 children with spastic cerebral palsy. Pediatr Neurol. 31(3):172-6, 2004
7. Mancini GM et al: Hereditary porencephaly: clinical and MRI findings in two Dutch families. Eur J Paediatr Neurol. 8(1):45-54, 2004
8. Prayson RA et al: Clinicopathologic findings in patients with infantile hemiparesis and epilepsy. Hum Pathol. 35(6):734-8, 2004
9. Burneo JG et al: Temporal lobectomy in congenital porencephaly associated with hippocampal sclerosis. Arch Neurol. 60(6):830-4, 2003
10. Moinuddin A et al: Intracranial hemorrhage progressing to porencephaly as a result of congenitally acquired cytomegalovirus infection--an illustrative report. Prenat Diagn. 23(10):797-800, 2003
11. Carreno M et al: Intractable epilepsy in vascular congenital hemiparesis: clinical features and surgical options. Neurology. 59(1):129-31, 2002
12. Vilain C et al: Neuroimaging fails to identify asymptomatic carriers of familial porencephaly. Am J Med Genet. 112(2):198-202, 2002
13. Aprile I et al: Analysis of cystic intracranial lesions performed with fluid-attenuated inversion recovery MR imaging. AJNR Am J Neuroradiol. 20(7):1259-67, 1999
14. Raybaud C: Destructive lesions of the brain. Neuroradiology. 25(4):265-91, 1983

# PORENCEPHALIC CYST

## IMAGE GALLERY

### Typical

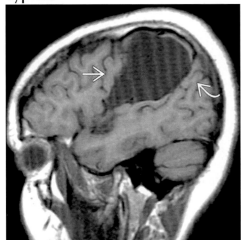
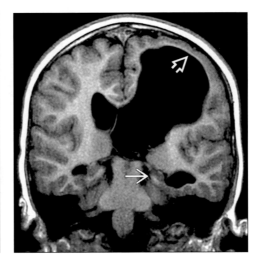

*(Left)* Sagittal T1WI MR shows porencephaly that matches territory of parietal branches of MCA between motor strip ➡ and angular gyrus ➡. These are usually caused by antenatal events. *(Right)* Coronal T1WI MR shows massive destruction of white matter but preservation of dysplastic cortex & U-fibers ➡. Result of grade 4 neonatal hemorrhage. Note hippocampal atrophy ➡.

### Typical

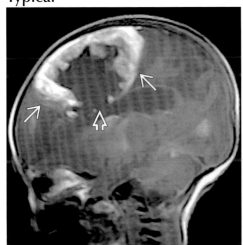
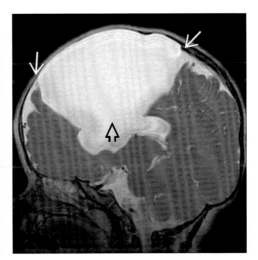

*(Left)* Sagittal T1WI MR in neonate shows massive white matter hemorrhage ➡ with hemorrhagic cavity opening into lateral ventricle ➡. Etiology was uncertain. *(Right)* Sagittal T2WI MR *(same child as previous image)* at 6 months shows complete liquefaction of cavity, wide connection with ventricle ➡. Preserved pial membranes ➡ bulge peripherally and remodel adjacent bone.

### Typical

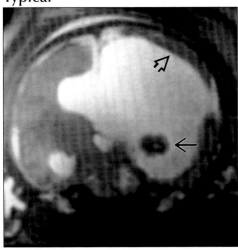
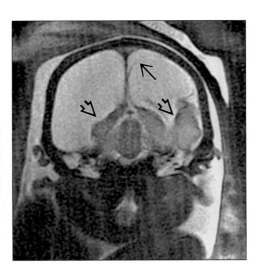

*(Left)* Coronal T2WI MR in fetus shows hydrocephalus & large, presumably hemorrhagic porencephaly with white matter destruction & preserved cortex ➡. Note hemorrhagic choroid plexus ➡. *(Right)* Coronal T2WI MR in fetus shows hydranencephaly with near complete replacement of hemispheres with vesicles (bordered by covering membrane ➡). Note part of temporal lobes preserved ➡.

# NEUROGLIAL CYST

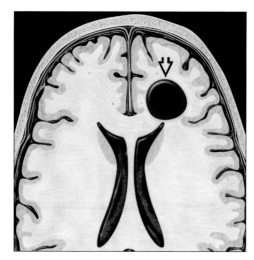

*Axial graphic shows a classic parenchymal neuroglial cyst: Well-delineated unilocular, homogeneous, spherical cystic lesion ⊳ containing clear fluid. Surrounding brain is normal.*

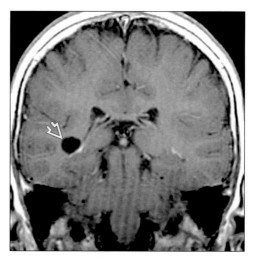

*Coronal T1 C+ MR shows same appearance as previous graphic: Paraventricular rounded lesion ⊳ with normal surrounding brain; its content has same signal as that of CSF. No enhancement.*

## TERMINOLOGY

### Abbreviations and Synonyms
- Neuroglial cyst (NGC), glioependymal cyst

### Definitions
- Benign cyst lined with neuroepithelium

## IMAGING FINDINGS

### General Features
- Best diagnostic clue: Nonenhancing CSF-like cyst with no surrounding signal abnormality
- Location: Ventricular, parenchymal, extra-axial (commonly suprasellar, ambient cistern, posterior fossa)
- Size: From a few mm up to several cm
- Morphology: Smooth, rounded, unilocular cyst

### CT Findings
- NECT: Well-delineated, unilocular, low density, no Ca++
- CECT: No enhancement

### MR Findings
- T1WI: Similar to CSF
- T2WI: Similar to CSF
- FLAIR: Hypointense, similar to CSF
- T2* GRE: No blooming
- DWI: Hyperintense (increased diffusivity)
- T1 C+: No enhancement

### Imaging Recommendations
- Best imaging tool: MR without, with contrast
- Protocol advice: Use FLAIR, DWI and contrast

## DIFFERENTIAL DIAGNOSIS

### Epidermoid
- Hyperintense on FLAIR and on DWI

### Parenchymal Cysts
- Porencephaly (gliosis), schizencephaly (lined with cortex), enlarged perivascular spaces (cluster of cavities)
- Cystic tumors (fluid different from CSF, enhancement), parasitic cysts (exposed area)

### DDx: Other Cysts

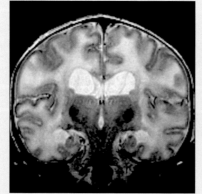

*Ependymal Cysts*

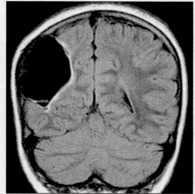

*Porencephalic Cyst*

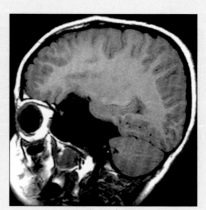

*Arachnoid Cyst*

# NEUROGLIAL CYST

## Key Facts

### Terminology
- Benign cyst lined with neuroepithelium

### Imaging Findings
- Best diagnostic clue: Nonenhancing CSF-like cyst with no surrounding signal abnormality
- Location: Ventricular, parenchymal, extra-axial (commonly suprasellar, ambient cistern, posterior fossa)

### Top Differential Diagnoses
- Epidermoid
- Cystic tumors (fluid different from CSF, enhancement), parasitic cysts (exposed area)

### Clinical Issues
- Most common signs/symptoms: Incidental finding
- Other signs/symptoms: Headaches, seizures, deficits
- Depends on size, location, stability

---

### Ventricular Cysts
- Cyst of choroid plexus (within plexus), subependymal cysts (located in ventricular walls, context)

### Extra-Axial Cysts
- Arachnoid cysts: Neuroglial cysts often have thicker wall; may be indistinguishable

## PATHOLOGY

### General Features
- General path comments: CSF-containing cyst lined with neuroepithelium resembling ependyma
- Etiology
  - Embryonic neural lining in developing white matter
  - Extra-axial: Neuroglial heterotopia postulated
- Epidemiology: Uncommon (< 1% of intracranial cysts)

### Gross Pathologic & Surgical Features
- Rounded, smooth, unilocular cyst, usually containing clear fluid resembling CSF

### Microscopic Features
- Varies from columnar (ependymal type) epithelium to low cuboidal cells resembling choroid plexus

## CLINICAL ISSUES

### Presentation
- Most common signs/symptoms: Incidental finding

- Other signs/symptoms: Headaches, seizures, deficits

### Demographics
- Age: Developmental: Any age
- Gender: M = F

### Natural History & Prognosis
- Depends on size, location, stability

### Treatment
- Observation vs. fenestration/drainage of cyst

## DIAGNOSTIC CHECKLIST

### Consider
- Rule out cystic tumor

### Image Interpretation Pearls
- Epidermoids have reduced diffusion

## SELECTED REFERENCES

1. Salzman KL et al: Giant tumefactive perivascular spaces. AJNR Am J Neuroradiol. 26(2):298-305, 2005
2. Tsuchida T et al: Glioependymal cyst in the posterior fossa. Clin Neuropathol. 16(1):13-6, 1997
3. Ismail A et al: Glioependymal cysts: CT and MR findings. J Comput Assist Tomogr. 16(6):860-4, 1992
4. Nakase H et al: Neuroepithelial cyst of the lateral ventricle. Clinical features & treatment. Surg Neurol. 37:94-100,1992
5. Friede RL: Developmental Neuropathology. Springer Wien, New York. 196-202, 1975

## IMAGE GALLERY

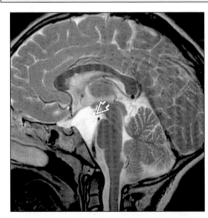 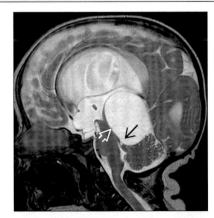 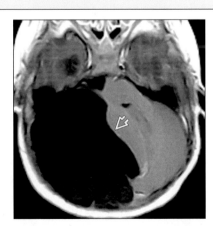

*(Left)* Sagittal T2WI MR shows closed supra-retrosellar cyst ➡ with mild mass effect on adjacent structures. This differs from common suprasellar cysts that grow upward, elevating 3rd ventricle. *(Center)* Sagittal oblique T2WI MR shows CSF-filled neuroglial cyst ➡ in ambient cistern, with aqueduct compression and hydrocephalus. Note the thick enclosing membrane ➡. *(Right)* Axial T1 C+ MR shows large CSF-filled cyst in lateral posterior fossa ➡ with mass effect on cerebellum and brainstem. Usually called arachnoid, such cysts are typically neuroglial on pathology.

# CONGENITAL CMV

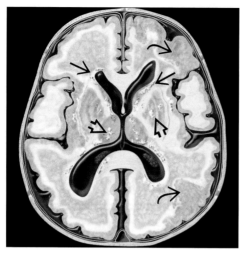

Axial graphic shows periventricular ⊡ and basal ganglia ⊡ calcification. Note regions of cortical dysplasia ⊡. Ventricular dilation reflects adjacent WM volume loss.

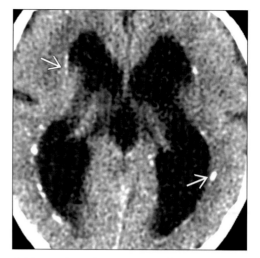

Axial NECT shows scattered periventricular calcifications ➡. Also note the dilatation of the lateral ventricles which reflects periventricular WM volume loss.

## TERMINOLOGY

### Abbreviations and Synonyms
- Congenital cytomegalovirus (CMV) encephalitis

### Definitions
- Congenital infection caused by transplacental transmission of human herpes virus
  - Most common cause of intrauterine infection in the United States
  - Spectrum of brain injury is possible depending upon timing of the fetal infection

## IMAGING FINDINGS

### General Features
- Best diagnostic clue
  - Microcephaly
  - Cerebral calcification (40-70%)
    - Periventricular (subependymal)
  - Cortical gyral abnormalities
    - Agyria ↔ pachygyria ↔ diffuse polymicrogyria ↔ focal polymicrogyria

- Cerebellar hypoplasia
- Myelin delay or destruction
- Location: Dystrophic periventricular Ca++ has predilection for germinal matrix
- Gestational age at time of infection determines pattern of central nervous system (CNS) injury
  - Prior to 18 wks → reduction in neurons and glia, lissencephaly, small cerebellum, ventriculomegaly
  - 18-24 wks → cortical gyral abnormalities, frontal > temporal
  - Third trimester → myelin delay or destruction, periventricular cysts
  - Perinatal infection → delay in myelin maturation, focal white matter (WM) injury (astrogliosis)

### CT Findings
- NECT
  - Cerebral parenchymal Ca++ (40-70%)
    - Periventricular (subependymal)
  - Ventricular dilatation and WM volume loss
  - Focal regions of WM low attenuation
  - Cortical gyral abnormalities
  - Cerebellar hypoplasia

## DDx: Neonatal Periventricular Calcification

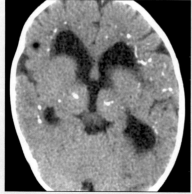

Lymphocytic Choriomeningitis

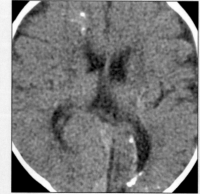

Toxoplasmosis

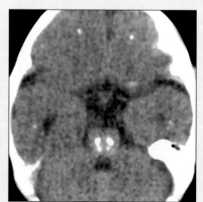

Pseudo-TORCH

## Key Facts

### Imaging Findings
- Microcephaly
- Cerebral parenchymal Ca++ (40-70%)
- Cerebellar hypoplasia
- Cortical gyral abnormalities
- Echogenic periventricular foci (Ca++)
- Branching basal ganglia and thalamic echoes (lenticulostriate vasculopathy)
- Cranial sonography for neonatal screening
- NECT when clinically suspected
- MR brain to completely characterize abnormalities

### Top Differential Diagnoses
- Congenital Lymphocytic Choriomeningitis (LCM)
- Toxoplasmosis
- Pseudo-TORCH Syndromes

### Pathology
- Most common cause of intrauterine infection
- CMV is a ubiquitous DNA virus of the herpes-virus family
- Affects ≈ 1% of all newborns
- Cytomegaly (25-40 microns) with viral nuclear and cytoplasmic inclusions

### Clinical Issues
- Most infected newborns appear normal

### Diagnostic Checklist
- Consider congenital CMV in the developmentally delayed, microcephalic infant with SNHL

## MR Findings
- T1WI
  - Periventricular subependymal foci of T1 shortening due to Ca++
  - Ventricular dilatation and periventricular WM volume loss
  - Cerebellar hypoplasia
- T2WI
  - Cortical gyral abnormalities
    - Ranging from agyria to focal polymicrogyria
  - Myelination delay or destruction
  - Periventricular pseudocysts
  - Focal WM lesions with ↑ T2 (gliosis) predominately in parietal deep WM
  - Hippocampal dysplasia (vertical orientation)
  - Temporal tip cystic changes frequent
  - Late T2 signal changes affect WM between juxta-cortical and periventricular layers
- FLAIR: Focal, patchy, or confluent regions of increased signal due to gliosis
- T2* GRE: Periventricular ↓ signal due to Ca++
- MRS: ↓ NAA/Cr ratio due to loss of neuronal elements, ↑ myoinositol (gliosis)

## Ultrasonographic Findings
- Grayscale Ultrasound
  - Ring-like regions of periventricular lucency may precede Ca++
  - Echogenic periventricular foci (Ca++)
  - Branching basal ganglia and thalamic echoes (lenticulostriate vasculopathy)
  - Periventricular pseudocysts and ventricular adhesions
  - Cerebellar hypoplasia

## Imaging Recommendations
- Best imaging tool
  - Cranial sonography for neonatal screening
  - NECT when clinically suspected
  - MR brain to completely characterize abnormalities
- Protocol advice
  - NECT for detecting periventricular Ca++
  - T2* GRE to detect subtle calcification or hemorrhage

## DIFFERENTIAL DIAGNOSIS

### Congenital Lymphocytic Choriomeningitis (LCM)
- Rodent borne Arenavirus
  - Carried by the feral house mouse and hamster
- Produces a necrotizing ependymitis leading to aqueductal obstruction
  - Macrocephaly (43%) > microcephaly (13%)
- NECT may perfectly mimic CMV

### Toxoplasmosis
- Protozoan parasite
  - Maternal risk factors include
    - Exposure to cat excreta during pregnancy
    - Eating raw or undercooked meat
- 1/10th as common as CMV
- Macrocrania > microcephaly
- Neuronal migration abnormalities less common
- Cerebral calcifications: Random locations

### Pseudo-TORCH Syndromes
- Baraister-Reardon, Aicardi-Goutieres [cerebrospinal fluid (CSF) pleocytosis, ↑ CSF alpha interferon]
  - Auto recessive
  - Progressive cerebral and cerebellar demyelination
  - Basal ganglia Ca++
  - +/- Periventricular Ca++

## PATHOLOGY

### General Features
- General path comments
  - Most common cause of intrauterine infection
  - Mechanism of fetal infection
    - Mother has primary infection during pregnancy
    - Mother has reactivation of latent infection
  - Mechanism of neonatal infection
    - Mother infected at delivery

# CONGENITAL CMV

- Transmission of virus in breast milk
- Blood transfusion
- Etiology
  - CMV is a ubiquitous DNA virus of the herpes-virus family
  - Hematogenously seeds the choroid plexus
  - Replicates in ependyma, germinal matrix, and capillary endothelia
  - Capillary involvement leads to thrombosis and ischemia
  - Chronic ischemia from placentitis leading to secondary perfusion insufficiency
- Epidemiology
  - Affects ≈ 1% of all newborns
    - 10% of these have CNS or systemic signs and symptoms
  - 40% of mothers who acquire infection during pregnancy transmit virus to fetus

## Gross Pathologic & Surgical Features

- Micrencephaly
- Early gestational infection
  - Germinal zone necrosis
  - Diminished number of neurons and glial cells
  - White matter volume loss → ventriculomegaly

## Microscopic Features

- Hallmark of CMV infection
  - Cytomegaly (25-40 microns) with viral nuclear and cytoplasmic inclusions
- Patchy and focal cellular necrosis (particularly germinal matrix cells)
- Vascular inflammation and thrombosis
- Vascular and subependymal dystrophic Ca++

## Staging, Grading or Classification Criteria

- Timing of gestational infection determines insult
  - Neuronal formation between 8-20 weeks
  - Neuron migration until 24-26 weeks
  - Astrocyte generation begins near end of neuronal production
  - Maximal size of germinal zones at 26 weeks
  - Oligodendrocytes produced during first half of third trimester

## CLINICAL ISSUES

### Presentation

- Most common signs/symptoms
  - Most infected newborns appear normal
  - 10% have systemic signs of disease
    - Hepatosplenomegaly (52%), petechiae (51%), chorioretinitis, jaundice, and intrauterine growth retardation (IUGR)
  - 55% with systemic disease have CNS involvement
    - Microcephaly, parenchymal Ca++, hearing loss, seizures, hypotonia or hypertonia
- Clinical Profile: Seronegative women are at greatest risk for vertical transmission
- Methods of diagnosis
  - Shell-vial assay for CMV (urine)
  - Late diagnosis with polymerase-chain-reaction (PCR) for CMV-DNA

## Natural History & Prognosis

- Three prognostic groups
  - Newborns with CNS manifestations (microcephaly, periventricular Ca++)
    - Up to 95% have major neurodevelopmental sequelae
  - Newborns with only systemic manifestations (hepatosplenomegaly, petechiae, jaundice)
    - Have better prognosis but still significantly affected
  - Infected newborns with neither CNS or systemic manifestations
    - Have best prognosis
    - At risk for: Developmental delay, motor deficits, and SNHL (most common)
  - Mortality ≈ 5%

## Treatment

- Ganciclovir may benefit infected infants

## DIAGNOSTIC CHECKLIST

### Consider

- Consider congenital CMV in the developmentally delayed, microcephalic infant with SNHL

### Image Interpretation Pearls

- Congenital CMV encephalitis should be considered when MR shows
  - Cerebellar hypoplasia
  - Cortical gyral abnormalities (particularly agyria with thin cortex)
  - Myelin delay or destruction
  - Microcephaly
- When NECT is classic for CMV encephalitis but the work-up for TORCH infection is negative, consider
  - Lymphocytic choriomeningitis (LCM)
  - Pseudo TORCH syndromes (most are autosomal recessive)

## SELECTED REFERENCES

1. Tatli B et al: Not a new leukodystrophy but congenital cytomegalovirus infection. J Child Neurol. 20(6):525-7, 2005
2. de Vries LS et al: The spectrum of cranial ultrasound and magnetic resonance imaging abnormalities in congenital cytomegalovirus infection. Neuropediatrics. 35(2):113-9, 2004
3. van der Knaap MS et al: Pattern of white matter abnormalities at MR imaging: use of polymerase chain reaction testing of Guthrie cards to link pattern with congenital cytomegalovirus infection. Radiology. 230(2):529-36, 2004
4. El Ayoubi M et al: Lenticulostriate echogenic vessels: clinical and sonographic study of 70 neonatal cases. Pediatr Radiol. 33(10):697-703, 2003
5. Wright R et al: Congenital lymphocytic choriomeningitis virus syndrome: A disease that mimics congenital toxoplasmosis or cytomegalovirus infection. Pediatrics. 100:1-6, 1997
6. Barkovich AJ et al: Congenital cytomegalovirus infections of the brain: imaging analysis and embryologic considerations. AJNR. 15:703-15, 1994

# CONGENITAL CMV

## IMAGE GALLERY

### Typical

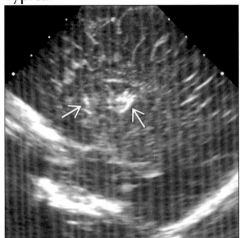
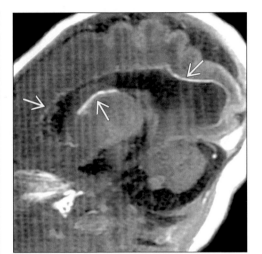

*(Left)* Sagittal oblique ultrasound shows linear and branching foci of hyperechogenicity consistent with lenticulostriate vasculopathy ➡. *(Right)* Sagittal T1WI MR shows T1 shortening secondary to calcification that lines the walls of the lateral ventricle ➡.

### Typical

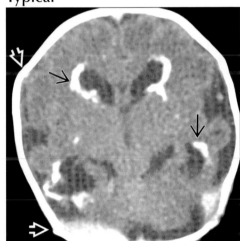
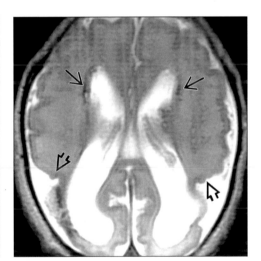

*(Left)* Axial NECT shows extensive calcification lining the walls of the lateral ventricles ➡. Note the overlap of the cranial sutures ⇨ reflecting atrophy in this microcephalic neonate. *(Right)* Axial T2WI MR shows hypointense periventricular calcification ➡. Note the primitive sulcation pattern and diffuse polymicrogyric cortex ➡.

### Variant

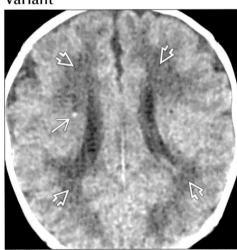
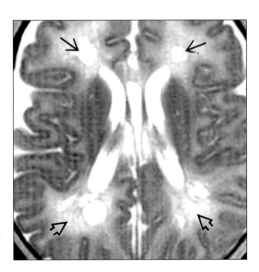

*(Left)* Axial NECT shows sparse periventricular calcification ➡. Periventricular WM attenuation is symmetrically diminished ⇨. *(Right)* Axial T2WI MR shows bilateral periventricular cavitary cysts ➡. Note the delay in myelination in this 10 month old term infant ➡.

# CONGENITAL HIV

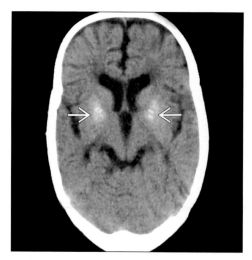
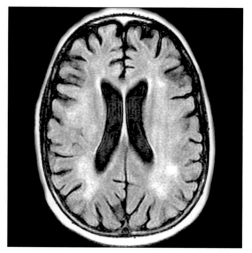

Axial NECT shows diffuse mild to moderate atrophy and calcifications ➡ of the basal ganglia (primarily the globus pallidus) in a 2 year old with vertically acquired HIV.

Axial FLAIR MR in a 13 year old with HIV leukoencephalopathy shows diffuse volume loss and increased hyperintensity in the cerebral white matter, corpus callosum.

## TERMINOLOGY

### Abbreviations and Synonyms
- Congenital AIDS, maternally transmitted AIDS

### Definitions
- Vertical HIV infection early inutero/late pregnancy, at delivery or by breastfeeding

## IMAGING FINDINGS

### General Features
- Best diagnostic clue: Basal ganglia (BG) Ca++, atrophy

### CT Findings
- NECT
  - Atrophy (57-86%), frontal > BG > diffuse
  - Mineralizing microangiopathy (> 8 weeks of age)
  - BG Ca++ (30-85%) > frontal WM > cerebellum
  - Lymphadenopathy, benign lymphoepithelial parotid cysts
- CECT: May show faint enhancement of BG prior to appearance of Ca++

### MR Findings
- T1WI: Atrophy
- T2WI: High signal in subcortical WM (demyelination) with progressive encephalopathy
- T2* GRE: May accentuate Ca++
- T1 C+: Faint BG enhancement initially
- MRA: Fusiform vasculopathy (late)
- MRS: ↓ NAA, ↑ Cho/Cr; progressive encephalopathy

### Imaging Recommendations
- Best imaging tool: MR
- Protocol advice
  - Baseline NECT
  - MR in symptomatic patients

## DIFFERENTIAL DIAGNOSIS

### Cytomegalovirus
- Periventricular Ca++, microcephaly, neuronal migration anomalies, cortical dysplasias

### Congenital Toxoplasmosis
- Scattered Ca++, hydrocephalus

## DDx: Cerebral Calcifications in Children

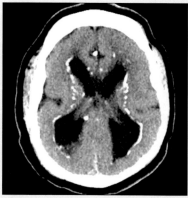
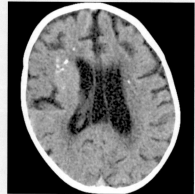
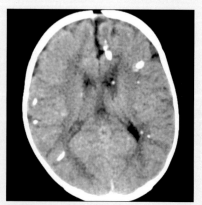

Cytomegalovirus

Aicardi Goutieres

Toxoplasmosis

## Key Facts

### Terminology
- Vertical HIV infection early inutero/late pregnancy, at delivery or by breastfeeding

### Imaging Findings
- Best diagnostic clue: Basal ganglia (BG) Ca++, atrophy
- Atrophy (57-86%), frontal > BG > diffuse
- Lymphadenopathy, benign lymphoepithelial parotid cysts
- MRA: Fusiform vasculopathy (late)

### Top Differential Diagnoses
- Cytomegalovirus
- Congenital Toxoplasmosis
- Other Etiologies of BG Calcifications

### Diagnostic Checklist
- Consider HIV if bilateral symmetrical calcifications in BG are found in a child > than 2 months

### Other Etiologies of BG Calcifications
- Endocrine (parathyroid), metabolic (mitochondrial), developmental (Cockayne syndrome), toxic (radiation, methotrexate)

### Microscopic Features
- HIV encephalitis: Microglial nodules, multinucleated giant cells, perivascular mononuclear cells
- HIV leukoencephalopathy: Myelin loss, astrogliosis

## PATHOLOGY

### General Features
- Etiology
  - HIV in microglial cells and macrophages
  - Viral proteins/neurotoxins → inflammation
- Epidemiology
  - Most acquired at birth, 3rd trimester, via breast feeding
  - Risk of HIV infection in infants of HIV-infected mothers: 30% if mother untreated; 2% with maternal treatment, C-section
  - In the past 15 years, new cases/year in the USA decreased from 2,500 to 400-600

### Gross Pathologic & Surgical Features
- Microcephaly
- Hemorrhage → arteriopathy, infarct, HIV-induced thrombocytopenia/clotting
- Calcific vasculitis (90%) of medium/small arteries
- Cerebrovascular disease
  - Infarctions, fusiform aneurysms
  - Diffuse fibrosing/sclerosing vasculopathy

## CLINICAL ISSUES

### Presentation
- Encephalopathy, developmental delay: Common
- Opportunistic infections: Less common in children

### Demographics
- Age: Symptoms begin at 12 weeks of life, some asymptomatic until 10 years of age

### Natural History & Prognosis
- Infected children survive longer with therapy
- If symptomatic in 1st year of life → 20% die in infancy

## DIAGNOSTIC CHECKLIST

### Image Interpretation Pearls
- Consider HIV if bilateral symmetrical calcifications in BG are found in a child > than 2 months

## SELECTED REFERENCES

1. Brady MT: Pediatric human immunodeficiency virus-1 infection. Adv Pediatr. 52:163-93, 2005

## IMAGE GALLERY

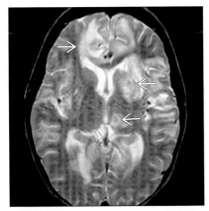 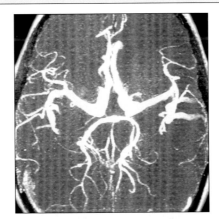 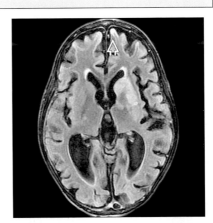

*(Left) Axial T2WI MR shows extensive toxoplasmosis. Multiple inflammatory masses ➡ with surrounding edema are evident in the left basal ganglia, thalamus, and the subcortical WM. (Center) Axial MRA in a 12 year old shows marked fusiform dilatation of the arteries of the circle of Willis. The distal ICA, the M1 and A1 segments are most affected. (Right) Axial FLAIR MR shows an acute infarct in the left BG. Bifrontal cortical laminar infarction is also evident ➡ (bright cortical ribbon). Diffuse cerebral atrophy with enlarged ventricles, sulci.*

# ABSCESS

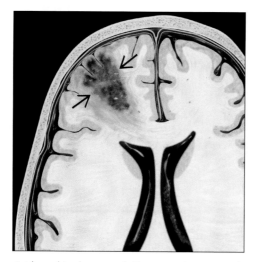

*Axial graphic shows cerebritis stage prior to capsule formation. There is breakdown of brain tissue, resulting in necrosis ➜ in the center of a larger area of infected, edematous brain.*

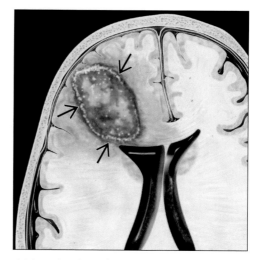

*Axial graphic shows later stage of abscess formation. The area of necrosis has grown, and there is an increase in mass effect and edema. A capsule ➜ has formed around central pus.*

## TERMINOLOGY

### Definitions
- Focal pyogenic infection of the brain parenchyma, typically bacterial; fungal or parasitic less common
- Four pathologic stages: Early cerebritis, late cerebritis, early capsule, late capsule

## IMAGING FINDINGS

### General Features
- Best diagnostic clue
  - Imaging varies with stage of abscess development
  - Smooth T2 hypointense ring-enhancing lesion with central decreased diffusion (bright DWI)
- Location
  - Typically supratentorial
  - Neonate: Frontal and parietal lobes, periventricular white matter most common
  - Children: Subcortical white matter and basal ganglia
- Size: Neonate: Large and multiple; child: Variable, 5 mm-several cm
- Morphology: Smooth, ring-enhancing lesion

- Gas-containing abscess rare

### CT Findings
- NECT
  - Early cerebritis: May be normal early; ill-defined hypodense subcortical lesion with mass effect
  - Late cerebritis: Central low density area; peripheral edema, increased mass effect
  - Early capsule: Hypodense mass with moderate vasogenic edema and mass effect
  - Late capsule: Edema, mass effect diminish
- CECT
  - Early cerebritis: ± Mild patchy enhancement
  - Late cerebritis: Irregular rim enhancement
  - Early capsule: Low density center with thin enhancing capsule
  - Late capsule: Cavity shrinks, capsule thickens, ± "daughter" abscesses, loculations

### MR Findings
- T1WI
  - Early cerebritis: Poorly marginated, mixed hypo/isointense mass
  - Late cerebritis: Hypointense center, iso/mildly hyperintense rim

## DDx: Ring-Enhancing Lesions

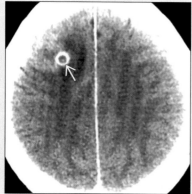

*Neurocysticercosis*

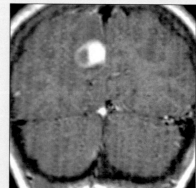

*Tumor*

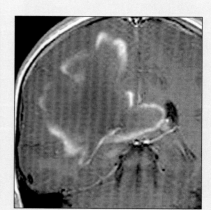

*Demyelination*

# ABSCESS

## Key Facts

### Terminology
- Four pathologic stages: Early cerebritis, late cerebritis, early capsule, late capsule

### Imaging Findings
- Imaging varies with stage of abscess development
- Early capsule: T2 Hypointense rim (due to collagen, hemorrhage, or paramagnetic free radicals)
- ↑ DWI signal in cerebritis and abscess
- Early capsule: Well-defined, thin-walled enhancing rim thicker on side near cortex
- Resolving abscess: T2 hypointense rim resolves, central ADC increases, enhancement resolves last

### Top Differential Diagnoses
- Cysticercosis
- Neoplasm
- Demyelination
- Resolving Hematoma

### Clinical Issues
- Child: Headache lethargy, vomiting, seizure, focal neurological deficit
- Surgical drainage and/or excision primary therapy
- Antibiotics only if small (< 2.5 cm) or early phase of cerebritis

### Diagnostic Checklist
- DWI, MRS helpful in distinguishing abscess from mimics
- Search for local cause such as sinusitis, otitis media, or mastoiditis
- T2 hypointense abscess rim resolves before enhancement in successfully treated patients

---

  - Early capsule: Rim iso/hyperintense to white matter; center hyperintense to CSF
  - Late capsule: Cavity shrinks, capsule thickens
- T2WI
  - Early cerebritis: Ill-defined hyperintense mass
  - Late cerebritis: Hyperintense center, hypointense rim; hyperintense edema
  - Early capsule: T2 Hypointense rim (due to collagen, hemorrhage, or paramagnetic free radicals)
  - Late capsule: Edema and mass effect diminish
- DWI
  - ↑ DWI signal in cerebritis and abscess
  - ADC markedly decreased in abscess
- T1 C+
  - Early cerebritis: No to patchy enhancement
  - Late cerebritis: Intense but irregular rim enhancement
  - Early capsule: Well-defined, thin-walled enhancing rim thicker on side near cortex
  - Late capsule: Cavity collapses, thickened enhancement of capsule especially side near cortex
- MRS: ± Lactate, lipids, acetate, alanine, succinate, pyruvate, and amino acids centrally
- Resolving abscess: T2 hypointense rim resolves, central ADC increases, enhancement resolves last

### Nuclear Medicine Findings
- PET: Abscess

### Imaging Recommendations
- Best imaging tool: Contrast-enhanced MR
- Protocol advice: DWI; MRS may be helpful

## DIFFERENTIAL DIAGNOSIS

### Cysticercosis
- Scolex, ± punctate calcifications

### Neoplasm
- Irregular enhancement, incomplete T2 rim, DWI not bright

### Demyelination
- Incomplete ring of enhancement, no surrounding edema, minimal mass effect

### Resolving Hematoma
- History of trauma, prior surgery or vascular lesion, blood products

### Subacute Infarct
- History of stroke, gyriform enhancement

### Tuberculoma
- ADC values not as low (mildly decreased to increased)

## PATHOLOGY

### General Features
- General path comments
  - Cerebritis: Unencapsulated zone of vessels, inflammatory cells, edema; necrotic foci gradually coalesce
  - Capsule (neonate): Poor capsule formation, large, often multiple
  - Capsule (child): Well-defined capsule develops around necrotic core; as abscess matures, edema/mass effect decrease
- Etiology
  - Neonatal: 2/3 associated with meningitis
  - Right-to-left shunts (congenital cardiac malformations)
  - Hematogenous from extracranial location (e.g., generalized sepsis)
  - Direct extension from a calvarial or meningeal infection
    - Paranasal sinus, middle ear, throat (via valveless emissary veins)
  - Penetrating trauma (bone fragments > > metal)
  - Post-operative
  - 5-15% have no identifiable source (cryptogenic)
- Epidemiology
  - Uncommon

○ Neonates (2/3 of pediatric abscesses): Citrobacter, Proteus, Pseudomonas, Serratia, Staphylococcus aureus (2° to meningitis)
○ Bacterial: Staphylococcus, Streptococcus, Pneumococcus
○ Post-transplant: Nocardia, Aspergillus, Candida
○ AIDS: Toxoplasmosis, mycobacterium tuberculosis

## Gross Pathologic & Surgical Features

- Early cerebritis (3-5 days)
  ○ Infection is focal but not localized
  ○ Unencapsulated mass of PMNs, edema, scattered foci of necrosis and petechial hemorrhage
- Late cerebritis (4-5 days up to 2 weeks)
  ○ Necrotic foci coalesce
  ○ Rim of inflammatory cells, macrophages, granulation tissue, fibroblasts surrounds central necrotic core
  ○ Vascular proliferation, surrounding vasogenic edema
- Early capsule (begins at around 2 weeks)
  ○ Well-delineated collagenous capsule except in neonates
  ○ Liquified necrotic core, peripheral gliosis
- Late capsule (weeks to months)
  ○ Central cavity shrinks
  ○ Thick wall (collagen, granulation tissue, macrophages, gliosis)

## Microscopic Features

- Early cerebritis: Hyperemic tissue with PMNs, necrotic blood vessels, microorganisms
- Late cerebritis: Progressive necrosis of the neuropil, destruction of PMNs, and inflammatory cells
- Early capsule: Proliferation of granulation tissue about necrotic core
- Late capsule: Multiple layers of collagen and fibroblasts

# CLINICAL ISSUES

## Presentation

- Most common signs/symptoms
  ○ Neonates: Seizure, increased intracranial pressure, meningitis
  ○ Child: Headache lethargy, vomiting, seizure, focal neurological deficit
  ○ Fever usually present
  ○ Increased erythrocyte sedimentation rate (ESR), elevated WBC often present
- Clinical Profile: Potentially fatal but treatable if diagnosed early
- Variable prognosis, depending on
  ○ Size, location of abscess, virulence of infecting organism(s)
  ○ Systemic conditions

## Demographics

- Age: Average age 7 years, 12% < 1 year (neonatal average age 9 days)
- Gender: M:F = 1.7:1

## Natural History & Prognosis

- Complications of inadequately or untreated abscesses

○ Intraventricular rupture, ventriculitis (may be fatal)
  ▪ Ventricular debris with irregular fluid level
  ▪ Hydrocephalus
  ▪ Ependymal enhancement typical
○ Meningitis, "daughter" lesions
○ Mass effect, herniation
- Stereotactic surgery + medical therapy have greatly reduced mortality
- Neonate: At least 15% mortality, 75% cognitive deficits, 60% epilepsy
- Child: 0-20% mortality, 30% epilepsy

## Treatment

- Surgical drainage and/or excision primary therapy
- Antibiotics only if small (< 2.5 cm) or early phase of cerebritis
- Steroids to treat edema and mass effect
- Lumbar puncture hazardous, pathogen often can't be determined from CSF unless 2° to meningitis

# DIAGNOSTIC CHECKLIST

## Consider

- DWI, MRS helpful in distinguishing abscess from mimics

## Image Interpretation Pearls

- Search for local cause such as sinusitis, otitis media, or mastoiditis
- T2 hypointense abscess rim resolves before enhancement in successfully treated patients

# SELECTED REFERENCES

1.  Fanning NF et al: Serial diffusion-weighted MRI correlates with clinical course and treatment response in children with intracranial pus collections. Pediatr Radiol. 36(1):26-37, 2006
2.  Gary M et al: Brain abscess: etiologic catheterization with vivo proton MR spectroscopy. Radiol. 230:519-27, 2004
3.  Kao PT et al: Brain abscess: clinical analysis of 53 cases. J Microbiol Immunol Infect. 36(2):129-36, 2003
4.  Guzman R et al: Use of diffusion-weighted magnetic resonance imaging in differentiating purulent brain processes from cystic brain tumors. J Neurosurg. 97(5):1101-7, 2002
5.  Lai PH et al: Brain abscess and necrotic brain tumor: discrimination with proton MR spectroscopy and diffusion-weighted imaging. AJNR Am J Neuroradiol. 23(8):1369-77, 2002
6.  Leuthardt EC et al: Diffusion-weighted MR imaging in the preoperative assessment of brain abscesses. Surg Neurol. 58(6):395-402; discussion 402, 2002
7.  Hartmann M et al: Restricted diffusion within ring enhancement is not pathognomonic for brain abscess. AJNR Am J Neuroradiol. 22(9):1738-42, 2001
8.  Rushing EJ et al: Infections of the nervous system. Neuroimaging Clin N Am. 11(1):1-13, 2001
9.  Verlicchi A et al: From diagnostic imaging to management of brain abscesses. Riv di Neuroradiol. 14: 267-74, 2001
10. Falcone S et al: Encephalitis, cerebritis, and brain abscess: pathophysiology and imaging findings. Neuroimaging Clin N Am. 10(2):333-53, 2000
11. Wong TT et al: Brain abscesses in children--a cooperative study of 83 cases. Childs Nerv Syst. 5(1):19-24, 1989

# ABSCESS

## IMAGE GALLERY

### Typical

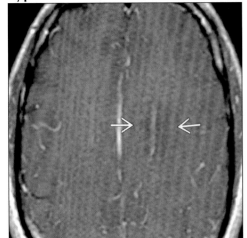
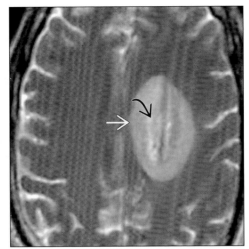

*(Left)* Axial T1 C+ MR shows a case of early cerebritis. The lesion ➡ is poorly defined with indistinct edges. No enhancement of the rim is seen in this early stage. *(Right)* Axial T2WI MR (same patient as previous image) shows a region of increased T2 signal (edema ➡) without a rim of low T2 signal. Central hyperintensity ⇗ is brain tissue undergoing necrosis.

### Typical

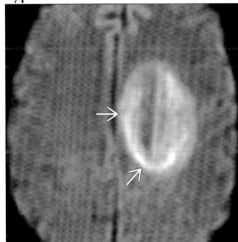
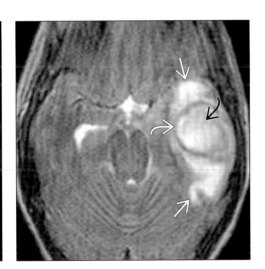

*(Left)* Axial DWI MR (same patient as previous image) shows a rim of bright signal ➡ in a patient with early cerebritis. On ADC map only the rim had decreased diffusion. *(Right)* Axial T2WI MR shows an abscess with a low signal intensity rim ➡ around more hypointense pus ⇗ in this pyogenic abscess, surrounded by hyperintense edema ➡.

### Typical

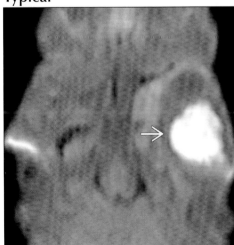
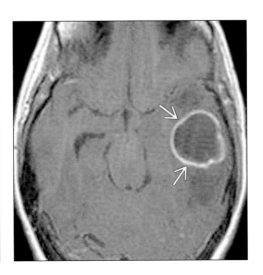

*(Left)* Axial DWI MR (same patient as previous image) shows the pus within the abscess to be extremely hyperintense ➡. This helps distinguish abscess from other masses. *(Right)* Axial T1 C+ MR (same patient as previous image) shows a smooth uniform rim of contrast enhancement ➡ around central pus in this pyogenic abscess.

# HERPES ENCEPHALITIS

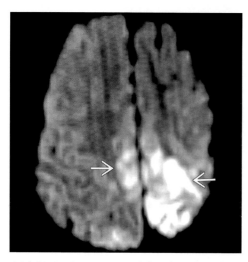

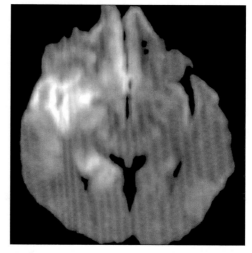

*Axial DWI MR in an encephalopathic infant shows increased signal ➡ due to decreased diffusion and increased T2 signal in the left > right parietal cortex.*

*Axial DWI MR in this child shows the classic distribution of increased DWI in the cortex involving primarily the right limbic system: Insula, temporal lobe and inferior frontal lobe cortex.*

## TERMINOLOGY

### Abbreviations and Synonyms
• Herpes simplex encephalitis (HSE)

### Definitions
• Meningoencephalitis caused by herpes simplex virus type 1 (HSV-1) or type 2 (HSV-2)

## IMAGING FINDINGS

### General Features
• Best diagnostic clue: Focal or multifocal DWI abnormalities in setting of acute neurological deterioration
• Location
  ○ Neonate: Focal or multifocal, any lobe
  ○ Infants and young children: Focal or multifocal vascular distribution, any lobe
  ○ Children: Primarily limbic system (medial temporal and inferior frontal lobes, insula and cingulate gyri)
    ▪ Typically bilateral disease, but asymmetric
    ▪ Basal ganglia usually spared

    ▪ Rarely, may affect midbrain and pons (mesenrhombencephalitis)
  ○ Rarely can present as acute hemorrhagic leukoencephalitis

### CT Findings
• NECT
  ○ Often normal early
  ○ Neonate: Diffuse, focal or multifocal low attenuation ± cortical hyperintensity from hemorrhage progressing to multicystic encephalomalacia
  ○ Child: Low attenuation, mild mass effect in medial temporal lobes, insula, hemorrhage usually a late feature
• CECT
  ○ Neonate: Ill-defined patchy enhancement
  ○ Child: Patchy or gyral enhancement of temporal lobes a late feature

### MR Findings
• T1WI: May see regions of bright T1 signal due to subacute hemorrhage
• T2WI

## DDx: Reduced Diffusion in Cortex

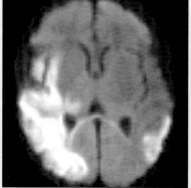

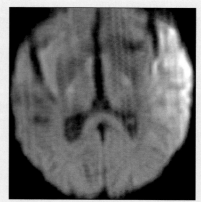

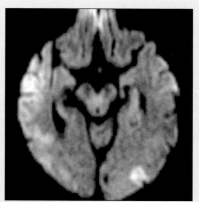

*Neonatal Strokes*   *MELAS*   *Status Epilepticus*

# HERPES ENCEPHALITIS

## Key Facts

### Terminology
- Meningoencephalitis caused by herpes simplex virus type 1 (HSV-1) or type 2 (HSV-2)

### Imaging Findings
- Neonate: Focal or multifocal, any lobe
- Children: Primarily limbic system (medial temporal and inferior frontal lobes, insula and cingulate gyri)
- Typically bilateral disease, but asymmetric

### Top Differential Diagnoses
- Arterial Ischemic Stroke
- Inborn Errors of Metabolism
- Status Epilepticus
- Other Encephalitides
- Limbic Encephalitis

### Pathology
- HSV-1 causes 95% of all herpes encephalitis
- HSV-2 causes 75-90% of congenital herpes encephalitis
- Most common cause of fatal sporadic encephalitis
- Hemorrhagic, necrotizing encephalitis of gray and white matter

### Clinical Issues
- Mortality ranges from 50-70%
- Antiviral therapy with intravenous Acyclovir

### Diagnostic Checklist
- IV Acyclovir therapy started immediately if herpes encephalitis is suspected!
- DWI is the most sensitive sequence but can be negative if acyclovir started early

---

- Neonate: Diffuse, focal or multifocal cerebral swelling with increased T2
- Child: Increased signal in gray, subcortical white matter, typically bilateral but asymmetric
- May see acute cortical hemorrhage as low signal or subacute hemorrhage as increased signal
- PD/Intermediate: Similar to T2
- FLAIR
  - Neonate: Diffuse, focal or multifocal cerebral swelling ± increased signal
  - Child: Hyperintense swollen cortex/subcortical white matter
- T2* GRE: If hemorrhagic regions of hypointensity on T2 "bloom"
- DWI
  - Hyperintense (decreased diffusivity) early
  - DWI findings may precede T2 changes
- T1 C+
  - Neonate: May see mild, patchy enhancement early
  - Child: Gyral enhancement usually seen 1 week after initial symptoms
  - Meningeal enhancement occasionally seen

### Imaging Recommendations
- Best imaging tool: MR
- Protocol advice: DWI, T2* GRE, contrast

## DIFFERENTIAL DIAGNOSIS

### Arterial Ischemic Stroke
- Typically vascular distribution but typically does not progress
- Cortical and subcortical white matter bright on DWI

### Inborn Errors of Metabolism
- Similar bright DWI in cortex
- No cortical hemorrhage; CSF profile not one of infection

### Status Epilepticus
- Similar bright DWI in cortex

- No cortical hemorrhage, CSF profile not one of infection

### Other Encephalitides
- Neonate: Citrobacter often bifrontal and subcortical; TORCH not bright DWI
- Child: Limbic system not selectively involved

### Infiltrating Neoplasm
- Onset usually indolent and DWI rarely bright

### Limbic Encephalitis
- Rare paraneoplastic syndrome associated with a primary tumor more common in adults but reports in teenagers
- Predilection for limbic system, often bilateral, but no hemorrhage
- Symptom onset usually weeks to months (vs. acute in HSE)

## PATHOLOGY

### General Features
- General path comments
  - Neonates: HSV-2 more common than HSV-1
  - Infants and young children: HSV-1
  - Children: HSV-1
  - HSV-1 and 2 are DNA viruses
  - Viruses are obligate intracellular pathogens
  - Herpes viruses include: HSV-1, HSV-2, Epstein-Barr virus (EBV), cytomegalovirus (CMV), varicella-zoster virus (VZV), B virus, HSV-6, HSV-7
- Etiology
  - HSV-1
    - Initial infection usually in oronasopharynx through contact with infected secretions
    - Invades along cranial nerves (via lingual nerve, a division of the trigeminal nerve) to ganglia
    - Dormant in the trigeminal ganglion
    - New infection with genetically distinct HSV > reactivation of dormant virus (entry probably via CN1)

# HERPES ENCEPHALITIS

- Reactivation may occur spontaneously or be precipitated by local trauma, immunosuppression, hormonal fluctuations, emotional stress
  - Infants and young children may not show classic pattern of involvement; in these cases the etiology is not known
  ○ HSV-2
    - Usually acquired by fetus as passing through infected birth canal
- Epidemiology
  ○ HSV-1 causes 95% of all herpes encephalitis
  ○ HSV-2 causes 75-90% of congenital herpes encephalitis
  ○ Most common cause of fatal sporadic encephalitis
  ○ Most common nonepidemic cause of viral meningoencephalitis
  ○ Incidence: 1-3 cases/million

## Gross Pathologic & Surgical Features
- Hemorrhagic, necrotizing encephalitis of gray and white matter
- Severe edema and massive tissue necrosis with hemorrhage typical
- Neonate: Focal or multifocal but no limbic predilection
- Infant and young child: Focal or multifocal lobar involvement with no limbic predilection
- Children: Involvement of temporal lobes, insular cortex, and orbital surface of frontal lobes common

## Microscopic Features
- Intense perivascular cuffing and interstitial lymphocytic inflammation
- Intranuclear inclusion bodies in infected cells (neurons, glia, endothelial cells)
  ○ Typically eosinophilic Cowdry A nuclear inclusions
- Immunohistochemistry shows viral antigens, antibodies to HSV-1 or HSV-2
- Chronic cases, microglial nodules form

# CLINICAL ISSUES

## Presentation
- Most common signs/symptoms
  ○ Neonates: Lethargy, stupor, irritability, seizures
  ○ Children often present with nonspecific symptoms
    - Behavioral changes, fever, headaches, seizures
    - Altered mental status, focal or diffuse neurologic deficit (< 30%)
  ○ May progress to coma and death
- Clinical Profile
  ○ CSF studies show a lymphocytic pleocytosis and elevated protein
  ○ Polymerase chain reaction (PCR) of CSF, most useful for diagnosis
    - Sensitivity/specificity of approximately 95-100% in CSF
  ○ Neonate: EEG shows paroxysmal periodic or quasiperiodic repetitive sharp-slow wave complexes
  ○ Children: EEG shows temporal lobe activity

## Demographics
- Age
  ○ Occurs at any age
  ○ Highest incidence of HSV-1 in adolescents and young adults
    - Approximately 30% of patients are less than 20 years old
  ○ HSV-2 only in neonates
- Gender: No gender predominance

## Natural History & Prognosis
- Rapid diagnosis, early treatment with antiviral agents can decrease mortality and improve outcome
- Mortality ranges from 50-70%
- Despite Acyclovir therapy, approximately 50% of patients have neurological disabilities
- Neonate: Often devastating particularly if HSV-2
- Child: Survival complicated by memory difficulties, hearing loss, medically intractable epilepsy, personality changes

## Treatment
- Antiviral therapy with intravenous Acyclovir

# DIAGNOSTIC CHECKLIST

## Consider
- IV Acyclovir therapy started immediately if herpes encephalitis is suspected!
- At all ages may mimic stroke, history often helpful!
- Teenagers: Rare paraneoplastic limbic encephalitis should be considered if clinical tests for herpes negative and subacute onset of symptoms

## Image Interpretation Pearls
- MR is most sensitive for diagnosis
- DWI is the most sensitive sequence but can be negative if acyclovir started early
- Imaging is often key in diagnosis!

# SELECTED REFERENCES

1. Kabakus N et al: Acute hemorrhagic leukoencephalitis manifesting as intracerebral hemorrhage associated with herpes simplex virus type I. J Trop Pediatr. 51:245-9, 2005
2. Kuker W et al: Diffusion-weighted MRI in herpes simplex encephalitis: a report of three cases. Neuroradiology. 46(2):122-5, 2004
3. Toth C et al: Neonatal herpes encephalitis: a case series and review of clinical presentation. Can J Neurol Sci. 30(1):36-40, 2003
4. Cakirer S et al: MR imaging in epilepsy that is refractory to medical therapy. Eur Radiol. 12(3):549-58, 2002
5. Kleinschmidt-DeMasters BK et al: The expanding spectrum of herpesvirus infections of the nervous system. Brain Pathol. 11(4):440-51, 2001
6. Teixeira J et al: Diffusion imaging in pediatric central nervous system infections. Neuroradiology. 43(12):1031-9, 2001
7. Leonard JR et al: MR imaging of herpes simplex type 1 encephalitis in infants and young children: a separate pattern of findings. AJR Am J Roentgenol. 174(6):1651-5, 2000
8. Domingues RB et al: Diagnosis of herpes simplex encephalitis by magnetic resonance imaging and polymerase chain reaction assay of cerebrospinal fluid. J Neurol Sci. 157(2):148-53, 1998

# HERPES ENCEPHALITIS

## IMAGE GALLERY

### Typical

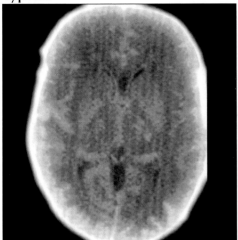
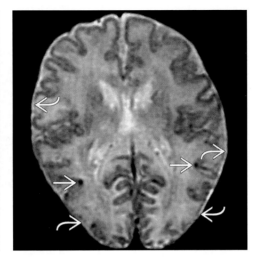

*(Left)* Axial NECT in this neonate presenting subacutely shows diffuse low attenuation in the white matter and deep gray matter with cortical hyperintensity secondary to hemorrhage. *(Right)* Axial T2WI MR in neonate with subacute neonatal herpes encephalitis shows diffuse increased T2 signal in white matter, cortical necrosis ➔ and foci ➔ of cortical hemorrhage.

### Typical

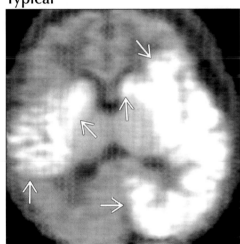
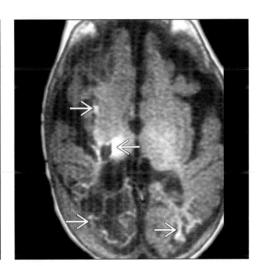

*(Left)* Axial DWI MR in this encephalopathic neonate shows multifocal areas ➔ of increased signal due to cortical and subcortical injury. Diffuse or multifocal involvement is typical in neonates. *(Right)* Axial T1WI MR in this neonate shows chronic sequelae of neonatal herpes encephalitis with multicystic encephalomalacia and regions of increased T1 ➔ suggesting calcium or blood products.

### Typical

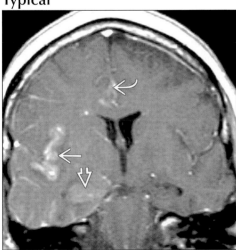
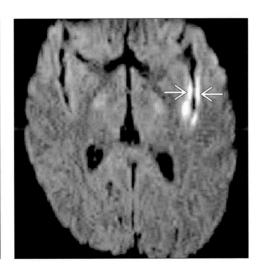

*(Left)* Coronal oblique T1 C+ MR in this child shows multifocal cortical enhancement in the right cingulate gyrus ➔, insula ➔, and the hippocampus ➔. *(Right)* Axial DWI MR in a patient with encephalopathy and seizures shows ➔ increased DWI signal indicating early necrosis in the insula and adjacent temporal lobe cortex. This is a common location for HSE.

# RASMUSSEN ENCEPHALITIS

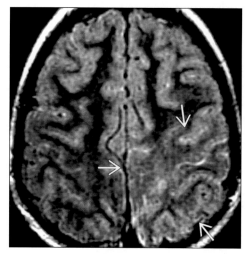

Axial FLAIR MR shows increased T2 signal ➔ in the cortex and subcortical white matter of the left parietal lobe. This is the appearance of stage 1 Rasmussen encephalitis.

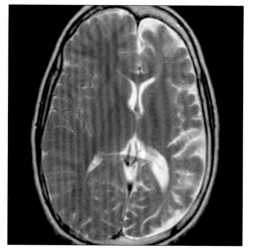

Axial T2WI MR shows diffuse left hemispheric cerebral atrophy with small left hemicalvarium and thickening of the ipsilateral diploic space secondary to stage 4 Rasmussen encephalitis.

## TERMINOLOGY

### Abbreviations and Synonyms
- Rasmussen syndrome (RS)
- Chronic focal encephalitis (new term)

### Definitions
- Chronic, progressive, relentless, unilateral inflammation of brain of uncertain etiology
- Characterized by hemispheric volume loss and difficult to control focal seizure activity

## IMAGING FINDINGS

### General Features
- Best diagnostic clue
  - Unilateral progressive cortical atrophy
  - CT/MR often normal initially
    - Cortical swelling, then atrophy ensue
    - Most brain damage subsequently identified occurs in first 12 months of disease
- Location
  - Cerebral hemisphere

- Usually unilateral
  - Precentral, inferior frontal atrophy
  - Unilateral cerebellar progressive volume loss
- Size: Variable but usually lobar, occasionally entire hemisphere affected
- Morphology
  - Focal abnormality "spreads across hemisphere"
  - Becomes progressively more diffuse, extensive

### CT Findings
- NECT: Atrophy
- CECT
  - Usually no enhancement
  - RARE transient cortical enhancement may occur

### MR Findings
- T1WI: Blurring of cortical ribbon during early swelling
- T2WI
  - Early focal swelling of gyri
    - Gray, underlying white matter mildly hyperintense
    - ± Basal ganglia, hippocampi involved
  - Caudate atrophy may occur early
  - Late: Atrophy of involved cerebral hemisphere or lobe

## DDx: Atrophy

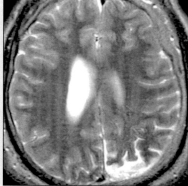

*Sturge-Weber*

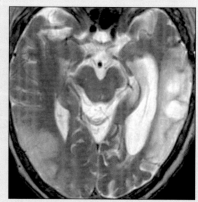

*MELAS (Chronic L, Acute R)*

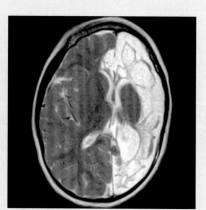

*Perinatal Infection*

# RASMUSSEN ENCEPHALITIS

## Key Facts

### Terminology

- Chronic, progressive, relentless, unilateral inflammation of brain of uncertain etiology
- Characterized by hemispheric volume loss and difficult to control focal seizure activity

### Imaging Findings

- Unilateral progressive cortical atrophy
- Early focal swelling of gyri
- Caudate atrophy may occur early
- Late: Atrophy of involved cerebral hemisphere or lobe

### Top Differential Diagnoses

- Sturge-Weber Syndrome
- Mitochondrial Encephalopathy, Lactic Acidosis, and Stroke-like Episodes (MELAS)
- Other Causes of Dyke-Davidoff-Masson Syndrome

### Pathology

- Three theories
- 1. Autoimmune theory
- 2. Immune mediated triggered by viral infection
- 3. Viral infection
- 50% preceded by inflammatory episode

### Clinical Issues

- Age: Usually begins in childhood between 18 months and 14 years (peak 6-8)
- Refractory to antiepileptic medications

### Diagnostic Checklist

- In patient with progressive intractable epilepsy with normal MR or progressive atrophy of one hemisphere and high T2 signal consider Rasmussen encephalitis

---

- PD/Intermediate: Same as T2WI
- FLAIR
  - Small areas of hyperintensity that progressively increase over time
  - Late: Atrophic, encephalomalacic/gliotic residual brain
- T2* GRE
  - Typically normal
  - Nonhemorrhagic
- DWI: Subtle high signal on ADC maps
- T1 C+: Usually no enhancement
- MRS
  - ↓ N-acetyl-aspartate (NAA) and choline; ↑ myo-inositol, ↑ glutamine/glutamate
  - MRS findings may precede structural abnormalities

### Nuclear Medicine Findings

- Tc-99m HMPAO nuclear scintigraphy: Early ↓ perfusion even if normal MR
- PET and SPECT
  - Decreased cerebral perfusion/metabolism
  - Crossed cerebellar diaschisis
  - Transient hypermetabolism may be related to recent seizures (rare)
    - 11C methionine shows increased multifocal uptake

### Imaging Recommendations

- Best imaging tool: MR PLUS appropriate EEG findings
- Protocol advice: MR with contrast, PET

## DIFFERENTIAL DIAGNOSIS

### Sturge-Weber Syndrome

- Progressive hemispheric atrophy
- Cortical Ca++
- Port wine facial nevus and enhancement of pial angioma

### Mitochondrial Encephalopathy, Lactic Acidosis, and Stroke-like Episodes (MELAS)

- Acute: May cause cortical hyperintensity (parieto-occipital most common)
- Chronic: Cortical atrophy, lacunes (basal ganglia, thalami)

### Other Causes of Dyke-Davidoff-Masson Syndrome

- Unilateral brain atrophy
- Compensatory calvarial thickening
- Elevation of the petrous ridge and hyperaeration of the paranasal sinuses
- Congenital and acquired causes; other than Rasmussen, acquired causes include trauma, infection, ischemia and hemorrhage

## PATHOLOGY

### General Features

- General path comments: Diffuse hemispheric atrophy
- Genetics: Possibly viral trigger of genetic predisposition to immunodysfunction
- Etiology
  - Three theories
  - 1. Autoimmune theory
    - Glutamate is excitatory neurotransmitter
    - Glutamate antibodies cross damaged blood-brain barrier
    - Antibodies bind and activate glutamate receptors GluR3
    - Nerve cells stimulated and seizures induced
  - 2. Immune mediated triggered by viral infection
  - 3. Viral infection
- Epidemiology
  - 50% preceded by inflammatory episode
    - Tonsillitis, upper respiratory infection, otitis media
  - Extremely rare

# RASMUSSEN ENCEPHALITIS

## Gross Pathologic & Surgical Features
- Hemispheric cortical atrophy

## Microscopic Features
- Robitaille classification
  - Group 1 (pathologically active): Ongoing inflammatory process
    - Microglial nodules, ± neuronophagia, perivascular lymphocytes (T-cells)
  - Group 2 (active and remote disease): Acute on chronic
    - Above plus at least one gyral segment of complete necrosis and cavitation including full-thickness cortex
  - Group 3 (less active "remote" disease)
    - Neuronal loss/gliosis and fewer microglial nodules
  - Group 4 (burnt out)
    - Nonspecific scarring with little active inflammation

## Staging, Grading or Classification Criteria
- Classification and staging: MR (T2WI)
  - Stage 1: Swelling/hyperintense signal
  - Stage 2: Normal volume/hyperintense signal
  - Stage 3: Atrophy/hyperintense signal
  - Stage 4: Progressive atrophy and normal signal

# CLINICAL ISSUES

## Presentation
- Most common signs/symptoms
  - Three phases
  - 1. Prodrome (first ~ 7 months or more): Low seizure frequency, mild hemiparesis
  - 2. Second phase (median duration 8 months): Acute increase in seizures, 50% with epilepsia partialis continua and progressive hemiplegia, atrophy develops
  - 3. Third phase: Permanent, stable hemiparesis
  - Cognitive decline common
- Other signs/symptoms: Other symptoms: Homonomous hemianopsia, sensory deficits, dysarthria, dysphasia
- Clinical Profile
  - 20% present in status epilepticus
  - EEG: Early: Slow focal activity; late: Epilepsia partialis continua
  - CSF: ± Oligoclonal bands
  - Other: ± GluR3 antibodies (50%), but not specific

## Demographics
- Age: Usually begins in childhood between 18 months and 14 years (peak 6-8)
- Gender: M = F
- Ethnicity: No predilection

## Natural History & Prognosis
- Hemiplegia and cognitive deterioration in most cases
- Older age at onset have longer prodromal stage and protracted course
- Prognosis is poor
- Hemiplegia is inevitable with or without treatment

- Three patterns of MR evolution
  - 1. Normal MR to increasing T2 signal and progressive cortical atrophy over time
  - 2. Initial focal increased T2 signal followed by decreased in extent and degree of T2 abnormality
  - 3. Initial increased T2 signal with no change over time

## Treatment
- Refractory to antiepileptic medications
- ± Transient improvement with plasma exchange, ganciclovir, steroids, immunoadsorption
- Surgical options
  - Hemispherectomy
  - Functional hemispherectomy/central disconnection

# DIAGNOSTIC CHECKLIST

## Consider
- Rasmussen if previously normal child with increasing frequency of partial seizures and post ictal defects

## Image Interpretation Pearls
- In patient with progressive intractable epilepsy with normal MR or progressive atrophy of one hemisphere and high T2 signal consider Rasmussen encephalitis

# SELECTED REFERENCES

1. Bien CG et al: Pathogenesis, diagnosis and treatment of Rasmussen encephalitis: a European consensus statement. Brain. 128(Pt 3):454-71, 2005
2. Deb P et al: Neuropathological spectrum of Rasmussen encephalitis. Neurol India. 53(2):156-60; discussion 160-1, 2005
3. Takahashi Y et al: Autoantibodies and cell-mediated autoimmunity to NMDA-type GluRepsilon2 in patients with Rasmussen's encephalitis and chronic progressive epilepsia partialis continua. Epilepsia. 46 Suppl 5:152-8, 2005
4. Tubbs RS et al: Long-term follow-up in children with functional hemispherectomy for Rasmussen's encephalitis. Childs Nerv Syst. 21(6):461-5, 2005
5. Cook SW et al: Cerebral hemispherectomy in pediatric patients with epilepsy: comparison of three techniques by pathological substrate in 115 patients. J Neurosurg. 100(2 Suppl Pediatrics):125-41, 2004
6. Pardo CA et al: The pathology of Rasmussen syndrome: stages of cortical involvement and neuropathological studies in 45 hemispherectomies. Epilepsia. 45(5):516-26, 2004
7. Granata T et al: Experience with immunomodulatory treatments in Rasmussen's encephalitis. Neurology. 61(12):1807-10, 2003
8. Maeda Y et al: Rasmussen syndrome: multifocal spread of inflammation suggested from MRI and PET findings. Epilepsia. 44(8):1118-21, 2003
9. Bien CG et al: Diagnosis and staging of Rasmussen's encephalitis by serial MRI and histopathology. Neurology. 58(2):250-7, 2002
10. Kim SJ et al: A longitudinal MRI study in children with Rasmussen syndrome. Pediatr Neurol. 27(4):282-8, 2002
11. Fiorella DJ et al: (18)F-fluorodeoxyglucose positron emission tomography and MR imaging findings in Rasmussen encephalitis. AJNR Am J Neuroradiol. 22(7):1291-9, 2001

## IMAGE GALLERY

### Variant

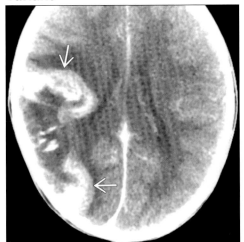
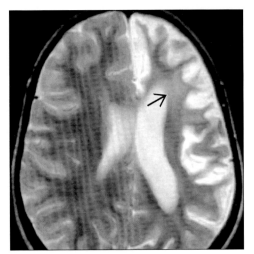

*(Left)* Axial CECT shows an unusual variant of stage 1 Rasmussen encephalitis. Note the presence of marked gyral enhancement ➡ in the right frontal and parietal cortex. *(Right)* Axial T2WI MR shows striking enlargement of sulci in left frontal lobe and ipsilateral lateral ventricle with increased signal ➡ in the underlying white matter (likely gliosis). Stage 3.

### Typical

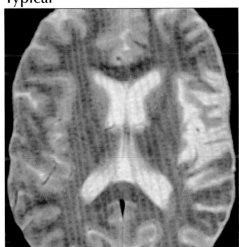
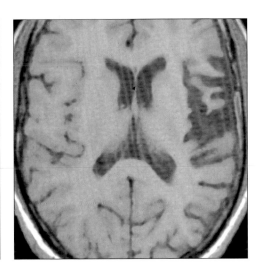

*(Left)* Axial T2WI MR shows focal atrophy involving the left temporal lobe. Note the enlargement of the sylvian fissure with prominent perisylvian sulci. Chronic focal Rasmussen encephalitis. *(Right)* Axial T1WI MR (same patient as previous image) shows the focal atrophy involving the left frontal and temporal lobes and enlargement of the ipsilateral lateral ventricle.

### Typical

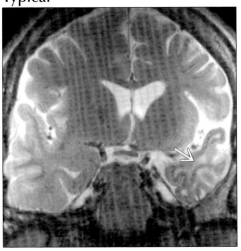
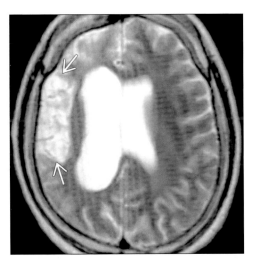

*(Left)* Coronal T2WI MR (same patient as previous Image) shows enlarged left hemispheric sulci and increased signal in the anterior temporal lobe white matter ➡ consistent with astrogliosis. *(Right)* Axial T2WI MR shows ➡ a focal area of encephalomalacia involving the right hemisphere and marked enlargement of the ipsilateral lateral ventricle in stage 4 Rasmussen encephalitis.

# SUBACUTE SCLEROSING PANENCEPHALITIS

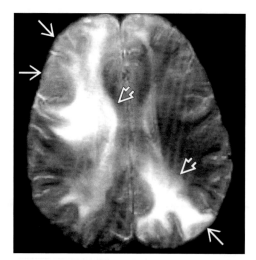

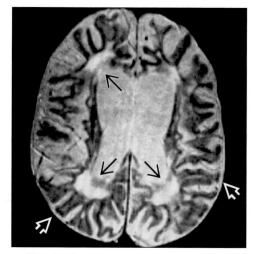

*Axial PD/Intermediate MR shows large bilateral asymmetrical areas of inhomogeneous high signal involving white matter ⇒ as well as cortex ⇒. Brain biopsy disclosed diagnosis of SSPE.*

*Axial T2WI MR shows major brain atrophy in late stage of SSPE. White matter has vanished and is replaced with gliosis ⇒. Ulegyric cortical ribbon seems relatively better preserved ⇒.*

## TERMINOLOGY

### Abbreviations and Synonyms
- Subacute sclerosing panencephalitis (SSPE), Dawson encephalitis

### Definitions
- Rare, progressive measles virus-mediated encephalitis

## IMAGING FINDINGS

### General Features
- Best diagnostic clue: Nonspecific leukoencephalopathy

### CT Findings
- NECT: Normal or nonspecific

### MR Findings
- T1WI: Normal or atrophy
- T2WI
  - Often normal when scanned early
  - Develops into mild asymmetric leukoencephalopathy; extends to cortex, basal ganglia, thalami

- Late: Diffuse atrophy & high signal of WM
- DWI: Gliosis: ↑ Diffusivity, ↑ ADC, ↓ FA
- MRS: Active inflammation: ↓ NAA/Cr, ↑ Cho/Cr, ↑ Ins/Cr, ↑ Lac-Lip

### Imaging Recommendations
- Best imaging tool: MR
- Protocol advice: Add MRS

## DIFFERENTIAL DIAGNOSIS

### Post-Infectious Progressive Encephalitides
- Subacute measles encephalitis & measles inclusion body encephalitis
- Progressive rubella panencephalitis: SSPE-like, but post congenital rubella infection
- Progressive multifocal leukoencephalopathy (PML): Subcortical demyelination in immunodeficient patients (cancer, HIV)
- Human immunodeficiency virus (HIV): Ill-defined areas of ↑ T2 signal in WM, no mass effect

### Other Progressive Encephalopathies
- Metabolic diseases: Typically symmetric involvement

## DDx: Other Non-Specific Leukoencephalopathies

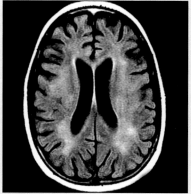

*Human Immunodeficiency Virus*

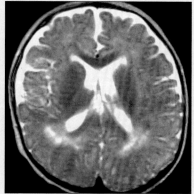

*Fetal Rubella*

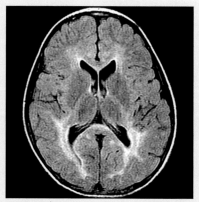

*Unknown Leukodystophy*

# SUBACUTE SCLEROSING PANENCEPHALITIS

## Key Facts

### Imaging Findings
- Best diagnostic clue: Nonspecific leukoencephalopathy
- MRS: Active inflammation: ↓ NAA/Cr, ↑ Cho/Cr, ↑ Ins/Cr, ↑ Lac-Lip
- Best imaging tool: MR
- Protocol advice: Add MRS

### Top Differential Diagnoses
- Post-Infectious Progressive Encephalitides

- Other Progressive Encephalopathies

### Clinical Issues
- Clinical Profile: Child who had measles in infancy

### Diagnostic Checklist
- Consider SSPE in non-specific leukoencephalopathy with history previous infantile measles
- MR findings correlate poorly with clinical stages

## PATHOLOGY

### General Features
- General path comments: Measles virus dormant in brain induces inflammation & apoptosis
- Etiology: Mutated measles virus persisting in brain tissue escapes immune defenses
- Epidemiology: Countries with no measles vaccination

### Gross Pathologic & Surgical Features
- Early inflammation; late atrophy, demyelination & sclerosis

### Microscopic Features
- Chronic encephalitis: Infiltration by lymphocytes and macrophages
  - Microglial hyperplasia, astrocytosis, neuronal loss
- Inclusions: Sharply defined intranuclear eosinophilic bodies
- Alzheimer-type neurofibrillary tangles

## CLINICAL ISSUES

### Presentation
- Most common signs/symptoms: Behavior changes → myoclonus, spasticity, ataxia & loss of language, seizures → dementia → progressive coma
- Clinical Profile: Child who had measles in infancy

### Demographics
- Age: Late childhood, early adolescence; rare in adults

- Gender: M:F = 2:1

### Natural History & Prognosis
- Invariably fatal

### Treatment
- Early treatment may delay clinical course
  - Intraventricular interferon-alpha and ribavirin

## DIAGNOSTIC CHECKLIST

### Consider
- Consider SSPE in non-specific leukoencephalopathy with history previous infantile measles

### Image Interpretation Pearls
- MR findings correlate poorly with clinical stages

## SELECTED REFERENCES

1. Teksam M et al: Proton MR spectroscopy in the diagnosis of early-stage subacute sclerosing panencephalitis. Diagn Interv Radiol. 12(2):61-3, 2006
2. Trivedi R et al: Assessment of white matter damage in subacute sclerosing panencephalitis using quantitative diffusion tensor MR imaging. AJNR Am J Neuroradiol. 27(8):1712-6, 2006
3. Schneider-Schaulies J et al: Measles infection of the central nervous system. J Neurovirol. 9(2):247-52, 2003
4. Brismar J et al: Subacute sclerosing panencephalitis: evaluation with CT and MR. AJNR Am J Neuroradiol. 17(4):761-72, 1996

## IMAGE GALLERY

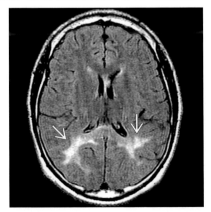 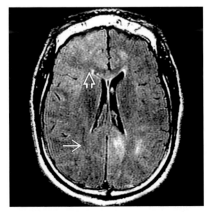 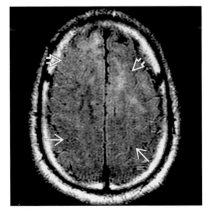

*(Left)* Axial FLAIR MR shows non-specific periventricular changes ➡ in a rapidly deteriorating child. History of measles at 1 year; diagnosis of early stage SSPE confirmed biologically. *(Center)* Axial FLAIR MR in same child as previous image, one year later, with new deterioration shows better-looking periventricular white matter ➡ but new changes in right frontal white matter ➡. *(Right)* Axial FLAIR MR in same patient as previous image shows bilateral asymmetrical white matter changes in frontal lobes ➡ and loss of gray/white contrast in parietal lobes ➡.

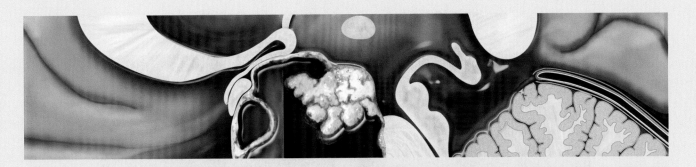

# SECTION 2: Sella/Suprasellar

# PITUITARY DEVELOPMENT

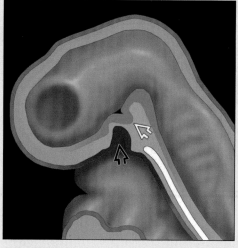

*Lateral graphic shows Rathke pouch ⬇, an infolding of pharyngeal ectoderm (red), invaginating toward the ventral diencephalon (blue), and inducing downward folding of incipient neurohypophysis ⬇.*

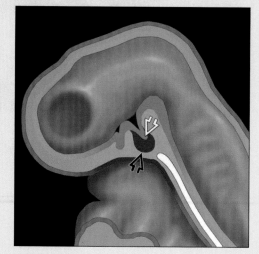

*Lateral graphic shows Rathke cleft ⬇ surrounding neurohypophysis, influenced to become anterior pituitary, pars intermedia, and pars tuberalis. Diencephalic extension ⬇ becomes neurohypophysis.*

## IMAGING ANATOMY

### General Anatomic Considerations
- Pituitary gland lies in sella turcica at base of skull
- Connects via infundibulum (stalk) to hypothalamus at median eminence

### Critical Anatomic Structures
- Pituitary gland, adenohypophysis (AH), anterior lobe
  - Anatomy
    - 80% of pituitary gland (Pit)
    - Includes pars anterior (pars distalis or glandularis), pars intermedia, pars tuberalis
  - Cell types
    - Corticotropes produce proopiomelanocortin (POMC), cleave it into adrenocorticotropic hormone (ACTH) ⇒ glucocorticoid synthesis in adrenal gland
    - Melanotropes produce POMC, cleave it into melanocyte-stimulating hormone-α ⇒ pigment formation, feeding regulation
    - Somatotropes produce growth hormone ⇒ cell proliferation
    - Lactotropes make prolactin ⇒ milk production, uterine contractions
    - Gonadotropes synthesize LH and FSH ⇒ gonad growth and development
- Pituitary gland, pars intermedia (PI)
  - Small (< 5% of Pit), between adeno-, neurohypophysis
  - Origin = Rathke cleft (pharyngeal ectoderm)
  - Function: Axons from hypothalamus pass through stalk, terminate, carry releasing hormones to AH
- Pituitary gland, neurohypophysis (NH), posterior lobe
  - Anatomy
    - Posteromedial 20% of Pit
    - Includes pars posterior (pars nervosa, posterior or neural lobe), infundibulum (stalk) and median eminence of tuber cinereum
    - Contains pituicytes, hypothalamohypophyseal tract
  - Origin = embryonic forebrain (diencephalon)
  - Function: Vasopressin, oxytocin transported from hypothalamus along hypothalamohypophyseal tract in stalk, stored in NH

### Anatomic Relationships
- Vessels, cavernous sinus (CS)
  - Internal carotid artery (ICA), branches
    - Meningohypophyseal trunk (MHT) supplies CS, tentorium, pituitary
    - Inferolateral trunk (ILT) supplies tentorium, CNs 3/4/6, Gasserian ganglion, CN V3; extensive anastomoses with ECA
    - Inferior hypophyseal arteries supply NH
- Vessels, suprasellar cistern
  - Supraclinoid ICA
    - Superior hypophyseal arteries supply median eminence, stalk, NH
  - Circle of Willis (COW); surrounds suprasellar cistern
- Nerves, cavernous sinus
  - Oculomotor nerve (CN 3) = superior lateral dural wall
  - Trochlear nerve (CN 4) = dural wall below CN 3
  - Abducens nerve (CN 6) = inside CS, adjacent to ICA
  - Trigeminal nerve (CN 5)
    - CN V1 = lateral dural wall above CN V2, exits superior orbital fissure as ophthalmic nerve
    - CN V2 = lateral dural wall below CN 4, exits through foramen rotundum as maxillary nerve
  - Sympathetic plexus (surrounds cavernous ICA)
- Cerebrospinal fluid (CSF) spaces, suprasellar cistern: Contiguous with interpeduncular, ambient cisterns, medial sylvian fissure
- CSF spaces, 3rd ventricle: Optic recess (rounded, in front of infundibulum)
- Bone, basisphenoid
  - Sphenoid sinus variably aerated, septated
  - Sphenooccipital synchondrosis
  - Craniopharyngeal canal (midline, almost vertical conduit in basisphenoid contains dura, some vessels; 10% persist into childhood)
- Mammillary bodies
- Hypothalamus
  - Tuber cinereum (from stalk to mamillary bodies)

# PITUITARY DEVELOPMENT

## Differential Diagnosis

### Pseudolesions

- Physiologic hypertrophy (normal in adolescence, pregnancy)
- End-organ failure (e.g., hypothyroidism)
- Pit enlargement secondary to venous congestion (intracranial hypotension, dAVF)

### Congenital

- Arachnoid cyst (intra- or suprasellar)
- Epidermoid/dermoid tumor
- Rathke cleft cyst, pars intermedia cyst
- Ectopic NH
- Duplicated stalk/gland
- Tuber cinereum (hypothalamic) hamartoma
- Lipoma (tuber cinereum)
- Cephalocele

### Infectious/Inflammatory

- Meningitis (bacterial, fungal, TB)
- Hypophysitis (lymphocytic)
- Histiocytosis, sarcoidosis
- Pseudotumor

### Vascular

- Aneurysm
- Hemochromatosis (causes very hypointense pituitary)

### Neoplasm

- Craniopharyngioma
- Astrocytoma
- Germinoma
- Adenoma (macro-, microadenoma)
- Lymphoma, leukemia

- ○ Median eminence, where stalk originates
- ○ Supraoptic, paraventricular nuclei (secrete vasopressin, oxytocin)
- ○ Stalk, NH are part of hypothalamus
- Meninges
  - ○ Dura (lines sellar floor, forms diaphragma sellae)
  - ○ Arachnoid (may protrude inferiorly through diaphragma sellae)

## ANATOMY-BASED IMAGING ISSUES

### Key Concepts or Questions

- MR general modality of choice in imaging pituitary, hypothalamic disorders
- Coronal plane minimizes volume averaging
  - ○ Begin with 2 mm, small FOV precontrast T1-, T2WIs
  - ○ From lamina terminalis through mamillary bodies
- Sagittal plane also necessary
  - ○ ≤ 3 mm images, small FOV, pre- and post-contrast T1WIs
  - ○ Completely through both cavernous sinuses
  - ○ FOV to include corpus callosum and nasopharynx
- 20-30% of microadenomas seen only with "dynamic" MR C+
  - ○ Rapid bolus contrast infusion
  - ○ Scans obtained q 10-12 seconds, sorted by slice

### Imaging Pitfalls

- Normal variants
  - ○ Physiologic hypertrophy of adenohypophysis (puberty, pregnancy)
    - ■ Decrease of 10% in size after delivery of baby
  - ○ "Empty sella"
    - ■ Protrusion of arachnoid, CSF into sella
    - ■ Normal pituitary flattened against sellar floor
    - ■ Rarely symptomatic (may be associated with pseudotumor cerebri)
- Variation during development
  - ○ AH is T1 hyperintense and large in neonate
  - ○ Decreases in size, signal intensity during 6 weeks post birth

- ○ By 2 months has normal childhood appearance ⇒ small, hypointense
- ○ At puberty, gland increases markedly in size
- Anatomic pitfalls
  - ○ 20% of imaged pituitary glands in children have "filling defects" (probably cysts, many transient)

### Normal Measurements

- Size/height/configuration of normal Pit varies with gender, age
  - ○ Children = 6 mm
  - ○ Males, post-menopausal females = 8 mm
  - ○ Adolescent females = 10 mm (can bulge upwards)
  - ○ Pregnant, lactating females = 12 mm

## EMBRYOLOGY

### Embryologic Events

- Pituitary gland- an amalgam of two tissues
  - ○ Finger of ectoderm (midline of anterior neural ridge, to become Rathke pouch) grows upward from the roof of the pharynx, invaginates into ventral diencephalon, will develop into the AH (anterior pituitary)
    - ■ 1: Extrinsic signals cause cell proliferation and determination of tissue as pituitary
    - ■ 2: Intrinsic signaling gradients within Rathke pouch activate core group of transcription factors
    - ■ 3: Cells commit to particular lineages through combinatorial associations of transcription factors
  - ○ Second finger of ectodermal tissue evaginates ventrally from the embryonic diencephalon to become the NH (posterior pituitary)
  - ○ Two tissues grow into one another, their growth factors influence cell differentiation
    - ■ Structures become tightly apposed, but their structures remain distinct

### Practical Implications

- Developmental anomalies of hypothalamus usually associated with pituitary anomalies

# PITUITARY DEVELOPMENT

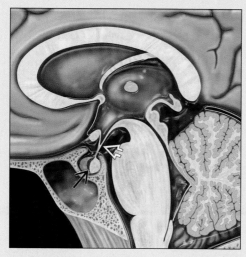

*Sagittal graphic shows normal mature sella, pituitary gland. Anterior and posterior glands contribute to infundibulum, which arises from median eminence ➡. Pars intermedia ➡ lies between AH and PH.*

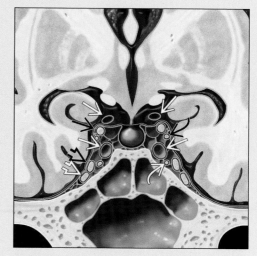

*Coronal graphic shows coronal relationships of pituitary, cavernous sinuses (CN3 ➡, 4 ➡, V1 ➡, V2 ➡ in wall of sinus and 6 ➡ inside sinus), stalk, and carotid arteries ➡.*

## CLINICAL IMPLICATIONS

### Clinical Importance
- Pituitary dwarfism
  - Usually developmental
  - Primary AH dysfunction (hypoplasia)
  - Ectopic NH ("bright spot" in hypothalamus)
  - Discontinuous or absent stalk
- Precocious puberty
  - Secondary sexual development > 2.5 SD below mean
  - Central = premature activation of hypothalamic-pituitary-gonadal axis
    - Neoplasms of hypothalamus/optic chiasm
    - Tuber cinereum abnormalities (hamartoma)
  - Peripheral = gonadotropin-independent
- Central diabetes insipidus
  - Hypothalamic-neurohypophyseal axis dysfunction
    - Trauma (post-op, transection)
    - Infection/inflammation (meningitis, hypophysitis, granulomatous disease)
    - Neoplasm (germinoma, histiocytosis, lymphoma)
- Hypersecretion syndromes: Named for hormones (e.g., prolactin with prolactinoma)

- Craniopharyngioma (enhancing wall)
- Dilated 3rd V (obstructive hydrocephalus)
- Pituitary abscess (rare)

### Infundibular Mass
- Ectopic posterior pituitary (pituitary dwarf)
- Histiocytosis
- Germinoma
- Leukemia
- Neurohypophysitis

### Suprasellar "Bright Spot" (on T1WI)
- Ectopic NH
- Lipoma
- Dermoid

### Cavernous Sinus Syndrome
- Infection (CS thrombophlebitis, fungal infection)
- Inflammation (Tolosa-Hunt, inflammatory pseudotumor)
- Vascular (ICA aneurysm, C-C fistula)
- Neoplasm (meningioma, schwannoma, metastasis, neurofibroma, lymphoma, hemangioma)
- Abscess (rare)

## CUSTOM DIFFERENTIAL DIAGNOSIS

### Intrasellar Mass
- Hyperplasia: Physiological in adolescence
- Microadenoma (rare in children)
- Nonneoplastic cyst (Rathke, occasionally colloid)
- Craniopharyngioma (truly intrasellar rare)

### Suprasellar Mass
- Craniopharyngioma (adamantinomatous type)
- Astrocytoma (optic chiasm, hypothalamus)
- Germinoma (primary or spread from pineal)
- Arachnoid cyst
- Tuber cinereum hamartoma

### Cystic-Appearing Intra- or Suprasellar Mass
- Arachnoid cyst
- Epidermoid

## RELATED REFERENCES

1. Argyroupoulou MI et al: MRI of the hypothalamic-pituitary axis in children. Pediatr Radiol. 35(4):1045-55, 2005
2. Miki Y et al: The pituitary gland: changes on MR images during the 1st year after delivery. Radiology. 235(6):999-1004, 2005
3. Iaconetta G et al: The sphenopetroclival venous gulf: a microanatomical study. J Neurosurg. 99(2):366-75, 2003
4. Lee JH et al: Cavernous sinus syndrome: clinical features and differential diagnosis with MR imaging. AJR Am J Roentgenol. 181(2):583-90, 2003
5. Robinson DH et al: Embolization of meningohypophyseal and inferolateral branches of the cavernous internal carotid artery. AJNR Am J Neuroradiol. 20(6):1061-7, 1999
6. Cox TD et al: Normal pituitary gland: changes in shape, size and signal intensity during the 1st year of life at MR imaging. Radiology. 179:721-4, 1991
7. Renn WH et al: Microsurgical anatomy of the sellar region. J Neurosurg. 43(3):288-98, 1975

## IMAGE GALLERY

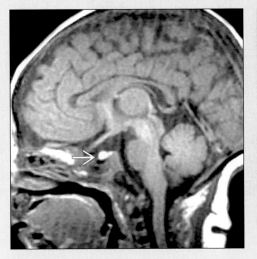

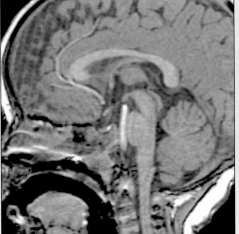

*(Left)* Sagittal T1WI MR shows normal neonatal pituitary gland with large adenohypophysis ➔ that is bright on T1WI. *(Right)* Sagittal T1WI MR shows normal pituitary gland in a child. Adenohypophysis is isointense to gray matter, relatively small. Neurohypophysis shows T1 hyperintensity. Stalk is well seen.

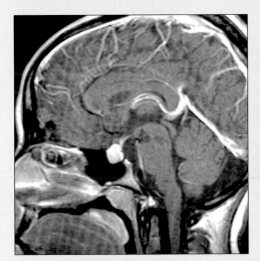

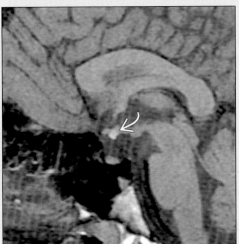

*(Left)* Sagittal T1 C+ MR shows adolescent gland with large adenohypophysis with convex superior margin. The normal gland is homogeneous with homogeneous enhancement. *(Right)* Sagittal T1WI MR shows ectopic posterior pituitary gland. The hyperintense neurohypophysis ➔ sits at the median eminence of the hypothalamus, does not suppress. The adenohypophysis is small.

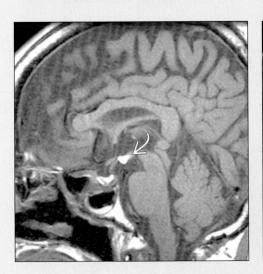

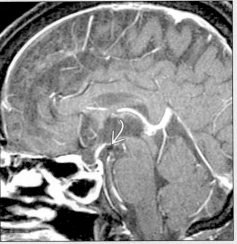

*(Left)* Sagittal T1WI MR shows hypothalamic lipoma ➔. Note that the lipoma is situated behind the median eminence within the tuber cinereum. Pituitary is normal in size. *(Right)* Sagittal T1 C+ FS MR shows that the lipoma ➔ (same patient as previous image) becomes hypointense when the fat suppression pulse is applied. Ectopic neurohypophysis will not suppress.

# PITUITARY ANOMALIES

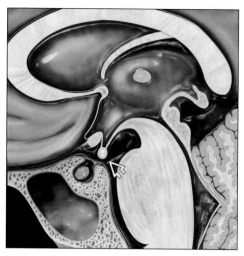

*Sagittal graphic shows ectopia of the posterior pituitary gland ➡ at the distal end of a truncated pituitary stalk. The sella turcica and adenohypophysis are small.*

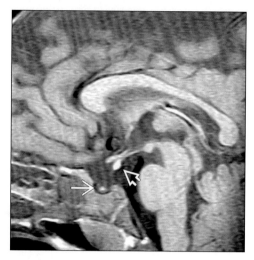

*Sagittal T1WI MR shows ectopic posterior pituitary gland ➡ located within a truncated infundibulum, similar to graphic. The adenohypophysis ➡ is small.*

## TERMINOLOGY

### Abbreviations and Synonyms
- Posterior pituitary ectopia (PPE)
- Duplicated pituitary gland/stalk (DP)

### Definitions
- Congenital anomalies of pituitary stalk may indicate potential hypothalamic/pituitary axis malfunction

## IMAGING FINDINGS

### General Features
- Best diagnostic clue
  - PPE: Absent (or tiny) pituitary stalk; ectopic posterior pituitary gland (EPPG) on mid-sagittal view
  - DP: 2 pituitary stalks on coronal view, tubo-mamillary fusion on mid-sagittal view
- Location
  - PPE: EPPG located along median eminence of tuber cinereum or truncated stalk
  - DP: Paired **lateral** stalks, glands, bony fossae
- Size

- PPE: Anterior pituitary (adenohypophysis) small
- DP: Each pituitary gland normal in size
- Morphology
  - PPE: Adenohypophysis **and** bony sella small
  - DP: Each pituitary gland **and** bony sella normal in morphology, just laterally located

### CT Findings
- CTA
  - PPE: Medial deviation of juxtasellar/supraclinoid carotid arteries, "kissing carotids"
  - DP: Duplicated basilar artery, ± widely separated juxtasellar/supraclinoid carotid arteries
- NECT
  - PPE: Narrow pituitary fossa & skull base structures, clivus, ± persistent sphenopharyngeal foramen
  - DP: Two widely separated pituitary fossae, ± midline basisphenoid cleft or frontonasal dysplasia

### MR Findings
- T1WI
  - PPE: Absent, truncated or thread-like pituitary stalk (axial and coronal); small adenohypophysis
    - EPPG located along truncated stalk or median eminence of tuber cinereum

## DDx: Tuber Cinereum Lesions

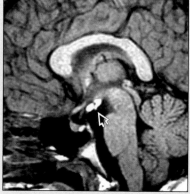

*TC Lipoma*

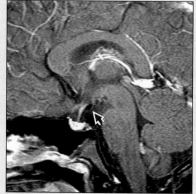

*TC Lipoma Fat-Sat*

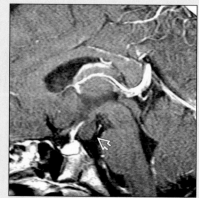

*TC Hamartoma*

# PITUITARY ANOMALIES

## Key Facts

### Terminology
- Posterior pituitary ectopia (PPE)
- Duplicated pituitary gland/stalk (DP)
- Congenital anomalies of pituitary stalk may indicate potential hypothalamic/pituitary axis malfunction

### Imaging Findings
- PPE: Absent (or tiny) pituitary stalk; ectopic posterior pituitary gland (EPPG) on mid-sagittal view
- DP: 2 pituitary stalks on coronal view, tubo-mamillary fusion on mid-sagittal view
- DP: Each pituitary gland normal in size
- PPE: Medial deviation of juxtasellar/supraclinoid carotid arteries, "kissing carotids"
- DP: Duplicated basilar artery, ± widely separated juxtasellar/supraclinoid carotid arteries

### Pathology
- PPE: Genetic mutation leads to defective neuronal migration during embryogenesis
- Midline CNS anomalies common in both
- DP: Fused tuber cinereum, mamillary bodies and incompletely migrated hypothalamic nuclear cells

### Clinical Issues
- PPE: Short stature (growth hormone deficiency), ± multiple endocrine deficiencies
- DP: ± Facial midline anomalies; oral mass
- Outcome unrelated to pituitary function

### Diagnostic Checklist
- PPE: Assess optic and olfactory nerves, frontal cortex
- DP: Oral tumors compromise airway

---

- EPPG usually ↑ on T1WI (phospholipids/secretory granules)
- Bright spot may "dim over time" as patient outgrows available hormone levels
- Chiari 1 (20%), ± olfactory hypoplasia, frontal lobe dysgenesis/migration anomalies
- ± Absent septum pellucidum, ocular dysgenesis or hypoplastic optic nerves/chiasm
- DP: Mass-like thickening tuber cinereum on sagittal view signals duplicated pituitary axis
  - Mamillary bodies fused with tuber cinereum into thickened 3rd ventricle (3rd V) floor
  - Two normal pituitary glands/stalks
  - Brain anomalies: Callosal dysgenesis, duplicated anterior 3rd V; cleft brainstem; Dandy-Walker
  - Cranial nerve anomalies: Olfactory nerve and optic nerve hypoplasia
  - Oral tumors: Epignathus (giant teratoma) or dermoid mixed signal; lipoma ↑ T1WI
- T2WI
  - PPE: Variable signal posterior pituitary bright spot
  - DP: Normal signal of glands, stalk, fusion mass
- T1 C+
  - BOTH: Stalks & remnants enhance (absent blood-brain barrier)
  - PPE: Bright spot absent if multiple endocrine anomalies/diabetes insipidus (if so, enhance to find neurohypophysis)
- MRA
  - PPE: Supraclinoid carotid arteries medially deviated, "kiss" in midline; rare absent carotid artery/canal
  - DP: Partial split (common) or total duplication (rare) of basilar artery (BA); widely separated juxtasellar carotid arteries
- MRV: Defines torcular and straight sinus anomalies if midline posterior fossa anomaly present

### Radiographic Findings
- Radiography
  - PPE: Small sella turcica on lateral radiography
  - DP: Astute may find two fossae on AP view; craniofacial/craniocervical anomalies common

### Angiographic Findings
- Conventional
  - PPE: Variable deviation "kissing carotids" 37%
  - DP: Split/duplicated BA, ± lateral deviation carotids

### Imaging Recommendations
- Best imaging tool: MR, multiplanar T1WI
- Protocol advice
  - Both: Sagittal and coronal T1WI of hypothalamic/pituitary axis
  - PPE: Assess olfactory nerves, anterior frontal lobes with coronal FSE T2WI
  - DP: 3D CT of skull base & face in selected patients

## DIFFERENTIAL DIAGNOSIS

### PPE: Central DI; Stalk Transection; Lipoma
- Central diabetes insipidus (absent posterior pituitary hyperintensity, but normal location stalk & gland)
- Surgical or traumatic stalk transection allows build-up of neurosecretory granules along stump
- Bright spot doesn't "fat-sat"; lipoma does

### DP: Dilated Infundibular Recess of 3rd Ventricle ("Pseudoduplication"); Hamartoma Tuber Cinereum
- Dilated infundibular recess simulates duplicated stalk, but only one gland and one pituitary fossa
- Hamartoma tuber cinereum (TC) has round mass of 3rd V floor, but one midline pituitary stalk/gland

## PATHOLOGY

### General Features
- General path comments
  - PPE: Disorder of midline prosencephalic development; multiple pituitary hormone deficiencies common
  - DP: Rarely symptomatic from pituitary causes
  - Embryology-anatomy: PPE

# PITUITARY ANOMALIES

- Adenohypophysis grows up from stomodeal ectoderm (Rathke pouch)
- Neurohypophysis grows down from diencephalic neuroectoderm, should remain attached by stalk
- Antidiuretic hormone & oxytocin transported to neurohypophysis via neurosecretory cells along infundibular stalk
- Hypothalamic releasing hormones reach adenohypophysis via infundibular portal system
- Anterior pituitary dysfunction in PPE likely related to absent infundibulum
  - Embryology-anatomy: DP
    - Theory: Duplicated prechordal plate and tip of rostral notochord ⇒ duplicated pituitary primordium
- Genetics
  - PPE: Mutations in genes encoding developmental transcription factors allow maldevelopment
    - HESX1 (homeobox gene), PIT1, PITX2, LHX3, LHX4, PROP1, SF1, and TPIT
  - DP: Gene mutation unknown
- Etiology
  - PPE: Genetic mutation leads to defective neuronal migration during embryogenesis
  - DP: Congenital anomaly, presumed genetic duplication of stomodeal origin structures
- Epidemiology
  - PPE: 1:4,000 to 1:20,000
  - DP: Extremely rare (reported in 20+ patients)
- Associated abnormalities
  - Midline CNS anomalies common in both
    - PPE: ± Lobar holoprosencephaly, septooptic dysplasia, Joubert syndrome, Kallman
    - PPE: ± Anomalies of structures formed at same time (pituitary, forebrain, eyes, olfactory bulbs)
    - DP: Callosal dysgenesis, Dandy-Walker continuum, frontonasal dysplasia
    - DP: Craniofacial clefting and duplication anomalies: Frontonasal dysplasia; clefts/duplication of skull base, face, jaw
  - DP: Midline tumors: Oral, nasopharyngeal, palate
    - Epignathus, teratomas, dermoids, lipomas
  - DP: Spinal anomalies: Segmentation/fusion anomalies, schisms, hydromyelia, enteric cysts
  - DP: Rib & cardiac anomalies; Pierre-Robin anomaly

## Gross Pathologic & Surgical Features

- PPE: Hypoplastic anterior lobe, truncation or aplasia of stalk; sella may be covered over with dura
- DP: Tubo-mamillary fusion; 2 normal glands/stalks

## Microscopic Features

- PPE: Ectopic pituitary cells in stalk or sphenoid bone
- DP: Normal, but duplicated, pituitary glands
- DP: Fused tuber cinereum, mamillary bodies and incompletely migrated hypothalamic nuclear cells

## CLINICAL ISSUES

## Presentation

- Most common signs/symptoms
  - PPE: Short stature

- DP: Often unsuspected finding on craniofacial imaging
- Clinical Profile
  - PPE: Short stature (growth hormone deficiency), ± multiple endocrine deficiencies
    - Peak growth hormone levels < 3 g/L more likely to have abnormal MR
    - ± Anosmia, poor vision, seizures (cortical malformations)
    - Neonatal hypoglycemia or jaundice, micropenis, single central incisor
  - DP: ± Facial midline anomalies; oral mass
    - Face: ± Hypertelorism or frontonasal dysplasia
    - Craniocervical segmentation and fusion anomalies
    - Airway or oral obstruction from pharyngeal tumor

## Demographics

- Age
  - PPE: Disorder becomes apparent in childhood with early growth failure
  - DP: Usually discovered in infant with complicated facial anomalies
- Gender
  - PPE: M > F
  - DP: M < F
- Ethnicity: None identified in either diagnosis

## Natural History & Prognosis

- PPE: Stable if no pituitary/hypothalamic crises; growth may be normal for a while
  - Severity and number of hormone deficiencies predicted by degree of hypoplasia of stalk and gland
- DP: Usually significant intracranial, upper airway or cranio-cervical malformations, some lethal
  - Outcome unrelated to pituitary function

## Treatment

- Assess/treat endocrine malfunction (especially PPE)

## DIAGNOSTIC CHECKLIST

## Consider

- PPE: Assess optic and olfactory nerves, frontal cortex
- DP: Oral tumors compromise airway

## Image Interpretation Pearls

- Both: Thin sagittal, coronal views required

## SELECTED REFERENCES

1. Slavotinek A et al: Craniofacial defects of blastogenesis: duplication of pituitary with cleft palate and orophgaryngeal tumors. Am J Med Genet A. 135(1):13-20, 2005
2. Shroff M et al: Basilar artery duplication associated with pituitary duplication: a new finding. AJNR Am J Neuroradiol. 24(5):956-61, 2003
3. Cushman LJ et al: Genetic defects in the development and function of the anterior pituitary gland. Ann Med. 34(3):179-91, 2002
4. Hamilton J et al: MR imaging in idiopathic growth hormone deficiency. AJNR Am J Neuroradiol. 19(9):1609-15, 1998

# PITUITARY ANOMALIES

## IMAGE GALLERY

### Typical

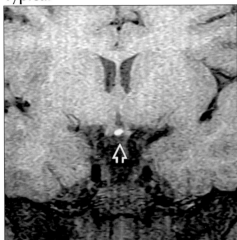 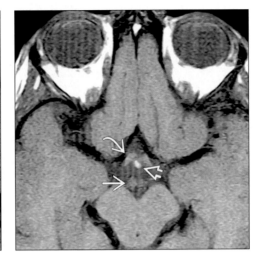

*(Left) Coronal T1WI FS MR confirms that the small increased signal mass ⊳ tucked between the post-chiasmatic optic nerves is not a lipoma, as it does not suppress. (Right) Axial T1WI MR in same patient as previous image better localizes the ectopic posterior pituitary gland ⊳ in the median eminence of the hypothalamus, between the mamillary bodies ➔ and the chiasm ➔.*

### Typical

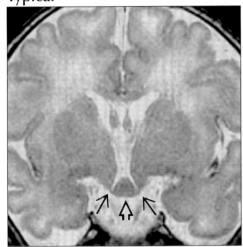 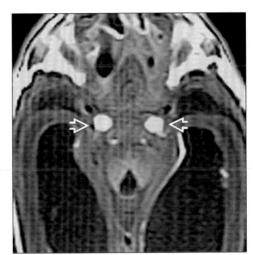

*(Left) Coronal T2WI MR shows duplication of the infundibular recess ➔ on either side of a thickened mass-like structure, which is comprised of fused mammillary bodies and tuber cinereum ⊳. (Right) Axial T1WI MR in same neonate as previous image shows pituitary gland ⊳ within each of the duplicated sella turcica. Entire pituitary gland is increased signal in newborns due to maternal stimulation.*

### Typical

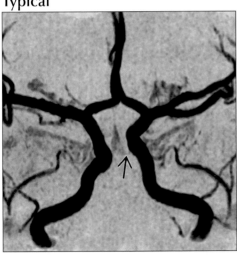 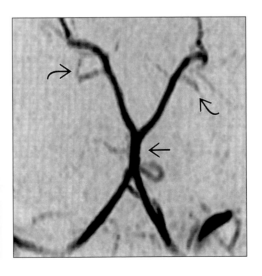

*(Left) Anteroposterior MRA shows medial deviation ➔ of the juxtasellar/supraclinoid internal carotid arteries in posterior pituitary ectopia. Medial deviation is associated with a narrow sella. (Right) Anteroposterior MRA shows a short basilar artery ➔ with partial duplication in association with pituitary duplication. A superior cerebellar artery ➔ arises from each basilar artery.*

# CRANIOPHARYNGIOMA

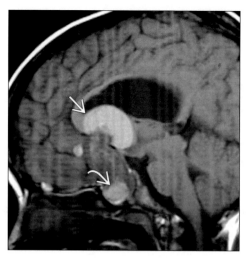

Sagittal T1WI MR shows hyperintense signal in superior ➡ and inferior ➡ cystic components of a craniopharyngioma that projects into the foramina of Monro and causes hydrocephalus.

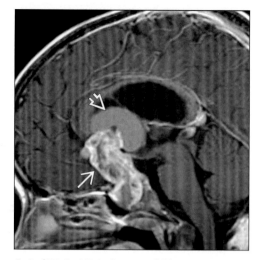

Sagittal T1 C+ MR in the same child as previous image shows heterogeneous enhancement of the stalk-like solid component ➡; as a result, the cyst contents now appear less hyperintense ➡.

## TERMINOLOGY

### Abbreviations and Synonyms
- Craniopharyngioma (CrP), craniopharyngeal duct tumor, Rathke pouch tumor, adamantinoma

### Definitions
- Histologically benign epithelial tumor arising from squamous rests along involuted hypophyseal-Rathke duct

## IMAGING FINDINGS

### General Features
- Best diagnostic clue: Cystic suprasellar mass with calcifications (Ca++) and enhancement of a mural nodule or cyst wall
- Location
  - Suprasellar ⇒ 75%
  - Mixed suprasellar + intrasellar ⇒ 21%
  - Intrasellar ⇒ 4%
  - Larger tumors can extend into multiple cranial fossae

- Term "monstrous craniopharyngioma" has been proposed for these
  - Rare ectopic locations
    - Third ventricle, nasopharynx, sphenoid sinus
  - Distinction of retro-chiasmatic vs. pre-chiasmatic key for surgical approach
- Size
  - Often large at presentation (> 5 cm)
    - Cyst is typically largest component
- Morphology: Complex cystic mass, often lobulated

### CT Findings
- 90% percent rule
  - 90% are cystic
  - 90% have calcifications
  - 90% enhance (wall and solid portions)
- May present with obstructive hydrocephalus from compression on 3rd ventricle and foramen of Monro
- CT can sometimes detect recurrence before MR because of sensitivity for Ca++

### MR Findings
- T1WI
  - Cyst contents hyperintense to cerebrospinal fluid (CSF)

## DDx: Sellar and Suprasellar Masses

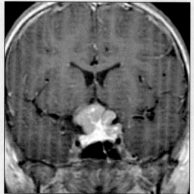

Germinoma

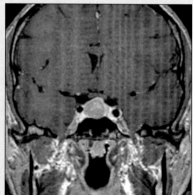

Macroadenoma

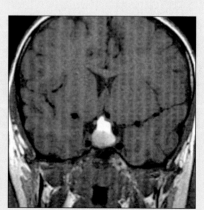

Rathke Cleft Cyst

## Key Facts

### Terminology
- Histologically benign epithelial tumor arising from squamous rests along involuted hypophyseal-Rathke duct

### Imaging Findings
- Best diagnostic clue: Cystic suprasellar mass with calcifications (Ca++) and enhancement of a mural nodule or cyst wall
- 90% are cystic
- 90% have calcifications
- 90% enhance (wall and solid portions)
- Most often vessels are displaced by cysts
- Circle of Willis vessels may be encased by solid components
- Rarely narrowed
- Important to identify displacement of chiasm

### Top Differential Diagnoses
- Rathke Cleft Cyst (RCC)
- Germinoma, Brain
- Arachnoid Cyst

### Pathology
- Adamantinomatous subtype
- Classic calcified cyst with mural nodule
- Squamous-papillary subtype
- Most common non-glial pediatric intracranial tumor
- 6-9% of all pediatric intracranial tumors

### Clinical Issues
- 64-96% overall 10 year survival
- Recurrence much more frequent with adamantinomatous histology than with papillary
- Treatment associated with high rate of morbidity

---

- Often very bright ⇒ reflects protein, cholesterol, and/or blood products in fluid
    - Solid component heterogeneous
- T2WI
    - Solid component heterogeneous
        - Hypointensity from Ca++, blood products, cholesterol
    - ± Hyperintense signal in adjacent brain
        - Tumor invasion, reactive gliosis/edema
- FLAIR: Cyst contents typically hyperintense
- T2* GRE: Ca++ components markedly hypointense
- DWI: Variable depending upon the character of cyst fluid
- T1 C+
    - Solid portions enhance heterogeneously
    - Cyst wall enhances
- MRA
    - Most often vessels are displaced by cysts
    - Circle of Willis vessels may be encased by solid components
        - Rarely narrowed
- MRS: Cyst contents show broad lipid spectrum at 0.9-1.5 ppm

### Radiographic Findings
- Skull radiographs
    - Sellar enlargement, erosion of clinoids
    - Suprasellar calcifications

### Imaging Recommendations
- Best imaging tool: Thin sagittal and coronal T1 C+ MR
- Protocol advice
    - Contrast-enhanced MR, with thin post-contrast sagittal and coronal imaging
    - MRA to aid in surgical planning
    - Important to identify displacement of chiasm

## DIFFERENTIAL DIAGNOSIS

### Rathke Cleft Cyst (RCC)
- Not calcified, generally nonenhancing
- No solid component

- Cyst more homogeneous

### Dermoid and Epidermoid Cysts
- Epidermoids are solid lesions that mimic cysts
- Suprasellar lesions are rare in children
- Minimal enhancement

### Germinoma, Brain
- Solid components larger than cystic
- Associated with diabetes insipidus

### Pituitary Adenoma
- Solid tumor that is isointense with brain, enhances strongly
- Cystic adenomas very rare in children

### Hypothalamic-Chiasmatic Glioma
- More solid and homogeneous
- Extension into prechiasmatic optic nerves, optic tracts/radiations
- Infiltrate/enlarge chiasm instead of displacing it

### Arachnoid Cyst
- Thin/imperceptible wall
- Cyst contents follow CSF

### Aneurysm
- "Onion skin" layers of aging blood products
- Bright enhancement of residual lumen

## PATHOLOGY

### General Features
- General path comments
    - Adamantinomatous subtype
        - Classic calcified cyst with mural nodule
        - Diagnosed in children
    - Squamous-papillary subtype
        - Mostly solid tumor
        - Almost exclusively found in adults
    - 15% of tumors have mixed histology ⇒ behave like adamantinomatous
- Etiology

# CRANIOPHARYNGIOMA

I

2

12

- ○ Arise from rests of epithelial cells
- ○ Two proposed sites of origin
  - In the pars tuberalis at the distal aspect of infundibulum
  - Along tract of involuted craniopharyngeal duct
- • Epidemiology
  - ○ Most common non-glial pediatric intracranial tumor
    - 6-9% of all pediatric intracranial tumors
  - ○ 0.5-2.5 new cases per million per year
  - ○ Comprise over half of all pediatric suprasellar region tumors
  - ○ Second peak of incidence in 5-7th decade
    - Squamous-papillary subtype
- • Embryology
  - ○ Rathke pouch (hypophyseal duct) is an invagination of the primitive stomatodeum
  - ○ Rathke pouch forms the pars tuberalis and adenohypophysis

## Gross Pathologic & Surgical Features
- • Cyst fluid is usually straw-colored and thick ⇒ "crankcase oil"
- • Adamantinomatous
  - ○ Mixed cystic and solid tumor
  - ○ Cysts > > solid components
- • Papillary
  - ○ Solid > > cysts
- • Epithelial fronds invade adjacent structures, hampering resection

## Microscopic Features
- • Adamantinomatous
  - ○ Cyst walls of simple stratified squamous epithelium, with a collagenous basement membrane
  - ○ Peripheral cellular palisading and stellate reticulum
  - ○ Nodules of "wet" keratin
  - ○ Dystrophic Ca++
- • Papillary
  - ○ Formation of papillae
  - ○ Ca++ or necrotic debris rare

## Staging, Grading or Classification Criteria
- • Both adamantinomatous and squamous-papillary are WHO Grade I

# CLINICAL ISSUES

## Presentation
- • Most common signs/symptoms
  - ○ Headache, vomiting
  - ○ Hydrocephalus and papilledema
    - Up to 50% at presentation
  - ○ Visual disturbance (bitemporal hemianopsia), decline in school performance
- • Other signs/symptoms
  - ○ Hormonally-mediated symptoms in at least 1/3 of cases
    - Due to mass effect on pituitary/hypothalamus
    - Growth hormone deficiency, hypothyroidism, diabetes insipidus

## Demographics
- • Age

- ○ Peak at 8-12 years
  - Peak for squamous-papillary at 40-60 years
- • Gender: M = F

## Natural History & Prognosis
- • Slow-growing and benign tumor
- • High rate of recurrence
  - ○ 20% recurrence rate if < 5 cm
  - ○ 83% recurrence rate if > 5 cm
  - ○ Can recur up to 30 years after resection
  - ○ Occasional ectopic sites of recurrence
- • 64-96% overall 10 year survival
- • Recurrence much more frequent with adamantinomatous histology than with papillary

## Treatment
- • Surgical
  - ○ Gross total resection
    - Limited by tumor size, adherence to vessels and hypothalamus
  - ○ Limited resection
    - Radiation therapy
    - Intracavitary radiation
- • Treatment associated with high rate of morbidity
  - ○ Peri-operative hyperthermia
  - ○ Vascular injury and pseudoaneurysm
  - ○ Hypopituitarism
  - ○ Long term hypothalamic syndrome
    - Morbid obesity from compulsive eating

# DIAGNOSTIC CHECKLIST

## Consider
- • RCC can be identical to small CrP
  - ○ RCC has no Ca++ and is more homogeneous
  - ○ Use NECT to identify Ca++ in CrP
- • Be sure to identify displacement of chiasm for surgical planning

# SELECTED REFERENCES

1. Chakrabarti I et al: Long-term neurological, visual, and endocrine outcomes following transnasal resection of craniopharyngioma. J Neurosurg. 102(4):650-7, 2005
2. Karavitaki N et al: Craniopharyngiomas in children and adults: systematic analysis of 121 cases with long-term follow-up. Clin Endocrinol (Oxf). 62(4):397-409, 2005
3. Ullrich NJ et al: Craniopharyngioma therapy: long-term effects on hypothalamic function. Neurologist. 11(1):55-60, 2005
4. Tavangar SM et al: Craniopharyngioma: a clinicopathological study of 141 cases. Endocr Pathol. 15(4):339-44, 2004
5. Barua KK et al: Treatment of recurrent craniopharyngiomas. Kobe J Med Sci. 49(5-6):123-32, 2003
6. Tominaga JY et al: Characteristics of Rathke's cleft cyst in MR imaging. Magn Reson Med Sci. 2(1):1-8, 2003
7. Sartoretti-Schefer S et al: MR differentiation of adamantinous and squamous-papillary craniopharyngiomas. AJNR Am J Neuroradiol. 18(1):77-87, 1997
8. Sutton LN et al: Proton spectroscopy of suprasellar tumors in pediatric patients. Neurosurgery. 41(2):388-94; discussion 394-5, 1997

# CRANIOPHARYNGIOMA

## IMAGE GALLERY

### Typical

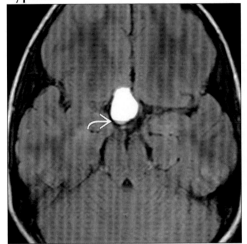
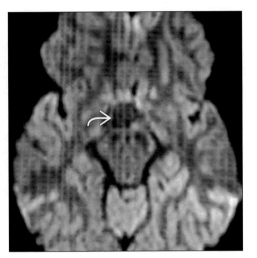

*(Left) Axial FLAIR MR shows hyperintense cyst contents in a craniopharyngioma. Note the fluid-fluid level at the posterior aspect of the tumor ⮡. (Right) Axial DWI MR shows no restricted diffusion in the same lesion ⮡, despite the complex contents of the fluid. As a result, DWI is inconsistent in its ability to differentiate craniopharyngioma from RCC.*

### Typical

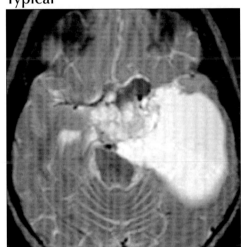
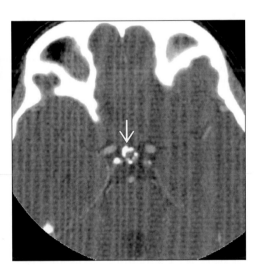

*(Left) Axial T2WI MR shows a heterogeneous CrP with a large cyst extending into the left middle cranial fossa. Some have advocated the term "monstrous" craniopharyngioma to describe these tumors. (Right) Axial CECT shows dense Ca++ in the suprasellar cistern ➡ of an adolescent with a small CrP. CT can be more sensitive and specific than MR in identification of the calcifications of CrP.*

### Typical

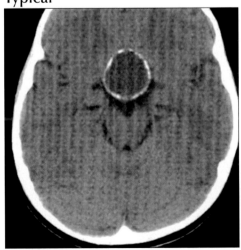
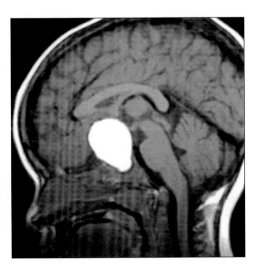

*(Left) Axial NECT shows characteristic irregular calcifications in the wall of a cystic craniopharyngioma. (Right) Sagittal T1WI MR in the same child as previous image shows the homogeneous bright signal of the cyst contents. This hyperintensity may hamper identification of enhancement in the wall of the tumor.*

# TUBER CINEREUM HAMARTOMA

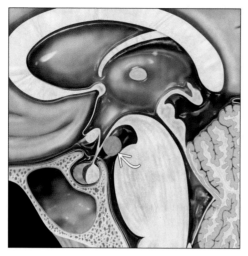

Sagittal graphic shows a pedunculated mass ➔ interposed between the infundibulum anteriorly and the mammillary bodies posteriorly. Mass resembles gray matter. Classic tuber cinereum hamartoma.

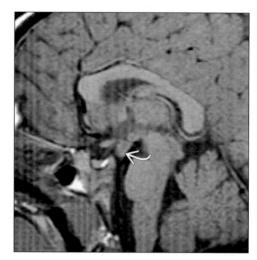

Sagittal T1WI MR shows a pedunculated mass ➔ arising from the floor of the third ventricle between the pituitary stalk and the mamillary bodies.

## TERMINOLOGY

### Abbreviations and Synonyms

- Hypothalamic hamartoma, diencephalic hamartoma

### Definitions

- Non-neoplastic congenital collection of heterotopic neurons and glia originating from tuber cinereum (floor of 3rd ventricle), characterized clinically by luteinizing hormone-releasing hormone (LHRH) dependent central precocious puberty at a very young age and/or gelastic seizures

## IMAGING FINDINGS

### General Features

- Best diagnostic clue: Small (typically ~1 cm), round, nonenhancing mass contiguous with tuber cinereum
- Location: Floor of 3rd ventricle → ventricle or suprasellar cistern
- Size: Variable, few millimeters to giant (3-5 cm)
- Morphology: Sessile or pedunculated round mass, similar in density/intensity to gray matter

### CT Findings

- NECT
  ○ Homogeneous suprasellar mass
    ■ Between the cerebral peduncles and the optic chiasm on axial views
    ■ Isodense or slightly ↓ density to brain
    ■ Less common: Cysts, Ca++
    ■ Associated patent craniopharyngeal canal is very rare
- CECT: Nonenhancing

### MR Findings

- T1WI
  ○ Isointense or slightly hypointense to gray matter
    ■ Between mammillary bodies and infundibular stalk on coronal and sagittal
    ■ May sit in floor of or ventral to 3rd ventricle
    ■ Anecdotal cases contain fat or cysts (RARE, look for other diagnosis)
- T2WI: Iso or slightly ↑ signal intensity (occasionally ↑↑ due to fibrillary gliosis)
- PD/Intermediate: Hyperintense to cerebrospinal fluid (CSF), slightly ↑ signal than gray matter
- FLAIR: +/- Bright

## DDx: Suprasellar Masses

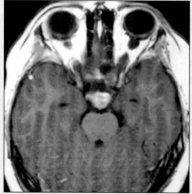

Astrocytoma, Enhancing

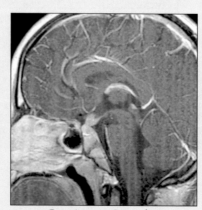

Germinoma, Spreading

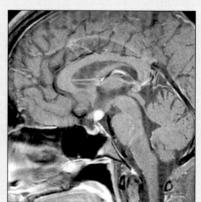

Histiocytosis, Enhancing

# TUBER CINEREUM HAMARTOMA

## Key Facts

### Terminology
- Non-neoplastic congenital collection of heterotopic neurons and glia originating from tuber cinereum (floor of 3rd ventricle), characterized clinically by luteinizing hormone-releasing hormone (LHRH) dependent central precocious puberty at a very young age and/or gelastic seizures

### Imaging Findings
- Best diagnostic clue: Small (typically ~1 cm), round, nonenhancing mass contiguous with tuber cinereum
- Isointense or slightly hypointense to gray matter
- T2WI: Iso or slightly ↑ signal intensity (occasionally ↑↑ due to fibrillary gliosis)
- T1 C+: Nonenhancing (if enhances, look for other diagnosis)

### Top Differential Diagnoses
- Craniopharyngioma
- Hypothalamic/Chiasmatic Astrocytoma
- Suprasellar Germinoma
- Langerhans Cell Histiocytosis

### Pathology
- Shape and size of lesion reported to predict symptoms
- Of histologically verified lesions: 3/4 precocious puberty, 1/2 seizures
- Found in up to 33% of patients with precocious puberty

### Clinical Issues
- Infant with gelastic seizures, precocious puberty

---

- T1 C+: Nonenhancing (if enhances, look for other diagnosis)
- MRS
  - Long echo time (TE): ↓ N-acetyl-aspartate (NAA), minimally ↑ choline
  - (Short TE): ↑ Myoinositol

## Radiographic Findings
- Radiography: Occasional suprasellar calcifications, eroded dorsum, enlarged sella

## Angiographic Findings
- Conventional: Avascular lesion

## Imaging Recommendations
- Best imaging tool: MRI
- Protocol advice: Thin (3 mm) sagittal and coronal T2 and T1 C+ MR

# DIFFERENTIAL DIAGNOSIS

## Craniopharyngioma
- Most common suprasellar mass in children
- Contains increased or decreased signal cysts (90%), Ca++ (90%), enhancement (90%)

## Hypothalamic/Chiasmatic Astrocytoma
- 2nd most common pediatric suprasellar mass (+/- NF1)
- Enhancement heterogeneous and often vigorous; +/- optic tract extension

## Lipoma
- Contains fat

## Suprasellar Germinoma
- Often multicentric masses: Suprasellar, pineal, thalamus, basal ganglia
- Early leptomeningeal metastatic dissemination; lack precocious puberty
- Causes early diabetes insipidus

## Langerhans Cell Histiocytosis
- Enhances

- Often causes diabetes insipidus

# PATHOLOGY

## General Features
- General path comments
  - Shape and size of lesion reported to predict symptoms
    - Large sessile lesions ⇒ seizures
    - Small pedunculated lesions ⇒ central precocious puberty (CPP)
    - In fact, presentation with both seizures and CPP common
  - Embryology: Disturbed embryogenesis between gestational days 33-41
- Genetics
  - Pallister-Hall syndrome (GLI3 frameshift mutations, chromosome 7p13)
    - Hamartoma of tuber cinereum
    - Digital malformations (short metacarpals, syndactyly, polydactyly)
    - Other midline (epiglottis/larynx) and cardiac/renal/anal anomalies
  - Often reported with facial or congenital cerebral midline anomalies
  - Other central nervous system (CNS) plus skeletal/visceral syndromes: Cerebroacrovisceral-early lethality, Smith-Lemli-Opitz, Meckel, oro-facial-digital, holoprosencephaly-polydactyly, hydrolethalis, Laurence-Moon-Biedl, Varadi
- Etiology
  - Neuronal migration anomaly
  - Pathogenesis of precocious puberty-induced sexual precocity
    - +/- LHRH granules in hamartoma/connecting axons in some
    - Activating astroglial-derived factors in tumors may stimulate endogenous LHRH secretion if no intra-tumoral LHRH granules
- Epidemiology

- ○ Of histologically verified lesions: 3/4 precocious puberty, 1/2 seizures
- ○ Found in up to 33% of patients with precocious puberty

## Gross Pathologic & Surgical Features
- Mature neuronal ganglionic tissue project from hypothalamus, tuber cinereum or mamillary bodies; rarely lie free in interpeduncular fossa
- Pedunculated or sessile, rounded or nodular; lack invasion

## Microscopic Features
- May be considered as heterotopia
- Resembles gray matter with neurons similar to hypothalamus
- Myelinated/unmyelinated axons and variable amounts of fibrillary gliosis
- Rare reports of cysts, necrosis, calcifications and fat
- Hamartoblastomas include more primitive undifferentiated cells

## Staging, Grading or Classification Criteria
- Valdueza classification
  - ○ Pedunculated, central precocious puberty or asymptomatic
    - ▪ Originates tuber cinereum
    - ▪ Originates mamillary bodies
  - ○ Sessile, hypothalamus displaced, seizures
    - ▪ More hypothalamic dysfunction and abnormal behavior

## CLINICAL ISSUES

### Presentation
- Most common signs/symptoms
  - ○ Gelastic seizures at onset in majority of patients
    - ▪ Gelastic seizures may also occur in other hypothalamic tumors
- Clinical Profile
  - ○ Infant with gelastic seizures, precocious puberty
  - ○ Precocious puberty, tall, overweight, and advanced bone age
  - ○ May result in acromegaly
- Seizures (gelastic type: Laughing/crying spells) with larger hamartomas
  - ○ Some children present with partial complex epilepsy
- Other seizure types frequent, but only gelastic originate in or near hamartoma and thalamus
  - ○ Gelastic seizures may progress to partial epilepsy, partial complex seizures, generalized tonic clonic seizures
- Patients with seizures have deterioration in behavior (aggression, psychiatric comorbidity) and cognition (speech and learning impairment)
- As high as 33% in young patients with central precocious puberty
- Rare: May secrete releasing hormone

### Demographics
- Age: Usually present between 1-3 years of age
- Gender: No predilection, some report M > F
- Ethnicity: No predilection

## Natural History & Prognosis
- Lack of growth; if growth is detected, surgery/biopsy indicated
- Pedunculated lesions are less likely to be symptomatic
- Sessile lesions are almost always symptomatic
- Syndromic patients do poorly, may not survive their other malformations

## Treatment
- Hormonal suppressive therapy (LHRH agonist therapy); treat seizures
  - ○ Hormonal suppressive therapy is successful in most patients
- Surgery if failure of medical therapy or rapid growth of lesion
  - ○ Stereotatic thermocoagulation
  - ○ Gamma knife surgery
- Microsurgical approach with total resection
  - ○ Good response expected if seizures originate in or near mass
  - ○ Location of lesion has significant risk of hypothalamic complications

## DIAGNOSTIC CHECKLIST

### Consider
- Hypothalamic astrocytoma, histiocytosis, germ cell tumor (all show some contrast-enhancement)

### Image Interpretation Pearls
- Nonenhancing mass in hypothalamus, isointense to gray matter on T1, slightly ↑ signal on T2 images

## SELECTED REFERENCES

1. Voyadzis J M et al: Hypothalamic hamartoma secreting corticotropin-releasing hormone. Case report J Neurosurg. 100.212-6, 2004
2. Kremer S et al: Epilepsy and hypothalamic hamartoma: look at the hand Pallister-Hall syndrome. Epileptic Disord. 5:27-30, 2003
3. Martin DD et al: MR imaging and spectroscopy of a tuber cinereum hamartoma in a patient with growth hormone deficiency and hypogonadotropic hypogonadism. AJNR. 24:1177-80, 2003
4. Mullatti N et al: The clinical spectrum of epilepsy in children and adults with hypothalamic hamartoma. Epilepsia. 44:1310-19, 2003
5. Luo s et al: Microsurgical treatment for hypothalamic hamartoma in children with precocious puberty. Surg Neurol. 57:356-62, 2002
6. Debeneix C et al: Hypothalamic hamartoma: comparison of clinical presentation and magnetic resonance images. Horm Res. 56:12-18, 2001
7. Tsugo H et al: Hypothalamic hamartoma associated with multiple congenital abnormalities. Two patients and a review of reported cases. Pediatr Neurosurg. 29(6):290-6, 1998
8. Valdueza JM et al: Hypothalamic hamartomas: With special reference to gelastic epilepsy and surgery. Neurosurgery. 34(6):949-58, 1994
9. Boyko OB et al: Hamartomas of the tuber cinereum: CT, MR and pathologic findings. AJNR. 12:309-14, 1991

# TUBER CINEREUM HAMARTOMA

## IMAGE GALLERY

### Typical

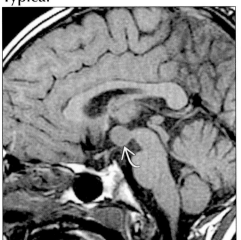
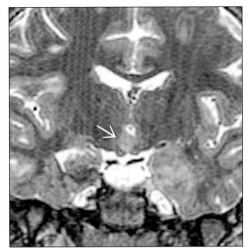

*(Left)* Sagittal T1WI MR shows a hamartoma ➡ within the third ventricle. Hamartomas may extend inferiorly into the suprasellar or interpeduncular cistern or upward into the third ventricle. *(Right)* Coronal T2WI MR shows a hamartoma ➡ that is isointense to cortex, sitting asymmetrically within the floor of the 3rd ventricle. Hamartomas within the 3rd often are asymmetric to the side.

### Typical

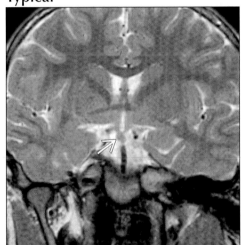
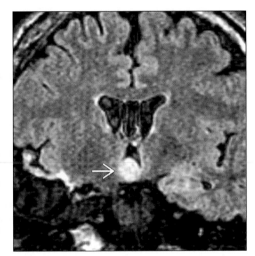

*(Left)* Coronal T2WI MR shows a small pedunculated hamartoma ➡ in the suprasellar cistern. Note that the lesion hangs from the floor of the ventricle and is isointense to cortex. *(Right)* Coronal FLAIR MR shows a hamartoma ➡ sitting asymmetrically in the inferior 3rd ventricle. On FLAIR and proton density images, hamartomas are often slightly hyperintense.

### Variant

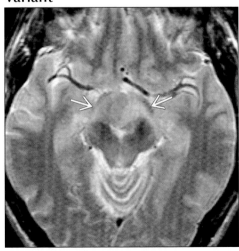
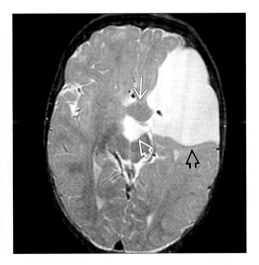

*(Left)* Axial T2WI MR shows a large hamartoma ➡ splaying the cerebral peduncles and sitting in the suprasellar and interpeduncular cisterns. Large hamartomas can be heterogeneous secondary to gliosis. *(Right)* Axial T2WI MR shows hamartoma ➡ in suprasellar cistern associated with large cysts in the interpeduncular cistern ➡ and sylvian cistern ➡.

# LYMPHOCYTIC HYPOPHYSITIS

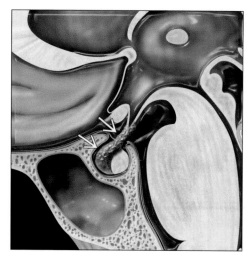

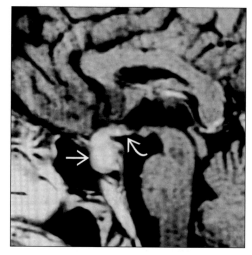

*Lateral graphic shows panhypophysitis with the inflammatory process (blue, ➡) involving the anterior pituitary and extending up the stalk to the median eminence of the hypothalamus.*

*Sagittal T1 C+ MR shows panhypophysitis with enlarged pituitary gland ➡ and thickened stalk ➡ extending upward to the median eminence of the hypothalamus.*

## TERMINOLOGY

### Abbreviations and Synonyms
- Lymphocytic hypophysitis (LH); lymphocytic panhypophysitis, primary hypophysitis; stalkitis

### Definitions
- Idiopathic, autoimmune inflammation of the pituitary gland and stalk

## IMAGING FINDINGS

### General Features
- Best diagnostic clue: Thick nontapered stalk, +/- pituitary, hypothalamic mass
- Location: Supra- or intrasellar, infundibulum, median eminence of hypothalamus
- Size: Anterior pituitary usually < 10 mm but may be up to 2-3 cms
- Morphology
  - Rounded pituitary gland with thickened, nontapering or bulbous infundibulum

- Stalk/hypothalamus may be involved in isolation (infundibuloneurohypophysitis)
- Gland, stalk, and hypothalamus all involved (panhypophysitis)

### CT Findings
- NECT: Thick/bulbous stalk, +/- enlarged pituitary gland
- CECT: Suprasellar mass/thick stalk with intense uniform enhancement

### MR Findings
- T1WI
  - Thick stalk (> 2 mm + loss of normal "top to bottom" tapering)
  - Adenohypophysis ⇒ enlarged pituitary gland
    - Cystic in 5%
  - Infundibuloneurohypophysitis ⇒ mass in stalk, median eminence of hypothalamus
  - Panhypophysitis ⇒ mass in pituitary gland, stalk, median eminence of hypothalamus
  - 75% show loss of posterior pituitary "bright spot"
- T2WI: Iso/hypointense with gray matter
- T1 C+

## DDx: Mimics of Lymphocytic Hypophysitis

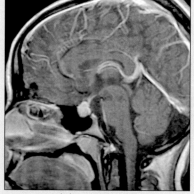

*Adolescent Pituitary*

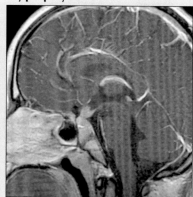

*Suprasellar Germinoma*

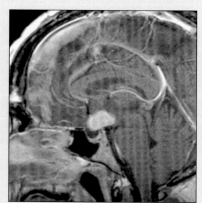

*Langerhans Cell Histiocytosis*

# LYMPHOCYTIC HYPOPHYSITIS

## Key Facts

### Terminology
- Lymphocytic hypophysitis (LH); lymphocytic panhypophysitis, primary hypophysitis; stalkitis

### Imaging Findings
- Best diagnostic clue: Thick nontapered stalk, +/- pituitary, hypothalamic mass
- Location: Supra- or intrasellar, infundibulum, median eminence of hypothalamus

### Top Differential Diagnoses
- Pituitary Hyperplasia
- Macroadenoma (Prolactinoma)
- Suprasellar Germinoma
- Langerhans Cell Histiocytosis

### Pathology
- Three forms of disease ⇒
- Adenohypophysitis (anterior pituitary): Association with pregnancy
- Infundibuloneurohypophysitis (stalk, posterior pituitary, +/- hypothalamus)
- Panhypophysitis (involves anterior and posterior pituitary and stalk)

### Clinical Issues
- Adenohypophysitis ⇒ headache, visual impairment
- May mimic pituitary apoplexy
- Infundibuloneurohypophysitis ⇒ DI
- Panhypophysitis ⇒ combination of anterior and posterior pituitary signs/symptoms

---

○ Affected regions enhance intensely, usually uniformly
○ May have adjacent dural, cavernous sinus thickening, sphenoid sinus mucosal thickening

### Imaging Recommendations
- Best imaging tool: MRI
- Protocol advice
  ○ Pre-contrast thin-section (< 3 mm) sagittal, coronal T1- and T2WIs
  ○ Coronal "dynamic" T1 C+ (may show delayed pituitary enhancement)

## DIFFERENTIAL DIAGNOSIS

### Pituitary Hyperplasia
- Stalk usually normal
- Seen during adolescence, later stages of pregnancy, post-partum

### Macroadenoma (Prolactinoma)
- Diabetes insipidus (DI) is common in LH, rare with adenomas
- Posterior pituitary "bright spot" absent or displaced/deformed; sella enlarged/eroded
- Adenoma may be off midline; LH is midline

### Suprasellar Germinoma
- Diabetes insipidus develops before imaging abnormality
- Enhancing mass in 3rd ventricle floor, stalk

### Langerhans Cell Histiocytosis
- Involves infundibulum, neurohypophysis
- Associated with calvarial, skull base lesions
- May have multiple central nervous system (CNS) lesions

### Suprasellar Astrocytoma
- Mass does not involve pituitary gland
- Usually extends into optic pathways
- DI is uncommon, only late in disease

### Ectopic Posterior Pituitary Gland
- Stalk may appear short and "stubby"
- Anterior pituitary often small

### Sarcoid: Uncommon in Pediatrics
- Evidence for systemic disease often (but not invariably) present
- Other granulomatous hypophysitis (Wegener) can mimic LH

## PATHOLOGY

### General Features
- General path comments
  ○ Rare idiopathic inflammatory disorder of pituitary/hypothalamus
  ○ Pituitary inflammation can be 2° to neighboring lesion: Germinoma, craniopharyngioma: "Secondary hypophysitis"
  ○ Differs from granulomatous hypophysitis seen with sarcoidosis, Wegner granulomatosis, tuberculosis
- Etiology
  ○ Autoimmune disorder with unknown trigger
  ○ Adenohypophysitis ⇒ strong temporal association with pregnancy
  ○ Antibodies to pituicytes often found
- Epidemiology: Rare (1-2% of sellar lesions)

### Gross Pathologic & Surgical Features
- Diffusely enlarged stalk/pituitary gland
- Three forms of disease ⇒
  ○ Adenohypophysitis (anterior pituitary): Association with pregnancy
  ○ Infundibuloneurohypophysitis (stalk, posterior pituitary, +/- hypothalamus)
  ○ Panhypophysitis (involves anterior and posterior pituitary and stalk)

### Microscopic Features
- Acute
  ○ Dense infiltrate of B-, T-lymphocytes, plasma cells, occasionally eosinophils; +/- lymphoid follicles

- ○ No granulomas, giant cells or organisms; no evidence for neoplasm
- Chronic may demonstrate extensive fibrosis

## CLINICAL ISSUES

### Presentation
- Most common signs/symptoms
  - ○ Adenohypophysitis ⇒ headache, visual impairment
    - ■ Vision: Bitemporal hemianopsia, diplopia
    - ■ May mimic pituitary apoplexy
  - ○ Infundibuloneurohypophysitis ⇒ DI
    - ■ Common cause of DI in childhood
    - ■ Other important causes: Germinoma, Langerhans cell histiocytosis
    - ■ DI may be masked by hypercortisolism
  - ○ Panhypophysitis ⇒ combination of anterior and posterior pituitary signs/symptoms
- Other signs/symptoms: Amenorrhea/galactorrhea 2° to stalk compression: Uncommon
- Clinical Profile: Peripartum female with headache, visual complaints, multiple endocrine deficiencies

### Demographics
- Age
  - ○ More common in adolescents than younger children
  - ○ Mean age at presentation for F = 35 y, M = 45 y
- Gender
  - ○ Overall female predominance
    - ■ Adenohypophysitis: M:F = 1:6
    - ■ Infundibuloneurohypophysitis: M:F = 1:1
    - ■ Panhypophysitis: M:F = 1:1.8

### Natural History & Prognosis
- Infundibuloneurohypophysitis ⇒ symptoms may develop before radiologic abnormality
- Unrecognized, untreated LH can result in death from panhypopituitarism

### Treatment
- Diagnosis established by imaging or biopsy
- Biopsy plus endocrine replacement
- Glucocorticoids: Prednisone, hydrocortisone, methylprednisolone
- Subtotal surgical resection, chiasm decompression if mass effect but risk is impaired endocrine function
- Rarely radiation

## DIAGNOSTIC CHECKLIST

### Consider
- Other findings present (e.g., thickened meninges, enlarged cavernous sinus)?
- Ensure absence of other, inciting lesions (germinoma, craniopharyngioma)

### Image Interpretation Pearls
- Adenohypophysitis can mimic adenoma
- Infundibuloneurohypophysitis can mimic germinoma, histiocytosis

## SELECTED REFERENCES

1. Caturegli P et al: Autoimmune Hypophysitis. Endocrine Reviews. 26(5):599-614, 2005
2. Huang CH et al: A case of lymphocytic hypophysitis with masked diabetes insipidus unveiled by glucocorticoid replacement. Am J Kidney Dis. 45(1):197-200, 2005
3. Leung GK et al: Primary hypophysitis: a single-center experience in 16 cases. J Neurosurg. 101(2):262-71, 2004
4. Lidove O et al: Lymphocytic hypophysitis with lachrymal, salivary and thyroid gland involvement. Eur J Intern Med. 15(2):121-124, 2004
5. Wong RW et al: Lymphocytic hypophysitis with a long latent period before development of a pituitary mass. Can J Neurol Sci. 31(3):406-8, 2004
6. Lee MS et al: Apoplectic lymphocytic hypophysitis. Case report. J Neurosurg. 98(1):183-5, 2003
7. Ng WH et al: Lymphocytic hypophysitis. J Clin Neurosci. 10(4):409-13, 2003
8. Dan NG et al: Pituitary apoplexy in association with lymphocytic hypophysitis. J Clin Neurosci. 9(5):577-80, 2002
9. Flanagan DE et al: Inflammatory hypophysitis - the spectrum of disease. Acta Neurochir (Wien). 144(1):47-56, 2002
10. Hashimoto K et al: A case of lymphocytic infundibuloneurohypophysitis associated with systemic lupus erythematosus. Endocr J. 49(6):605-10, 2002
11. Tashiro T et al: Spectrum of different types of hypophysitis: a clinicopathologic study of hypophysitis in 31 cases. Endocr Pathol. 13(3):183-95, 2002
12. Buxton N et al: Lymphocytic and granulocytic hypophysitis: a single centre experience. Br J Neurosurg. 15(3):242-5, discussion 245-6, 2001
13. Tubridy N et al: Infundibulohypophysitis in a man presenting with diabetes insipidus and cavernous sinus involvement. J Neurol Neurosurg Psychiatry. 71(6):798-801, 2001
14. Sato N et al: Hypophysitis: endocrinologic and dynamic MR findings. AJNR Am J Neuroradiol. 19(3):439-44, 1998
15. Sato N et al: Hypophysitis: endocrinologic and dynamic MR findings. AJNR Am J Neuroradiol. 19(3):439-44, 1998
16. Cemeroglu AP et al: Lymphocytic hypophysitis presenting with diabetes insipidus in a 14-year-old girl: case report and review of the literature. Eur J Pediatr. 156(9):684-8, 1997
17. Heinze HJ et al: Acquired hypophysitis in adolescence. J Pediatr Endocrinol Metab. 10(3):315-21, 1997
18. Mizokami T et al: Hypopituitarism associated with transient diabetes insipidus followed by an episode of painless thyroiditis in a young man. Intern Med. 35(2):135-41, 1996
19. Patel MC et al: Peripartum hypopituitarism and lymphocytic hypophysitis. QJM. 88(8):571-80, 1995
20. Powrie JK et al: Lymphocytic adenohypophysitis: magnetic resonance imaging features of two new cases and a review of the literature. Clin Endocrinol. 42:315-22, 1995

# LYMPHOCYTIC HYPOPHYSITIS

## IMAGE GALLERY

### Typical

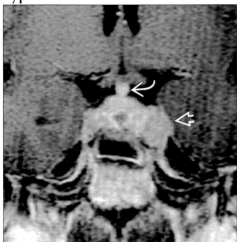 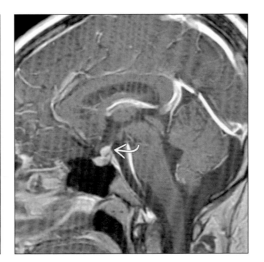

*(Left)* Coronal T1 C+ MR shows adenohypophysitis with involvement of the left cavernous sinus ➡ which is expanded. The anterior pituitary is enlarged and the infundibulum ➡ is thickened. *(Right)* Sagittal T1 C+ MR shows infundibuloneurohypophysitis with normal adenohypophysis, thick stalk, and mass at the median eminence of the hypothalamus ➡ in this adolescent girl.

### Typical

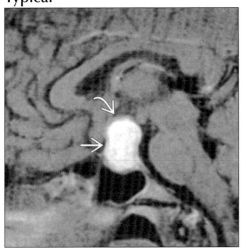 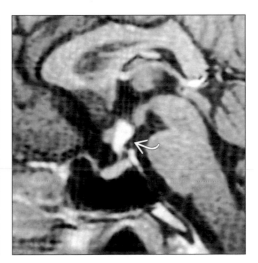

*(Left)* Sagittal T1 C+ MR shows adenohypophysitis with a large enhancing anterior pituitary mass ➡ extending upward into the suprasellar cistern and upwardly displacing the optic chiasm ➡. *(Right)* Sagittal T1 C+ MR shows infundibuloneurohypophysitis, with a uniformly enhancing focus of inflammation ➡ situated in and posterior to the median eminence of the hypothalamus.

### Variant

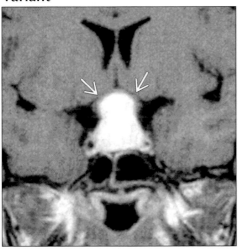 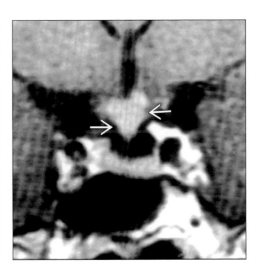

*(Left)* Coronal T1 C+ MR shows adenohypophysitis with a markedly expanded anterior pituitary gland extending into the suprasellar cistern and displacing/compressing the optic chiasm ➡. *(Right)* Coronal T1 C+ MR shows infundibuloneurohypophysitis, with a homogeneously enhancing mass ➡ at the median eminence of the hypothalamus and extending into the infundibulum.

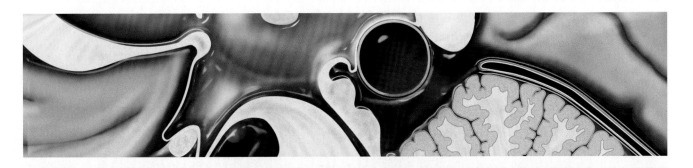

# SECTION 3: Pineal Region

# GERMINOMA

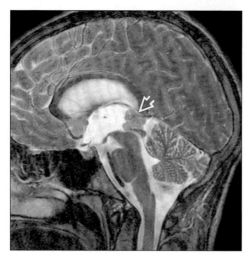

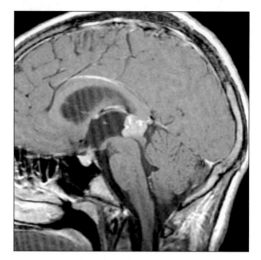

*Sagittal T2WI MR shows a homogeneous pineal germinoma flattening the tectum and obstructing the cerebral aqueduct ➡. These tumors commonly present with hydrocephalus or Parinaud syndrome.*

*Sagittal T1 C+ MR (same patient as previous image) shows the mildly heterogeneous and diffuse enhancement of the tumor. Germinomas account for up to 50% of pineal region tumors in childhood.*

## TERMINOLOGY

### Abbreviations and Synonyms
- Dysgerminoma, extra-gonadal seminoma, formerly called atypical teratoma

### Definitions
- Tumor of primordial germs cells, essentially identical to seminoma or dysgerminoma in the gonads or mediastinum
- Non-germinomatous germ cell tumors (NGGCTs) include teratomas, endodermal sinus tumors, embryonal cell carcinomas, and choriocarcinomas

## IMAGING FINDINGS

### General Features
- Best diagnostic clue
  - Pineal region mass that "engulfs" the pineal gland
  - Suprasellar mass with diabetes insipidus (DI)
- Location
  - Central nervous system (CNS) germinomas have a propensity to hug the midline near the 3rd ventricle
    - Suprasellar ~ 50-60%
    - Pineal region ~ 30-40%
    - Thalamic or basal ganglia tumors in up to 14%
- Size
  - 1-3 cm
  - Relatively small pineal region germinoma may present with ventricular obstruction
  - Tiny or inapparent suprasellar germinoma may cause DI
- Morphology: Often well-delineated, lobular

### CT Findings
- NECT
  - Sharply circumscribed high attenuation mass (hyperdense to gray matter)
    - Drapes around posterior 3rd ventricle or "engulfs" pineal gland
    - Suprasellar mass without dominant cyst
  - Pineal Ca++ pattern
    - Pineal germinoma rumored to "displace" pineal Ca++
    - Pineoblastomas rumored to "engulf" pineal Ca++
    - In practice, this is not a helpful differentiation
- CECT

## DDx: Pineal Region Masses

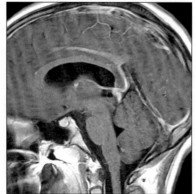

*Pineal Cyst*

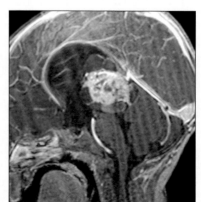

*Pineoblastoma*

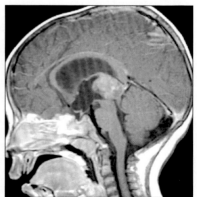

*ATRhT*

# GERMINOMA

## Key Facts

### Terminology
- Tumor of primordial germs cells, essentially identical to seminoma or dysgerminoma in the gonads or mediastinum
- Non-germinomatous germ cell tumors (NGGCTs) include teratomas, endodermal sinus tumors, embryonal cell carcinomas, and choriocarcinomas

### Imaging Findings
- Central nervous system (CNS) germinomas have a propensity to hug the midline near the 3rd ventricle
- Suprasellar ~ 50-60%
- Pineal region ~ 30-40%
- Thalamic or basal ganglia tumors in up to 14%
- Avid enhancement
- Often "speckled"

### Top Differential Diagnoses
- Other Germ Cell Tumors (NGGCTs)
- Pineoblastoma (Pineal PNET)
- Pineal Cyst
- Craniopharyngioma (Suprasellar)
- Langerhans Cell Histiocytosis (LCH, Suprasellar)

### Clinical Issues
- Germinomas are most commonly seen in adolescents
- Intracranial NGGCTs are more common in younger children

### Diagnostic Checklist
- Child or adolescent with DI
- Expect absence of posterior pituitary bright spot
- Repeat MR imaging with contrast in 3-6 months in children with DI and no identified lesion

- ○ Avid enhancement
- ○ Look for enhancing subarachnoid metastases

### MR Findings
- T1WI
  - ○ Sharply demarcated round or lobulated mass
  - ○ Isointense or hyperintense to GM
  - ○ Absent posterior pituitary bright spot in children with DI (suprasellar)
    - ■ No tumor may be apparent at presentation
- T2WI
  - ○ Iso- to hyperintense to GM
  - ○ Hyperintense cystic or necrotic foci
    - ■ Hypointense foci from blood or Ca++ rare
- FLAIR: Hyperintense to GM
- DWI: Restricted diffusion
- T1 C+
  - ○ Avid enhancement
    - ■ Often "speckled"
  - ○ Look for enhancing subarachnoid metastases
- MRS: ↑ Choline, ↓ NAA, ± lactate

### Radiographic Findings
- Radiography
  - ○ Pineal Ca++ on skull radiographs before age 10?
    - ■ Not a useful sign in CT era: Look for mass!
    - ■ Physiologic pineal Ca++ reported in children younger than 6 yrs old
    - ■ If no associated mass, pineal Ca++ of doubtful significance

### Imaging Recommendations
- Best imaging tool: Enhanced MR of brain and spine
- Protocol advice
  - ○ MR evaluation of entire neuraxis before surgery
  - ○ **Negative MR in child with DI does not exclude germinoma!**
    - ■ Repeat study in 3-6 months to assess for growing suprasellar tumor

## DIFFERENTIAL DIAGNOSIS

### Other Germ Cell Tumors (NGGCTs)
- Heterogeneous, with Ca++, fat, and hemorrhage

### Pineoblastoma (Pineal PNET)
- Aggressive tumor of primitive poorly differentiated cells
- Much worse prognosis than germinoma

### Atypical Teratoid Rhabdoid Tumor (ATRhT)
- Aggressive tumor of young children
- Mimics PNET in appearance and behavior

### Pineal Cyst
- Atypical features (> 1 cm, heterogeneous enhancement, ± tectal compression)
- Repeat imaging in 9-12 months to show stability if no other findings

### Tectal Astrocytoma
- Little or no enhancement
- Blends into tectal plate

### Craniopharyngioma (Suprasellar)
- Cystic, solid, and Ca++ components

### Hypothalamic/Chiasmatic Astrocytoma
- Rarely associated with DI

### Langerhans Cell Histiocytosis (LCH, Suprasellar)
- Thickened infundibulum
- Small enhancing lesion
- Associated calvarial, cerebellar lesions

## PATHOLOGY

### General Features
- General path comments
  - ○ Unencapsulated solid mass, soft and friable, tan-white coloration, ± cystic foci
  - ○ Necrosis, calcification and hemorrhage uncommon

# GERMINOMA

- Genetics
  - Cytogenetics ~ ↑ risk of CNS germ cell neoplasms
    - Extra X chromosome (Klinefelter syndrome)
    - Alterations of chromosome 1 (1q21-1qter region)
    - Over-representation of chromosome 12 (12p duplication)
    - Other chromosomes: 8q, 13q, 18q, 9q, 11q
  - Molecular genetics ~ ↑ risk of CNS germ cell neoplasms
    - P53 tumor suppressor gene mutations (exons 5-8)
    - MDM2 gene amplification
- Etiology
  - Germ cell tumors are found in the gonads, mediastinum, parasellar, and pineal regions
    - Regions where primordial germ cells migrate during embryogenesis
  - Primordial germ cells persist, maldifferentiate into germinoma or NGGCTs
- Epidemiology
  - 3-8% of pediatric CNS tumors
  - Germinomas ~ 65-70% of all CNS germ cell tumors
  - Germinomas ~ 40% of pineal region neoplasms
- Associated abnormalities
  - Klinefelter syndrome (47XXY)
  - Down syndrome
  - Neurofibromatosis type I (NF1)
  - Laboratory derangements
    - Elevated placental alkaline phosphatase (PLAP)
    - ± Elevation of serum and cerebrospinal fluid (CSF) human chorionic gonadotropin (HCG)

## Gross Pathologic & Surgical Features
- Soft and friable, tan-white mass, ± necrosis

## Microscopic Features
- Sheets of large polygonal primitive germ cells
  - Large vesicular nuclei & prominent nucleoli
  - Clear, glycogen-rich cytoplasm (PAS-positive)
- Lymphocytic infiltrates along fibrovascular septa

## Staging, Grading or Classification Criteria
- Multiple site involvement (pineal, suprasellar, basal ganglia, thalamus) is considered metastatic in USA but synchronous in Canada and Europe

# CLINICAL ISSUES

## Presentation
- Most common signs/symptoms
  - Pineal region germinoma
    - Headache due to tectal compression and hydrocephalus
    - Parinaud syndrome (upward gaze paralysis and altered convergence)
    - Precocious puberty or DI (associated with infiltration into 3rd ventricle floor)
  - Suprasellar germinoma
    - Diabetes insipidus ⇒ can be present for an extended period prior to MR abnormalities
    - Visual loss
    - Hypothalamic-pituitary dysfunction (↓ growth, precocious puberty)

## Demographics
- Age
  - Germinomas are most commonly seen in adolescents
    - Peak age: 10-12 years
  - Intracranial NGGCTs are more common in younger children
    - Teratoma is the most common congenital brain tumor
- Gender
  - Pineal region and thalamic germinoma have a strong male predominance
  - Suprasellar germinoma may be slightly more common in females
- Ethnicity
  - CNS GCTs much more prevalent in Asia
    - 9-15% of all CNS tumors in Japan
  - Basal ganglia and thalamic germinomas also more common in Japan and Korea

## Natural History & Prognosis
- Pure germinoma has favorable prognosis
  - Low secretion of HCG (< 50) ⇒ favorable
- Relatively good prognosis: Sensitivity to radiation and chemotherapy

## Treatment
- Radiotherapy ± adjuvant chemotherapy
- 5 year survival > 90%

# DIAGNOSTIC CHECKLIST

## Consider
- Adolescent boy with pineal mass ⇒ germinoma
- Young child with pineal mass
  - Heterogeneous and complex ⇒ NGGCT or PNET
  - Homogeneous ⇒ germinoma or PNET
- Child or adolescent with DI
  - Expect absence of posterior pituitary bright spot
  - Thickened and enhancing infundibulum ⇒ LCH or germinoma
  - Lobular enhancing mass ⇒ germinoma
  - No enhancing lesion ⇒ could still be germinoma

## Image Interpretation Pearls
- Repeat MR imaging with contrast in 3-6 months in children with DI and no identified lesion

# SELECTED REFERENCES

1. Oyama N et al: Bilateral germinoma involving the basal ganglia and cerebral white matter. AJNR Am J Neuroradiol. 26(5):1166-9, 2005
2. Kanagaki M et al: MRI and CT findings of neurohypophyseal germinoma. Eur J Radiol. 49(3):204-11, 2004
3. Wellons JC 3rd et al: Neuroendoscopic findings in patients with intracranial germinomas correlating with diabetes insipidus. J Neurosurg Spine. 100(5):430-6, 2004
4. Gomori E et al: Cytogenetic profile of primary pituitary germinoma. J Neurooncol. 50(3):251-5, 2000
5. Sano K: Pathogenesis of intracranial germ cell tumors reconsidered. J Neurosurg. 90(2):258-64, 1999

# GERMINOMA

## IMAGE GALLERY

### Typical

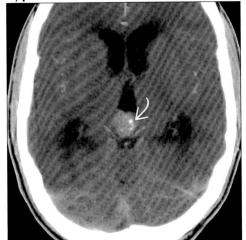

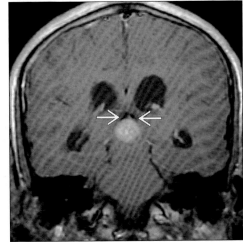

*(Left)* Axial CECT shows a pineal germinoma in a teenage male with hydrocephalus. Note the punctate calcification ➡, likely arising from the pineal gland itself, rather than formed by the tumor. *(Right)* Coronal T1 C+ MR (same patient as previous image) shows the mild lateral displacement of the internal cerebral veins ➡ by tumor. Pineal germinomas are up to 10x more common in males than females.

### Typical

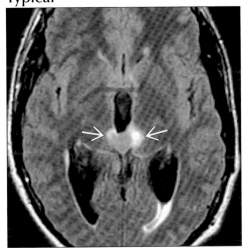

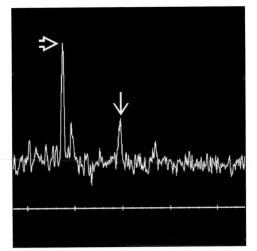

*(Left)* Axial FLAIR MR shows a pineal germinoma, isointense to gray matter, with some infiltration ➡ into the adjacent posterior thalamic nuclei. *(Right)* MRS (same lesion as previous image) shows a markedly elevated choline resonance ➡, with diminished NAA ➡. Despite this aggressive metabolite pattern, this tumor is very amenable to treatment with radiotherapy and chemotherapy.

### Typical

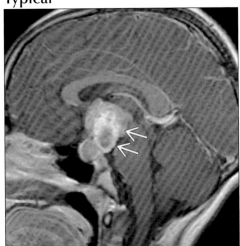

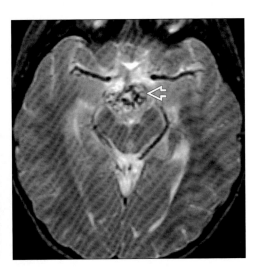

*(Left)* Sagittal T1 C+ MR shows a large, heterogeneous, enhancing suprasellar germinoma ➡ in a female with diabetes insipidus. Suprasellar tumors are more common than pineal region germ cell tumors. *(Right)* Axial T2WI MR (same tumor as previous image) shows punctate calcifications ➡. The strong male predominance for pineal region germinomas is not duplicated for those found in the suprasellar region.

# EMBRYONAL CARCINOMA

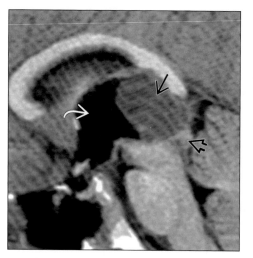

Sagittal T1WI MR shows a hypointense pineal region mass ➡. Note tectal compression ⊳ and dilated third ventricle ➡ secondary to aqueductal obstruction.

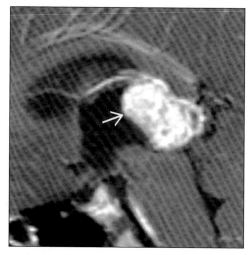

Sagittal T1 C+ MR in same patient as previous image shows the pineal region embryonal carcinoma ➡ to enhance robustly.

## TERMINOLOGY

### Abbreviations and Synonyms
• Malignant germ cell tumor (GCT)

### Definitions
• Malignant tumor composed of undifferentiated epithelial cells

## IMAGING FINDINGS

### General Features
• Best diagnostic clue: Heterogeneous pineal or suprasellar mass in adolescent
• Location: Hugs midline as do other CNS GCTs
• Size: Tumors in suprasellar, pineal region tend to be smaller
• Morphology: Typically well-circumscribed or lobulated

### CT Findings
• NECT: Heterogeneous, ± cysts and hemorrhage
• CECT: Variable enhancement

### MR Findings
• T1WI: Hypo- or isointense to GM, T1 shortening from blood, fat or protein
• T2WI: Isointense to slightly hyperintense to GM
• T2* GRE: Dephasing from hemorrhagic foci
• DWI: Solid portions have low diffusivity
• T1 C+: Heterogeneous enhancement, ± CSF spread
• MRS: ↑ Choline, ↑ lipid and lactate, ↓ NAA

### Imaging Recommendations
• Best imaging tool: MR of brain and spine with contrast
• Protocol advice: Pre-operative enhanced MR of entire neuraxis

## DIFFERENTIAL DIAGNOSIS

### Other Intracranial Germ Cell Tumors
• Germinoma, mixed germ cell tumor, yolk sac, teratoma

### Supratentorial PNET
• Typically intra-axial, lacking peritumoral edema

## DDx: Pediatric Pineal Region Masses

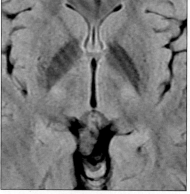

*Astrocytoma*

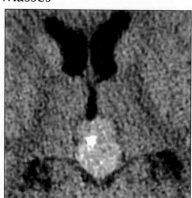

*Germinoma*

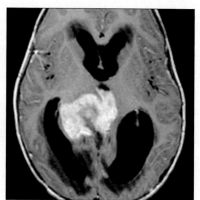

*Pineoblastoma*

# EMBRYONAL CARCINOMA

## Key Facts

### Imaging Findings
- Best diagnostic clue: Heterogeneous pineal or suprasellar mass in adolescent
- Location: Hugs midline as do other CNS GCTs
- T1 C+: Heterogeneous enhancement, ± CSF spread
- Best imaging tool: MR of brain and spine with contrast

### Top Differential Diagnoses
- Other Intracranial Germ Cell Tumors

- Supratentorial PNET

### Pathology
- Typically part of a mixed malignant germ cell tumor

### Diagnostic Checklist
- Embryonal carcinoma with heterogeneous pineal or suprasellar mass, metastasis from testicle tumor
- Difficult to differentiate from other CNS GCTs

## Other Tumors
- Astrocytoma, pineoblastoma, pineocytoma, dermoid

## PATHOLOGY

### General Features
- General path comments: Solid mass often with cysts and hemorrhage
- Genetics: Reports of near triploid complex karyotypes
- Etiology: Aberrations in: Histogenesis, germ cell migration, or stem cells
- Epidemiology: Rare (< 1% of all CNS tumors)
- Associated abnormalities: Klinefelter syndrome (47XXY)

### Gross Pathologic & Surgical Features
- Soft, often friable mass

### Microscopic Features
- Undifferentiated epithelial cells

### Staging, Grading or Classification Criteria
- Typically part of a mixed malignant germ cell tumor
  - Mixed tumor with benign tumor types ⇒ much better prognosis than mixed with largely malignant

## CLINICAL ISSUES

### Presentation
- Most common signs/symptoms: ↑ ICP, endocrine disturbance, Parinaud syndrome
- Clinical Profile: Lab: PLAP and cytokeratin markers

### Demographics
- Age: Peripubertal patients, rare < 4 years
- Gender: Males show slight increased incidence
- Ethnicity: More common in Asians

### Natural History & Prognosis
- Local invasive and metastatic potential

### Treatment
- Surgical resection → chemotherapy → radiation

## DIAGNOSTIC CHECKLIST

### Consider
- Embryonal carcinoma with heterogeneous pineal or suprasellar mass, metastasis from testicle tumor

### Image Interpretation Pearls
- Difficult to differentiate from other CNS GCTs

## SELECTED REFERENCES
1. Liang L et al: MRI of intracranial germ-cell tumours. Neuroradiology. 44(5):382-8, 2002

## IMAGE GALLERY

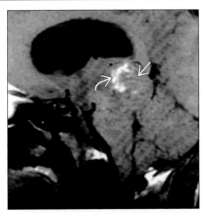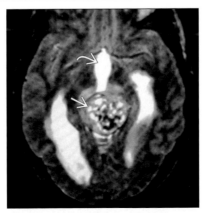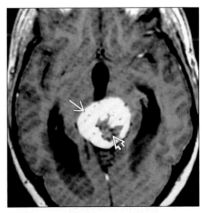

*(Left)* Sagittal T1WI MR shows a heterogeneous pineal region tumor ➡ that compresses the aqueduct and grows into the 3rd ventricle. Foci of T1 shortening ➡ correspond to intratumoral hemorrhage. *(Center)* Axial T2WI MR shows a heterogeneous pineal region embryonal carcinoma ➡. Note the 3rd ventricular enlargement ➡ secondary to aqueductal obstruction from tectal compression. *(Right)* Axial T1 C+ MR shows vibrant tumor enhancement ➡. The necrotic, hemorrhagic core ➡ lacks enhancement.

# TERATOMA

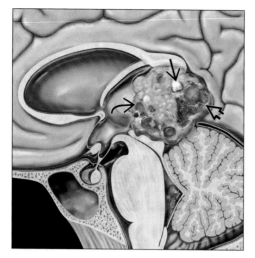
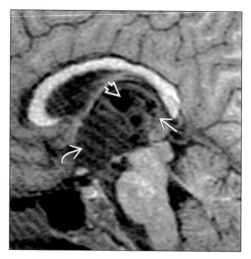

*Sagittal graphic shows a heterogeneous pineal region teratoma. There are fatty (yellow), cystic ➜, and solid ➤ elements. Also, note the calcific component ➤ of the tumor.*

*Sagittal T1WI MR shows a heterogeneous pineal region teratoma with cystic ➤ and solid ➤ components. Note the large suprasellar cystic element ➜ within anterior 3rd ventricle.*

## TERMINOLOGY

### Abbreviations and Synonyms
- Intracranial teratoma
- Benign germ cell tumor
- Congenital intracranial teratoma
- Intracranial germ cell tumor (GCT)

### Definitions
- Tridermal mass originating from
  - Displaced primordial germ cells
  - Embryonic stem cells become embedded in midline structures of: Head, mediastinum, sacrococcygeal regions
  - Divided into three subtypes
    - Mature teratoma
    - Immature teratoma
    - Teratoma with malignant transformation or malignant teratoma
- 2nd most common pineal tumor in children of all ages
- Congenital intracranial teratomas constitute 1/3-1/2 of all congenital brain tumors

## IMAGING FINDINGS

### General Features
- Best diagnostic clue
  - Midline mass containing: Ca++, soft tissue, cysts, and fat
  - Immature and malignant teratomas have smaller cystic elements, may have adjacent edema
- Location
  - Hugs midline
  - Two most common sites
    - Pineal region
    - Suprasellar region
  - Majority are supratentorial
- Size: Variable; holocranial teratomas are huge
- Morphology: Smaller tumors rounded ⇒ lobulated

### CT Findings
- NECT: Fat, soft tissue, Ca++, cystic attenuation
- CECT: Soft tissue components may enhance

### MR Findings
- T1WI
  - ↑ Signal from fat, variable signal from Ca++

## DDx: Mimics of Midline Intracranial Teratomas

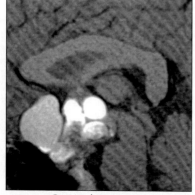
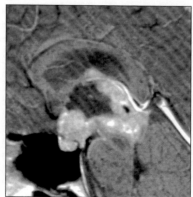
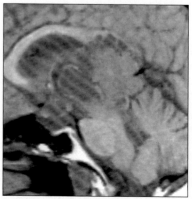

*Craniopharyngioma*

*Germinoma*

*Pineocytoma*

# TERATOMA

## Key Facts

### Terminology
- Intracranial teratoma
- Congenital intracranial teratoma
- Intracranial germ cell tumor (GCT)

### Imaging Findings
- Midline mass containing: Ca++, soft tissue, cysts, and fat
- Hugs midline
- Majority are supratentorial
- CECT: Soft tissue components may enhance
- ↑ Signal from fat, variable signal from Ca++
- Heterogeneous mass with internal shadowing (Ca++)
- In-utero ultrasound: Hydrocephalus, polyhydramnios, complex intracranial mass with shadowing (Ca++) elements
- CT demonstrates: Soft tissue, fat, and Ca++

### Top Differential Diagnoses
- Craniopharyngioma
- Dermoid
- Germinoma
- Non-Germinoma GCT
- Pineoblastoma

### Pathology
- Lobulated tridermal mass, tan-cream colored

### Clinical Issues
- HCG normal in mature teratoma

### Diagnostic Checklist
- Think teratoma in newborn with holocranial tumor
- Congenital intracranial teratoma when prenatal US shows a complex mass with calcifications

---

  - ○ Difficult to distinguish mature from immature by imaging
- T2WI: Soft tissue components iso- to hyperintense
- FLAIR: ↓ Signal from cysts, ↑ signal from solid tissue
- T2* GRE: ↓ Signal from Ca++
- T1 C+: Variable soft tissue enhancement
- MRS: ↑ Lipid moieties on short echo

### Ultrasonographic Findings
- Heterogeneous mass with internal shadowing (Ca++)
- In-utero ultrasound: Hydrocephalus, polyhydramnios, complex intracranial mass with shadowing (Ca++) elements

### Imaging Recommendations
- Best imaging tool
  - ○ CT demonstrates: Soft tissue, fat, and Ca++
  - ○ MR
    - Characterizes relationship of teratoma to midline structures
    - Identifies other associated anomalies
- Protocol advice: MR, + fat suppression helps to confirm fat content

## DIFFERENTIAL DIAGNOSIS

### Craniopharyngioma
- Partially Ca++/cystic/solid; no fat

### Dermoid
- Minimal to no enhancement

### Germinoma
- Increased attenuation on NECT
  - ○ Boys-pineal region, girls-suprasellar

### Non-Germinoma GCT
- Yolk sac tumor
- Embryonal carcinoma

### Other Mimics of Midline Intracranial Teratomas
- Pineoblastoma

- PNET
- Astrocytoma (rarely calcify)

## PATHOLOGY

### General Features
- General path comments
  - ○ Teratomas differentiate along ectodermal, endodermal, and mesodermal lines
  - ○ Mature teratomas are composed exclusively of fully differentiated, "adult-type" tissue elements that may be arranged in a pattern resembling normal tissue relationships; mitotic activity is low or absent
  - ○ Immature teratomas are composed of incompletely differentiated tissues resembling fetal tissues
  - ○ Malignant teratomas reflect a generic designation for a teratomatous neoplasm that contains an additional malignant component of conventional somatic type
  - ○ Lobulated tridermal mass, tan-cream colored
  - ○ ↑ AFP if tumor contains enteric glandular elements
    - Yolk sac or embryonal elements
- Genetics
  - ○ Diploid or near diploid
  - ○ Molecular biology of germ cell tumors
    - Loss of Ch 4, 9p, 11q, 13q, 18q
    - Gain of Ch 8q, 21, 1q, 12p
- Etiology
  - ○ Originates during 3rd and 4th week of fetal development
  - ○ Mis-migration of primordial germ cells
  - ○ Anomalous development of primitive streak or its derivatives
- Epidemiology
  - ○ 2-4% of intracranial tumors < 15 years of age
  - ○ 33% of intracranial tumors in the neonate
- Associated abnormalities: Klinefelter syndrome and sex chromosome aberration

### Gross Pathologic & Surgical Features
- Mature teratomas ⇒ fully differentiated tissue
  - ○ Ectoderm, endoderm, mesoderm

# TERATOMA

- Immature teratoma ⇒ resembles fetal tissues
- Malignant teratoma may include elements of
  - Adenocarcinoma, squamous cell carcinoma, sarcoma, or mesenchymal carcinoma

## Microscopic Features
- Mature teratoma ⇒ mature tridermal tissue
  - Neuroectodermal elements: Neuroepithelial rosettes and tubules
  - Mesodermal elements: Immature cartilage, primitive stroma, muscle
  - Endodermal elements: Respiratory and enteric epithelium
- Immature or malignant ⇒ mitotically active stroma, + primitive neuroectodermal elements

## Staging, Grading or Classification Criteria
- WHO classification
  - Mature; immature, or malignant transformation

# CLINICAL ISSUES

## Presentation
- Most common signs/symptoms
  - Pineal lesions ⇒ Parinaud syndrome
  - Macrocephaly, secondary obstructive hydrocephalus, diabetes insipidus
- Other signs/symptoms
  - HCG normal in mature teratoma
  - Elevated HCG in blood and CSF typically means a mixed germ cell tumor
    - Embryonal and/or choriocarcinoma components
  - Elevated AFP indicates yolk sac and/or embryonal components
- Clinical Profile: In-utero demonstration of hydrocephalus and heterogeneous mass

## Demographics
- Age
  - Congenital intracranial teratoma detected in-utero or as neonate
  - Non-neonatal form has presentation younger than germinoma
- Gender: Males > females (3:1 to 10:1)
- Ethnicity
  - More common among Asians
    - In Japan and Taiwan, GCTs account for 11% of intracranial tumors

## Natural History & Prognosis
- Varies with size, location and classification
- Mature teratoma
  - 5 year survival approaches 100% if lesion is resectable
  - Holocranial form of congenital intracranial teratoma has a high mortality rate
- Immature teratoma
  - If serum HCG and AFP are elevated, prognosis is less favorable
  - 5 year survival ~ 67%
- Malignant teratoma
  - Chance of survival at 5 years 18-50%

- Congenital intracranial teratoma may cause death from brainstem compression
- Growth of congenital intracranial teratoma may be rapid

## Treatment
- Mature teratoma
  - Surgical resection, operative mortality ~ 20%
- Immature teratoma: Surgery and adjunctive therapy
- Malignant teratoma: Surgery and aggressive adjunctive chemoradiation

# DIAGNOSTIC CHECKLIST

## Consider
- Think teratoma in newborn with holocranial tumor
- Congenital intracranial teratoma when prenatal US shows a complex mass with calcifications

## Image Interpretation Pearls
- Midline tumor containing: Fat, soft tissue, and Ca++

# SELECTED REFERENCES

1. Erman T et al: Congenital intracranial immature teratoma of the lateral ventricle: a case report and review of the literature. Neurol Res. 27(1):53-6, 2005
2. Woodward PJ et al: From the archives of the AFIP: a comprehensive review of fetal tumors with pathologic correlation. Radiographics. 25(1):215-42, 2005
3. Yokoi K et al: RNA expression analysis of a congenital intracranial teratoma. Pediatr Blood Cancer. 44(5):516-20, 2005
4. Isaacs H Jr: Perinatal (fetal and neonatal) germ cell tumors. J Pediatr Surg. 39(7):1003-13, 2004
5. Sandow BA et al: Best cases from the AFIP: congenital intracranial teratoma. Radiographics. 24(4):1165-70, 2004
6. Yagi K et al: Growing teratoma syndrome in a patient with a non-germinomatous germ cell tumor in the neurohypophysis--case report. Neurol Med Chir (Tokyo). 44(1):33-7, 2004
7. Cavalheiro S et al: Fetal brain tumors. Childs Nerv Syst. 19(7-8):529-36, 2003
8. Im SH et al: Congenital intracranial teratoma: prenatal diagnosis and postnatal successful resection. Med Pediatr Oncol. 40(1):57-61, 2003
9. Isaacs H Jr: I. Perinatal brain tumors: a review of 250 cases. Pediatr Neurol. 27(4):249-61, 2002
10. Jaing TH et al: Intracranial germ cell tumors: a retrospective study of 44 children. Pediatr Neurol. 26(5):369-73, 2002
11. Liang L et al: MRI of intracranial germ-cell tumours. Neuroradiology. 44(5):382-8, 2002
12. Rodriguez-Mojica W et al: Prenatal sonographic evaluation of two intracranial teratomas. P R Health Sci J. 21(1):43-5, 2002
13. Ortega-Aznar A et al: Neonatal tumors of the CNS: a report of 9 cases and a review. Clin Neuropathol. 20(5):181-9, 2001

# TERATOMA

## IMAGE GALLERY

### Typical

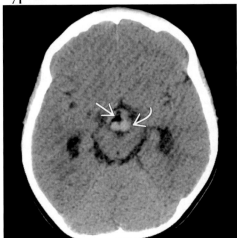

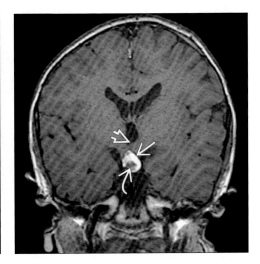

*(Left)* Axial NECT shows a small suprasellar teratoma with low attenuation fat ➜ and calcific ⟿ elements. Also note the temporal horn dilation secondary to 3rd ventricular compression. *(Right)* Coronal T1WI MR shows the hyperintense fatty ➜ and hypointense calcific ➜ components of the suprasellar teratoma. Note the compression of the lower 3rd ventricle ➜.

### Variant

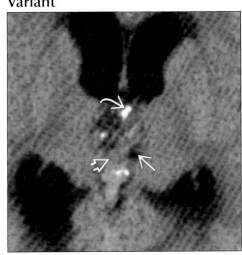

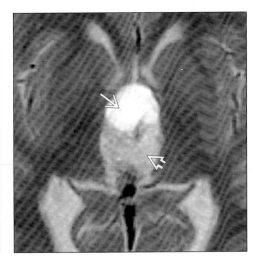

*(Left)* Axial NECT shows an immature teratoma of the pineal region with fatty ➜, calcific ➜, and solid ➜ elements. Note the ventricular obstruction and periventricular interstitial edema. *(Right)* Axial T2WI MR shows a partially cystic ➜, and solid ➜, immature teratoma of the pineal region. The dominant cystic component ➜ grows anteriorly into the suprasellar cistern.

### Variant

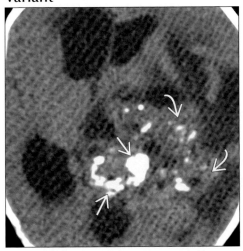

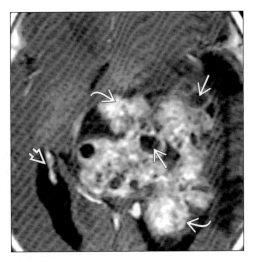

*(Left)* Axial NECT shows a heavily calcified ➜ predominantly solid ➜ immature teratoma which arose within the left thalamus leading to ventricular compression and subfalcial herniation. *(Right)* Axial T1 C+ MR shows a heterogeneous enhancing principally solid ➜, partially cystic ➜ immature teratoma. There is subfalcial herniation and right lateral ventricular obstruction ➜.

# PINEOBLASTOMA

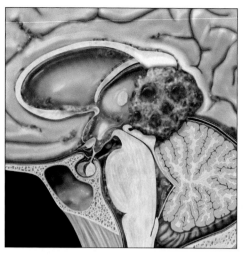

Sagittal graphic shows large, heterogeneous pineal mass with areas of hemorrhage and necrosis. Note compression of adjacent structures, hydrocephalus, and diffuse CSF seeding.

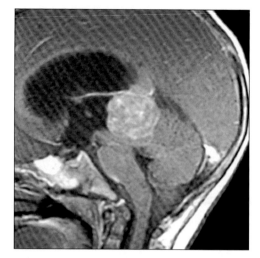

Sagittal T1 C+ MR shows a heterogeneously enhancing pineal mass consistent with PB. Proximity of the lesion to the cerebral aqueduct causes hydrocephalus, seen in nearly all cases of PB.

## TERMINOLOGY

### Abbreviations and Synonyms
- Pineoblastoma (PB)
- Primitive neuroectodermal tumor (PNET) of pineal gland

### Definitions
- Highly malignant, primitive embryonal tumor of pineal gland

## IMAGING FINDINGS

### General Features
- Best diagnostic clue
  ○ Large, heterogeneous, enhancing pineal mass with hydrocephalus
    ▪ "Exploded" peripheral Ca++ on CT classic
    ▪ Solid portion hyperdense on CT, iso- hypointense on T2
- Location
  ○ Pineal gland

- ○ Frequent extension/invasion into third ventricle, thalamus, midbrain, cerebellar vermis
- ○ Proximity to cerebral aqueduct accounts for hydrocephalus in nearly 100%
- Size: Large; most ≥ 3 cm
- Morphology: Lobular mass with ill-defined margins

### CT Findings
- NECT
  ○ Mixed density; solid portion frequently hyperdense
  ○ Peripheral, "exploded" Ca++ classic
- CECT: Weak to moderate heterogeneous enhancement

### MR Findings
- T1WI: Solid portion iso- to hypointense (compared to cortical gray matter)
- T2WI
  ○ Solid portion iso- to hypointense
  ○ Frequent necrosis; occasional hemorrhage
  ○ Mild peritumoral edema characteristic
- T2* GRE: Ca++, hemorrhage may bloom
- DWI: Solid portion frequently hyperintense
- T1 C+: Moderate, heterogeneous enhancement
- MRS
  ○ ↑ Cho, ↓ NAA

### DDx: Pediatric Pineal Region Lesions

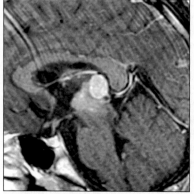

*Germinoma*

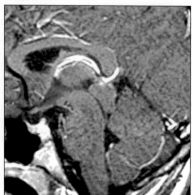

*Tectal Glioma*

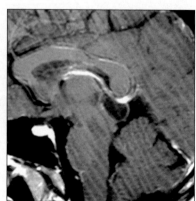

*Pineal Cyst*

# PINEOBLASTOMA

## Key Facts

### Terminology
- Highly malignant, primitive embryonal tumor of pineal gland

### Imaging Findings
- Large, heterogeneous, enhancing pineal mass with hydrocephalus

### Top Differential Diagnoses
- Germ Cell Tumors (GCTs)
- Astrocytoma
- Pineal Cyst
- Pineocytoma
- Meningioma
- Epidermoid/Dermoid

### Pathology
- PBs largely undifferentiated, similar to other PNETs

### Clinical Issues
- Elevated ICP: Headache, nausea, vomiting, lethargy, papilledema, abducens nerve palsy
- Prognosis
- Poor: Median post-surgical survival = 24-30 months

### Diagnostic Checklist
- Both PBs and germinomas frequently hyperdense on CT and prone to CSF dissemination
- Peripheral "exploded" Ca++ in PB and central "engulfed" Ca++ in germinoma: Classic but variable

---

- Prominent glutamate and taurine peak (~ 3.4 ppm) described at TE 20 ms

## Nuclear Medicine Findings
- PET: Increased F-18 FDG uptake

## Angiographic Findings
- Variable: Hyper- and hypovascular mass described

## Imaging Recommendations
- Best imaging tool: Contrast-enhanced MR
- Protocol advice
  - Image entire neuraxis
  - Sagittal images ideal for pineal region anatomy

## DIFFERENTIAL DIAGNOSIS

### Germ Cell Tumors (GCTs)
- 1% CNS tumors in Western population; 4% in Asia
- 2nd decade presentation
- Germinoma
  - Most common GCT and pineal region tumor (PRT)
  - M >> F
  - Homogeneous, hyperdense (iso-/hypointense T2WI) mass with intense uniform enhancement
    - Central, "engulfed" Ca++ classic
  - Coexistent suprasellar mass pathognomonic
  - Elevation of CSF/serum placental alkaline phosphatase (PLAP) characteristic
- Mature teratoma
  - 2nd most common GCT & PRT; M >> F
  - Heterogeneous mass with cysts, Ca++ and fat density
- Choriocarcinoma, endodermal sinus tumor, embryonal cell carcinoma
  - Uncommon, highly malignant tumors
  - Nonspecific imaging appearance but characteristic elevation of serum tumor markers
    - Choriocarcinoma: β-hCG
    - Endodermal sinus tumor: AFP
    - Embryonal cell carcinoma: β-hCG and AFP
- 10% of GCTs are mixed histology (mixed GCT)

### Astrocytoma
- Usually arises from thalamus or midbrain tectum
- Pilocytic astrocytoma (WHO grade I) most common
- Tectal astrocytoma
  - Nonenhancing, expansile tectal mass
- Thalamic astrocytoma
  - Enhancing solid mass or cyst with nodule

### Pineal Cyst
- Small cyst with no to minimal rim enhancement
- Frequent incidental finding
- Rare large cyst can cause hydrocephalus

### Pineocytoma
- More common in 3rd and 4th decades
- Differentiated tumor arising from pineal gland parenchyma
- Well-defined, round, homogeneous mass with peripheral or central homogeneous enhancement

### Meningioma
- Uncommon in pediatric age group
- Intensely enhancing dural based mass

### Epidermoid/Dermoid
- Pineal location uncommon in pediatric age group
- Nonenhancing, cyst-like lesion, hyperintense on diffusion (epidermoid) or with fat density (dermoid)

### Metastases
- Pineal gland metastases uncommon in children
- Adenocarcinoma reported

## PATHOLOGY

### General Features
- General path comments
  - Three pineal parenchymal tumors (PPTs) distinguished by WHO based on degree of differentiation: Pineocytoma, PPT of intermediate differentiation, PB

# PINEOBLASTOMA

- PBs largely undifferentiated, similar to other PNETs
  - PPTs may have photosensory, astrocytic, neuronal or mixed differentiation
    - Photosensory differentiation unique to PPTs and retinal tumors
- Genetics
  - No TP53 mutations
  - Genetically distinct from infratentorial PNET (medulloblastoma)
  - Trilateral retinoblastoma has PB-like pineal PNET
- Etiology
  - Derived from embryonic precursors of pineal parenchymal cells (pinealocytes)
  - Pinealocyte = cell with photosensory, neuroendocrine function
  - Common phylogenetic origin of retina and pineal gland as light-sensing organs
- Epidemiology
  - PPTs comprise 15% of pineal region neoplasms
  - PBs comprise 30-45% of PPTs

## Gross Pathologic & Surgical Features
- Soft, friable, poorly marginated, infiltrative tumor
- CSF dissemination at autopsy frequent

## Microscopic Features
- Patternless sheets of densely packed, small, undifferentiated cells with round hyperchromatic nuclei and high nuclear:cytoplasmic ratio
  - Identical to other PNETs
  - Accounts for dense/T2 hypointense appearance
- Occasional Homer-Wright or Flexner-Wintersteiner rosettes
- Necrosis and hemorrhage common
- Mitoses common, MIB-1 elevated
- Immunohistochemistry: Variable immunolabeling for synaptophysin, neuronal specific enolase, neurofilaments, chromogranin A, class III beta-tubulin, and retinal S antigen

## Staging, Grading or Classification Criteria
- WHO grade IV
- New prognostic grading system for PPTs
  - Grade 1 = pineocytoma (WHO II)
  - Grade 2 and 3 = PPTs with intermediate differentiation
    - Grade 2: < 6 mitoses and (+) immunolabeling for neurofilaments
    - Grade 3: ≥ 6 mitoses or < 6 mitoses but (-) immunolabeling for neurofilaments
  - Grade 4 = PB

# CLINICAL ISSUES

## Presentation
- Most common signs/symptoms
  - Elevated ICP: Headache, nausea, vomiting, lethargy, papilledema, abducens nerve palsy
  - Parinaud syndrome, ataxia
- Clinical Profile
  - Young child with signs/symptoms of elevated ICP and Parinaud syndrome

  - No elevation of CSF/serum tumor markers

## Demographics
- Age: Children > adults; up to 40% occur in infants
- Gender: Slight male preponderance
- Ethnicity: Equal to slightly greater incidence in Western population compared to Asia

## Natural History & Prognosis
- Natural History
  - CSF seeding
    - 16-45% present with spinal CSF dissemination
  - Rare reports hematogenous metastases to bone
- Prognosis
  - Poor: Median post-surgical survival = 24-30 months
  - Age ≤ 1, CSF dissemination, and occurrence in context of trilateral retinoblastoma associated with particularly poor prognosis

## Treatment
- Third ventriculostomy or VP shunt for hydrocephalus
- Surgical resection of tumor plus cranial/spinal radiation and chemotherapy
- No radiation therapy in young children
- High dose chemotherapy with stem cell rescue may improve survival particularly in high risk patients, young children

# DIAGNOSTIC CHECKLIST

## Consider
- Could pineal region mass be GCT (more common)?

## Image Interpretation Pearls
- Both PBs and germinomas frequently hyperdense on CT and prone to CSF dissemination
- Peripheral "exploded" Ca++ in PB and central "engulfed" Ca++ in germinoma: Classic but variable
- Clinical pearl: Pineal region astrocytomas typically do not present with Parinaud syndrome

# SELECTED REFERENCES

1. Cuccia V et al: Pinealoblastomas in children. Childs Nerv Syst. 2006
2. Li MH et al: Molecular genetics of supratentorial primitive neuroectodermal tumors and pineoblastoma. Neurosurg Focus. 2005
3. Parwani AV et al: Pineal gland lesions: a cytopathologic study of 20 specimens. Cancer. 105(2):80-6, 2005
4. Bruce JN et al: Surgical strategies for treating patients with pineal region tumors. J Neurooncol. 69(1-3):221-36, 2004
5. Gururangan S et al: High-dose chemotherapy with autologous stem-cell rescue in children and adults with newly diagnosed pineoblastomas. J Clin Oncol. 2003
6. Konovalov AN et al: Principles of treatment of the pineal region tumors. Surg Neurol. 59(4): 250-68, 2003
7. Korogi Y et al: MRI of pineal region tumors. J Neurooncol. 54(3):251-61, 2001
8. Jouvet A et al: Pineal parenchymal tumors: a correlation of histological features with prognosis in 66 cases. Brain Pathol. 10(1):49-60, 2000
9. Nakamura M et al: Neuroradiological characteristics of pineocytoma and pineoblastoma. Neuroradiology. 42(7):509-14, 2000

# PINEOBLASTOMA

## IMAGE GALLERY

### Typical

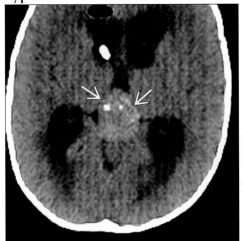
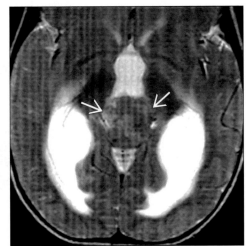

*(Left)* Axial NECT status post stereotactic biopsy shows a hyperdense pineal region mass ➡. Peripheral ("exploded") calcifications are classic, but variable findings for PB. *(Right)* Axial T2WI MR shows a mildly heterogeneous pineal region tumor ➡ causing hydrocephalus. The solid portion of tumor is hypointense to cortex. Both PB and germinoma can have this appearance.

### Typical

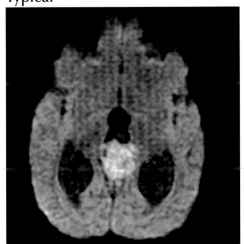
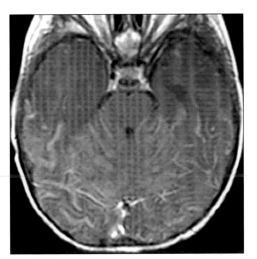

*(Left)* Axial DWI MR shows reduced diffusivity (hyperintensity) within a PB. The increased cellularity and high nuclear:cytoplasmic ratio account for the imaging appearance of PB on T2 and DWI. *(Right)* Axial T1 C+ MR shows diffuse leptomeningeal tumor dissemination in an infant five months after presentation. Prognosis in infants with PB is particularly poor.

### Variant

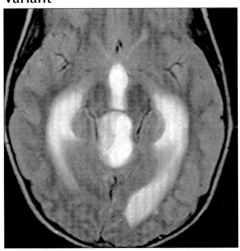
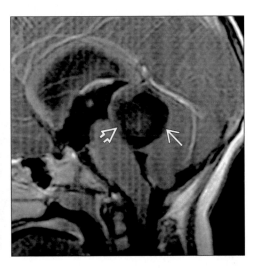

*(Left)* Axial T2WI MR shows a predominantly cystic tumor in the pineal region. While PBs are heterogeneous with multiple small areas of necrosis, a large dominant cyst, as in this case, is unusual. *(Right)* Sagittal T1 C+ MR (same patient as previous image) shows the PB with a dominant, large cyst. Note mass effect of the lesion on the cerebellum ➡ and tectal plate ➡.

# PINEAL CYST

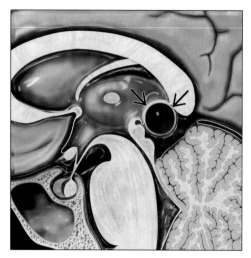

Sagittal graphic shows a small cystic lesion within the pineal gland ➡. Small benign pineal cysts (PCs) are often found incidentally at autopsy or imaging.

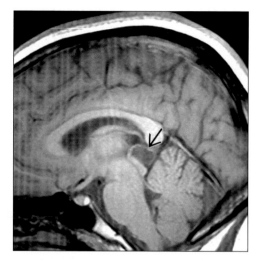

Sagittal T1WI MR shows large pineal cyst ➡. Note that despite the large size of the lesion and the apparent compression of the superior colliculus, there is no hydrocephalus.

## TERMINOLOGY

### Abbreviations and Synonyms
- Pineal cyst (PC); glial cyst of pineal gland

### Definitions
- Non-neoplastic intrapineal glial-lined cyst

## IMAGING FINDINGS

### General Features
- Best diagnostic clue: 5 mm or larger fluid-filled mass within pineal gland
- Location: Above tectum, below internal cerebral veins (ICVs)
- Size: Most are small (5-10 mm) but can be 20 mm or more
- Morphology
  - Round/ovoid, relatively thin-walled cyst
    - May flatten tectum (especially superior colliculus), occasionally compress aqueduct
    - May be uni- or multiloculated

### CT Findings
- NECT
  - Sharply-demarcated, smooth cyst behind 3rd ventricle
    - Fluid iso-/slightly hyperdense to CSF
    - 25% Ca++ in cyst wall but Ca++ rare if < 5 years old
    - Rare: Very hyperdense cyst with acute hemorrhage ("pineal apoplexy")
- CECT: Rim or nodular enhancement

### MR Findings
- T1WI
  - 55-60% slightly hyperintense to CSF on T1WI
  - 40% isointense
  - 1-2%: Hemorrhage (heterogeneous or fluid-fluid level)
- T2WI: Iso-/hyperintense to CSF
- PD/Intermediate: Majority hyperintense to CSF
- FLAIR: Hyperintense to CSF
- T2* GRE: Occasionally blooming caused by old or recent hemorrhage
- DWI: Typically not bright; similar to CSF
- T1 C+

## DDx: Mimics

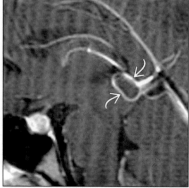

Pineocytoma

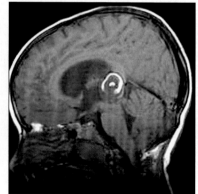

Teratoma

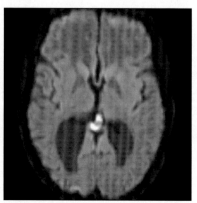

Epidermoid Cyst

# PINEAL CYST

## Key Facts

### Terminology
- Non-neoplastic intrapineal glial-lined cyst

### Imaging Findings
- Best diagnostic clue: 5 mm or larger fluid-filled mass within pineal gland
- 55-60% slightly hyperintense to CSF on T1WI
- FLAIR: Hyperintense to CSF
- Thin (< 2 mm) rim of enhancement typical but can be nodular

### Top Differential Diagnoses
- Pineocytoma
- Trilateral Retinoblastoma
- Epidermoid
- Arachnoid Cyst

### Clinical Issues
- Large cysts (> 1 cm) may (rarely) become symptomatic
- Small cysts very common at ages 0-10 years
- Gender: M:F = 1:3
- Cysts can form or involute over time
- If > 1 cm, nodularity, or associated clinical symptoms ⇒ recommend short interval follow-up

### Diagnostic Checklist
- Asymptomatic pineal cysts are a common incidental finding
- Some literature ⇒ benign pineal cyst can't be distinguished from neoplasm (pineocytoma) by imaging alone

---

  - Thin (< 2 mm) rim of enhancement typical but can be nodular
    - Enhancing tissue is pineal gland
  - Cystic areas may fill in on delayed scans, resembling solid tumor
- MRV: Internal cerebral veins (ICVs) may be elevated by large lesions

### Imaging Recommendations
- Best imaging tool: MR with/without contrast
- Protocol advice: Use sagittal thin sections (3 mm) or volumetric imaging

## DIFFERENTIAL DIAGNOSIS

### Pineocytoma
- Usually solid but rarely cystic tumors occur
- Consider if enhancing cyst wall > 2 mm thick
- May be indistinguishable from benign pineal cyst on imaging, require histology for definitive diagnosis
- Both pineal cyst, indolent pineocytoma may not change on serial imaging
- Uncommon in children but do occur (average age 34)

### Trilateral Retinoblastoma
- Pineal cysts may occur with increased incidence in bilateral retinoblastoma
- True pineal retinoblastoma are mass-like, not cysts

### Epidermoid
- Quadrigeminal cistern relatively rare location
- "Cauliflower" configuration
- Bright on DWI

### Arachnoid Cyst
- No Ca++ or enhancement
- Follows CSF attenuation, signal intensity

### Germinoma
- Typically solid but cystic variants can occur, consider if precocious puberty

### Teratoma
- Solid and cystic mass, fat typically present

### Astrocytoma
- Solid and cystic mass

### Choroid Plexus Papilloma
- Rare (one case report), cystic and solid enhancing mass

## PATHOLOGY

### General Features
- General path comments
  - Embryology
    - Primitive pineal diverticulum divides into pineal recess, cavum pineal
    - Cavum pineal: Patent cavity within gland lined by ependyma communicating with 3rd ventricle
    - Cavum pineal usually obliterated by glial fibers
    - Incomplete obliteration may leave residual cavity
- Genetics: None known
- Etiology
  - Etiology-pathogenesis: Major theories
    - Enlargement of embryonic pineal cavity
    - Ischemic glial degeneration ± hemorrhagic expansion
    - Small pre-existing cysts enlarge with hormonal influences
    - Degeneration of cells that differentiate into ependyma or neuroglia
- Epidemiology
  - 0.6% prevalence of cysts 5 mm or greater in children on MR (24% if include < 5 mm)
  - 25-40% have cysts < 1.0 cm at autopsy (adults and children, includes cysts < 5 mm)
- Associated abnormalities: Hydrocephalus (uncommon, cyst usually > 2 cm)

### Gross Pathologic & Surgical Features
- Smooth, soft, tan to yellow cyst wall
- Fluid contents vary from clear yellow (most common) to hemorrhagic

# PINEAL CYST

- 80% < 10 mm
- Can be large (reported up to 4.5 cm)

## Microscopic Features
- Outer thin leptomeningeal fibrous layer
- Middle layer of pineal parenchyma, with/without Ca++
- Inner layer of glial tissue
- Hemorrhage may be present

## CLINICAL ISSUES

### Presentation
- Most common signs/symptoms
  - Vast majority incidental
  - Large cysts (> 1 cm) may (rarely) become symptomatic
    - 50% headache (aqueduct compression, hydrocephalus)
    - 10% Parinaud syndrome (tectal compression)
    - Vertigo
    - Visual symptoms
- Other signs/symptoms: Very rare: "Pineal apoplexy" with intracystic hemorrhage, acute hydrocephalus, sudden death
- Clinical Profile: Young female with nonfocal headache

### Demographics
- Age
  - Cysts > 5 mm: Low incidence 0-10 years, 3% incidence 11-20 years, 3.4% 21-30 years, decreasing to < 0.5 at 70 years
  - Males: Little change with age; peak 11-20 years
  - Females: Significant age variation; peak 21-30 years
  - Small cysts very common at ages 0-10 years
- Gender: M:F = 1:3
- Ethnicity: None known

### Natural History & Prognosis
- Cysts can form or involute over time
- Size generally remains unchanged in males
- Cystic expansion of pineal in some females begins in adolescence, decreases with aging
- Rare: Sudden expansion, hemorrhage ("pineal apoplexy")
- Single case report of choroid plexus papilloma arising in pineal cyst

### Treatment
- Usually none
- Atypical/symptomatic lesions may require stereotactic aspiration or biopsy/resection
- If > 1 cm, nodularity, or associated clinical symptoms ⇒ recommend short interval follow-up

## DIAGNOSTIC CHECKLIST

### Consider
- Asymptomatic pineal cysts are a common incidental finding

- MR appearance varies from uncomplicated nonenhancing cyst to heterogeneous nodular or ring-like enhancing cyst

### Image Interpretation Pearls
- Some literature ⇒ benign pineal cyst can't be distinguished from neoplasm (pineocytoma) by imaging alone
- Area of controversy: Are pineocytomas over diagnosed at biopsy?

## SELECTED REFERENCES

1. Beck Popovic M et al: Benign pineal cysts in children with bilateral retinoblastoma: a new variant of trilateral retinoblastoma? Pediatr Blood Cancer. 46(7):755-61, 2006
2. Karatza EC et al: Pineal cyst simulating pinealoblastoma in 11 children with retinoblastoma. Arch Ophthalmol. 124(4):595-7, 2006
3. Patel AJ et al: Pineal cyst apoplexy: case report and review of the literature. Neurosurgery. 57(5):E1066; discussion E1066, 2005
4. Hayashida Y et al: Pineal cystic germinoma with syncytiotrophoblastic giant cells mimicking MR imaging findings of a pineal cyst. AJNR Am J Neuroradiol. 25(9):1538-40, 2004
5. Mandera M et al: Pineal cysts in childhood. Childs Nerv Syst. 19(10-11):750-5, 2003
6. Michielsen G et al: Symptomatic pineal cysts: clinical manifestations and management. Acta Neurochir (Wien). 144(3):233-42; discussion 242, 2002
7. Petitcolin V et al: [Prevalence and morphology of pineal cysts discovered at pituitary MRI: review of 1844 examinations] J Radiol. 83(2 Pt 1):141-5, 2002
8. Barboriak DP et al: Serial MR imaging of pineal cysts: implications for natural history and follow-up. AJR Am J Roentgenol. 176(3):737-43, 2001
9. Korogi Y et al: MRI of pineal region tumors. J Neurooncol. 54(3):251-61, 2001
10. Engel U et al: Cystic lesions of the pineal region--MRI and pathology. Neuroradiology. 42(6):399-402, 2000
11. Tartara F et al: Glial cyst of the pineal gland: case report and considerations about surgical management. J Neurosurg Sci. 44(2):89-93, 2000
12. Kang HS et al: Large glial cyst of the pineal gland: a possible growth mechanism. Case report. J Neurosurg. 88(1):138-40, 1998
13. Steven DA et al: A choroid plexus papilloma arising from an incidental pineal cyst. AJNR Am J Neuroradiol. 17(5):939-42, 1996
14. Sawamura Y et al: Magnetic resonance images reveal a high incidence of asymptomatic pineal cysts in young women. Neurosurgery. 37(1):11-5; discussion 15-6, 1995
15. Sener RN: The pineal gland: a comparative MR imaging study in children and adults with respect to normal anatomical variations and pineal cysts. Pediatr Radiol. 25(4):245-8, 1995
16. Fain JS et al: Symptomatic glial cysts of the pineal gland. J Neurosurg. 80(3):454-60, 1994
17. Fleege MA et al: Benign glial cysts of the pineal gland: unusual imaging characteristics with histologic correlation. AJNR Am J Neuroradiol. 15(1):161-6, 1994
18. Di Costanzo A et al: Pineal cysts: an incidental MRI finding? J Neurol Neurosurg Psychiatry. 56(2):207-8, 1993
19. Golzarian J et al: Pineal cyst: normal or pathological? Neuroradiology. 35(4):251-3, 1993
20. Mamourian AC et al: Enhancement of pineal cysts on MR images. AJNR Am J Neuroradiol. 12(4):773-4, 1991

# PINEAL CYST

## IMAGE GALLERY

### Variant

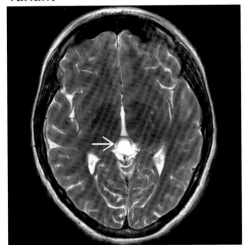
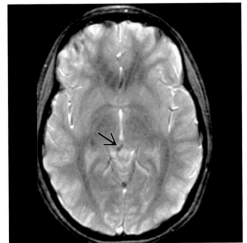

*(Left)* Axial T2WI MR shows large pineal cyst ➡ to remain isointense to CSF. No associated ventriculomegaly is present. *(Right)* Axial T2* GRE MR shows blooming ➡ anteromedial to the cyst. The blooming is likely due to hemosiderin or, more likely, calcification in the adjacent pineal gland.

### Typical

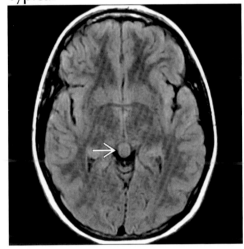
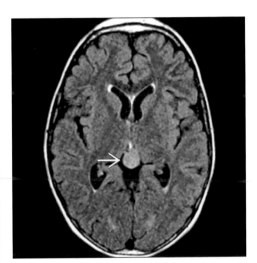

*(Left)* Axial FLAIR MR shows pineal cyst ➡ that is isointense to brain. This suggests the presence of protein or hemorrhage within the cyst. *(Right)* Axial FLAIR MR shows pineal cyst ➡ to be hyperintense with respect to brain and some periventricular hyperintensity. Contrast should be administered to ensure that this is not a tumor.

### Typical

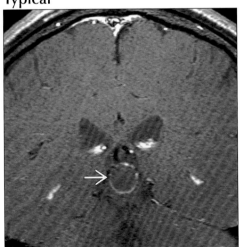
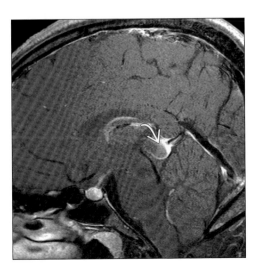

*(Left)* Coronal T1 C+ MR shows thin enhancing rim ➡, confirming the diagnosis of pineal cyst. Enhancing rim is normal pineal tissue. Tumors show more extensive enhancement. *(Right)* Sagittal T1 C+ MR (same patient as previous image) shows thin enhancing rim is slightly thicker posteriorly, resulting from cyst being asymmetric within the gland. Some contrast is leaking into cyst ➡.

I

3

19

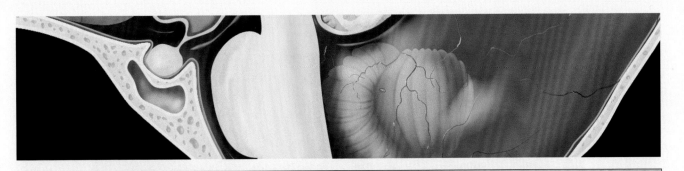

# SECTION 4: Cerebellum/Brain Stem

# BRAINSTEM TUMORS

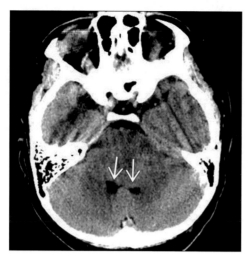

Axial NECT shows low attenuation and marked expansion of the pons with compression and posterior displacement of the fourth ventricle ➡.

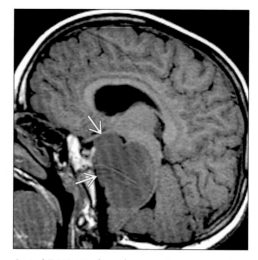

Sagittal T1WI MR shows large pontine tumor, pushing midbrain up and pontomedullary junction down. Anterior exophytic ➡ portion extends into suprasellar and prepontine cisterns.

## TERMINOLOGY

### Abbreviations and Synonyms
- Brain stem tumors (BST), brain stem glioma (BSG), pontine glioma, diffuse pontine glioma (DPG), midbrain glioma, medullary glioma, dorsally exophytic medullary glioma

### Definitions
- BST distinguished by location and imaging/histology characteristics of tumor
  - Medullary, pontine, mesencephalic, or tectal
  - Diffuse or focal
  - Most large pontine tumors are fibrillary astrocytomas
    - Nonenhancing, poorly marginated, expansile
  - Primitive neuroectodermal tumors (PNET), pilocytic astrocytomas (PA), glioblastomas (GBM) can occur
    - PA more likely to be dorsally exophytic, medullary or cervicomedullary
    - GBM usually rim-enhancing
    - PA has best prognosis, GBM worst
    - All histologies occur in midbrain
- Tectal gliomas are distinct

  - Present with hydrocephalus in 6-10 year olds
  - Rarely progressive
  - Shunting is often only treatment required
- BST associated with Neurofibromatosis type I ⇒ another distinct group
  - Rarely enlarge, often asymptomatic

## IMAGING FINDINGS

### General Features
- Best diagnostic clue
  - Pons is most common location
    - Typically nonenhancing expansile mass
- Location
  - Cervico-medullary junction to cerebral peduncles
    - Separate into medullary, pontine, mesencephalic, and tectal tumors
- Size: Any size
- Morphology
  - Depends on histology; focal vs. large/infiltrative
    - Sometimes exophytic
    - Invasion of midbrain or medulla ⇒ higher grade

## DDx: Brain Stem Tumor

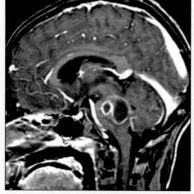

Brain Stem Abscess

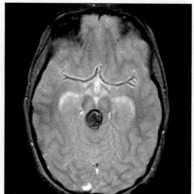

Cavernoma

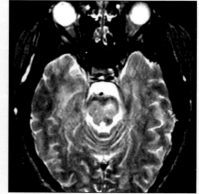

Demyelination

# BRAINSTEM TUMORS

## Key Facts

### Terminology
- BST distinguished by location and imaging/histology characteristics of tumor
- Most large pontine tumors are fibrillary astrocytomas
- Primitive neuroectodermal tumors (PNET), pilocytic astrocytomas (PA), glioblastomas (GBM) can occur
- Tectal gliomas are distinct

### Imaging Findings
- Pons is most common location
- Invasion of midbrain or medulla ⇒ higher grade
- Foci of reduced diffusion may reflect necrosis or higher grade
- GBM ⇒ often rim-enhancement
- Include sagittal T2 or FLAIR images ⇒ tumor extent

### Top Differential Diagnoses
- Brainstem Encephalitis, Rhombencephalitis, Abscess
- Acute Disseminated Encephalomyelitis (ADEM)
- Neurofibromatosis Type 1 (NF1)
- Cavernoma

### Pathology
- ~ 15% Of pediatric brain tumors

### Clinical Issues
- Cranial nerve palsies with long tract signs
- Age: Peak incidence ~ 3-10 years old
- Median survival ~ 1 year

### Diagnostic Checklist
- Flattening of floor of 4th ventricle on CT ⇒ proceed to MR with contrast

## CT Findings
- NECT
  - Decreased attenuation and enlargement of affected region
  - Pontine tumors ⇒ flattening of anterior border of 4th ventricle
    - Streak artifact from petrous pyramids can hamper detection
- CECT: Mild to absent enhancement

## MR Findings
- T1WI
  - Mildly to moderately hypo-intense
  - Central areas of preserved signal may reflect preserved white matter (WM) tracts
- T2WI
  - Bright signal, slightly heterogeneous
  - Edema vs. infiltrating tumor
  - Exophytic component can engulf basilar artery, vertebral arteries
- FLAIR
  - High signal
    - Sometimes better defined than on T2WI
- DWI
  - Most infiltrating gliomas do not have reduced diffusion
    - Hampers distinction of tumor from surrounding edema
  - Foci of reduced diffusion may reflect necrosis or higher grade
  - Diffusion tractography (DTI) can show displacement of white matter tracts by tumor
    - Caveat ⇒ tracts typically preserved
- T1 C+
  - Fibrillary tumors ⇒ variable enhancement, usually minimal
    - Enhancement at presentation ⇒ worse prognosis (higher grade) except PA
  - GBM ⇒ often rim-enhancement
  - PA ⇒ solid portion enhances
    - May be solid, cystic with nodule, or rim-enhancing

  - Development of enhancement during treatment ⇒ response to therapy?
    - Decrease in enhancement during therapy may reflect steroid effect on blood-brain barrier; not necessarily a decrease in tumor
- MRA: Basilar artery engulfed by tumor but not typically narrowed
- MRS
  - Preservation of NAA may indicate less aggressive course
  - Elevated choline: NAA ratio typically implies more aggressive tumor
  - Presence of lactate implies necrosis

## Imaging Recommendations
- Best imaging tool: MR with contrast
- Protocol advice
  - Include sagittal T2 or FLAIR images ⇒ tumor extent
  - Consider use of DTI, but be cautious with conclusions

## DIFFERENTIAL DIAGNOSIS

### Brainstem Encephalitis, Rhombencephalitis, Abscess
- Listeria monocytogenes often implicated
  - Viral agents ⇒ West Nile virus, adenovirus, Epstein-Barr, herpes
- More acute clinical course
- Febrile

### Acute Disseminated Encephalomyelitis (ADEM)
- Other sites ⇒ supratentorial, spinal cord (transverse myelitis)
- Delayed onset after viral prodrome or vaccination

### Neurofibromatosis Type 1 (NF1)
- Asymptomatic poorly defined foci of bright signal on T2WI in brain stem, cerebellum (Cb)
  - Probably areas with dysplastic myelin

# BRAINSTEM TUMORS

- Increase in early childhood and diminish as adolescence approaches
- Cb WM involvement more common than pons
  - Globus pallidus very frequently affected

## Cavernoma
- Low flow vascular malformation
- Present acutely with cranial neuropathy, long tract signs/symptoms
- T2* hypointensity, often associated with venous malformation

## Histiocytosis
- Langerhans cell histiocytosis (LCH)
- Hemophagocytic lymphohistiocytosis (HLH)
- May cause signal abnormalities in pons and cerebellum
- Often associated with other sites of disease

# PATHOLOGY

## General Features
- General path comments: No metastases outside central nervous system (CNS)
- Genetics
  - Mutations of p53 tumor suppressor gene
  - Progression to higher grade gliomas associated with
    - Inactivation of tumor suppressor gene (p53)
    - Loss of heterozygosity of chromosomes 10, 17p
- Epidemiology
  - ~ 15% of pediatric brain tumors
  - 20-30% of pediatric posterior fossa tumors
- Associated abnormalities
  - NF1
    - Better prognosis when associated with NF1
    - Medulla is most common site in NF1

## Gross Pathologic & Surgical Features
- Swollen pons
  - Diffuse tumor infiltration
  - Craniocaudal extension along fiber tracts

## Microscopic Features
- Increased cellularity, mitoses
- Pleomorphism, nuclear atypia
- Endothelial proliferation
- Necrosis

## Staging, Grading or Classification Criteria
- Astrocytomas, WHO I-IV, PNETs

# CLINICAL ISSUES

## Presentation
- Most common signs/symptoms
  - Cranial nerve palsies with long tract signs
  - Headache, nausea, vomiting, ataxia
- Other signs/symptoms: Dysarthria, nystagmus, sleep apnea

## Demographics
- Age: Peak incidence ~ 3-10 years old
- Gender: M = F

## Natural History & Prognosis
- Most have poor prognosis
  - Dissemination occurs in 50% prior to death
- Median survival ~ 1 year
- 20% survival at 2 years
- Better prognosis in NF1 and PA (dorsally exophytic)

## Treatment
- Radiation therapy if > 3 years old
- Experimental chemotherapy

# DIAGNOSTIC CHECKLIST

## Consider
- Rapid onset symptoms: Abscess
- Blood: Cavernoma
- Lesions in other locations: Infection or demyelination
- Atypical appearance ⇒ consider biopsy

## Image Interpretation Pearls
- CT is rarely adequate for evaluation of cranial nerve palsies
  - Flattening of floor of 4th ventricle on CT ⇒ proceed to MR with contrast

# SELECTED REFERENCES

1. Laprie A et al: Longitudinal multivoxel MR spectroscopy study of pediatric diffuse brainstem gliomas treated with radiotherapy. Int J Radiat Oncol Biol Phys. 62(1):20-31, 2005
2. Moffat BA et al: Functional diffusion map: a noninvasive MRI biomarker for early stratification of clinical brain tumor response. Proc Natl Acad Sci U S A. 102(15):5524-9, 2005
3. Carrie C et al: Diffuse medulla oblongata and pontine gliomas in childhood. A review of 37 cases. Bull Cancer. 91(6):E167-83, 2004
4. Jallo GI et al: Brainstem gliomas. Childs Nerv Syst. 20(3):143-53, 2004
5. Reddy AT et al: Pediatric high-grade gliomas. Cancer J. 9(2):107-12, 2003
6. Tummala RP et al: Application of diffusion tensor imaging to magnetic-resonance-guided brain tumor resection. Pediatr Neurosurg. 39(1):39-43, 2003
7. Farmer JP et al: Brainstem Gliomas. A 10-year institutional review. Pediatr Neurosurg. 34(4):206-14, 2001
8. Chenevert TL et al: Diffusion magnetic resonance imaging: an early surrogate marker of therapeutic efficacy in brain tumors. J Natl Cancer Inst. 92(24):2029-36, 2000
9. Fisher PG et al: A clinicopathologic reappraisal of brain stem tumor classification. Identification of pilocystic astrocytoma and fibrillary astrocytoma as distinct entities. Cancer. 89(7):1569-76, 2000
10. Donahue B et al: Patterns of recurrence in brain stem gliomas: evidence for craniospinal dissemination. Int J Radiat Oncol Biol Phs. 40(3):677-80, 1998
11. Rubin G et al: Pediatric brain stem gliomas: an update. Child's Nerv Syst .14:167-73, 1998
12. Broniscer A et al: Brain stem involvement in children with neurofibromatosis type 1: role of magnetic resonance imaging and spectroscopy in the distinction from diffuse pontine glioma. Neurosurgery. 40(2):331-7, 1997
13. Raffel C: Molecular biology of pediatric gliomas. J Neurooncol. 28(2-3):121-8, 1996

# BRAINSTEM TUMORS

## IMAGE GALLERY

### Variant

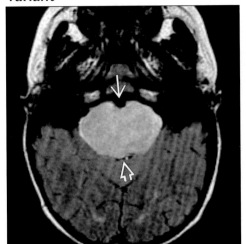
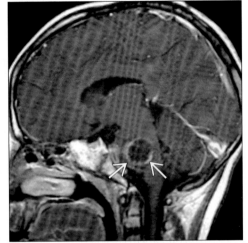

*(Left)* Axial FLAIR MR shows typical pontine tumor: Large hyperintense mass expanding the pons, posteriorly displacing, compressing the fourth ventricle ➡, engulfing the basilar artery ➡. *(Right)* Sagittal T1 C+ MR shows irregular rim-enhancement and central necrosis in pontine mass ➡. Biopsy showed glioblastoma multiforme.

### Variant

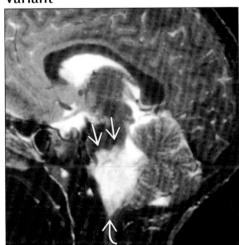
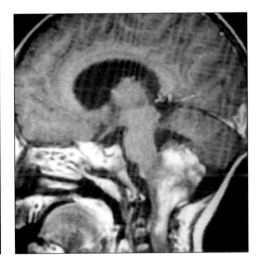

*(Left)* Sagittal T2WI MR shows originating in and involving all of medulla while extending rostrally into pons ➡ and caudally into cervical spinal cord ➡, findings suggesting high grade tumor. *(Right)* Sagittal T1 C+ MR shows large enhancing medullary mass that is dorsally exophytic, displacing and elevating the cerebellum. Surgery showed pilocytic astrocytoma.

### Variant

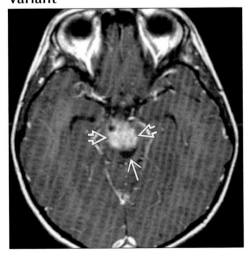
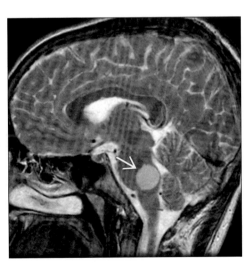

*(Left)* Axial T1 C+ MR shows well-demarcated, enhancing midbrain mass ➡ with small posterior cystic component ➡. Biopsy showed pilocytic astrocytoma. *(Right)* Sagittal T2WI MR shows a well-defined mass ➡ in the inferior, dorsal aspect of the pons. The mass has intensity of gray matter and did not enhance. Biopsy showed PNET.

# PILOCYTIC ASTROCYTOMA

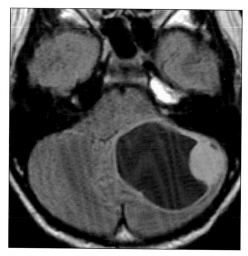 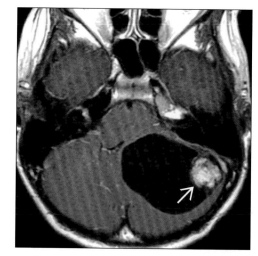

*Axial FLAIR MR shows classic "cyst with mural nodule" morphology of cerebellar pilocytic astrocytoma. Cyst contents are only slightly hyperintense to CSF.*

*Axial T1 C+ MR in the same child as previous image shows avid enhancement of the mural nodule ➡, but no enhancement of cyst wall. Pilocytic astrocytoma is the most common brain tumor diagnosed in children.*

## TERMINOLOGY

### Abbreviations and Synonyms
- Pilocytic astrocytoma (PA), juvenile pilocytic astrocytoma (JPA)

### Definitions
- Pilocytic astrocytoma: Well-circumscribed tumor, often cystic, slow growing
  - May be solid, necrotic, or cystic with mural nodule

## IMAGING FINDINGS

### General Features
- Best diagnostic clue
  - Cystic cerebellar mass with enhancing mural nodule
  - Enlarged optic nerve/chiasm/tract with variable enhancement
- Location: Cerebellum (60%) > optic nerve/chiasm (25-30%) > adjacent to 3rd ventricle > brainstem
- Size: Cerebellar lesions are large (> 3 cm) at diagnosis
- Morphology: Overall morphology often determined by cystic component

### CT Findings
- NECT
  - Mixed cystic/solid mass
  - Variable surrounding edema
  - Solid component hypodense to gray matter (GM)
  - Ca++ 20%, hemorrhage rare
  - Often causes obstructive hydrocephalus
    - May be a greater clinical management problem than tumor itself
- CECT
  - > 95% enhance (patterns vary)
    - 50% nonenhancing cyst, strongly enhancing mural nodule
    - 40% solid with necrotic center, heterogeneous enhancement
    - 10% solid, homogeneous
    - Cyst may accumulate contrast on delayed images
    - Cyst wall may have some enhancement

### MR Findings
- T1WI
  - Solid portions iso/hypointense to GM
  - Cyst contents iso- to slightly hyperintense to cerebrospinal fluid (CSF)

## DDx: Posterior Fossa Masses

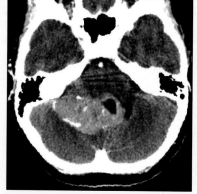 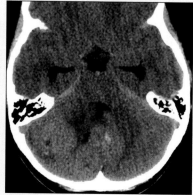 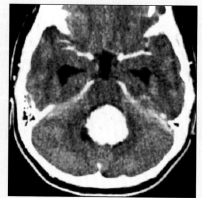

*Ependymoma*     *Medulloblastoma*     *Choroid Plexus Papilloma*

# PILOCYTIC ASTROCYTOMA

## Key Facts

### Imaging Findings
- Cystic cerebellar mass with enhancing mural nodule
- Location: Cerebellum (60%) > optic nerve/chiasm (25-30%) > adjacent to 3rd ventricle > brainstem
- Paradoxical finding: MRS does not accurately reflect clinical behavior of tumor

### Top Differential Diagnoses
- Medulloblastoma (PNET-MB)
- Ependymoma
- Choroid Plexus Papilloma (CPP)
- Pleomorphic Xanthoastrocytoma (PXA)
- Optic neuritis in acute multiple sclerosis (MS), acute disseminated encephalomyelitis, pseudotumor, or sarcoid can mimic optic nerve glioma

### Pathology
- 15% of NF1 patients develop PAs, most commonly in optic pathway
- Up to 1/3 of patients with optic pathway PAs have NF1
- Most common primary brain tumor in children
- WHO grade I
- Prototypical grade I neoplasm

### Diagnostic Checklist
- Differentiate cerebellar lesions from medulloblastoma
- Medulloblastoma arises from vermis and fills/expands 4th ventricle
- PA arises from hemisphere, compresses 4th ventricle
- Enhancement, MRS characteristics misleading

- T2WI
  - Solid portions hyperintense to GM
  - Cyst contents iso- to slightly hyperintense to CSF
- FLAIR
  - Solid portions hyperintense to GM
  - Cyst contents moderately hyperintense relative to CSF
- DWI: Solid tumor has similar diffusivity to GM
- T1 C+
  - Intense but heterogeneous enhancement of solid portion
  - Cyst wall occasionally enhances; suggests tumor
  - Rare leptomeningeal metastases
- MRS
  - Aggressive-appearing metabolite pattern
    - High choline, low NAA, high lactate
  - Paradoxical finding: MRS does not accurately reflect clinical behavior of tumor

## Ultrasonographic Findings
- Grayscale Ultrasound
  - Solid components are hyperechoic relative to brain parenchyma
  - Cysts may contain debris

## Nuclear Medicine Findings
- PET
  - 18F-fluorodeoxyglucose (FDG) studies show increased tumor metabolism
  - Paradoxical finding: PET does not accurately reflect clinical behavior of tumor

## Angiographic Findings
- Conventional
  - Avascular mass
    - Occasional neovascularity seen in solid portion

## Imaging Recommendations
- Best imaging tool: Contrast-enhanced MR
- Protocol advice
  - Multiplanar or 3D volume post-contrast imaging key to showing point of origin and degree of extension
  - MRS pattern is contradictory to clinical behavior

## DIFFERENTIAL DIAGNOSIS

### Medulloblastoma (PNET-MB)
- Hyperdense (on CT) midline mass fills 4th ventricle
- Younger patient age (2-6 years)

### Ependymoma
- "Plastic" tumor, extends through 4th ventricle foramina
- Ca++, cysts, hemorrhage common; heterogeneous enhancement

### Atypical Teratoid-Rhabdoid Tumor
- Large mass with cyst or necrosis
- Variable enhancement pattern
- PNET-MB mimic

### Choroid Plexus Papilloma (CPP)
- Avidly enhancing 4th ventricular mass in an infant
- More common in lateral ventricle in children

### Pilomyxoid Astrocytoma
- Chiasmatic/hypothalamic tumor in infants
- Solid and enhancing
- More likely to disseminate, more aggressive

### Ganglioglioma
- Solid/cystic, cortically-based enhancing mass
- Ca++ common

### Dysembryoplastic Neuroepithelial Tumor (DNET)
- Cortical lesion
- May remodel overlying skull

### Pleomorphic Xanthoastrocytoma (PXA)
- Enhancing nodule abuts pia
- May remodel overlying skull

### Hemangioblastoma
- Large cyst with small enhancing mural nodule
- Adult tumor
- Associated with von Hippel Lindau disease

# PILOCYTIC ASTROCYTOMA

## Demyelination/Inflammation
- Optic neuritis in acute multiple sclerosis (MS), acute disseminated encephalomyelitis, pseudotumor, or sarcoid can mimic optic nerve glioma
- "Tumoral" MS may mimic hemispheric supratentorial PA

## PATHOLOGY

### General Features
- General path comments: Gross appearance and clinical impact varies with location
- Genetics
  - Syndromic: Association with neurofibromatosis type 1 (NF1)
    - 15% of NF1 patients develop PAs, most commonly in optic pathway
    - Up to 1/3 of patients with optic pathway PAs have NF1
  - Sporadic: No definite loss of tumor suppressor gene identified
- Etiology: Astrocytic precursor cell
- Epidemiology
  - Most common primary brain tumor in children
    - Close to 25% of total
  - Analysis often divides into subtypes based on location
- Associated abnormalities
  - Major source of morbidity in NF1
  - Frequently causes obstructive hydrocephalus

### Gross Pathologic & Surgical Features
- Well-circumscribed, soft, gray mass +/- cyst

### Microscopic Features
- Classic "biphasic" pattern of two astrocyte populations
  - Compacted bipolar cells with Rosenthal fibers
    - Rosenthal fibers = electron dense glial fibrillary acidic protein (GFAP) staining cytoplasmic inclusions
  - Loose-textured multipolar cells with microcysts, eosinophilic granular bodies
- MIB-1 (histological marker of cellular proliferation) = 0-3.9% (mean 1.1%)
- Rare development of malignant features
  - Some association with prior radiation therapy

### Staging, Grading or Classification Criteria
- WHO grade I
  - Prototypical grade I neoplasm
  - May resolve spontaneously in adulthood

## CLINICAL ISSUES

### Presentation
- Most common signs/symptoms
  - Headache, nausea and vomiting
  - Visual loss (optic pathway lesions)
  - Ataxia, cerebellar signs (cerebellar lesions)
- Other signs/symptoms
  - "Middle-aged" child, 5-15 years old

- Prolonged duration of symptoms (months to years) on close inquiry

### Demographics
- Age
  - > 80% under 20 years
  - Peak incidence: 5-15 years of age
    - Older than children with medulloblastoma

### Natural History & Prognosis
- Slowly growing
  - Mass effect tolerated due to accommodation
  - May involute spontaneously after partial resection or biopsy
- Tumor may spread through subarachnoid space in rare cases (but is still WHO grade I)
- > 94% survival at 10 years

### Treatment
- Cerebellum or cerebral hemisphere: Resection
  - Adjuvant chemotherapy or radiation only if residual progressive unresectable tumor
- Optic chiasm/hypothalamus
  - Stable or slowly progressive tumors watched
  - Debulking or palliative surgery considered after vision loss
  - Radiation or chemotherapy for rapidly progressive disease

## DIAGNOSTIC CHECKLIST

### Consider
- Cerebellar or suprasellar cyst with enhancing mural mass in "middle age" child ⇒ PA

### Image Interpretation Pearls
- Differentiate cerebellar lesions from medulloblastoma
  - Medulloblastoma arises from vermis and fills/expands 4th ventricle
  - PA arises from hemisphere, compresses 4th ventricle
- Enhancement, MRS characteristics misleading

## SELECTED REFERENCES

1. Arai K et al: MR signal of the solid portion of pilocytic astrocytoma on T2-weighted images:is it useful for differentiation from medulloblastoma? Neuroradiology. 2006
2. Steinbok P et al: Spontaneous regression of cerebellar astrocytoma after subtotal resection. Childs Nerv Syst. 2006
3. Suarez JC et al: Management of child optic pathway gliomas: new therapeutical option. Childs Nerv Syst. 2006
4. Koeller KK et al: From the archives of the AFIP: pilocytic astrocytoma: radiologic-pathologic correlation. Radiographics. 24(6):1693-708, 2004
5. Fernandez C et al: Pilocytic astrocytomas in children: prognostic factors--a retrospective study of 80 cases. Neurosurgery. 53(3):544-53; discussion 554-5, 2003
6. Hwang JH et al: Proton MR spectroscopic characteristics of pediatric pilocytic astrocytomas. AJNR. 19:535-540, 1998

# PILOCYTIC ASTROCYTOMA

## IMAGE GALLERY

### Typical

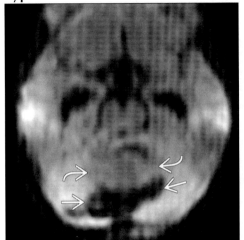 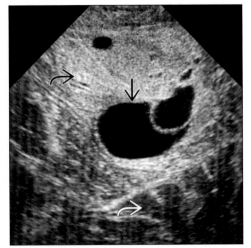

*(Left)* Axial DWI MR shows diffusivity similar to normal cerebellum in the solid ⮕ component of this vermian pilocytic astrocytoma. Diffusivity similar to CSF is seen in the cyst ⮕. *(Right)* Intra-operative ultrasound of a cerebellar pilocytic astrocytoma show increased echogenicity of solid tumor ⮕ relative to normal parenchyma ⮕, with hypoechoic tumor cysts ⮕.

### Typical

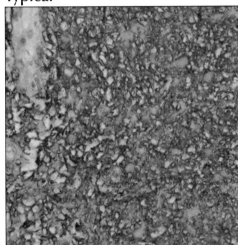 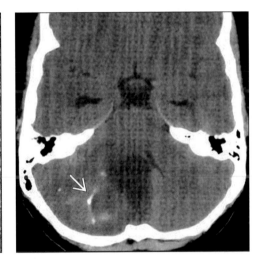

*(Left)* Micropathology, high power with GFAP stain shows diffuse positivity (brown-orange staining). Pilocytic astrocytomas will express GFAP prominently in regions of high cellular density. *(Right)* Axial NECT shows irregular calcification in a right cerebellar PA ⮕. Calcification is seen in up to 20% of PA, which is more common than in medulloblastoma, but less common than in ependymoma.

### Typical

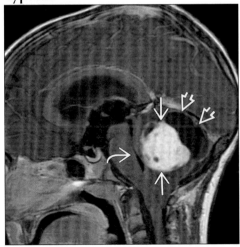 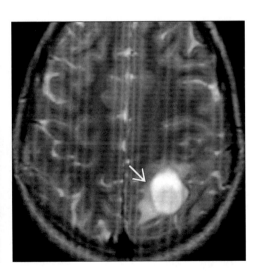

*(Left)* Sagittal T1 C+ MR shows midline cerebellar PA with solid ⮕ and cystic ⮕ regions. Although usually hemispheric, some cerebellar PAs are found in the vermis. 4th ventricle ⮕ is compressed. *(Right)* Axial T2WI MR shows a PA of the left parietal lobe ⮕ with some surrounding edema. These tumors are much less frequently found in the cerebral hemispheres than in the posterior fossa.

# MEDULLOBLASTOMA

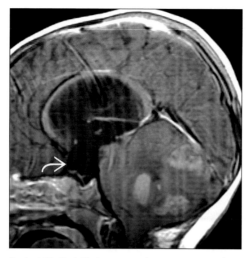

Sagittal T1 C+ MR shows an enhancing posterior fossa tumor compressing the 4th V and causing obstructive hydrocephalus, with depression of the optic recess of the 3rd V ⤳.

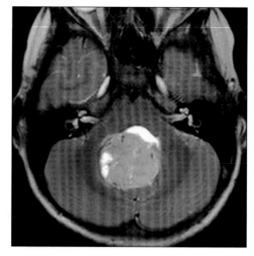

Axial T2WI MR shows a gray matter intensity fourth ventricular medulloblastoma in a 7 year old with 2 weeks of vomiting and several days of double vision.

## TERMINOLOGY

### Abbreviations and Synonyms
- Medulloblastoma (MB), posterior fossa PNET, PNET-MB

### Definitions
- Malignant, invasive, highly cellular embryonal tumor

## IMAGING FINDINGS

### General Features
- Best diagnostic clue: Round, dense, 4th ventricle (V) mass
- Location
  - Arises from roof (superior medullary velum) of 4th V
    - Helps distinguish it from ependymoma, which typically arises from floor of 4th V
  - Lateral origin (cerebellar hemisphere) more common in older children and adults
    - May indicate desmoplastic sub-type
- Size: Variable, usually 1-3 cm
- Morphology: Spherical, pushes brain away on all sides

### CT Findings
- NECT
  - Solid mass in 4th V
    - 90% hyperdense
    - Ca++ in up to 20%; hemorrhage rare
    - Small intratumoral cysts/necrosis in 40-50%
  - Hydrocephalus common (95%)
- CECT
  - > 90% enhance
    - Relatively homogeneous
    - Occasionally patchy (may fill in slowly)

### MR Findings
- T1WI
  - Hypointense to gray matter (GM)
  - Dilated lateral and 3rd V
- T2WI
  - Near GM signal intensity
  - Often rim of CSF on one or more sides of mass
- PD/Intermediate: Hyperintense to GM
- FLAIR
  - Hyperintense to brain
  - Good differentiation of tumor from CSF in 4th V
- DWI: Reduced diffusion compared to parenchyma

## DDx: Posterior Fossa Masses in Children

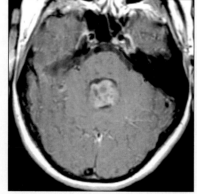

Ependymoma

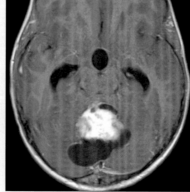

Pilocytic Astrocytoma

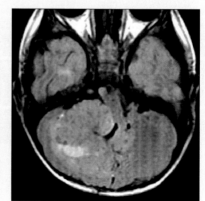

Atypical Teratoid/Rhabdoid Tumor

# MEDULLOBLASTOMA

## Key Facts

### Terminology
- Medulloblastoma (MB), posterior fossa PNET, PNET-MB
- Malignant, invasive, highly cellular embryonal tumor

### Imaging Findings
- Arises from roof (superior medullary velum) of 4th V
- > 90% enhance
- Contrast essential to detect CSF dissemination

### Top Differential Diagnoses
- Ependymoma
- Atypical Teratoid/Rhabdoid Tumor (AT/RhT)
- Cerebellar Pilocytic Astrocytoma (PA)
- Dorsally Exophytic Brainstem Glioma

### Pathology
- 15-20% of all pediatric brain tumors
- 30-40% of posterior fossa tumors in children
- WHO grade IV

### Clinical Issues
- Headache, ataxia, vomiting
- Relatively short (< 1 month) duration of symptoms
- Most common tumor in children 6-11 years old
- Up to a third have subarachnoid metastatic disease at presentation
- Surgical excision, adjuvant chemotherapy

### Diagnostic Checklist
- Remember AT/RhT in patients under 3 years
- 4th V tumor arising from roof = PNET-MB
- 4th V tumor arising from floor = ependymoma

- T1 C+
  - > 90% enhance
  - Often heterogeneous
  - Contrast essential to detect CSF dissemination
    - Linear icing-like enhancement over brain surface: "Zuckerguss"
    - Extensive "grape-like" tumor nodules less common
  - Contrast-enhanced MR of spine (entire neuraxis)
    - Image pre-op to avoid false (+) post-op: Blood in spinal canal may mimic or mask metastases
- MRS
  - ↓↓ NAA
  - ↑↑ Choline
  - Lactate usually present

## Radiographic Findings
- Radiography: Hyperdense bone metastases may occur late in disease course (rare)

## Nuclear Medicine Findings
- PET
  - Increased uptake on FDG PET
    - Correlates with poor survival

## Imaging Recommendations
- Best imaging tool: Contrast-enhanced MR
- Protocol advice
  - Sagittal images pre- and post-contrast to show site of origin (roof vs. floor)
  - Quality of spine MR better if performed as a separate exam

## DIFFERENTIAL DIAGNOSIS

### Ependymoma
- More heterogeneous, Ca++ and hemorrhage more common
- Extension through 4th V foramina/foramen magnum: "Plastic tumor"

### Atypical Teratoid/Rhabdoid Tumor (AT/RhT)
- Indistinguishable by imaging
- Younger children

### Cerebellar Pilocytic Astrocytoma (PA)
- Older children
- Hemispheric lesion
- Cyst with enhancing nodule

### Choroid Plexus Papilloma (CPP)
- Much less common in 4th V
- Vigorous and homogeneous enhancement
- Less mass effect

### Dorsally Exophytic Brainstem Glioma
- Use MR to show origin from brainstem

## PATHOLOGY

### General Features
- General path comments
  - Most common posterior fossa tumor in children
  - Four major PNET-MB subtypes recognized
    - Classic
    - Desmoplastic
    - Extensively nodular with advanced neuronal differentiation
    - Large cell
- Genetics
  - "Patched-1" and "smoothened" genes implicated in tumor development
  - Neoplasm and germline mutations (isochromosomes 17q, p53)
  - Sonic hedgehog (SHH) activation in desmoplastic MB
- Etiology
  - Two cell lines suspected as source
    - Cell rests of posterior medullary velum (roof of 4th V)
    - External granular layer of cerebellum
- Epidemiology
  - 15-20% of all pediatric brain tumors
  - 30-40% of posterior fossa tumors in children
  - Rare in adults
- Associated abnormalities

# MEDULLOBLASTOMA

- o Association with familial cancer syndromes
  - ▪ Gorlin (nevoid basal cell carcinoma) syndrome
  - ▪ Li-Fraumeni syndrome
  - ▪ Turcot syndrome
  - ▪ Gardner syndrome
  - ▪ Cowden syndrome
  - o Also associated with Taybi and Coffin-Siris syndromes

## Microscopic Features
- Densely packed hyperchromatic cells with scanty cytoplasm
- Frequent mitoses
- Anaplasia 24%
- Neuronal/neuroblastic differentiation manifests as pale islands or Homer-Wright rosettes
  - o Homer Wright rosette = central stellate zone of fibrillar processes coming from tumor cells
  - o Neuronal/neuroblastic differentiation often causes nodular growth pattern
- Desmoplastic subtype has abundant connective tissue between tumor cells
- Immunohistochemistry: +/- Synaptophysin, vimentin
  - o Some have glial differentiation (+ GFAP staining)

## Staging, Grading or Classification Criteria
- WHO grade IV

# CLINICAL ISSUES

## Presentation
- Most common signs/symptoms
  - o Headache, ataxia, vomiting
  - o Macrocephaly in infants with open sutures
- Other signs/symptoms
  - o Relatively short (< 1 month) duration of symptoms
  - o Cranial nerve palsies (less common than in brainstem astrocytomas)

## Demographics
- Age
  - o 75% < 10 years
  - o Most common tumor in children 6-11 years old
- Gender: M > F = 2-4:1

## Natural History & Prognosis
- Rapid growth with early subarachnoid spread
  - o Up to a third have subarachnoid metastatic disease at presentation
- Initial positive response to treatment reflects high mitotic activity
- "Standard risk" clinical profile
  - o No metastases or gross residual tumor s/p resection
  - o With ERBB-2 tumor protein negative = high 5 year survival rate (100%)
  - o With ERBB-2 tumor protein positive = low 5 year survival rate (54%)
- "High risk" clinical profile
  - o 5 year survival rate is ≈ 20%
  - o Gross residual tumor after surgery
  - o Documented metastatic disease
- Desmoplastic sub-type has better long-term outcome but often has greater peri-operative morbidity

- Adult presentation slightly better outcome
  - o May be due to higher percentage of lateral lesions leading to easier resectability
  - o May be due to higher percentage of desmoplastic variant

## Treatment
- Surgical excision, adjuvant chemotherapy
- Craniospinal irradiation if > 3 years
- Complications of treatment
  - o Endocrinopathy, growth failure
  - o Leukoencephalopathy
  - o Mineralizing microangiopathy
  - o Hearing loss

# DIAGNOSTIC CHECKLIST

## Consider
- Remember AT/RhT in patients under 3 years
- Pre-operative evaluation of entire neuraxis and post-operative evaluation of surgical bed are keys to prognosis

## Image Interpretation Pearls
- 4th V tumor arising from roof = PNET-MB
- 4th V tumor arising from floor = ependymoma

# SELECTED REFERENCES

1. Arai K et al: MR signal of the solid portion of pilocytic astrocytoma on T2-weighted images:is it useful for differentiation from medulloblastoma? Neuroradiology. 48(4):233-7, 2006
2. Thompson MC et al: Genomics Identifies Medulloblastoma Subgroups That Are Enriched for Specific Genetic Alterations. J Clin Oncol. 2006
3. Ribi K et al: Outcome of medulloblastoma in children: long-term complications and quality of life. Neuropediatrics. 36(6):357-65, 2005
4. Gajjar A et al: Clinical, histopathologic, and molecular markers of prognosis: toward a new disease risk stratification system for medulloblastoma. J Clin Oncol. 22(6):984-93, 2004
5. Gururangan S et al: [18F]Fluorodeoxyglucose-Positron Emission Tomography in Patients with Medulloblastoma. Neurosurgery. 55(6):1280-9, 2004
6. Koeller K et al: Medulloblastoma: a comprehensive review with radiologic-pathologic correlation. RadioGraphics. 23:1613-37, 2003
7. Pramanik P et al: A comparative study of classical vs. desmoplastic medulloblastomas. Neurol India. 51(1):27-34, 2003
8. Sarkar C et al: Are childhood and adult medulloblastomas different? A comparative study of clinicopathological features, proliferation index and apoptotic index. J Neurooncol. 59(1):49-61, 2002
9. Meyers SP et al: Postoperative evaluation for disseminated medulloblastoma involving the spine. Am J Neuroradiol. 21:1757-65, 2000

# MEDULLOBLASTOMA

## IMAGE GALLERY

### Variant

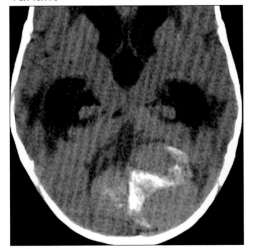
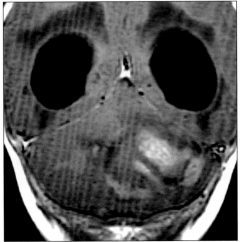

*(Left)* Axial NECT shows dense calcification in a desmoplastic medulloblastoma centered in the left cerebellar hemisphere of a 1 year old. Calcifications are found in up to 20% of medulloblastomas. *(Right)* Coronal T1 C+ MR in the same infant as previous image shows irregular, heterogeneous enhancement. This sub-type of medulloblastoma has a better long term prognosis, but frequent peri-operative complications.

### Variant

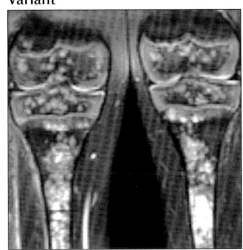
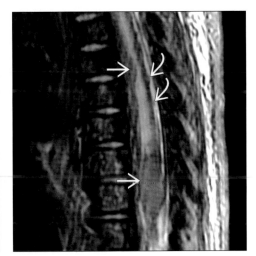

*(Left)* Coronal T1 C+ FS MR of the knees shows diffuse osseous metastases in a child with metastatic medulloblastoma. PNET-MB is one of the few primary brain tumors that will cause skeletal metastases. *(Right)* Sagittal T2WI MR of the spine in the same child as previous image shows multiple intramedullary ➡ and surface ⇗ metastatic lesions.

### Typical

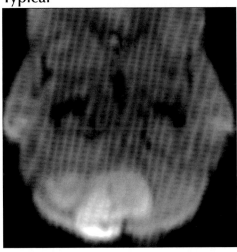
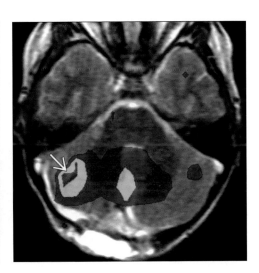

*(Left)* Axial DWI MR shows bright signal in a medulloblastoma in a 10 year old with 1 month of headache. Many aggressive tumors in children will have reduced diffusion. *(Right)* Tri-color choline map from multivoxel MRS shows elevated choline in residual medulloblastoma tissue as red signal ➡ on the periphery of the right cerebellar hemisphere surgical cavity.

# INFRATENTORIAL EPENDYMOMA

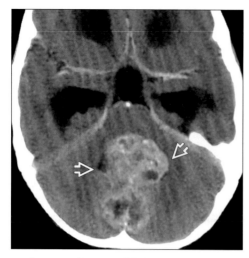

Axial CECT shows a lobulated, heterogeneously enhancing mass centered in the 4th ventricle ➡ in this 9 year old with vomiting and headache due to obstructive hydrocephalus.

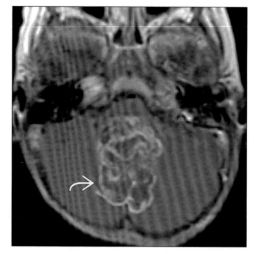

Axial T1 C+ MR (same child as previous) shows the markedly heterogeneous pattern of enhancement typical of ependymoma. Note growth of the tumor posteriorly through the foramen of Magendie ➡.

## TERMINOLOGY

### Abbreviations and Synonyms
- Ependymoma
- Subtypes: Cellular, myxopapillary, subependymoma

### Definitions
- Slow-growing tumor of ependymal cells

## IMAGING FINDINGS

### General Features
- Best diagnostic clue
  - Soft or "plastic" tumor: Squeezes out through 4th ventricle foramina into cisterns
  - Indistinct interface with floor of 4th ventricle
  - Heterogeneous signal
- Location
  - 2/3rds of intracranial ependymomas are infratentorial
    - Arise from floor of 4th ventricle
    - Project through foramina into cerebellopontine angle (CPA) cisterns

- Sometimes lie wholly in the CPA cistern, with no 4th ventricle component
  - 1/3rd are supratentorial
    - Periventricular white matter of parietal lobes
  - Spinal tumors are much more common in adults than in children
    - Spinal cord astrocytoma is more common than spinal cord ependymoma in children
- Size: 2-4 cm
- Morphology: Irregular: Accommodates to shape of ventricle or cisterns

### CT Findings
- NECT
  - Heterogeneous
    - Ca++ common (50%)
    - + Cysts
    - ± Hemorrhage
  - Hydrocephalus common
- CECT: Variable heterogeneous enhancement

### MR Findings
- T1WI
  - Heterogeneous
    - Usually iso- to hypointense

## DDx: Posterior Fossa Masses

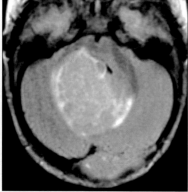

*Medulloblastoma*

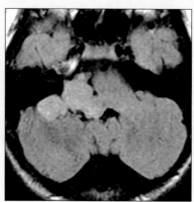

*Schwannoma*

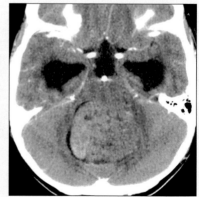

*Exophytic Glioma*

I
4

14

# INFRATENTORIAL EPENDYMOMA

## Key Facts

### Imaging Findings
- Soft or "plastic" tumor: Squeezes out through 4th ventricle foramina into cisterns
- 2/3rds of intracranial ependymomas are infratentorial
- Ca++ common (50%)
- Hydrocephalus common
- MR spectroscopy alone does not reliably differentiate ependymoma from astrocytoma or PNET-MB
- High quality sagittal imaging can distinguish point of origin as floor vs. roof of 4th ventricle

### Top Differential Diagnoses
- Medulloblastoma (PNET-MB)
- Choroid Plexus Papilloma (CPP)
- Cerebellar Pilocytic Astrocytoma (PA)

### Pathology
- Third most common posterior fossa tumor in children (after PA and PNET-MB)

### Clinical Issues
- Usually older than medulloblastoma
- Overall 5 year survival for brain lesions: 60-70%
- Surgical resection is key element of treatment

### Diagnostic Checklist
- Surveillance imaging to detect asymptomatic recurrence can increase survival
- Indistinct interface with floor of 4th ventricle = ependymoma
- Indistinct interface with roof of 4th ventricle = PNET-MB

- Cystic foci slightly hyperintense to cerebrospinal fluid (CSF)
- Hyperintense Ca++, blood products
- T2WI
  - Heterogeneous
    - Usually iso- to hyperintense
  - Hyperintense cystic foci
  - Hypointense Ca++, blood products
- FLAIR
  - Can show sharp interface between tumor and CSF
  - Tumor cysts very hyperintense to CSF
- T2* GRE: "Blooming" of hypointense Ca++ foci
- DWI
  - Typically iso-intense
  - May see restricted diffusion in cystic or necrotic components
- T1 C+: Mild to moderate heterogeneous enhancement
- MRS
  - NAA ↓ Cho ↑
  - Lactate ↑ especially in necrotic regions
  - NAA: Cho ratio higher than in PNET-MB
    - Choline elevation may not be as high due to slower growth of ependymoma
  - MR spectroscopy alone does not reliably differentiate ependymoma from astrocytoma or PNET-MB

### Nuclear Medicine Findings
- PET
  - Increased F-18-fluorodeoxyglucose (FDG) uptake
  - May help differentiate recurrent tumor from radiation necrosis

### Imaging Recommendations
- Best imaging tool: MR with contrast
- Protocol advice
  - MR with contrast, CT, MRS before surgery
  - Need a combination of imaging & clinical findings to distinguish from PNET-MB
  - High quality sagittal imaging can distinguish point of origin as floor vs. roof of 4th ventricle

## DIFFERENTIAL DIAGNOSIS

### Medulloblastoma (PNET-MB)
- Hyperdense homogeneous mass on NECT
- Arises from roof of 4th ventricle
  - More distinct interface with floor

### Brainstem Glioma
- Infiltrating mass expanding brainstem
- May project into 4th ventricle

### Atypical Teratoid Rhabdoid Tumor
- Rare aggressive primitive tumor of young children
- 50% infratentorial
- Restricted diffusion

### Choroid Plexus Papilloma (CPP)
- 4th ventricle location more common in adults

### Cerebellar Pilocytic Astrocytoma (PA)
- Cyst with mural nodule
- Solid portion enhances vigorously

### Schwannoma
- Vestibular lesions centered in the CPA
- Uncommon in children; may be associated with NF2

## PATHOLOGY

### General Features
- General path comments
  - 4 subtypes encountered in brain
    - Cellular: Most common type in 4th ventricle and in spinal cord
    - Papillary: Extensive epithelial surface
    - Clear-cell: Microscopic features of oligodendroglioma
    - Tanycytic: Elongated cells resembling pilocytic astrocytoma
  - No difference in clinical outcome between the 4 subtypes

○ Myxopapillary ependymoma nearly exclusive to filum terminale
- Genetics
  ○ Intracranial tumors associated with aberrations on chromosomes 1q, 6q, 9, 13, 16, 17, 19, 20, 22
  ○ Spinal lesions associated with chromosome 7, 22 abnormalities
    ▪ Chromosome 22 abnormalities associated with neurofibromatosis 2 (NF2)
- Etiology
  ○ Arise from ependymal cells or ependymal rests
    ▪ Periventricular ependymal rests account for supratentorial tumors
- Epidemiology
  ○ 15% of posterior fossa tumors in children
    ▪ Third most common posterior fossa tumor in children (after PA and PNET-MB)

## Gross Pathologic & Surgical Features
- Well demarcated soft, lobulated, grayish-red mass
- ± Cysts, necrosis, hemorrhage
- Extrudes through 4th V outlet foramina

## Microscopic Features
- Ependymoma
  ○ Perivascular pseudorosettes
  ○ Moderately cellular with low mitotic activity and occasional nuclear atypia
  ○ Immunohistochemistry: S-100, glial fibrillary acidic protein (GFAP), vimentin positive
- Anaplastic ependymoma
  ○ High cellularity, nuclear atypia, hyperchromatism
  ○ Occasional pseudopalisading or necrosis in most malignant lesions

## Staging, Grading or Classification Criteria
- Standard cellular type: WHO grade II
- Anaplastic: WHO grade III
- Subependymoma: WHO grade I
- Myxopapillary: WHO grade I
- Mitotic index and MIB-1 labeling index correlate with survival

# CLINICAL ISSUES

## Presentation
- Most common signs/symptoms
  ○ Headache, nausea, vomiting
  ○ Clinical history may be prolonged
    ▪ Reflecting slow growth of tumor
- Other signs/symptoms
  ○ Ataxia, hemiparesis, visual disturbances, neck pain, torticollis, dizziness
  ○ Infants: Irritability, lethargy, developmental delay, vomiting, macrocephaly

## Demographics
- Age
  ○ Usually older than medulloblastoma
    ▪ Peak at 1-5 years, but many cases in adolescents
- Gender: Slight male predominance

## Natural History & Prognosis
- 3-17% CSF dissemination
- Overall 5 year survival for brain lesions: 60-70%
  ○ Worse with ↑ grade
    ▪ Greater tendency for CSF dissemination
- Can have delayed recurrence after many years of disease-free survival
- Younger age at diagnosis associated with worse outcome

## Treatment
- Surgical resection is key element of treatment
  ○ Gross total resection + XRT correlates with improved survival
  ○ ± Chemotherapy and radiation therapy (XRT)
  ○ 5 year survival after recurrence = 15%
- Surgical resection of 4th V tumors often difficult due to adherence and infiltrating nature

# DIAGNOSTIC CHECKLIST

## Consider
- Much less common than PNET-MB or PA
- Gross total resection has greater impact on survival than in PNET-MB or PA
- Surveillance imaging to detect asymptomatic recurrence can increase survival

## Image Interpretation Pearls
- Indistinct interface with floor of 4th ventricle = ependymoma
- Indistinct interface with roof of 4th ventricle = PNET-MB

# SELECTED REFERENCES

1.  Kurt E et al: Identification of relevant prognostic histopathologic features in 69 intracranial ependymomas, excluding myxopapillary ependymomas and subependymomas. Cancer. 106(2):388-95, 2006
2.  Kawabata Y et al: Long-term outcome in patients harboring intracranial ependymoma. J Neurosurg. 103(1):31-7, 2005
3.  Chen CJ et al: Imaging predictors of intracranial ependymomas. J Comput Assist Tomogr. 28(3):407-13, 2004
4.  Jaing TH et al: Multivariate analysis of clinical prognostic factors in children with intracranial ependymomas. J Neurooncol. 68(3):255-61, 2004
5.  Korshunov A et al: Gene expression patterns in ependymomas correlate with tumor location, grade, and patient age. Am J Pathol. 163(5):1721-7, 2003
6.  Good CD et al: Surveillance neuroimaging in childhood intracranial ependymoma: how effective, how often, and for how long? J Neurosurg. 94(1):27-32, 2001
7.  Akyuz C et al: Intracranial ependymomas in childhood--a retrospective review of sixty-two children. Acta Oncol. 39(1):97-100, 2000
8.  Merchant TE et al: Pediatric low-grade and ependymal spinal cord tumors. Pediatr Neurosurg. 32(1):30-6, 2000
9.  Palma L et al: The importance of surgery in supratentorial ependymomas. Long-term survival in a series of 23 cases. Childs Nerv Syst. 16(3):170-5, 2000
10. Lonjon M et al: Intramedullary spinal cord ependymomas in children: treatment, results and follow-up. Pediatr Neurosurg. 29(4):178-83, 1998

# INFRATENTORIAL EPENDYMOMA

## IMAGE GALLERY

### Variant

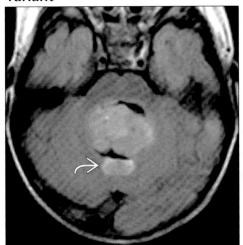

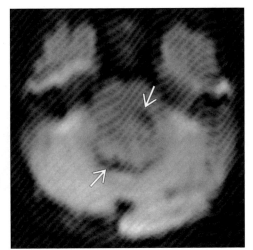

*(Left) Axial FLAIR MR in a 2 year old who presented with 2 weeks of vomiting shows the slightly heterogeneous, hyperintense signal of an ependymoma. There is some posterior vermis invasion ➡. (Right) Axial DWI MR (same patient as previous) shows the tumor diffusivity to be similar to that in white matter. Increased diffusivity ➡ may reflect regions of tumor necrosis or adjacent ventricle.*

### Typical

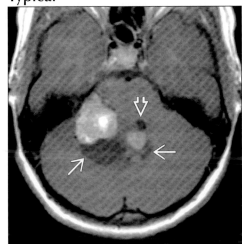

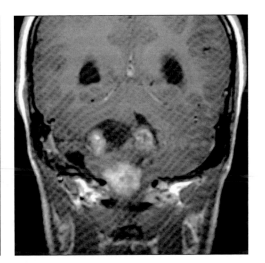

*(Left) Axial T1 C+ MR shows several enhancing nodules in an infratentorial ependyma. Note that the cystic regions of the tumor ➡ have brighter signal than CSF in the 4th ventricle ➡. (Right) Coronal T1 C+ MR of the same tumor shows the "plastic pattern" of growth typical of infratentorial ependymoma. This characteristic makes surgical extirpation more difficult.*

### Typical

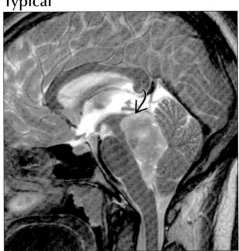

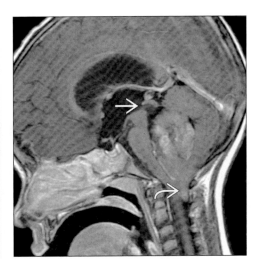

*(Left) Sagittal T2WI MR shows an infratentorial ependymoma pushing the vermis dorsally and elevating the tectum while obstructing flow at the caudal aqueduct ➡. (Right) Sagittal T1 C+ MR in another child shows a 4th ventricular tumor widening the cerebral aqueduct ➡, and projecting through the foramen magnum ➡.*

# CEREBELLAR HYPOPLASIA

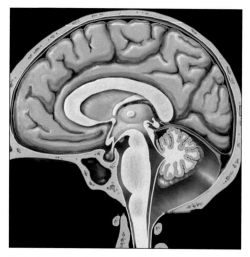

Sagittal graphic shows hypoplasia of the vermis and hemispheres with a large surrounding CSF space. The posterior fossa and brain stem are normal in size.

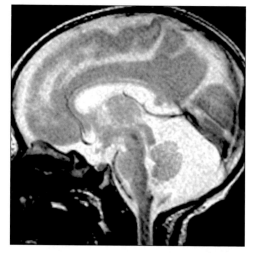

Sagittal T2WI MR shows a normal sized brainstem and hypoplastic cerebellum. Lobulation is normal, but vermian craniocaudal height measures small when compared to normal controls.

## TERMINOLOGY

### Abbreviations and Synonyms
- Microcerebellum, cerebellar (CBLL) hypogenesis

### Definitions
- Inherited or acquired condition, isolated or syndromic/malformative
- Characterized by ↓ or arrested CBLL embryogenesis or ↑ apoptosis

## IMAGING FINDINGS

### General Features
- Best diagnostic clue: Small CBLL hemispheres and vermis
- Location
  - ± Isolated to posterior fossa structures or may include supratentorial brain malformation
  - Holo-CBLL, vermian, or hemispheric hypoplasia
- Size: Variable
- Morphology
  - Isolated CBLL hypoplasia
    - Symmetric holo-CBLL hypoplasia with normal sized fissures & interfoliate sulci
    - Some have disorganized gyri
  - CBLL with brainstem hypoplasia (pontocerebellar hypoplasia)
    - Common association
  - CBLL hypoplasia associated with CNS malformation
    - Dandy-Walker continuum, molar-tooth deformity, rhombencephalosynapsis
  - Focal or hemi-CBLL hypoplasia often (not always) acquired

### CT Findings
- NECT: Bony posterior fossa variable in size

### MR Findings
- T1WI
  - Small CBLL
    - ± Pontine hypoplasia or clefting
    - ± Vermian hypogenesis, anomalous fissuration, cortical dysplasias, infra/supratentorial malformations
- T2WI: ± Hypomyelination
- FLAIR: Gliosis should suggest atrophy rather than hypogenesis

## DDx: Small Cerebellum

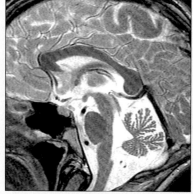

Cerebellar Atrophy

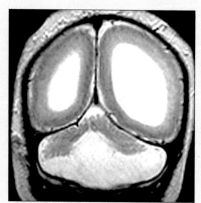

Microlissencephaly

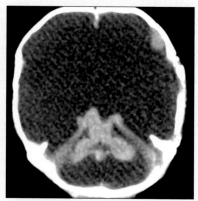

Hydranencephaly

# CEREBELLAR HYPOPLASIA

## Key Facts

### Terminology
- Microcerebellum, cerebellar (CBLL) hypogenesis
- Inherited or acquired condition, isolated or syndromic/malformative

### Imaging Findings
- Best diagnostic clue: Small CBLL hemispheres and vermis
- Size: Variable
- Protocol advice: MR brain, 3D reconstructions of cerebellar surface useful

### Pathology
- Early (genetic or acquired) insults lead to pontocerebellar "hypoplasia"

### Clinical Issues
- Isolated CBLL hypoplasia: Non-progressive congenital ataxia (may be mild or severe), hypotonia, tremor or titubation, strabismus, nystagmus, cognitive and speech delays
- Pontocerebellar hypoplasias (PCH) often progressive

### Diagnostic Checklist
- Beware! Terms CBLL hypoplasia and CBLL atrophy often used indiscriminately
- May be difficult to differentiate atrophy from hypoplasia if damaged in-utero or if due to inherited disorder of metabolism with intra-uterine onset
- Additional features important to make useful diagnosis

## Imaging Recommendations
- Best imaging tool: MR brain
- Protocol advice: MR brain, 3D reconstructions of cerebellar surface useful

## DIFFERENTIAL DIAGNOSIS

### Cerebellar Atrophy
- Loss of CBLL tissue after formation
  - ± Gliosis, focal volume loss, enlarged CBLL fissures/interfoliate sulci
- Progressive inborn errors of metabolism or neurodegenerative
  - Partial list: GM2, congenital disorders of glycosylation type 1, ataxia-telangiectasia (ATM), infantile neuraxonal dystrophy, CoEnzyme Q deficiency, spinocerebellar atrophy, olivopontocerebellar atrophy

## PATHOLOGY

### General Features
- General path comments
  - Early (genetic or acquired) insults lead to pontocerebellar "hypoplasia"
  - Later ones may affect external granular cell layer (GCL) in isolation
  - Selective destruction of granular cell precursors = GCL hypoplasia
  - Selective destruction of granular cells = GCL necrosis/atrophy
- Genetics
  - Non-progressive CBLL hypoplasias: Many
    - Familial neo-CBLL hypoplasias: X-linked (OPHN1, DCK1) and autosomal recessive forms
    - Aneuploidy: Trisomies 18, 21; Cornelia de Lange, etc.
  - Pontocerebellar hypoplasias (PC)
    - Inherited: Congenital disorder of glycosylation (CDG) type 1, PCH types 1 & 2, PEHO syndrome

- Lissencephalies
  - Congenital muscular dystrophies: Walker-Warburg syndrome (WWS), muscle-eye-brain (MEB), Fukuyama
  - LCH: Lissencephaly with cerebellar hypoplasia/dysplasia (LIS1, DCX, RELN, VLDLR mutations)
  - Vermian malformations and hypoplasias
    - Dandy-Walker continuum (ZIC1/4); Joubert and molar tooth syndromes (JBTS1-4; AHI1); rhombencephalosynapsis
- Etiology
  - Genetic mutations OR acquired insults disturb embryogenesis
  - Acquired insults
    - Focal ischemia, diffuse hypoxia (NICU, premature), irradiation
    - Post inflammatory (STORCH): Rubella, Parvovirus and CMV in particular have all been implicated in cases of cerebellar or pontocerebellar "arrest"
- Epidemiology: Extremely heterogeneous
- Associated abnormalities
  - Many associations CBLL hypoplasia
    - And quadripedal locomotion: Chr 17p
    - And endosteal sclerosis, oligodontia, microcephaly
    - And pachygyria: Goldberg-Shprintzen syndrome (KIAA1279 gene)
    - And pancreatic agenesis: PTF1A
    - And microcephaly, Hutterite form: VLDLR mutation
    - And ophthalmoplegia: Xp11.21-q24
    - And pancytopenia: Hoyeraal and Hreidarsson, DKC1 mutation
    - Or agenesis and digital anomalies: Oropalatodigital syndrome (OPD2)
- Embryology-anatomy
  - CBLL development occurs under direction of "isthmic organizer" and homeotic patterning genes
    - Cell-rich inverted "V" (rhombic-lip) thickens to form rudimentary cerebellum, which grows and covers 4th ventricular roof

# CEREBELLAR HYPOPLASIA

- Rhombic-lip also contributes neurons to pontine nuclei
  - Fissuration
    - Primary fissure forms later, separating anterior and posterior lobes of vermis
  - Cellular layers: 4 layers present in full-term newborn
    - External granular, molecular, single-cell Purkinje cell, internal granular cell
    - External granular cells divide and migrate inward to join internal granular layer throughout first year of life, 3 layers remain

## Gross Pathologic & Surgical Features
- Neocerebellar, ± pontine hypoplasia, ± fissuration anomalies

## Microscopic Features
- Decreased number of cerebellar cortical neurons
- ± Dentate nucleus disorganized
- ± Nuclear grey matter of brainstem hypoplastic or absent
- ± Heterotopic islands within white matter or cortical heterotopias

## Staging, Grading or Classification Criteria
- Total CBLL aplasia: Extremely rare
- Isolated holo-CBLL hypoplasia
- Vermian (common) or hemispheric hypoplasia
- Focal CBLL hypoplasia (unilateral hemisphere)
- Refine grading by assessing additional features: ± CBLL dysplasia, supratentorial malformation, hypomyelination, extra-CNS

# CLINICAL ISSUES

## Presentation
- Most common signs/symptoms
  - Isolated CBLL hypoplasia: Non-progressive congenital ataxia (may be mild or severe), hypotonia, tremor or titubation, strabismus, nystagmus, cognitive and speech delays
  - Pontocerebellar hypoplasia
    - PCH type 1: Profound muscle weakness (spinal muscular atrophy)
    - PCH type 2: Severe feeding difficulties and psychomotor delay, extrapyramidal dyskinesia
    - Congenital disorder of glycosylation 1a: Unusual fat deposition, variable mental retardation, parkinsonian, ataxia, kyphoscoliosis
    - PEHO: Progressive encephalopathy, hypsarrhythmia, optic atrophy
- Other signs/symptoms: Renal, ocular, hepatic or cardiac malformations may be clue to specific diagnosis
- Clinical Profile: Variable hypotonia, ataxia (may be mild or severe), tremor or titubation, strabismus, nystagmus, cognitive and speech delays

## Demographics
- Age: Infancy and early childhood
- Ethnicity: Population isolates: Hutterite variant, Cayman Island variant

## Natural History & Prognosis
- Isolated CBLL hypoplasia: Non-progressive congenital ataxia, cognitive impairment in up to 85%
- Pontocerebellar hypoplasias (PCH) often progressive
  - IF PCH associated with anterior horn cell disease (PCH 1), severe muscle weakness and lifespan only a few months

## Treatment
- Supportive

# DIAGNOSTIC CHECKLIST

## Consider
- Beware! Terms CBLL hypoplasia and CBLL atrophy often used indiscriminately

## Image Interpretation Pearls
- May be difficult to differentiate atrophy from hypoplasia if damaged in-utero or if due to inherited disorder of metabolism with intra-uterine onset
  - Serial imaging may be helpful
- Additional features important to make useful diagnosis

# SELECTED REFERENCES

1. Ventura P et al: Mental retardation and epilepsy in patients with isolated cerebellar hypoplasia. J Child Neurol. 21(9):776-81, 2006
2. Adamsbaum C et al: MRI of the fetal posterior fossa. Pediatr Radiol. 35(2):124-40, 2005
3. Glass HC et al: Autosomal recessive cerebellar hypoplasia in the Hutterite population. Dev Med Child Neurol. 47(10):691-5, 2005
4. Messerschmidt A et al: Disruption of cerebellar development: potential complication of extreme prematurity. AJNR Am J Neuroradiol. 26(7):1659-67, 2005
5. Ozgen HM et al: Cerebellar hypoplasia-endosteal sclerosis: a long term follow-up. Am J Med Genet A. 134(2):215-9, 2005
6. Yapici Z et al: Non-progressive congenital ataxia with cerebellar hypoplasia in three families. Acta Paediatr. 94(2):248-53, 2005
7. Yapici Z et al: Non-progressive congenital ataxia with cerebellar hypoplasia in three families. Acta Paediatr. 94(2):248-53, 2005
8. Boltshauser E. Related Articles et al: Cerebellum-small brain but large confusion: a review of selected cerebellar malformations and disruptions. Am J Med Genet A. 126(4):376-85, 2004
9. Soto Ares G et al: [Cerebellar cortical dysplasia: MRI aspects and significance] J Radiol. 85(6 Pt 1):729-40, 2004
10. Soto-Ares G: Analysis and classification of cerebellar malformations. AJNR Am J Neuroradiol. 24(1):153; author reply 153, 2003
11. Wassmer E et al: Clinical spectrum associated with cerebellar hypoplasia. Pediatr Neurol. 28(5):347-51, 2003
12. Patel S et al: Analysis and classification of cerebellar malformations. AJNR Am J Neuroradiol. 23(7):1074-87, 2002
13. Ramaekers VT et al: Genetic disorders and cerebellar structural abnormalities in childhood. Brain. 120 ( Pt 10):1739-51, 1997
14. al Shahwan SA et al: Non-progressive familial congenital cerebellar hypoplasia. J Neurol Sci. 128(1):71-7, 1995

## IMAGE GALLERY

### Typical

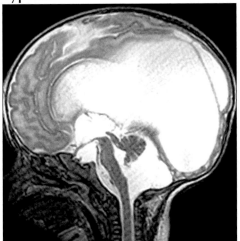
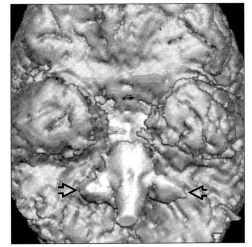

*(Left) Sagittal T2WI MR in an ex-premature infant with a complicated NICU course shows hydrocephalus and acquired hypoplasia of cerebellum and pons. (Right) Axial oblique 3D surface reconstruction of MR shows small, hypoplastic cerebellar hemispheres ⊃ in an otherwise normal-sized brain.*

### Variant

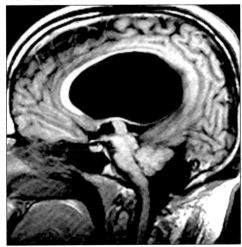
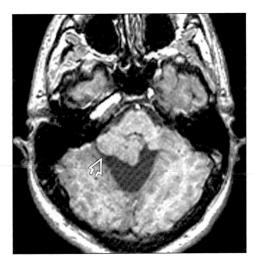

*(Left) Sagittal T1WI MR shows ventriculomegaly and a hypoplastic cerebellum with disorganized vermian lobulation. Note small 4th ventricle and small pons. (Right) Axial T1WI MR in the same patient as previous image shows asymmetric hypoplasia of the cerebellar hemispheres and confirms abnormal hemispheric foliation ⊃.*

### Variant

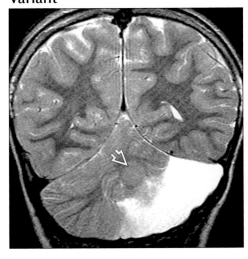
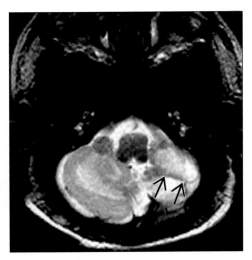

*(Left) Coronal T2WI MR shows hemi-CBLL hypoplasia and dysplasia. A large nodule of heterotopic gray matter ⊃ is situated in the hypoplastic hemisphere. These conditions are often acquired. (Right) Axial T2WI MR shows hemi-CBLL, with destruction and atrophy → of the left cerebellar hemisphere following hemorrhagic infarction during the newborn period.*

# DANDY WALKER SPECTRUM

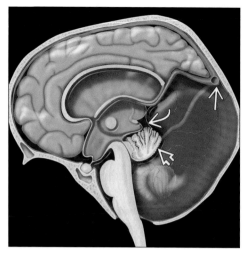

*Sagittal graphic shows enlarged posterior fossa, elevated torcular Herophili ➡, superior rotation of hypoplastic cerebellar vermis ➡ over expanded 4th ventricle with thin wall ➡.*

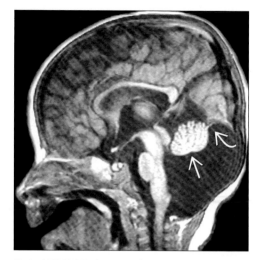

*Sagittal T1WI MR shows moderate DWM. Hypoplastic, rotated vermis with hypoplastic fastigial crease ➡, absent primary fissure, visible cyst wall ➡, moderately expanded posterior fossa.*

## TERMINOLOGY

### Abbreviations and Synonyms
- Dandy Walker (DW) continuum; "classic" DW malformation (DWM), hypoplastic vermis with rotation (HVR), Blake pouch cyst (BPC), mega cisterna magna (MCM)

### Definitions
- DW spectrum represents spectrum of cystic posterior fossa (PF) malformations
  - 4th ventriculocele variant of DWM
    - Large 4th ventricle (V) erodes occipital bone ⇒ "encephalocele"
  - "Classic" DWM
    - Cystic dilatation of 4th V ⇒ enlarged PF (torcular-lambdoid inversion), superiorly rotated, hypoplastic vermis
  - HVR (formerly called DW variant)
    - Vermian hypoplasia ± upward rotation
  - BPC
    - Fastigial recess and primary fissure present, "open" 4th V
  - MCM

- Enlarged pericerebellar cisterns communicate with basal subarachnoid spaces

## IMAGING FINDINGS

### General Features
- Best diagnostic clue
  - DWM: PF enlarged (torcular elevated) by huge 4th V, hypoplastic vermis
  - BPC: Failure of "closure" of 4th V, enhancing choroid plexus in cyst wall
- Location: Posterior fossa
- Size: Varies from slightly enlarged cisterna magna to huge PF cyst
- Morphology
  - From most to least severe
    - DWM + 4th ventriculocele (10-15% of cases)
    - "Classic" DWM: Small hypoplastic vermis superiorly rotated by expanded 4th V, torcular arrested in fetal position (cyst mechanically hinders descent)
    - HVR: Variable vermian hypoplasia, mild vermis rotation, normal sized PF/brainstem

## DDx: Dandy Walker Look-Alikes

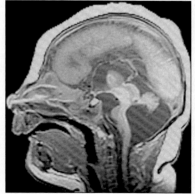
*Cerebellar Hypoplasia*

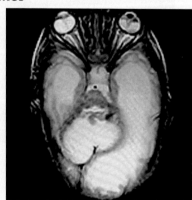
*Cerebellum Destroyed*

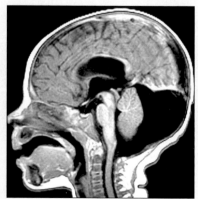
*Retrocerebellar Cyst*

# DANDY WALKER SPECTRUM

## Key Facts

### Terminology
- Dandy Walker (DW) continuum; "classic" DW malformation (DWM), hypoplastic vermis with rotation (HVR), Blake pouch cyst (BPC), mega cisterna magna (MCM)
- DW spectrum represents spectrum of cystic posterior fossa (PF) malformations
- 4th ventriculocele variant of DWM

### Imaging Findings
- DWM: PF enlarged (torcular elevated) by huge 4th V, hypoplastic vermis
- BPC: Failure of "closure" of 4th V, enhancing choroid plexus in cyst wall

### Top Differential Diagnoses
- PF Arachnoid Cyst (Retrocerebellar, Supravermian or in Cerebellopontine Angle)
- Molar Tooth Deformity (Prototype = Joubert Anomaly)
- Isolated 4th Ventricle

### Pathology
- Associated abnormalities: 2/3 have associated CNS/extracranial anomalies

### Clinical Issues
- DWM: Macrocephaly, bulging fontanel, etc.
- Classic DWM: Early death common (up to 44%)
- Cognitive outcome dependent upon associated syndromes or supratentorial anomalies/hydrocephalus and completeness of residual vermis

- BPC: Mild expansion of 4th V under vermis; enhancing choroid plexus in cyst wall
- MCM: Large PF, normal vermis/4th ventricle, cistern crossed by falx cerebelli, tiny veins

### CT Findings
- NECT
  - DWM: Large posterior fossa
    - Enlarged 4th V fills PF
    - Torcular-lambdoid inversion (torcular above lambdoid suture)
  - Occipital bone may appear scalloped, remodeled with all posterior fossa cysts, including MCM

### MR Findings
- T1WI
  - Sagittal DWM
    - Floor 4th V present
    - 4th V expands dorsally to variable-sized CSF cyst
    - Cyst wall difficult to discern
    - Hypoplastic vermis (variable presence of fastigium, fissures) rotated up, over cyst
    - ± Remnant fused to tentorium
    - Elevated torcular with high/steeply sloping tentorium (classic)
  - Sagittal HVR
    - Smaller PF ± mildly enlarged 4th V
    - 4th V "open" with partial rotation vermis; fastigium and fissures variable
  - Sagittal BPC
    - Rotated but normal-appearing vermis, normal fastigium and primary fissure
    - 4th V expands into infravermian region
    - Basal cisterns compressed posteriorly or effaced
  - Sagittal MCM
    - Normal vermis (not rotated/hypoplastic)
    - 4th V is "closed"
- T2WI
  - Associated anomalies
    - Callosal anomalies, cortical dysplasia, heterotopia, myelination delays (rare)
- FLAIR: Very slight differentiation between cyst, compressed basal cisterns may be present

- T1 C+: Assesses position of 4th ventricular choroid plexus
- MRV: Elevated torcular Herophili (DWM)
- MR Cine: ± Sagittal 3D FIESTA to visualize cyst wall

### Radiographic Findings
- Radiography
  - Enlarged calvarium, particularly posterior fossa
  - DWM: Lambdoid-torcular inversion (transverse sinus grooves elevated above lambda)
    - Sinuses are originally above lambda in fetus, cyst mechanically hinders descent

### Ultrasonographic Findings
- Grayscale Ultrasound: Fetal diagnosis of DWM possible

### Non-Vascular Interventions
- Myelography: Cisternography to visualize cyst wall, but rarely used

### Imaging Recommendations
- Best imaging tool: MR best characterizes severity, associated anomalies
- Protocol advice: Thin sagittal views crucial

## DIFFERENTIAL DIAGNOSIS

### Hypoplastic Vermis with Rotation
- Formerly called "Dandy Walker variant"

### PF Arachnoid Cyst (Retrocerebellar, Supravermian or in Cerebellopontine Angle)
- Included in DW spectrum by some authors
- Normal 4th V compressed or displaced
- AC not traversed by falx cerebelli, tiny veins
- ACs lined by arachnoid cells/collagen

### Molar Tooth Deformity (Prototype = Joubert Anomaly)
- Episodic hyperpnea, oculomotor apraxia, retinal dystrophy; +/- renal cysts, hepatic fibrosis

# DANDY WALKER SPECTRUM

- Split vermis, "bat-wing" 4th V, mesencephalon shaped like "molar-tooth"

## Isolated 4th Ventricle
- Inferior 4th ventricle "closed" versus "open" in DWM/HVR on sagittal view

## PATHOLOGY

### General Features
- General path comments
  ○ Embryology
    ▪ Common association DWM/HVR with facial, cardiovascular anomalies suggests onset between formation, migration of neural crest cells (3rd-4th post-ovulatory week)
- Genetics
  ○ Majority sporadic, X-linked DWM reported
  ○ Some have interstitial deletions of 3q2 encompassing ZIC1 + ZIC4 genes
  ○ Many, many syndromes with DW spectrum
    ▪ Chromosomal or midline anomalies; PHACE (facial hemangiomas, coarctation, DW in 81%)
- Etiology
  ○ Rhombencephalic roof divides into cephalic (anterior membranous area AMA) and caudal (posterior membranous area PMA)
    ▪ AMA invaded by neural cells ⇒ becomes cerebellum
    ▪ PMA expands then disappears to form outlet foramina of 4th V
  ○ Hindbrain development arrest
    ▪ Defective formation AMA and PMA ⇒ DWM
    ▪ Defective PMA only ⇒ BPC
- Epidemiology
  ○ 1:25,000-100,000 births
  ○ Accounts for 1-4% of all hydrocephalus cases
- Associated abnormalities: 2/3 have associated CNS/extracranial anomalies

### Gross Pathologic & Surgical Features
- DWM: Large posterior fossa, large 4th V (cyst)
  ○ Inferior vermian margin continuous with cyst wall
  ○ 4th V choroid plexus absent or laterally displaced

### Microscopic Features
- DWM: Outer cyst wall layer continuous with leptomeninges
  ○ Intermediate stretched neuroglial layer is continuous with vermis
  ○ Inner layer lined with ependyma/ependymal nests
  ○ Anomalies of inferior olivary nuclei/corticospinal tract crossings

### Staging, Grading or Classification Criteria
- DWM with 4th ventriculocele (most severe) ⇒ classic DWM ⇒ HVR ⇒ BPC ⇒ MCM (mildest)
- Stage by amount of residual vermis, presence of fastigium, primary fissure

## CLINICAL ISSUES

### Presentation
- Most common signs/symptoms
  ○ DWM: Macrocephaly, bulging fontanel, etc.
  ○ MCM: Incidental finding
- Clinical Profile: Sporadic > > genetic, clinical heterogeneity

### Demographics
- Age: DWM: 80% diagnosed by 1 y
- Gender: M ≤ F

### Natural History & Prognosis
- Classic DWM: Early death common (up to 44%)
- Cognitive outcome dependent upon associated syndromes or supratentorial anomalies/hydrocephalus and completeness of residual vermis
  ○ Intelligence normal in 35 to 50% of classic DWM
    ▪ Small vermis without fissures or fastigium: Seizures, motor and cognitive delay
    ▪ Large vermis with normal lobulation and fastigium and normal supratentorial brain: Good outcome even in classic DWM if no associated syndrome

### Treatment
- CSF diversion if hydrocephalus: VP shunt ± cyst shunt/marsupialization

## DIAGNOSTIC CHECKLIST

### Consider
- Many associated syndromes, "look-alikes"

### Image Interpretation Pearls
- Presence of fastigium/vermian lobulation predicts better outcome if no associated syndrome

## SELECTED REFERENCES

1. Grinberg I et al: Heterozygous deletion of the linked genes ZIC1 and ZIC4 is involved in Dandy-Walker malformation. Nat Genet. 36(10):1053-5, 2004
2. Boddaert N et al: Intellectual prognosis of the Dandy-Walker malformation in children: the importance of vermian lobulation. Neuroradiology. 45(5):320-4, 2003
3. Klein O et al: Dandy-Walker malformation: prenatal diagnosis and prognosis. Childs Nerv Syst. 19(7-8):484-9, 2003
4. ten Donkelaar HJ et al: Development and developmental disorders of the human cerebellum. J Neurol. 250(9):1025-36, 2003
5. Patel S et al: Analysis and classification of cerebellar malformations. AJNR Am J Neuroradiol. 23(7):1074-87, 2002
6. Calabro F et al: Blake's pouch cyst: an entity within the Dandy-Walker continuum. Neuroradiology. 42(4):290-5, 2000
7. Tortori-Donati P et al: Cystic malformations of the posterior cranial fossa originating from a defect of the posterior membranous area. Mega cisterna magna and persisting Blake's pouch: two separate entities. Childs Nerv Syst. 12(6):303-8, 1996

# DANDY WALKER SPECTRUM

## IMAGE GALLERY

### Typical

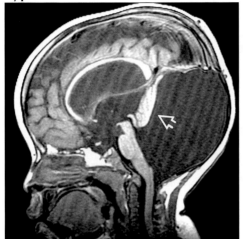

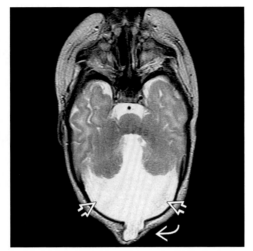

*(Left)* Sagittal T1WI MR shows very large posterior fossa, large 4th ventricle (cyst), and cephalad rotation of hypoplastic vermis ➡. All are features of classic Dandy Walker malformation. *(Right)* Axial T2WI MR shows large posterior fossa, large 4th ventricle and vallecula, small cerebellar hemispheres and a 4th ventriculocele ➡. Cyst ➡ is expanded 4th ventricle.

### Typical

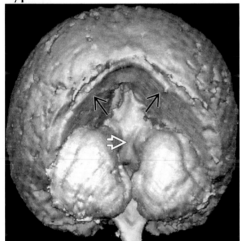

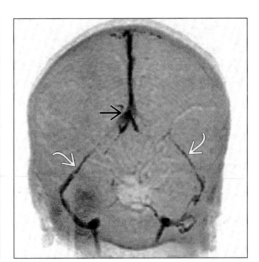

*(Left)* Anteroposterior 3D reconstruction from MR shows typical tentorial elevation ➡ and separation of cerebellar hemispheres. The undersurface of the vermian remnant is seen ➡. *(Right)* Anteroposterior MRV shows torcular-lambdoid inversion. The transverse sinuses ➡ are angled upwards towards the torcular ➡. The cyst has prevented normal fetal torcular descent.

### Variant

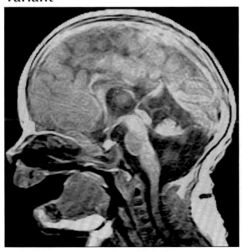

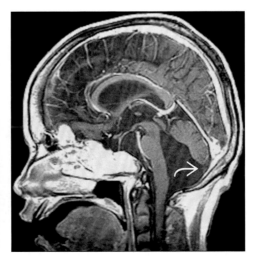

*(Left)* Sagittal T1WI MR shows moderate cyst and hypoplastic vermis without fastigial recess. There is no torcular lambdoid inversion. This condition is best termed vermian hypoplasia with rotation. *(Right)* Sagittal T1 C+ MR shows an "open 4th ventricle" (increased tegmento-vermian angle). The vermis is rotated, but normal sized. Choroid plexus ➡ marks cyst wall in this Blake pouch cyst.

# COWDEN-LHERMITTE-DUCLOS (COLD) SYNDROME

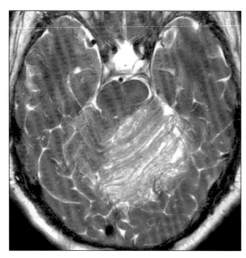

*Axial T2WI MR shows enlarged left cerebellar hemisphere. The affected portion has a gyriform or striated appearance cortical thickening and subcortical increased T2.*

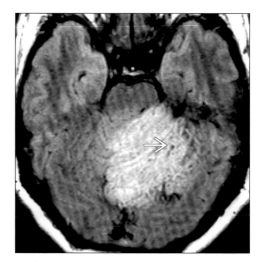

*Axial FLAIR MR (same patient as previous image) shows similar findings to those on T2WI image, but areas of hypointense subarachnoid space ➡ can be differentiated from hyperintense white matter.*

## TERMINOLOGY

### Abbreviations and Synonyms
- Cowden syndrome (CS) → multiple hamartoma syndrome, multiple hamartoma-neoplasia syndrome
- Lhermitte-Duclos disease (LDD)
  - ○ Hamartoma of cerebellum
  - ○ Hamartoblastoma
  - ○ Granule cell hypertrophy, granular cell hypertrophy, granulomolecular hypertrophy
  - ○ Diffuse ganglioneuroma of cerebellar cortex
  - ○ Neurocytic blastoma
  - ○ Myelinated neurocytoma
  - ○ Purkingeoma
  - ○ Dysplastic cerebellar gangliocytoma, gangliocytoma dysplasticum
  - ○ Diffuse cerebellar hypertrophy
- Cowden-Lhermitte-Duclos syndrome (COLD)

### Definitions
- COLD is considered a new phakomatosis
  - ○ Lhermitte-Duclos disease
  - ○ Cowden syndrome
    - ■ Mucocutaneous lesions

- ■ Multiple hamartomas/neoplasias in breast/thyroid
- ■ Gastrointestinal tract polyps
- ■ Genitourinary malignancies
- ■ Diagnosis of CS determined clinically by presence of pathognomonic mucocutaneous lesions or a combination of major and minor criteria (LDD is a major criteria)

## IMAGING FINDINGS

### General Features
- Best diagnostic clue: Relatively well-defined cerebellar mass with a striated or "gyriform" pattern
- Location: Cerebellum
- Size
  - ○ Varies in size/extent
  - ○ May be large → mass effect
- Morphology: Relatively well-defined mass with a "gyriform" pattern

### CT Findings
- NECT
  - ○ Hypodense cerebellar mass with/striations of ↑ attenuation

## DDx: Mass Effect and Striated or Unusual T2 Appearance

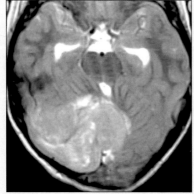

*Medulloblastoma*

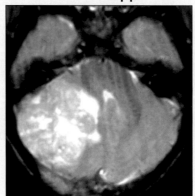

*Desmoplastic Medulloblastoma*

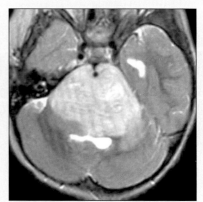

*Glioma*

# COWDEN-LHERMITTE-DUCLOS (COLD) SYNDROME

## Key Facts

### Terminology
- COLD is considered a new phakomatosis

### Imaging Findings
- Best diagnostic clue: Relatively well-defined cerebellar mass with a striated or "gyriform" pattern
- ↑ Signal, striations are iso- to hypointense (newborns may not have obvious striations since not myelinated)
- May have a very bizarre gyriform appearance
- T1 C+: ± Enhancement (corresponds to increased vascularity in molecular layer and leptomeninges, predominantly venous)
- ↑ Lactate

### Top Differential Diagnoses
- Medulloblastoma
- Pilocytic Astrocytoma

### Pathology
- > ½ patients w/LDD have CS

### Clinical Issues
- Vague neurological findings related to ↑ intracranial pressure, brainstem and cerebellar findings (cranial nerve palsies, ataxia)
- Surgical resection in symptomatic patients

### Diagnostic Checklist
- Search for other features of CS when a LDD is diagnosed and vice versa
- If COLD: Long term cancer screening for detection of malignancies (particularly breast in women, thyroid in men and women)

- o Relatively well-demarcated, no edema
- o Variable mass effect and resulting hydrocephalus
- o Calcifications rare, typically associated with increased vascularity
- CECT: Enhancement → rare
- CT perfusion

### MR Findings
- T1WI
  - o Hypointense mass with striations ("corduroy" or "tiger-striped" pattern)
  - o Signal similar to gray matter (GM)
  - o Generally affects one hemisphere but commonly extends to involve vermis
- T2WI
  - o ↑ Signal, striations are iso- to hypointense (newborns may not have obvious striations since not myelinated)
  - o May have a very bizarre gyriform appearance
  - o Rarely the signal abnormality may extend to involve the brainstem
- FLAIR: Similar to T2WI
- DWI: Generally bright on trace images but ADC not decreased
- T1 C+: ± Enhancement (corresponds to increased vascularity in molecular layer and leptomeninges, predominantly venous)
- MRS
  - o ↓ NAA
  - o Normal or ↓ choline
  - o ↑ Lactate

### Other Modality Findings
- Perfusion MR may show areas of ↑ rCBV
- SPECT may show ↑ levels of 201-Tl uptake

### Imaging Recommendations
- Best imaging tool: MR
- Protocol advice: Routine MR (include T1 C+, coronal T2 may be helpful)

## DIFFERENTIAL DIAGNOSIS

### Medulloblastoma
- Lateral "desmoplastic" type may have somewhat striated appearance
- Nearly all show moderate enhancement and marked elevation of Cho/NAA

### Pilocytic Astrocytoma
- 50-80% cystic and almost all have enhancing nodules

### Glioma
- May have striated appearance but typically involves brainstem

### Ganglioglioma
- Ganglioglioma may have bizarre appearance simulating Lhermitte-Duclos disease

### Cerebellar Stroke
- Marked ADC decrease, acute onset of symptoms

## PATHOLOGY

### General Features
- General path comments
  - o Very rare, benign mass-like lesion of cerebellum
  - o May produce mass-effect, cause hydrocephalus
- Genetics: Some patients: Mutations of PTEN/MMAC 1 gene at 10q23.3 (phosphatase/tensin homologue, a tumor suppressor gene)
- Etiology
  - o Unclear if hamartomatous or neoplastic
  - o Evidence of non-proliferation/absence of malignant transformation → favors hamartomatous nature
- Epidemiology
  - o Generally M = F but in some series M < F
  - o ↑ Degree of penetrance in family members
- Associated abnormalities
  - o CS
    - Macrocephaly
    - Benign breast, skin lesions

- Oral papillomas
- Benign thyroid lesions (adenomas)
- Gastrointestinal tract polyps/hamartomas
- Cataracts
- Genitourinary neoplasias
○ CS also have 1,000x risk of developing meningiomas
○ > ½ patients w/LDD have CS
○ CS → associated to other hamartoma syndromes such as the Bannayan-Zonana syndrome
○ Associated systemic AVMs and retinal angiomas are rare

## Gross Pathologic & Surgical Features
- Markedly enlarged cerebellar hemisphere/vermis with thick folia
- Pale appearing mass

## Microscopic Features
- Inner granule cell layer: Abnormal ganglion cells
- Middle Purkinje cell layer: Loss of Purkinje cell bodies
- Outer molecular cell layer: Thickened, hypermyelination
- ↓ Volume of white matter
- Histologically may be confused with ganglion cell tumor

## Staging, Grading or Classification Criteria
- WHO grade 1 but also classified as cerebellar malformation

## CLINICAL ISSUES

### Presentation
- Most common signs/symptoms
  ○ Vague neurological findings related to ↑ intracranial pressure, brainstem and cerebellar findings (cranial nerve palsies, ataxia)
  ○ Chronic hydrocephalus
  ○ CS may have
    - Multiple facial trichilemmomas
    - Oral mucosa papillomatosis
    - Palmoplantar keratosis
    - Gastrointestinal polyposis
- Clinical Profile
  ○ Onset of symptoms most common during 3rd-4th decades of life
  ○ LDD → very rare, all patients must be screened for CS; in patients w/CS LD must be excluded

### Demographics
- Age
  ○ Any age, birth-60 years but 30-40 most common
  ○ Congenital lesions have been reported
- Gender: M ≤ F
- Ethnicity: No predilection

### Natural History & Prognosis
- Many lesions do not grow or grow slowly
- If mass effect is not relieved → prognosis is poor
- Post-surgery recurrences are rare but occur

### Treatment
- Options, risks, complications
  ○ Surgical resection in symptomatic patients

○ Borders of lesion blend into normal surrounding cerebellum → total resection is difficult

## DIAGNOSTIC CHECKLIST

### Consider
- Search for other features of CS when a LDD is diagnosed and vice versa
- If COLD: Long term cancer screening for detection of malignancies (particularly breast in women, thyroid in men and women)

### Image Interpretation Pearls
- Solitary mass in cerebellum containing striations of intensity similar to GM → Lhermitte-Duclos disease

## SELECTED REFERENCES

1. Robinson S et al: Cowden disease and Lhermitte-Duclos disease: an update. Case report and review of the literature. Neurosurg Focus. 20(1):E6, 2006
2. Van Calenbergh F et al: Lhermitte-Duclos disease: 11C-methionine positron emission tomography data in 4 patients. Surg Neurol. 65(3):293-6; discussion 296-7, 2006
3. Abel TW et al: Lhermitte-Duclos disease: a report of 31 cases with immunohistochemical analysis of the PTEN/AKT/mTOR pathway. J Neuropathol Exp Neurol. 64(4):341-9, 2005
4. Lok C et al: Brain magnetic resonance imaging in patients with Cowden syndrome. Medicine (Baltimore). 84(2):129-36, 2005
5. Turnbull MM et al: Arteriovenous malformations in Cowden syndrome. J Med Genet. 42(8):e50, 2005
6. Derrey S et al: Association between Cowden syndrome and Lhermitte-Duclos disease: report of two cases and review of the literature. Surg Neurol. 61(5):447-54; discussion 454, 2004
7. Perez-Nunez A et al: Lhermitte-Duclos disease and Cowden disease: clinical and genetic study in five patients with Lhermitte-Duclos disease and literature review. Acta Neurochir (Wien). 146(7):679-90, 2004
8. Buhl R et al: Dysplastic gangliocytoma of the cerebellum: rare differential diagnosis in space occupying lesions of the posterior fossa. Acta Neurochir (Wien). 145(6):509-12; discussion 512, 2003
9. Capone Mori A et al: Lhermitte-Duclos disease in 3 children: a clinical long-term observation. Neuropediatrics. 34(1):30-5, 2003
10. Gicquel JJ et al: Retinal angioma in a patient with Cowden disease. Am J Ophthalmol. 135(3):400-2, 2003
11. Okunaga T et al: [A case report of Lhermitte-Duclos disease with systematic AVMs] No To Shinkei. 55(3):251-5, 2003
12. Spaargaren L et al: Contrast enhancement in Lhermitte-Duclos disease of the cerebellum: correlation of imaging with neuropathology in two cases. Neuroradiology. 45(6):381-5, 2003
13. Nowak DA et al: Lhermitte-Duclos disease (dysplastic cerebellar gangliocytoma): a malformation, hamartoma or neoplasm? Acta Neurol Scand. 105(3):137-45, 2002
14. Klisch J et al: Lhermitte-Duclos disease: assessment with MR imaging, positron emission tomography, single-photon emission CT, and MR spectroscopy. AJNR Am J Neuroradiol. 22(5):824-30, 2001
15. Robinson S et al: Cowden disease and Lhermitte-Duclos disease: characterization of a new phakomatosis. Neurosurgery. 46(2):371-83, 2000

# COWDEN-LHERMITTE-DUCLOS (COLD) SYNDROME

## IMAGE GALLERY

### Typical

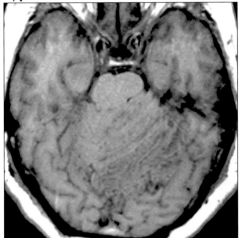
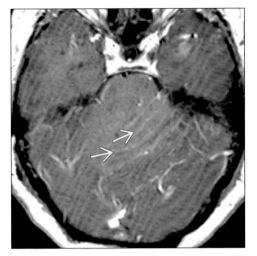

*(Left)* Axial T1WI MR (same patient as previous image) shows normal cortical intensity but hypointensity of the affected subcortical white matter with mild mass effect in the left cerebellar hemisphere. *(Right)* Axial T1 C+ MR (same patient as previous image) shows subtle contrast-enhancement ➡ of the molecular layer and probable compressed veins in the cerebellar fissures.

### Typical

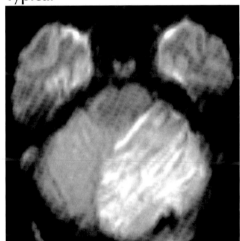
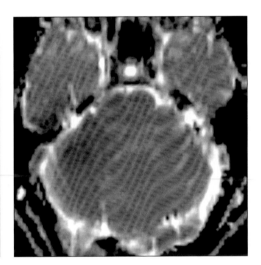

*(Left)* Axial DWI MR (same patient as previous image) shows linear areas of increased signal in the left cerebellum, probably as a result of decreased diffusion and T2 "shine through". *(Right)* Axial ADC (same patient as previous image), corresponding to the DWI on the left, shows normal diffusivity in the cerebellar cortex but increased diffusivity in the subcortical white matter.

### Typical

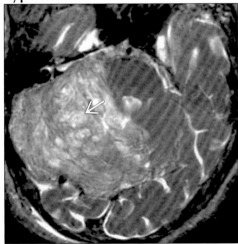
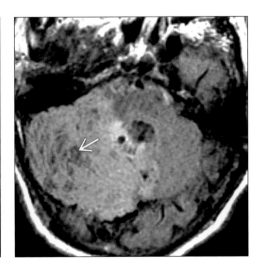

*(Left)* Axial T2WI MR shows shows gyriform or striated appearance of the right cerebellum with mild mass effect and vermian involvement and ➡ regions with almost a cystic appearance. *(Right)* Axial FLAIR MR shows increased signal and a gyriform or striated appearance to the right cerebellum and mild mass effect with vermian involvement and ➡ areas that appear almost cystic.

# RHOMBENCEPHALOSYNAPSIS

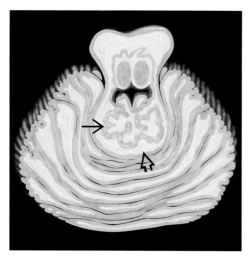

Axial graphic shows absence of vermis. There is fusion of folia, interfoliate sulci, dentate nuclei ➡ and cerebellar white matter ⊳ across the midline.

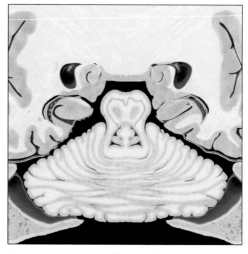

Coronal graphic shows fusion of folia and interfoliate sulci across the midline.

## TERMINOLOGY

### Abbreviations and Synonyms
- Rhombencephalosynapsis (RES)

### Definitions
- Congenital fusion of cerebellar hemispheres, dentate nuclei, and superior cerebellar peduncles; vermian agenesis

## IMAGING FINDINGS

### General Features
- Best diagnostic clue: Hypoplastic, single lobed cerebellum
- Location: Midline posterior fossa
- Size: Narrowed transverse diameter of cerebellum
- Morphology: One hemisphere, not two

### CT Findings
- NECT
  - Cerebellar hemispheric fusion
  - Narrow diamond or "keyhole" shaped 4th ventricle

- Narrowed transverse diameter of cerebellum

### MR Findings
- T1WI
  - Coronal
    - Fused cerebellar hemispheres: Total or partial
    - Absent or severely hypoplastic vermis
    - +/- Septooptic dysplasia or holoprosencephaly
  - Sagittal
    - Absent primary fissure (usually easy to find in normal cerebellum)
    - +/- Fastigial recess of 4th ventricle appears upwardly rounded
    - +/- Aqueductal stenosis ⇒ hydrocephalus
    - +/- Corpus callosum dysgenesis (especially posterior)
  - Axial
    - Narrow diamond or "keyhole" shaped 4th ventricle
    - +/- Holoprosencephaly
- T2WI
  - Transverse folia
  - Absent posterior cerebellar notch and vallecula
  - Fused horseshoe-shaped dentate nuclei

---

### DDx: Transverse Folia

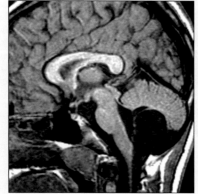

Rhombencephalosynapsis and Cyst

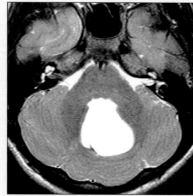

Rhombencephalosynapsis and Cyst

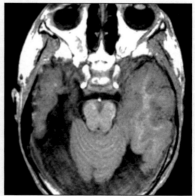

Partial Rhombencephalosynapsis

# RHOMBENCEPHALOSYNAPSIS

## Key Facts

### Terminology
- Rhombencephalosynapsis (RES)
- Congenital fusion of cerebellar hemispheres, dentate nuclei, and superior cerebellar peduncles; vermian agenesis

### Imaging Findings
- Best diagnostic clue: Hypoplastic, single lobed cerebellum
- Size: Narrowed transverse diameter of cerebellum
- Morphology: One hemisphere, not two
- Narrow diamond or "keyhole" shaped 4th ventricle
- +/- Septooptic dysplasia or holoprosencephaly

### Top Differential Diagnoses
- Chronic Shunting
- Severe Congenital Vermian Hypoplasia

### Pathology
- Likely genetic defect resulting in abnormal dorso-ventral patterning
- Extremely rare but increasingly recognized on MR
- Prosencephalic and midline facial anomalies common

### Clinical Issues
- Short lifespan usual
- Occasional survival to adult life

### Diagnostic Checklist
- Isolated rhombencephalosynapsis less common than rhombencephalosynapsis with supratentorial anomalies
- Remember to define associated supratentorial anomalies

- May be "apposed, not fused" in mild cases
  - +/- Cortical dysplasias
- FLAIR: No gliosis
- T2* GRE: Occasional TORCH-related or dystrophic Ca++ of supratentorial white matter
- DWI
  - Diffusion tensor imaging reveals absence of normal transverse fibers in vermis
    - Deep cerebellar nuclei and proximal superior cerebellar peduncles more medially oriented
- MRA
  - Azygous anterior cerebral artery (if holoprosencephaly present)
  - No posterior circulation arterial anomalies described

## Radiographic Findings
- Radiography
  - Bilateral lambdoid synostosis ⇒ "flattened" occiput
  - Occasionally associated with holoprosencephaly ⇒ hypotelorism or midline facial anomalies/clefts

## Ultrasonographic Findings
- Grayscale Ultrasound: Has been reported in fetal sonography (rare)

## Imaging Recommendations
- Best imaging tool: MR (fetal or postnatal)
- Protocol advice: Multiplanar MR

## DIFFERENTIAL DIAGNOSIS

### Chronic Shunting
- Distortions especially in Chiari II malformation with rotation or unilateral herniation

### Severe Congenital Vermian Hypoplasia
- Vermian agenesis or hypogenesis, but cerebellar hemispheres not fused

### Syndromic vs. Non-Syndromic Rhombencephalosynapsis
- Complicated midline anomaly syndromes

- Gomez-Lopez-Hernandez (cerebellotrigeminal dermal dysplasia)
  - Rhombencephalosynapsis
  - Trigeminal anesthesia
  - Midface hypoplasia
  - Scalp: Bilateral bands of alopecia

## PATHOLOGY

### General Features
- General path comments
  - Embryology-anatomy
    - Failure of dorsal induction/differentiation of normal midline structures
    - Lateral structures relatively preserved
- Genetics
  - Likely genetic defect resulting in abnormal dorso-ventral patterning
    - FGF8 and LMX1A genes being considered
    - Other dorsalizing factors: Bone morphogenic proteins, ZIC2
  - Gomez-Lopez-Hernandez syndrome
    - Likely under-recognized
    - Inheritance unknown
  - Anecdotal reports
    - Interstitial deletion chromosome 2q
    - Parental consanguinity
- Etiology
  - Disturbed early cerebellar development (genetic or acquired): 33-34 days gestation
  - Maternal environment
    - Hyperpyrexia
    - Diabetes
    - Phencyclidine or alcohol
- Epidemiology
  - Extremely rare but increasingly recognized on MR
  - Greater than 50 cases reported
- Associated abnormalities
  - Prosencephalic and midline facial anomalies common
  - Occasional associated extracranial anomalies

# RHOMBENCEPHALOSYNAPSIS

- Segmentation and fusion anomalies in spine
- Cardiovascular (conotruncal) anomalies reported
- Variable respiratory, GU anomalies reported
- Musculoskeletal anomalies common: Phalangeal and radial-ray

## Gross Pathologic & Surgical Features
- Usual
  - Fused cerebellar hemispheres
  - Fused cerebellar white matter ⇒ large corpus medullare
  - Absent posterior cerebellar incisura, vallecula
  - Horseshoe-shaped dentate nuclei
  - Agenesis or hypogenesis anterior vermis, velum medullare anterior and nuclei fastigii
  - Hypoplastic posterior vermis: Nodulus may form
- Often
  - Supratentorial midline anomalies
    - Commissural (corpus callosum, anterior commissure) dysgenesis/hypoplasia
    - Holoprosencephaly or septooptic dysplasia
    - Fused inferior colliculi; absent dorsal olivary nuclei
  - Aqueductal stenosis-related hydrocephalus
  - Craniosynostosis (especially lambdoid)
- Rare
  - Aventriculy (also called synencephaly or telencephalosynapsis); encysted 4th ventricle

## Staging, Grading or Classification Criteria
- Isolated or involves supratentorial midline structures
- Fusion can be partial or total

# CLINICAL ISSUES

## Presentation
- Most common signs/symptoms
  - Variable neurological signs
    - Ataxia, gait abnormalities
    - Involuntary head movement
    - Developmental delay
    - Seizures
    - Cerebral palsy
    - Compulsive self-injurious behavior common
    - Rare: Near normal patients have been discovered at autopsy
- Clinical Profile
  - Ataxia
  - Developmental delay
  - Variable growth hormone deficiency (depends on supratentorial midline anomalies)

## Demographics
- Age
  - Usually found during early infancy or childhood
  - Rare incidental finding in adults
- Gender: No gender predilection
- Ethnicity: Gomez-Lopez-Hernandez (cerebellotrigeminal dermal dysplasia) reported more commonly in Brazil

## Natural History & Prognosis
- Short lifespan usual

- Occasional survival to adult life
  - Developmental delay
  - Psychiatric disorders (self-injurious, bipolar, hyperactive)
  - Rare normal or near-normal adults with RES and no other intracranial anomaly
- Additional midline supratentorial anomalies and hydrocephalus ⇒ worse prognosis

## Treatment
- Treat related hydrocephalus, monitor hypothalamic-pituitary axis

# DIAGNOSTIC CHECKLIST

## Consider
- Isolated rhombencephalosynapsis less common than rhombencephalosynapsis with supratentorial anomalies
- Remember to define associated supratentorial anomalies

## Image Interpretation Pearls
- Can be simulated by mechanically induced cerebellar deformation in chronically shunted patients

# SELECTED REFERENCES

1. Widjaja E et al: Diffusion tensor imaging of midline posterior fossa malformations. Pediatr Radiol. 36(6):510-7, 2006
2. Demaerel P et al: Partial rhombencephalosynapsis. AJNR. 25(1):29-31, 2004
3. Napolitano M et al: Prenatal magnetic resonance imaging of rhombencephalosynapsis and associated brain anomalies: report of 3 cases. J Comput Assist Tomogr. 28(6):762-5, 2004
4. Patel S et al: Analysis and classification of cerebellar malformations. AJNR. 23:1074-87, 2002
5. Toelle SP et al: Rhombencephalosynapsis: clinical findings and neuroimaging in 9 children. Neuropediatrics. 33:209-14, 2002
6. Yachnis AT: Rhombencephalosynapsis with massive hydrocephalus: case report and pathogenetic considerations. Acta Neuropathol. 103(3):305-6, 2002
7. Brocks D et al: Gomez-Lopez-Hernandez syndrome: expansion of the phenotype. Am J Med Genet. 94(5):405-8, 2000
8. Takanashi J et al: Partial midline fusion of the cerebellar hemispheres with vertical folia: a new cerebellar malformation. AJNR. 20(6):1151-3, 1999
9. Utsonomiya H et al: Rhombencephalosynapsis: cerebellar embryogenesis. AJNR. 19(3):547-9, 1998
10. Romanengo M et al: Rhombencephalosynapsis with facial anomalies and probable autosomal recessive inheritance: a case report. Clin Genet. 52(3):184-6, 1997
11. Isaac M et al: Two cases of agenesis of the vermis of cerebellum, with fusion of the dentate nuclei and cerebellar hemispheres. Acta Neuropathol. 74(3):278-80, 1987
12. Lopez-Hernandez A: craniosynostosis, ataxia, trigeminal anaesthesia and parietal alopecia with pons-vermis fusion anomaly (atresia of the fourth ventricle). Report of two cases. Neuropediatrics. 13(2):99-102, 1982

# RHOMBENCEPHALOSYNAPSIS

## IMAGE GALLERY

### Typical

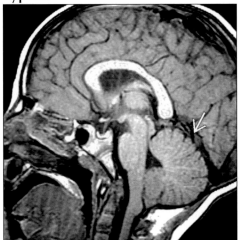 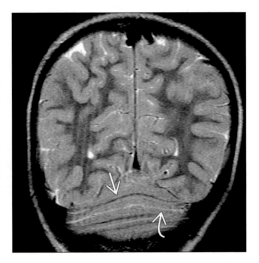

*(Left) Sagittal T1WI MR shows absence of the primary fissure ➡ in a child with isolated RES. Foliation is that of the cerebellar hemisphere as no vermis is present. (Right) Coronal T2WI MR shows transverse folia ➡ and interfoliate sulci ➡ in the same child as previous image. RES is complete in this child, but may be partial in others.*

### Typical

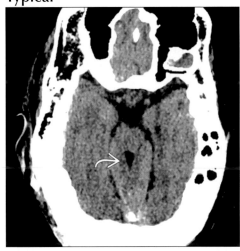 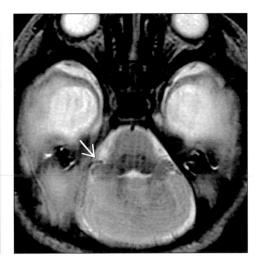

*(Left) Axial NECT shows a narrow cerebellum and a key-hole shaped 4th ventricle ➡. Fusion of the white matter across the midline is present. (Right) Axial T2WI MR shows a narrow cerebellum with transverse folia in a different child. The flocculi ➡ remain as separate structures.*

### Variant

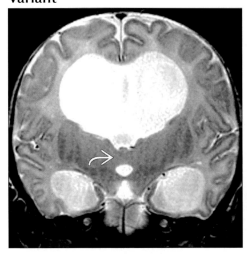 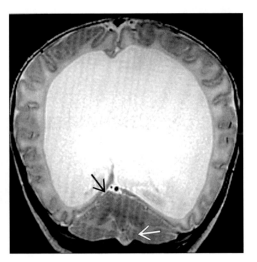

*(Left) Coronal T2WI MR shows fused thalami ➡ and absent septi pellucidi, common findings in rhombencephalosynapsis. (Right) Coronal T2WI MR shows partial rhombencephalosynapsis in same infant. There is no midline cleft superiorly ➡, but the cerebellar hemispheres are separate inferiorly ➡.*

# MOLAR TOOTH MALFORMATIONS (JOUBERT)

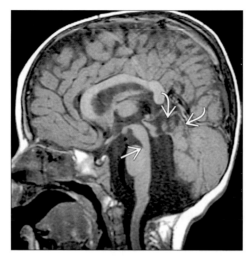

Sagittal T1WI MR shows classic MTM. Midbrain is elongated and narrow at isthmus ➡. Vermis ➡ is small and dysplastic (abnormal foliation). 4th ventricle is high, at pons-midbrain junction.

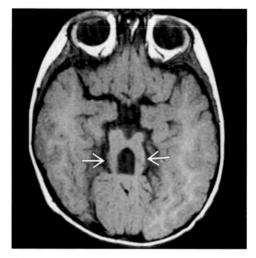

Axial T1WI MR shows molar tooth sign. Midbrain is narrow in midline due to absent decussation of SCPs. SCPs ➡ are large and horizontal, forming the "roots" of the molar tooth.

## TERMINOLOGY

### Abbreviations and Synonyms
- Molar tooth malformations (MTM), Joubert syndrome related disorders
- Includes Joubert, Dekaban-Arima, COACH, Senior-Loken, Varadi-Papp, Joubert-polymicrogyria syndromes

### Definitions
- Midbrain-hindbrain malformation characterized by small, dysplastic vermis with midline cleft, large rounded superior cerebellar peduncles, and absence of decussation of white matter pathways in brain stem

## IMAGING FINDINGS

### General Features
- Best diagnostic clue: "Molar tooth" appearance of midbrain on axial images
- Location: Midbrain, cerebellar vermis, other midline structures of posterior fossa
- Size

- ○ Vermis is small
- ○ Superior cerebellar peduncles (SCPs) are big
- Morphology
  - ○ Small, dysplastic vermis with midline sagittal cleft
    - 4th ventricle situated high, at midbrain-pons junction
  - ○ Large, horizontal superior cerebellar peduncles
  - ○ Absent septum pellucidum
  - ○ Supratentorial anomalies
    - Absent septum pellucidum
    - Fused fornices
    - Ventriculomegaly
    - Occasional polymicrogyria

### CT Findings
- NECT
  - ○ Vermis not seen on lower posterior fossa sections
  - ○ 4th ventricle has "bat-wing" configuration

### MR Findings
- T1WI
  - ○ Sagittal
    - Small dysplastic vermis with abnormal foliation
    - Narrow isthmus at ponto-mesencephalic junction

## DDx: Vermian Atrophy, Hypoplasia, Dysplasia

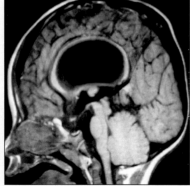

Rhombencephalosynapsis

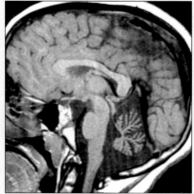

Vermian Atrophy

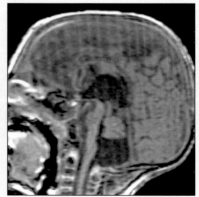

Pontocerebellar Hypoplasia

# MOLAR TOOTH MALFORMATIONS (JOUBERT)

## Key Facts

### Terminology
- Molar tooth malformations (MTM), Joubert syndrome related disorders

### Imaging Findings
- Best diagnostic clue: "Molar tooth" appearance of midbrain on axial images
- 4th ventricle situated high, at midbrain-pons junction
- Small dysplastic vermis with abnormal foliation
- Midline cleft in vermis
- Thick, rounded superior cerebellar peduncles
- Molar tooth appearance of midbrain ⇒ narrow anterior-posterior midline diameter, large superior cerebellar peduncles
- Prenatal sonography shows small vermis, large cisterna magna

### Top Differential Diagnoses
- Cerebellar Vermian Hypoplasia
- Rhombencephalosynapsis
- Pontocerebellar Hypoplasia
- Cerebellar Vermian Atrophy
- Cong Disorders of Glycosylation Type 1

### Clinical Issues
- Most common signs/symptoms: Hypotonia (severe), ataxia, oculomotor apraxia, developmental delay

### Diagnostic Checklist
- If vermis looks small on sagittal MR, check axial images for molar tooth appearance of midbrain, check coronal images for midline cleft in superior vermis

---

- High 4th ventricle with fastigium at upper pons/pontomesencephalic junction
- Elongated midbrain in some patients
- Thin corpus callosum in some patients
  - Coronal
    - Midline cleft in vermis
    - Thick, rounded superior cerebellar peduncles
    - Apposition of cerebellar hemispheres below small vermis
    - May show absent septum pellucidum, fused fornices
  - Axial
    - Molar tooth appearance of midbrain ⇒ narrow anterior-posterior midline diameter, large superior cerebellar peduncles
    - Small vermis ⇒ triangular mid-4th ventricle, "bat-wing" superior 4th ventricle
    - Apposition of cerebellar hemispheres below small vermis
    - Polymicrogyria
- T2WI
  - Best for showing cerebral polymicrogyria if present
  - Normal signal intensity of small vermis ⇒ dysplasia, not atrophy

### Ultrasonographic Findings
- Prenatal sonography shows small vermis, large cisterna magna
  - May show supernumerary digits, absence of septum pellucidum, if present

### Imaging Recommendations
- Best imaging tool: MR
- Protocol advice: 3 mm images in sagittal, coronal, axial planes

## DIFFERENTIAL DIAGNOSIS

### Cerebellar Vermian Hypoplasia
- Vermis is small, but normally formed
- Normal cerebellar peduncles, midbrain

### Rhombencephalosynapsis
- Cerebellar hemispheres are fused without vermis
- Marked ventriculomegaly
- Fused thalami

### Pontocerebellar Hypoplasia
- Patients have anterior horn cell dysfunction or extrapyramidal signs/symptoms
- Pons is hypoplastic
- Vermis foliation is nearly normal; no midline vermian cleft
- Normal cerebellar peduncles

### Cerebellar Vermian Atrophy
- Midbrain, cerebellar peduncles normal
- Normal vermian foliation with enlarged fissures

### Cong Disorders of Glycosylation Type 1
- Vermis is atrophic and small, but foliation is normal
- Midbrain, cerebellar peduncles normal

## PATHOLOGY

### General Features
- Genetics
  - AHI1 gene at 6q23 (part of JBST3 locus), NPHP1 gene at 2q12
    - NPHP1 mutations have more subtle neuroimaging findings, severe renal disease
    - AHI1 mutations have severe cerebellar and midbrain-hindbrain malformation, ± polymicrogyria
  - Loci at 9q34.3 (JBTS1), 11p11.2-q12.3 (JBTS2) and 6q23 (JBTS3) identified
    - JBST1 largely pure cerebellar and midbrain-hindbrain involvement
    - JBST2 multiorgan involvement of kidney, retina, and liver as well as central nervous system (CNS)
    - JBST3 has cerebral polymicrogyria in addition to cerebellum and brain stem
  - Probably the result of several different processes
    - Exact features depend on specific mutation

# MOLAR TOOTH MALFORMATIONS (JOUBERT)

- Etiology: Genetic mutations
- Associated abnormalities
  - Supratentorial anomalies
    - Absent septum pellucidum
    - Fused fornices
    - Sometimes polymicrogyria
    - Hypothalamic hamartomas
  - Lack of decussation of corticospinal tracts, superior cerebellar peduncles
  - Juvenile nephronophthisis or multicystic dysplastic kidney
  - Ocular anomalies (retinal dysplasias and colobomata)
  - Hepatic fibrosis and cysts
  - Polydactyly

## Gross Pathologic & Surgical Features
- Small, dysplastic cerebellar vermis with midline clefting
- Thick, horizontal superior cerebellar peduncles

## Microscopic Features
- Absence of decussation of superior cerebellar peduncles
- Near total absence of pyramidal decussations
- Dysplasias and heterotopia of cerebellar nuclei
- Structural anomalies in multiple locations
  - Inferior olivary nuclei
  - Descending trigeminal tract
  - Solitary fascicle
  - Dorsal column nuclei

# CLINICAL ISSUES

## Presentation
- Most common signs/symptoms: Hypotonia (severe), ataxia, oculomotor apraxia, developmental delay
- Other signs/symptoms
  - Nystagmus, neonatal alternating apnea, hyperpnea (Joubert syndrome), seizures
  - Characteristic facial features
    - Large head
    - Prominent forehead
    - High, rounded eyebrows
    - Epicanthal folds
    - Upturned nose with evident nostrils
    - Tongue protrusion and rhythmic tongue motions
  - Retinal anomalies
    - Congenital retinal dystrophy
    - Pigmentary retinopathy
    - Chorioretinal colobomata
    - Fundus flavus

## Demographics
- Age: Infancy and childhood; isolated oculomotor apraxia may present later
- Gender: M = F

## Natural History & Prognosis
- Older children ⇒ problems with temperament, hyperactivity, aggressiveness, and dependency
- Most affected children are severely impaired

## Treatment
- Genetic counseling, physical therapy, occupational therapy

# DIAGNOSTIC CHECKLIST

## Consider
- Look for molar tooth malformations whenever scanning infants/children with severe hypotonia and ocular anomalies

## Image Interpretation Pearls
- If vermis looks small on sagittal MR, check axial images for molar tooth appearance of midbrain, check coronal images for midline cleft in superior vermis

# SELECTED REFERENCES

1. Parisi MA et al: AHI1 mutations cause both retinal dystrophy and renal cystic disease in Joubert syndrome. J Med Genet. 43(4):334-9, 2006
2. Valente EM et al: AHI1 gene mutations cause specific forms of Joubert syndrome-related disorders. Ann Neurol. 59(3):527-34, 2006
3. Chodirker BN et al: Another case of Varadi-Papp Syndrome with a molar tooth sign. Am J Med Genet A. 136(4):416-7, 2005
4. Kroes HY et al: Cerebral, cerebellar, and colobomatous anomalies in three related males: Sex-linked inheritance in a newly recognized syndrome with features overlapping with Joubert syndrome. Am J Med Genet A. 135(3):297-301, 2005
5. Valente EM et al: Distinguishing the four genetic causes of Jouberts syndrome-related disorders. Ann Neurol. 57(4):513-9, 2005
6. Gleeson JG et al: Molar tooth sign of the midbrain-hindbrain junction: occurrence in multiple distinct syndromes. Am J Med Genet A. 125(2):125-34; discussion 117, 2004
7. Kumandas S et al: Joubert syndrome: review and report of seven new cases. Eur J Neurol. 11(8):505-10, 2004
8. Marsh SE et al: Neuroepithelial cysts in a patient with Joubert syndrome plus renal cysts. J Child Neurol. 19(3):227-31, 2004
9. Valente EM et al: Description, nomenclature, and mapping of a novel cerebello-renal syndrome with the molar tooth malformation. Am J Hum Genet. 73(3):663-70, 2003
10. Aslan H et al: Prenatal diagnosis of Joubert syndrome: a case report. Prenat Diagn. 22(1):13-6, 2002
11. Chance PF et al: Clinical nosologic and genetic aspects of Joubert and related syndromes. J Child Neurol. 14(10):660-6; discussion 669-72, 1999
12. Maria BL et al: Clinical features and revised diagnostic criteria in Joubert syndrome. J Child Neurol. 14(9):583-90; discussion 590-1, 1999
13. Quisling RG et al: Magnetic resonance imaging features and classification of central nervous system malformations in Joubert syndrome. J Child Neurol. 14(10):628-35; discussion 669-72, 1999
14. Satran D et al: Cerebello-oculo-renal syndromes including Arima, Senior-Loken and COACH syndromes: more than just variants of Joubert syndrome. Am J Med Genet. 86(5):459-69, 1999
15. Maria BL et al: Molar tooth sign in Joubert syndrome: clinical, radiologic, and pathologic significance. J Child Neurol. 14 (2): 368-76

# MOLAR TOOTH MALFORMATIONS (JOUBERT)

## IMAGE GALLERY

### Typical

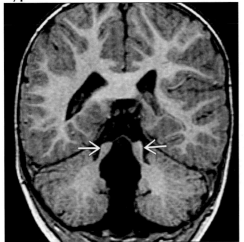 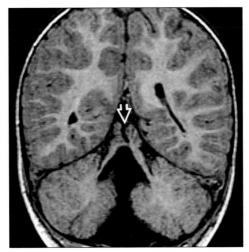

*(Left) Coronal T1WI MR shows thickened superior cerebellar peduncles ➡. The cerebellar hemispheres are widely split without intervening vermis. (Right) Coronal T1WI MR shows midline sagittally oriented cleft ➡ in the cerebellar vermis, another manifestation of the vermian dysplasia seen in molar tooth malformations.*

### Typical

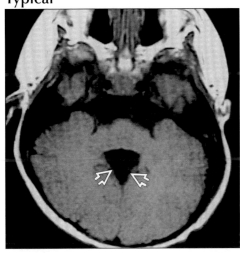 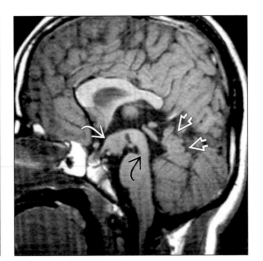

*(Left) Axial T1WI MR shows the triangular shaped inferior portion of the 4th ventricle ➡ resulting from the absence of the vermis inferiorly. (Right) Sagittal T1WI MR shows typical features of MTM (narrow isthmus ➡, small dysplastic vermis ➡) and a hypothalamic hamartoma ➡ that is characteristic of the Varadi-Papp syndrome.*

### Variant

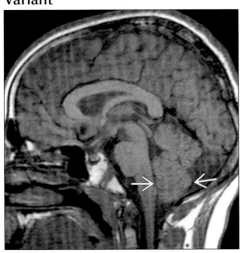 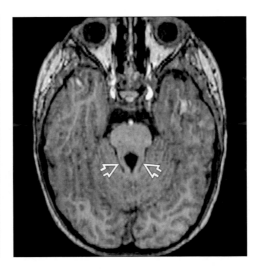

*(Left) Sagittal T1WI MR shows subtle MTM with slightly high 4th ventricle and small vermis. The cerebellar hemisphere ➡ is seen to come into the midline below the abnormal vermis. (Right) Axial T1WI MR shows that the molar tooth is not as characteristic in this patient, but the superior cerebellar peduncles ➡ are too thick and horizontal, confirming the diagnosis.*

# CEREBELLAR DYSPLASIAS (UNCLASSIFIED)

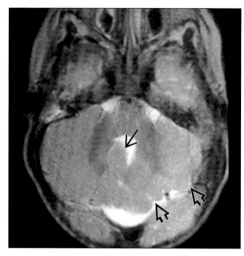

*Axial T2WI MR shows focal dysplasia: Small, dysplastic left cerebellar hemisphere with abnormal outer contour ⊳. The left cerebellar tonsil is absent, causing the right one ➡ to look like a mass.*

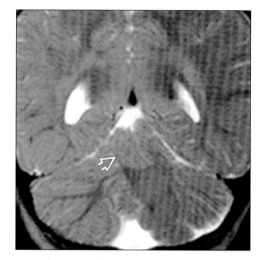

*Coronal T2WI MR shows abnormally oriented vermian fissures (⊡, should be horizontal) and lack of radial orientation of hemispheric fissures in dysmorphic inferior left hemisphere.*

## TERMINOLOGY

### Abbreviations and Synonyms
- Cerebellar dysgenesis, cerebellar heterotaxias, cerebellar polymicrogyria, cerebellar schizencephaly

### Definitions
- Developmental abnormality of the cerebellar cortex, not otherwise classified
  - Can be focal or diffuse
  - Focal dysplasias can be vermian, hemispheric, or both
  - Diffuse dysplasias usually associated with supratentorial anomalies
    - Congenital muscular dystrophies, lissencephalies, polymicrogyria

## IMAGING FINDINGS

### General Features
- Best diagnostic clue: Asymmetry of cerebellar hemispheres with abnormal foliation
- Location: Cerebellar vermis, hemisphere, or both

- Size: Affected structure (hemisphere or vermis) is usually small
- Morphology
  - Abnormal shape of hemispheric or vermian lobules
  - Abnormal orientation of fissures and lobules
  - Abnormal fissuration (sulcation)
  - Can be single, multiple, uni- or bilateral

### CT Findings
- NECT
  - Small cerebral hemisphere
  - Abnormal shape of 4th ventricle

### MR Findings
- T1WI
  - Sagittal ⇒ vermis usually small or has abnormal foliation
  - Coronal ⇒ distortion of normal radial orientation of fissures
    - Abnormal contour of hemisphere
    - Gray matter-lined cleft may be present
  - Axial ⇒ abnormal contour of affected hemisphere
    - Vermis usually small
    - Asymmetric, abnormally shaped 4th ventricle
- T2WI

## DDx: Cerebellar Dysplasia

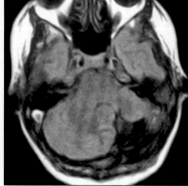

*Hemispheric Hypoplasia*

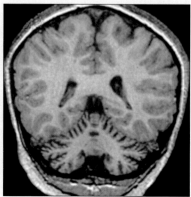

*Cerebellar Atrophy*

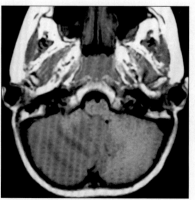

*Medulloblastoma*

# CEREBELLAR DYSPLASIAS (UNCLASSIFIED)

## Key Facts

### Terminology
- Developmental abnormality of the cerebellar cortex, not otherwise classified
- Focal dysplasias can be vermian, hemispheric, or both
- Diffuse dysplasias usually associated with supratentorial anomalies

### Imaging Findings
- Best diagnostic clue: Asymmetry of cerebellar hemispheres with abnormal foliation

- Abnormal shape of hemispheric or vermian lobules
- Abnormal orientation of fissures and lobules
- Best imaging tool: High-resolution MR in three orthogonal planes

### Top Differential Diagnoses
- Neoplasm (Medulloblastoma, Ependymoma)
- Prior Injury or Infarction
- Vermian or Hemispheric Hypoplasia
- Vermian or Hemispheric Atrophy

○ Normal signal intensity of cortex and white matter
○ Coronal ⇒ white matter bundles have abnormal orientation

### Ultrasonographic Findings
- Difficult to detect subtle anomalies with ultrasound

### Imaging Recommendations
- Best imaging tool: High-resolution MR in three orthogonal planes
- Protocol advice
  ○ Thin-section (1.5-3 mm) T1 and T2 weighted images with maximum gray-white contrast
  ○ Give intravenous contrast to rule out neoplasm

## DIFFERENTIAL DIAGNOSIS

### Neoplasm (Medulloblastoma, Ependymoma)
- Can be difficult to differentiate hypoplastic tonsil on one side from nonenhancing tumor on the other side
- Contrast administration can be useful

### Prior Injury or Infarction
- Continuous cortex around hemisphere suggests congenital lesion

### Vermian or Hemispheric Hypoplasia
- Hypoplasia has normal foliation
- Dysplasia has abnormal foliation

### Vermian or Hemispheric Atrophy
- Normal lobules, folia are present but shrunken

## PATHOLOGY

### Gross Pathologic & Surgical Features
- One of four types of cerebellar dysplasia identified by Friede (1989): Others are 1) heterotopia, 2) dysplasias of cerebellar nuclei, 3) trivial dysplasias in neonates

### Microscopic Features
- Affected cortex is abnormally smooth, thicker than normal
  ○ Interlacing nests of granular and molecular layers; Purkinje cells present irregularly at borders
  ○ Absence of gliosis, scarring, atrophy

## SELECTED REFERENCES

1. Jissendi Tchofo P et al: Supratentorial functional disturbances in two children with cerebellar cortical dysplasia. J Neuroradiol. 31(5):399-405, 2004
2. Soto Ares G et al: [Cerebellar cortical dysplasia: MRI aspects and significance] J Radiol. 85(6 Pt 1):729-40, 2004
3. Patel S et al: Analysis and classification of cerebellar malformations. AJNR Am J Neuroradiol. 23(7):1074-87, 2002
4. Soto-Ares G et al: Neuropathologic and MR imaging correlation in a neonatal case of cerebellar cortical dysplasia. AJNR Am J Neuroradiol. 23(7):1101-4, 2002
5. Soto-Ares G et al: Cerebellar cortical dysplasia: MR findings in a complex entity. AJNR Am J Neuroradiol. 21(8):1511-9, 2000

I

4

39

## IMAGE GALLERY

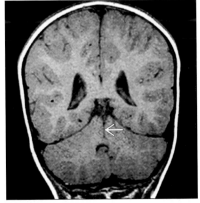 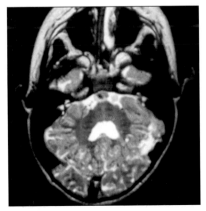 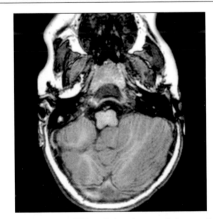

*(Left)* Coronal T1WI MR shows focal dysplasia with dysplastic vermis. Note the abnormal sagittally oriented cleft ➡ and the abnormal shape of the 4th ventricle. *(Center)* Axial T2WI MR shows diffuse cerebellar dysplasia, with abnormal folial pattern involving both cerebellar hemispheres and the vermis. *(Right)* Axial T1WI MR shows focal cerebellar hemispheric dysplasia: Abnormal orientation and depth of fissures, dysplastic orientation of folia, decreased hemispheric size.

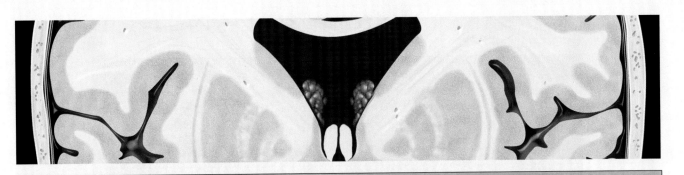

## SECTION 5: Ventricular System

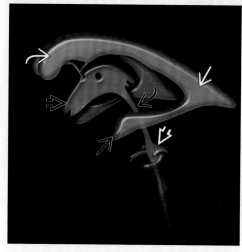

*Lateral graphic shows the ventricular system: Frontal horns ➤, trigones ➤, temporal horns →, third ventricle ➤, aqueduct ↗, and fourth ventricle ➤ with outlet foramina.*

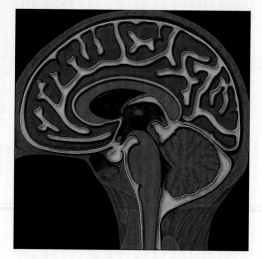

*Lateral graphic shows the subarachnoid spaces (yellow), which are filled with CSF and surround the brain and spinal cord, supporting and bathing the structures of the CNS.*

## TERMINOLOGY

### Definitions
- Two major intracranial CSF-containing compartments = ventricles, subarachnoid space (SAS)

## IMAGING ANATOMY
- Lateral ventricles
  - Paired CSF-containing, ependymal-lined spaces curve from temporal horns around/above thalami
  - Frontal (anterior) horns
    - Triangle-shaped, indented by caudate heads (some asymmetry common)
    - Extend from genu/rostrum of corpus callosum posteriorly to pillars of fornix, foramina of Monro
    - Separated by septum pellucidum (may contain CSF)
  - Bodies
    - Axial: Course laterally as curve posteriorly
    - Coronal: Flattened triangles with inferomedial concavity formed by caudate, thalamus
    - Lateral: Roughly triangular shaped from CC to fornix in midline section; C-shaped with indentation from pulvinar of thalamus off-midline
  - Atria (trigones): Confluence of body, occipital and temporal horns; contain choroid plexus glomus
  - Occipital horns
    - Extend posteriorly from atrium, bordered medially by forceps major, laterally by tapetum and occipital radiations
    - Contain only CSF (when patient is supine, choroid plexus glomus may "dangle" into occipital horn)
    - Elevations on medial wall = upper (bulb), lower (calcar avis), accessory intraventricular prominence caused by hippocampal tail
  - Temporal (inferior) horns

- Axial: Curve laterally, then anteromedially into slit-like termination between hippocampus and amygdala
- Coronal: Slit-like, pial-lined choroid fissure appears to join ependymal-lined temporal horn as it curves over pes hippocampus
- Sagittal: Finger-like CSF space with medial indentation formed by collateral eminence of hippocampus
- Interventricular foramen (of Monro)
  - Y-shaped, with upper "arms" of Y into each lateral ventricle
  - Common stem opens into roof of 3rd V
  - Bounded anteriorly by fornices, posteriorly by choroid plexus, thalamostriate veins, and thalami
- Third ventricle
  - Axial: Single, midline; lateral borders are hypothalami (anterior, inferior), thalami (posterior)
    - 75% show interthalamic adhesion (massa intermedia)
  - Sagittal
    - Anterior border formed by lamina terminalis, anterior commissure
    - Recesses: Optic (between optic chiasm and lamina terminalis); infundibular (points down towards center of pituitary stalk); suprapineal (rounded posterior diverticulum above pineal gland); pineal (posterior diverticulum points into stalk of pineal gland, bordered inferiorly by posterior commissure)
  - Coronal
    - Roof bordered by pial-lined tela choroidea of velum interpositum (contains choroid plexus, internal cerebral veins)
    - CSF flow artifacts common, especially adjacent to foramen of Monro
- Aqueduct of Sylvius
  - Narrow tube-like structure that joins 3rd and 4th ventricles
  - Traverses midbrain, surrounded by periaqueductal gray matter

# VENTRICULAR ANATOMY & IMAGING ISSUES

## Disorders of Ventricles, Cisterns

### Congenital Variants, Malformations
- Cavum Septi Pellucidi, Cavum Vergae
- Septo-optic dysplasia, holoprosencephaly variants
- Callosal anomalies (high-riding 3rd V)
- Chiari II (elongated 4th V, fastigium usually absent)

### Trauma
- IVH ± choroid plexus hematoma

### Infection/Inflammation
- Ventriculitis ± choroid plexitis
- Pyocephalus (fluid-debris level; often fatal)
- Histiocytosis

### Nonneoplastic Cysts
- CSF-containing (arachnoid, ependymal) cyst

- Germinolytic cyst (frontal horns, genetic/metabolic disease)
- Parasitic (e.g., neurocysticercosis)
- Colloid cyst (at foramen of Monro)

### Benign Neoplasm
- Choroid plexus papilloma (usually in atrium, temporal horn, 4th ventricle)
- Astrocytoma (usually giant cell, pilocytic)
- Meningioma (atrium most common site)
- Subependymoma (F of Monro, 4th V obex)

### Malignant Neoplasm
- Astrocytoma (WHO II-IV)
- Ependymoma (4th V most common site)
- Medulloblastoma (4th V)
- Germinoma (hypothalamus, 3rd V)

○ Roof formed by tectum (quadrigeminal plate), floor by tegmentum
- 4th ventricle
  ○ Complex configuration with rhomboid-shaped floor, tented roof
  ○ Sagittal
    ▪ Funnel-shaped expansion from aqueduct into body of 4th V
    ▪ Roof formed by superior medullary velum, a thin sheet of tissue stretching between the superior cerebellar peduncles
    ▪ Triangular-shaped dorsal projection (fastigium) points towards vermis
    ▪ Floor appears smooth, formed by dorsal surface of pons, medulla
    ▪ Narrows gently inferiorly (calamus scriptorius) into foramen of Magendie at obex
  ○ Axial: Bean-shaped; posterior indentation formed by vermis
  ○ Coronal
    ▪ Diamond-shaped with upper point into aqueduct, lower toward F. of Magendie
    ▪ Recesses: Posterosuperior (blind wing-like pouches that curve over cerebellar tonsils)
    ▪ Recesses: Lateral (curve around pons under major cerebellar peduncles)
    ▪ Foramina: Luschka (opening of lateral recesses into cerebellopontine angle cisterns; contains choroid plexus that protrudes through lateral apertures into CPA)
    ▪ Foramina: Magendie (medial aperture = midline opening into cisterna magna)
    ▪ Foramina are the ONLY normal connections between ventricular system, SAS
- Choroid plexus and CSF production/resorption
  ○ Approximately 75% of CSF is produced by ventricular choroid plexus (remainder by other sites known and unknown)
    ▪ Choroid plexus lacks BBB, enhances intensely
    ▪ May contain cysts or xanthogranulomas
    ▪ In embryo, CSF carries chemicals critical to cortex development

○ Produced at rate of one-third to one-half ml/minute or approximately 500 ml/day in adults
○ Total CSF volume in ventricles, SAS = approximately 125-150 ml in adults
○ Bulk removal of CSF occurs through venous system, arachnoid granulations (AGs) in dural sinuses
  ▪ If ventricular system is blocked (most often at FOM, aqueduct, 4th V foramina), intraventricular hydrocephalus (HCP) ensues
  ▪ If venous resorption of CSF impaired, extraventricular HCP ensues
○ Arachnoid granulations most prominent in large (transverse, superior sagittal) sinuses
○ Variant: "Giant" arachnoid granulations
  ▪ CSF attenuation/signal intensity
  ▪ Seen as "filling defects" within intensely enhancing venous sinuses
  ▪ Don't mistake for thrombus!
- SAS and CSF cisterns
  ○ Numerous; most prominent are suprasellar and CPA cisterns (discussed in separate sections)
  ○ Are usually prominent in infants (less than 2 years): DON'T mistake for HCP

## ANATOMY-BASED IMAGING ISSUES

### Key Concepts or Questions
- Ventricles, cisterns contain CSF
- Interstitial fluid (ISF) is found in brain parenchyma and within the perivascular (Virchow-Robin) spaces
- CSF and ISF look grossly similar on imaging studies but are slightly different in chemical composition

### Imaging Pitfalls
- Ventricular volume/size
  ○ Prominent ventricles and cisterns in infancy
- Asymmetry
  ○ Asymmetry of the frontal, occipital horns is common, should not be mistaken for disease
  ○ Volume of right lateral, 3rd V larger in right-handed; left lateral ventricle in left-handed individuals
  ○ No gender differences

# VENTRICULAR ANATOMY & IMAGING ISSUES

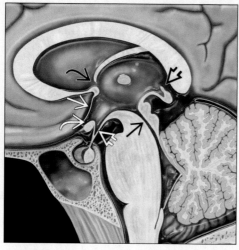

Sagittal graphic shows anatomy of the third ventricle: Foramen of Monro ➴, lamina terminalis ➡, chiasmatic recess ➘, infundibular recess ➡, suprapineal recess ➘, aqueduct ➡.

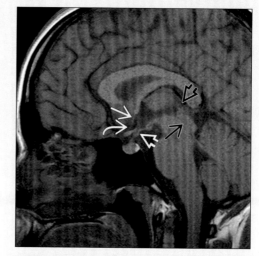

Sagittal T1WI MR shows anatomy of 3rd ventricle: Lamina terminalis ➡, chiasmatic recess ➴, infundibular recess ➘, suprapineal recess ➘, aqueduct ➡.

- CSF flow
  - Pulsatile, but net flow essentially one-way within ventricles
  - Pulsatile flow may cause bizarre artifacts on MR
    - Mass-like mimics may occur (e.g., flow at F of M can mimic colloid cyst or tuber)
    - Mismapped flow may appear as parenchymal lesion

## Normal Measurements
- Atrium of fetal lateral ventricles at 22 wks or later = 10-12 mm

## CLINICAL IMPLICATIONS

### Clinical Importance
- Significant variation, ventricular asymmetry is common
- Actual size or change in size of ventricles is not reliable predictor of increased intracranial pressure
- Ventricular volume relatively large in infants and healthy aging adults > 60 y

## CUSTOM DIFFERENTIAL DIAGNOSIS

### Mass in Frontal Horn of Lateral Ventricle
- Subependymal giant cell astrocytoma (patients with tuberous sclerosis)
- Astrocytoma (fibrillary)
- Heterotopion

### Mass in Body of Lateral Ventricle
- Astrocytoma
- PNET

### Mass in Atrium of Lateral Ventricle
- Choroid plexus cysts (nonenhancing)
- Choroid plexus papilloma (children < 5 y)
- Meningioma

### Mass in 3rd Ventricle
- Astrocytoma (hypothalamus, optic chiasm)

- Germ cell tumor
- Pituitary adenoma, craniopharyngioma (intraventricular rare)
- Choroid plexus papilloma (rare location)
- Colloid cyst (rare in children)

### Mass in 4th Ventricle
- Medulloblastoma (superior medullary velum)
- Ependymoma
- Dorsally exophytic brainstem tumor
- Choroid plexus papilloma
- Epidermoid cyst
- Subependymoma (obex; adults)

## RELATED REFERENCES

1. Barkovich AJ: Pediatric Neuroimaging 4th Ed, Lippincott Williams & Wilkins, Philadelphia, 659-703, 2005
2. Duffner F et al: Anatomy of the cerebral ventricular system for endoscopic neurosurgery: a magnetic resonance study. Acta Neurochir (Wien). 145(5):359-68, 2003
3. Encha-Razavi F et al: Features of the developing brain. Childs Nerv Syst. 19(7-8):426-8, 2003
4. Garel C et al: Ventricular dilatations. Childs Nerv Syst. 19(7-8):517-23, 2003
5. Jamous M et al: Frontal and occipital horn width ratio for the evaluation of small and asymmetrical ventricles. Pediatr Neurosurg. 39(1):17-21, 2003
6. Jodicke A et al: Virtual endoscopy of the cerebral ventricles based on 3-D ultrasonography. Ultrasound Med Biol. 29(2):339-45, 2003
7. Joseph VB et al: MR ventriculography for the study of CSF flow. AJNR Am J Neuroradiol. 24(3):373-81, 2003
8. Karachi C et al: Hydrocephalus due to idiopathic stenosis of the foramina of Magendie and Luschka. Report of three cases. J Neurosurg. 98(4):897-902, 2003
9. Miyan JA et al: Development of the brain: a vital role for cerebrospinal fluid. Can J Physiol Pharmacol. 81(4):317-28, 2003
10. Resnick SM et al: Longitudinal magnetic resonance imaging studies of older adults: a shrinking brain. J Neurosci. 23(8):3295-301, 2003

## IMAGE GALLERY

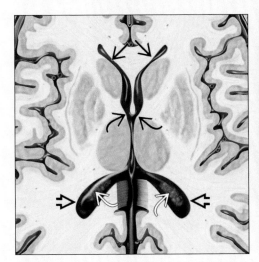
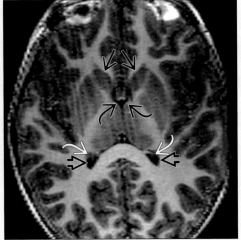

(Left) Axial graphic shows anatomy of lateral ventricles: Frontal horns ➡, atria (trigones ➡), glomus of choroid plexus ➡, foramina of Monro ➡. (Right) Axial graphic shows frontal horns ➡, atria (trigones) ➡, glomus of choroid plexus ➡, foramina of Monro ➡.

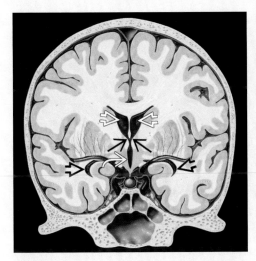
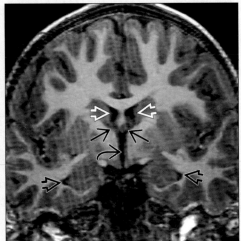

(Left) Coronal graphic shows frontal horns ➡ extending into third ventricle ➡ via foramina of Monro ➡. Fornices form medial borders of the foramina. Temporal horns ➡ wrap around hippocampi. (Right) Coronal T1WI MR shows frontal horns ➡ extending into third ventricle ➡ via foramina of Monro ➡ (with choroid plexus in them). Temporal horns ➡ wrap around hippocampi.

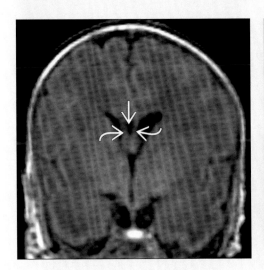
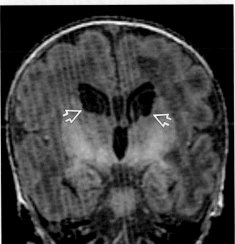

(Left) Coronal T1WI MR shows cavum septi pellucidi in a prematurely born infant. The cavum ➡ is filled with CSF and lies between the septal leaves ➡. Note the dark, unmyelinated white matter. (Right) Coronal T1WI MR shows germinolytic cysts ➡ in the frontal horns of both lateral ventricles in this neonate with Zellweger syndrome.

# CAVUM SEPTI PELLUCIDI (CSP)

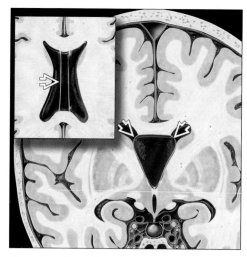

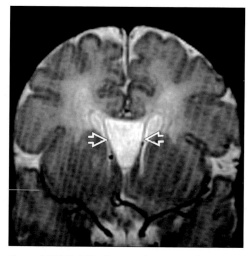

*Coronal graphic with axial insert shows classic cavum septi pellucidi (CSP) with cavum Vergae (CV) ➡. Note finger-like CSF collection between lateral ventricles.*

*Coronal T2WI MR shows a large CSF fluid space between the leaves of the SP ➡, below the corpus callosum.*

## TERMINOLOGY

### Abbreviations and Synonyms
- Cavum septi pellucidi (CSP), cavum Vergae (CV)

### Definitions
- CSF cavity within septum pellucidum (SP) ± posterior continuation (CV)

## IMAGING FINDINGS

### General Features
- Best diagnostic clue: Elongated finger-shaped CSF collection between septal leaves/lateral ventricles
- Location: CSP = between frontal horns of lateral ventricles, CV = posterior extension between fornices
- Size: From slit-like to several mm, occasionally > 1 cm
- Morphology: Elongated, finger-like

### CT Findings
- NECT: CSF collection between leaves of SP

### MR Findings
- T1WI
  - Axial: Finger-like CSF space between lateral ventricles
  - Sagittal: CSP-CV from rostrum to splenium of corpus callosum above, ICVs below; pure CSP restricted to SP; pure CV restricted to fornices
- T2WI: Isointense with CSF
- FLAIR: Isointense with CSF

### Ultrasonographic Findings
- Grayscale Ultrasound: Always present in fetus; enlarges from 19-27 weeks, plateaus, closes in rostral direction from 28 weeks to term

### Imaging Recommendations
- Best imaging tool: US in fetus, infant; MR later, CT not bad
- Protocol advice: Triplanar, multiple sequence imaging ensuring that it is CSF

## DIFFERENTIAL DIAGNOSIS

### Cavum Velum Interpositum (CVI)
- Triangular in axial plane; behind foramen of Monro

## DDx: Other Midline Cysts and Abnormalities

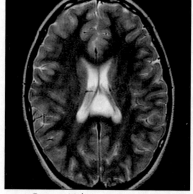

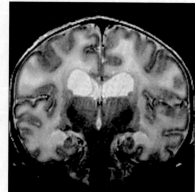

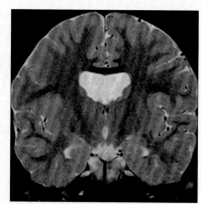

*Cavum Velum Interpositum*

*Ependymal Cysts*

*Absent Septum Pellucidum*

# CAVUM SEPTI PELLUCIDI (CSP)

## Key Facts

### Imaging Findings
- Best diagnostic clue: Elongated finger-shaped CSF collection between septal leaves/lateral ventricles
- Size: From slit-like to several mm, occasionally > 1 cm
- Sagittal: CSP-CV from rostrum to splenium of corpus callosum above, ICVs below; pure CSP restricted to SP; pure CV restricted to fornices

- Grayscale Ultrasound: Always present in fetus; enlarges from 19-27 weeks, plateaus, closes in rostral direction from 28 weeks to term
- Best imaging tool: US in fetus, infant; MR later, CT not bad

### Diagnostic Checklist
- CSP common in metabolic disorders of the brain

## Ependymal Cyst
- Lateral, in body/atrium of lateral ventricle

## Absent Septum Pellucidum (SP)
- Looks like CSP/CV on sagittal (coronal: Absent SP)

## PATHOLOGY

### General Features
- General path comments: CSP, CV are not ventricles, but may communicate
- Etiology: Fetal SP fails to obliterate, reason unknown
- Epidemiology
  - CSP: In 100% of premature, 85% term infants, 1% up to 15-20% of adults
  - CV: In 100% at 6 months fetal, 30% term, < 1% adults

### Gross Pathologic & Surgical Features
- CSP, CV may/may not communicate with other CSF spaces

### Staging, Grading or Classification Criteria
- Shaw and Ellsworth classification for CSP, CV
  - Asymptomatic cavum (communicating or not)
  - Symptomatic, pathological, non-communicating cavum (cyst of the cavum)
    - Uncomplicated vs. headaches, hydrocephalus

## CLINICAL ISSUES

### Presentation
- Most common signs/symptoms
  - Usually asymptomatic, incidental
  - Headache common: Intermittent occlusion of foramina of Monro?
  - Expanding CSP: Visual, behavioral, autonomic symptoms

### Natural History & Prognosis
- Rarely enlarge (cyst) ⇒ obstruction, hydrocephalus

### Treatment
- Usually none (may be fenestrated/drained/shunted)

## DIAGNOSTIC CHECKLIST

### Consider
- CSP common in metabolic disorders of the brain

## SELECTED REFERENCES
1. Sencer A et al: Cerebrospinal fluid dynamics of the cava septi pellucidi and vergae. Case report. J Neurosurg. 94(1):127-9, 2001

## IMAGE GALLERY

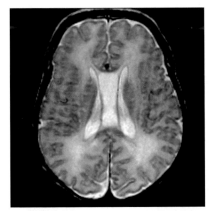 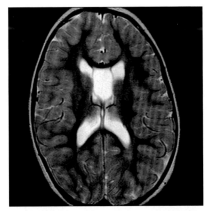 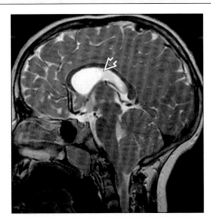

*(Left)* Axial T2WI MR shows that this "finger-like" CSF filled space continues posteriorly for the whole length of the corpus callosum and that therefore it corresponds to a CSP-CV. *(Center)* Axial T2WI MR shows a pure CSP separating the septal leaves anteriorly without posterior extension to the CV. *(Right)* Sagittal T2WI MR shows the posterior boundary of this pure CSP ➡; a pure cavum Vergae is rare and would be located behind this boundary.

# CAVUM VELUM INTERPOSITUM (CVI)

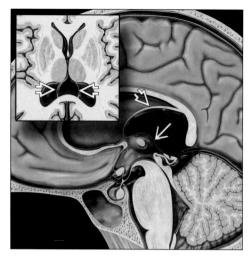

Sagittal graphic with axial insert shows a CVI. Elevated, splayed fornices ⇨, internal cerebral veins and 3rd ventricle lowered ⇨.

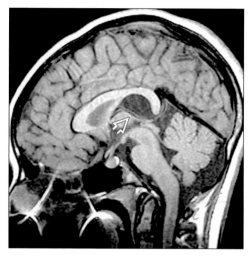

Sagittal T1WI MR shows CSF-filled cavity ⇨ between fornix and posterior corpus callosum above, 3rd ventricular tela choroidea and pineal gland below.

## TERMINOLOGY

### Abbreviations and Synonyms
- Cavum velum interpositum (CVI); cavum velum triangulare; cyst of velum interpositum (VI)

### Definitions
- Cystic dilation of the cistern of the VI

## IMAGING FINDINGS

### General Features
- Best diagnostic clue: Triangular cerebrospinal fluid (CSF) space between lateral ventricles on axial MR/CT
- Location: Between lateral ventricles, below fornix, above 3rd ventricular tela choroidea/internal cerebral veins (ICV), behind foramen of Monro
- Size: Fetal: Range = 10-30 mm; postnatal varies
- Morphology: Triangle, apex anterior, base at splenium

### CT Findings
- NECT: Triangular CSF space between fornices
- CECT: Does not enhance

### MR Findings
- T1WI
  - Axial: CSF-filled triangle between lateral ventricles, behind foramen of Monro, anterior to splenium
  - Sagittal: Round/ovoid CSF collection between fornix and 3rd ventricle
  - Coronal: Below callosal splenium, splaying fornices
- T2WI: Isointense with CSF
- FLAIR: Low intensity (like CSF)
- DWI: High diffusivity (like CSF)

### Ultrasonographic Findings
- Color Doppler
  - Hypoechoic midline interhemispheric cyst
  - Inverted "helmet shape" on sagittal sonograms
  - Internal cerebral veins (ICVs) pushed downward

### Imaging Recommendations
- Best imaging tool: MR without contrast
- Protocol advice: FLAIR, DWI to rule out an epidermoid

## DDx: Other Midline Fluid-Filled Cavities

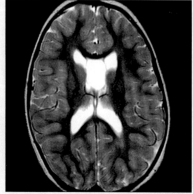

*Anterior Pure CSP*

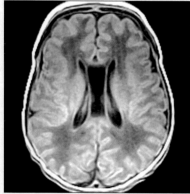

*Global CSP-CV*

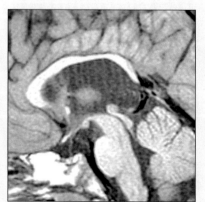

*Enlarged SPR*

# CAVUM VELUM INTERPOSITUM (CVI)

## Key Facts

### Terminology
- Cystic dilation of the cistern of the VI

### Imaging Findings
- Best diagnostic clue: Triangular cerebrospinal fluid (CSF) space between lateral ventricles on axial MR/CT
- T2WI: Isointense with CSF

### Top Differential Diagnoses
- Cavum Septi Pellucidi (CSP), Vergae (CV)
- Enlarged Supra-Pineal Recess (SPR)
- Epidermoid

### Pathology
- General path comments: CSF-filled space in roof of 3rd ventricle, between ICVs and fornices

### Diagnostic Checklist
- Deep midline epidermoid cyst may mimic a CSF collection; use FLAIR/DWI to differentiate

## DIFFERENTIAL DIAGNOSIS

### Cavum Septi Pellucidi (CSP), Vergae (CV)
- CSP/CV elongated CSF space (CVI triangular)

### Enlarged Supra-Pineal Recess (SPR)
- Bulging posterior 3rd ventricle

### Epidermoid
- Hyperintense on FLAIR, DWI

## PATHOLOGY

### General Features
- General path comments: CSF-filled space in roof of 3rd ventricle, between ICVs and fornices
- Genetics: No known association
- Etiology: As fetal cerebral hemispheres expand, pia-arachnoid infolding along deep transverse fissure forms VI cistern that may become encysted
- Epidemiology: Uncommon
- Associated abnormalities: Hydrocephalus, rare

### Gross Pathologic & Surgical Features
- Slit-like pial-lined arachnoid, CSF-filled space

### Microscopic Features
- May contain glia and scattered neurons

## CLINICAL ISSUES

### Presentation
- Most common signs/symptoms: Asymptomatic, relation to headaches unclear

### Demographics
- Age: Any age, prevalence decreases with age
- Gender: M = F

### Natural History & Prognosis
- Prenatal: Isolated, single CVI, stable in size, has favorable postnatal outcome

### Treatment
- Symptomatic cysts should be fenestrated

## DIAGNOSTIC CHECKLIST

### Consider
- Deep midline epidermoid cyst may mimic a CSF collection; use FLAIR/DWI to differentiate

## SELECTED REFERENCES

1. Eisenberg VH et al: Prenatal diagnosis of cavum velum interpositum cysts: significance and outcome. Prenat Diagn. 23(10):779-83, 2003
2. Vergani P et al: Ultrasonographic differential diagnosis of fetal intracranial interhemispheric cysts. Am J Obstet Gynecol. 180(2 Pt 1):423-8, 1999

## IMAGE GALLERY

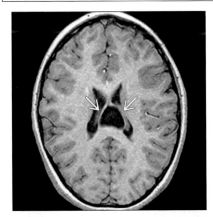
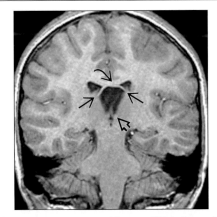
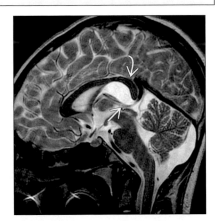

*(Left) Axial T1WI MR shows triangular CSF-filled space between crura of fornices ➡, in front of splenium of corpus callosum. (Center) Coronal T1WI MR shows enlarged space below the fornices ➡ and corpus callosum ➡, above pineal gland ➡. (Right) Sagittal T2WI MR shows the CSF-intensity CVI above the ICV ➡ and below the corpus callosum ➡.*

# SEPTOOPTIC DYSPLASIA

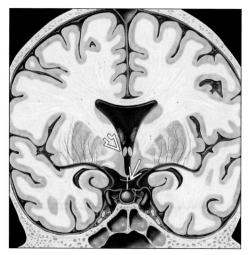

Coronal graphic depicts flat-roofed anterior horns & absence of midline septum pellucidum. Anterior horns are draped inferiorly around fornices ➡. Optic chiasm ➡ small.

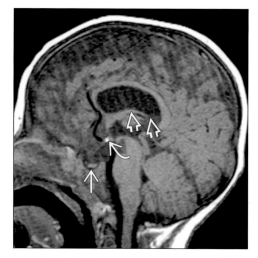

Sagittal T1WI MR shows ectopic posterior pituitary gland ➡. Pituitary stalk isn't clearly identified and anterior pituitary ➡ is too small. Fornices ➡ are too low.

## TERMINOLOGY

### Abbreviations and Synonyms
- Septooptic dysplasia (SOD)
- De Morsier syndrome
- Kaplan-Grumbach-Hoyt syndrome
- Septooptic-pituitary dysgenesis
- SOD plus: Abnormal optic nerves/chiasm, septum pellucidum, pituitary gland, + cortical dysplasias

### Definitions
- SOD = heterogeneous disorder characterized by hypoplasia of optic nerves/tract, absent septum pellucidum, (usually) hypothalamic-pituitary dysfunction
- De Morsier (1956): Described 7 patients with SOD
- Hoyt (1978): Described the association of SOD with hypopituitarism
- Some consider SOD a mild form of lobar holoprosencephaly

## IMAGING FINDINGS

### General Features
- Best diagnostic clue: Absent septum pellucidum, small optic chiasm
- Location: Optic nerves, pituitary gland, septum pellucidum
- Size
  - Small optic nerves
  - Small pituitary gland, sometimes with ectopic posterior lobe
- Morphology
  - Sagittal and coronal imaging shows
    - Absent septum pellucidum
    - Low and sometimes fused fornices

### CT Findings
- NECT
  - Absent septum pellucidum
  - Small bony optic foramina on axial and coronal imaging

### MR Findings
- T1WI

## DDx: Septooptic Dysplasia

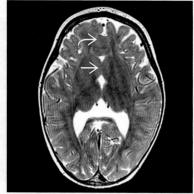

Semilobar Holoprosencephaly

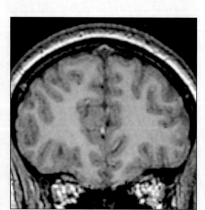

Kallmann Syndrome

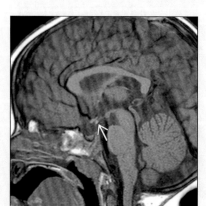

Ectopic Posterior Pituitary

# SEPTOOPTIC DYSPLASIA

## Key Facts

### Terminology
- De Morsier syndrome
- SOD = heterogeneous disorder characterized by hypoplasia of optic nerves/tract, absent septum pellucidum, (usually) hypothalamic-pituitary dysfunction

### Imaging Findings
- Absent septum pellucidum (remnants may be present)
- Flat roof of frontal horns, inferior aspect of frontal horns "point down"
- Small optic chiasm/nerve(s) (fat-sat aides visualization of optic nerves)
- ± Thin pituitary stalk
- Best imaging tool: MR

### Top Differential Diagnoses
- Kallmann Syndrome
- Lobar Holoprosencephaly
- Isolated Ectopic Posterior Pituitary Lobe

### Pathology
- Optic nerve hypoplasia (ONH)
- 60% have brain abnormalities (not just schizencephaly)
- 62-88% have pituitary insufficiency
- Frequently associated with other cerebral anomalies
- Schizencephaly or polymicrogyria in up to 35%
- Midline malformations (callosal dysgenesis, etc.)
- Ocular anomalies (coloboma, anophthalmia, microphthalmia)
- Olfactory tract/bulb hypoplasia

---

- Three planes crucial to identify all findings
  - Absent septum pellucidum (remnants may be present)
  - Flat roof of frontal horns, inferior aspect of frontal horns "point down"
  - Small optic chiasm/nerve(s) (fat-sat aides visualization of optic nerves)
  - ± Thin pituitary stalk
  - Small anterior pituitary, posterior pituitary ectopia
  - Callosal-forniceal continuation or fused midline fornices
  - Thin corpus callosum
  - Vertical hippocampi
  - ± Hypoplastic/absent olfactory nerves
  - ± Schizencephaly
  - ± Heterotopia, cortical dysplasias
- T2WI: Deficient falx (esp anteriorly); ± hypomyelination
- T1 C+
  - Better shows thin infundibulum when posterior pituitary lobe is ectopic
  - Delayed enhancement of anterior pituitary lobe on dynamic MR

### Imaging Recommendations
- Best imaging tool: MR
- Protocol advice
  - Coronal, sagittal thin-sections through sella/orbits
  - Use fat-sat to better visualize optic nerves

## DIFFERENTIAL DIAGNOSIS

### Syndromes Overlapping with Septooptic Dysplasia
- Optic-infundibular dysplasia (OID), normal septum
- Schizencephaly: Usually bilateral, frontal, temporal, or parietal

### Kallmann Syndrome
- Absent or dysplastic olfactory nerves, olfactory sulci
- Hypogonadotropic hypogonadism
- ± Visual, septal, pituitary abnormalities

### Lobar Holoprosencephaly
- Similar to SOD but has lack of separation ("fusion") of cerebral hemispheres
- Many consider SOD a milder form of same disorder

### Isolated Ectopic Posterior Pituitary Lobe
- Normal chiasm/nerves, septum pellucidum

## PATHOLOGY

### General Features
- General path comments
  - Sudden death reported from hypothalamic-pituitary axis malfunction
  - Embryology-anatomy
    - Disorder of midline ventral prosencephalic development (6th wk gestation): Pituitary gland, forebrain, optic nerves, olfactory bulbs
    - HESX1 (homeobox gene): Needed for pituitary/forebrain development: Possibly implicated
- Genetics
  - Most cases sporadic
  - Some are autosomal dominant or recessive
  - A few cases have mutations in HESX1 gene
    - Homozygous mutations = full syndrome
    - Heterozygous mutations = milder pituitary phenotypes
  - Inactivation of HESX1 (3p21.2-3p21.2) by an Arg53Cys substitution leads to deficient anterior pituitary lobe (doesn't occur in sporadic SOD)
- Etiology
  - Theories
    - Genetic ventral midline defect (possibly mild holoprosencephaly variant)
    - Or secondary degeneration of optic nerve fibers due to cerebral lesion
    - Or vascular disruption (field defect) during brain development (unlikely)
    - Teratogens: Cytomegalovirus (CMV), antiepileptic drugs, ethanol alcohol (ETOH), maternal diabetes

# SEPTOOPTIC DYSPLASIA

- Epidemiology
  - 1 in 50,000 live births
  - Optic nerve hypoplasia (ONH)
    - 60% have brain abnormalities (not just schizencephaly)
    - 62-88% have pituitary insufficiency
    - 30% have both of the above
    - 25-50% have absent septum pellucidum
  - SOD
    - 75-90% have brain abnormalities; 45% have pituitary insufficiency
    - Bilateral optic nerve hypoplasia 70%
- Associated abnormalities
  - Frequently associated with other cerebral anomalies
    - Schizencephaly or polymicrogyria in up to 35%
    - Midline malformations (callosal dysgenesis, etc.)
    - Ocular anomalies (coloboma, anophthalmia, microphthalmia)
    - Olfactory tract/bulb hypoplasia
    - Gray matter heterotopia
  - Overlapping syndromes with optic, septal, frontal lobe, midline, olfactory deficiencies

## Gross Pathologic & Surgical Features
- Small optic chiasm/nerves
- Small or absent geniculate nucleus
- Deficient/absent septum pellucidum
- Forniceal columns (± fused) ⇒ run along roof of 3rd ventricle
- Common: Hypoplasia pituitary, olfactory lobes

## Microscopic Features
- Lateral geniculate nucleus (if found): Disorganized layering of small neurons

## Staging, Grading or Classification Criteria
- Isolated ONH: Visual defect only; intelligence and growth normal
- ONH and deficient septum: Same as isolated
- ONH with septal and pituitary deficiency: May have developmental delay
- Above plus malformation of cortical development: Plus seizures

# CLINICAL ISSUES

## Presentation
- Most common signs/symptoms
  - Newborns: Hypoglycemic seizures, apnea, cyanosis, hypotonia, prolonged conjugated jaundice, (and microphallus in boys)
  - Abnormal endocrine function (60%): Look for multiple pituitary deficiencies
  - Normal endocrine function (40%): Usually have schizencephaly or heterotopia, seizures
- Clinical Profile
  - Child with short stature, endocrine dysfunction
  - Vision can be normal or color blindness, visual loss, nystagmus, strabismus
  - ± Mental retardation, spasticity, microcephaly, anosmia

## Demographics
- Age
  - Generally detected in infants
  - More common among younger mothers & first-born
- Gender: M = F
- Ethnicity: All groups equally affected

## Natural History & Prognosis
- Hypothalamic and pituitary crises; sudden death (hypocortisolism)
- Depends upon severity of associated brain and pituitary malformations

## Treatment
- Hormonal replacement therapy

# DIAGNOSTIC CHECKLIST

## Consider
- SOD in small stature pediatric patient with absent septum pellucidum

## Image Interpretation Pearls
- Small optic nerves, + small anterior pituitary or ectopic posterior pituitary lobe, + absent septum pellucidum = SOD

# SELECTED REFERENCES

1. Polizzi A et al: Septo-optic dysplasia complex: a heterogeneous malformation syndrome. Pediatr Neurol. 34(1):66-71, 2006
2. Rainbow LA et al: Mutation analysis of POUF-1, PROP-1 and HESX-1 show low frequency of mutations in children with sporadic forms of combined pituitary hormone deficiency and septo-optic dysplasia. Clin Endocrinol (Oxf). 62(2):163-8, 2005
3. Camino R et al: Septo-optic dysplasia plus. Lancet Neurol. 2(7):436, 2003
4. Campbell CL: Septo-optic dysplasia: a literature review. Optometry. 74(7):417-26, 2003
5. Tajima T et al: Sporadic heterozygous frameshift mutation of HESX1 causing pituitary and optic nerve hypoplasia and combined pituitary hormone deficiency in a Japanese patient. J Clin Endocrinol Metab. 88(1):45-50, 2003
6. Wakeling EL et al: Septo-optic dysplasia, subglottic stenosis and skeletal abnormalities: a case report. Clin Dysmorphol. 12(2):105-7, 2003
7. Antonini SR et al: Cerebral midline developmental anomalies: endocrine, neuroradiographic and ophthalmological features. J Pediatr Endocrinol Metab. 15(9):1525-30, 2002
8. Dattani M: Structural hypothalamic defects. J Pediatr Endocrinol Metab. 15 Suppl 5:1423-4, 2002
9. Orrico A et al: Septo-optic dysplasia with digital anomalies associated with maternal multidrug abuse during pregnancy. Eur J Neurol. 9(6):679-82, 2002
10. Dattani ML et al: Molecular genetics of septo-optic dysplasia. Horm Res. 53 Suppl 1:26-33, 2000
11. Miller SP et al: Septo-optic dysplasia plus: a spectrum of malformations of cortical development. Neurology. 54(8):1701-3, 2000
12. Barkovich AJ et al: Septo-optic dysplasia: MR imaging. Radiology. 171(1):189-92, 1989

# SEPTOOPTIC DYSPLASIA

Typical

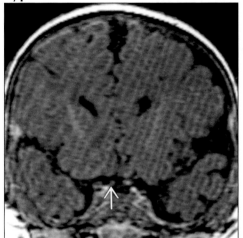
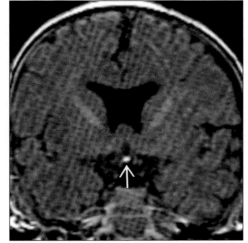

*(Left) Coronal T1WI MR shows very small (hypoplastic) right optic nerve ➡ and shallow olfactory sulci. (Right) Coronal T1WI MR shows complete absence of the septum pellucidum and the ectopic posterior pituitary gland ➡ in the median eminence of the hypothalamus.*

Typical

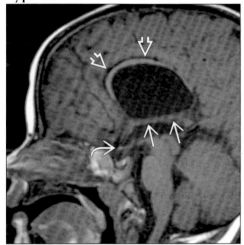
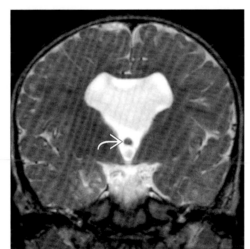

*(Left) Sagittal T1WI MR shows small optic chiasm ➡, low fornices ➡, and thin, hypoplastic corpus callosum ➡. Note the pituitary gland is normal in this case. (Right) Coronal T2WI MR shows large lateral ventricles secondary to diminished cerebral white matter, fused fornices ➡ and absent septum pellucidum.*

Typical

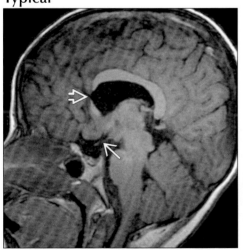
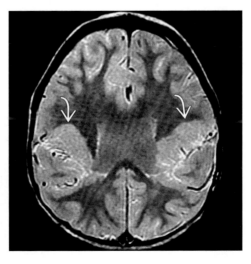

*(Left) Sagittal T1WI MR shows a very small optic chiasm ➡, low-lying fornices, and a dysplastic corpus callosum, with absence of part of the genu ➡. The posterior pituitary gland is absent. (Right) Axial PD/Intermediate MR shows absent septum pellucidum and bilateral schizencephalic clefts ➡. Up to 35% of SOD cases have associated malformations of cortical development.*

# HYDROCEPHALUS

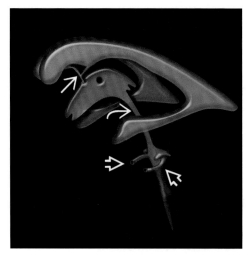

Graphic of ventricular system illustrates key locations where lesions cause obstructive hydrocephalus; foramen of Monro ➡, cerebral aqueduct ➔, and 4th ventricle outlet foramina ➡.

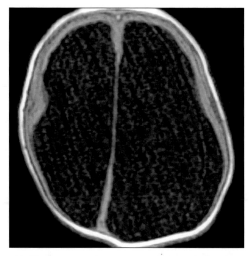

Axial T1WI MR shows severe hydrocephalus from aqueductal stenosis. It is important to distinguish this diagnosis from hydranencephaly in the neonate with ventriculomegaly.

## TERMINOLOGY

### Abbreviations and Synonyms

- Obstructive hydrocephalus, intraventricular obstructive hydrocephalus (IVOH)
- Communicating hydrocephalus, external hydrocephalus, extraventricular obstructive hydrocephalus (EVOH)
  - Not covered in this discussion

### Definitions

- Excess vol of intracranial cerebrospinal fluid (CSF)
- Can be due to obstruction within ventricular system, over production of CSF, or decreased resorption
  - Many will assume obstruction and increased pressure when the term hydrocephalus is used
- Ventriculomegaly does not equal hydrocephalus!
  - Ventriculomegaly describes enlarged ventricles only
    - Not necessarily associated with increased pressure
  - May reflect decreased parenchymal volume

## IMAGING FINDINGS

### General Features

- Best diagnostic clue
  - Enlarged ventricles with decreased extra-axial spaces
  - In children with open sutures, hydrocephalus results in macrocrania
    - Macrocrania accommodates increasing CSF volume with less increase in pressure
  - In children with closed sutures, hydrocephalus results in increased intracranial pressure (ICP)
    - Associated herniation of brain tissue
- Location
  - Obstructing lesions at key points in ventricular system
    - Foramen of Monro, posterior 3rd ventricle, cerebral aqueduct, 4th ventricle
    - Temporal horn "trapped" by mass effect on trigone
- Size
  - Early onset and slow progression of obstructive hydrocephalus can lead to massive ventriculomegaly
    - May mimic hydranencephaly or holoprosencephaly

## DDx: Non-Obstructive Ventriculomegaly

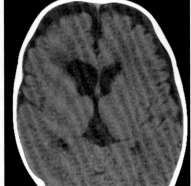

EVOH

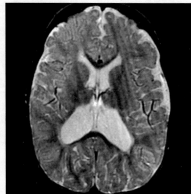

End Stage PVL

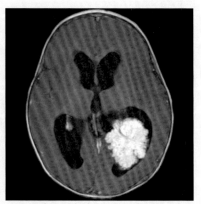

Choroid Plexus Papilloma

# HYDROCEPHALUS

## Key Facts

### Terminology
- Excess vol of intracranial cerebrospinal fluid (CSF)
- Ventriculomegaly does not equal hydrocephalus!

### Imaging Findings
- In children with open sutures, hydrocephalus results in macrocrania
- Shunt series is mainstay of evaluating integrity of ventricular drainage systems
- Periventricular halo of low attenuation ⇒ interstitial edema
- MRV: Increased ICP can flatten transverse sinuses
- NECT (reduced radiation dose) most efficient and consistent means of evaluating ventricle size

### Top Differential Diagnoses
- Obstructing Tumors

- Congenital Malformations
- Periventricular leukomalacia (PVL)
- EVOH

### Pathology
- General path comments: Hydrocephalus results from the loss of homeostasis of CSF production and resorption
- Classical theory holds that there is net migration of CSF from the ventricles to SAS
- IVOH reverses normal pressure gradient from interstitium to ventricles

### Diagnostic Checklist
- Always correlate ventriculomegaly with head circumference in neonates and infants

---

- Distinguished by thin rim of remaining cortical mantle
- Morphology
  - As ventricles enlarge, angular margins become rounded
  - Anterior recesses of 3rd ventricle dilate early
  - Trigones enlarge first when lateral ventricles obstructed
    - Laplace law ⇒ as pressure increases, regions with larger surface area (assuming similar compliance) are subject to more pressure and preferentially dilate

### CT Findings
- NECT
  - Enlarged and rounded ventricles
  - Periventricular halo of low attenuation ⇒ interstitial edema
  - Basal cisterns and sulci compressed

### MR Findings
- T1WI
  - Enlarged and rounded ventricles
  - Corpus callosum thinned, stretched upward
  - Anterior recesses of 3rd ventricle enlarge, herniate downward
  - Ventricular "entrapment"
    - Localized hydrocephalus caused by strategically placed lesion
    - Absence of dilation of entire system may result in atypical clinical symptoms
    - Temporal horns can be entrapped by mass effect on occipital horn or trigone of ventricle
    - 4th ventricle can become entrapped if all adjacent foramina (Magendie, Luschka, aqueduct) are obstructed
- FLAIR
  - Interstitial edema
    - Hyperintense "stain" in periventricular white matter
    - May reduce or resolve in chronic obstruction (compensated)
- MRV: Increased ICP can flatten transverse sinuses

- MR Cine
  - Ideal for demonstrating patency of 3rd ventriculostomy fenestration
    - Third ventriculostomy ⇒ hole created in floor of 3rd ventricle via ventriculoscope
    - Allows passage of CSF from 3rd ventricle into subarachnoid space (SAS)

### Radiographic Findings
- Shunt series is mainstay of evaluating integrity of ventricular drainage systems
  - Anteroposterior (AP) and lateral skull, AP chest, and AP abdomen radiographs

### Ultrasonographic Findings
- Transcranial US ideal for identifying ventriculomegaly in infants with macrocrania and patent anterior fontanelle

### Other Modality Findings
- Contrast-enhanced ventriculography (CT or MR) can identify webs and other subtle obstructing lesions

### Imaging Recommendations
- Best imaging tool
  - NECT (reduced radiation dose) most efficient and consistent means of evaluating ventricle size
  - Fast and/or motion-reducing MR sequences may be a reasonable alternative to CT
- Protocol advice
  - CT studies should be acquired at consistent levels and angles
    - Surveillance exams should be performed with reduced radiation technique

---

## DIFFERENTIAL DIAGNOSIS

### Obstructing Tumors
- Tectal glioma ⇒ cerebral aqueduct
- Medulloblastoma, ependymoma ⇒ 4th ventricle
- Subependymal giant cell astrocytoma (SEGA) ⇒ foramen of Monro
- Colloid cyst ⇒ foramen of Monro

- Choroid plexus papilloma (CPP)
  - Can over-produce or obstruct CSF

## Inflammatory Disease
- Neurocysticercosis
- Meningitis and ventriculitis

## Congenital Malformations
- Typically have a combination of dysmorphic ventriculomegaly and obstructive hydrocephalus
  - Chiari 2, Dandy-Walker malformation, callosal anomalies
- Hydranencephaly
  - Pre-natal loss of parenchymal in bilateral carotid distribution
- Open-lip schizencephaly
- Vein of Galen malformation (VGAM)
  - ↑ Pressure in dural sinuses impairs CSF resorption
  - Varix can obstruct CSF flow at cerebral aqueduct

## Ventriculomegaly from Parenchymal Volume Loss
- Periventricular leukomalacia (PVL)
  - In-utero injury to oligodendrocyte-rich periventricular white matter
  - White matter is resorbed ⇒ ex-vacuo ventriculomegaly
- Diffuse enlargement of sulci, cisterns
- Normal to small head circumference

## EVOH
- Prior meningitis or intracranial hemorrhage
- Idiopathic

## Benign Macrocrania
- Self-limited form of EVOH common in children 6-24 months of age
- No associated neurologic symptoms

## PATHOLOGY

### General Features
- General path comments: Hydrocephalus results from the loss of homeostasis of CSF production and resorption
- Genetics
  - X-linked aqueductal stenosis is due to a mutation of the L1CAM gene located at Xq28
    - Associated with malformations of cortical development, thalamic fusion
- Etiology
  - Majority of CSF is produced by choroid
  - Remainder is interstitial fluid of brain and spinal cord parenchyma
    - Functions analogous to lymph in extra-CNS solid organs
    - Some drains into lymphatics around cranial nerves
  - Classical theory holds that there is net migration of CSF from the ventricles to SAS
  - CSF is resorbed into dural sinuses via veins, arachnoid granulations
  - Bulk flow of CSF requires

- Normal CSF pulsatility with systole and diastole
- Normal elasticity of ventricles and SAS
- Normal (low) pressure in dural sinuses
  - IVOH reverses normal pressure gradient from interstitium to ventricles
    - Fluid "backs up" into white matter surrounding ventricles
    - Accentuated at acute angles of ventricles, where multiple channels converge onto a small ependymal surface area
    - Associated with reduced blood flow and metabolic rate in periventricular white matter
- Epidemiology: Most common neurosurgical procedure in children = CSF shunting for hydrocephalus

### Microscopic Features
- Ependymal lining damaged or lost
- Choroid becomes fibrotic

## CLINICAL ISSUES

### Presentation
- Most common signs/symptoms
  - Macrocrania, headache, papilledema
  - Nausea, irritability, seizures
- Other signs/symptoms: Transtentorial herniation can cause "blown" pupil

### Demographics
- Age: Variable, usually a disease of childhood
- Gender: Some congenital causes (X-linked aqueductal stenosis), tumors (germinoma) are gender biased

### Natural History & Prognosis
- Typically fatal, but untreated hydrocephalus may become compensated
- Massive macrocrania can result if process begins when sutures are open

### Treatment
- CSF diversion (shunt), third ventriculostomy, fenestration of septae

## DIAGNOSTIC CHECKLIST

### Consider
- Consider MR for routine assessment to reduce life-long radiation dose to patients with shunts

### Image Interpretation Pearls
- Always correlate ventriculomegaly with head circumference in neonates and infants
- Size of ventricles generally correlates poorly with intracranial pressure

## SELECTED REFERENCES

1. Bargallo N et al: Functional analysis of third ventriculostomy patency by quantification of CSF stroke volume by using cine phase-contrast MR imaging. AJNR Am J Neuroradiol. 26(10):2514-21, 2005
2. Joseph VB et al: MR ventriculography for the study of CSF flow. AJNR Am J Neuroradiol. 24(3):373-81, 2003

# HYDROCEPHALUS

## IMAGE GALLERY

### Typical

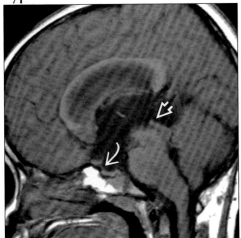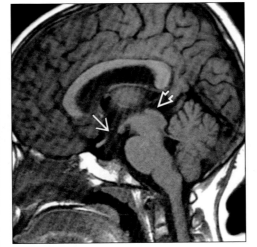

*(Left) Sagittal T1WI MR in a child with NF1 and aqueductal stenosis shows flattening of rostral tectum due to dilation of posterior 3rd ventricle ➡. Note anterior bowing of infundibulum ➡. (Right) Sagittal T1WI MR (same child as previous image) 3 months later shows normalization of tectal morphology ➡ and of third ventricle size as a result of a 3rd ventriculostomy ➡.*

### Typical

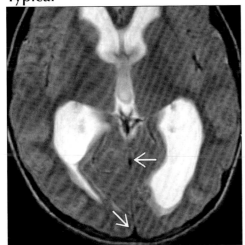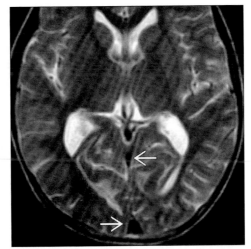

*(Left) Axial T2WI MR shows very small caliber of the straight sinus and the sagittal sinus ➡ in this child with obstructive hydrocephalus from a 4th ventricular tumor. (Right) Axial T2WI MR in the same child as previous image after tumor resection shows normalization of the size of the sinuses ➡. When ICP is greater than venous pressure, sinus compression can exacerbate hydrocephalus.*

### Typical

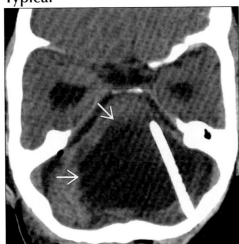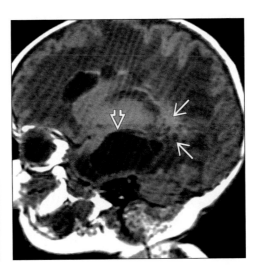

*(Left) Axial NECT shows "trapped" 4th ventricle ➡. The adjacent drainage catheter was not functioning. The outlet foramina of the 4th ventricle can all become obstructed by webs and adhesions. (Right) Sagittal T1WI MR through the temporal lobe shows entrapment of the temporal horn ➡ due to adhesions ➡ in this child with a history of meningitis and ventriculitis.*

# AQUEDUCTAL STENOSIS

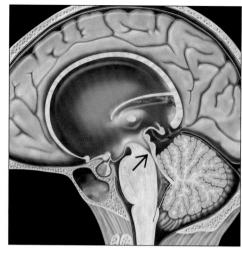

*Sagittal graphic shows obstructive hydrocephalus with massively enlarged ventricles, callosal thinning, "funnel" shaped aqueduct of Sylvius ⊒ and herniation of floor of 3rd ventricle.*

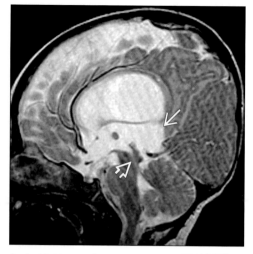

*Sagittal T2WI MR shows a marked ventricular marked dilation (dilated supra-pineal recess ⊒) and bowed corpus callosum; funnel dilation and occlusion of the posterior aqueduct ⊒.*

## TERMINOLOGY

### Abbreviations and Synonyms
- Aqueductal stenosis (AS)

### Definitions
- Focal reduction in aqueduct size (diameter), either congenital or benign acquired

## IMAGING FINDINGS

### General Features
- Best diagnostic clue
  - Funnel-shaped aqueduct of Sylvius
  - "Ballooned" ventricles (lateral, third) and foramina of Monroe proximal to obstruction
  - Normal 4th ventricle and outlets distal to obstruction
  - Interstitial edema with indistinct ("blurred") ventricular margins when decompensated (absent if AS chronic or "arrested")

- Location: Narrowing/obstruction at cerebral aqueduct, either at level of the superior colliculi or at intercollicular sulcus
- Size: Normal mean cross-sectional area of aqueduct at birth is 0.2-1.8 mm²
- Morphology
  - Typically funnel-shaped aqueduct of Sylvius
  - May rarely see "aqueductal forking" or branching of aqueduct into channels
  - Aqueductal forking often accompanied by fusion of quadrigeminal bodies, third nerve nuclei or tectal beaking

### CT Findings
- NECT
  - Enlarged ventricles supratentorially, large head
    - Lateral and third disproportionately enlarged compared to 4th ventricle
  - No obstructing midbrain mass
- CECT: No pathologic enhancement

### MR Findings
- T1WI
  - Lateral ventricles enlarged, rounded temporal horns with hippocampi compressed medially

## DDx: Other Aqueductal Occlusions

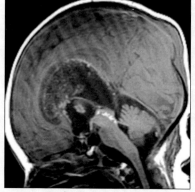

*Clot in Aqueduct*

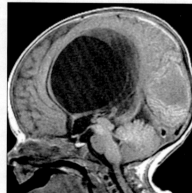

*Tectal Mass*

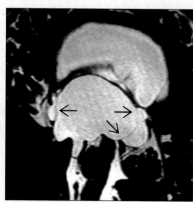

*Ventricular Cyst*

# AQUEDUCTAL STENOSIS

## Key Facts

### Terminology
- Focal reduction in aqueduct size (diameter), either congenital or benign acquired

### Imaging Findings
- Funnel-shaped aqueduct of Sylvius
- "Ballooned" ventricles (lateral, third) and foramina of Monroe proximal to obstruction
- Normal 4th ventricle and outlets distal to obstruction
- Corpus callosum (CC) thinned, stretched upward
- Carefully scrutinize posterior 3rd ventricle, tectum and tegmentum for presence of mass

### Top Differential Diagnoses
- Obstructing Extraventricular Midbrain (Tectal) Pathology
- Obstructing Intraventricular Pathology

- Post Inflammatory Gliosis (Aqueductal Gliosis) as Etiology

### Pathology
- AS obstructs CSF flow; increases resistance, lateral/3rd ventricular fluid pressure increases
- AS responsible for approximately 20% of congenital hydrocephalus

### Clinical Issues
- Hormonal deficiency
- Decompensated hydrocephalus: Headache, papilledema, 6th nerve palsy, bulging fontanelles
- Sun-setting eyes (Parinaud syndrome, lid retraction & tonic downgaze) in infants

---

- ○ Corpus callosum (CC) thinned, stretched upward
- ○ Septum pellucidum may be fenestrated in congenital cases
- ○ Dilated 3rd ventricle with floor displaced downward into the interpeduncular cistern (bulging tuber cinereum)
- T2WI
  - ○ When compensated, little or no periventricular edema
  - ○ When decompensated, "fingers" of cerebrospinal fluid (CSF)-like hyperintensity extend outwards from ventricles into brain (including CC)
  - ○ Interstitial edema most striking around ventricular horns
  - ○ Disturbed/turbulent CSF flow in ventricles
  - ○ Absent aqueductal "flow void" common, but may be present in incomplete occlusion (severe narrowing)
  - ○ Proximal stenosis ⇒ more severe hydrocephalus; distal stenosis ⇒ less severe
- T1 C+
  - ○ Helps to differentiate benign AS from neoplastic AS
  - ○ Hydrocephalus can induce leptomeningeal vascular stasis, mimics meningitis or metastases!
  - ○ Carefully scrutinize posterior 3rd ventricle, tectum and tegmentum for presence of mass
- MRV: Downward displacement of internal cerebral veins
- Cardiac-gated cine-MR: Lack of significant CSF flow in aqueduct
- 3D constructive interference in steady state (CISS, FIESTA) ⇒ outstanding depiction of CSF pathway obstruction

### Ultrasonographic Findings
- Grayscale Ultrasound
  - ○ Mastoid (posterolateral) fontanelle imaging in newborn may help differentiate AS from other pathologic conditions
  - ○ Dilated lateral, 3rd; normal 4th ventricles
  - ○ Prenatal sonography ⇒ same findings

### Imaging Recommendations
- Best imaging tool: Sagittal MR

- Protocol advice: High definition T2 imaging (CISS, Fiesta) allows better delineation of ventricular contour, septa and better differential

## DIFFERENTIAL DIAGNOSIS

### Obstructing Extraventricular Midbrain (Tectal) Pathology
- Neoplasm
  - ○ Tectal astrocytoma, especially neurofibromatosis 1
  - ○ Pineal region tumors
- Vascular malformation
- Paracollicular arachnoid cyst

### Obstructing Intraventricular Pathology
- Suprasellar/3rd ventricular floor cysts (rounded 3rd ventricle)
- Neurocysticercosis with aqueductal cyst

### Post Inflammatory Gliosis (Aqueductal Gliosis) as Etiology
- Post inflammatory process that is usually secondary to a perinatal infection or hemorrhage
- Increasing in prevalence as newborns with bacterial meningitis or ICH survive at increasing rates
- As in "benign" AS, the onset of symptoms (those of hydrocephalus) is insidious
- Ependymal lining of aqueduct is destroyed; marked fibrillary gliosis of adjacent tissue is present
- On imaging studies, differentiation of AS from aqueductal gliosis is not possible

## PATHOLOGY

### General Features
- General path comments: Congenital or early occurring stenosis at level of aqueduct of Sylvius
- Genetics

# AQUEDUCTAL STENOSIS

- o Cell adhesion molecule L1 (L1CAM) only gene recognized to cause human hydrocephalus, located on X chromosome (Xq28)
- o Overexpression of some growth factors [tumor growth factor(TGF)], mutated Otx2 (head organizer during morphogenesis) reported
- Etiology
  - o Aqueductal lumen normally decreases in relative size beginning 2nd week of fetal life until birth
    - Caused by growth pressures from adjacent mesencephalic structures
  - o AS obstructs CSF flow; increases resistance, lateral/3rd ventricular fluid pressure increases
  - o Ventricles expand, compress adjacent parenchyma, stretch corpus callosum, may rupture/open ependymal cell junctions
  - o Subependymal veins compressed and periventricular interstitial fluid increases
  - o Some cases of AS may be secondary to communicating hydrocephalus and secondary (external) compression of quadrigeminal plate by dilated cerebral hemispheres
- Epidemiology
  - o AS responsible for approximately 20% of congenital hydrocephalus
  - o 0.5-1 per 1,000 births, with recurrence rate in siblings of 1-4.5%
- Associated abnormalities
  - o CRASH: Callosal hypoplasia, mental retardation, adducted thumbs, spastic paraplegia and X-linked hydrocephalus
  - o Bickers-Adam syndrome: X-linked hydrocephalus accounts for 7% cases in males
    - Stenosis of aqueduct, severe mental retardation, 50% with adduction-flexion deformity of thumb

## Gross Pathologic & Surgical Features
- Generalized lateral and 3rd ventricular enlargement

## Microscopic Features
- Increased periventricular extracellular space, peri-ependymal fibrosis/sclerosis, demyelination, loss of fibers

# CLINICAL ISSUES

## Presentation
- Most common signs/symptoms
  - o Macrocephaly
  - o Hormonal deficiency
- Other signs/symptoms: Symptoms are insidious, may occur at any time from birth to adulthood, depend upon age of patient at time of onset
- Decompensated hydrocephalus: Headache, papilledema, 6th nerve palsy, bulging fontanelles
- Sun-setting eyes (Parinaud syndrome, lid retraction & tonic downgaze) in infants

## Demographics
- Age: Presentation anytime from birth to adulthood; depends on severity of stenosis and adaptation of the brain
- Gender: M:F = 2:1

## Natural History & Prognosis
- Usually progressive with loss of brain substance unless treated
- May rarely stabilize as "arrested hydrocephalus"

## Treatment
- Classical: CSF shunt diversion (most common neurosurgical procedure in children)
- Today: Endoscopic 3rd ventriculostomy (bulging tuber cinereum)

# DIAGNOSTIC CHECKLIST

## Consider
- Post inflammatory gliosis (aqueductal gliosis) as etiology
- Communicating hydrocephalus may present with a small 4th ventricle
- Most common cause of obstruction at aqueduct in children is a pineal region tumor

## Image Interpretation Pearls
- Tectal astrocytomas large enough to obstruct aqueduct can be missed on routine CT scanning
- All patients with suspected AS should be scrutinized for presence of an obstructing mass!
- Severe hydrocephalus ⇒ usually stenosis in proximal aqueduct, at level of superior colliculi or immediately inferior to posterior commissure
- In mild hydrocephalus, obstruction is more often in distal portion of aqueduct

# SELECTED REFERENCES

1. Tisell M et al: Neurological symptoms and signs in adult aqueductal stenosis. Acta Neurol Scand. 107(5):311-7, 2003
2. Fukuhara T et al: Clinical features of late-onset idiopathic aqueductal stenosis. Surg Neurol. 55(3):132-6; discussion 136-7, 2001
3. Partington MD: Congenital hydrocephalus. Neurosurg Clin N Am. 12(4):737-42, ix, 2001
4. Senat MV et al: Prenatal diagnosis of hydrocephalus-stenosis of the aqueduct of Sylvius by ultrasound in the first trimester of pregnancy. Report of two cases. Prenat Diagn. 21(13):1129-32, 2001
5. Schroeder HW et al: Endoscopic aqueductoplasty: technique and results. Neurosurgery. 45(3):508-15; discussion 515-8, 1999
6. Blackmore CC et al: Aqueduct compression from venous angioma: MR findings. AJNR Am J Neuroradiol. 17(3):458-60, 1996
7. Castro-Gago M et al: Autosomal recessive hydrocephalus with aqueductal stenosis. Childs Nerv Syst. 12(4):188-91, 1996
8. Kadowaki C et al: Cine magnetic resonance imaging of aqueductal stenosis. Childs Nerv Syst. 11(2):107-11, 1995
9. Villani R et al: Long-term outcome in aqueductal stenosis. Childs Nerv Syst. 11(3):180-5, 1995
10. Oka K et al: Flexible endoneurosurgical therapy for aqueductal stenosis. Neurosurgery. 33(2):236-42; discussion 242-3, 1993

# AQUEDUCTAL STENOSIS

## IMAGE GALLERY

### Typical

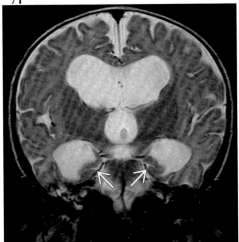

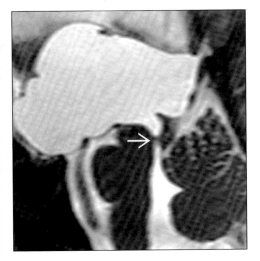

*(Left) Coronal T2WI MR shows tri-ventricular dilation with rounding of the ventricles and medial displacement of the hippocampi ➡. (Right) Sagittal T2\* GRE MR shows precise depiction of the AS ➡ with high definition T2\* (CISS); the tuber cinereum bulges in the suprasellar cistern (site of 3rd ventriculostomy).*

### Variant

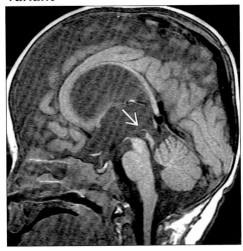

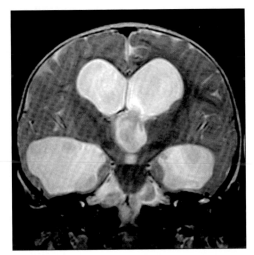

*(Left) Sagittal T1WI MR shows tri-ventricular hydrocephalus resulting from an undetermined, presumably congenital, cystic structure at the cranial opening of the aqueduct ➡. (Right) Coronal T2WI MR shows a huge tri-ventricular hydrocephalus with CSF turbulence, manifested as swirls of hypointensity within the ventricles.*

### Variant

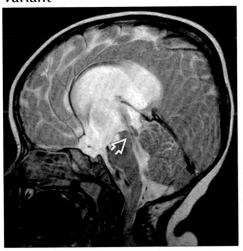

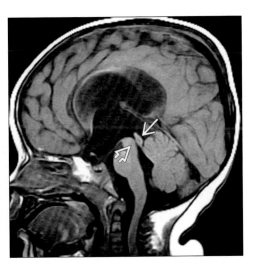

*(Left) Sagittal T2WI MR (same patient as previous image) shows a marked flow void through the aqueduct ➡, presumably patent. (Right) Sagittal T1WI MR shows concentric narrowing ➡ that explains the increased resistance to and increased velocity of, CSF flow, associated with abnormal tectal plate ➡.*

# COMMUNICATING HYDROCEPHALUS

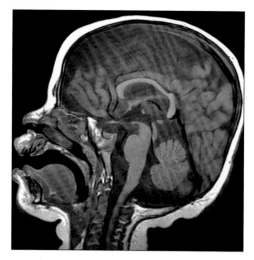

Sagittal T1WI MR shows macrocephaly, dilatation of the subarachnoid spaces, including the 4th ventricle, cisterna magna, prepontine cistern. Aqueduct is open. Corpus callosum is normal thickness for 8 month old.

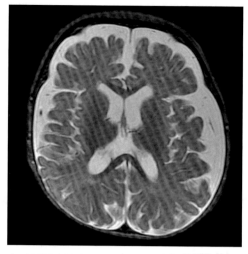

Axial T2WI MR shows moderate enlargement of lateral ventricles, extra-axial subarachnoid spaces. Myelination is normal for an 8 month old.

## TERMINOLOGY

### Abbreviations and Synonyms
- Obstructive extraventricular hydrocephalus

### Definitions
- Ventriculomegaly without a definable area of stenosis or obstruction as seen on MR

## IMAGING FINDINGS

### General Features
- Best diagnostic clue
  - Dilatation of all ventricular cavities, with or without enlargement of the basilar cisterns and cortical sulci, in a child with macrocephaly
    - 4th ventricle ⇒ normal size in 25% of cases
- Morphology
  - Diffuse expansion of ventricles usually out of proportion to amount of subarachnoid space (SAS) enlargement

- When severe, both enlarged temporal horns can compress the dorsal midbrain & quadrigeminal plate with resultant secondary compression of the aqueduct
- Diagnostic challenge ⇒ identify co-existent diffuse cerebral atrophy

### CT Findings
- NECT
  - Ventriculomegaly with rounded frontal and temporal horns, enlargement and ballooning of the third ventricle
  - When 4th ventricle enlarged, 4th ventricular outlets usually do not bulge
  - Basilar cisterns, SAS can be normal or diffusely enlarged

### MR Findings
- T1WI
  - Enlargement of lateral, third, ± 4th ventricle
  - Increased height of lateral ventricles; corpus callosum bowed, forms an arch
  - Meningeal enhancement in cases of infectious or carcinomatous meningitis

## DDx: Communicating Hydrocephalus

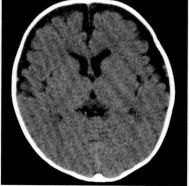

Benign Hygromas of Infancy

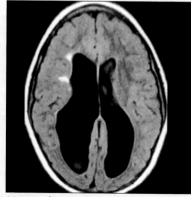

Ventriculomegaly w/o Macrocephaly

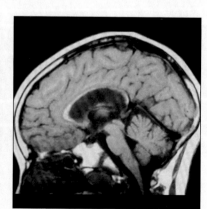

Ventriculomegaly w/o Macrocephaly

# COMMUNICATING HYDROCEPHALUS

## Key Facts

### Terminology
- Obstructive extraventricular hydrocephalus
- Ventriculomegaly without a definable area of stenosis or obstruction as seen on MR

### Imaging Findings
- Dilatation of all ventricular cavities, with or without enlargement of the basilar cisterns and cortical sulci, in a child with macrocephaly
- 4th ventricle ⇒ normal size in 25% of cases
- Diagnostic challenge ⇒ identify co-existent diffuse cerebral atrophy
- Basilar cisterns, SAS can be normal or diffusely enlarged

### Top Differential Diagnoses
- Benign Enlargement of the SASs in Infants (Benign External Hydrocephalus)
- Cerebral Atrophy
- Ventriculomegaly without Macrocephaly
- X-Linked Hydrocephalus
- Normal Pressure Hydrocephalus

### Diagnostic Checklist
- When atrophy and gliosis present, consider if they are the primary abnormality or the result of the hydrocephalus
- In patients with CH and craniosynostosis or anomalies of craniocervical junction, look for venous stenosis (sigmoid sinus, jugular bulb) on MRV

---

- In general, bacterial meningitis produces cerebral cortical arachnoiditis; granulomatous/parasitic meningitides produce cisternal obstruction
- T2WI
  - Patent aqueduct/aqueductal "flow void"
  - Periventricular high signal, primarily anterior to frontal horns (interstitial edema) occasionally seen
  - Post hemorrhage: May see T2 dark signal of the parenchyma or meninges (superficial siderosis)
- Dilatation of optic and infundibular recesses of anterior 3rd ventricle and downward displacement of hypothalamus
- Decreased cerebral volume, gliosis, delayed myelination can be signs of secondary atrophy
- MR venography (MRV) useful to assess venous patency, exclude sinovenous stenosis or thrombosis

### Imaging Recommendations
- Best imaging tool: CT = MR in most cases
- Protocol advice
  - Do MR when 4th ventricle, SAS not enlarged
  - MRV when venous stenosis suspected, especially when craniosynostosis or cranio-cervical junction anomaly (including Chiari 1) present

## DIFFERENTIAL DIAGNOSIS

### Benign Enlargement of the SASs in Infants (Benign External Hydrocephalus)
- Transient developmental phenomenon of macrocephaly and prominence of SAS ± mild ventricular enlargement
- Usually presents between 2nd and 7th month of life
- Enlargement of anterior SAS (frontal, temporal, anterior interhemispheric, sylvian)
- Must differentiate from abnormal subdural fluid collections (rule out non-accidental trauma)

### Cerebral Atrophy
- Diffuse, symmetric enlargement of ventricles, sulci
- Decreased cerebral volume, decreased thickness of corpus callosum

- Head circumference normal or small

### Ventriculomegaly without Macrocephaly
- Diffuse ex vacuo enlargement of lateral ventricles
- Low volume cerebral white matter, thin corpus callosum, ± white matter gliosis
- Third trimester damage to oligodendrocytes results in periventricular white matter injury

### X-Linked Hydrocephalus
- Part of CRASH syndrome: Corpus callosum hypoplasia, mental retardation, adducted thumbs, spasticity, hydrocephalus
- Etiology of hydrocephalus unknown: Primary aqueductal vs. communicating hydrocephalus causing secondary compression of the aqueduct
- Corticospinal tracts hypoplastic with absent medullary pyramids: Best assessed with diffusion imaging

### Normal Pressure Hydrocephalus
- CT/MR features similar to communicating hydrocephalus

## PATHOLOGY

### General Features
- General path comments
  - Pathogenesis of communicating hydrocephalus (CH) multifactorial
  - Abnormal thickening of the arachnoid membranes or meninges leads to obstruction of SAS or villi
  - Actual mechanism and site of cerebrospinal fluid (CSF) resorption controversial
    - Arachnoid granulations in sagittal/transverse sinuses vs. post capillary venules in cerebral parenchyma vs. nasal lymphatics at base of cribriform plate
- Etiology
  - CH common following infection, trauma, prior subarachnoid hemorrhage

- CSF tumor seeding (carcinomatous meningitis) most common with medulloblastoma, germinoma, leukemia, lymphoma
- Elevation of venous pressure
  - Absorption of CSF ceases if the pressure of blood in the superior sagittal sinus is greater than CSF pressure
  - Occlusion of intracranial dural sinuses, jugular foramen stenosis, jugular vein thrombosis, superior vena cava thrombosis, pulmonary hypertension
  - In children < 18 months, increase in venous pressure results in hydrocephalus; in children > 3 years, pseudotumor cerebri results
  - Common in complex craniosynostosis, achondroplasia
- In congenital muscular dystrophy syndromes, caused by over migration of neuronal and glial elements into the leptomeninges
  - Over migrated cells cause obliteration of SAS
  - Seen in Walker-Warburg, Fukuyama, muscle-eye-brain diseases
- Can be caused by mass lesions in the spine, especially upper cervical: Altered CSF flow dynamics vs. elevation of CSF protein
- Epidemiology: Represents approximately 30% of all childhood hydrocephalus

## Gross Pathologic & Surgical Features
- Enlarged ventricles, elevated CSF pressure

## Microscopic Features
- Arachnoid villi traditionally seen as primary site of CSF absorption
  - Evagination of the SAS into the lumen of the dural and venous sinuses
  - Act as one-way valves, with opening pressure between 20 and 50 mm of water
  - In traditional theory of CSF flow, CSF drainage occurs at the level of arachnoid villi and is determined by hydrostatic pressure differences between CSF and venous sinuses
- Facts that challenge traditional theory of CSF flow
  - Arachnoid villi absent until cranial sutures fuse (after 1 year of age)
  - Flow sensitive MR does not demonstrate net flow between the cisterna magna and the sagittal sinus
  - Extracellular spaces of the brain are in open contact with SAS and with capillaries within cerebral tissues
- Alternative ("new") theory of CSF flow
  - In the SAS, CSF is mixed and dispersed evenly by pulsation (systolic expansion) of the intracranial extracerebral arteries
  - CSF absorbed throughout the brain and spinal cord via their capillaries, not through arachnoid villi

## CLINICAL ISSUES

### Presentation
- Most common signs/symptoms
  - Increased head circumference/macrocrania in infants and young children
  - Headache, lethargy, vomiting

- Rapid head circumference growth evidenced by serial measurements of increasing head circumference ⇒ most important indication of progressive hydrocephalus
- Other signs/symptoms
  - Pediatric form of normal pressure hydrocephalus
    - Subtle mental deterioration manifested by poor or decreasing scholar performance
    - Anomalies in gait manifested by delay in walking (infants) or repeated falling spells (older children)
    - Anomalies of micturition with delayed bladder control
    - Also encountered with chronic shunt malfunction
- Clinical Profile: Treatable cause of macrocrania

### Demographics
- Age: All pediatric ages
- Gender: M = F
- Ethnicity: No racial predilection

### Natural History & Prognosis
- Progressive macrocrania with worsening vomiting, lethargy; neurologic and intellectual disabilities
- Can become arrested (asymptomatic)

### Treatment
- Placement of extracranial shunt in most cases

## DIAGNOSTIC CHECKLIST

### Consider
- When atrophy and gliosis present, consider if they are the primary abnormality or the result of the hydrocephalus

### Image Interpretation Pearls
- In patients with CH and craniosynostosis or anomalies of craniocervical junction, look for venous stenosis (sigmoid sinus, jugular bulb) on MRV

## SELECTED REFERENCES
1. Papaiconomou C et al: Reassessment of the pathways responsible for cerebrospinal fluid absorption in the neonate. Childs Nerv Syst. 20(1):29-36, 2004
2. Taylor WJ et al: Enigma of raised intracranial pressure in patients with complex craniosynostosis: the role of abnormal intracranial venous drainage. J Neurosurg. 94(3):377-85, 2001
3. Rollins N et al: MR venography in children with complex craniosynostosis. Pediatr Neurosurg. 32(6):308-15, 2000
4. Greitz D et al: A proposed model of cerebrospinal fluid circulation: observations with radionuclide cisternography. AJNR Am J Neuroradiol. 17(3):431-8, 1996
5. Bret P et al: Chronic ("normal pressure") hydrocephalus in childhood and adolescence. A review of 16 cases and reappraisal of the syndrome. Childs Nerv Syst. 11(12):687-91, 1995
6. Rosman NP et al: Hydrocephalus caused by increased intracranial venous pressure: a clinicopathological study. Ann Neurol. 3(5):445-50, 1978

I
5
24

# COMMUNICATING HYDROCEPHALUS

## IMAGE GALLERY

Typical

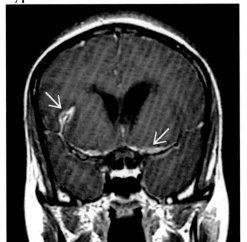
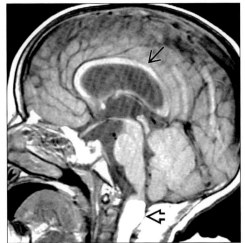

*(Left)* Coronal T1 C+ MR shows enlarged frontal horns and communicating hydrocephalus in child with tuberculous meningitis. Note inflammatory exudates in the basal cisterns ➡. *(Right)* Sagittal T1WI MR shows dilated lateral ventricles (bowed corpus callosum ➡) and distended basilar cisterns. Hydrocephalus caused by a large subpial lipoma completely filling the upper cervical canal ➡.

Typical

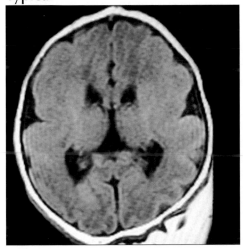
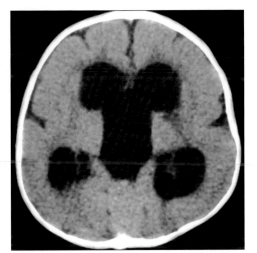

*(Left)* Axial T1WI MR in a newborn with Walker-Warburg muscular dystrophy. Cobblestone lissencephaly anomaly of the cerebral cortex and mild ventricular prominence. *(Right)* Axial NECT (same patient as previous image), now 8 months old, shows severe communicating hydrocephalus is now evident.

Typical

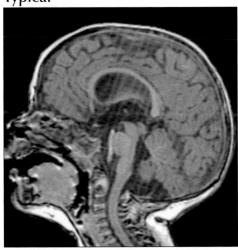
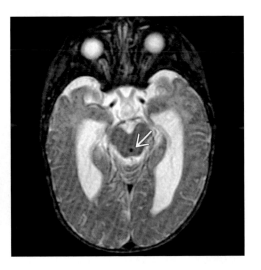

*(Left)* Sagittal T1WI MR shows bowed corpus callosum, enlarged CSF spaces. Typical findings of communicating hydrocephalus but infant presents with normal pressure hydrocephalus. *(Right)* Axial T2WI MR (same infant as previous image) shows bulging temporal horns and a prominent aqueductal flow void ➡.

# CSF SHUNTS AND COMPLICATIONS

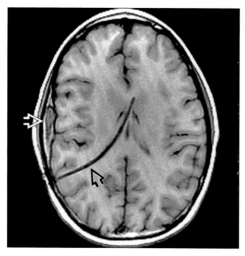
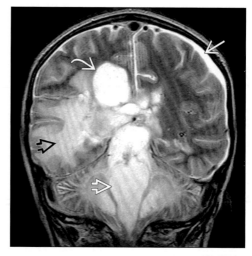

*Axial T1WI MR shows acute right-sided epidural hematoma ➡ and ventricular collapse following shunt catheter ➡ placement.*

*Coronal T2WI MR shows brain edema ➡, left subdural collection ➡, isolated lateral ➡ and 4th ventricles ➡ following IVH, shunting and subsequent ventriculitis.*

## TERMINOLOGY

### Abbreviations and Synonyms
- Ventriculo-peritoneal (VP), ventriculo-atrial (VA), ventriculo-pleural (VPL), lumbo-peritoneal (LP)

### Definitions
- CSF shunt establishes an accessory drainage pathway to bypass obstructed natural pathways
- Varied pediatric disorders necessitate CSF diversion
- Shunting obstructed ventricles restores vascular compliance and normal trans-parenchymal drainage

## IMAGING FINDINGS

### General Features
- Best diagnostic clue: Dilated ventricles + fluid/edema "blurring" margin around valve/ventricles
- Location
  - Proximal catheter in cerebral ventricles (common), intracranial subarachnoid space, or thecal sac (rare)
  - Unidirectional valve prevents reflux back into ventricles; reservoir attached to valve is optional
  - Catheter tunneled in subcutaneous tissue
  - Distal shunt in peritoneal cavity (common), cardiac atrium or pleural cavity (rare)
- Size: Distal tip long enough to allow for growth
- Morphology: Usually constructed from silicone

### CT Findings
- NECT
  - Ventricular dilatation (diffuse or loculated)
    - Isolated ventricles may follow infection or hemorrhage
  - Periventricular interstitial fluid "blurs" ventricles
  - Previous studies for comparison needed
  - +/- Subdural fluid or bleed with acute overdrainage
  - Small, "slit" ventricles occur with non-compliant ventricle syndrome, chronic overdrainage
- CECT
  - +/- Ependymal enhancement
  - May identify meningitis, neoplasm, etc.

### MR Findings
- T1WI: Assess ventricular size
- T2WI: Periventricular interstitial fluid
- FLAIR: "Fingers" of CSF within periventricular white matter common

## DDx: Shunt Complications

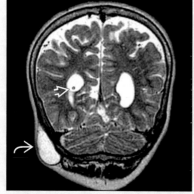
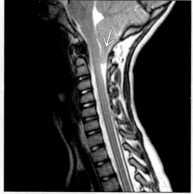
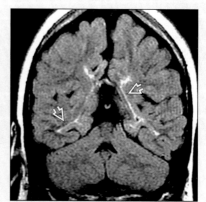

*Peri-Shunt Fluid*  *LP Shunt Slump*  *Slit Ventricles*

# CSF SHUNTS AND COMPLICATIONS

## Key Facts

### Terminology

- Varied pediatric disorders necessitate CSF diversion
- Shunting obstructed ventricles restores vascular compliance and normal trans-parenchymal drainage

### Imaging Findings

- Best diagnostic clue: Dilated ventricles + fluid/edema "blurring" margin around valve/ventricles

### Top Differential Diagnoses

- Shunt Failure with Normal Ventricles or Lack of Interstitial Edema
- Acquired Chiari I/Tonsillar Ectopia
- Non-Compliant ("Slit") Ventricle Syndrome

### Pathology

- Common complications include shunt obstruction/breakage, infection, overdrainage
- Shunts, valves/devices ⇒ specific complications

### Clinical Issues

- Most: Headache, vomiting, lethargy, altered LOC with obstruction
- 50% fail in first 2 years, 80% fail by 10 years
- Acute shunt obstruction may lead to death

### Diagnostic Checklist

- Not all shunt + headache = obstruction: Remember sinusitis, trauma, sinovenous thrombosis!
- Comparison with baseline studies crucial!

---

- T2* GRE: Assess hemorrhagic shunt tracts, shunt
- DWI: Increased diffusion in interstitial edema
- T1 C+: Always enhance first scan of hydrocephalus to identify occult neoplasm
- MRA: Stretched arteries with hydrocephalus
- MRV: Venous thrombosis may precede hydrocephalus or follow shunting
- MRS: Small lactate resonances can be detected in up to 20% of CSF, even if no hydrocephalus
- 2D PC MR flow studies confirm obstruction (e.g., aqueduct) or patency of CSF pathways/ventriculostomy stoma

### Radiographic Findings

- Radiography
  - Plain films: Evaluate shunt continuity/integrity
    - Shunt fractures/separation (13%)
    - Shunt migration (rare = bowel perforation)

### Ultrasonographic Findings

- Grayscale Ultrasound: Sonography for ventricular size possible with open fontanelle
- Pulsed Doppler: Resistive indices increase with shunt obstruction and raised intracranial pressure (ICP)
- Color Doppler: Research studies document flow within shunt tubing and aqueduct

### Nuclear Medicine Findings

- PET: Cerebral vascular reserve (CVR) measurement aids in selection of shunt candidates
- Radionuclide studies
  - Can confirm distal obstruction, rarely needed

### Non-Vascular Interventions

- Myelography: Myelography/cisternography rarely needed, but may define loculations

### Fluoroscopic Findings

- Contrast shuntograms define site of obstructions (radionuclide shuntograms more common)

### Imaging Recommendations

- Best imaging tool: CT easiest to obtain in setting of acute obstruction

- Protocol advice
  - CT or MR to evaluate ventricles/CSF flow
    - Consider fast MR (HASTE or SSFSE)
  - Always enhance the first imaging study of hydrocephalus (occult neoplasm) and fever (ventriculitis)
  - Baseline CT/MR following shunt insertion, follow-up at 1 year, then as needed
  - Plain films to identify shunt fracture or dislocation

## DIFFERENTIAL DIAGNOSIS

### Shunt Failure with Normal Ventricles or Lack of Interstitial Edema

- Look for fluid along shunt catheter or reservoir as only sign of malfunction

### Acquired Chiari I/Tonsillar Ectopia

- Functioning LP shunt causes tonsillar descent

### Non-Compliant ("Slit") Ventricle Syndrome

- Older child (shunted in infancy), small ventricles + intermittent signs of shunt obstruction
- Ventricles may appear normal/small even if shunt is malfunctioning!
- Can be caused by shunt-induced sutural ossification

## PATHOLOGY

### General Features

- General path comments
  - Infected shunts 5-10%, especially younger than 6 months or within 3 months insertion
  - Ventricular loculation or isolation 6%
  - Overshunting 3% (leads to subdural effusions/hematomas and occasionally to parenchymal hemorrhage)
  - Shunt migration: Caudal > > cephalic
- Etiology
  - CSF production 0.35 mL/min

# CSF SHUNTS AND COMPLICATIONS

- ○ 500 mL (adults), 250 mL (children) produced/absorbed in 24 hour period
- ○ Absorption requires > 6.8 mm $H_2O$ pressure to overcome sinovenous pressure
- ○ Impaired CSF absorption allows accumulation and increased intraventricular/intracranial pressure
- ○ CSF diversion via shunt restores/maintains normal intracranial pressure
- • Epidemiology
  - ○ CSF shunts in USA = 125,000 total
    - ▪ 33,000 per year (nearly half are revisions)
  - ○ 160,000 shunts implanted each year worldwide
- • Associated abnormalities
  - ○ Shunts in infants younger than 6 months carry increased risk of infection
  - ○ Shunts in presence of blood or protein content > 1 g/dL prone to failure, early blockage

## Gross Pathologic & Surgical Features
- • Transventricular ependymal adhesions
- • Ependymal "scar" restricts ventricular expansion
- • Extracranial shunt tubing calcifications

## Microscopic Features
- • Gliosis along tract

## Staging, Grading or Classification Criteria
- • Shunt complication rate 25-37%
- • Common complications include shunt obstruction/breakage, infection, overdrainage
- • Shunts, valves/devices ⇒ specific complications
  - ○ VP abdominal complications: CSF pseudocyst/ascites, bowel perforation
  - ○ VA: Shunt nephritis, cor pulmonale, pulmonary embolus
  - ○ LP: Arachnoiditis, cerebellar tonsillar herniation, high migration rate
  - ○ Internal 3rd ventricle to spinal SAS (Lapras catheter) no external access, no way to check flow
  - ○ Shuntless CSF diversion: 3rd ventriculostomy, 4th ventricle outlet fenestration 70% patency
  - ○ Anti-siphon devices: Capsule forms, obstructs
  - ○ Flanged catheters: Choroid plexus occludes
  - ○ Programmable shunt: Reprogram after MR!
  - ○ One piece shunt decreased obstruction rate, but increased slit ventricle/SDH rate
  - ○ VPL (if peritoneum contaminated or cardiac complicated) can lead to pleural effusion
  - ○ Pressure regulating shunts prone to overdrainage
  - ○ Flow regulating valves prone to obstruction
- • Late complications
  - ○ Child outgrows peritoneal tubing
  - ○ Material degradation/fatigue, mechanical stress: Especially craniocervical junction, inferior ribs

## CLINICAL ISSUES

### Presentation
- • Most common signs/symptoms
  - ○ Most: Headache, vomiting, lethargy, altered LOC with obstruction
  - ○ Also: Seizures, diplopia, neuropsychologic, cognitive or behavioral difficulties
- ○ Infants: Bulging fontanelle, increased head circumference
- • Clinical Profile: Dependent upon diagnosis leading to CSF diversion and to number of complications

### Demographics
- • Age
  - ○ Peak age for shunt within first few weeks of life for myelomeningocele and congenital hydrocephalus
  - ○ Later shunting follows trauma, meningitis, tumor

### Natural History & Prognosis
- • Hydrocephalus: Mortality 80% without CSF diversion
- • Following shunting: 70% normal or relatively normal intelligence if no anomalies, complications
- • Epilepsy: Incidence up to 47% if shunt follows meningitis, hemorrhage
- • Most shunts eventually fail
  - ○ 50% fail in first 2 years, 80% fail by 10 years
  - ○ 50% multiple revisions, progressively shorter intervals to next failure
- • Acute shunt obstruction may lead to death
- • Shunt related mortality: Malfunction (30%), infection (20%), pulmonary embolus (7%)

### Treatment
- • Lengthen distal shunt as child grows
- • Change intraventricular component/valve if proximal obstruction
- • Alter pressure valve if over/under-draining
- • Subtemporal decompression/3rd ventriculostomy for non-compliant ventricle syndrome
- • Catheters impregnated with antimicrobial agents may decrease shunt infections

## DIAGNOSTIC CHECKLIST

### Consider
- • Not all shunt + headache = obstruction: Remember sinusitis, trauma, sinovenous thrombosis!

### Image Interpretation Pearls
- • Comparison with baseline studies crucial!
- • Fluid tracking along shunt may be only sign of obstruction, even if normal or unchanged ventricles

## SELECTED REFERENCES

1. Browd SR et al: Failure of cerebrospinal fluid shunts: part I: Obstruction and mechanical failure. Pediatr Neurol. 34(2):83-92, 2006
2. Browd SR et al: Failure of Cerebrospinal Fluid Shunts: Part II: Overdrainage, Loculation, and Abdominal Complications. Pediatr Neurol. 34(3):171-176, 2006
3. de Aquino HB et al: Nonfunctional abdominal complications of the distal catheter on the treatment of hydrocephalus: an inflammatory hypothesis? Experience with six cases. Childs Nerv Syst. 2006
4. Braun KP et al: 1H MRS in human hydrocephalus. J MRI. 17(3):291-99, 2003
5. Drake JM et al: CSF shunts 50 years on past, present and future. Childs Nerv Syst. 16:800-4, 2000

# CSF SHUNTS AND COMPLICATIONS

## IMAGE GALLERY

### Typical

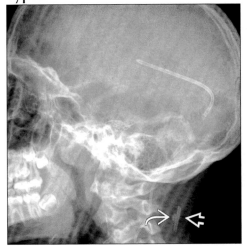
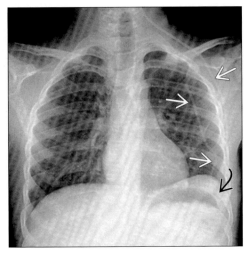

*(Left)* Lateral radiograph shows small catheter fragment ➡ with associated dystrophic calcification ➡. Calcification commonly occurs along extracranial shunt, almost never intracranially. *(Right)* Anteroposterior radiograph shows ventriculopleural shunt ➡. Subpulmonic fluid collection ➡ seen above gastric bubble.

### Variant

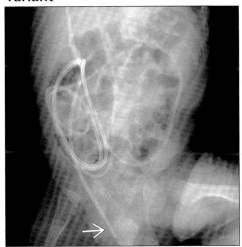
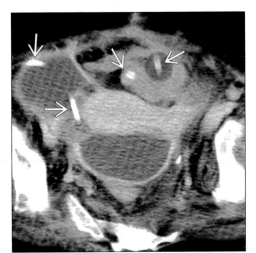

*(Left)* Anteroposterior radiograph shows shunt tubing coiled in the abdomen and extending into a right hydrocele ➡ in an infant. Extra tubing length often placed to accommodate growth of child. *(Right)* Axial CECT shows complicated loculated and infected pelvic CSF collections associated with shunt tubing ➡ with shunt obstruction and fever.

### Variant

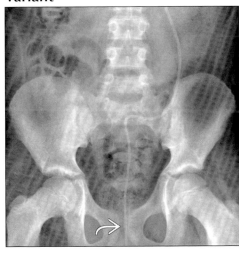
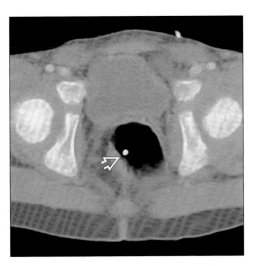

*(Left)* Anteroposterior radiograph shows single VP shunt ➡ extending through rectum in 10 year old. Proximal shunt was fractured in the neck. *(Right)* Axial CECT shows distal shunt tubing ➡ inside rectal lumen in 4 year old.

# ENLARGED SUBARACHNOID SPACES

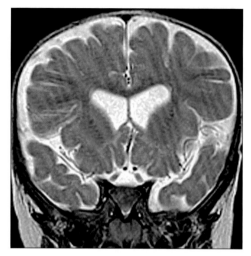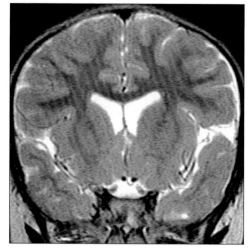

*Coronal T2WI MR shows mild enlargement of ventricles and subarachnoid space in 10 month old with macrocephaly.*

*Coronal T2WI MR shows resolution of subarachnoid space enlargement (same child as previous image) now 3 years of age. Macrocephaly persists.*

## TERMINOLOGY

### Abbreviations and Synonyms
- External hydrocephalus, physiologic extraventricular obstructive hydrocephalus (EVOH)
- Physiologic subarachnoid space (SAS) enlargement, benign macrocephaly of infancy

### Definitions
- Idiopathic enlargement of SAS during first year of life

## IMAGING FINDINGS

### General Features
- Best diagnostic clue: Enlarged SAS and increased head circumference (HC) (> 95%)
- Location
  - SAS
    - Craniocortical: Widest vertical distance between brain and calvarium
    - Sinocortical: Widest distance between lateral wall of superior sagittal sinus and brain surface
    - Interhemispheric: Widest distance between hemispheres
- Size
  - ≥ 5 mm widening bifrontal craniocortical/anterior interhemispheric SAS
  - Note normal maximum width peaks at 28 postnatal weeks (7 months) of life
- Morphology
  - CSF space follows (not flattens) gyral contour
  - Right and left subarachnoid spaces symmetric

### CT Findings
- NECT
  - ≥ 5 mm widening bifrontal/anterior interhemispheric SAS
  - Enlarged cisterns (especially suprasellar/chiasmatic)
  - Mildly enlarged ventricles (66%)
  - Sulci generally normal (especially posteriorly)
  - Postural unilateral lambdoid flattening common
  - Posterior fossa normal
- CECT
  - Demonstrates veins traversing SAS
  - No abnormal enhancement of meninges

## DDx: Large Subarachnoid Spaces

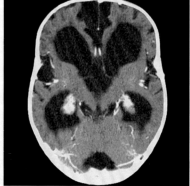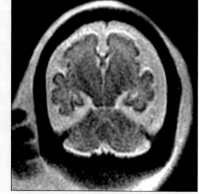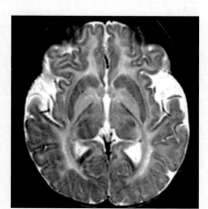

*CSF Overproduced*  *Fetus Small Head Circumference*  *Glutaric Aciduria Type 1*

# ENLARGED SUBARACHNOID SPACES

## Key Facts

### Terminology
- External hydrocephalus, physiologic extraventricular obstructive hydrocephalus (EVOH)
- Physiologic subarachnoid space (SAS) enlargement, benign macrocephaly of infancy
- Idiopathic enlargement of SAS during first year of life

### Imaging Findings
- Best diagnostic clue: Enlarged SAS and increased head circumference (HC) (> 95%)
- ≥ 5 mm widening bifrontal craniocortical/anterior interhemispheric SAS
- After diagnosis, best follow-up = tape measure, not imaging!

### Top Differential Diagnoses
- Atrophy

- Acquired Extraventricular Obstructive Hydrocephalus (EVOH)
- Inflicted "Nonaccidental" Trauma (NAT)

### Pathology
- Immature CSF drainage pathways

### Clinical Issues
- Macrocrania: Head circumference > 95%
- Family history of benign macrocephaly common
- Age: Detected typically between ages 3 and 8 months
- Self-limited; SAS enlargement resolves without therapy between 12-24 months
- Macrocephaly often persists
- Normal outcome (developmental delay resolves as prominent SAS resolves)

## MR Findings
- T1WI: Similar to NECT
- T2WI
  - No abnormal brain tissue nor signal abnormalities
  - Single layer of fluid (SAS) with traversing vessels
  - Normal flow in aqueduct
- FLAIR: Cerebrospinal fluid (CSF) homogeneously hypointense
- T2* GRE: No blood products
- DWI: Normal diffusivity
- T1 C+: Enhancing veins traverse SAS
- Fetal MR: Seen in fetus with distribution fluid/ventricular prominence related to positioning
  - Usually frontal prominence after birth due to position of child lying on back for scan

## Radiographic Findings
- Radiography: Macrocephaly, frontal bossing

## Ultrasonographic Findings
- Grayscale Ultrasound
  - Enlarged SAS ≥ 5 mm
  - Veins as "dots" floating in SAS
- Pulsed Doppler: Increased cerebral blood flow may identify "progressive" cases
- Color Doppler: Veins traverse SAS

## Nuclear Medicine Findings
- Isotope cisternography
  - Accumulation of CSF in 4th and lateral ventricles similar to extraventricular hydrocephalus

## Angiographic Findings
- Conventional: Widened space between skull and arteries of brain surface

## Non-Vascular Interventions
- Myelography: Cisternography confirms communication of SAS, but not necessary

## Imaging Recommendations
- Best imaging tool: MR to exclude chronic subdural collections

- Protocol advice
  - Doppler sonography: Documents veins traversing SAS
  - MR or CECT: To exclude underlying etiology
  - MR: To exclude chronic subdural collections
    - SAS isointense with CSF on all sequences if benign
  - PC MR shows normal intraventricular CSF flow
  - After diagnosis, best follow-up = tape measure, not imaging!

# DIFFERENTIAL DIAGNOSIS

## Atrophy
- Atrophy: Small head circumference (HC)
  - Forehead "pointed" due to metopic fusion
- Benign SAS enlargement has large head
  - Forehead "flat" due to frontal bossing
- Knowledge of HC critical for diagnosis

## Acquired Extraventricular Obstructive Hydrocephalus (EVOH)
- Hemorrhagic/post inflammatory/neoplastic
  - Density of extra-axial collection does not = CSF
- Achondroplasia and other skull base anomalies
  - Narrow foramen magnum/jugular foramina
- Intermittent intracranial pressure waves

## Inflicted "Nonaccidental" Trauma (NAT)
- Predisposition to bleed with minor trauma controversial
  - Possible if SAS ≥ than 6 mm
  - Venous "stretching" implicated

## Glutaric Aciduria Type 1
- Enlarged Sylvian fissures
- ↑ T2 basal ganglia
- Delayed myelination

# ENLARGED SUBARACHNOID SPACES

## PATHOLOGY

### General Features
- General path comments: Clear CSF
- Genetics
  - No documented genetic predisposition, although common in benign familial macrocrania families
    - Family history of macrocephaly > 80%
- Etiology
  - Immature CSF drainage pathways
    - CSF primarily drained via extracellular space ⇒ capillaries
    - Pacchionian granulations (PGs) don't mature until 18 months
    - PGs are then displaced into veins (as Starling-type resistors)
    - PGs regulate pulse pressure/venous drainage CSF after fontanels close
    - Benign SAS enlargement usually resolves at that time
  - Large SAS are normal in infancy
    - Only detected if macrocephaly is present
- Epidemiology: Reported on 2-65% of neuroimaging for macrocrania < 1 year old
- Associated abnormalities: Anecdotal

### Gross Pathologic & Surgical Features
- Deep/prominent but otherwise normal-appearing SAS
- No pathologic membranes

### Microscopic Features
- Ependymal damage not seen in benign SAS enlargement

### Staging, Grading or Classification Criteria
- Danger signs
  - Elevated intracranial pressure (ICP)
  - Rapid enlargement of head circumference
  - > > > 6 mm width SAS
  - Onset or persistence > 1 year old

## CLINICAL ISSUES

### Presentation
- Most common signs/symptoms
  - Macrocrania: Head circumference > 95%
  - Frontal bossing
  - Mild developmental delay in 50% (motor > > language)
    - Motor "delay" is usually due to large head size
  - No signs of elevated ICP; normal pressure on lumbar puncture
- Clinical Profile
  - Family history of benign macrocephaly common
  - Male infants, sometimes "late to walk"

### Demographics
- Age: Detected typically between ages 3 and 8 months
- Gender: 80% male

### Natural History & Prognosis
- Enlarged SAS ⇒ ↑ suture/calvarial malleability/compliance ⇒ predisposes to posterior plagiocephaly
- Self-limited; SAS enlargement resolves without therapy between 12-24 months
  - Spontaneous resolution of spaces and symptoms
- Calvarium grows faster than brain
  - Brain eventually "catches up"
- Macrocephaly often persists
- Theory: May result in NPH in late adult life

### Treatment
- No treatment necessary
- Normal outcome (developmental delay resolves as prominent SAS resolves)

## DIAGNOSTIC CHECKLIST

### Consider
- Nonaccidental injury if enlarged SAS atypical in any way

### Image Interpretation Pearls
- Crucial: Know head circumference!
- Always enhance CT (veins traverse SAS in benign enlarged SAS) and search for membranes (chronic subdural)

## SELECTED REFERENCES

1. Bradley WG et al: Increased intracranial volume: a clue to the etiology of idiopathic normal-pressure hydrocephalus? AJNR Am J Neuroradiol. 25(9):1479-84, 2004
2. Cosan TE et al: Cerebral blood flow alterations in progressive communicating hydrocephalus: transcranial Doppler ultrasonography assessment in an experimental model. J Neurosurg. 94(2):265-9, 2001
3. Girard NJ et al: Ventriculomegaly and pericerebral CSF collection in the fetus: early stage of benign external hydrocephalus? Childs Nerv Syst. 17(4-5):239-45, 2001
4. Lam WW et al: Ultrasonographic measurement of subarachnoid space in normal infants and children. Pediatr Neurol. 25(5):380-4, 2001
5. Papasian NC et al: A theoretical model of benign external hydrocephalus that predicts a predisposition towards extra-axial hemorrhage after minor head trauma. Pediatr Neurosurg. 33(4):188-93, 2000
6. Greitz D et al: The pathogenesis and hemodynamics of hydrocephalus: proposal for a new understanding. IJNR. 3:367-75, 1997
7. Chen CY et al: Pericerebral fluid collection: differentiation of enlarged subarachnoid spaces from subdural collections with color Doppler US. Radiology. 201(2):389-92, 1996
8. Prassopoulos P et al: The size of the intra- and extraventricular cerebrospinal fluid compartments in children with idiopathic benign widening of the frontal subarachnoid space. Neuroradiology. 37(5):418-21, 1995
9. Wilms G et al: CT and MR in infants with pericerebral collections and macrocephaly: benign enlargement of the subarachnoid spaces versus subdural collections. AJNR Am J Neuroradiol. 14(4):855-60, 1993
10. Maytal J et al: External hydrocephalus: radiologic spectrum and differentiation from cerebral atrophy. AJR Am J Roentgenol. 148(6):1223-30, 1987

# ENLARGED SUBARACHNOID SPACES

## IMAGE GALLERY

Typical

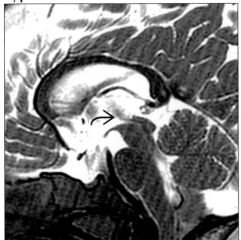 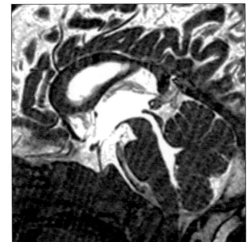

*(Left)* Sagittal T2WI MR shows flow void across the aqueduct ⇗ into the 4th ventricle in this 10 month old with moderate EVOH. Note prominent interhemispheric subarachnoid space. *(Right)* Sagittal T2WI MR FIESTA in same patient confirms widely patent aqueduct.

Typical

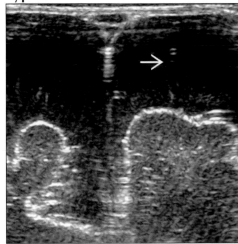 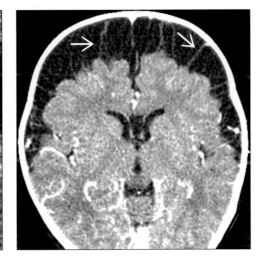

*(Left)* Coronal ultrasound shows marked enlargement of subarachnoid spaces with greater than 1 cm widening of bifrontal craniocortical CSF spaces. Traversing vessels are present ➡. *(Right)* Axial CECT shows marked enlargement of the subarachnoid spaces (same 7 month old as previous image) with macrocrania. Traversing veins ➡ are demonstrated with contrast-enhancement.

Typical

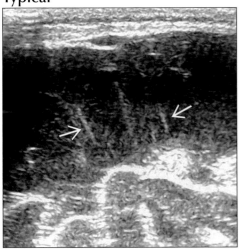 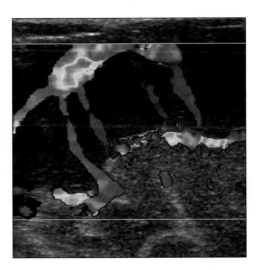

*(Left)* Sagittal ultrasound shows multiple linear structures ➡ traversing enlarged subarachnoid space. *(Right)* Sagittal ultrasound with Doppler confirms that venous origin (color coded blue) of vessels traversing subarachnoid space.

# VENTRICULITIS

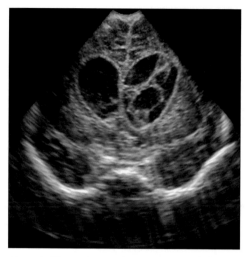

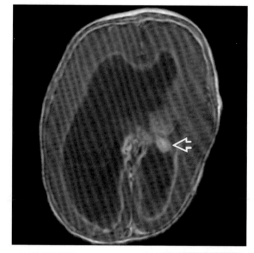

*Coronal oblique ultrasound in a neonate with seizures and obtundation shows significant ventriculomegaly, with irregular intraventricular septations and debris.*

*Axial T1 C+ MR in an infant with secondary bacterial infection shows enhancing ventricular wall and irregular, clumped choroid plexus ➡.*

## TERMINOLOGY

### Abbreviations and Synonyms
• Pyogenic ventriculitis, ependymitis

### Definitions
• Inflammation of ventricular ependyma 2° to infection

## IMAGING FINDINGS

### General Features
• Best diagnostic clue: Irregular debris/septations
• Location: Lateral ventricles most common

### CT Findings
• NECT: Irregular debris, septations, ventriculomegaly
• CECT: ± Enhancement of ventricular margins

### MR Findings
• T1WI: Ventriculomegaly
• T2WI: High signal in periventricular white matter
• FLAIR: Irregular debris/septations within ventricles, periventricular increased signal
• T2* GRE: Intraventricular debris does not bloom
• DWI: Intraventricular debris iso- to hyperintense
• T1 C+: ± Ependymal enhancement, ± enlarged intensely enhancing choroid plexus (CP)

### Ultrasonographic Findings
• Grayscale Ultrasound: Ventriculomegaly with irregular echogenic debris or septations, increased periventricular echogenicity

### Imaging Recommendations
• Best imaging tool
  ○ Neonates: US for debris, MR for complications
  ○ Children: MR
• Protocol advice: MR with FLAIR, contrast, DWI and MRV

## DIFFERENTIAL DIAGNOSIS

### Inflammation due to IVH in Neonate
• Debris not as irregular

### Ependymal Tumor Spread
• Nodular enhancement

---

## DDx: Ventricular Loculation/Enhancement

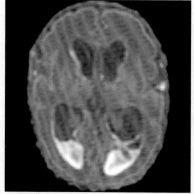

*Grade III IVH*

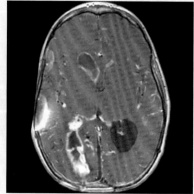

*Ependymal Tumor Spread*

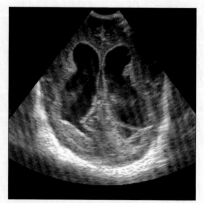

*Grade III IVH*

# VENTRICULITIS

## Key Facts

### Imaging Findings
- Best diagnostic clue: Irregular debris/septations
- FLAIR: Irregular debris/septations within ventricles, periventricular increased signal
- T2* GRE: Intraventricular debris does not bloom
- DWI: Intraventricular debris iso- to hyperintense
- T1 C+: ± Ependymal enhancement, ± enlarged intensely enhancing choroid plexus (CP)

### Top Differential Diagnoses
- Inflammation due to IVH in Neonate
- Ependymal Tumor Spread

### Clinical Issues
- Neonate: Death or severe morbidity in up to 54%

### Diagnostic Checklist
- Irregular debris can occur without enhancement

---

## Radiation/Chemotherapy Changes
- No debris

## PATHOLOGY

### General Features
- General path comments: Pathogens include bacteria, fungi, viruses, parasites
- Etiology
  - Commonly bacterial
  - Neonates: Hematogenous seeding to CP
  - Children: Complication of meningitis, empyema, cerebral abscess, neurosurgical procedure
- Epidemiology
  - 80-90% of neonates with meningitis, up to 30% of children with meningitis
  - Bacterial after trauma or neurosurgical procedures
  - Fungal or viral in immunosuppressed patients

### Gross Pathologic & Surgical Features
- Inflammation, proteinaceous debris

### Microscopic Features
- Congestion, macrophages, lymphocytes

## CLINICAL ISSUES

### Presentation
- Most common signs/symptoms

  - Neonate (< 1 week, early onset): Sepsis, respiratory symptoms
  - Neonate (> 1 week, late onset): Lethargy, seizures, coma
  - Child: Irritability, lethargy, vomiting, fever
- Clinical Profile: Neonate (< 1 week): Obstetrical complications, prematurity

### Natural History & Prognosis
- Neonate: Death or severe morbidity in up to 54%

### Treatment
- Antibiotics vs. surgical irrigation and drainage

## DIAGNOSTIC CHECKLIST

### Image Interpretation Pearls
- Irregular debris can occur without enhancement

## SELECTED REFERENCES

1. Pezzullo JA et al: Diffusion-weighted MR imaging of pyogenic ventriculitis. AJR Am J Roentgenol. 180(1):71-5, 2003
2. Fukui MB et al: CT and MR imaging features of pyogenic ventriculitis. AJNR Am J Neuroradiol. 22(8):1510-6, 2001
3. Rypens E et al: Hyperechoic thickened ependyma: sonographic demonstration and significance in neonates. Pediatr Radiol. 24(8):550-3, 1994
4. Barloon TJ et al: Cerebral ventriculitis: MR findings. J Comput Assist Tomogr. 14(2):272-5, 1990

## IMAGE GALLERY

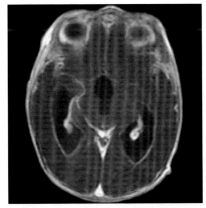 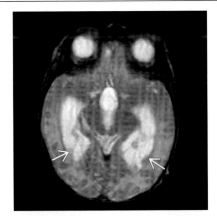 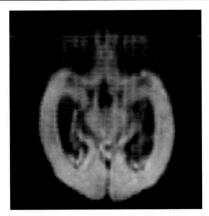

*(Left)* Axial T1 C+ MR in a 3 week old with group B meningitis shows diffuse ependymal, choroid plexus and leptomeningeal enhancement. *(Center)* Axial T2WI MR in the same neonate as previous image shows irregular intraventricular debris ➡ and multiple septae. *(Right)* Axial DWI MR in same neonate as previous image shows that the intraventricular debris has decreased diffusion relative to normal CSF.

# INTRACRANIAL HYPOTENSION

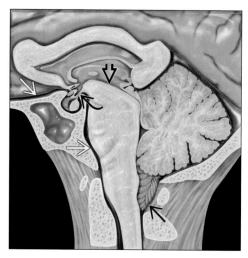

Sagittal graphic shows intracranial hypotension with dural venous engorgement ➡, "sagging midbrain" ⇒, tonsillar herniation ⇾, hypothalamus displaced downwards ⇾.

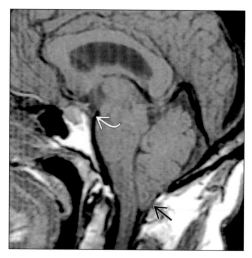

Sagittal T1WI MR shows slumping brain stem and vermis, herniated tonsils ⇾, enlarged pituitary, and hypothalamus ➡ drooping over dorsum sella.

## TERMINOLOGY

### Abbreviations and Synonyms
- Intracranial hypotension (IH)

### Definitions
- Frequently misdiagnosed syndrome of headache caused by reduced intracranial CSF pressure

## IMAGING FINDINGS

### General Features
- Best diagnostic clue
  - Classic imaging triad: Diffuse dural thickening/enhancement, downward displacement of brain through incisura ("slumping" brain), subdural hygromas/hematomas
  - Lack of one classic finding does not preclude diagnosis!
- Location
  - Pachymeninges (dura)
    - Both supra-, infratentorial
    - Primarily affects inner (meningeal) layer

- May extend into internal auditory canals (IACs)
- Spinal dura, epidural venous plexuses may be involved
  - Third ventricle, brain stem, cerebellum
    - "Slump" toward foramen magnum
- Size: Dural thickening varies from none/minimal to striking (several mm)
- Morphology: Dural enhancement smooth, not nodular or "lumpy-bumpy"

### CT Findings
- NECT
  - Relatively insensitive; may appear normal
  - +/- Thick dura
  - +/- Subdural fluid collections
    - Usually bilateral
    - Can be CSF (hygroma) or blood (hematoma)
  - Suprasellar cistern may appear obliterated
  - Atria of lateral ventricles may appear deviated medially, abnormally close ("tethered") to midline
- CECT: Diffuse dural thickening, enhancement

### MR Findings
- T1WI
  - Sagittal shows brain descent in 40-50% of cases

## DDx: Intracranial Hypotension Mimics

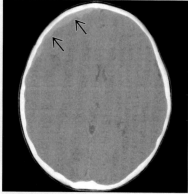

Traumatic SDH

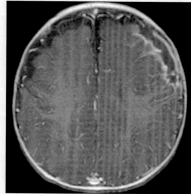

Subdural Empyema

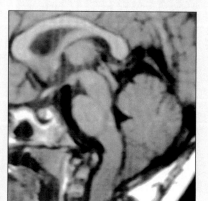

Chiari 1 Malformation

# INTRACRANIAL HYPOTENSION

## Key Facts

### Terminology
- Frequently misdiagnosed syndrome of headache caused by reduced intracranial CSF pressure

### Imaging Findings
- Sagittal shows brain descent in 40-50% of cases
- Caudal displacement of tonsils in 25-75%
- Bilateral subdural fluid collections in 15%
- FLAIR: Hyperintense dura, subdural fluid
- T1 C+: Diffuse, intense dural enhancement in 85%

### Top Differential Diagnoses
- Meningitis
- Subdural Hematoma
- Dural Sinus Thrombosis with Venous Engorgement
- Post-Surgical Dural Thickening
- Chiari I Malformation

### Pathology
- Common cause of IH = spontaneous spinal CSF leak

### Clinical Issues
- Severe headache (can be orthostatic, persistent, pulsatile or even associated with nuchal rigidity)
- Gender: M < F in patients with spontaneous IH
- Most IH cases resolve spontaneously
- Dural thickening, enhancement disappears; midline structures return (ascend) to normal position

### Diagnostic Checklist
- In children, look for occult skull base meningocele
- Not all findings must be present for diagnosis of IH

---

- - "Sagging" 3rd ventricle, brain stem (midbrain displaced inferiorly below level of dorsum sellae; pons may be compressed against clivus)
  - Caudal displacement of tonsils in 25-75%
  - Optic chiasm, hypothalamus draped over sella
  - Enlarged pituitary gland, venous sinuses
  - Axial
    - Suprasellar cistern crowded/effaced
    - Midbrain, pons appear elongated ("fat midbrain")
    - Temporal lobes herniated over tentorium, into incisura
    - Lateral ventricles small, often distorted (atria pulled medially by downward displacement of midbrain)
  - Bilateral subdural fluid collections in 15%
    - 70% have hygromas (clear fluid collects within dural border cell layer)
    - 10% have hematomas (blood of variable signal intensity)
- T2WI
  - Thickened dura usually hyperintense
  - Subdural fluid usually hyperintense (variable, depending on age of hematoma)
- PD/Intermediate: Thickened dura usually hyperintense
- FLAIR: Hyperintense dura, subdural fluid
- T2* GRE: May bloom if hemorrhage present
- T1 C+: Diffuse, intense dural enhancement in 85%

## Ultrasonographic Findings
- Color Doppler: Enlarged superior ophthalmic veins with higher mean maximum flow velocity

## Nuclear Medicine Findings
- Radionuclide cisternography (RNC)
  - Direct findings: Focal accumulation of radioactivity outside of subarachnoid space at leakage site
  - Indirect findings
    - Rapid washout from subarachnoid space
    - Early appearance in kidneys, urinary bladder
    - Poor migration of isotope over convexities

## Non-Vascular Interventions
- Myelography

- - May demonstrate epidural contrast extravasation +/- precise site
    - Dynamic CT myelogram may show extradural contrast
  - Caution: Myelography may facilitate CSF leak, worsen symptoms

## Imaging Recommendations
- Best imaging tool
  - Contrast-enhanced cranial MR for diagnosis
  - RNC or CT myelogram if localization required
- Protocol advice
  - Search for actual leakage site only if
    - Two adequate blood patches have failed
    - Post-traumatic leak is suspected

## DIFFERENTIAL DIAGNOSIS

### Meningitis
- Dura-arachnoid enhancement pattern less common than pia-subarachnoid space

### Dural/Calvarial Metastases
- Usually thicker, more irregular ("lumpy-bumpy")

### Subdural Hematoma
- Enhancing membranes enclosing blood products common
- No "sagging midbrain"

### Dural Sinus Thrombosis with Venous Engorgement
- Look for thrombosed sinus ("empty" delta sign, etc.)

### Post-Surgical Dural Thickening
- Look for other post-operative findings (e.g., burr holes)
- May occur almost immediately after surgery, persist for months/years

### Chiari I Malformation
- Headache occipital, not orthostatic
- No slumping of hypothalamus, brain stem
- Often abnormal skull base, pointed tonsils

# INTRACRANIAL HYPOTENSION

## PATHOLOGY

### General Features
- General path comments: Normal-appearing skin and dura (no identifiable connective tissue abnormalities)
- Genetics: Abnormalities in COL5A1/2 in E-DII; FBN1 usually normal in patients with isolated skeletal features of Marfan
- Etiology
  - Common cause of IH = spontaneous spinal CSF leak
    - Weak dura +/- arachnoid diverticula common
    - Look for occult meningocele (temporal bone, sphenoid bone)
    - May be provoked by vigorous exercise, violent coughing
  - Other causes: Reduced CSF
    - Surgery (CSF overshunting) or trauma (including trivial fall)
    - Diagnostic lumbar puncture
    - Spontaneous dural tear, ruptured arachnoid diverticulum
    - Severe dehydration
    - Disc herniation or osteophyte (rare)
  - Pathophysiology = CSF and intracranial blood volume vary inversely
    - In face of low CSF pressure, dural venous plexuses dilate
- Associated abnormalities
  - Dilated cervical epidural venous plexus, spinal hygromas, retrospinal fluid collections
  - Low opening pressure (< 6 cm H2O), pleocytosis, increased protein on lumbar puncture
  - Stigmata of systemic connective tissue disorder found in up to 2/3 of patients
    - Marfan, Ehlers-Danlos type II
    - Clinical findings: Minor skeletal features, small-joint hypermobility, etc; may be subtle

### Gross Pathologic & Surgical Features
- Skull: Basilar meningoceles leak into temporal, sphenoid bones
- Spine: Meningeal diverticula (often multiple), dural holes/rents common
- No specific leakage site identified at surgery in at least 50%

### Microscopic Features
- Meningeal surface normal
- Inner surface
  - Layer of numerous delicate thin-walled dilated vessels often attached to inner surface
  - May show marked arachnoidal, dural fibrosis if long-standing
  - Nests of meningothelial cells may be prominent, should not be misinterpreted as meningioma

## CLINICAL ISSUES

### Presentation
- Most common signs/symptoms
  - Severe headache (can be orthostatic, persistent, pulsatile or even associated with nuchal rigidity)

  - Less common: Cranial nerve palsy (e.g., abducens), visual disturbances
  - Rare: Severe encephalopathy with disturbances of consciousness
- Clinical Profile: Young to middle-aged adult with orthostatic headache, often of acute onset

### Demographics
- Age: Any age; peak in third, fourth decades
- Gender: M < F in patients with spontaneous IH

### Natural History & Prognosis
- Most IH cases resolve spontaneously
  - Dural thickening, enhancement disappears; midline structures return (ascend) to normal position
- Rare: Coma, death from severe intracranial herniation

### Treatment
- Aimed at restoring CSF volume (fluid replacement, bedrest)
  - Initial: Lumbar or directed epidural blood patch
  - Emergent intrathecal saline infusion if patient severely encephalopathic, obtunded
- Surgery if blood patch fails (usually large dural tear) or subdural hematoma (SDHs) with acute clinical deterioration

## DIAGNOSTIC CHECKLIST

### Consider
- Frequently misdiagnosed; imaging is key to diagnosis
- In children, look for occult skull base meningocele

### Image Interpretation Pearls
- Not all findings must be present for diagnosis of IH
- Look for enlarged spinal epidural venous plexus
- Retrospinal fluid at C1-2 level does not necessarily indicate site of CSF leak!

## SELECTED REFERENCES

1. Rai A et al: Epidural blood patch at C2: diagnosis and treatment of spontaneous intracranial hypotension. AJNR Am J Neuroradiol. 26(10):2663-6, 2005
2. Schievink WI et al: Spectrum of subdural fluid collections in spontaneous intracranial hypotension. J Neurosurg. 103(4):608-13, 2005
3. Weindling SM et al: Spontaneous craniospinal hypotension. J Magn Reson Imaging. 22(6):804-9, 2005
4. Schievink WI et al: Connective tissue disorders with spontaneous spinal cerebral spinal fluid leaks and intracranial hypotension: A prospective study. Neurosurg 54: 65-71, 2004
5. Schievink WI et al: False localizing sign of C1-2 cerebrospinal fluid leak in spontaneous intracranial hypotension. J Neurosurg 100:639-44, 2004
6. de Noronha RJ et al: Subdural haematoma: a potentially serious consequence of spontaneous intracranial hypotension. J Neurol Neurosurg Psychiatry. 74(6):752-5, 2003
7. Koss SA et al: Angiographic features of spontaneous intracranial hypotension. AJNR Am J Neuroradiol. 24(4):704-6, 2003

# INTRACRANIAL HYPOTENSION

## IMAGE GALLERY

### Typical

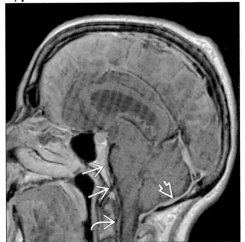 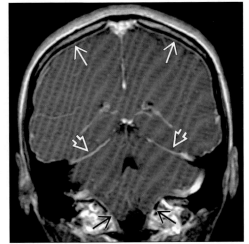

*(Left)* Sagittal T1 C+ MR shows dilated clival venous plexus ➡ extending into cervical spine ➡ and dilated venous plexus ➡ posterior and inferior to slumping cerebellum. *(Right)* Coronal T1 C+ MR shows enhancing dilated dura over the cerebral convexities ➡ and dilated enhancing tentorial leaves ➡. The cerebellar tonsils ➡ herniate below the foramen magnum.

### Typical

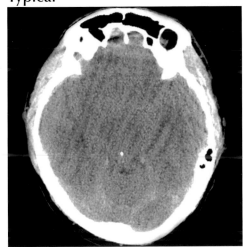 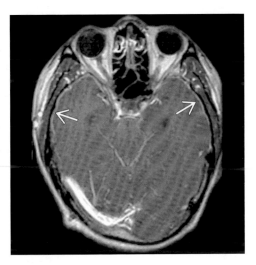

*(Left)* Axial NECT shows inability to visualize the suprasellar cistern or the perimesencephalic cisterns due to slumping of the brain downward through the tentorial incisura. *(Right)* Axial T1 C+ MR shows the same patient as previous image with marked compression of the midbrain, which appears elongated from anterior to posterior by the lateral compression. Dural enhancement is seen in the middle cranial fossae ➡.

### Typical

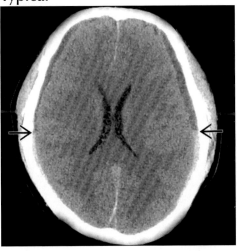 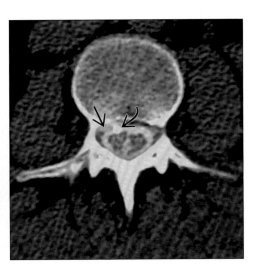

*(Left)* Axial NECT (same patient as previous 2 images) shows frank subdural hematomas, with hematocrit effect ➡ on each side. Note the abnormal configuration of the ventricles due to brain slumping. *(Right)* Axial myelography shows local leakage of contrast ➡ into extradural space resulting from meningeal tear due to the presence of the adjacent indwelling subarachnoid catheter ➡.

# CHOROID PLEXUS CYST

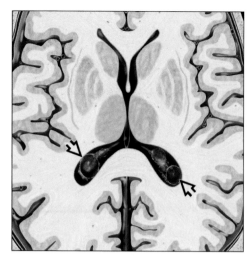

Axial graphic shows multiple cystic masses in the choroid plexus glomi ⇗, often seen incidentally on scans of middle-aged and older adults. Most are degenerated xanthogranulomas.

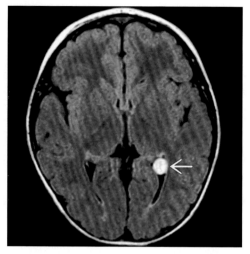

Axial FLAIR MR shows an incidental hyperintense choroid plexus cyst ➡ located in the glomus of the left lateral ventricular choroid plexus.

## TERMINOLOGY

### Abbreviations and Synonyms
- Choroid plexus cyst (CPC)

### Definitions
- Benign cysts (> 2 mm) of the choroid plexus

## IMAGING FINDINGS

### General Features
- Best diagnostic clue: > 2 mm cyst within choroid plexus
- Location
  ○ Atria of lateral ventricles most common site
    ▪ Attached to or within choroid plexus
    ▪ Unilateral or bilateral
  ○ Less common: 3rd ventricle
- Size
  ○ Variable
    ▪ Usually small (2-20 mm)
    ▪ Large cysts (> 20 mm) rare

- Morphology: Cystic mass within choroid plexus, either single or multiple, uniloculate or multiloculated

### CT Findings
- NECT: Iso- or slightly hyperdense compared to cerebrospinal fluid (CSF)
- CECT: Surrounding choroid plexus enhances

### MR Findings
- T1WI: Iso- to slightly hyperintense compared to CSF
- T2WI: Isointense compared to CSF
- PD/Intermediate: Iso- to hyperintense compared to CSF
- FLAIR: Iso- to hyperintense compared to CSF
- T2* GRE: Blooms only if intracystic hemorrhage (rare)
- DWI: Iso to slightly hyperintense to CSF with ADC similar to slightly lower than CSF
- T1 C+
  ○ Surrounding choroid plexus enhances
  ○ Delayed scans may show filling in of contrast within cysts

### Ultrasonographic Findings
- Grayscale Ultrasound
  ○ US

## DDx: Intraventricular Cystic Lesions and Choroid Plexus Lesions

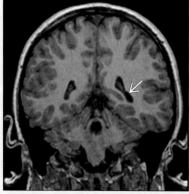

Ependymal Cyst

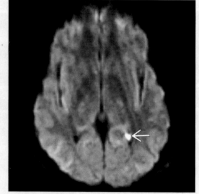

CP Xanthogranuloma

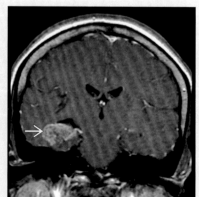

CP Papilloma

# CHOROID PLEXUS CYST

## Key Facts

### Terminology
- Benign cysts (> 2 mm) of the choroid plexus

### Imaging Findings
- Best diagnostic clue: > 2 mm cyst within choroid plexus
- Large cysts (> 20 mm) rare
- NECT: Iso- or slightly hyperdense compared to cerebrospinal fluid (CSF)
- FLAIR: Iso- to hyperintense compared to CSF
- DWI: Iso to slightly hyperintense to CSF with ADC similar to slightly lower than CSF
- Surrounding choroid plexus enhances
- Delayed scans may show filling in of contrast within cysts

### Top Differential Diagnoses
- Ultrasound "Pseudolesion"
- Arachnoid Cyst
- Ependymal Cyst
- Infectious/Inflammatory Cysts

### Pathology
- Fetal choroid plexus cysts associated with increased risk of trisomy 21 or 18 if additional risk factors

### Diagnostic Checklist
- Communicate with referring physician to determine risk
- Isolated CPC in fetus not associated with significant increase in risk for chromosomal abnormality
- CPC after birth only a concern if large and in location where obstructive hydrocephalus a risk

---

- > 2 mm cyst within or attached to echogenic choroid
- May see double wall

## Imaging Recommendations
- Best imaging tool
  - Child: MR
  - Neonate: US or MR
  - Fetus: Maternal US
- Protocol advice
  - MR: T1, T2 FSE, FLAIR, gradient echo, DWI and consider contrast
  - US: Must visualize in at least 2 planes

# DIFFERENTIAL DIAGNOSIS

## Ultrasound "Pseudolesion"
- Tiny anechoic areas < 2 mm in fetal choroid are normal, not CPC
- "Split" or "truncated" choroid can mimic CPC

## Arachnoid Cyst
- Not within choroid plexus

## Ependymal Cyst
- Not within choroid plexus
- Usually unilateral
- Histopathology shows immunoreactivity for GFAP

## Xanthogranuloma or Xanthoma
- Benign, degenerative change, often bilateral
- May be bright on DWI
- Rare in children

## Infectious/Inflammatory Cysts
- Neurocysticercosis (NCC)
  - 4th > lateral > 3rd ventricle
  - May be migratory
  - Look for other signs of NCC (e.g., other parenchymal cysts with scolex or Ca++)

## Neoplasm
- Choroid plexus papilloma or carcinoma (enhancing mass although may have cystic components)
- Meningioma (enhancing mass although may have cystic components)
- Cystic astrocytoma (exophytic from cerebral hemisphere)
- Metastasis (rare unless known metastatic disease and rarely cystic)

## Epidermoid Cyst
- Intraventricular location rare (4th > > lateral ventricle)
- "Cauliflower", insinuating pattern, with internal structure on FLAIR, bright on DWI, ADC similar to brain

# PATHOLOGY

## General Features
- General path comments: Benign cysts of choroid plexus lined by low cuboidal epithelium
- Genetics
  - Fetal choroid plexus cysts associated with increased risk of trisomy 21 or 18 if additional risk factors
    - Presence of additional abnormalities on US increases risk
    - Advanced maternal age and abnormal maternal serum triple-screen increase risk
    - Size > 10 mm greater risk of chromosomal abnormalities in some studies but controversial
- Etiology: Unknown
- Epidemiology
  - 1% of all 2nd trimester pregnancies on routine US (range 0.6-3.6%)
  - 28.5% (2nd trimester) to 50% (midgestation) of fetuses with T18
  - Small asymptomatic CPCs found incidentally in > 1/3 of all autopsied adults
- Associated abnormalities
  - Fetal CPC (if additional risk factors present)
    - Trisomy 18

# CHOROID PLEXUS CYST

- Trisomy 21

## Gross Pathologic & Surgical Features
- Cyst associated with choroid plexus epithelium

## Microscopic Features
- Positive immunostaining for EMA, transthyretin and S-100 protein, not for GFAP

## CLINICAL ISSUES

### Presentation
- Most common signs/symptoms
  - Fetal CPC: Detected on screening US
  - Pediatric CPC
    - Typically incidental
    - Rarely presents with hydrocephalus due to ventricular obstruction

### Demographics
- Age
  - Fetus
    - Prevalence 1% of all 2nd trimester pregnancies on routine US (range 0.6-3.6%)
    - Prevalence decreases after 2nd trimester
  - Neonate: Prevalence up to 3%
  - Child: Prevalence unknown

### Natural History & Prognosis
- Fetal CPC
  - Typically resolve in 3rd trimester even if associated with chromosomal abnormality
  - CPC and other US abnormalities or other risk factors increases risk for chromosomal abnormality
- Pediatric CPC
  - Incidental finding

### Treatment
- Fetal CPC
  - Must know status of additional risk factors for accurate counseling
  - Most centers consider isolated CPC (no additional risk factors) clinically insignificant
- Pediatric CPC
  - Almost always none
  - Rarely shunt for hydrocephalus due to ventricular obstruction by large cyst

## DIAGNOSTIC CHECKLIST

### Consider
- Fetus: If no additional US abnormalities
  - Communicate with referring physician to determine risk
  - Follow-up MR or US in 3rd trimester to better detect additional abnormalities
- Fetus: If additional US abnormalities consider genetic counseling
- Neonate and child: Follow-up only if large and in location where obstructive hydrocephalus a risk

## Image Interpretation Pearls
- Resolution of CPC in 3rd trimester occurs whether or not a chromosomal abnormality is present
- Isolated CPC in fetus not associated with significant increase in risk for chromosomal abnormality
- CPC after birth only a concern if large and in location where obstructive hydrocephalus a risk

## SELECTED REFERENCES

1. Epelman M et al: Differential diagnosis of intracranial cystic lesions at head US: correlation with CT and MR imaging. Radiographics. 26(1):173-96, 2006
2. Kinoshita T et al: Clinically silent choroid plexus cyst: evaluation by diffusion-weighted MRI. Neuroradiology. 47(4):251-5, 2005
3. Bronsteen R et al: Second-trimester sonography and trisomy 18: the significance of isolated choroid plexus cysts after an examination that includes the fetal hands. J Ultrasound Med. 23(2):241-5, 2004
4. Liebeskind DS et al: Infarction of the choroid plexus. AJNR Am J Neuroradiol. 25(2):289-90, 2004
5. Sahinoglu Z et al: Second trimester choroid plexus cysts and trisomy 18. Int J Gynaecol Obstet. 85(1):24-9, 2004
6. Enriquez G et al: Potential pitfalls in cranial sonography. Pediatr Radiol. 33(2):110-7, 2003
7. Turner SR et al: Sonography of fetal choroid plexus cysts: detection depends on cyst size and gestational age. J Ultrasound Med. 22(11):1219-27, 2003
8. Kraus I et al: Some observations of the structure of the choroid plexus and its cysts. Prenat Diagn. 22(13):1223-8, 2002
9. Pettenati MJ et al: Prenatal diagnosis of complete sole trisomy 1q. Prenat Diagn. 21(6):435-40, 2001
10. Boockvar JA et al: Symptomatic lateral ventricular ependymal cysts: criteria for distinguishing these rare cysts from other symptomatic cysts of the ventricles: case report. Neurosurgery. 46(5):1229-32; discussion 1232-3, 2000
11. Mendez-Martinez OE et al: Symptomatic bilateral xanthogranulomas of choroid plexus in a child. Br J Neurosurg. 14(1):62-4, 2000
12. Behnke M et al: Cranial ultrasound abnormalities identified at birth: their relationship to perinatal risk and neurobehavioral outcome. Pediatrics. 103(4):e41, 1999
13. Brown T et al: A role for maternal serum screening in detecting chromosomal abnormalities in fetuses with isolated choroid plexus cysts: a prospective multicentre study. Prenat Diagn. 19(5):405-10, 1999
14. Morcos CL et al: The isolated choroid plexus cyst. Obstet Gynecol. 92(2):232-6, 1998
15. Parizek J et al: Choroid plexus cyst of the left lateral ventricle with intermittent blockage of the foramen of Monro, and initial invagination into the III ventricle in a child. Childs Nerv Syst. 14(12):700-8, 1998
16. Peleg D et al: Choroid plexus cysts and aneuploidy. J Med Genet. 35(7):554-7, 1998
17. Gupta JK et al: Management of fetal choroid plexus cysts. Br J Obstet Gynaecol. 104(8):881-6, 1997
18. Gross SJ et al: Isolated fetal choroid plexus cysts and trisomy 18: a review and meta-analysis. Am J Obstet Gynecol. 172(1 Pt 1):83-7, 1995
19. Nava S et al: Significance of sonographically detected second-trimester choroid plexus cysts: a series of 211 cases and a review of the literature. Ultrasound Obstet Gynecol. 4(6):448-51, 1994
20. Riebel T et al: Choroid plexus cysts: a normal finding on ultrasound. Pediatr Radiol. 22(6):410-2, 1992

# CHOROID PLEXUS CYST

### Typical

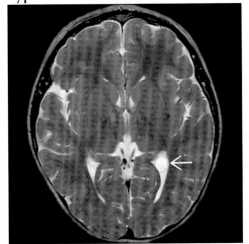 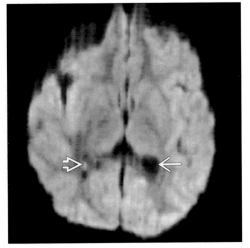

*(Left) Axial T2WI MR (same patient as previous FLAIR image) shows same incidental choroid plexus cyst ➡. Note cyst contents are isointense to CSF on T2. (Right) Axial DWI MR in same patient as previous image shows left cyst ➡ isointense and right cyst ➡ iso- to hyperintense compared to CSF.*

### Typical

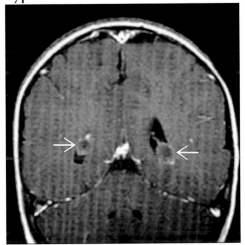 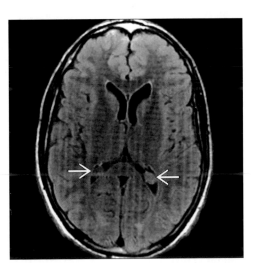

*(Left) Coronal T1 C+ MR in same patient as previous image shows enhancement of the choroid plexus ➡ surrounding the cysts. (Right) Axial FLAIR MR shows bilateral choroid plexus cysts ➡. Note only mildly increased signal of cyst contents.*

### Typical

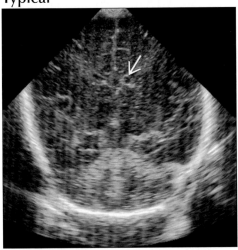 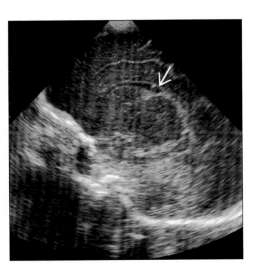

*(Left) Coronal oblique ultrasound shows a well-defined choroid plexus cyst ➡ in the left lateral ventricle. Note absence of internal echoes. (Right) Sagittal oblique ultrasound in same patient as previous image confirms the choroid plexus cyst ➡ seen on the coronal oblique image.*

# EPENDYMAL CYST

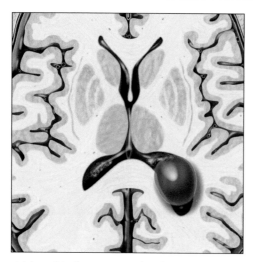

*Axial graphic shows an ependymal cyst arising in the wall and projecting into the lumen of the lateral ventricle.*

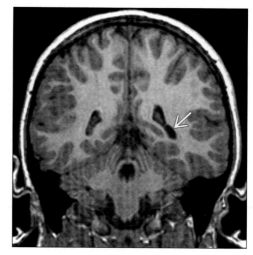

*Coronal T1WI MR in a 12 year old boy with headaches and a single seizure thought to be unrelated to this finding. An incidental CSF intensity lesion ➔ is seen in the right lateral ventricle.*

## TERMINOLOGY

### Abbreviations and Synonyms
- Neuroepithelial cyst (less favored)

### Definitions
- Congenital, benign ependymal-lined cyst

## IMAGING FINDINGS

### General Features
- Best diagnostic clue: Nonenhancing thin-walled cyst similar to cerebrospinal fluid (CSF) on all sequences
- Location
  - Central white matter of temporoparietal and frontal lobes, often near the ventricles
  - Intraventricular (typically lateral ventricle)
  - Subarachnoid space, mesencephalon rare
- Size: Variable, typically small; range 2-3 mm to 8-9 cm
- Morphology: Rounded or multiseptated

### CT Findings
- NECT: Isodense to CSF; Ca++ extremely rare
- CECT: No enhancement

### MR Findings
- T2WI: Iso- to slightly hyperintense to CSF
- FLAIR: Iso- to slightly hyperintense to CSF
- DWI: Isointense to CSF
- T1 C+: No enhancement

### Imaging Recommendations
- Best imaging tool: MR
- Protocol advice: MR with FLAIR, DWI and contrast

## DIFFERENTIAL DIAGNOSIS

### Choroid Plexus Cyst
- Within or attached to choroid plexus glomus

### Arachnoid Cyst
- Much more common in subarachnoid space

### Epidermoid Cyst
- Lobulated; bright on DWI

### Parasitic Cyst
- Scolex often seen in cysticercosis

## DDx: Cystic Lesions

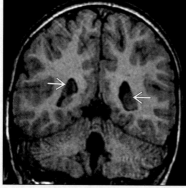

*Choroid Plexus Cysts*

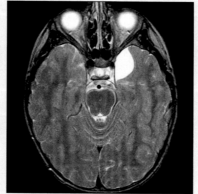

*Arachnoid Cyst*

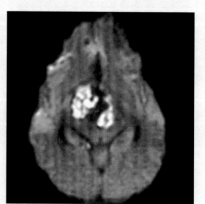

*Epidermoid*

# EPENDYMAL CYST

## Key Facts

### Imaging Findings
- Best diagnostic clue: Nonenhancing thin-walled cyst similar to cerebrospinal fluid (CSF) on all sequences
- Central white matter of temporoparietal and frontal lobes, often near the ventricles
- Intraventricular (typically lateral ventricle)

### Top Differential Diagnoses
- Choroid Plexus Cyst
- Arachnoid Cyst

- Epidermoid Cyst
- Parasitic Cyst
- Cystic Neoplasm

### Pathology
- General path comments: Congenital, benign cyst

### Clinical Issues
- Conservative management if asymptomatic

---

### Cystic Neoplasm
- Rarely CSF signal; associated mass ± enhancement

## PATHOLOGY

### General Features
- General path comments: Congenital, benign cyst
- Etiology: Sequestration of developing neuroectoderm
- Epidemiology: Unknown

### Gross Pathologic & Surgical Features
- Thin-walled cyst filled with clear serous liquid

### Microscopic Features
- Fluid-filled space lined by columnar or cuboidal cells, ± cilia, no goblet cells
- Immunohistochemistry positive for GFAP and S-100

## CLINICAL ISSUES

### Presentation
- Most common signs/symptoms: Asymptomatic
- Other signs/symptoms: Headache (hydrocephalus), seizure or neurological deficit

### Demographics
- Age: Any; typically young adults

### Natural History & Prognosis
- Typically stable if asymptomatic

### Treatment
- Surgical excision or endoscopic fenestration
- Conservative management if asymptomatic

## DIAGNOSTIC CHECKLIST

### Consider
- Need contrast to rule out cystic tumor

## SELECTED REFERENCES

1. Yano S et al: Third ventricular ependymal cyst presenting with acute hydrocephalus. Pediatr Neurosurg. 42(4):245-8, 2006
2. Hirano A et al: Benign cysts in the central nervous system: neuropathological observations of the cyst walls. Neuropathology. 24(1):1-7, 2004
3. Pawar SJ et al: Giant ependymal cyst of the temporal horn -- an unusual presentation. Case report with review of the literature. Pediatr Neurosurg. 34(6):306-10, 2001
4. Boockvar JA et al: Symptomatic lateral ventricular ependymal cysts: criteria for distinguishing these rare cysts from other symptomatic cysts of the ventricles: case report. Neurosurgery. 46(5):1229-32; discussion 1232-3, 2000
5. Guermazi A et al: Imaging findings of central nervous system neuroepithelial cysts. Eur Radiol. 8(4):618-23, 1998
6. Lustgarten L et al: Benign intracerebral cysts with ependymal lining: pathological and radiological features. Br J Neurosurg. 11(5):393-7, 1997

## IMAGE GALLERY

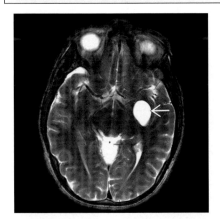
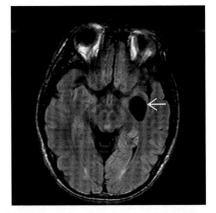
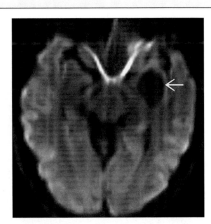

*(Left)* Axial T1WI MR in a 15 year old boy imaged due to loss of consciousness after head trauma. An incidental well-defined CSF intensity lesion ➡ is seen in the left temporal lobe. *(Center)* Axial FLAIR MR in the same child as previous image shows that the lesion ➡ remains isointense to CSF with no surrounding signal abnormality. *(Right)* Axial DWI MR in the same child as previous image shows the center of the lesion ➡ has rapid diffusion similar to CSF.

# SUBEPENDYMAL GIANT CELL ASTROCYTOMA

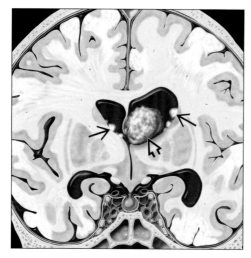

Coronal graphic shows early left lateral ventricular obstruction from a subependymal giant cell tumor arising near the left foramen of Monro ➥. Note the subependymal tubers ➡.

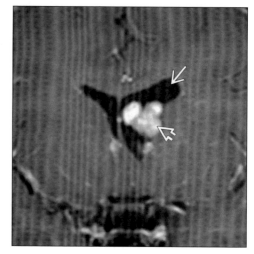

Coronal T1 C+ MR shows a lobulated strongly enhancing subependymal giant cell tumor ➥. Note the early left lateral ventricular obstruction ➡.

## TERMINOLOGY

### Abbreviations and Synonyms
- Subependymal giant cell astrocytoma (SGCA)
- Subependymal giant cell tumor (SGCT)
- Intraventricular astrocytoma of tuberous sclerosis (TS)

### Definitions
- Intraventricular glioneuronal tumor arising in ventricular wall, usually near the foramen of Monro

## IMAGING FINDINGS

### General Features
- Best diagnostic clue
  - Enlarging, enhancing intraventricular mass in patient with tuberous sclerosis complex (TSC)
  - Origin of mass from ventricular wall, typically near foramen of Monro
  - Other findings of TS (cortical tubers, SE nodules)
- Location: Almost always near foramen of Monro
- Size
  - Variable, slow growing
  - Often presents when 2-3 cm, causing obstructive hydrocephalus
- Morphology
  - Well marginated, often lobulated
  - Frond-like margins mimic choroid plexus tumor

### CT Findings
- NECT
  - Hypo- to isodense
  - Heterogeneous
  - Ca++ variable
  - Hydrocephalus
- CECT
  - Heterogeneous, strong enhancement
  - Growth suggests SGCT
- CT perfusion
  - May be mildly hypervascular

### MR Findings
- T1WI
  - Hypointense to isointense to GM
  - ± Ca++ (hyperintense to hypointense)
- T2WI
  - Heterogeneous
    - Isointense to hyperintense

## DDx: Foramen of Monro Region Neoplasms in Children

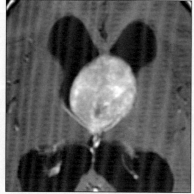

*Astrocytoma*

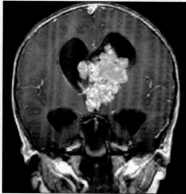

*Choroid Papilloma*

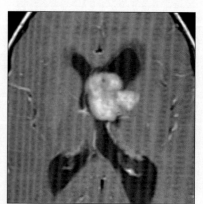

*PNET*

# SUBEPENDYMAL GIANT CELL ASTROCYTOMA

## Key Facts

### Imaging Findings

- Enlarging, enhancing intraventricular mass in patient with tuberous sclerosis complex (TSC)
- Location: Almost always near foramen of Monro
- Well marginated, often lobulated
- Heterogeneous, strong enhancement
- Growth suggests SGCT
- Enhancement alone does not allow discrimination from hamartoma
- FLAIR MR to detect subtle CNS features of TSC
- Recommend brain MR with contrast every 1-2 years for SGCT follow-up

### Top Differential Diagnoses

- Choroid Plexus Tumors
- Astrocytoma
- Germinoma
- Subependymoma

### Pathology

- Most common CNS neoplasm in TSC
- Does not seed CSF pathways
- WHO grade I

### Clinical Issues

- Increased ICP secondary to tumor obstructing foramen of Monro

### Diagnostic Checklist

- SGCT in tuberous sclerosis patient with worsening seizures and/or symptoms of ventricular obstruction

---

- ○ Ca++ foci hypointense
- ○ Hydrocephalus
- PD/Intermediate: Hyperintense
- FLAIR
  - ○ Heterogeneously hyperintense
  - ○ Periventricular interstitial edema from ventricular obstruction
- T2* GRE: Low signal from Ca++
- DWI: ADC values less than parenchymal hamartomas of TS
- T1 C+
  - ○ Robust enhancement
    - ■ Enhancement alone does not allow discrimination from hamartoma
  - ○ Enlarging foramen of Monro mass strongly suggests SGCT
  - ○ Size of intraventricular SGCT > 1.2 cm
  - ○ No predilection for CSF spread
- MRS: Less than "expected" ↓ NAA due to neuronal elements in tumor

## Ultrasonographic Findings

- Intra-operative
  - ○ Hyperechoic intraventricular mass
  - ○ Heterogeneous shadowing foci of Ca++

## Angiographic Findings

- Conventional
  - ○ Variable vascularity
  - ○ ± Stretched thalamostriate veins (hydrocephalus)

## Imaging Recommendations

- Best imaging tool: MR brain demonstrates extent of mass, delineates associated TSC features
- Protocol advice
  - ○ FLAIR MR to detect subtle CNS features of TSC
  - ○ Recommend brain MR with contrast every 1-2 years for SGCT follow-up

## DIFFERENTIAL DIAGNOSIS

### Choroid Plexus Tumors

- Papilloma and carcinoma
  - ○ Uncommon at foramen of Monro
  - ○ Vivid enhancement; ± CSF seeding
  - ○ Parenchymal invasion and peritumoral edema with choroid plexus carcinoma

### Astrocytoma

- Origin ⇒ septum pellucidum fornices or medial basal ganglia
  - ○ Common pediatric intra-axial neoplasm
  - ○ Variable enhancement, Ca++ rare

### Germinoma

- Hugs midline, often arises in/near third ventricle
- Early diabetes insipidus
- Early CSF spread

### Subependymoma

- Inferior fourth and frontal horn most common locations
- Nonenhancing mass
- Tumor of middle age and elderly

### Central Neurocytoma

- Well-defined, variably vascularized lobulated mass
- Origin near foramen of Monro or septum pellucidum
- Necrosis and cyst formation are common
- Seen in young adults

### Supratentorial PNET

- May exophytically extend into ventricle
- Lack of peritumoral edema
- Highly cellular tumor, isointense → slightly hyperintense on T2WI

## PATHOLOGY

### General Features

- General path comments

# SUBEPENDYMAL GIANT CELL ASTROCYTOMA

- ○ Benign, slow growing tumor
- ○ Most common CNS neoplasm in TSC
- ○ Rarely (if ever) arises in absence of TSC
- ○ Recurrence after resection rare
- ○ Ca++ and hemorrhage may be seen
- • Genetics
  - ○ 50% of TSC patients have positive family history
    - ▪ High rate of de novo mutations
  - ○ In affected kindreds
    - ▪ Inheritance: Autosomal dominant
    - ▪ High penetrance
    - ▪ Considerable phenotypic variability
  - ○ Molecular genetics
    - ▪ Two distinct TSC loci (chromosome 9q ⇒ TSC1 & 16p ⇒ TSC2)
    - ▪ TSC1 and TSC2 are likely tumor suppressor genes
    - ▪ Mammalian target of rapamycin mTOR is a key kinase, regulates growth and survival of SGCT cells
    - ▪ Signaling pathway of mTOR includes: Neurofibromin (NF1), hamartin (TSC1), and tuberin (TSC2)
    - ▪ Rapamycin (immunosuppressant) strongly inhibits mTOR
- • Etiology: SGCT probably arises from subependymal nodule
- • Epidemiology
  - ○ Incidence of SGCT ⇒ 5-20% of patients with TSC, M = F, age: 8-18 years
  - ○ 1.4% of all pediatric brain tumors
- • Associated abnormalities
  - ○ Other tumors are rare in TSC
    - ▪ Pilocytic astrocytoma, fibrillary astrocytoma, ganglioglioma

## Gross Pathologic & Surgical Features
- • Well marginated mass arising from lateral ventricular wall near foramen of Monro
  - ○ ± Cysts, Ca++, and hemorrhage
- • Does not seed CSF pathways

## Microscopic Features
- • Tumor cells of SGCTs show wide spectrum of astroglial phenotypes
  - ○ Giant pyramidal ganglioid astrocytes
  - ○ Perivascular pseudopalisading
- • Immunohistochemistry
  - ○ Variable immunoreactivity for GFAP and S 100 protein
  - ○ Some tumor cells express glial and neuronal antigens

## Staging, Grading or Classification Criteria
- • WHO grade I

# CLINICAL ISSUES

## Presentation
- • Most common signs/symptoms
  - ○ Increased ICP secondary to tumor obstructing foramen of Monro
    - ▪ Headache, vomiting, obtunded
  - ○ Other signs/symptoms

- ▪ Worsening epilepsy
- ▪ Massive spontaneous hemorrhage
- • Clinical Profile
  - ○ Patient with TSC develops signs and symptoms of ventricular obstruction
  - ○ Worsening of epilepsy

## Demographics
- • Age
  - ○ SGCT typically occurs during the first two decades
  - ○ Mean age 11 years
- • Gender: No gender predilection
- • Ethnicity: No race predilection

## Natural History & Prognosis
- • Solitary, slow growing benign tumor
  - ○ Rarely degenerate into malignant tumor
- • Symptoms from ventricular obstruction
- • Good outcome and low recurrence rate with complete resection
- • Rarely, massive spontaneous hemorrhage

## Treatment
- • Surgical resection (open vs. endoscopic)
- • Massive hemorrhage possible complication
- • Rapamycin causes regression of SGCTs

# DIAGNOSTIC CHECKLIST

## Consider
- • SGCT in tuberous sclerosis patient with worsening seizures and/or symptoms of ventricular obstruction

## Image Interpretation Pearls
- • Enlarging, enhancing intraventricular mass near the foramen of Monro in TSC patient

# SELECTED REFERENCES

1. Clarke MJ et al: Imaging characteristics and growth of subependymal giant cell astrocytomas. Neurosurg Focus. 20(1):E5, 2006
2. Ess KC et al: Developmental origin of subependymal giant cell astrocytoma in tuberous sclerosis complex. Neurology. 64(8):1446-9, 2005
3. Chan JA et al: Pathogenesis of tuberous sclerosis subependymal giant cell astrocytomas: biallelic inactivation of TSC1 or TSC2 leads to mTOR activation. J Neuropathol Exp Neurol. 63(12):1236-42, 2004
4. Goh S et al: Subependymal giant cell tumors in tuberous sclerosis complex. Neurology. 63(8):1457-61, 2004
5. Sharma M et al: Subependymal giant cell astrocytoma: a clinicopathological study of 23 cases with special emphasis on proliferative markers and expression of p53 and retinoblastoma gene proteins. Pathology. 36(2):139-44, 2004
6. Cuccia V et al: Subependymal giant cell astrocytoma in children with tuberous sclerosis. Childs Nerv Syst. 19(4):232-43, 2003
7. Koeller KK et al: From the archives of the AFIP. Cerebral intraventricular neoplasms: radiologic-pathologic correlation. Radiographics. 22(6):1473-505, 2002
8. Nishio S et al: Tumours around the foramen of Monro: clinical and neuroimaging features and their differential diagnosis. J Clin Neurosci. 9(2):137-41, 2002

# SUBEPENDYMAL GIANT CELL ASTROCYTOMA

## IMAGE GALLERY

### Typical

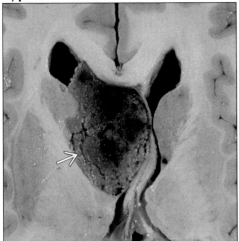

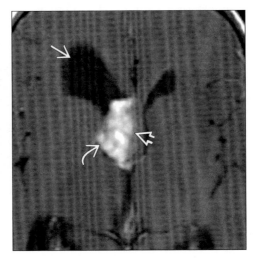

**(Left)** *Axial gross pathology shows subependymal giant cell tumor at the foramen of Monro in a patient with tuberous sclerosis ➡. (Courtesy R. Hewlett, MD). (Right) Axial T1 C+ MR shows an enhancing subependymal giant cell tumor ➡. At surgery, the tumor infiltrated the septum pellucidum ➡. Note the moderate right frontal horn obstruction ➡.*

### Typical

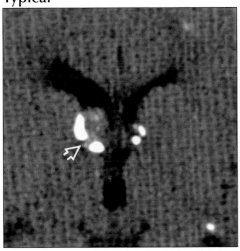

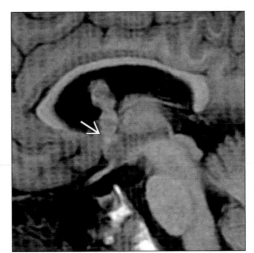

**(Left)** *Axial NECT shows a partially calcified right foramen of Monro region subependymal giant cell tumor ➡. (Right) Sagittal T1WI MR shows a slightly heterogeneous intraventricular component of a subependymal giant cell tumor originating from the foramen of Monro ➡.*

### Typical

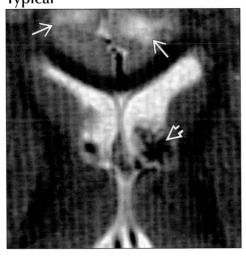

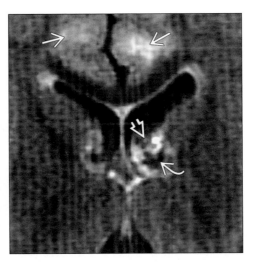

**(Left)** *Axial T2WI MR shows a predominantly hypointense (secondary to calcification) left foramen of Monro region subependymal giant cell tumor ➡. Note the bilateral frontal lobe tubers ➡. (Right) Axial FLAIR MR shows a heterogeneous subependymal giant cell tumor ➡. The central hypointense core ➡ corresponds to calcification on NECT. Note bilateral frontal lobe tubers ➡.*

# CHOROID PLEXUS PAPILLOMA

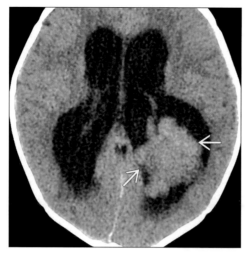

Axial NECT shows lobulated choroid plexus papilloma arising from glomus of left lateral ventricle ➡ with associated ventriculomegaly.

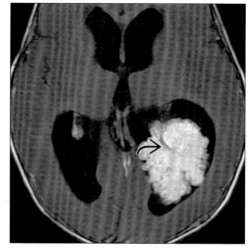

Axial T1 C+ MR in the same child shows diffuse and homogeneous enhancement of the tumor. Note prominent draining vein centrally located within tumor ➡.

## TERMINOLOGY

### Abbreviations and Synonyms
- Choroid plexus papilloma (CPP), choroid plexus tumor (CPT)

### Definitions
- Intraventricular, papillary neoplasm derived from choroid plexus epithelium

## IMAGING FINDINGS

### General Features
- Best diagnostic clue: Strongly enhancing, lobulated intraventricular mass
- Location
  - 70% ⇒ atrium of lateral ventricle
    - Left > right
  - 20% ⇒ fourth ventricle
    - Most common site of origin in adults
- Size: Often large at diagnosis
- Morphology: Lobulated fronds, some accommodation to ventricular morphology

### CT Findings
- NECT
  - Intraventricular lobular mass
  - 75% iso- or hyper-attenuating
  - 25% have calcification (Ca++)
  - Hydrocephalus
    - Overproduction of cerebrospinal fluid (CSF) by tumor
    - Sometimes due to tumor obstructing CSF pathways
    - Hemorrhage from tumor can hamper CSF resorption
- CECT
  - Intense, homogeneous enhancement
    - Heterogeneous enhancement may suggest carcinoma (CPCA)

### MR Findings
- T1WI
  - Well-delineated, lobulated mass
  - Iso- to hypointense
- T2WI
  - Iso- to hyperintense
  - ± Internal linear and branching vascular flow voids

## DDx: Intraventricular Tumors

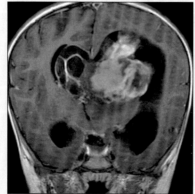

DIG

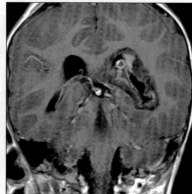

PNET

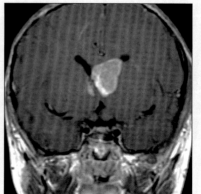

SEGA

# CHOROID PLEXUS PAPILLOMA

## Key Facts

### Terminology
- Choroid plexus papilloma (CPP), choroid plexus tumor (CPT)
- Intraventricular, papillary neoplasm derived from choroid plexus epithelium

### Imaging Findings
- Best diagnostic clue: Strongly enhancing, lobulated intraventricular mass
- 70% ⇒ atrium of lateral ventricle

### Top Differential Diagnoses
- Medulloblastoma
- Ependymoma
- Sturge-Weber

### Pathology
- CPP or CPCA may both show invasion into brain parenchyma
- Both may also have subarachnoid spread of tumor
- WHO grade I

### Clinical Issues
- One of the more common brain tumors in children less than 2 years of age
- 86% present by 5 years
- 5 year survival close to 100%

### Diagnostic Checklist
- Imaging alone cannot reliably distinguish CPP from CPCA

---

- o Large CPP may invade into brain parenchyma
  - ■ Extensive invasion suggests CPCA
- FLAIR
  - o Bright periventricular signal
    - ■ Transependymal interstitial edema due to ventricular obstruction
- T2* GRE: ± Foci of diminished signal if Ca++ and/or blood products are present
- T1 C+
  - o Robust homogeneous enhancement
  - o Occasional cysts and small foci of necrosis
  - o May spread through subarachnoid space
    - ■ Scan entire neuraxis
- MRA: Enlarged choroidal artery (trigonal mass)
- MRS
  - o Absent N-acetyl-aspartate (NAA), ↑ choline
  - o Lactate indicates necrosis ⇒ not necessarily more aggressive

### Ultrasonographic Findings
- Grayscale Ultrasound
  - o Hyperechoic mass with frond-like projections
  - o Echotexture similar to normal choroid plexus

### Nuclear Medicine Findings
- PET: 11C-Methionine ⇒ ↑ tumor-to-normal brain ratios in CPP compared to gliomas

### Angiographic Findings
- Conventional
  - o Enlarged choroidal artery
  - o Prolonged vascular stain
  - o Arteriovenous shunting

### Imaging Recommendations
- Best imaging tool: MR with contrast
- Protocol advice: Perform contrast-enhanced MR of entire neuraxis before surgery

## DIFFERENTIAL DIAGNOSIS

### Medulloblastoma
- Most common 4th ventricular neoplasm in a child

- More spherical than CPP

### Ependymoma
- Ependymoma and medulloblastoma are more common 4th ventricular masses than CPP
- More heterogeneous than CPP

### Supratentorial Primitive Neuroectodermal Tumor (PNET)
- Similar to medulloblastoma
- Hemispheric tumor that can invade ventricle

### Subependymal Giant-Cell Astrocytoma (SEGA)
- Characteristic tumor of Tuberous Sclerosis
- Arise at foramen of Monro

### Desmoplastic Infantile Ganglioglioma (DIG)
- Aggressive-appearing tumor of infants with typically benign clinical course

### Xanthogranuloma or Xanthoma
- Benign tumor of lipid laden cells in choroid glomus
- More common in adults
- Unrelated to juvenile xanthogranuloma (histiocytic skin lesion)

### Hematoma
- Intraventricular hemorrhage (IVH) can be a consequence of germinal matrix hemorrhage in the neonate
- Clot adherent to the choroid can be mass-like in appearance

### Sturge-Weber
- Enlargement of the choroid glomus ipsilateral to the pial venous malformation

## PATHOLOGY

### General Features
- General path comments
  - o Well-circumscribed lobulated intraventricular mass

# CHOROID PLEXUS PAPILLOMA

- ○ CPP or CPCA may both show invasion into brain parenchyma
  - ■ More extensive invasion ⇒ carcinoma
  - ○ Both may also have subarachnoid spread of tumor
- Genetics
  - ○ Li-Fraumeni and Aicardi syndromes (possible TP53 germline mutation)
  - ○ Association of CPP and duplication of short arm of chromosome 9
- Etiology: DNA sequences from simian virus 40 (SV40), have been found in CPT
- Epidemiology: 2-4% of all pediatric brain tumors

## Gross Pathologic & Surgical Features
- Pink or reddish-tan intraventricular mass
- Cauliflower-like surface
- ± Cysts, necrosis, and hemorrhage

## Microscopic Features
- Resembles non-neoplastic choroid plexus
- Fibrovascular connective tissue fronds, covered by cuboidal or columnar epithelium
- Mitotic activity, necrosis, and brain invasion typically absent
- Immunohistochemistry
  - ○ Cytokeratin and vimentin are expressed
  - ○ S-100 protein in 90%
  - ○ Some are positive for glial fibrillary acidic protein (GFAP)

## Staging, Grading or Classification Criteria
- WHO grade I

## CLINICAL ISSUES

### Presentation
- Most common signs/symptoms: Child in first two years of life with signs, symptoms of elevated ICP
- Other signs/symptoms: Macrocrania, bulging fontanelle, vomiting, headache, ataxia, seizure

### Demographics
- Age
  - ○ One of the more common brain tumors in children less than 2 years of age
  - ○ 86% present by 5 years
- Gender: M > F

### Natural History & Prognosis
- Benign, slowly growing
- May become anaplastic over time
  - ○ Reports of benign tumors at first surgery having malignant degeneration at second surgery

### Treatment
- Total surgical resection
- 5 year survival close to 100%

## DIAGNOSTIC CHECKLIST

### Consider
- Although relatively rare, CPP is still most likely enhancing mass in lateral ventricle of a child < 2

- 4th ventricular CPP is much less likely than ependymoma or medulloblastoma

## Image Interpretation Pearls
- Imaging alone cannot reliably distinguish CPP from CPCA
  - ○ Final diagnosis is histologic

## SELECTED REFERENCES

1. Kumar R et al: Childhood choroid plexus papillomas: operative complications. Childs Nerv Syst. 21(2):138-43, 2005
2. Fujimura M et al: Hydrocephalus due to cerebrospinal fluid overproduction by bilateral choroid plexus papillomas. Childs Nerv Syst. 20(7):485-8, 2004
3. Noguchi A et al: Choroid plexus papilloma of the third ventricle in the fetus. Case illustration. J Neurosurg. 100(2 Suppl Pediatrics):224, 2004
4. Phi JH et al: Temporal lobe epilepsy caused by choroid plexus papilloma in the temporal horn. Clin Neuropathol. 23(3):95-8, 2004
5. Strojan P et al: Choroid plexus tumors: a review of 28-year experience. Neoplasma. 51(4):306-12, 2004
6. D'Ambrosio AL et al: Villous hypertrophy versus choroid plexus papilloma: a case report demonstrating a diagnostic role for the proliferation index. Pediatr Neurosurg. 39(2):91-6, 2003
7. Heese O et al: Diffuse arachnoidal enhancement of a well differentiated choroid plexus papilloma. Acta Neurochir (Wien). 144(7):723-8, 2002
8. Koeller KK et al: From the archives of the AFIP. Cerebral intraventricular neoplasms: radiologic-pathologic correlation. Radiographics. 22(6):1473-505, 2002
9. Murphy M et al: Presentation of a choroid plexus papilloma mimicking an extradural haematoma after a head injury. Childs Nerv Syst. 18(8):457-9, 2002
10. Pianetti Filho G et al: Choroid plexus papilloma and Aicardi syndrome: case report. Arq Neuropsiquiatr. 60(4):1008-10, 2002
11. Sunada I et al: 18F-FDG and 11C-methionine PET in choroid plexus papilloma--report of three cases. Radiat Med. 20(2):97-100, 2002
12. Horska A et al: Proton magnetic resonance spectroscopy of choroid plexus tumors in children. J Magn Reson Imaging. 14(1):78-82, 2001
13. Levy ML et al: Choroid plexus tumors in children: significance of stromal invasion. Neurosurgery. 48(2):303-9, 2001
14. Shin JH et al: Choroid plexus papilloma in the posterior cranial fossa: MR, CT, and angiographic findings. Clin Imaging. 25(3):154-62, 2001
15. Aguzzi A et al: Choroid plexus tumors. In Kleihues P, Cavenee WK (eds): Tumors of the Nervous System. IARC Press. 84-6, 2000
16. Sarkar C et al: Choroid plexus papilloma: a clinicopathological study of 23 cases. Surg Neurol. 52(1):37-9, 1999

I 5 52

# CHOROID PLEXUS PAPILLOMA

## IMAGE GALLERY

### Typical

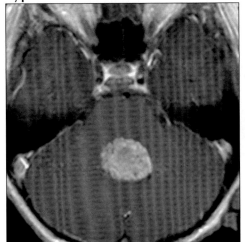
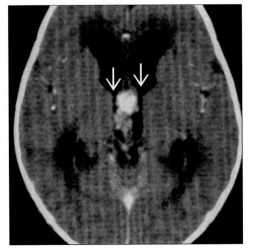

*(Left)* Axial T1 C+ MR shows homogeneously enhancing 4th ventricular choroid plexus papilloma. Ependymoma and medulloblastoma are more common 4th ventricular tumors in children. *(Right)* Axial CECT shows enhancing choroid plexus papilloma in the 3rd ventricle. The foramina of Monro are patent ⮕, but the tumor is causing ventriculomegaly by CSF overproduction.

### Typical

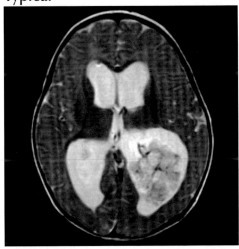
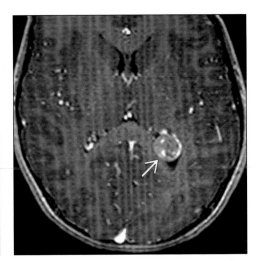

*(Left)* Axial T2WI MR shows choroid plexus papilloma in the left lateral ventricle with associated hydrocephalus. Lateral ventricular tumors can also cause hydrocephalus by overproduction of CSF. *(Right)* Axial T1 C+ MR shows partially enhancing choroid plexus papilloma in the glomus of the left lateral ventricle ⮕. Lateral ventricular tumors are more commonly found on the left side.

### Typical

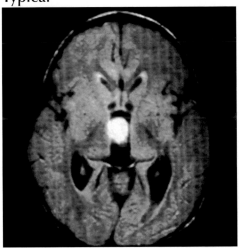
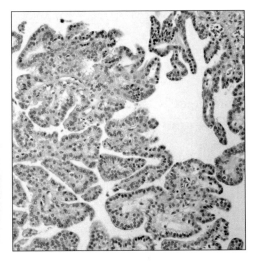

*(Left)* Axial FLAIR MR shows homogeneous hyperintense signal of a 3rd ventricular choroid plexus papilloma. *(Right)* Micropathology, low power, H&E shows characteristic fibrovascular connective tissue fronds covered by cuboidal epithelium. Note regular cellular morphology and absence of mitotic activity.

# CHOROID PLEXUS CARCINOMA

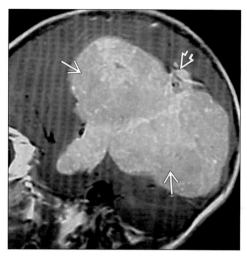
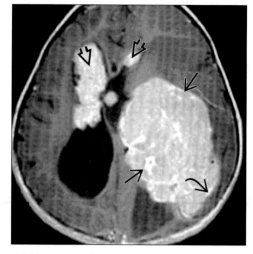

Sagittal T1 C+ MR shows a strongly enhancing lobulated lateral ventricular mass ➡. Note a focus of ependymal invasion ⮞.

Axial T1 C+ MR shows a large robustly enhancing left trigonal choroid plexus carcinoma ➡. There is a region of ependymal invasion ↗ and intraventricular tumor seeding ⮞.

## TERMINOLOGY

### Abbreviations and Synonyms
- Choroid plexus carcinoma (CPCA)

### Definitions
- Malignant tumor originating from epithelium of choroid plexus

## IMAGING FINDINGS

### General Features
- Best diagnostic clue
  - Child < 5 year, with enhancing intraventricular mass and ependymal invasion
  - Differentiation from choroid plexus papilloma (CPP) is histologic, not radiologic
- Location: Almost always arise in lateral ventricle
- Size: Variable
- Morphology
  - Cauliflower-like mass
  - Commonly with necrosis, cysts and hemorrhage

### CT Findings
- NECT
  - Iso- to hyperattenuating
  - Irregular contours
  - Necrosis, hemorrhage, and cysts
  - Ca++ (20-25%)
- CECT
  - Heterogeneous, strong enhancement
  - Peritumoral edema
  - ± Cerebrospinal fluid (CSF) tumor seeding

### MR Findings
- T1WI
  - Iso- to hypointense intraventricular mass
  - Lobulated or irregularly marginated, papillary appearance
  - Heterogeneous: Reflects necrosis, hemorrhage, or cysts
- T2WI
  - Mixed signal intraventricular mass, hypo- iso- or hyperintense
  - Heterogeneity reflects: Necrosis, hemorrhage, cysts and or calcification
  - May invade brain and incite edema

## DDx: Mimics of Choroid Plexus Carcinoma

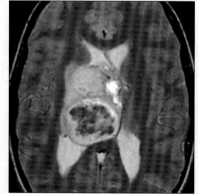
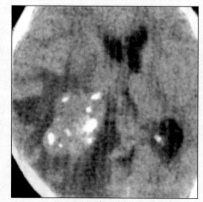
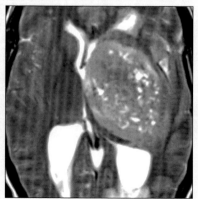

Glioblastoma Multiforme

Ependymoma

Primitive Neuroectodermal Tumor

# CHOROID PLEXUS CARCINOMA

## Key Facts

### Imaging Findings
- Child < 5 year, with enhancing intraventricular mass and ependymal invasion
- Differentiation from choroid plexus papilloma (CPP) is histologic, not radiologic
- Location: Almost always arise in lateral ventricle
- Commonly with necrosis, cysts and hemorrhage
- Irregular contours
- Necrosis, hemorrhage, and cysts
- Ca++ (20-25%)
- Lobulated or irregularly marginated, papillary appearance
- May invade brain and incite edema
- Heterogeneous
- DWI: Low apparent diffusion coefficient (ADC) values in solid components

- Heterogeneous enhancement
- Protocol advice: Enhanced MR of entire neuraxis prior to surgery

### Top Differential Diagnoses
- Choroid Plexus Papilloma (CPP)
- Ependymoma
- Subependymal Giant Cell Tumor

### Clinical Issues
- Nausea, vomiting, headache, obtundation
- Age: Between 2 and 4 years, median age ~ 26 months

### Diagnostic Checklist
- MR may not distinguish papilloma from carcinoma
- Heterogeneity, brain invasion, CSF spread favor CPCA

---

- PD/Intermediate
  - Heterogeneous
  - Internal vascular flow voids
- FLAIR
  - Tumor heterogeneity
  - Peritumoral edema in surrounding parenchyma
- T2* GRE: Low signal from hemorrhage
- DWI: Low apparent diffusion coefficient (ADC) values in solid components
- T1 C+
  - Heterogeneous enhancement
  - ± CSF tumor seeding in ventricles, cisterns
- MRS: ↓ NAA, ↑ choline, ± ↑ lactate

### Ultrasonographic Findings
- Grayscale Ultrasound: Hyperechoic intraventricular mass
- Pulsed Doppler: Bidirectional flow through diastole
- Color Doppler: Hypervascular mass

### Nuclear Medicine Findings
- PET: 11C-Methionine ⇒ ↑ tumor-to-normal brain ratios
- Tc-99m Sestamibi ⇒ ↑ in choroid plexus tumors (CPTs)

### Angiographic Findings
- Conventional: Enlarged choroidal artery & vascular stain

### Imaging Recommendations
- Best imaging tool: Contrast-enhanced MR of brain and spine
- Protocol advice: Enhanced MR of entire neuraxis prior to surgery

## DIFFERENTIAL DIAGNOSIS

### Choroid Plexus Papilloma (CPP)
- MR may not be able to distinguish papilloma from carcinoma by radiology
- Aggressive papillomas may seed through CSF pathways
- CPP may show minimal brain invasion

### Ependymoma
- In 4th ventricle more commonly
- Supratentorial tumors often deep hemispheric, periventricular, and heterogeneous

### Subependymal Giant Cell Tumor
- Associated central nervous system (CNS) findings of tuberous sclerosis
- Characteristic location near foramen of Monro
- Rarely elicit edema

### Astrocytic Tumors
- May arise from septum pellucidum, thalamus, or other periventricular tissues
- Borders of mass typically lack the papillary margins
- High grade tumors are necrotic, elicit edema

### Primitive Neuroectodermal Tumors (PNET)
- May arise deep in the hemisphere
- Peritumoral edema often lacking or minimal
- High nuclear-to-cytoplasmic composition of the tumor yields little T2 prolongation

### Atypical Teratoid/Rhabdoid Tumors
- Often large, heterogeneous, intra-axial mass
- Typically presenting < 2 years of age
- Solid portions have low diffusivity

### Central Neurocytoma
- Necrosis and cyst formation are common
- Arises from septum pellucidum
- Predominantly seen in adults

### Meningioma
- Uncommon in the pediatric age group, association with NF2
- Morphology of intraventricular tumor usually more well-delineated

### Vascular Lesions
- Arteriovenous malformation (AVM), cavernous malformation
- Use gradient echo sequence to identify blood products

# CHOROID PLEXUS CARCINOMA

## PATHOLOGY

### General Features
- General path comments
  - Comprises approximately 5% of supratentorial tumors in children
  - Comprises < 1% of all pediatric intracranial tumors
  - Most found in infants, young (typically < 5 years) children
  - Lobulated mass
- Genetics
  - Increased incidence in Li-Fraumeni & Aicardi syndromes
  - TP53 germline mutations
- Etiology: SV40 virus DNA sequences in 50% of CPTs
- Epidemiology: First 5 years of life, 80% arise in children
- Associated abnormalities: Diffuse hydrocephalus ⇒ mechanical obstruction, increased CSF production, decreased resorption

### Gross Pathologic & Surgical Features
- Well-circumscribed intraventricular mass
- Ependymal invasion

### Microscopic Features
- Hypercellular
- Pleomorphic
- Increased mitotic activity
- Cysts, necrosis, hemorrhage, microcalcifications
- Brain invasion
- Possible CSF seeding with aggressive papillomas or choroid plexus carcinoma

### Staging, Grading or Classification Criteria
- WHO grade III

## CLINICAL ISSUES

### Presentation
- Most common signs/symptoms
  - Nausea, vomiting, headache, obtundation
  - Focal neurologic signs and symptoms
- Clinical Profile: Infant or child with elevated intracranial pressure (ICP) and focal neuro deficits

### Demographics
- Age: Between 2 and 4 years, median age ~ 26 months
- Gender: Equal male/female distribution

### Natural History & Prognosis
- Grows rapidly, 40% 5 year survival
- Poor outcome with brain invasion, CSF seeding

### Treatment
- Gross total resection, chemotherapy, ± radiation

## DIAGNOSTIC CHECKLIST

### Consider
- CPCA in a child with heterogeneous intraventricular mass, surrounding parenchymal edema and focal neurologic signs

## Image Interpretation Pearls
- MR may not distinguish papilloma from carcinoma
- Heterogeneity, brain invasion, CSF spread favor CPCA
- Image spine prior to surgery

## SELECTED REFERENCES

1. Krutilkova V et al: Identification of five new families strengthens the link between childhood choroid plexus carcinoma and germline TP53 mutations. Eur J Cancer. 41(11):1597-603, 2005
2. Parwani AV et al: Atypical teratoid/rhabdoid tumor of the brain: cytopathologic characteristics and differential diagnosis. Cancer. 105(2):65-70, 2005
3. Strother D: Atypical teratoid rhabdoid tumors of childhood: diagnosis, treatment and challenges. Expert Rev Anticancer Ther. 5(5):907-15, 2005
4. Barreto AS et al: Papillomas and carcinomas of the choroid plexus: histological and immunohistochemical studies and comparison with normal fetal choroid plexus. Arq Neuropsiquiatr. 62(3A):600-7, 2004
5. Meyers SP et al: Choroid plexus carcinomas in children: MRI features and patient outcomes. Neuroradiology. 46(9):770-80, 2004
6. Strojan P et al: Choroid plexus tumors: a review of 28-year experience. Neoplasma. 51(4):306-12, 2004
7. Gupta N: Choroid plexus tumors in children. Neurosurg Clin N Am. 14(4):621-31, 2003
8. Cho KT et al: Pediatric brain tumors: statistics of SNUH, Korea (1959-2000). Childs Nerv Syst. 18(1-2):30-7, 2002
9. Connor SE et al: Preoperative and early postoperative magnetic resonance imaging in two cases of childhood choroid plexus carcinoma. Eur Radiol. 12(4):883-8, 2002
10. Carter AB et al: Choroid plexus carcinoma presenting as an intraparenchymal mass. J Neurosurg. 95(6):1040-4, 2001
11. Horska A et al: Proton magnetic resonance spectroscopy of choroid plexus tumors in children. J Magn Reson Imaging. 14(1):78-82, 2001
12. Levy ML et al: Choroid plexus tumors in children: significance of stromal invasion. Neurosurgery. 48(2):303-9, 2001
13. Taylor MB et al: Magnetic resonance imaging in the diagnosis and management of choroid plexus carcinoma in children. Pediatr Radiol. 31(9):624-30, 2001
14. Wolff JE et al: Detection of choroid plexus carcinoma with Tc-99m sestamibi: case report and review of the literature. Med Pediatr Oncol. 36(2):323-5, 2001
15. Guermazi A et al: Diagnostic imaging of choroid plexus disease. Clin Radiol. 55(7):503-16, 2000
16. McEvoy AW et al: Management of choroid plexus tumours in children: 20 years experience at a single neurosurgical centre. Pediatr Neurosurg. 32(4):192-9, 2000
17. Gaudio RM et al: Pathology of choroid plexus papillomas: a review. Clin Neurol Neurosurg. 100(3):165-86, 1998
18. Vital A et al: Astrocytomas and choroid plexus tumors in two families with identical p53 germline mutations. J Neuropathol Exp Neurol. 57(11):1061-9, 1998

# CHOROID PLEXUS CARCINOMA

## IMAGE GALLERY

### Typical

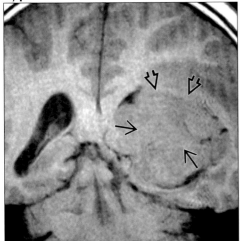

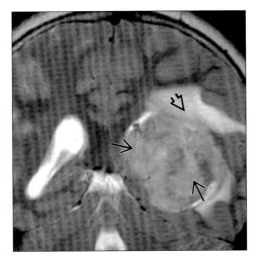

*(Left)* Coronal T1WI MR shows a slightly heterogeneous hypointense to white matter left trigonal tumor ➡. Note the indistinct superior interface of tumor and ependyma, reflecting early invasion ⮞. *(Right)* Coronal T2WI MR shows a heterogeneous left trigonal choroid plexus carcinoma ➡. Moderate peritumoral edema corresponded to parenchymal invasion at surgery ⮞.

### Typical

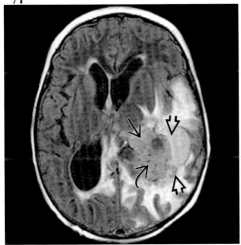

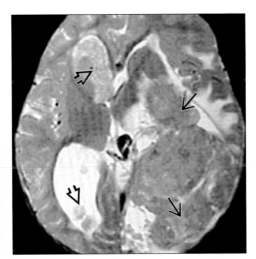

*(Left)* Axial FLAIR MR shows a heterogeneous tumor arising from the trigone ➡. Ependymal invasion and parenchymal edema is noted laterally ⮞. Numerous tumor vascular flow voids are demonstrated ➡. *(Right)* Axial T2WI MR shows a heterogeneous predominantly hypointense trigonal choroid plexus carcinoma with brain invasion ➡ and CSF tumor dissemination ⮞.

### Typical

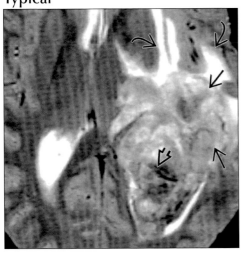

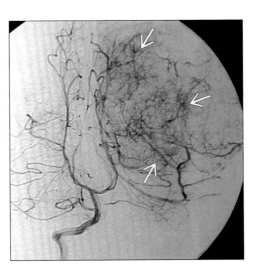

*(Left)* Axial T2WI MR shows a complex partially hemorrhagic ⮞ left trigonal tumor. There is lateral parenchymal invasion ➡. Note the peri-tumoral edema ➡. *(Right)* Anteroposterior angiography shows a hypervascular left trigonal choroid plexus carcinoma supplied by medial and lateral branches of the left superior cerebellar artery ➡.

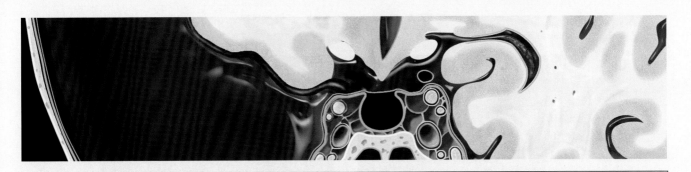

# SECTION 6: Meninges, Cisterns, Calvarium, Skull Base

# ARACHNOID CYST

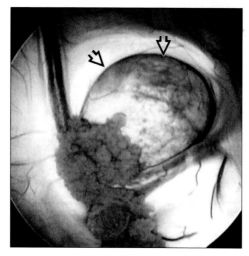

Intra-operative photograph shows an arachnoid cyst ⇨ projecting into the foramen of Monro. Arachnoid cysts in this location may cause "bobble-head doll syndrome".

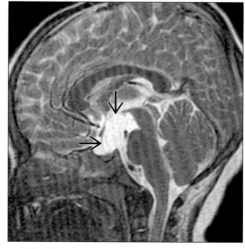

Sagittal T2WI MR shows the imaging appearance of a suprasellar AC ⇨ caused by upward herniation of the membrane of Liliequist. These lesions can be effectively treated endoscopically.

## TERMINOLOGY

### Abbreviations and Synonyms
- Arachnoid cyst (AC), subarachnoid cyst

### Definitions
- Pocket of cerebrospinal fluid (CSF) lined by arachnoid that does not directly communicate with ventricular system or subarachnoid space

## IMAGING FINDINGS

### General Features
- Best diagnostic clue: Extra-axial CSF collection with mass effect
- Location
  - 50-60% middle cranial fossa (MCF)
  - 10% cerebellopontine angle (CPA)
  - 10% suprasellar arachnoid cyst
- Size: Variable ⇒ likelihood of symptoms increases with cyst size
- Morphology
  - Sharply delineated
  - "Compromised" shape ⇒ partly accommodates to surrounding spaces

### CT Findings
- CTA: Displaces vessels
- NECT
  - Usually CSF attenuation
    - Intracystic hemorrhage may increase attenuation (rare)
  - Often thins or remodels calvaria

### MR Findings
- T1WI
  - Sharply-marginated extra-axial fluid collection isointense with CSF
  - Less than expected mass effect
    - Adjacent brain accommodates cyst
    - Reflects altered development of brain at the same time that cyst develops
- T2WI
  - Isointense with CSF
  - No edema in adjacent brain
- PD/Intermediate: Isointense with CSF
- FLAIR
  - Hypointense on FLAIR images

---

## DDx: Cystic Intracranial Lesions in Children

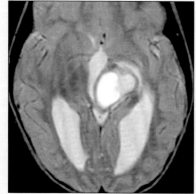

*Astrocytoma*

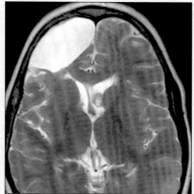

*Porencephaly*

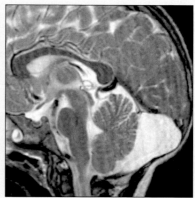

*Mega Cisterna Magna*

# ARACHNOID CYST

## Key Facts

### Terminology
- Arachnoid cyst (AC), subarachnoid cyst
- Pocket of cerebrospinal fluid (CSF) lined by arachnoid that does not directly communicate with ventricular system or subarachnoid space

### Imaging Findings
- Best diagnostic clue: Extra-axial CSF collection with mass effect
- 50-60% middle cranial fossa (MCF)
- Less than expected mass effect
- Adjacent brain accommodates cyst
- Hypointense on FLAIR images
- Reduced/absent flow artifact compared to subarachnoid CSF
- DWI: Similar to CSF

### Top Differential Diagnoses
- Epidermoid Cyst
- Subdural Hygroma
- Porencephalic Cyst
- Neuroepithelial Cyst

### Pathology
- 1% of all intracranial masses

### Clinical Issues
- Often asymptomatic, found incidentally
- 75% diagnosed in childhood

### Diagnostic Checklist
- FLAIR, DWI best sequences for differentiating arachnoid cyst from epidermoid or cystic tumor

---

  - Reduced/absent flow artifact compared to subarachnoid CSF
- DWI: Similar to CSF
- T1 C+: No enhancement
- MRA: Cortical vessels displaced away from calvaria
- MRV: Can demonstrate anomalies of venous drainage
- MR Cine: Can help distinguish AC from enlarged subarachnoid space
- MRS
  - No identifiable resonances
    - Can easily distinguish from other cystic intracranial masses

### Ultrasonographic Findings
- Grayscale Ultrasound: Anechoic

### Nuclear Medicine Findings
- SPECT
  - May show hypoperfusion in brain adjacent to cyst

### Non-Vascular Interventions
- CT cisternography can definitively distinguish arachnoid cyst from enlarged subarachnoid space (mega cisterna magna)

### Imaging Recommendations
- Best imaging tool: Non-contrast MR
- Protocol advice: Always use FLAIR, DWI

## DIFFERENTIAL DIAGNOSIS

### Epidermoid Cyst
- Does not follow CSF on all sequences
  - "Brighter" on CT and T1WI
  - Doesn't suppress on FLAIR
  - Shows restricted diffusion (bright) on DWI
- Engulfs vessels and nerves, doesn't displace them

### Chronic Subdural Hematoma
- Signal not identical to CSF
  - Hyperintense to CSF on FLAIR, PD, and T1WI
- May show enhancing membrane

### Subdural Hygroma
- Leakage of CSF from subarachnoid space into subdural space
  - 2-7 days after trauma
- Crescentic, often bilateral

### Porencephalic Cyst
- Result of trauma or stroke
- Surrounded by injured, not compressed/distorted, brain

### Neuroepithelial Cyst
- Benign cysts lined by "epithelium"
- Periventricular, intraventricular, choroid fissure

### Epidural Abscess
- Enhancing wall
- Elevated lactate on MRS
- Restricted diffusion (bright) on DWI

### Pilocytic Astrocytoma
- Enhancing mural nodule
- Intra-axial

### Mega Cisterna Magna (MCM)
- Tends to push vermis up from foramen magnum
  - Retrocerebellar AC pushes vermis forward

## PATHOLOGY

### General Features
- General path comments
  - Fluid-containing cyst with translucent membrane
  - Arachnoid layers contain CSF
- Genetics
  - Vast majority are sporadic
  - Rare reports of familial cases
    - Associated with deletion in the long arm of chromosome 16
    - Associated with polycystic kidney disease
- Etiology

# ARACHNOID CYST

- ○ Old concept = "splitting" or diverticulum of developing arachnoid
- ○ New concept (middle fossa ACs)
  - ▪ Frontal, temporal embryonic meninges (endomeninx) fail to merge as sylvian fissure forms
  - ▪ Remain separate, forming "duplicated" arachnoid
- ○ May rarely form as shunt complication
- ○ Suprasellar AC may reflect upward herniation of an obstructed membrane of Liliequist
- ○ Possible mechanisms for enlargement
  - ▪ Active fluid secretion by cyst wall
  - ▪ Slow distention by CSF pulsations
  - ▪ CSF accumulates by one-way (ball-valve) flow
- • Epidemiology
  - ○ 1% of all intracranial masses
    - ▪ Likely even more common ⇒ small MCF or convexity cysts may be missed
- • Associated abnormalities
  - ○ With MCF cysts, adjacent temporal lobe is often hypoplastic
  - ○ Subdural hematoma (increased prevalence, especially MCF)
  - ○ Syndromic ACs
    - ▪ Acrocallosal (cysts in 1/3), Aicardi, Pallister-Hall syndromes

## Gross Pathologic & Surgical Features
- • Bluish-gray arachnoid bulges around CSF-filled cyst

## Microscopic Features
- • Wall consists of flattened but normal arachnoid cells
- • No inflammation or neoplastic changes

## Staging, Grading or Classification Criteria
- • Galassi classification: ↑ With ↑ size/mass effect and ↓ communication with basal cisterns
  - ○ Type I: Small, spindle shaped, limited to anterior MCF
  - ○ Type II: Superior extent along sylvian fissure; temp lobe displaced
  - ○ Type III: Huge, fills entire MCF; frontal/temp/parietal displacement

# CLINICAL ISSUES

## Presentation
- • Most common signs/symptoms
  - ○ Often asymptomatic, found incidentally
  - ○ Associated symptoms vary with size, location of cyst
    - ▪ Headache, dizziness, sensorineural hearing loss, hemifacial spasm/tic
    - ▪ Suprasellar ACs may cause obstructive hydrocephalus, precocious puberty
- • Other signs/symptoms
  - ○ "Bobble-head doll syndrome" ⇒ continuous or episodic forward and backward head nodding
    - ▪ Associated with suprasellar or 3rd ventricle cysts

## Demographics
- • Age
  - ○ Can be found at any age
  - ○ 75% diagnosed in childhood

- • Gender: M:F = 3-5:1 especially middle cranial fossa

## Natural History & Prognosis
- • May (but usually don't) slowly enlarge

## Treatment
- • Treatment: Often none
  - ○ Morbidity from treatment may be greater than symptoms attributed to cyst
- • Resection/fenestration (may be endoscopic)
- • Shunt

# DIAGNOSTIC CHECKLIST

## Consider
- • Think of epidermoid when encountering CPA arachnoid cyst
  - ○ Concept that they are nearly identical is not supported with modern imaging techniques

## Image Interpretation Pearls
- • FLAIR, DWI best sequences for differentiating arachnoid cyst from epidermoid or cystic tumor

# SELECTED REFERENCES

1. Nowoslawska E et al: Neuroendoscopic techniques in the treatment of arachnoid cysts in children and comparison with other operative methods. Childs Nerv Syst. 22(6):599-604, 2006
2. Struck AF et al: Spontaneous development of a de novo suprasellar arachnoid cyst. Case report. J Neurosurg. 104(6 Suppl):426-8, 2006
3. Arriola G et al: Familial arachnoid cysts. Pediatr Neurol. 33(2):146-8, 2005
4. Eskandary H et al: Incidental findings in brain computed tomography scans of 3000 head trauma patients. Surg Neurol. 63(6):550-3; discussion 553, 2005
5. Sztriha L et al: Hippocampal dysgenesis associated with temporal lobe hypoplasia and arachnoid cyst of the middle cranial fossa. J Child Neurol. 20(11):926-30, 2005
6. Huang HP et al: Arachnoid cyst with GnRH-dependent sexual precocity and growth hormone deficiency. Pediatr Neurol. 30(2):143-5, 2004
7. Sinha S et al: Familial posterior fossa arachnoid cyst. Childs Nerv Syst. 20(2):100-3, 2004
8. Cokluk C et al: Spontaneous disappearance of two asymptomatic arachnoid cysts in two different locations. Minim Invasive Neurosurg. 46(2):110-2, 2003
9. Desai KI et al: Suprasellar arachnoid cyst presenting with bobble-head doll movements: a report of 3 cases. Neurol India. 51(3):407-9, 2003
10. Tamburrini G et al: Subdural hygroma: an unwanted result of Sylvian arachnoid cyst marsupialization. Childs Nerv Syst. 19(3):159-65, 2003
11. Alehan FK et al: Familial arachnoid cysts in association with autosomal dominant polycystic kidney disease. Pediatrics. 110(1 Pt 1):e13, 2002
12. Gosalakkal JA: Intracranial arachnoid cysts in children: a review of pathogenesis, clinical features, and management. Pediatr Neurol. 26(2):93-8, 2002
13. Sgouros S et al: Congenital middle fossa arachnoid cysts may cause global brain ischaemia: a study with 99Tc-hexamethylpropyleneamineoxime single photon emission computerised tomography scans. Pediatr Neurosurg. 35(4):188-94, 2001

# ARACHNOID CYST

### Variant

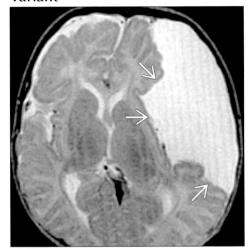
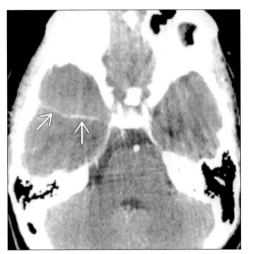

*(Left)* Axial T2WI MR shows a very large arachnoid cyst, expanding the sylvian fissure ➡. The congenital nature of the lesion results in few clinical manifestations, given its size. *(Right)* Axial CECT shows an essentially isodense arachnoid cyst of the right middle cranial fossa ➡; the increased attenuation relative to CSF is secondary to hemorrhage into the cyst.

### Typical

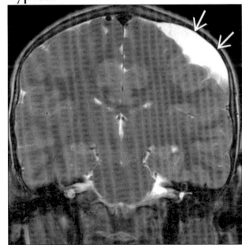
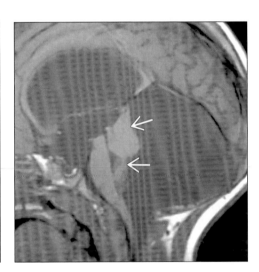

*(Left)* Coronal T2WI MR shows a moderate sized arachnoid cyst ➡ over the left cerebral convexity. This location is considerably less common than the middle cranial fossa. *(Right)* Sagittal T1WI MR shows a large retrocerebellar arachnoid cyst causing hydrocephalus and displacing the vermis ➡ anteriorly. Mega cisterna magna will cause less mass effect.

### Typical

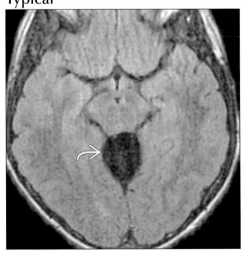
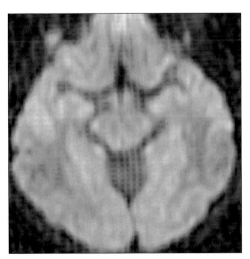

*(Left)* Axial FLAIR MR shows a classic arachnoid cyst of the supravermian cistern ➡. It is isointense to CSF in the ventricles and cisterns. *(Right)* Axial DWI MR (same patient as previous image) shows diffusivity identical to CSF in ventricles and cisterns, differentiating the lesion from an epidermoid cyst or exophytic glioma.

# ACUTE SUBDURAL HEMATOMA

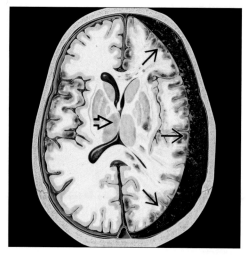

Axial graphic shows diffuse hemorrhagic extraparenchymal collection over left hemisphere ➡. Note that the collection crosses the sutures, and causes midline shift ⊳.

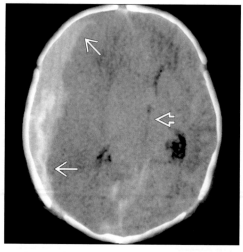

Axial NECT shows extensive SDH with partial clotting over left hemisphere ➡. Midline shift ⊠ is marked. Edema in the right hemisphere may be from trauma or compression of vascular bed.

## TERMINOLOGY

### Abbreviations and Synonyms
- Acute subdural hematoma (aSDH)

### Definitions
- Acute (< 3 days) hemorrhagic collection between parietal dura and arachnoid

## IMAGING FINDINGS

### General Features
- Best diagnostic clue: Crescent-shaped, homogeneously hyperdense on CT, extra-axial collection that spreads diffusely over brain
- Location
  - Between arachnoid & parietal layer of dura
  - Brain convexity, falx, tentorium, posterior fossa
  - Typically on contrecoup side
- Size
  - From few mm to several cm thickness
  - If extends diffusely around brain, thin collection in infant may contain large amount of blood

- Morphology
  - Crescent-shaped extra-axial dense collection
  - Crosses sutures, extends along falx, tentorium
  - Mass effect on underlying brain
  - Other hemorrhages, brain contusion, ischemia, edema common

### CT Findings
- NECT
  - Hyperacute SDH (< 6 hours) mostly hypodense (unclotted)
  - aSDH (± 6 hours-few days) typically homogeneously hyperdense to cortex
    - Mixed hyper-, hypodense → active bleeding ("swirl" sign), CSF accumulation, clot retraction, multilaminar bleed
    - Rarely isodense → coagulopathy, anemia (Hgb < 8-10 g/dl), dilution with CSF, or in previous chronic collection
    - Density decreases ± 1.5 HU/day as SDH evolves
  - Coronal, sagittal reformats
  - Associated lesions
    - Extracerebral: Epidural hematoma (EDH), subarachnoid hemorrhage (SAH)

## DDx: Other Pericerebral Hemorrhages

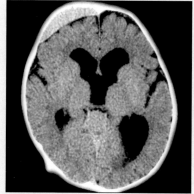

Chronic SDH Rebleed

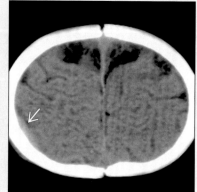

Small Epidural Hematoma

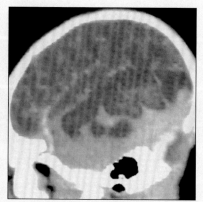

Subarachnoid Hemorrhage

# ACUTE SUBDURAL HEMATOMA

## Key Facts

### Terminology
- Acute (< 3 days) hemorrhagic collection between parietal dura and arachnoid

### Imaging Findings
- Best diagnostic clue: Crescent-shaped, homogeneously hyperdense on CT, extra-axial collection that spreads diffusely over brain
- CECT: Inward displacement of vessels against cortex
- T2* GRE: Hypointense signal in most cases

### Top Differential Diagnoses
- Acute Epidural Hematoma

### Pathology
- Bridging veins torn when entering dura
- Predisposing factors may favor venous tears

- Enlarged pericerebral CSF spaces (infantile external hydrocephalus); controversial
- Coagulopathy

### Clinical Issues
- Early evacuation prevents chronicity, improves brain blood supply in large SDH

### Diagnostic Checklist
- Always consider child abuse when described trauma does not explain brain lesions
- Wide window settings for CT increases conspicuity of subtle SDH
- FLAIR, T2* most sensitive sequences for SDH when thin or isointense on standard MR sequences

---

- Brain: Cortical contusion, intracerebral hemorrhage (ICH), diffuse axonal injury (DAI)
- Vascular lesions: Arterial infarction related to brain herniation, venous infarction related to venous tear, or compression
- Edema, swelling
- CECT: Inward displacement of vessels against cortex

### MR Findings
- T1WI
  - Hyperacute: Isointense to cortex
  - Acute: Iso- to moderately hyperintense
- T2WI
  - Hyperacute: Iso- to hyperintense
  - Acute: Hypointense
- FLAIR
  - Hyperintense to CSF
  - Acute hematomas most conspicuous on FLAIR
- T2* GRE: Hypointense signal in most cases
- DWI
  - Heterogeneous signal (non-specific)
  - Demonstrates areas of associated brain ischemia (vascular compression, stretching)
- T1 C+: Bridging veins displaced against cortex

### Angiographic Findings
- Conventional
  - Displacement, mass effect from extra-axial mass
  - Excludes vascular malformation in non-traumatic cases (rare in children)

### Imaging Recommendations
- Best imaging tool
  - NECT initial screen for aSDH, brain evaluation; coronal and sagittal reformats
  - MR for additional findings of traumatic brain injury
- Protocol advice: Wide window settings (150-200 HU) to see small SDH against calvarium on CT

## DIFFERENTIAL DIAGNOSIS

### Acute Epidural Hematoma
- Biconvex, crosses dural attachment, not sutures
- May be indistinguishable from aSDH when small: Risk of acute expansion

### Bleed into Arachnoid Space
- No tamponade, large amount of blood may accumulate
  - True aSDH may rupture into arachnoid cyst
  - Arachnoid cyst may rupture into SD space and behave as an aSDH

### Incidental Neonatal SDH
- Small, non-compressive, transient SDH may be observed along tentorium and falx in the neonates

### Other Subdural Collections
- New aSDH versus spontaneous rebleed in chronic SDH
- Subacute, chronic SDH; not hyperdense
- Clear fluid subdural collections ("hygroma", "effusion"); low CT density, no growth, no mass effect; but new bleeding may occur
- Empyema: Peripheral enhancement, reduced diffusion (infectious context)

### Pachymeningopathies (Thickened Contrast-Enhanced Dura)
- Subdural fibrosis (chronic shunted hydrocephalus)
- Intracranial hypotension ("slumping" midbrain, tonsillar herniation)
- Sarcoid (nodular, "lumpy-bumpy")

### Pachymeningeal Tumors (Contrast-Enhancement)
- Lymphoma, sarcoma, leukemia, metastases
- Dural based, enhancing mass
- ± Skull involved

# ACUTE SUBDURAL HEMATOMA

## PATHOLOGY

### General Features
- Etiology
  - Bridging veins torn when entering dura
    - High velocity trauma (HVT): Teenagers, boys; often associated with (complex) fractures
    - Documented minor head trauma: Intracranial injury in 15%, of which 20% aSDH
    - Non-accidental injury (NAI) with high energy rotational acceleration/deceleration common in infants and toddlers, occasionally in children
  - Difficult delivery
    - Breech, forceps instrumentation, cranial moulding, primiparous
    - Dural or dural sinus laceration, venous rupture, rupture of hematoma within SD space
    - Small tentorium, posterior falx & cisterna magna SDH: Common, clinically non-significant
  - Less common etiologies
    - Dissection of intraparenchymal hematoma into subarachnoid, then "subdural" (SD) space
    - Vascular malformations (rarely in children): Dural AVF, AVM, cavernoma
    - Ventricular shunt if low opening pressure
    - Rarely, lumbar puncture in children with coagulopathy
  - Predisposing factors may favor venous tears
    - Enlarged pericerebral CSF spaces (infantile external hydrocephalus); controversial
    - Coagulopathy
    - Arachnoid cyst: aSDH may rupture in cyst, (no tamponade); cyst may dissect SD space
- Epidemiology: aSDH represents 30% of traumatic intracranial injury (ICI) in children
- Associated abnormalities: 22% of ICI in children associated with EDH, SAH, parenchymal contusion, necrosis or edema

### Gross Pathologic & Surgical Features
- Not truly subdural; cleaving of innermost dural cell border layer/layers (laminar bleed)

### Microscopic Features
- Brain edema, shearing lacerations of parenchyma

## CLINICAL ISSUES

### Presentation
- Most common signs/symptoms
  - HVT (MVA): Teenagers, clear circumstances, altered consciousness (associated lesions), skull fracture
  - NAI: Infants, unclear circumstances, seizures, lethargy, headaches, vomiting, multiple bruising
  - Neonatal: Difficult delivery; failure to thrive, irritability, seizures, apnea, bradycardia, anemia

### Demographics
- Age
  - Infants ⇒ consider NAI
  - Older children ⇒ consider fall, MVA
- Gender: No predilection in young age; later, boys

### Natural History & Prognosis
- Can grow slowly over time, with increasing mass effect if untreated: Chronic SDH
- Prognosis in aSDH globally fair (62% good outcome), but worse when associated brain lesions (NAI, high velocity trauma)
- Spontaneous regression of small SDH possible

### Treatment
- Early evacuation prevents chronicity, improves brain blood supply in large SDH

## DIAGNOSTIC CHECKLIST

### Consider
- Always consider child abuse when described trauma does not explain brain lesions

### Image Interpretation Pearls
- Wide window settings for CT increases conspicuity of subtle SDH
- FLAIR, T2* most sensitive sequences for SDH when thin or isointense on standard MR sequences

## SELECTED REFERENCES

1. Salehi-Had H et al: Findings in older children with abusive head injury: does shaken-child syndrome exist? Pediatrics. 117(5):e1039-44, 2006
2. Hymel KP et al: Intracranial hemorrhage and rebleeding in suspected victims of abusive head trauma: addressing the forensic controversies. Child Maltreat. 7(4):329-48, 2002
3. Loh JK et al: Acute subdural hematoma in infancy. Surg Neurol. 58(3-4):218-24, 2002
4. Feldman KW et al: The cause of infant and toddler subdural hemorrhage: a prospective study. Pediatrics. 108(3):636-46, 2001
5. Simon B et al: Pediatric minor head trauma: indications for computed tomographic scanning revisited. J Trauma. 51(2):231-7; discussion 237-8, 2001
6. Herrera EJ et al: Postraumatic intracranial hematomas in infancy. a 16-year experience. Childs Nerv Syst. 16(9):585-9, 2000
7. Barlow KM et al: Magnetic resonance imaging in acute non-accidental head injury. Acta Paediatr. 88(7):734-40, 1999
8. Rao P et al: The acute reversal sign: comparison of medical and non-accidental injury patients. Clin Radiol. 54(8):495-501, 1999
9. Dias MS et al: Serial radiography in the infant shaken impact syndrome. Pediatr Neurosurg. 29(2):77-85, 1998
10. Gilles EE et al: Cerebral complications of nonaccidental head injury in childhood. Pediatr Neurol. 19(2):119-28, 1998
11. Perrin RG et al: Management and outcomes of posterior fossa subdural hematomas in neonates. Neurosurgery. 40(6):1190-9; discussion 1199-200, 1997
12. Steinbok P et al: Acute subdural hematoma associated with cerebral infarction in the full-term neonate. Pediatr Neurosurg. 23(4):206-15, 1995
13. Wilms G et al: CT and MR in infants with pericerebral collections and macrocephaly: benign enlargement of the subarachnoid spaces versus subdural collections. AJNR Am J Neuroradiol. 14(4):855-60, 1993
14. Menezes AH et al: Posterior fossa hemorrhage in the term neonate. Neurosurgery. 13(4):452-6, 1983

I

6

8

# ACUTE SUBDURAL HEMATOMA

## IMAGE GALLERY

### Typical

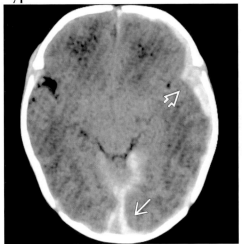 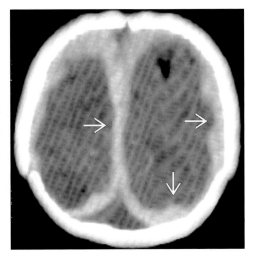

*(Left)* Axial NECT shows extensive SDH overlying tentorium, posterior falx ➡, and left convexity ➡ in neonate. This large blood accumulation in the subdural space caused anemia. *(Right)* Coronal NECT (same neonate as previous image) shows the accumulated subdural blood surrounding the posterior part of the hemispheres ➡, accounting for large blood volume loss.

### Typical

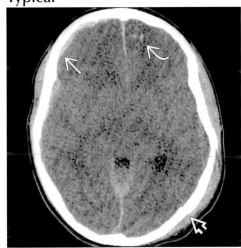 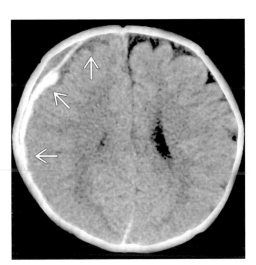

*(Left)* Axial NECT shows scalp contusion and fracture ➡ on left (coup), thin layer of SDH ➡ on right (contrecoup), parasagittal frontal shear hemorrhage ➡ and global brain swelling. *(Right)* Axial NECT after shaking injury shows different laminar attenuations in mixed aSDH ➡ reflecting blood in various clotting stages, likely with some blood/CSF dilution.

### Typical

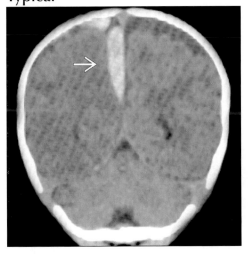 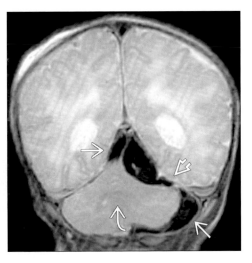

*(Left)* Coronal NECT shows typical location of sagittal parafalcine SDH in infant with NAI ➡; other features of NAI are non-consistent history, bilateral retinal hemorrhages, multifocal bruising. *(Right)* Coronal T2WI MR shows large posterior fossa aSDH ➡ in a neonate. Note probable tentorial tear ➡ (focal loss of low T2 signal of dura), significant shift of cerebellar midline ➡.

# EVOLVING SUBDURAL HEMATOMA

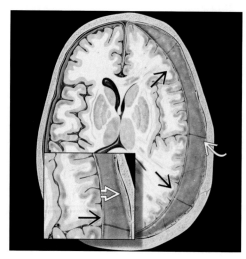

Axial graphic shows large convexity SDH ➡, with traversing septations ⇨ and compression of brain parenchyma. Magnified insert shows second juxta-osseous SDH compartment ⇥.

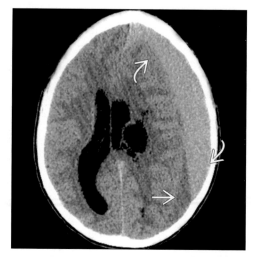

Axial NECT shows huge collection 3 months post-surgery (no recorded intervening trauma) with one isodense ⇨ and one hypodense ➡ components in two adjacent "subdural" (really dural) clefts.

## TERMINOLOGY

### Abbreviations and Synonyms
- Evolving subdural hematoma (SDH)

### Definitions
- Diverse presentations of SDH according to timing, dilution, recurrence of bleed

## IMAGING FINDINGS

### General Features
- Best diagnostic clue: Crescent-shaped extra-axial collection that spreads diffusely over affected hemisphere with various densities/signals
- Location: Within one or several cleavage planes within the innermost cell layer of dura
- Morphology
  - Crescent-shaped extra-axial fluid collection
  - Crosses sutures, not dural attachments, may extend along falx, tentorium
  - Displaces underlying cortex
  - CT density & MR signal intensity vary with timing, dilution, organization, recurrence of bleed

### CT Findings
- NECT
  - May be iso-, hyper-, hypodense or mixed in relation to cortex, at any stage of evolution
    - May be diverse in different locations
    - May be diverse in same location, in a laminar way (typically acute stage)
    - May be diverse in same location, in a patchy way (chronic, multi-loculated SDH)
    - May be diverse in same location, with dependent layering (chronic, bleed in hygroma)
  - May be CSF-clear: Proteinaceous/xanthochromic hygroma (a.k.a. hydroma, or sometimes effusion)
    - Directly from trauma, or from aging acute SDH
    - May develop early, evolves to chronic SDH with subsequent bleed in 20-50%
  - Late calcification of inner membrane possible
  - Gray-white junction displaced medially; may see line of displaced/compressed sulci as "dots" of CSF
- CECT
  - Dura, membranes enhance after acute stage

## DDx: Other Pericerebral Collections

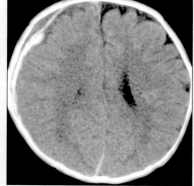

Acute Laminar SDH

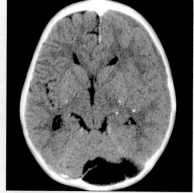

Extramedullary Hematopoiesis

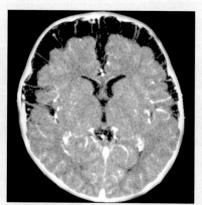

Subarachnoid Enlargement

# EVOLVING SUBDURAL HEMATOMA

## Key Facts

### Terminology
- Diverse presentations of SDH according to timing, dilution, recurrence of bleed

### Imaging Findings
- Best diagnostic clue: Crescent-shaped extra-axial collection that spreads diffusely over affected hemisphere with various densities/signals
- Location: Within one or several cleavage planes within the innermost cell layer of dura
- NECT initial screen, consider CECT for membranes/loculations
- MR more sensitive for thin SDH & additional findings of traumatic brain injury

### Top Differential Diagnoses
- Other Pericerebral Hemorrhages
- Other Subdural Collections
- Clear, CSF-Like Pericerebral Collections
- Subdural Collections in Metabolic Diseases

### Pathology
- Blood dissects the innermost cell layer of dura into one or several cleavage planes
- Acute SDH made of acute blood, but older SDH made of blood/fluid of various ages

### Clinical Issues
- Surgical evacuation/drainage if growing/symptomatic

### Diagnostic Checklist
- Guessing age of SDH from CT/MR appearance is highly deceptive!
- Age of blood is not age of hematoma, which is not age of trauma

---

- Inward displacement of enhanced cortical vessels

## MR Findings
- T1WI: Diverse signals depending on age, hemoglobin (Hb) oxidation, CSF dilution
- T2WI
  - Usually hyperintense to CSF, layering possible
  - Very low for recent blood or late hemosiderin
  - Vascular flow voids displaced inward
- FLAIR: Most conspicuous sequence; hyperintense compared to CSF
- T1 C+: Dura, membranes enhance after acute stage

## Imaging Recommendations
- Best imaging tool
  - NECT initial screen, consider CECT for membranes/loculations
  - MR more sensitive for thin SDH & additional findings of traumatic brain injury

## DIFFERENTIAL DIAGNOSIS

### Other Pericerebral Hemorrhages
- Epidural hemorrhage (EDH): May be isodense; limited by sutures, may cross insertion of falx, tentorium
- Acute subdural hemorrhage (SDH): May be of mixed density on CT
- Subarachnoid hemorrhage (SAH): "Cisternographic" appearance; often associated with EDH, SDH, contusions

### Other Subdural Collections
- Empyema: Pericerebral abscess, restricted diffusion

### Clear, CSF-Like Pericerebral Collections
- Benign subarachnoid enlargement (benign idiopathic external hydrocephalus)
  - Crossed by bridging veins, macrocephaly, infants-toddlers (not so benign if due to ↑ venous pressure)
  - Controversial: Predisposing factor for SDH
- Subdural effusion: CSF-like, typically associated with meningitis, may be initial stage for empyema

### Subdural Collections in Metabolic Diseases
- Menkes disease, glutaric aciduria type 1: Hygroma, hematoma

### Pachymeningopathies: Thickened Enhancing Dura
- Post-surgical (shunt, etc.)
- Intracranial hypotension
- Diffuse dural thickening & enhancement from chronic venous thrombosis
- Subdural fibrosis after hydrocephalus

### Tumors, Hemopathies
- Sarcoma, lymphoma, leukemia, extramedullary hematopoiesis
  - Dural based, enhancing mass, ± skull involved

## PATHOLOGY

### General Features
- Etiology
  - Traumatic stretching & tearing of bridging cortical veins as they cross meninges
    - Anatomically there is no subdural space, even virtual, between arachnoid and dura
    - Blood dissects the innermost cell layer of dura into one or several cleavage planes
    - Meningeal tears allow CSF to develop similar collections also, or to mix with hemorrhages
  - Past acute stage, vascularized membranes/septae develop that may bleed spontaneously
- Epidemiology
  - SDH found in 10-20% imaged & 30% autopsy cases following craniocerebral trauma
    - Accidental trauma (high velocity injury): Intensity and time of trauma well established
    - Non-accidental injury (NAI): Unclear circumstances, evolving subdural more common, prognosis often poor
    - Untreated neonatal acute SDHs tend to evolve into chronic SDH

# EVOLVING SUBDURAL HEMATOMA

○ Uncommon complication of surgery: Craniectomy, shunting
• Associated abnormalities: Be it non-accidental or accidental, SDH commonly associated with other intracranial lesions

## Gross Pathologic & Surgical Features
• CT, MR appearances: Depend on various factors
  ○ Clotted blood hyperdense to unclotted
  ○ Oxidation of Hb: Oxy-Hb (iso T1, high T2) vs. deoxy-Hb (iso T1, low T2)
  ○ Transition from ferrous Fe2+ to ferric Fe3+: Met-Hb (high T1, T2)
  ○ Late residual: Insoluble hemosiderin & soluble ferritin (low T2)
  ○ Fresh CSF mixing brings O2+ to Hb
  ○ CSF/blood dilution (secondary ingress of CSF in hemorrhage, or secondary bleed in hygroma)
• Staging
  ○ Acute blood (< 7 days)
    ▪ "Hyperacute" fresh unclotted blood: Isodense on CT, iso T1, high T2 on MR
    ▪ Acute clotted blood: Hyperdense on CT, iso T1, low T2 on MR
    ▪ Dilution apparent on CT mostly
    ▪ Association common (laminar SDH)
  ○ Subacute blood (7-22 days): Rapid, variable changes
    ▪ CT: Hypodensity more common (50%) than isodensity (40%); hyperdensity possible (10%)
    ▪ MR: Classically high T1, low T2 early, turning high T1, high T2
    ▪ Neomembranes, septations develop
  ○ Hygroma: CSF-like/CT, high T2/MR, may develop within days, either directly from trauma or from CSF ingress into acute SDH
  ○ Chronic blood (> 22 days): Features relate to aging collection and to re-bleeds from neomembranes
    ▪ Mostly secondary bleed in aging SDH/hygroma
    ▪ Predominantly isodense (87%), uncommonly hypodense (13%)
    ▪ Mixed loculated: Bleeds into septated collection
    ▪ Mixed with dependent layering: Bleed into pre-existing hygroma
    ▪ CT/MR changes further dependent on age of rebleeds
• Acute SDH made of acute blood, but older SDH made of blood/fluid of various ages

## Microscopic Features
• Membranes = hemorrhagic granulation tissue with resorbing blood products

# CLINICAL ISSUES

## Presentation
• Most common signs/symptoms
  ○ From asymptomatic to coma
  ○ ↑ ICP, seizures, irritability, neurological deficit, developmental delay

## Demographics
• Age
  ○ Teenagers: Sport, traffic accidents, violence
  ○ Infants: NAI mostly
  ○ Neonate: Perinatal injury
• Gender: Among teenagers, boys more than girls

## Natural History & Prognosis
• Tends to resolve spontaneously after acute stage, but not always
• Prognosis depends on trauma severity and circumstances → associated lesions
  ○ Death uncommon past acute period
  ○ Morbidity: 30-40%
• Developmental delay may result from neonatal SDH

## Treatment
• Surgical evacuation/drainage if growing/symptomatic

# DIAGNOSTIC CHECKLIST

## Consider
• Guessing age of SDH from CT/MR appearance is highly deceptive!
• Age of blood is not age of hematoma, which is not age of trauma

# SELECTED REFERENCES

1. Hobbs C et al: Subdural haematoma and effusion in infancy: an epidemiological study. Arch Dis Child. 90(9):952-5, 2005
2. Vinchon M et al: Imaging of head injuries in infants: temporal correlates & forensic implications for the diagnosis of child abuse. J Neurosurg. 101:44-52, 2004
3. Hymel KP et al: Intracranial hemorrhage and rebleeding in suspected victims of abusive head trauma: addressing the forensic controversies. Child Maltreat. 7(4):329-48, 2002
4. Loh JK et al: Acute subdural hematoma in infancy. Surg Neurol. 58(3-4):218-24, 2002
5. Feldman KW et al: The cause of infant and toddler subdural hemorrhage: a prospective study. Pediatrics. 108(3):636-46, 2001
6. Lee KS et al: The fate of traumatic subdural hygroma in serial computed tomographic scans. J Korean Med Sci. 15(5):560-8, 2000
7. Mori K et al: Delayed magnetic resonance imaging with GdD-DTPA differentiates subdural hygroma and subdural effusion. Surg Neurol. 53(4):303-10; discussion 310-1, 2000
8. Sharma RR et al: Symptomatic calcified subdural hematomas. Pediatr Neurosurg. 31(3):150-4, 1999
9. Dias MS et al: Serial radiography in the infant shaken impact syndrome. Pediatr Neurosurg. 29(2):77-85, 1998
10. Fujisawa H et al: Serum protein exudation in chronic subdural haematomas: a mechanism for haematoma enlargement? Acta Neurochir (Wien). 140(2):161-5; discussion 165-6, 1998
11. Lee KS et al: The computed tomographic attenuation and the age of subdural hematomas. J Korean Med Sci. 12(4):353-9, 1997
12. Park CK et al: Spontaneous evolution of posttraumatic subdural hygroma into chronic subdural haematoma. Acta Neurochir (Wien). 127(1-2):41-7, 1994
13. Destian S et al: Differentiation between meningeal fibrosis and chronic subdural hematoma after ventricular shunting: value of enhanced CT and MR scans. AJNR Am J Neuroradiol. 10(5):1021-6, 1989
14. Ohno K et al: Role of traumatic subdural fluid collection in developing process of chronic subdural hematoma. Bull Tokyo Med Dent Univ. 33(3):99-106, 1986

# EVOLVING SUBDURAL HEMATOMA

## IMAGE GALLERY

Typical

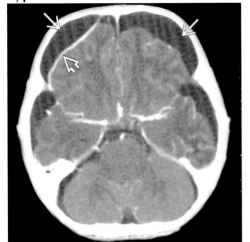

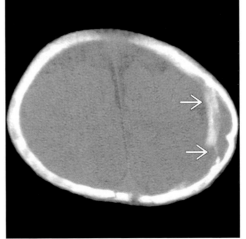

*(Left)* Axial CECT shows large bilateral CSF-like subdural collections ➡ displacing cortical vein ➡ inward. This collection developed during 13 days after trauma and minimal posterior SDH. *(Right)* Axial bone CT shows calcification of the inner membrane of SDH ➡ in infant who presented with acute SDH right after birth.

Typical

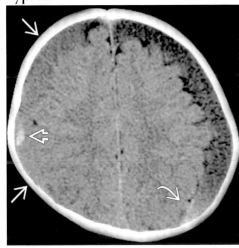

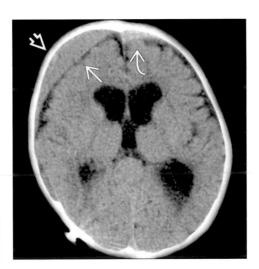

*(Left)* Axial NECT in a 10 month old infant with new neurologic symptoms shows large subdural collections, isodense ➡ with focal clot ➡ on right, and with layering on left ➡. *(Right)* Axial NECT (same child as previous image) two months after evacuation of SDHs, shows residual collections, larger right ➡ than left ➡, isodense to cortex with tiny focal bleed on right ➡.

I
6
13

Typical

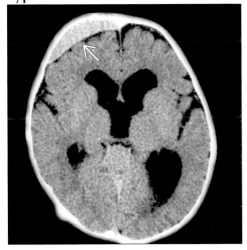

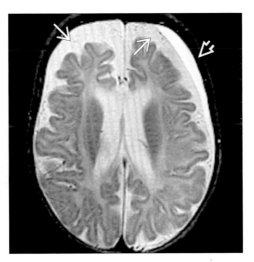

*(Left)* Axial NECT (same child as previous image) after one more month shows that SDH has disappeared on left while decreasing and becoming hyperdense on right ➡; it had disappeared altogether at 18 months. *(Right)* Axial T2WI MR in infant shows large idiopathic benign bilateral subarachnoid enlargement ➡, associated with small left SDH ➡, possibly facilitated by venous stretching (controversial).

# EPIDURAL HEMATOMA

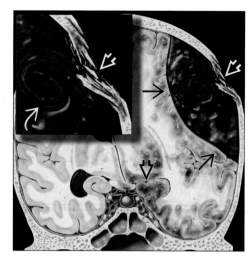

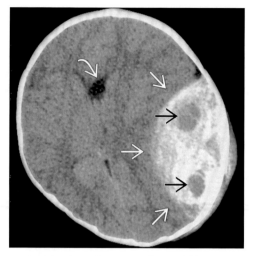

Coronal graphic shows epidural blood collection ➡, blood swirl ➡ from parietal fracture line ➡ (MMA course), gross mass effect, hemispheric contusion, uncal herniation ➡.

Axial NECT shows biconvex collection ➡ under left parietal squama. Also note mass effect with midline shift, trapped frontal horn ➡; low density ➡ means acute-ongoing bleed.

## TERMINOLOGY

### Abbreviations and Synonyms
- Epidural hematoma (EDH), extradural hematoma

### Definitions
- Blood collection within potential space between skull inner table & dura mater

## IMAGING FINDINGS

### General Features
- Best diagnostic clue: Biconvex hyperdense extra-axial collection on NECT in acute phase
- Location
  - Epidural space between skull & dura; because of different anatomical conditions, distribution in children different from adults
  - Nearly all EDH occur at impact ("coup") site
  - > 95% unilateral
  - 75-80% supratentorial
    - 50-55% parietal
    - 15% frontal, 5% temporal
  - 20-25% posterior fossa
  - Rarely at the vertex
- Size: Variable, most attain final size quickly
- Morphology
  - EDH
    - Biconvex or lentiform extra-axial collection at impact ("coup") site
    - Does not cross sutures
    - Can cross falx & tentorium (then venous rather than arterial)
    - Compresses & displaces underlying dura, subarachnoid space & brain
  - Venous EDH
    - EDH adjacent to venous sinus, sinus transgressed by fracture line
  - Other significant lesions
    - Skull fracture less common than in adults: 50-60%
    - Associated intracranial lesions in 30%: "Contrecoup" subdural hematoma, subarachnoid hemorrhage, cerebral contusions
    - Mass effect with secondary herniations common (subfalcine, transtentorial, foramen magnum)
    - In infants, extensive subperiosteal, subgaleal hemorrhages (anemia)

## DDx: Other Pericerebral Masses

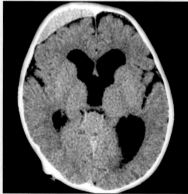

Focal Frontal Subdural Hematoma

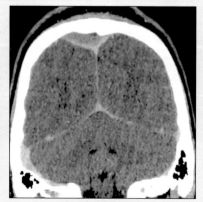

Ewing Sarcoma

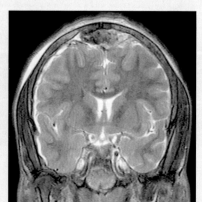

Sickle Cell Disease

# EPIDURAL HEMATOMA

## Key Facts

### Terminology
- Blood collection within potential space between skull inner table & dura mater

### Imaging Findings
- Best diagnostic clue: Biconvex hyperdense extra-axial collection on NECT in acute phase
- 20-25% posterior fossa
- Does not cross sutures
- Can cross falx & tentorium (then venous rather than arterial)
- Low density "swirl sign" = actively bleeding hematoma with unretracted semiliquid clot
- Coronal reformats not to miss vertex EDH; may show fracture lines better also
- Best imaging tool: NECT with appropriate windowing

### Clinical Issues
- Classic "lucid interval" uncommon in children
- Clinical symptoms commonly mild: Headache, vomiting, lethargy
- 50% of children with EDH have a Glasgow coma scale at 14-15 and normal examination
- Other signs/symptoms: Intense anemia, disseminated intravascular coagulation in neonates
- Generally good outcome if promptly recognized & treated

### Diagnostic Checklist
- NECT highly sensitive & widely available
- Involvement of dural sinuses: High risk of thrombosis

## CT Findings
- NECT
  - Acute EDH: 2/3 hyperdense, 1/3 mixed hyper/hypodense
    - Low density "swirl sign" = actively bleeding hematoma with unretracted semiliquid clot
    - Acutely extravasated = 30-50 HU; coagulated = 50-80 HU
  - Air in EDH suggests sinus or mastoid fracture
  - Coronal reformats not to miss vertex EDH; may show fracture lines better also
- CECT
  - Acute: Rarely contrast extravasation
  - Demonstrates associated sino-venous thrombosis
  - Chronic: Peripheral enhancement due to neovascularization & granulation

## MR Findings
- T1WI
  - Acute: Isointense
  - Subacute/early chronic: Hyperintense
  - Black line between EDH & brain = displaced dura
- T2WI
  - Acute: Variable hyper- to hypointense
  - Early subacute: Hypointense
  - Late subacute/early chronic: Hyperintense
  - Black line between EDH & brain = displaced dura
- T1 C+: Displaced vessels
- MRA: For associated arterial lesions: Spasm, pseudo-aneurysm, dissection (extra-, intracranial)
- MRV
  - Sino-venous tear, thrombosis
  - Venous sinus displaced or compressed by hematoma

## Radiographic Findings
- Radiography: Skull fracture in 50-60%

## Angiographic Findings
- Conventional
  - Avascular mass effect
    - Cortical arteries displaced away from skull
    - May displace dural venous sinus
  - Middle meningeal artery (MMA) laceration (rare), "tram-track" sign (AV fistula: Contrast extravasates from MMA into paired middle meningeal veins)
  - Arterial spasm, dissection, pseudo-aneurysm

## Imaging Recommendations
- Best imaging tool: NECT with appropriate windowing
- Protocol advice: Coronal reformat for vertex EDH

## DIFFERENTIAL DIAGNOSIS

### Subdural Hematoma
- Usually crescentic, but may also be biconvex
- Crosses sutures, does not cross falx
- Meningeal veins displaced but not the dura

### Neoplasm
- Any process originating in bone (e.g., Ewing); hemorrhage may be associated

### Extramedullary Hematopoiesis
- History of blood dyscrasia

## PATHOLOGY

### General Features
- Etiology
  - Trauma by far most common
    - Arterial: Mostly MMA, may be diploic arteries
    - Venous: Usually the dural sinuses or lakes, may be diploic also
  - Postsurgical
  - Neonatal
    - Young primiparous mother, term, instrumented vaginal delivery or C-section after failed instrumented vaginal delivery
  - Child abuse-related EDH considered uncommon
  - Non traumatic
    - Uncommon: Coagulopathy, skull neoplasm, hematologic disorder
- Epidemiology

# EPIDURAL HEMATOMA

- 2-3% of imaged head trauma children
- Fall in 50% (often mild, less than 5 feet), sport; MVA (more common in older children)
- Associated abnormalities
  - Skull fracture 50-60%, typically but not always across MMA groove or venous sinuses
  - Subdural, subarachnoid hemorrhages, contusion in 30% (worsens the prognosis)

## Gross Pathologic & Surgical Features
- Hematoma collects between calvarium and dura
  - Dural firm adhesion to sutures prevents hematoma from crossing them
  - Dural adherence to bone is stronger in children than in adults, EDH less common
- "Vertex" EDH
  - Usually venous: Linear or diastatic fracture crosses superior sagittal sinus
- At surgery or autopsy, 20% have blood in both epidural & subdural spaces

## Microscopic Features
- Tearing/laceration of dural, diploic and/or adjacent vessel

# CLINICAL ISSUES

## Presentation
- Most common signs/symptoms
  - Classic "lucid interval" uncommon in children
  - Clinical symptoms commonly mild: Headache, vomiting, lethargy
  - Clinical signs in 50%: Neurological deficits, signs of mass effect/herniation
  - 50% of children with EDH have a Glasgow coma scale at 14-15 and normal examination
- Other signs/symptoms: Intense anemia, disseminated intravascular coagulation in neonates

## Demographics
- Age
  - Fall more common in young children, better prognosis
  - High velocity trauma, MVA more common in older children, prognosis poorer
  - Skull fracture less common in children
  - Significant but not common complication of difficult delivery
- Gender: M:F = 1.5:1 to 2.5:1

## Natural History & Prognosis
- Factors affecting rate of EDH growth
  - Arterial vs. venous flow rate, arterial spasm
  - Decompression through fracture into scalp (mostly neonates)
  - Tamponade
- Delayed development or enlargement may occur
  - 10-25% of cases, usually within first 36 hours
- Spontaneous resorption possible with small EDH (careful CT surveillance)
- Generally good outcome if promptly recognized & treated

- Overall mortality < 5%: Mostly high ICP and circulatory arrest, major associated lesion, delayed treatment
  - In children, posterior fossa location of EDH, or neonatal occurrence, do not worsen prognosis
  - Permanent sequelae less than 10%
- Complications are usually secondary to EDH mass effect causing brain herniations

## Treatment
- Typically require prompt surgical evacuation
  - Poor outcome often related to delayed referral, diagnosis, or operation
- Small EDH may be followed without surgery
  - If stable, no radiolucency of current bleeding, < 15 mm, < 2 mm midline shift, no uncal herniation
  - Repeat CT to monitor for change: Stable or increase within 36 hours, resorption within few weeks
- In neonates, up to 50% EDH can be treated conservatively

# DIAGNOSTIC CHECKLIST

## Image Interpretation Pearls
- NECT highly sensitive & widely available
- Involvement of dural sinuses: High risk of thrombosis

# SELECTED REFERENCES

1. Radulovic D et al: Traumatic delayed epidural hematoma. Zentralbl Neurochir. 67(2):76-80, 2006
2. Heyman R et al: Intracranial epidural hematoma in newborn infants: clinical study of 15 cases. Neurosurgery. 57(5):924-9; discussion 924-9, 2005
3. Rocchi G et al: Traumatic epidural hematoma in children. J Child Neurol. 20(7):569-72, 2005
4. Yilmazlar S et al: Traumatic epidural haematomas of nonarterial origin: analysis of 30 consecutive cases. Acta Neurochir (Wien). 147(12):1241-8; discussion 1248, 2005
5. Berker M et al: Traumatic epidural haematoma of the posterior fossa in childhood: 16 new cases and a review of the literature. Br J Neurosurg. 17(3):226-9, 2003
6. Browne GJ et al: Isolated extradural hematoma in children presenting to an emergency department in Australia. Pediatr Emerg Care. 18(2):86-90, 2002
7. Simon B et al: Pediatric minor head trauma: indications for computed tomographic scanning revisited. J Trauma. 51(2):231-7; discussion 237-8, 2001
8. Singleton SD et al: Lenticular lesions: not always an epidural hematoma. Pediatr Emerg Care. 17(4):252-4, 2001
9. Harbury OL et al: Vertex epidural hematomas: imaging findings and diagnostic pitfalls. Eur J Radiol. 36(3):150-7, 2000
10. Shugerman RP et al: Epidural hemorrhage: is it abuse? Pediatrics. 97(5):664-8, 1996
11. Mohanty A et al: Prognosis of extradural haematomas in children. Pediatr Neurosurg. 23(2):57-63, 1995
12. Pillay R et al: Extradural haematomas in children. S Afr Med J. 85(7):672-4, 1995
13. Schutzman SA et al: Epidural hematomas in children. Ann Emerg Med. 22(3):535-41, 1993

# EPIDURAL HEMATOMA

## IMAGE GALLERY

### Typical

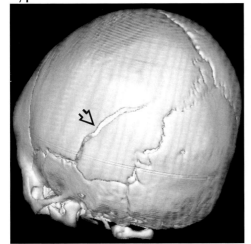
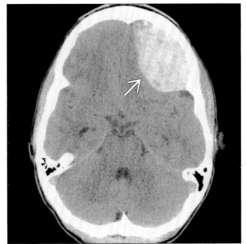

*(Left)* NECT after trauma from auto accident shows parietal fracture line ⊋ on surface rendering of calvarium. *(Right)* Axial NECT shows dense biconvex collection under frontal squama ➡. Frontal EDHs are relatively common in children, often associated with orbital fractures from falling forward.

### Typical

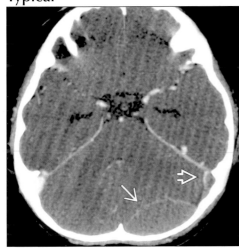
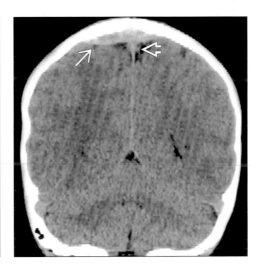

*(Left)* Axial CECT shows acute epidural collection under occipital squama ➡ that crossed transverse sinus upward. Note the thrombosis of the sigmoid sinus ⊋. *(Right)* Coronal NECT shows EDH at vertex ➡ displacing superior sagittal sinus ⊋. These are usually due to less active venous bleed, but risk of SVT is high. Coronal CT reformats or MR are useful.

### Typical

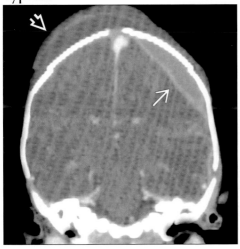
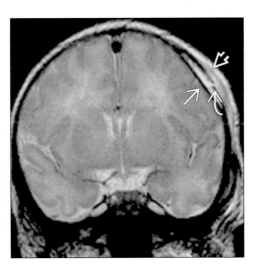

*(Left)* Coronal CECT in a neonate after instrumented delivery shows parietal EDH ➡. Anemia is a common feature when EDH is accompanied by subgaleal hematoma ⊋. *(Right)* Coronal T2WI MR shows small parietal EDH ➡. Note displaced low T2-signal dura; epidural blood goes through fracture line ➡ to subperiosteal hematoma ⊋, decompressing the brain.

# EMPYEMA

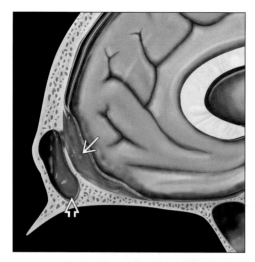

Sagittal graphic shows pus in frontal sinus ⇒, erosion of posterior sinus wall and extension of infection into anterior frontal epidural space ⇒.

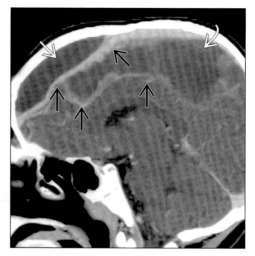

Sagittal CECT reformation shows large epidural empyema ⇒ adjacent to frontal sinus, with secondary subdural empyema along falx ⇒. Thick enhancing membrane → lines the collections.

## TERMINOLOGY

### Abbreviations and Synonyms
- Subdural empyema (SDE), epidural empyema (EDE), epidural abscess

### Definitions
- Collection of pus in subdural or epidural space, or both

## IMAGING FINDINGS

### General Features
- Best diagnostic clue: Extra-axial collection with rim enhancement
- Location
  - Supratentorial typical
    - SDE: Convexity in > 50%, parafalcine in 20%
    - EDE: Often adjacent to frontal sinus
  - Infratentorial, up to 10%
    - Often associated with mastoiditis
- Size: Variable, may become huge in infants
- Morphology
  - SDE: Crescentic typical; may be lentiform on coronal images
  - EDE: Biconvex, lens-shaped (lentiform)

### CT Findings
- NECT
  - Extra-axial collection, typically isodense to hyperdense to CSF
  - SDE: Crescentic iso/hyperdense collection, confined by falx (NB: Can be small, easily overlooked!)
    - Frequently bilateral
  - EDE: Biconvex low density collection between dura, calvarium, contained by cranial sutures
    - Often continuous across midline
  - Posterior fossa EDE
    - Typically at sinodural angle
    - Pus may extend into cerebellopontine angle
- CECT
  - Strong peripheral rim enhancement
  - Posterior fossa EDE
    - Look for sinovenous thrombosis
  - SDE: Crescentic collection, underlying brain may be hyperintense

## DDx: Other Pericerebral Collections

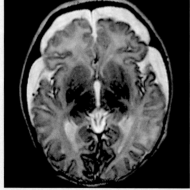

Clear Effusion

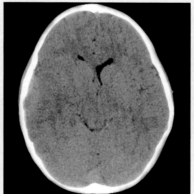

Isointense EDH

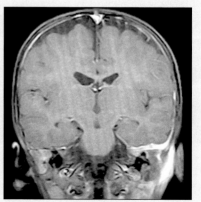

Acute Leukemia

# EMPYEMA

## Key Facts

### Terminology
- Collection of pus in subdural or epidural space, or both

### Imaging Findings
- Best diagnostic clue: Extra-axial collection with rim enhancement
- Best imaging tool: MR best to demonstrate presence, nature, extent, and complications
- Protocol advice: Contrast-enhanced multiplanar MR with DWI

### Top Differential Diagnoses
- Subdural Effusion
- Sterile, CSF-like collection associated with meningitis; may become infected → real SDE

### Pathology
- Infants, young children: Meningitis effusion which becomes superinfected
- Older children: Related to paranasal sinus disease in > 2/3, mastoiditis 20%

### Clinical Issues
- Mortality 10-15%

### Diagnostic Checklist
- SDE may go unrecognized without imaging in infantile meningitis
- If a patient has sinusitis and neurologic symptoms, look for empyema!
- DWI helps differentiate SDE from effusion, recognizes cortical ischemia

## MR Findings
- T1WI
  - Extra-axial collection, hyperintense to CSF
  - SDE: Crescentic extra-axial collection
  - EDE: Lens-shaped bifrontal or convexity collection
    - Inwardly displaced dura seen as hypointense line between collection and brain
    - May cross midline in frontal region
- T2WI
  - Isointense to hyperintense to CSF
    - EDE: Lens-shaped bifrontal or convexity collection
    - Inwardly displaced dura seen as hypointense line between collection and brain
- PD/Intermediate: Underlying brain may be hyperintense
- FLAIR
  - Hyperintense to CSF
  - SDE: Crescentic collection, underlying brain may be hyperintense
  - EDE: Lens-shaped bifrontal or convexity collection, underlying brain may be hyperintense
- DWI
  - SDE: Reduced diffusion (increased signal intensity) typical
    - Reduced diffusion in cortex: Involvement of pial vessels
  - EDE: Variable signal, may be mixed
- T1 C+
  - Prominent enhancement at margin related to granulomatous tissue and inflammation
    - SDE: Encapsulating membranes enhance strongly, may be loculated with internal fibrous strands
    - EDE: Strong enhancement of collection margins
  - May see enhancement of adjacent brain parenchyma (cerebritis/abscess)
  - Subgaleal phlegmon or abscess ("Pott puffy tumor")
- MRV: Venous thrombosis may be seen as lack of flow

## Ultrasonographic Findings
- Useful in infants
- Heterogeneous echogenic convexity collection with mass effect
  - Hyperechoic fibrous strands
  - Thick hyperechoic inner membrane
  - Increased echogenicity of pia-arachnoid and exudates in the subarachnoid space

## Imaging Recommendations
- Best imaging tool: MR best to demonstrate presence, nature, extent, and complications
- Protocol advice: Contrast-enhanced multiplanar MR with DWI

## DIFFERENTIAL DIAGNOSIS

### Chronic Subdural Hematoma
- MR shows blood products, may be loculated
- Often enhances along edge, typically thinner than SDE

### Subdural Effusion
- Sterile, CSF-like collection associated with meningitis; may become infected → real SDE
- Usually nonenhancing; may enhance mildly

### Subdural Hygroma
- Nonenhancing CSF collection, often trauma history

### Epidural Tumor, Hemopathy
- Solid epidural infiltrate, often enhancing

## PATHOLOGY

### General Features
- General path comments
  - Subdural empyema is more common than EDE
  - SDE are more commonly complicated by abscess and venous thrombosis, > 10% of patients
  - 15% of cases have both EDE, SDE
- Etiology
  - Infants, young children: Meningitis effusion which becomes superinfected
  - Older children: Related to paranasal sinus disease in > 2/3, mastoiditis 20%

# EMPYEMA

- Direct spread through posterior wall of frontal sinus
- Retrograde spread through valveless emissary veins of extra-, intracranial spaces
  - Complication of head trauma or neurosurgical procedure, rare
  - Causative organism: Streptococci, H. influenzae, S. aureus, S. epidermidis most common
  - Anaerobic or microaerophilic organisms (strep, bacteroides) common
- Epidemiology
  - Uncommon, occur 1/4 to 1/2 as often as abscess
    - Risk significant in infantile meningitis if antibiotics not efficient
  - SDE and EDE account for approximately 30% of intracranial infections
  - EDE: Sinusitis in 67%, mastoiditis in 10%

## Gross Pathologic & Surgical Features
- Encapsulated, yellowish, purulent collection
- Spreads widely but may be loculated
- Osteitis in 35%

## Microscopic Features
- Inflammatory infiltrate surrounded by granulomatous tissue

# CLINICAL ISSUES

## Presentation
- Most common signs/symptoms
  - From sinusitis, mastoiditis
    - Fever, headaches
    - Meningismus common, may mimic meningitis
    - Mass effect if large, sinovenous involvement
  - Infantile meningitis
    - Poor response to treatment: CT/MR show SDE
    - Adjacent cortical ischemia: Seizures, deficit
    - Mass effect ⇒ ↑ ICP
- Clinical Profile
  - Sinus or ear infection in > 75% of cases
    - Periorbital swelling may be seen
  - Frontal subgaleal abscess ("Pott puffy tumor") in up to 1/3
    - Typically adolescent males
- Clinical diagnosis often delayed, confused with meningitis
- Epidural, subdural empyemas are rare, yet highly lethal

## Demographics
- Age: Can occur at any age

## Natural History & Prognosis
- May progress rapidly, considered neurosurgical emergencies
- EDE may occasionally have an indolent course as the dura mater functions as a barrier between infection and brain
  - Much better prognosis than SDE
- Complications common
  - Cerebritis and brain abscess, approximately 5%

- Cortical vein, dural sinus thrombosis with secondary venous ischemia
  - Cerebral edema
  - Hydrocephalus (> 75% of infratentorial SDE)
- Mortality 10-15%

## Treatment
- Surgical drainage through wide craniotomy is gold standard
- Intravenous antibiotics
- Conservative management may be effective in small sinus-related EDE with adequate sinus drainage, antibiotics

# DIAGNOSTIC CHECKLIST

## Consider
- SDE may go unrecognized without imaging in infantile meningitis
- If a patient has sinusitis and neurologic symptoms, look for empyema!

## Image Interpretation Pearls
- MR with contrast and DWI is most sensitive; CT may miss small collections
- DWI helps differentiate SDE from effusion, recognizes cortical ischemia

# SELECTED REFERENCES

1. Fanning NF et al: Serial diffusion-weighted MRI correlates with clinical course and treatment response in children with intracranial pus collections. Pediatr Radiol. 36(1):26-37, 2006
2. Germiller JA et al: Intracranial complications of sinusitis in children and adolescents and their outcomes. Arch Otolaryngol Head Neck Surg. 132(9):969-76, 2006
3. Vinchon M et al: Postmeningitis subdural fluid collection in infants: changing pattern and indications for surgery. J Neurosurg. 104(6 Suppl):383-7, 2006
4. Adame N et al: Sinogenic intracranial empyema in children. Pediatrics. 116(3):e461-7, 2005
5. Leotta N et al: Intracranial suppuration. J Paediatr Child Health. 41(9-10):508-12, 2005
6. Chang CJ et al: Bacterial meningitis in infants: the epidemiology, clinical features, and prognostic factors. Brain Dev. 26(3):168-75, 2004
7. Wong AM et al: Diffusion-weighted MR imaging of subdural empyemas in children. AJNR Am J Neuroradiol. 25(6):1016-21, 2004
8. Heran NS et al: Conservative neurosurgical management of intracranial epidural abscesses in children. Neurosurgery. 53(4):893-7; discussion 897-8, 2003
9. Vazquez E et al: Imaging of complications of acute mastoiditis in children. Radiographics. 23(2):359-72, 2003
10. Bambakidis NC et al: Intracranial complications of frontal sinusitis in children: Pott's puffy tumor revisited. Pediatr Neurosurg. 35(2):82-9, 2001
11. Chen CY et al: Subdural empyema in 10 infants: US characteristics and clinical correlates. Radiology. 207(3):609-17, 1998
12. Chang YC et al: Risk factor of complications requiring neurosurgical intervention in infants with bacterial meningitis. Pediatr Neurol. 17(2):144-9, 1997

# EMPYEMA

## IMAGE GALLERY

### Typical

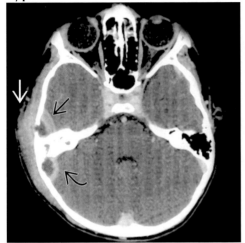

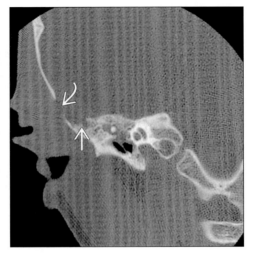

*(Left)* Axial CECT shows two epidural empyemas, one in temporal fossa ⟶, one in posterior fossa ⟶, associated with superficial soft tissue inflammation ⟶ and opacified mastoid cells. *(Right)* Coronal bone CT (same patient as previous image) shows mastoiditis with bone erosion of upper aspect of temporal bone ⟶ and temporal squama ⟶, explaining the extent of inflammation.

### Typical

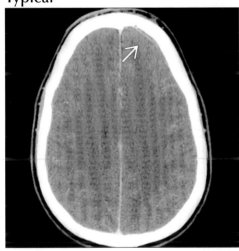

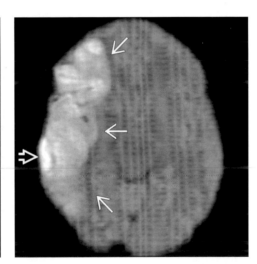

*(Left)* Axial CECT shows small epidural empyema over left frontal convexity ⟶, related to osteitis and supraorbital Pott puffy tumor. Such a lesion is impossible to detect on unenhanced CT. *(Right)* Axial DWI MR shows reduced diffusion ⟶ in small subdural empyema. Note the extensive MCA territory ischemia ⟶, which is likely due to meningitis-related vasculitis.

### Typical

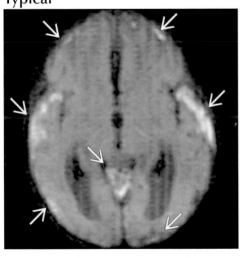

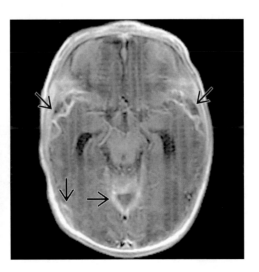

*(Left)* Axial DWI MR shows multiple pericerebral collections of reduced diffusion ⟶. These empyemas were associated with septic meningitis in this young infant. *(Right)* Axial T1 C+ MR (same patient as previous image, different obliquity) shows the hypointense collections ⟶ with marked enhancement of the thick limiting membranes on cortical side.

# TRAUMATIC SUBARACHNOID HEMORRHAGE

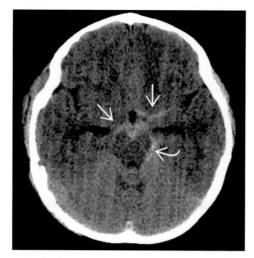

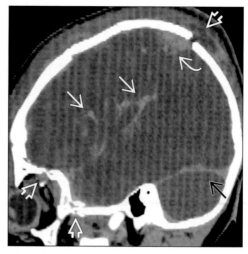

*Axial NECT shows hyperdense blood filling perimesencephalic ➔ and proximal sylvian ➔ cisterns, resulting in positive contrast cisternographic appearance of CSF spaces.*

*Sagittal NECT reformation shows fractures of calvarium and skull base ➔, cortical hemorrhagic contusion ➔, SDH along tentorium ➔, and SAH surrounding sulci of insular lobe ➔.*

## TERMINOLOGY

### Abbreviations and Synonyms
- Traumatic subarachnoid hemorrhage (tSAH)

### Definitions
- Traumatic bleed within subarachnoid spaces between pial & external arachnoid layer

## IMAGING FINDINGS

### General Features
- Best diagnostic clue: High density on CT, hyperintensity on FLAIR within sulci/cisterns in setting of trauma
- Location
  - Focally, adjacent to contusion, subdural hematoma (SDH), fracture, laceration
  - Diffusely throughout subarachnoid space &/or basal cisterns
  - Layering into interpeduncular or preculminal cisterns, in cisterna magna
- Morphology
  - Fills subarachnoid space; cisternographic appearance
    - Spreads into sulci
    - Horizontal fluid-fluid layering in cisterns

### CT Findings
- NECT
  - High density in subarachnoid space/cisterns
    - Molds the brain anatomy, enters sulci
    - Often dependent
    - When layering, horizontal dependent fluid-fluid level
  - Layering blood in interpeduncular cistern
    - May be only manifestation of subtle SAH
  - Location different from aneurysmal SAH
    - Adjacent to contusions, subdural hematomas
    - Convexity sulci > basal cisterns
  - Cortical vein sign = cortical veins evident crossing through hyperdense SAH

### MR Findings
- T1WI: Isointense with brain on T1WI ("dirty" CSF)
- T2WI
  - Isointense with brain on T2WI ("dirty" CSF)
  - Evolution of hemoglobin signal different from intracerebral hematoma

## DDx: Other Extracerebral Collections

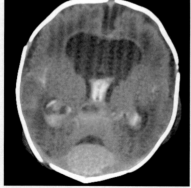
*SDH Cisterna Magna*

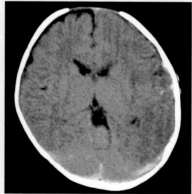
*SDH Posterior Falx, Tentorium*

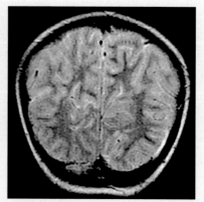
*Septic Meningitis*

# TRAUMATIC SUBARACHNOID HEMORRHAGE

## Key Facts

### Terminology
- Traumatic bleed within subarachnoid spaces between pial & external arachnoid layer

### Imaging Findings
- Best diagnostic clue: High density on CT, hyperintensity on FLAIR within sulci/cisterns in setting of trauma
- Fills subarachnoid space; cisternographic appearance
- FLAIR: Hyperintense sulci/cisterns

### Top Differential Diagnoses
- Subdural Hematoma
- Non-Traumatic SAH (ntSAH)
- Meningitis
- Pseudo-Subarachnoid Hemorrhage

### Pathology
- Trauma, not ruptured aneurysm, is most common cause of SAH in global population, still more in children
- Associated abnormalities: Contusions, subdural/epidural hematoma, diffuse axonal injury

### Clinical Issues
- SAH part of more complex traumatic brain injury (TBI)
- TBI associated with tSAH has poor prognosis

### Diagnostic Checklist
- Cisternographic appearance of SAH
- Hyperdense blood in interpeduncular cistern may be only manifestation of subtle SAH

---

- Progression much slower, likely because high ambient oxygen tension of CSF
- Dilution in CSF
- FLAIR: Hyperintense sulci/cisterns
- DWI
  - Useful for evaluation of effects of tSAH-induced spasm
    - Reduced diffusion (hyperintense) in areas of ischemia

### Angiographic Findings
- Conventional
  - DSA
    - Useful for evaluation of tSAH-induced spasm, but risk of ischemia increased
    - Rules out arterial tear, aneurysm; "beaded appearance" of vasospasm

### Imaging Recommendations
- Best imaging tool: CT > MR given its accessibility
- Protocol advice
  - NECT
  - FLAIR > CT in detection of small amounts of SAH

## DIFFERENTIAL DIAGNOSIS

### Subpial Hemorrhage
- Corresponds to the gyrus, spares sulcus, adjacent CSF
- Separates feeding/draining pial vessels from underlying cortex with resulting ischemia

### Subdural Hematoma
- Lining the posterior falx, tentorium, collecting in cisterna magna
  - No spreading into sulci
  - No horizontal fluid-fluid layering

### Non-Traumatic SAH (ntSAH)
- Ruptured aneurysm
  - Infrequent in children
  - Different clinical context
  - 80-90% ntSAH, identified on DSA, CTA, MRA in > 85%

- Arterio-venous malformation
  - Mostly intracerebral bleed
  - Nidus, related vessels: Flow voids, enhancement
  - 15% ntSAH, identified on DSA, CTA, MRA
- Perimesencephalic venous hemorrhage
  - Uncommon; often limited cisternal SAH, negative initial & repeat DSA
- Ruptured dissecting aneurysm
  - SAH and dissecting aneurysm may be two effects from same trauma
- Spinal vascular malformation
  - Diagnosis of exclusion with negative initial & repeat cerebral DSA
- Hypertensive hemorrhage
  - Exceptional in children (mostly intensive care setting)
- Cerebral infarction with reperfusion hemorrhage
  - Presence of known infarct
- Coagulation disorder
  - Anticoagulation therapy; clinical context
  - Blood dyscrasia; vitamin K deficiency in young infants

### Meningitis
- Proteinaceous CSF prevents FLAIR CSF nulling
- Contrast enhancement

### Carcinomatosis
- Cellular CSF prevents FLAIR CSF nulling
- Contrast enhancement

### Pseudo-Subarachnoid Hemorrhage
- Severe, diffuse cerebral edema → brain becomes diffusely hypodense, dura & circulating blood relatively "hyperdense"
- Gadolinium administration may cause CSF hyperintensity when lesion lined by CSF spaces
- Inspired 100% oxygen may affect nulling of CSF on FLAIR
- Incomplete nulling of CSF FLAIR signal 2° to propofol has been described

# TRAUMATIC SUBARACHNOID HEMORRHAGE

## PATHOLOGY

### General Features
- Genetics: Less favorable outcome in SAH patients who possess APOξ4 allele
- Etiology
  - Closed head injury: Most likely arises from tearing of veins in subarachnoid space
  - Penetrating head injury: Direct vascular lesion, subsequent pseudo-aneurysm may develop
  - In neonates: SAH often occurs in association with adjacent parenchymal hemorrhage; mechanism is uncertain (venous injury?)
- Epidemiology
  - Trauma, not ruptured aneurysm, is most common cause of SAH in global population, still more in children
  - 33% with moderate brain injury; nearly 100% at autopsy
  - tSAH-associated vasospasm 2-41% of cases
- Associated abnormalities: Contusions, subdural/epidural hematoma, diffuse axonal injury

### Gross Pathologic & Surgical Features
- Acute blood within sulci/cisterns

### Microscopic Features
- Late meningeal fibrosis

## CLINICAL ISSUES

### Presentation
- Most common signs/symptoms: Headache, emesis, ↓ consciousness, seizures
- Clinical Profile
  - SAH part of more complex traumatic brain injury (TBI)
  - Delivery

### Demographics
- Age: Mostly infants and teenagers
- Gender: Older boys more likely than girls to sustain traumatic brain injury (TBI)
- Populations at increased risk of sustaining TBI
  - Teenagers: Sport activities, MVA, bicycling
  - Infants: Incidence of SAH in child abuse is similar to that in accidental trauma
- Neonate: Intracranial hemorrhage in term neonates is mostly subdural or subarachnoid

### Natural History & Prognosis
- Natural history = clears in a few weeks from breakdown & resorption from CSF
- Acute hydrocephalus
  - Rare → usually obstruction of aqueduct or 4th ventricular outlet by clotted SAH
  - Obstructive, non-communicating hydrocephalus
- Delayed hydrocephalus
  - Fibrous changes in arachnoid, possibly in arachnoid granulations
  - Communicating hydrocephalus
- Vasospasm

---

- May develop quickly (2-3 days post-injury), peaks 7-10 days after injury
- Often with brain swelling
- Uncommon cause of post traumatic infarct
- TBI associated with tSAH has poor prognosis
  - Amount of tSAH on initial CT correlates with delayed ischemia, poor outcome
  - 46-78% of TBI involving tSAH result in severe disability, vegetative state, or death

### Treatment
- Supportive therapy
  - Intubation, supplemental oxygen, IV fluids, maintain BP/brain perfusion
- Nimodipine, a calcium channel blocker, may prevent vasospasm & its complications

## DIAGNOSTIC CHECKLIST

### Image Interpretation Pearls
- Cisternographic appearance of SAH
- Hyperdense blood in interpeduncular cistern may be only manifestation of subtle SAH
- tSAH often secondary to/associated with other injuries

## SELECTED REFERENCES

1. Chung et al: Critical score of Glasgow coma scale for pediatric traumatic brain injury. Pediatr Neurol. 34:379-87, 2006
2. Bechtel K et al: Characteristics that distinguish accidental from abusive injury in hospitalized young children with head trauma. Pediatrics. 114:165-8, 2004
3. Huang AH et al: Spontaneous superficial parenchymal and leptomeningeal hemorrhage in term neonates. AJNR Am J Neuroradiol. 25:469-75, 2004
4. Kay A et al: Temporal alterations in cerebrospinal fluid amyloid beta-protein and apolipoprotein E after subarachnoid hemorrhage. Stroke. 34(12):e240-3, 2003
5. Shih et al: Development of intracranial complications following transoral stab wounds in children. Report of two cases. Pediatr Neurosurg. 37:35-7, 2002
6. Filippi CG et al: Hyperintense signal abnormality in subarachnoid spaces and basal cisterns on MR images of children anesthetized with propofol: new fluid-attenuated inversion recovery finding. AJNR Am J Neuroradiol. 22(2):394-9, 2001
7. Gorrie et al: Extent and distribution of vascular brain injury in pediatric road fatalities. J Neurotrauma. 18:849-60, 2001
8. Simon B et al: Pediatric minor head trauma: indications for computed tomographic scanning revisited. J Trauma. 51:231-7, 2001
9. Taoka T et al: Sulcal hyperintensity on fluid-attenuated inversion recovery MR images in patients without apparent cerebrospinal fluid abnormality. AJR Am J Roentgenol. 176(2):519-24, 2001
10. Kim KA et al: Analysis of pediatric head injury from falls. Neurosurg Focus. 8:e3, 2000
11. Alvarez JA et al: Delayed rupture of traumatic intracranial pseudoaneurysm in a child following gunshot wound to the head. J Craniomaxillofac Trauma. 5:39-44, 1999
12. Aydinli N et al: Vitamin K deficiency-late onset intracranial hemorrhage. Eur J Paediatr Neurol. 2:199-203, 1998

## IMAGE GALLERY

Typical

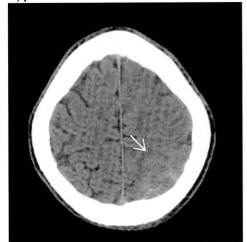
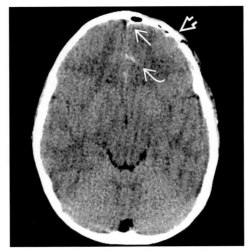

*(Left)* Axial NECT shows diffuse filling of parietal cortical sulci by mild SAH ➜. Sulcal pattern is preserved but CSF low attenuation replaced by high attenuation of hemorrhage. *(Right)* Axial NECT shows right frontal compound fracture ➡ with thin adjacent SDH ➜ extending to falx. Blood in calloso-marginal sulcus ➜ indicates presence of associated SAH.

Typical

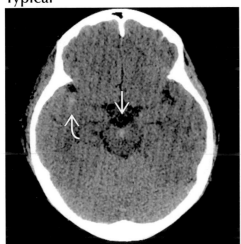
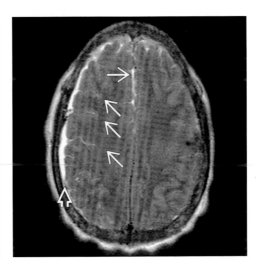

*(Left)* Axial NECT shows minimal amount of blood collected in interpeduncular cistern ➜. Note blood in anterior right temporal lobe ➡. Small hemorrhages were present in basal ganglia. *(Right)* Axial FLAIR MR shows high signal of subarachnoid blood within anterior interhemispheric and right convexity sulci ➜. Associated layer of SDH ➡ is indistinguishable from SAH.

Typical

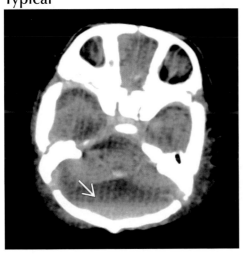
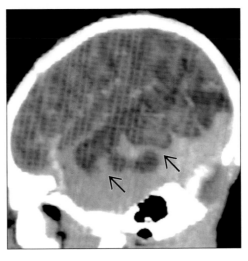

*(Left)* Axial NECT shows a blood-fluid layer ➜ in the cisterna magna. It was associated with intraventricular, parenchymal and SDH in neonate after a difficult delivery. *(Right)* Sagittal NECT shows massive pericerebral neonatal hemorrhage that is partly subdural, but blood surrounding the temporal sulci ➜ means that much is subarachnoid in location.

# BACTERIAL MENINGITIS

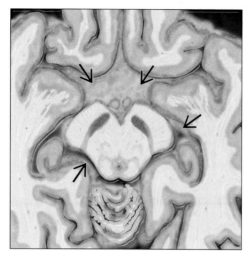

Axial graphic shows diffuse inflammatory exudate ➡ involving the leptomeninges, and filling the basal cisterns and sulci.

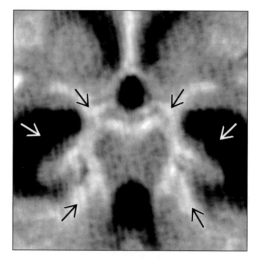

Axial CECT shows robust basilar cisternal enhancement ➡ in a patient with TB meningitis. There is associated obstructive hydrocephalus ➡. (Courtesy C. Glasier, MD).

## TERMINOLOGY

### Abbreviations and Synonyms
- Leptomeningitis

### Definitions
- Acute or chronic inflammation of predominantly the pia and arachnoid membranes
- Classified as
  - Acute pyogenic (bacterial), lymphocytic (viral), and chronic (granulomatous)

## IMAGING FINDINGS

### General Features
- Best diagnostic clue: + CSF by lumbar puncture
- Location: Predominantly: Pia, arachnoid, and subarachnoid space (SAS) of brain and spine

### CT Findings
- CTA: ± Arterial narrowing, ± vessel occlusion
- NECT
  - May be normal

- Increased attenuation in basilar cisterns or sylvian fissures due to inflammatory debris
- Ventricular dilatation secondary to hydrocephalus
- Subarachnoid space enlargement
- ± Subdural effusion (20-50 % in affected < 1 year)
- CECT
  - Variable meningeal enhancement
    - Bacterial meningitis usually involving the convexities
    - Basal enhancement more common in granulomatous meningitis
  - ± Empty delta sign if cortical venous thrombosis extends to dural sinus

### MR Findings
- T1WI: Detects mass effect and hemorrhage, exudate is hypo- to isointense
- T2WI
  - Delineates edema, infarction, and abscess ⇒ T2 hyperintensity
  - Exudate is hyperintense
- FLAIR
  - Hyperintense signal in sulci and cisterns

## DDx: Leptomeningeal Disease

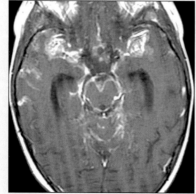

PNET Metastasis

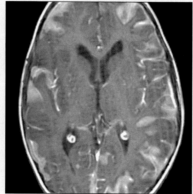

Leukemia

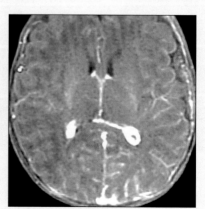

Sturge-Weber

# BACTERIAL MENINGITIS

## Key Facts

### Terminology
- Acute or chronic inflammation of predominantly the pia and arachnoid membranes
- Acute pyogenic (bacterial), lymphocytic (viral), and chronic (granulomatous)

### Imaging Findings
- Best diagnostic clue: + CSF by lumbar puncture
- Best imaging tool: MR brain with contrast and DWI ⇒ superior to CECT

### Top Differential Diagnoses
- Carcinomatous Meningitis
- Leukemia
- Sturge-Weber Syndrome

### Clinical Issues
- Neonate: Poor feeding, respiratory distress, temperature instability, bulging fontanel, apnea, and seizures
- Older Children: Fever, headache, photophobia, stiff neck, Kernig and Brudzinski signs
- Death can occur in ~ 5% of cases of pyogenic meningitis

### Diagnostic Checklist
- An imaging study is not the means by which the diagnosis of meningitis is made, LP is needed
- On NECT, ventricular dilatation (hydrocephalus) may be the only clue to meningitis
- Contrast-enhanced MR is more sensitive than CECT

---

  - Sensitive for early cerebral edema (cerebritis & ischemia)
  - FLAIR with MR contrast more sensitive than T1 C+
- T2* GRE: Sensitive in detecting hemorrhage
- DWI: Invaluable for detecting: Infarction, subdural empyema, and abscess
- T1 C+
  - Meninges and SAS typically enhance
  - Characterizes extent of inflammation and complications: Subdural empyema, cerebritis, abscess
- MRA: ± Arterial narrowing , ± vessel occlusion
- MRV: Thrombosis can affect deep veins, cortical veins, and venous sinuses
- MRS
  - Cerebritis ⇒ ↑ excitatory neurotransmitters, mild ↑ choline, mild ↓ NAA
  - Infarction ⇒ ↑ lactate, ↑ Choline and cytosolic amino acids, ↓ NAA
  - Cerebral abscess ⇒ NAA ↓, Choline ↑, products of fermentation (lactate, acetate, and succinate)

## Ultrasonographic Findings
- Grayscale Ultrasound
  - Early meningitis
    - Unexplained ventricular dilatation and subdural fluid accumulations
- Color Doppler: ± Dural venous sinus thrombosis

## Imaging Recommendations
- Best imaging tool: MR brain with contrast and DWI ⇒ superior to CECT
- Protocol advice: MR brain with contrast including DWI

## DIFFERENTIAL DIAGNOSIS

### Carcinomatous Meningitis
- More common with
  - PNET, atypical teratoid rhabdoid tumor (ATRT), ependymoma, germinoma, choroid plexus carcinoma, and anaplastic astrocytomas

### Leukemia
- May mimic subarachnoid hemorrhage
- Pachymeningitis may herald the diagnosis of leukemia
- AML more common to involve leptomeninges than ALL

### Sturge-Weber Syndrome
- Early seizure presentation may reveal subtle or no cerebral atrophy
- Unilateral leptomeningeal enhancement + ipsilateral engorged glomus of choroid plexus

### Neurosarcoidosis
- Lacy leptomeningeal enhancement, ± ventricular or dural based masses

## PATHOLOGY

### General Features
- General path comments
  - Acute meningitis typically bacterial
    - Usually purulent, exudate in subarachnoid space
    - Subarachnoid vessels are congested and brain is swollen
    - PMNs and fibrin accumulate in subarachnoid space
  - Chronic meningitis
    - Acute and chronic inflammatory cells, basilar predilection
  - Proximity of inflammatory reaction to dural veins and subarachnoid spaces may lead to
    - Hydrocephalus
    - Ventriculitis
    - Venous and arterial thrombosis
    - Subdural effusions may occur as complication of meningitis, most often sterile
- Genetics: HLA-B12, HLA-Bw 40
- Etiology
  - Congenital malformations of the neural tube provide portal for infection

- o Hematogenous spread to meninges and choroid plexus
- o Contiguous infections: Sinuses, mastoid air cells
- o Penetrating trauma
- Epidemiology
  - o Risk factors (neonate)
    - Premature rupture of membranes, maternal fever
    - Traumatic delivery
    - Prematurity and low birth weight
    - Disturbance in humoral or cell mediated immunity
  - o Risk factors (> 1 month)
    - African American, diabetes mellitus, sickle cell disease, Cushing syndrome, coma
    - Complement depleting diseases, properdin deficiency
  - o Organisms responsible (neonate)
    - Group B streptococcus
    - Escherichia coli
    - Enterobacteriaceae (gram negative)
    - Others: Listeria monocytogenes, nonenterococcal group D streptococci, Citrobacter
  - o Organisms responsible (> 1 month)
    - Streptococcus pneumoniae
    - Neisseria meningitidis
    - Haemophilus influenzae; vaccination programs have markedly decreased incidence
- Associated abnormalities: Congenital malformations of the neural tube

## Gross Pathologic & Surgical Features

- Cisterns and sulci fill with cloudy CSF, then purulent exudate
- Pia-arachnoid is congested, may mimic subarachnoid hemorrhage
- Cerebral cortex often edematous

## Microscopic Features

- Meningeal exudate: PMNs, fibrin, bacteria
- Virchow-Robin spaces surrounding penetrating arteries
  - o Act as conduits for infection to reach brain parenchyma (cerebritis, abscess)
- Infection also spreads by direct invasion through the pia
- Inflammation infiltrates walls of arterioles and veins ⇒ focal necrosis → thrombosis → infarction
- Meningitis associated brain injury
  - o Cytokines, reactive nitrogen species, hippocampal apoptosis

## CLINICAL ISSUES

### Presentation

- Most common signs/symptoms
  - o Neonate: Poor feeding, respiratory distress, temperature instability, bulging fontanel, apnea, and seizures
  - o Older Children: Fever, headache, photophobia, stiff neck, Kernig and Brudzinski signs
- Other signs/symptoms: SIADH, cranial neuropathies, deafness, venous and arterial strokes
- Clinical Profile: Meningitis is a clinical-laboratory diagnosis

- Laboratory
  - o ↑ Neutrophils, ↑ protein, ↓ glucose
  - o Gram-stained smear of the CSF, 80% positive with culture proven pyogenic meningitis

## Demographics

- Age
  - o Neonatal meningitis
    - 0.2-0.5 cases per 1000 live term newborns
    - 1.4-2.3 cases per 1000 live preterm newborns
  - o Beyond the newborn
    - 0.1-6.6 cases per 100,000 population
- Gender: Male > female, males more susceptible to gram negative enteric bacilli
- Ethnicity: African American

## Natural History & Prognosis

- Death can occur in ~ 5% of cases of pyogenic meningitis
- Morbility in up to 30%
- Poor prognosticating factors
  - o Seizures > 72 hours, coma, need for inotropes, leukopenia
  - o Slow to clear CSF of bacteria, CSF protein > 500 mg/dL
  - o High concentrations of the K1 antigen with E. coli infections

## Treatment

- Intravenous antibiotics are the mainstay of therapy
- Specific therapy based on culture and sensitivity
- ± Adjunctive surgical drainage of empyema, and abscess
- TB meningitis requires combination therapy

## DIAGNOSTIC CHECKLIST

### Consider

- An imaging study is not the means by which the diagnosis of meningitis is made, LP is needed
- On NECT, ventricular dilatation (hydrocephalus) may be the only clue to meningitis

### Image Interpretation Pearls

- Neuroimaging studies are indicated
  - o If the diagnosis is unclear
  - o Clinical findings of ↑ ICP or neurologic deterioration
  - o Clinical course is unexpectedly slow
- Contrast-enhanced MR is more sensitive than CECT

## SELECTED REFERENCES

1. Meyer S et al: Tuberculous meningitis. Lancet. 367(9523):1682, 2006
2. Chavez-Bueno S et al: Bacterial meningitis in children. Pediatr Clin North Am. 52(3):795-810, vii, 2005
3. Hoffman JA et al: Streptococcus pneumoniae infections in the neonate. Pediatrics. 112(5):1095-102, 2003
4. Jan W et al: Diffusion-weighted imaging in acute bacterial meningitis in infancy. Neuroradiology. 45(9):634-9, 2003
5. Saez-Llorens X et al: Bacterial meningitis in children. Lancet. 361(9375):2139-48, 2003

# BACTERIAL MENINGITIS

## IMAGE GALLERY

### Typical

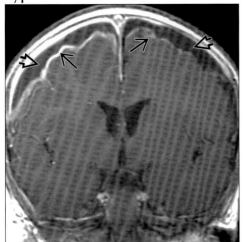 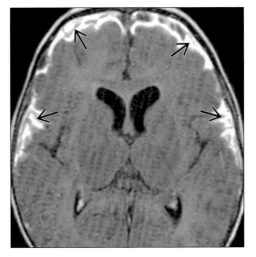

*(Left)* Coronal T1 C+ MR shows robust leptomeningeal enhancement ➔ and bilateral convexity subdural effusions ⇗ in a patient with Streptococcus pneumoniae meningitis. *(Right)* Axial FLAIR MR following contrast shows vivid leptomeningeal and subarachnoid space enhancement ➔ in a patient with streptococcus pneumoniae meningitis.

### Variant

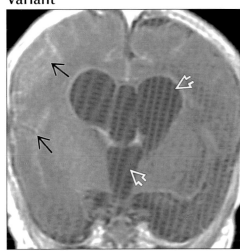 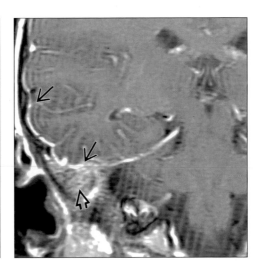

*(Left)* Coronal T1 C+ MR shows peripheral leptomeningeal enhancement ➔ in a neonate with E. coli meningitis. Obstructive hydrocephalus ⇗ results from inflammatory aqueductal debris. *(Right)* Coronal T1 C+ MR shows leptomeningeal enhancement ➔ secondary to meningitis in a patient with otomastoiditis ⇗ resulting from infection with Haemophilus influenzae.

### Variant

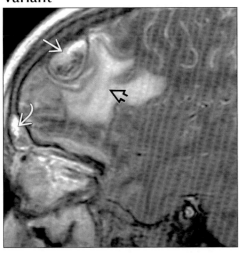 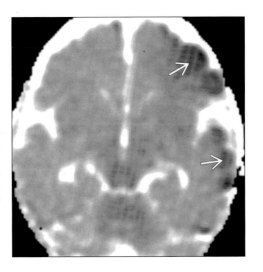

*(Left)* Sagittal T2WI MR shows a right frontal epidural empyema ➔ and cerebritis ⇗ in a patient with mixed bacterial meningitis secondary to complicated frontal sinusitis ➔. *(Right)* Axial ADC shows reduced diffusivity ➔ in the left frontal and temporal lobes secondary to venous infarction in a neonate with Group B Streptococcus sepsis and meningitis.

# NEUROCUTANEOUS MELANOSIS

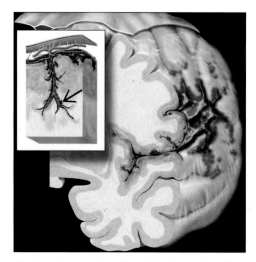

Graphic shows dark (melanotic) pigmentation of the leptomeninges. Inset demonstrates extension into the brain substance along the Virchow-Robin spaces ⇥.

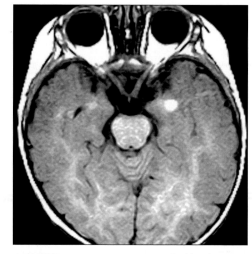

Axial T1WI screening MR in a 9-month old with GCMN shows parenchymal melanosis (PM): Small hyperintense foci without mass effect in the amygdala. PM is typically asymptomatic.

## TERMINOLOGY

### Abbreviations and Synonyms
- Neurocutaneous melanosis (NCM)

### Definitions
- Rare phakomatosis characterized by giant or multiple cutaneous melanocytic nevi (GCMN) and benign and malignant melanocytic lesions of the leptomeninges
  - Benign CNS disease
    - Melanosis: Excess of benign melanocytes in the leptomeninges or parenchyma
    - Melanocytes often confined to Virchow-Robin (VR) spaces in parenchymal melanosis (PM) although extension into brain does occur
  - Malignant CNS disease
    - Degeneration of PM and leptomeningeal (LM) melanosis into melanoma

## IMAGING FINDINGS

### General Features
- Best diagnostic clue

- Small, T1 hyperintense foci in amygdala or cerebellum without mass effect
- GCMN + diffuse LM enhancement
- Location
  - PM: Amygdala, cerebellum, basis pontis, thalami
  - LM disease (melanosis or melanoma): Diffuse > focal
  - Melanoma (parenchymal, MM)
    - Least common manifestation of NCM
    - Temporal lobe most common site
- Size
  - PM: < 1 cm
  - MM: Several cms
- Morphology
  - PM: Round or oval
  - LM disease: Linear or nodular
  - MM: Hemorrhagic/necrotic mass with mass effect
- Hydrocephalus: 64% symptomatic (sx) patients
  - Communicating > non-communicating; usually seen in association with diffuse LM enhancement
  - Occasionally secondary to Dandy-Walker complex
- Other findings
  - Dandy-Walker complex (10%)
  - Arachnoid cyst, mega cisterna magna

## DDx: Diffuse Leptomeningeal Enhancement

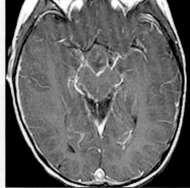

PNET-MB Mets

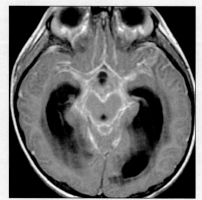

TB Meningitis

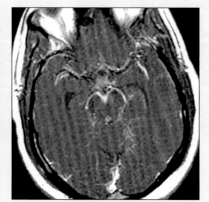

Sarcoidosis

# NEUROCUTANEOUS MELANOSIS

## Key Facts

### Terminology
- Neurocutaneous melanosis (NCM)
- Rare phakomatosis characterized by giant or multiple cutaneous melanocytic nevi (GCMN) and benign and malignant melanocytic lesions of the leptomeninges

### Imaging Findings
- Small, T1 hyperintense foci in amygdala or cerebellum without mass effect
- GCMN + diffuse LM enhancement

### Top Differential Diagnoses
- T1 Hyperintense Mass
- Diffuse Leptomeningeal Enhancement

### Pathology
- NCM: Rare; 100+ reported cases

- Sx NCM: 2-5% patients with GCMN
- Asx NCM: 25-30% patients with GCMN

### Clinical Issues
- Signs/sx related to hydrocephalus (rapidly increasing head circumference, seizures, vomiting, headache, CN6 palsy, irritability, lethargy)
- Detection PM on screening MR in symptom-free infant/child with GCMN
- Age: Sx NCM: Majority manifest by age 2-3
- Sx NCM: Dismal; median survival 6.5 months after sx onset

### Diagnostic Checklist
- MR appearance diagnostic in appropriate clinical setting
- Normal MR does not exclude diagnosis NCM

---

  - Spine (20%): LM enhancement, syrinx, arachnoiditis, cyst, lipoma, tethered cord

## CT Findings
- NECT
  - PM: Normal or hyperdense
  - MM: Heterogeneous mass with edema, mass effect
- CECT
  - PM: No enhancement
  - LM melanosis: Normal or LM enhancement
  - LM melanoma: LM enhancement
  - MM: Heterogeneous enhancement

## MR Findings
- T1WI
  - PM: Hyperintense
    - More difficult to detect after myelin maturation
  - LM disease: ± Iso- to hyperintense sulci, cisterns
  - MM: Heterogeneous; frequently hyperintense
  - T1 shortening caused by stable free radicals melanin
- T2WI
  - PM: Hypointense; no edema, mass effect
  - LM disease: ± Hypointense sulci, cisterns
  - MM: Heterogeneous with edema, mass effect
- FLAIR: LM disease: ± Hyperintense sulci, cisterns
- T2* GRE: "Blooming" of hemorrhage and melanin
- T1 C+
  - PM: No enhancement
  - LM melanosis: Normal or LM enhancement
  - LM melanoma: LM enhancement
  - MM: Avid enhancement, often heterogeneous

## Imaging Recommendations
- Best imaging tool: MR C+ brain and spine
- Protocol advice: MR screen for asymptomatic (asx) infants with GCMN

## DIFFERENTIAL DIAGNOSIS

### T1 Hyperintense Mass
- Lipoma/dermoid: Midline, extra-axial; chemical shift artifact

- Subacute hemorrhage: More pronounced T2 changes; mass effect; neurological deficit
- Hemorrhagic neoplasm: Enhancement; marked T2 hypointensity; mass effect/edema; neurological deficit

### Diffuse Leptomeningeal Enhancement
- Carcinomatous meningitis/CSF seeding: History 1° malignancy; linear/nodular LM enhancement
- Infectious meningitis: Basal cisterns; signs/symptoms meningitis; (+) CSF cultures
- Non-infectious inflammation (sarcoidosis, Wegener granulomatosis): Linear/nodular enhancement; other disease-related findings

## PATHOLOGY

### General Features
- General path comments
  - Embryology
    - Neural crest-derived primordial cells differentiate into melanocytes in epidermis and pia mater
    - Melanocytes in epidermis at 8-10 wks gestation
    - Melanocytes in pia mater at ~ 23 wks gestation
  - Anatomy
    - Normal distribution melanocytes in pia mater: Convexities, base cerebrum/cerebellum, ventral brainstem, cervical and lumbosacral spinal cord
    - Melanocytes normally surround blood vessels but do not extend into VR spaces
- Genetics
  - Sporadic
    - Theory: Survival of autosomal lethal gene by somatic mosaicism
- Etiology
  - Hypotheses
    - Abnormal migration melanocyte precursor cells
    - Abnormal expression melanin producing genes
    - Proliferation normal melanin-producing cells
  - Deregulation hepatocyte growth factor/scatter factor and receptor (Met) may play role
  - Hydrocephalus: Melanocyte-infiltrated leptomeninges or arachnoid villi obstruct CSF flow

# NEUROCUTANEOUS MELANOSIS

- Epidemiology
  - NCM: Rare; 100+ reported cases
  - GCMN: 1:20,000 live births
    - Sx NCM: 2-5% patients with GCMN
    - Asx NCM: 25-30% patients with GCMN
- Associated abnormalities
  - Strong association Dandy-Walker complex (10%)
    - Melanocyte-infiltrated LMs interfere with normal hindbrain development
  - Rare: Sturge-Weber, NF-1

## Gross Pathologic & Surgical Features
- PM: Focal, abnormal pigmentation within the brain
- LM disease: Darkly pigmented, thickened pia mater
- MM: Pigmented mass, ± necrosis, hemorrhage

## Microscopic Features
- PM: Pathologic extension melanocytes & melanin laden macrophages into VR spaces, parenchyma
- LM melanosis: ↑ Number melanocytes in pia mater
- LM melanoma
  - Difficult to differentiate from LM melanosis
  - Indicators of malignancy: Necrosis, hemorrhage, basal lamina invasion, cellular atypia, frequent mitoses, presence of annulate lamellae
- Immunohistochemistry: (+) Vimentin, S100, HMB45
- GCMN: Melanocytic nevi > compound nevi
  - Cells in reticular dermis, occasionally subcutis

## Staging, Grading or Classification Criteria
- Criteria for diagnosis
  - Giant or multiple (≥ 3) cutaneous melanocytic nevi
    - Child: 6 cm body, 9 cm head maximal diameter
    - Adult: 20 cm maximal diameter
  - Cutaneous melanoma only in patients with benign CNS disease
  - CNS melanoma only in patients with benign cutaneous lesions

# CLINICAL ISSUES

## Presentation
- Most common signs/symptoms
  - Signs/sx related to hydrocephalus (rapidly increasing head circumference, seizures, vomiting, headache, CN6 palsy, irritability, lethargy)
    - Referred to as "sx NCM"
    - Occurs with LM melanosis or melanoma; MM less common
    - Focal neurological deficit, psychiatric disturbance reported in rare older child/young adult presentation
  - Detection PM on screening MR in symptom-free infant/child with GCMN
    - Referred to as "asx NCM"
    - Rare reports seizure, development delay, spasticity
- Clinical Profile
  - Asx infant with GCMN (PM)
  - Infant/child with GCMN + signs/sx hydrocephalus
- CSF (sx NCM): ↑ Protein, ↓ glucose, ± benign/malignant melanocytes
- GCMN: Giant or multiple pigmented, hairy nevi
  - Giant nevi (66% of NCM)

- Lumbosacral > occipital, upper back
- Involvement of head & neck occurs in 94%
- Multiple nevi (34% of NCM)

## Demographics
- Age: Sx NCM: Majority manifest by age 2-3
- Gender: M = F

## Natural History & Prognosis
- Natural History
  - Asx NCM (PM): Unknown; often stable
    - Reports of regression and degeneration into MM
- Prognosis
  - Asx NCM: Unknown; at risk of developing sx NCM
  - Sx NCM: Dismal; median survival 6.5 months after sx onset
    - Prognosis equally poor for sx LM melanosis, LM melanoma, or MM
- GCMN
  - 5-15% lifetime risk of cutaneous melanoma
  - Risk factors for NCM
    - Nevi ≥ 50 cm maximal diameter
    - Posterior axis location; > 20 satellite lesions

## Treatment
- Asx NCM: Screening MR at 4 months of age
- Sx NCM: Shunt hydrocephalus (filter prevents peritoneal seeding)
  - Surgery, XRT, systemic/intrathecal chemotherapy
    - Palliative; no significant alteration course of NCM

# DIAGNOSTIC CHECKLIST

## Consider
- Utility of routine screening MRs in a disease with an unknown prognosis and no effective treatment

## Image Interpretation Pearls
- MR appearance diagnostic in appropriate clinical setting
- Normal MR does not exclude diagnosis NCM
- Diffuse LM enhancement seen in both LM melanosis and LM melanoma
  - Clinically irrelevant since sx LM melanosis and LM melanoma have equally poor prognosis

# SELECTED REFERENCES

1. Acosta FL Jr et al: Neurocutaneous melanosis presenting with hydrocephalus. Case report and review of the literature. J Neurosurg. 102(1 Suppl):96-100, 2005
2. Agero AL et al: Asymptomatic neurocutaneous melanocytosis in patients with large congenital melanocytic nevi: a study of cases from an Internet-based registry. J Am Acad Dermatol. 53(6):959-65, 2005
3. Plikaitis CM et al: Neurocutaneous melanosis: clinical presentations. J Craniofac Surg. 16(5):921-5, 2005
4. Foster RD et al: Giant congenital melanocytic nevi: the significance of neurocutaneous melanosis in neurologically asymptomatic children. Plast Reconstr Surg. 107(4):933-41, 2001
5. Byrd SE et al: MR imaging of symptomatic neurocutaneous melanosis in children. Pediatr Radiol. 27(1):39-44, 1997

# NEUROCUTANEOUS MELANOSIS

## IMAGE GALLERY

### Typical

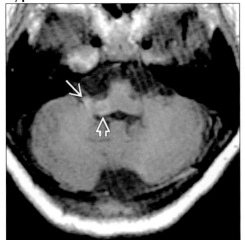
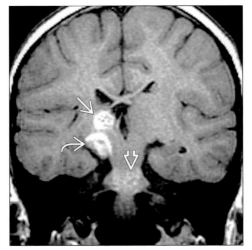

*(Left)* Axial T1WI MR shows findings of PM. Hyperintense foci without mass effect are seen in the right cerebellum ➡ and medulla ➡. Note mega cisterna magna dorsal to the vermis. *(Right)* Coronal T1WI MR shows PM and leptomeningeal (LM) melanosis in a 6 year old with seizures. Hyperintense foci are seen in the thalamus ➡, pons ➡, ambient cistern ➡.

### Typical

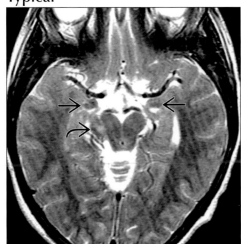
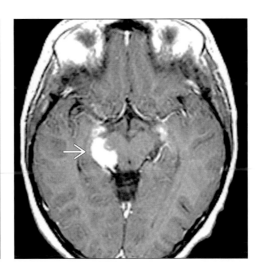

*(Left)* Axial T2WI MR in same patient as previous image shows hypointense appearance of amygdala ➡ and cisternal ➡ melanosis on T2. Focal, bulky LM melanosis is unusual. *(Right)* Axial T1 C+ MR in same patient as previous image shows enhancing LM melanosis ➡. Although patient has seizures, this is not considered "sx NCM" typified by diffuse LM enhancement, hydrocephalus.

### Typical

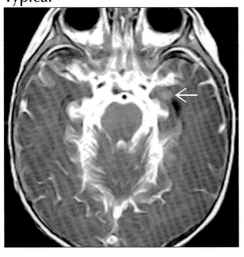
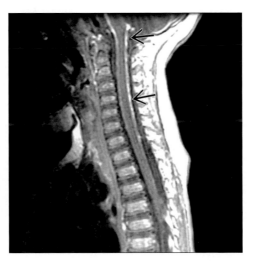

*(Left)* Axial T1 C+ MR shows typical findings seen in sx NCM: Diffuse, thick LM enhancement and hydrocephalus. Regardless of histology, prognosis of sx NCM is dismal. Note PM in amygdala ➡. *(Right)* Sagittal T1 C+ MR in same patient as previous image shows diffuse LM enhancement along the spinal cord ➡.

# MENINGIOANGIOMATOSIS

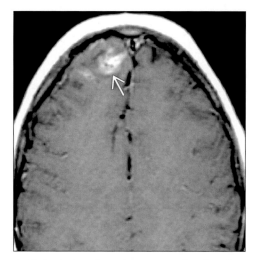

Axial T1 C+ MR shows leptomeningeal and gyriform cortical enhancement ➡ in the right superior frontal gyrus, likely due to proliferation of blood vessels and meningothelial cells.

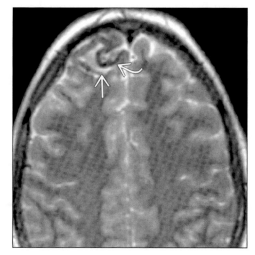

Axial T2WI MR shows focal curvilinear cortical hypointensity ➡ that corresponded to calcification on NECT. Note underlying edema ➡ in the subcortical white matter.

## TERMINOLOGY

### Definitions
- Hamartomatous lesion/malformation

## IMAGING FINDINGS

### General Features
- Best diagnostic clue: Cortical mass with enhancement, Ca++ but little mass effect
- Location
  - Cortex (frontal and temporal lobes), right > left
  - Rare: 3rd ventricle, thalami, brainstem, cerebellum
- Size: Generally small lesions (1-3 cm)

### CT Findings
- NECT
  - Leptomeningeal ± cortical mass(es) & Ca++ (nodular, linear or gyriform)
  - Rare: Hemorrhage & cysts
- CECT: Leptomeningeal ± cortical enhancement

### MR Findings
- T1WI: Isointense with areas of signal void (Ca++)
- T2WI: Hypointense cortex with areas of signal void (Ca++) with variable surrounding hyperintensity
- T2* GRE: Accentuates Ca++
- T1 C+: Leptomeningeal and cortical enhancement

### Imaging Recommendations
- Best imaging tool: MR and CT
- Protocol advice: CT for Ca++, C+ MR for lesion

## DIFFERENTIAL DIAGNOSIS

### Lesions with Enhancement & Ca++
- Sturge-Weber disease, oligodendroglioma, meningitis, meningioma

## PATHOLOGY

### General Features
- General path comments: Slow growing, no malignant degeneration

## DDx: Tumors with Ca++ and Leptomeningeal Enhancement

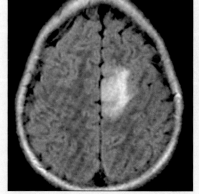

Oligodendroglioma

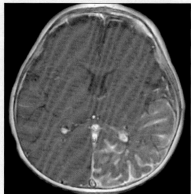

Sturge-Weber

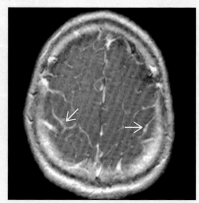

Bacterial Meningitis

# MENINGIOANGIOMATOSIS

## Key Facts

### Imaging Findings
- Best diagnostic clue: Cortical mass with enhancement, Ca++ but little mass effect

### Top Differential Diagnoses
- Lesions with Enhancement & Ca++
- Sturge-Weber disease, oligodendroglioma, meningitis, meningioma

### Pathology
- NF2 in ~ ½ of patients
- Proliferation of blood vessels and meningothelial cells around vessels in meninges, cortex, and underlying white matter

### Clinical Issues
- Intractable seizures, headaches (particularly sporadic)
- Often incidental (particularly NF2)

---

- Genetics
  - Germline alterations of the NF2 gene predispose to meningioangiomatosis
  - Sporadic not related to NF2 gene
- Etiology: Uncertain
- Epidemiology: Children, young adults
- Associated abnormalities
  - NF2 in ~ ½ of patients
  - Meningioma

### Gross Pathologic & Surgical Features
- Psammomatous Ca++ or dense osteoid
- Serpentine blood vessels overlying lesion

### Microscopic Features
- Proliferation of blood vessels and meningothelial cells around vessels in meninges, cortex, and underlying white matter
- Ca++, fibrocartilage and/or bone formation
- Gliotic cortex
- Absent MIB1

## CLINICAL ISSUES

### Presentation
- Most common signs/symptoms
  - Intractable seizures, headaches (particularly sporadic)
  - Often incidental (particularly NF2)

### Demographics
- Age: Children, young adults
- Gender: M > F

### Natural History & Prognosis
- Excellent with excision

### Treatment
- Surgery

## DIAGNOSTIC CHECKLIST

### Consider
- Leptomeningeal/cortical enhancement in patient with seizures, especially if NF2

### Image Interpretation Pearls
- Relatively little mass effect given size

## SELECTED REFERENCES

1. Kim NR et al: Childhood meningiomas associated with meningioangiomatosis: report of five cases and literature review. Neuropathol Appl Neurobiol. 28(1):48-56, 2002
2. Moreno A et al: Neuronal and mixed neuronal glial tumors associated to epilepsy. A heterogeneous and related group of tumours. Histol Histopathol. 16(2):613-22, 2001
3. Scroop R et al: Meningioangiomatosis. Australas Radiol. 44(4):460-3, 2000
4. Park MS et al: Multifocal meningioangiomatosis: a report of two cases. AJNR Am J Neuroradiol. 20(4):677-80, 1999

## IMAGE GALLERY

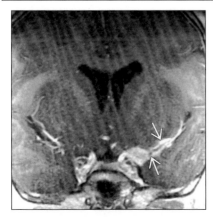
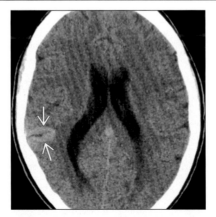
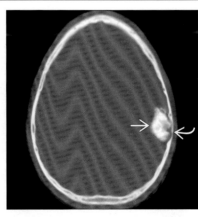

*(Left)* Coronal T1 C+ MR shows enhancement ➡ of the leptomeninges and in the subarachnoid space along the left Sylvian fissure. *(Center)* Axial NECT shows mildly increased attenuation ➡ localized to the cortex of a single gyrus. This increased attenuation was found to represent calcification. *(Right)* Axial NECT shows dense calcification ➡ just deep to the inner table of the left parietal bone. Note the significant scalloping ➡ of the adjacent inner table.

# DERMOID AND EPIDERMOID CYSTS

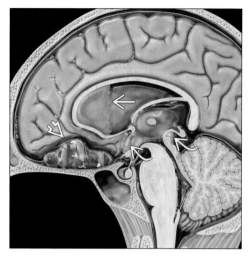

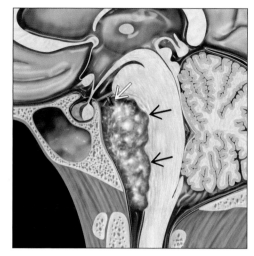

*Sagittal graphic shows complex dermoid → on planum sphenoidale, with fat globules → and fat-fluid levels → in the cisterns and ventricles, due to rupture.*

*Sagittal graphic shows a pre-pontine epidermoid cyst. Note encasement of basilar artery →, and irregular interface → with brainstem. Intracranial epidermoids are rare in children.*

## TERMINOLOGY

### Abbreviations and Synonyms
- Ectodermal inclusion cyst, cholesteatoma, epidermal inclusion cyst, dermolipoma
- (Epi)dermoid ⇔ epidermoid and dermoid

### Definitions
- Dermoids and epidermoids are inclusions of ectodermal tissue within the central nervous system (CNS)
- Epidermoids consist of squamous epithelium
- Dermoids contain squamous epithelium and associated dermal appendages
  - Sebaceous glands, dental enamel, hair follicles

## IMAGING FINDINGS

### General Features
- Best diagnostic clue
  - Dermoid ⇒ fat signal/attenuation droplets in cisterns, sulci, ventricles if ruptured

- Epidermoid ⇒ cerebrospinal fluid (CSF)-like mass that envelops vessels and nerves
- Location
  - Dermoids most commonly found in suprasellar and frontonasal regions
    - Less commonly in posterior fossa, midline vermis & 4th ventricle
  - Epidermoids most commonly found in cerebellopontine angle (CPA), around 4th ventricle, parasellar
  - Both can be found in association with closure defects of neural tube
    - Acquired lesions from trauma, lumbar puncture (LP)
  - Orbit ⇒ "dermolipoma" at zygomatico-frontal suture line
  - Subgaleal dermoids are occasionally found at anterior fontanelle or at osseous sutures
- Morphology
  - Dermoids ⇒ usually well-circumscribed
  - Epidermoids ⇒ more amorphous

### CT Findings
- NECT

## DDx: Cystic Intracranial Masses in Children

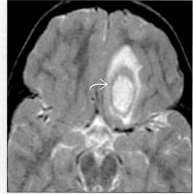

*Abscess*

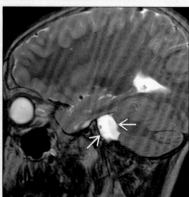

*Arachnoid Cyst*

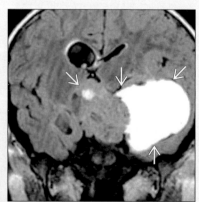

*Craniopharyngioma*

# DERMOID AND EPIDERMOID CYSTS

## Key Facts

### Terminology
- Dermoids and epidermoids are inclusions of ectodermal tissue within the central nervous system (CNS)
- Epidermoids consist of squamous epithelium
- Dermoids contain squamous epithelium and associated dermal appendages

### Imaging Findings
- Dermoids typically hyperintense on T1WI
- Epidermoids only slightly hyperintense to CSF on T1WI
- Epidermoids hyperintense on FLAIR; obvious distinction from CSF
- (Epi)dermoids ⇒ minimal marginal enhancement or none at all

### Top Differential Diagnoses
- Craniopharyngioma
- Arachnoid Cyst
- Lipoma

### Pathology
- Rare lesions: < 1% of primary intracranial tumors
- Although more common in adults, intracranial epidermoids are less common in pediatric population

### Diagnostic Checklist
- Contrast-enhancement distinguishes suprasellar dermoid from craniopharyngioma
- Striated appearance classic for dermoid
- Epidermoids easily distinguished from arachnoid cysts with MR

---

- ○ Dermoids have striking fat density on NECT ⇒ mimics air
  - With rupture, fat disseminates as globules in cisterns, may ⇒ fat-fluid level within ventricles
  - Ca++ in 20%
  - Skull/scalp dermoid expands diploe
- ○ Epidermoids usually resemble CSF on NECT
  - Ca++ in 10-25%
- ○ Rare dense dermoid/epidermoid is hyperattenuating on CT
- CECT: Generally no enhancement

### MR Findings
- T1WI
  - ○ Dermoids typically hyperintense on T1WI
    - Not as uniformly bright as lipomas
    - Heterogeneous, with a striated appearance
    - Go "dark" with fat suppression, but not as cleanly as lipoma
    - Droplets from rupture rise to non-dependent regions (frontal horns, convexities) and appear as fat-fluid levels
  - ○ Epidermoids only slightly hyperintense to CSF on T1WI
    - Mimic complex arachnoid cyst
    - Small septations or lobules may be visible
    - "White" epidermoids ⇒ hyperintense to brain (rare)
- T2WI
  - ○ Dermoids typically heterogeneous
    - Striated or "layered" appearance more easily seen
    - Chemical shift artifact in frequency encoding direction
    - Rare "dense" posterior fossa dermoid: Very hypointense
  - ○ Epidermoids iso- to hyperintense to CSF
    - Rare "dense" epidermoid: Very hypointense
- FLAIR
  - ○ Epidermoids hyperintense on FLAIR; obvious distinction from CSF
    - Easy distinction on proton density, constructive interference in steady-state (CISS) sequences also
- DWI

- ○ (Epi)dermoids have reduced diffusion
  - Distinction of epidermoid from CSF easier on DWI than on ADC image
- T1 C+
  - ○ (Epi)dermoids ⇒ minimal marginal enhancement or none at all
  - ○ Exception ⇒ ruptured dermoid will cause chemical ventriculitis and ependymal enhancement
- MRA: Vessels encased by epidermoid may be narrowed
- MRS: (Epi)dermoids show very strong and broad resonances from mobile lipids at 0.9 and 1.3 ppm

### Radiographic Findings
- Sutural dermoids often incidentally seen on skull radiographs as small lucencies at base of coronal suture or at zygomatico-frontal suture line

### Non-Vascular Interventions
- Cisternography can be used to distinguish epidermoid from arachnoid cyst
  - ○ Lobular "cauliflower-like" surface of epidermoid becomes apparent
  - ○ FLAIR/CISS/DWI have made cisternography unnecessary

### Imaging Recommendations
- Best imaging tool: MR, especially in setting of rupture
- Protocol advice
  - ○ Use fat suppression, DWI, and FLAIR
  - ○ Look for chemical shift artifact, especially with rupture

## DIFFERENTIAL DIAGNOSIS

### Craniopharyngioma
- Can have nearly identical imaging characteristics as suprasellar dermoid
  - ○ Difference is in nature of cells lining walls
- Distinguishing characteristic ⇒ enhancement in over 90%
- Much more common than dermoid

# DERMOID AND EPIDERMOID CYSTS

## Arachnoid Cyst
- Myth ⇒ arachnoid cysts and epidermoids can be identical
- Similar, but epidermoids always have more "character" of signal
- Much more common than epidermoids, except in spine

## Lipoma
- Fatty signal/attenuation more homogeneous
- Ca++ less frequent than in dermoids
- Similar etiology ⇒ mesodermal "inclusion"

## Teratoma
- Germ cell tumor that contains two or more embryologic layers
- Pituitary and pineal region
- Usually has enhancing components

## Abscess
- Can resemble dermoid on pre-contrast imaging
- Similar restricted diffusion
- Ring-enhancement and edema easily distinguished

## PATHOLOGY

### General Features
- General path comments
  - Rare dense dermoids have been reported in posterior fossa
    - Thought to result from saponification of lipid/keratinized debris
  - Although temporal bone epidermoids (cholesteatoma) will erode bone, intracranial lesions accommodate to surrounding structures
- Etiology
  - Inclusion of cutaneous ectoderm during neural tube closure
  - Acquired ⇒ displacement of epithelium into CNS during LP, trauma, surgery
- Epidemiology
  - Rare lesions: < 1% of primary intracranial tumors
  - Although more common in adults, intracranial epidermoids are less common in pediatric population
- Associated abnormalities
  - Dermal sinuses (> 50% associated with inclusion cysts)
  - Goldenhar syndrome (a.k.a. oculoauriculovertebral dysplasia)

### Gross Pathologic & Surgical Features
- Dermoids contain a mixture of greasy lipid, cholesterol debris
  - Often contain hair and may contain enamel
- Epidermoids often have shiny "mother of pearl" appearance to surface
  - Cyst contents ⇒ soft, waxy flaky material

### Microscopic Features
- Dermoid ⇒ outer wall of fibrous connective tissue, inner lining of keratinized squamous epithelium, dermal appendages
  - Desquamated keratin, cellular debris in cyst
- Epidermoid ⇒ wall of simple stratified cuboidal squamous epithelium
  - Solid crystalline cholesterol, keratin in cyst

## CLINICAL ISSUES

### Presentation
- Most common signs/symptoms
  - Dermoid: Headache, seizure
    - Rupture ⇒ acute severe headache, collapse
    - Causes chemical meningitis
  - Epidermoid: Headache, cranial nerve neuropathies
    - Chemical meningitis rare
- Other signs/symptoms: Hypopituitarism, diabetes insipidus, visual symptoms

### Demographics
- Age
  - Both lesions more commonly diagnosed in adults
    - Exception ⇒ periorbital/sutural dermoids

### Natural History & Prognosis
- Slowly growing, often asymptomatic
- Dermoid rupture can cause significant morbidity/mortality
- Dermoid + dermal sinus may cause infection
- Rare malignant transformation into squamous cell carcinoma (adults)

### Treatment
- Complete microsurgical excision
  - Residual capsule may lead to recurrence
  - Subarachnoid dissemination of contents may occur

## DIAGNOSTIC CHECKLIST

### Image Interpretation Pearls
- Contrast-enhancement distinguishes suprasellar dermoid from craniopharyngioma
- Striated appearance classic for dermoid
- Epidermoids easily distinguished from arachnoid cysts with MR
  - Use FLAIR, DWI, MRS, CISS

## SELECTED REFERENCES

1. Bonneville F et al: T1 signal hyperintensity in the sellar region: spectrum of findings. Radiographics. 26(1):93-113, 2006
2. Hashiguchi K et al: Subgaleal dermoid tumors at the anterior fontanelle. Pediatr Neurosurg. 41(1):54-7, 2005
3. Caldarelli M et al: Intracranial midline dermoid and epidermoid cysts in children. J Neurosurg. 100(5 Suppl Pediatrics):473-80, 2004
4. Brown JY et al: Unusual imaging appearance of an intracranial dermoid cyst. AJNR Am J Neuroradiol. 22(10):1970-2, 2001
5. Martinez-Lage JF et al: Extradural dermoid tumours of the posterior fossa. Arch Dis Child. 77(5):427-30, 1997
6. Higashi S et al: Occipital dermal sinus associated with dermoid cyst in the fourth ventricle. AJNR Am J Neuroradiol. 16(4 Suppl):945-8, 1995

# DERMOID AND EPIDERMOID CYSTS

## IMAGE GALLERY

### Typical

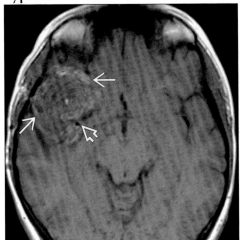
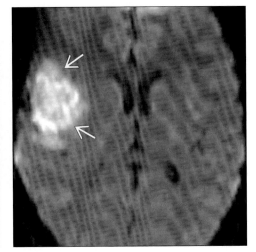

*(Left)* Axial T1WI MR shows the heterogeneous striated signal ➡ characteristic of a dermoid. The extraparenchymal tumor displaces the branches of the right middle cerebral artery ⇨. *(Right)* Axial DWI MR (same lesion as previous image) shows it to be hyperintense ➡. DWI is one of several MR sequences that help to distinguish dermoids and epidermoids from other cystic intracranial masses.

### Typical

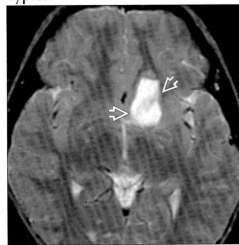
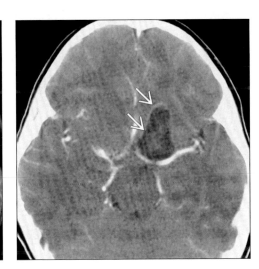

*(Left)* Axial T2WI MR shows an epidermoid tumor ⇨ situated at the base of the left frontal lobe. Epidermoids are more homogeneous than dermoids and do not contain fat. *(Right)* Axial CECT (same lesion as previous image). Note displacement of adjacent vessel ➡ and the sharply defined walls that give a clue to the extraparenchymal location of the mass.

### Typical

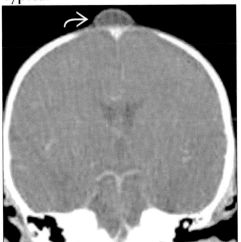
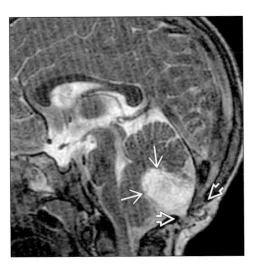

*(Left)* Coronal CECT shows a subgaleal dermoid ➡ situated at the anterior fontanelle, a very common location. Surgical excision of these lesions is readily performed and curative. *(Right)* Sagittal T2WI MR shows a heterogeneous dermoid ➡ extending from a defect in the occipital bone ⇨ into the vermis. Superficial tracts are seen more in dermoids than epidermoids.

I
6
39

# NEUROBLASTOMA, METASTATIC

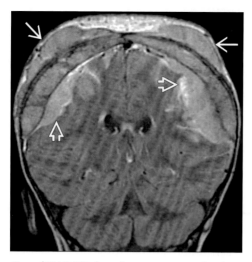

Coronal FLAIR MR shows large masses extending down into the cranium ⟹ and out into the scalp ⟹ from expanded parietal bones in this child with widely metastatic neuroblastoma.

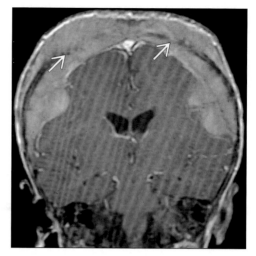

Coronal T1 C+ MR (same infant as previous) shows contiguity of the process ⟹ from the subcutaneous space through bone into the extradural (and sometimes subdural) spaces.

## TERMINOLOGY

### Abbreviations and Synonyms
- NBL, NBT, neuroblastic tumors (NT)

### Definitions
- Malignant tumor of the sympathetic nervous system arising from primordial neural crest cell derivatives

## IMAGING FINDINGS

### General Features
- Best diagnostic clue: Spiculated periorbital bone expansion in a child with "raccoon eyes"
- Location
  - Nearly always extradural calvarial-based mass
  - Often around orbit and sphenoid wings
  - Intra-axial lesions rare
- Size: Variable
- Morphology: Crescentic or lenticular, following contour of bone
- Classic imaging appearance
  - "Hair-on-end" spiculated periostitis of orbits & skull

### CT Findings
- NECT
  - NECT best modality for demonstrating fine spicules of periosteal bone projecting off skull or sphenoid wings
  - Soft tissue mass isodense to hyperdense relative to brain
    - Mimics epidural or subdural hematomas
  - May project through both inner and outer tables of skull
- CECT: Soft tissue masses enhance vigorously

### MR Findings
- T1WI
  - Slightly heterogeneous
  - Isointense to gray matter
- T2WI
  - Heterogeneous
  - Hypointense to brain
- PD/Intermediate
  - Heterogeneous
  - Iso- and hypointense to brain
- FLAIR
  - Heterogeneous

## DDx: Dural-Based Masses

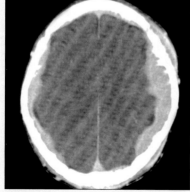

Leukemia

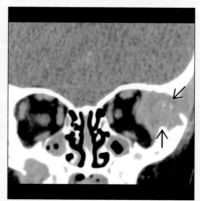

Langerhans Cell Histiocytosis

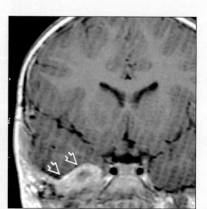

Ewing Sarcoma

# NEUROBLASTOMA, METASTATIC

## Key Facts

### Terminology
- Malignant tumor of the sympathetic nervous system arising from primordial neural crest cell derivatives

### Imaging Findings
- "Hair-on-end" spiculated periostitis of orbits & skull
- NECT best modality for demonstrating fine spicules of periosteal bone projecting off skull or sphenoid wings
- May project through both inner and outer tables of skull
- Bone scan essential for differentiating stage IV disease from stage IV-S in children < 1 year
- FDG-PET may identify recurrence when MIBG is negative due to de-differentiation

### Top Differential Diagnoses
- Leukemia
- Langerhans Cell Histiocytosis (LCH)
- Extra-Axial Hematoma

### Pathology
- 35% of primary neuroblastomas have deletion of distal short arm of chromosome 1
- Most common solid extracranial tumor in childhood
- 8-10% of all childhood cancer
- Calvarial metastases indicate Stage IV disease

### Clinical Issues
- Ocular involvement in 20% at presentation (poor prognostic indicator)
- Median age diagnosis = 22 months

---

- o Hyperintense to brain
- T2* GRE: Hypointense
- T1 C+: Vigorously enhances
- MRV: Assess effect of tumor upon dural sinuses

## Radiographic Findings
- Radiography
  - o Cranial suture widening
  - o Periosteal new bone

## Nuclear Medicine Findings
- PET
  - o FDG-PET imaging has shown high sensitivity and specificity for recurrent tumor in small numbers of cases
  - o FDG-PET may identify recurrence when MIBG is negative due to de-differentiation
- Bone Scan
  - o Meta-iodobenzylguanidine (MIBG)
    - Avid uptake by neural crest tumors
    - Labeled with iodine-131 or iodine-123
    - 85-95% sensitivity in detecting NBT, 100% specificity
  - o Tc-99m-MDP (methylene diphosphonate)
    - Distinguishes bony from marrow disease
    - Bone scan essential for differentiating stage IV disease from stage IV-S in children < 1 year

## Imaging Recommendations
- Best imaging tool
  - o CT/MR to evaluate primary tumor
  - o Nuclear medicine MIBG scan and Tc-99m-MDP bone scan
  - o Brain/orbit CT performed if nuclear medicine studies indicate disease
- Protocol advice: MR with contrast and fat-saturation technique complementary to CT

## DIFFERENTIAL DIAGNOSIS

### Leukemia
- Dural or calvarial based masses

- More frequent parenchymal masses
- Less heterogeneous on MR

### Langerhans Cell Histiocytosis (LCH)
- Lytic bone lesions without periosteal new bone
- Often accompanied by diabetes insipidus

### Extra-Axial Hematoma
- Subdural or epidural hematoma
- Bleeding disorder or child abuse to be considered

### Ewing Sarcoma
- < 1% of cases involve skull
- Aggressive bone destruction
- Spiculated periosteal reaction

### Osteosarcoma
- Rarely primary in calvarium

### Beta Thalassemia Major
- Diffuse "hair-on-end" calvarial expansion
- Not focal or destructive like NBL

## PATHOLOGY

### General Features
- General path comments
  - o Small round blue cell tumor
  - o NBL is the most common and aggressive of the neuroblastic tumors
    - Ganglioneuroblastoma: Malignant
    - Ganglioneuroma: Benign tumor of mature ganglion cells
  - o Embryology-anatomy
    - Primitive neural crest cell origin
    - Arise at sites of sympathetic ganglia
- Genetics
  - o 35% of primary neuroblastomas have deletion of distal short arm of chromosome 1
  - o Multiple other gene loci have been associated
    - Most important chromosomal marker is MYCN oncogene on chromosome 2

# NEUROBLASTOMA, METASTATIC

○ High association with chromosome 17 translocations
○ 1-2% of cases inherited
- Etiology: Arise from pathologically maturing neural crest progenitor cells
- Epidemiology
  ○ Most common solid extracranial tumor in childhood
  ○ 8-10% of all childhood cancer
- Associated abnormalities
  ○ Some association with neurocristopathy syndromes
  ○ Beckwith-Wiedemann syndrome (uncommon)

## Gross Pathologic & Surgical Features
- Well-demarcated gray-tan soft nodules without capsule
- Calcifications

## Microscopic Features
- Undifferentiated round blue cells with scant cytoplasm and hyperchromatic nuclei
- Ganglioneuroblastoma has interspersed mature ganglion cells
  ○ Different regions of same tumor may have ganglioneuroblastoma or NBL

## Staging, Grading or Classification Criteria
- Calvarial metastases indicate Stage IV disease
- Evans anatomic staging system
  ○ Stage I: Confined to organ of interest (13.5%)
  ○ Stage II: Extension beyond organ but not crossing midline (11%)
  ○ Stage III: Extension crossing midline (include vertebral column) (8.4%)
  ○ Stage IV: Systemic with widespread distal metastases (> 50%)
  ○ Stage IV-S: < 1 year at diagnosis, stage I plus metastatic disease confined to skin, liver, or bone marrow (7%)
    ■ May spontaneously regress

## CLINICAL ISSUES

### Presentation
- Most common signs/symptoms
  ○ "Raccoon eyes"
  ○ Palpable calvarial masses
- Other signs/symptoms
  ○ Opsoclonus, myoclonus, and ataxia (OMA)
    ■ Myoclonic encephalopathy of infancy (MEI)
    ■ Up to 4% of NBL patients
  ○ Elevated vasoactive intestinal peptides (VIP)
    ■ Diarrhea, hypokalemia, achlorhydria
  ○ Elevated homovanillic acid and vanillylmandelic acid in urine in > 90%
- Clinical Profile
  ○ Palpable abdominal or paraspinal mass
  ○ Cranial metastatic disease rarely occurs in isolation
  ○ Ocular involvement in 20% at presentation (poor prognostic indicator)
    ■ Bilateral periorbital discoloration/ecchymoses: "Raccoon eyes"
    ■ Horner syndrome

## Demographics
- Age
  ○ Median age diagnosis = 22 months
  ○ 40% < 1 year
  ○ 35% 1-2 years
  ○ 25% > 2 years
- Gender: M:F = 1.2:1

## Natural History & Prognosis
- 5 year survival
  ○ 83% for infants < 1
  ○ 55% for children 1-5
  ○ 40% for children > 5
- Good prognostic indicators: Localized disease, stage IV-S, ↓ n-myc gene amplification
- Bad prognostic indicators: Stage IV disease, ocular involvement, chromosome 1 deletion

## Treatment
- Stage IV-S may not require treatment: Follow for spontaneous regression
- Surgical resection
- Chemotherapy
- Bone marrow transplant
- Targeted 131I-MIBG therapy

## DIAGNOSTIC CHECKLIST

### Consider
- Abdominal imaging to identify primary tumor site

### Image Interpretation Pearls
- CT without contrast can help identify bone spicules, eliminating LCH from differential

## SELECTED REFERENCES

1. Papaioannou G et al: Neuroblastoma in childhood: review and radiological findings. Cancer Imaging. 5:116-27, 2005
2. Barai S et al: Does I-131-MIBG underestimate skeletal disease burden in neuroblastoma? J Postgrad Med. 50(4):257-60; discussion 260-1, 2004
3. Levitt GA et al: 4S neuroblastoma: the long-term outcome. Pediatr Blood Cancer. 43(2):120-5, 2004
4. Scanga DR et al: Value of FDG PET imaging in the management of patients with thyroid, neuroendocrine, and neural crest tumors. Clin Nucl Med. 29(2):86-90, 2004
5. Jaing TH et al: Brain metastases in children with neuroblastoma--a single-institution experience. Med Pediatr Oncol. 41(6):570-1, 2003
6. Matthay KK et al: Central nervous system metastases in neuroblastoma: radiologic, clinical, and biologic features in 23 patients. Cancer. 98(1):155-65, 2003
7. Pfluger T et al: Integrated imaging using MRI and 123I metaiodobenzylguanidine scintigraphy to improve sensitivity and specificity in the diagnosis of pediatric neuroblastoma. AJR Am J Roentgenol. 181(4):1115-24, 2003
8. Lonergan GJ et al: Neuroblastoma, ganglioneuroblastoma, and ganglioneuroma: radiologic-pathologic correlation. Radiographics. 22(4):911-34, 2002
9. Okuyama C et al: Utility of follow-up studies using meta-[123 I]iodobenzylguanidine scintigraphy for detecting recurrent neuroblastoma. Nucl Med Commun. 23(7):663-72, 2002

# NEUROBLASTOMA, METASTATIC

## IMAGE GALLERY

### Typical

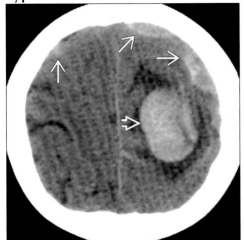
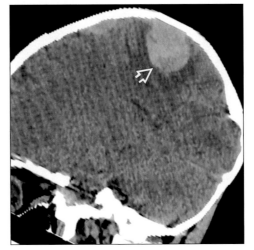

*(Left)* Axial NECT in a child with stage IV neuroblastoma shows multiple dural metastases ➡ with the dominant mass ⬧ extending into the brain parenchyma, eliciting edema. *(Right)* Sagittal NECT (same child as previous) shows that the dominant lesion ➡ is still extra-axial. These tumors may invade brain parenchyma, but true intra-axial metastases are quite rare.

### Typical

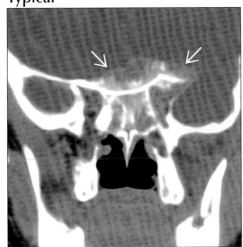
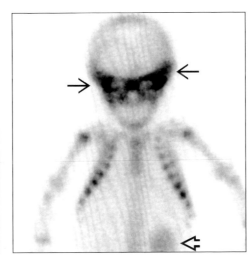

*(Left)* Coronal NECT shows metastatic neuroblastoma infiltrating and expanding the sphenoid bone, with spiculated new bone ➡ radiating out from the cortical surface. *(Right)* Anteroposterior bone scan shows extensive skull base uptake ➡ from metastatic neuroblastoma, as well as multiple rib metastases. Note uptake in primary left adrenal tumor ⬧.

### Typical

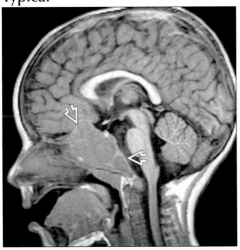
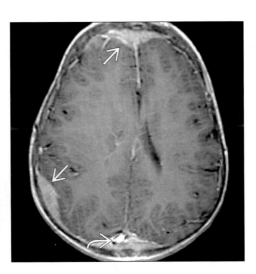

*(Left)* Sagittal T1WI MR shows marked expansion and abnormal signal throughout the clivus ⬧ in this 2 year old with stage IV disease. *(Right)* Axial T1 C+ MR shows multiple extradural metastases ➡. Note how the posterior lesion elevates the sagittal sinus ➡ off of the calvarial margin without compression.

# EXTRAMEDULLARY HEMATOPOIESIS, BRAIN

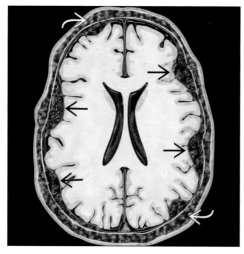

Axial graphic shows increased red marrow diffusely within the diploic space ➡. Multiple regions of hematopoietic tissue ⤇ are present in the intracranial space, displacing brain.

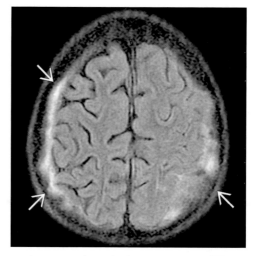

Axial FLAIR MR shows dural/subdural infiltrates ➡ with high FLAIR signal, consistent with EMH in child with chronic anemia and myelosclerosis. Note mass effect on left hemisphere.

## TERMINOLOGY

### Abbreviations and Synonyms
- EMH; extramedullary erythropoiesis

### Definitions
- Compensatory formation of blood elements due to decreased medullary hematopoiesis

## IMAGING FINDINGS

### General Features
- Best diagnostic clue: Juxta-osseous smooth homogeneous masses in patients with chronic anemias or marrow depletion
- Location: Dural/epidural, skull and spine

### CT Findings
- NECT
  - CT: Smooth homogeneous isodense masses
    - Mimics subdural hematoma
  - May show osseous findings of underlying disease
  - Soft tissue filling paranasal sinus(es)
- CECT: Homogeneous enhancement

### MR Findings
- T1WI: Iso- to slightly hyperintense to cortex
- T2WI: Slightly hypointense to cortex
- FLAIR: No underlying parenchymal edema
- T1 C+: Homogeneous enhancement

### Nuclear Medicine Findings
- Uptake by Tc-99m sulfur colloid

### Imaging Recommendations
- Best imaging tool: Contrast-enhanced MR
- Protocol advice: Contrast always

## DIFFERENTIAL DIAGNOSIS

### Pericerebral Collections
- Subdural hematoma: Trauma history, does not enhance (but subdural fibrosis does)
- Empyema: Infectious context

### Epidural Tumors, Other Hemopathies
- Infiltrative, skull invasion

## DDx: Other Pericerebral Lesions

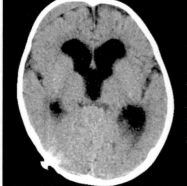

Isodense Subdural Hematoma

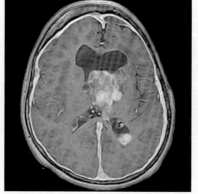

Subdural Fibrosis

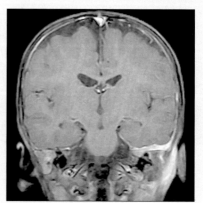

Acute Leukemia

# EXTRAMEDULLARY HEMATOPOIESIS, BRAIN

## Key Facts

### Terminology
- Compensatory formation of blood elements due to decreased medullary hematopoiesis

### Imaging Findings
- CT: Smooth homogeneous isodense masses
- Mimics subdural hematoma
- T1WI: Iso- to slightly hyperintense to cortex
- T2WI: Slightly hypointense to cortex
- T1 C+: Homogeneous enhancement

- Best imaging tool: Contrast-enhanced MR

### Top Differential Diagnoses
- Pericerebral Collections
- Epidural Tumors, Other Hemopathies

### Diagnostic Checklist
- EMH in unexplained SDH-appearing lesion in child with anemia

## PATHOLOGY

### General Features
- General path comments
  - Primarily in patients with congenital hemoglobinopathies
    - Thalassemia, sickle cell disease, hereditary spherocytosis, hemorrhagic thrombocytopenia
  - May be seen in any myelosclerosis
- Etiology
  - May be secondary to depleted, infiltrated or hyperactive bone marrow
  - After granulocyte-colony stimulating factor therapy
  - Occasionally no etiology found
- Epidemiology: Rare

### Microscopic Features
- Hematogenous stem cell spread

## CLINICAL ISSUES

### Presentation
- Most common signs/symptoms: Seizures; cranial nerve deficit(s); ↑ intracranial pressure
- Clinical Profile: Hemolytic anemia

### Demographics
- Age: Generally adult, may be seen in young individuals

### Natural History & Prognosis
- Most dependent on primary underlying disease, focal compression possible

### Treatment
- Low-dose radiotherapy, surgical resection

## DIAGNOSTIC CHECKLIST

### Consider
- EMH in unexplained SDH-appearing lesion in child with anemia

### Image Interpretation Pearls
- Contrast-enhancement

## SELECTED REFERENCES

1. Koch CA et al: Nonhepatosplenic extramedullary hematopoiesis: associated diseases, pathology, clinical course, and treatment. Mayo Clin Proc. 78(10):1223-33, 2003
2. Chourmouzi D et al: MRI findings of extramedullary haemopoiesis. Eur Radiol. 11(9):1803-6, 2001
3. Aydingoz U et al: Spinal cord compression due to epidural extramedullary haematopoiesis in thalassaemia: MRI. Neuroradiology. 39(12):870-2, 1997
4. Dibbern DA Jr et al: MR of thoracic cord compression caused by epidural extramedullary hematopoiesis in myelodysplastic syndrome. AJNR Am J Neuroradiol. 18(2):363-6, 1997

## IMAGE GALLERY

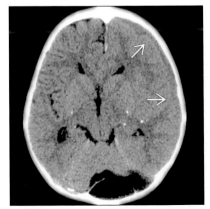 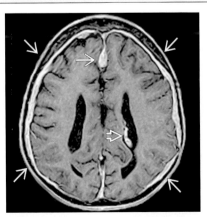 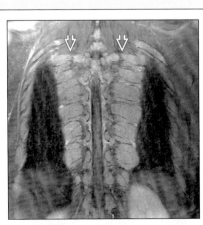

*(Left)* Axial NECT shows isodense subdural "collection" overlying left hemisphere ➡ in child with brain Ca++, callosal dysgenesis and chronic anemia. Surgery disclosed unsuspected EMH. *(Center)* Axial T1 C+ MR shows dural/subdural enhancement ➡ consistent with EMH in child with chronic anemia and myelodysplasia. Note enlarged choroid plexus as well ➡. *(Right)* Coronal T1 C+ FS MR of spine shows diffuse, massive costo-vertebral EMH ➡ in child with thalassemia intermedia; masses extended into spinal canal in epidural space.

# ENCEPHALOCELES

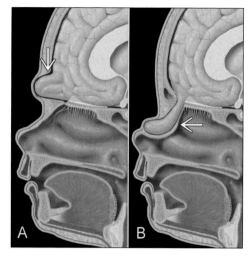

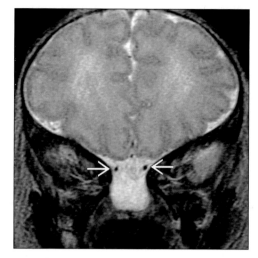

Sagittal graphic images of the two varieties of sincipital encephalocele; the frontonasal (A) extends into the glabella ➡, while the nasoethmoidal (B) projects into the nasal cavity ➡.

Coronal T2WI MR shows a sphenoethmoidal encephalocele projecting inferiorly into the posterior nasopharynx. Note the anterior cerebral arteries at the lateral margins of the defect ➡.

## TERMINOLOGY

### Abbreviations and Synonyms
- Cephalocele, meningocele, meningoencephalocele, gliocele

### Definitions
- Congenital herniation of one or more intracranial structures through a defect in the skull
  - Meningocele ⇒ herniation of meninges and cerebrospinal fluid (CSF)
  - Meningoencephalocele ⇒ meninges, CSF, and brain
  - Atretic parietal cephalocele (APC) ⇒ meninges, fibrous tissue
  - Gliocele ⇒ CSF-filled glial-lined cyst

## IMAGING FINDINGS

### General Features
- Best diagnostic clue: Cranial defect with mass projecting through it and distortion of subjacent brain parenchyma
- Location

- Nearly always midline
- Occipito-cervical (Chiari 3), occipital, parietal, frontonasal, fronto-ethmoidal, spheno-maxillary, spheno-orbital, nasopharyngeal
  - Sincipital encephaloceles ⇒ frontonasal and fronto-ethmoidal
- Size: APCs are flat, some lesions are larger than entire cranium

### CT Findings
- CTA
  - CTA/CTV single best modality to demonstrate vascular and bony anatomy around defect
    - Ideal for surgical planning
    - Clearly defines relationship of dural sinuses to skull defect
    - Clearly demonstrates displacement of vascular structures into encephalocele
  - Complementary with MR
- NECT
  - Distortion of brain morphology
    - Posterior (occipital, occipito-cervical) encephaloceles cause morphology similar to the Chiari 2 malformation

## DDx: Congenital Facial Masses

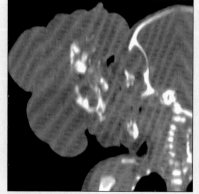

Teratoma

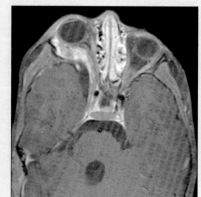

Neurofibromatosis

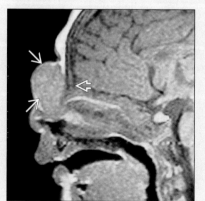

Nasal Glioma

# ENCEPHALOCELES

## Key Facts

### Terminology
- Congenital herniation of one or more intracranial structures through a defect in the skull
- Meningocele ⇒ herniation of meninges and cerebrospinal fluid (CSF)
- Meningoencephalocele ⇒ meninges, CSF, and brain
- Atretic parietal cephalocele (APC) ⇒ meninges, fibrous tissue

### Imaging Findings
- Posterior (occipital, occipito-cervical) encephaloceles cause morphology similar to the Chiari 2 malformation
- Use caution in evaluating the cribriform plate in infants
- CTA/CTV single best modality to demonstrate vascular and bony anatomy around defect

- Clearly demonstrates displacement of vascular structures into encephalocele
- Single best sequence for definition of encephalocele in neonate
- Sagittal thin profile imaging is key
- Best imaging tool: MR and CTA are complementary tools in evaluation of encephaloceles

### Pathology
- Occipital lesions are the most common in North America and Europe: 80%
- Fronto-ethmoidal lesions are more common in Southeast Asia

### Diagnostic Checklist
- Consider cryptic encephalocele when encountering recurrent meningitis

---

  - Microcephaly
    - Displaced neural tissue reduces volume of intracranial contents
  - Use caution in evaluating the cribriform plate in infants
    - Mostly cartilaginous at birth
    - Does not fully ossify until after 2 years of age

## MR Findings
- T1WI
  - Displacement of neural structures, vessels, ventricles into encephalocele
  - Bony margins may be difficult to resolve
- T2WI
  - Single best sequence for definition of encephalocele in neonate
    - Distinction of neural tissue from CSF and vessels more clear than T1WI
    - Key sequence for fetal MR imaging of encephaloceles
  - Sagittal thin profile imaging is key
  - Distinction of vascular structures from bone may be problematic (both hypointense)
  - APC ⇒ elevation of straight sinus and elongation of supra-vermian cistern
- T2* GRE: Can show hemorrhagic complications of delivery, surgery
- T1 C+: Key for differentiating nasopharyngeal tumors (they enhance) from nasopharyngeal encephaloceles (they don't)
- MRA
  - Can show vascular anatomy, displacement of arteries into encephalocele
  - Sometimes limited in neonate by rapid or turbulent flow, small vessel size
- MRV
  - Can show vascular anatomy, displacement of veins into encephalocele
  - Sometimes limited in neonate by rapid or turbulent flow, small vessel size

## Radiographic Findings
- Radiography: Midline skull defect of variable size

## Ultrasonographic Findings
- Large lesions characteristically identified in utero
  - Occipito-cervical encephalocele can mimic cystic hygroma
- Further evaluation with fetal MR may be warranted

## Non-Vascular Interventions
- Cisternography with CT
  - Sometimes used in inferior-anterior lesions (fronto-ethmoidal, nasopharyngeal) to assess contiguity of sac with subarachnoid space
    - Chance of false-negative if flow is intermittent
    - Need to keep head/face down after instillation of contrast
    - Low volumes of iso-osmolar water soluble agent

## Imaging Recommendations
- Best imaging tool: MR and CTA are complementary tools in evaluation of encephaloceles
- Protocol advice
  - Studies may need to be performed in unusual positions in neonates with large lesions who cannot lie supine
    - Volumetric (3D) acquisitions key for sorting out anatomy
  - Thin slice T2WI can define relationship of defect to remaining intracranial contents
  - CTA is ideal for demonstrating relationship of dural sinuses to bony defect
    - Sinus is frequently located right along margin of bone defect
    - Vascular/osseous anatomy more clearly shown than with MRV/MRA

---

## DIFFERENTIAL DIAGNOSIS

### Nasal Dermoid
- Intracranial involvement in 25%
  - Wide foramen cecum, bifid cristae galli
- DWI: Restricted diffusion (best sign)
- May have associated sinus tract

# ENCEPHALOCELES

## Capillary Hemangioma of Infancy
- Most common pediatric frontonasal mass, strawberry
- Faint macular stain ("stork bite") ⇒ rapid postnatal growth
- Can also occur along sagittal suture
  - Mimic of APC

## Nasal Glioma
- "Encephaloceles that have lost their intracranial connection"
- Persistent fibrovascular stalk in 15-20%
- Mixed signal intensity, variable enhancement

## Nasopharyngeal Neoplasms
- Rhabdomyosarcoma, lymphoma, nasopharyngeal carcinoma
- Juvenile nasopharyngeal angiofibroma, nasopharyngeal teratoma
- Nearly all enhance ⇒ easily distinguished on MR

## Orbital Neurofibroma and Sphenoid Defect in NF1
- Mimics orbito-frontal encephalocele
- Pulsatile exophthalmos

## Posterior Skull/Scalp Tumors
- Angiosarcoma, osteosarcoma ⇒ enhance strongly, bone destruction

## PATHOLOGY

### General Features
- General path comments: Occasionally reported with amniotic banding syndrome
- Etiology: Disturbed separation of surface ectoderm and neuroectoderm in midline after closure of neural folds (4th gestational week)
- Epidemiology
  - Occipital lesions are the most common in North America and Europe: 80%
  - Fronto-ethmoidal lesions are more common in Southeast Asia
    - 1:5,000 live births (1:35,000 live births North America)
- Associated abnormalities
  - High association with midline face and brain anomalies
  - Parietal, occipital ⇒ Chiari 2, Dandy-Walker, callosal dysgenesis
  - Nasopharyngeal ⇒ 80% callosal dysgenesis

### Gross Pathologic & Surgical Features
- Variable amounts of fibrotic, gliotic, dysplastic tissue in sac

## CLINICAL ISSUES

### Presentation
- Most common signs/symptoms
  - Occipital, parietal ⇒ clinically obvious mass
  - Fronto-ethmoidal ⇒ nasal stuffiness, nasal mass, nasal pit (dermal sinus)

- Midline facial features typical: Hypertelorism, broad nasal bridge
  - Nasopharyngeal ⇒ nasopharyngeal mass, obligatory mouth-breathing, nasal stuffiness
  - APC ⇒ hairless patch or scab
- Other signs/symptoms
  - Recurrent meningitis
  - Neurologic deficit, seizure, developmental delay (from associated malformation)

### Demographics
- Ethnicity
  - Anterior lesions much more common in Asia
  - Occipital lesions much more common in Europeans

### Natural History & Prognosis
- Worse prognosis with large amount of herniated tissue
- Worse prognosis in presence of other intracranial anomalies

### Treatment
- Surgery: Combined approach with ENT, plastic surgery and neurosurgery

## DIAGNOSTIC CHECKLIST

### Consider
- Consider cryptic encephalocele when encountering recurrent meningitis
- Don't forget encephalocele when considering ethmoid mucocele on CT

### Image Interpretation Pearls
- Use CTA and MR together for pre-surgical definition of lesions

## SELECTED REFERENCES

1. Garg P et al: CSF Rhinorrhea and recurrent meningitis caused by transethmoidal meningoencephaloceles. Indian Pediatr. 42(10):1033-6, 2005
2. Agrawal D et al: Giant occipital encephalocele with microcephaly and micrognathia. Pediatr Neurosurg. 40(4):205-6, 2004
3. Moron FE et al: Lumps and bumps on the head in children: use of CT and MR imaging in solving the clinical diagnostic dilemma. Radiographics. 24(6):1655-74, 2004
4. Rahbar R et al: Nasal glioma and encephalocele: diagnosis and management. Laryngoscope. 113(12):2069-77, 2003
5. Formica F et al: Transsphenoidal meningoencephalocele. Childs Nerv Syst. 18(6-7):295-8, 2002
6. Mahapatra AK et al: Anterior encephaloceles: a study of 92 cases. Pediatr Neurosurg. 36(3):113-8, 2002
7. Schlosser RJ et al: Three-dimensional computed tomography of congenital nasal anomalies. Int J Pediatr Otorhinolaryngol. 65(2):125-31, 2002
8. Lowe LH et al: Midface anomalies in children. Radiographics. 20(4):907-22; quiz 1106-7, 1112, 2000
9. Patterson RJ et al: Atretic parietal cephaloceles revisited: an enlarging clinical and imaging spectrum? AJNR Am J Neuroradiol. 19(4):791-5, 1998
10. Both nasal cerebral heterotopia and encephalocele in the same patient: Cleft Palate Craniofac J. 2006 Jan;43(1):112-6.

# ENCEPHALOCELES

Typical

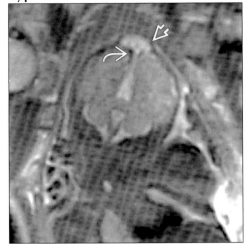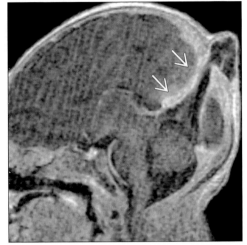

*(Left)* Coronal T2WI MR from a fetal study shows a small parietal encephalocele at the vertex ➡. Note that the lesion passes to the left of the sagittal sinus ➡. *(Right)* Sagittal T1 C+ MR shows a parietal encephalocele with elevation of the straight sinus ➡. Because this lesion contained only meninges and CSF, it is best termed a meningocele.

Typical

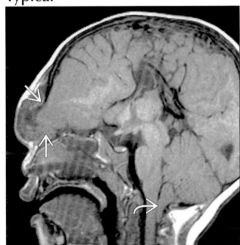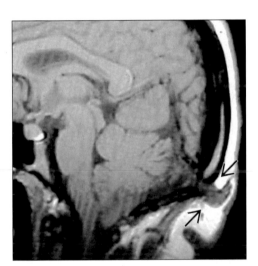

*(Left)* Sagittal T1WI MR of frontonasal encephalocele with brain tissue passing through persistent fonticulus frontalis between the frontal and nasal bones ➡. Note callosal agenesis and Chiari 1 ➡. *(Right)* Sagittal T1WI MR shows an atretic posterior cephalocele passing into the subcutaneous tissues through a defect in the superior occipital bone ➡.

Typical

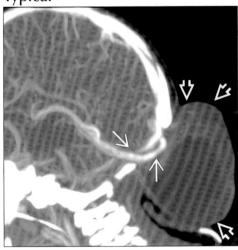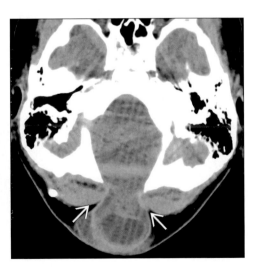

*(Left)* Sagittal reconstruction from a CTA study shows the flattened straight sinus ➡ passing through a defect in the occipital bone into an occipital meningoencephalocele ➡. *(Right)* Axial NECT shows herniation of meninges, CSF, and brain tissue into an occipitocervical meningoencephalocele, or Chiari 3 malformation ➡.

# ATRETIC CEPHALOCELE

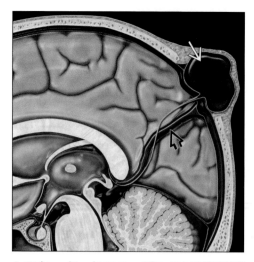

Sagittal graphic shows a midline sub-scalp atretic parietal cephalocele ➡. Note the vertically oriented persistent primitive falcine vein ⇨. The cranial defect is often small.

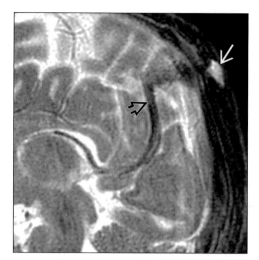

Sagittal T2WI MR shows an atretic parietal cephalocele as a hyperintense sub-scalp mass ➡. The cranium bifidum was < 1 cm. Note the associated primitive falcine vein ⇨.

## TERMINOLOGY

### Abbreviations and Synonyms
- Atretic parietal cephalocele (APC)

### Definitions
- Sub-scalp cephalocele connected to dura via cranium bifidum

## IMAGING FINDINGS

### General Features
- Best diagnostic clue: CSF tract & vertical falcine vein "points to" sub-scalp mass
- Location: Superior to lambda, midline, interparietal
- Size: Usually < 15 mm
- Morphology: Skin covered vertex sub-scalp mass

### CT Findings
- NECT: Cranium bifidum superior to lambda + sub-scalp mass
- CECT: Persistent primitive falcine vein, ± sagittal sinus fenestration

### MR Findings
- T1WI: Heterogeneous sub-scalp mass adjacent to cranium bifidum
- T2WI
  - Heterogeneous mass extends through cranium to or through dura
  - Spinning-top configuration of incisura (axial)
  - Prominent: Superior cerebellar cistern and suprapineal recess
- STIR: Sub-scalp cephalocele is hyperintense
- T1 C+: Vertical primitive falcine vein
- MRV: ± Bifid sagittal sinus

### Imaging Recommendations
- Best imaging tool: MR & MRV
- Protocol advice: MR: Thin, small FOV, sagittal T1 & T2 with fat-sat and contrast

## DIFFERENTIAL DIAGNOSIS

### (Epi) Dermoid Cyst
- Scallops outer table, ± thin enhancing wall

---

## DDx: Midline Parietal Sub-Scalp Masses

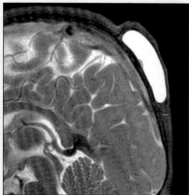

*Dermoid Cyst*

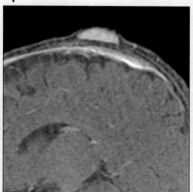

*Hemangioma*

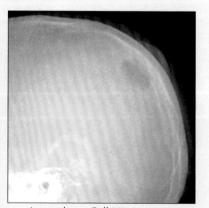

*Langerhans Cell Histiocytosis*

# ATRETIC CEPHALOCELE

## Key Facts

### Terminology
- Atretic parietal cephalocele (APC)

### Imaging Findings
- NECT: Cranium bifidum superior to lambda + sub-scalp mass
- Heterogeneous mass extends through cranium to or through dura
- T1 C+: Vertical primitive falcine vein

### Top Differential Diagnoses
- (Epi) Dermoid Cyst
- Proliferating Hemangioma
- Langerhans Cell Histiocytosis (LCH)

### Pathology
- Associated abnormalities: Cortical dysplasia

### Clinical Issues
- Age: Newborn, infants and young children

### Proliferating Hemangioma
- Lobulated mass, vivid enhancement

### Langerhans Cell Histiocytosis (LCH)
- ± Multiple lesions, beveled-edge defect

## PATHOLOGY

### General Features
- General path comments: Involuted true meningoceles or encephaloceles, 7-10 weeks of fetal life
- Genetics: Typically sporadic, if syndromic ⇒ midline anomalies (holoprosencephaly, CC agenesis)
- Etiology
  - Overdistended rhombencephalic vesicle
  - Folate deficiency, valproic acid exposure
- Epidemiology: APCs ⇒ 10x more common than parietal encephaloceles
- Associated abnormalities: Cortical dysplasia

### Gross Pathologic & Surgical Features
- Sub-scalp mass, with fibrous tract to dura
  - CSF tract to supracerebellar, suprapineal or quadrigeminal cistern

### Microscopic Features
- Meningeal and vestigial neural tissue, CSF tract ependymal lined

## CLINICAL ISSUES

### Presentation
- Most common signs/symptoms: Interparietal sub-scalp mass with cranium bifidum, ± enlarges with crying

### Demographics
- Age: Newborn, infants and young children
- Gender: Girls slightly more common
- Ethnicity: More common in Western hemisphere

### Natural History & Prognosis
- Outcome determined by associated anomalies

### Treatment
- Surgical

## DIAGNOSTIC CHECKLIST

### Consider
- APC in child with midline parietal sub-scalp mass

### Image Interpretation Pearls
- Persistent falcine vein points to cephalocele

## SELECTED REFERENCES

1. Patterson RJ et al: Atretic parietal cephaloceles revisited: an enlarging clinical and imaging spectrum? AJNR Am J Neuroradiol. 19(4):791-5, 1998

I

6

51

## IMAGE GALLERY

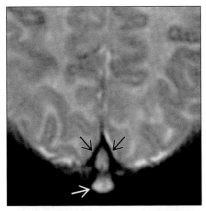 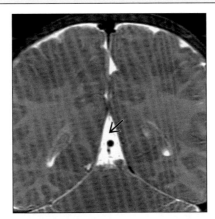 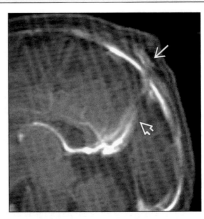

*(Left) Axial T2WI MR shows a small midline atretic parietal cephalocele ➡. Note the divided appearance of the hypointense sagittal venous sinus ➡ by the hyperintense CSF tract. (Center) Coronal T2WI MR shows a peaked appearance of the tentorium and a prominent tentorial incisura ➡. CSF tracts superiorly to split the sagittal sinus at the site of the APC. (Right) Sagittal T1 C+ MR shows patchy enhancement of the sub-scalp atretic parietal cephalocele ➡. Note the enhancing, vertical primitive falcine vein ➡.*

# CONGENITAL CALVARIAL DEFECTS

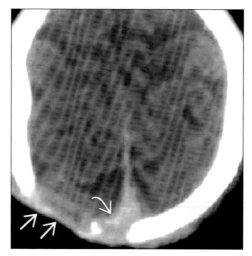

Axial CECT shows large bony defect ➡ in the right parietal bone; cutis aplasia was present in the overlying scalp. Note the close association of the defect with the superior sagittal sinus ➡.

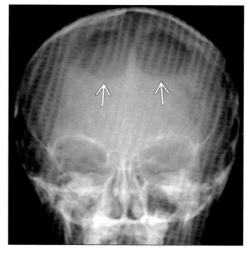

Anteroposterior radiograph shows bilateral giant parietal foramina ➡, separated by a bar of midline bone. PFM may be as large as 5 cm in diameter.

## TERMINOLOGY

### Abbreviations and Synonyms
- Calvarial deficiencies (CD), giant parietal foramina (PFM) also called foramina parietalis permagna, fenestrae parietals symmetricae

### Definitions
- Regions of congenitally missing bone in calvarium, often associated with overlying abnormalities of scalp or with vascular anomalies of the calvarium or underlying dura

## IMAGING FINDINGS

### General Features
- Best diagnostic clue: Absence of a portion of the calvarium on skull X-ray or CT
- Location
  - CD: Near midline, between anterior and posterior fontanelles
  - PFM: Symmetric, rounded areas on either side of sagittal suture
- Size
  - CD: Variable size, from < 1 cm to 10 cm
  - PFM: Size usually > 1 cm, < 5 cm
- Morphology
  - CD: Usually irregular ovoid lesions in continuity with suture or fontanelle
  - PFM: Usually round to oval
    - Sometimes in continuity across calvarial midline

### CT Findings
- CTA
  - CD: Rarely associated with vascular malformations
  - PFM: May be associated with anomalies of dural venous sinuses
- NECT
  - CD: Defect in the calvarium, typically adjacent to fontanelle
  - PFM: Bilateral symmetric oval to round defects in parietal bones
- CECT: CD: Close to superior sagittal sinus; hemorrhage may occur

### MR Findings
- T1WI
  - CD: Normal brain

## DDx: Calvarial Holes

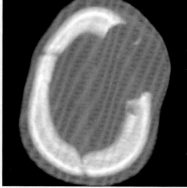

*Langerhans Cell Histiocytosis*

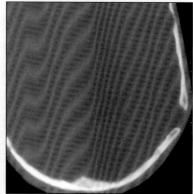

*Leptomeningeal Cyst*

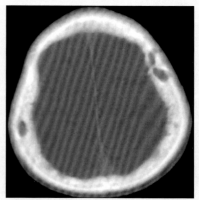

*Neuroblastoma*

# CONGENITAL CALVARIAL DEFECTS

## Key Facts

### Terminology

- Regions of congenitally missing bone in calvarium, often associated with overlying abnormalities of scalp or with vascular anomalies of the calvarium or underlying dura

### Imaging Findings

- Best diagnostic clue: Absence of a portion of the calvarium on skull X-ray or CT
- CD: Near midline, between anterior and posterior fontanelles
- PFM: Symmetric, rounded areas on either side of sagittal suture
- CD: Variable size, from < 1 cm to 10 cm
- PFM: Size usually > 1 cm, < 5 cm

### Top Differential Diagnoses

- Langerhans Cell Histiocytosis (LCH)
- Leptomeningeal Cyst
- Metastases (E.g., from Neuroblastoma, Leukemia)
- Amniotic Band Syndrome

### Pathology

- CD: Cutis aplasia, rare vascular malformations
- PFM: Craniosynostosis, vertebral anomalies, digital anomalies

### Clinical Issues

- CD: Defect in skin and subcutaneous tissue over vertex of skull ± dysmorphic features
- PFM: May be detected incidentally or found during work-up for associated anomalies

---

- o PFM: Sometimes associated with abnormal sulcation of medial parietal lobe
  - Gyri "droop" into tentorial incisura
- T2WI: PFM: Sometimes T2 prolongation in underlying cerebrum
- MRV: PFM: May be associated with anomalies of dural venous sinuses

## Angiographic Findings

- DSA
  - o CD: Rarely see vascular malformations
  - o PFM: Anomalies of dural venous sinuses

## Imaging Recommendations

- Best imaging tool: CT scan
- Protocol advice: Noncontrast with 3D reformation, post-contrast with identification of venous sinuses

## DIFFERENTIAL DIAGNOSIS

### Langerhans Cell Histiocytosis (LCH)

- Sharply demarcated lesions of the calvarium
- Soft tissue mass within calvarial defect
- May be associated with cerebral parenchymal lesions

### Leptomeningeal Cyst

- Due to skull fracture in infancy
  - o Meninges prevent fracture from healing
- Encephalomalacia in underlying brain

### Metastases (E.g., from Neuroblastoma, Leukemia)

- Malignancy is usually known
- Associated soft tissue mass in calvarial defect or underlying dura

### Amniotic Band Syndrome

- Typically associated with major facial clefts
  - o Clefts not associated with embryonic fusion lines
- Up to 33% of amniotic bands involve craniofacial region

- Often associated with major neural defects ⇒ cephaloceles, anencephaly

## PATHOLOGY

### General Features

- Genetics
  - o CD: Both autosomal dominant and autosomal recessive inheritance reported
  - o PFM: Autosomal dominant inheritance
    - Mutations of ALX4 (chromosome 11p11.2, causes PFM type 2), MSX2 (chromosome 5q34-35, causes PFM type 1)
    - Both genes encode paired-related homeodomain transcription factors that lead to intramembranous skull vault ossification
- Etiology
  - o CD: Possible fetal infarcts, injuries, infections, neural tube defects
  - o PFM: Ossification defect
- Epidemiology
  - o CD: Prevalence unknown; more than 500 cases reported
  - o PFM: Prevalence 1 in 15,000 live births
- Associated abnormalities
  - o CD: Cutis aplasia, rare vascular malformations
  - o PFM: Craniosynostosis, vertebral anomalies, digital anomalies
    - ALX4 and MSX2 ⇒ craniofacial dysostosis, cleidocranial dysplasia, posterior fossa abnormalities
    - ALX4 ⇒ medial cerebral cortex malformations, hypoplastic straight sinus, high insertion tentorium
    - CDAGS syndrome (chromosome 22q12-q13): C = craniosynostosis and clavicular hypoplasia; D = delayed closure of the fontanel, cranial defects, and deafness; A = anal anomalies (anterior placement of the anus, imperforate anus); G = genitourinary malformations; S = skin eruption

# CONGENITAL CALVARIAL DEFECTS

## Gross Pathologic & Surgical Features
- CD
  - 80% are midline
  - Average size 1-2 cm; may be > 10 cm
  - Associated with cutis aplasia of overlying scalp
    - 20% of neonates with cutis aplasia will have underlying osseous defects
- PFM
  - Symmetric parasagittal lesions up to 5 cm in diameter
  - Small parietal foramina contain emissary veins (of Santorini), connecting occipital veins with superior sagittal sinus
    - May also contain anastomoses between middle meningeal and occipital arteries
  - PFM only variably contain these vessels
  - Dura densely adherent to surrounding bone

## Microscopic Features
- CD
  - Layer of thin fibrous membrane
  - Composed of dermal collagen
  - Absence of overlying epithelium or adnexal structures
  - Marked absence of elastic fibers
- PFM
  - Failure of completion of ossification within parietal bones
    - Normal parietal bone ossification begins in two centers of parietal bones during the 8th and 9th weeks
    - Ossification normally complete by 7th month

## CLINICAL ISSUES

### Presentation
- Most common signs/symptoms
  - CD: Defect in skin and subcutaneous tissue over vertex of skull ± dysmorphic features
    - Involved area covered by thin membrane covering prominent veins
  - PFM: May be detected incidentally or found during work-up for associated anomalies

### Demographics
- Age
  - CD: Detected in infancy
  - PFM: Any age; size of foramina decrease with age at presentation

### Natural History & Prognosis
- CD
  - Defect in overlying skin may ⇒ infection, meningitis
  - Exposure of sagittal sinus may ⇒ hemorrhage
- PFM
  - Mostly related to associated anomalies (if present)

### Treatment
- CD
  - Small lesions ⇒ nonsurgical treatment; ointments and dressings
  - Large lesions ⇒ skin grafts and calvarial reconstructions or cranioplasty if natural osteogenesis insufficient
- PFM
  - Many decrease in size spontaneously; bone grafts, cranioplasty may be necessary

## DIAGNOSTIC CHECKLIST

### Consider
- Consider calvarial defects, dermal sinuses in patients with cutis aplasia of scalp

### Image Interpretation Pearls
- Look for cerebral cortical malformations, posterior fossa anomalies, anomalies of dural venous sinuses in children with giant parietal foramina
- Look for multiple midline bone defects in patients with PFM

## SELECTED REFERENCES

1. Mavrogiannis LA et al: Enlarged parietal foramina caused by mutations in the homeobox genes ALX4 and MSX2: from genotype to phenotype. Eur J Hum Genet. 14(2):151-8, 2006
2. Mendoza-Londono R et al: Characterization of a new syndrome that associates craniosynostosis, delayed fontanel closure, parietal foramina, imperforate anus, and skin eruption: CDAGS. Am J Hum Genet. 77(1):161-8, 2005
3. Perlyn CA et al: Congenital scalp and calvarial deficiencies: principles for classification and surgical management. Plast Reconstr Surg. 115(4):1129-41, 2005
4. Rice DP: Craniofacial anomalies: from development to molecular pathogenesis. Curr Mol Med. 5(7):699-722, 2005
5. Moore FO et al: Autogenous orbital reconstruction in a child with congenital abnormalities of the orbital roof and vertical orbital dystopia. J Craniofac Surg. 15(6):930-3, 2004
6. Tubbs RS et al: Duane's syndrome and giant parietal foramina. Pediatr Neurol. 30(1):75-6, 2004
7. Valente M et al: Malformation of cortical and vascular development in one family with parietal foramina determined by an ALX4 homeobox gene mutation. AJNR Am J Neuroradiol. 25(10):1836-9, 2004
8. Chen G et al: A novel locus for parietal foramina maps to chromosome 4q21-q23. J Hum Genet. 48(8):420-4, 2003
9. de Heer IM et al: Parietal bone agenesis and associated multiple congenital anomalies. J Craniofac Surg. 14(2):192-6, 2003
10. Garcia-Minaur S et al: Parietal foramina with cleidocranial dysplasia is caused by mutation in MSX2. Eur J Hum Genet. 11(11):892-5, 2003
11. Kortesis B et al: Surgical management of foramina parietalia permagna. J Craniofac Surg. 14(4):538-44, 2003
12. Tubbs RS et al: Parietal foramina are not synonymous with giant parietal foramina. Pediatr Neurosurg. 39(4):216-7, 2003
13. Steinbok P: Repair of a congenital cranial defect in a newborn with autologous calvarial bone. Childs Nerv Syst. 16(4):247-9; discussion 250, 2000
14. Wilkie AO et al: Functional haploinsufficiency of the human homeobox gene MSX2 causes defects in skull ossification. Nat Genet. 24(4):387-90, 2000
15. Fein JM et al: Evolution and significance of giant parietal foramina. Report of five cases in one family. J Neurosurg. 37(4):487-92, 1972

# CONGENITAL CALVARIAL DEFECTS

## IMAGE GALLERY

### Typical

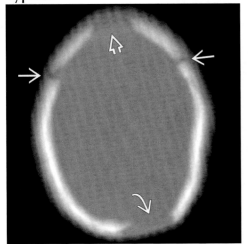 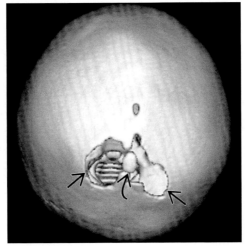

*(Left)* Axial NECT shows calvarial defect ➔ immediately to the left of midline in the left parietal bone. Note the normal coronal sutures ➔ and anterior fontanelle ➔. *(Right)* NECT 3D reformation of calvarium in PFM shows the bilateral parietal foramina ➔ with small intervening bar ➔ of midline bone.

### Typical

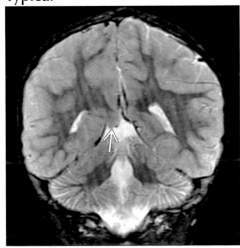 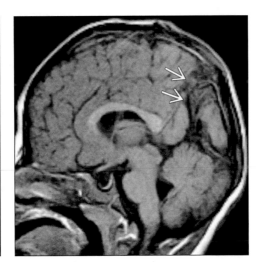

*(Left)* Coronal T2WI MR shows abnormal sulcation of the medial cerebral hemispheres in PFM with a small dysmorphic gyrus ➔ "dangling" from the medial parietal lobe into the tentorial incisura. *(Right)* Sagittal T1WI MR shows abnormal venous system in PFM with persistent falcine sinus ➔, usually a fetal anastomosis between the deep and superficial venous systems.

### Variant

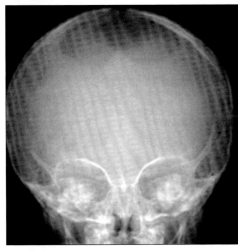 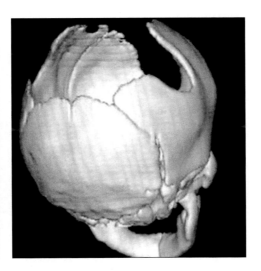

*(Left)* Anteroposterior radiograph shows giant parietal foramina in a neonate. The central strip of midline bone is often not yet ossified in neonates. *(Right)* NECT 3D reformation of calvarium shows PFM associated with coronal suture synostosis and enlarged anterior and posterior fontanelles in patient with CDAGS syndrome.

# FIBROUS DYSPLASIA

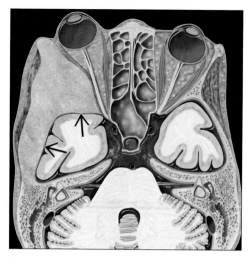

Axial graphic shows expansion of lateral orbital wing and temporal squamosa ➔ by fibrous dysplasia. There is exophthalmos and stretching of the ipsilateral optic nerve.

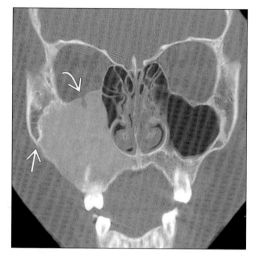

Coronal bone CT shows maxillary sinus expansion by monostotic fibrous dysplasia. There is extension to zygomaticomaxillary synchondrosis ➔ and infraorbital nerve engulfment ➔.

## TERMINOLOGY

### Abbreviations and Synonyms

- Fibrous dysplasia (FD); craniofacial fibrous dysplasia (CFD); osteitis fibrosa; osteodystrophie fibrosia
- McCune-Albright syndrome (MAS): One of the most common FD syndromes
- Jaffe-Lichtenstein dysplasia (monostotic FD)

### Definitions

- Congenital disorder characterized by expanding lesions, mixture of fibrous tissue and woven bone
- Defect in osteoblastic differentiation and maturation
- One of the most common of the fibro-osseous lesions

## IMAGING FINDINGS

### General Features

- Best diagnostic clue: "Ground-glass" matrix
- Location
  - May involve any aspect of the skull
  - CFD: Majority have more than one bone involved

- Maxilla, orbit, frontal bone most common in one series; ethmoids and sphenoids in another
- Size: Small focal lesion to extensive skull involvement

### CT Findings

- NECT
  - Imaging patterns relate to relative content of fibrous and osseous tissue
  - Expansile bone lesion, widened diploic space
  - CT shows "ground-glass", sclerotic, cystic or mixed bone changes
    - If cystic may have thick sclerotic "rind"

### MR Findings

- T1WI: Usual: ↓ T1WI signal
- T2WI
  - Usual: ↓ T2WI signal (if solid) or in rind (if "cystic")
  - ↑ Clinical-pathologic activity ⇒ ↑ signal
- T1 C+: Variable enhancement depends on lesion pattern (rim, diffuse, or none)

### Radiographic Findings

- Radiography
  - Expanded bone with "ground-glass" appearance
  - CFD: Dental malocclusions in 20%

## DDx: Craniofacial Fibrous Dysplasia Mimics

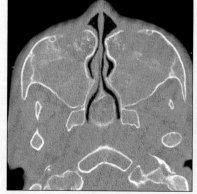

Thalassemia

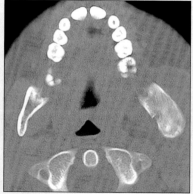

Garré Osteitis

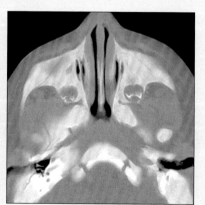

Osteopetrosis

# FIBROUS DYSPLASIA

## Key Facts

### Terminology
- Fibrous dysplasia (FD); craniofacial fibrous dysplasia (CFD); osteitis fibrosa; osteodystrophie fibrosia
- McCune-Albright syndrome (MAS): One of the most common FD syndromes
- Congenital disorder characterized by expanding lesions, mixture of fibrous tissue and woven bone
- Defect in osteoblastic differentiation and maturation

### Imaging Findings
- Best diagnostic clue: "Ground-glass" matrix
- Usual: ↓ T2WI signal (if solid) or in rind (if "cystic")
- Best imaging tool: Bone scan to stage
- CT or MR to define local extent

### Top Differential Diagnoses
- Garré Sclerosing Osteomyelitis

- Jaffe-Campanacci (J-C) Syndrome
- Craniometaphyseal Dysplasia
- Thalassemia: Maxillary sinus involvement typical; "hair-on-end" skull
- Osteopetrosis: Involvement of all bones

### Clinical Issues
- Most common signs/symptoms: Painless swelling or deformity
- Rare progression to fibro-, osteo-, chondro- and mesenchymal sarcoma

### Diagnostic Checklist
- Monostotic and polyostotic FD likely on same spectrum of phenotypic expression, consider checking for gene to predict complications

## Nuclear Medicine Findings
- PET: Accumulation (11C) MET
- Bone Scan
  - Radionuclide uptake: Perfusion/delayed phases
  - Nonspecific; sensitive to extent of skeletal lesions in polyostotic FD

## Imaging Recommendations
- Best imaging tool: Bone scan to stage
- Protocol advice
  - CT or MR to define local extent
  - Bone scan to search for additional lesions

# DIFFERENTIAL DIAGNOSIS

## Paget Disease
- Pagetoid ground-glass FD mimics Paget disease
- Paget: Calvarium, not craniofacial; "cotton wool" CT; adults

## Garré Sclerosing Osteomyelitis
- Bony expansion, but inhomogeneous sclerotic pattern; ± dehiscent bone cortex; ± periosteal reaction

## Jaffe-Campanacci (J-C) Syndrome
- Non-ossifying fibromas, axillary freckling and café-au-lait (lacks neurofibromas)
- Mimics polyostotic forms FD
  - J-C café-au-lait: Coast of California (like NF1)
  - McCune-Albright café-au-lait: Coast of Maine

## Craniometaphyseal Dysplasia
- Hyperostosis and sclerosis of craniofacial bones ⇒ facial distortion, cranial nerve compression
- Abnormal modelling of long bone metaphyses; paranasal "bossing"
- Mutations in transmembrane protein ANK on Chr 5p

## Meningioma
- Resulting hyperostosis mimics FD
- MRS: Characteristic alanine peak

## Other Disorders with Expanded Bone & Abnormal Bony Density
- Thalassemia: Maxillary sinus involvement typical; "hair-on-end" skull
- Osteopetrosis: Involvement of all bones
- Langerhans cell histiocytosis: Bony cortex frequently "disappears" during active phase
- Neurocutaneous disorders: Osteitis fibrosa cystica in tuberous sclerosis and NF1
- Renal osteodystrophy may simulate leontiasis ossea
- Morgagni syndrome of hyperostosis frontalis interna: Post-menopausal women, limited to frontal bone

# PATHOLOGY

## General Features
- General path comments: Any bone can be involved
- Genetics
  - GNAS1 gene mutations in monostotic, polyostotic and MAS
  - Cherubism: Autosomal dominant; mutations in the c-Abl-binding protein SH3BP2
- Etiology: Presence of activating mutation of Gs-α in osteoblastic progenitor cells ⇒ ↑ proliferation; abnormal differentiation
- Epidemiology
  - Actual incidence unknown
  - Monostotic FD is 6 times more common than polyostotic FD
  - Calvarial involvement differs: Polyostotic FD > monostotic FD
    - Monostotic FD (70%): Found in skull & face 25%
    - Polyostotic FD (25%): Found in skull & face 50%
- Associated abnormalities: Syndromic specific features such as endocrinopathy, intramuscular myxoma, failure to thrive

## Gross Pathologic & Surgical Features
- Tan-yellow to white lesion; soft/rubbery to gritty/firm
- Consistency depends upon fibrous vs. osseous make-up

# FIBROUS DYSPLASIA

- Woven immature bone structurally weak, prone to fractures

## Microscopic Features
- Fibrous stroma: Myxofibrous tissue of mixed vascularity
- Osseous metaplasia: Bone trabeculae made up of immature, woven bone seen as peculiar shapes floating in fibrous stroma
  - Looks like "Chinese letters" or "alphabet soup"

## Staging, Grading or Classification Criteria
- Monostotic vs. polyostotic
- Specific lesion type (Pagetoid, sclerotic, cystic) relates to disease activity
  - Cystic, Pagetoid and sclerotic FD proposed to represent (in order) the most active to least active
    - Cystic FD (11-21%): Hypodense (CT) except rind
    - Pagetoid mixed FD (56%): "Ground-glass" plus cystic change
    - Homogeneous sclerotic FD (23-34%)

# CLINICAL ISSUES

## Presentation
- Most common signs/symptoms: Painless swelling or deformity
- Clinical Profile
  - Proptosis, cranial neuropathy (diplopia, hearing loss, blindness), atypical facial pain or numbness, headache
  - Endocrinopathies if McCune-Albright
- Presentations: Monostotic, polyostotic, craniofacial (CFD) and syndromic (many known syndromes)
  - Monostotic FD
    - 70% of all FD cases; single osseous site is affected
    - Older children and young adults (75% present before the age 30)
    - Skull and face involved in 25%; maxilla (especially zygomatic process) and mandible (molar area) > > frontal > ethmoid & sphenoid > temporal > occipital bones
  - Polyostotic FD
    - 25% of all FD cases; involves ≥ 2 separate sites
    - Skull and face involved in 50%
    - Younger group, 2/3 have symptoms by 10 years
  - CFD
    - Autosomal dominant, stabilizes with skeletal maturity
  - McCune-Albright syndrome (MAS)
    - Subtype of unilateral polyostotic FD: Clinical triad of polyostotic FD, hyperfunctioning endocrinopathies, café-au-lait spots
    - 5% of FD cases; appears earlier; affects more bones more severely
    - Renal phosphate wasting (50%) associated with elevation of circulating factor FGF-23; may result in rickets and osteomalacia
  - Mazabraud syndrome
    - Polyostotic FD and intramuscular myxoma
    - ↑ Risk malignant transformation FD lesions
  - Cherubism: Familial bilateral FD of jaw

- "Mulibrey" nanism: Primarily Finland; severe, progressive growth failure; pericardial constriction
  - (MU)scle, (LI)ver, (BR)ain, (EY)e = triangular face; yellow ocular fundi pigment; hypoplastic tongue; peculiar high voice; nevae flammei 65%
  - Peroxisomal disorder with mutation TRIM37 gene
  - FD of long bones in 25%

## Demographics
- Age: < 6 years (39%), 6-10 years (27%), > 10 years (39%)
- Gender: MAS usually, but not exclusively, female

## Natural History & Prognosis
- Rare progression to fibro-, osteo-, chondro- and mesenchymal sarcoma
  - 0.5% (Netherlands Committee on Bone Tumors)
  - Usually polyostotic/syndromic forms
  - Nearly half arise following irradiation (marked increase in malignant potential)
- Monostotic CFD has an excellent prognosis
- Most spontaneously "burn out" in their teens and 20s
- Polyostotic FD rarely life threatening, but poorer prognosis is present

## Treatment
- Aggressive resection reserved for visual loss, severe deformity ("vault" more accessible than skull base)
- No radiation therapy ⇒ malignant progression
- Bisphosphonate ameliorates course (pain, fractures) in polyostotic and monostotic forms
- Treat precocious puberty and renal phosphate wasting

# DIAGNOSTIC CHECKLIST

## Consider
- Monostotic and polyostotic FD likely on same spectrum of phenotypic expression, consider checking for gene to predict complications

## Image Interpretation Pearls
- "Ground-glass" appearance on PF or CT and homogeneously decreased signal on T2WI characteristic

# SELECTED REFERENCES

1. Hoshi M et al: Malignant change secondary to fibrous dysplasia. Int J Clin Oncol. 11(3):229-35, 2006
2. Shah ZK et al: Magnetic resonance imaging appearances of fibrous dysplasia. Br J Radiol. 78(936):1104-15, 2005
3. Karlberg N et al: Mulibrey nanism: clinical features and diagnostic criteria. J Med Genet. 41(2):92-8, 2004
4. MacDonald-Jankowski DS: Fibro-osseous lesions of the face and jaws. Clin Radiol. 59(1):11-25, 2004
5. Chattopadhyay A et al: Hypophosphatemic rickets and osteomalacia in polyostotic fibrous dysplasia. J Pediatr Endocrinol Metab. 16(6):893-6, 2003
6. Riminucci M et al: FGF-23 in fibrous dysplasia of bone and its relationship to renal phosphate wasting. J Clin Invest. 112(5):683-92, 2003
7. Bianco P et al: Mutations of the GNAS1 gene, stromal cell dysfunction, and osteomalacic changes in non-McCune-Albright fibrous dysplasia of bone. J Bone Miner Res. 15(1):120-8, 2000

# FIBROUS DYSPLASIA

## IMAGE GALLERY

### Typical

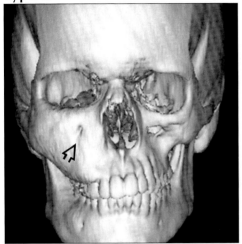

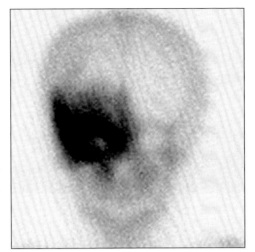

*(Left)* Anteroposterior bone CT with 3D reconstructions shows expansion of the maxillary bone. Again note typical infraorbital nerve engulfment ⊳ and distortion of the alveolar ridge. *(Right)* Anteroposterior bone scan in another child shows markedly increased uptake of the affected bones in the sphenoid wings, maxilla and orbital roof.

### Variant

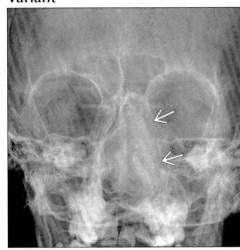

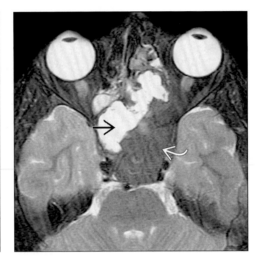

*(Left)* Anteroposterior radiograph shows the ground-glass appearance of central skull base fibrous dysplasia →. There is replacement of the left nasal cavity and sphenoethmoid air cells. *(Right)* Axial T2WI MR in same teen as previous image shows surgically confirmed cystic foci → and homogeneously decreased signal of ground glass foci →. Cysts and mucoceles may occur in tandem.

I
6
59

### Variant

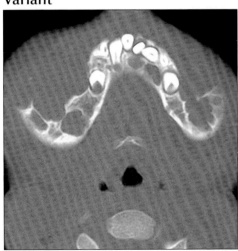

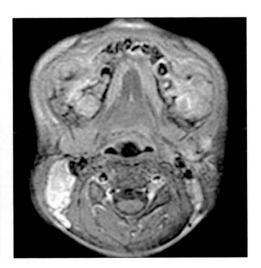

*(Left)* Axial bone CT shows expansion of mandible by extensive, bilateral involvement in cherubism. *(Right)* Axial T1 C+ FS MR shows extensive involvement of the mandible. Enhancement is inhomogeneous. Teeth, as on CT, are displaced and "floating".

# CRANIOSTENOSES

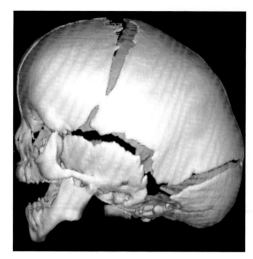

Sagittal NECT 3D reconstruction shows marked scaphocephaly in infant with sagittal synostosis.

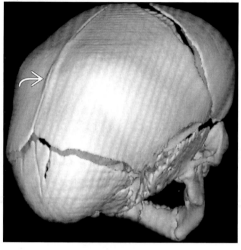

Sagittal oblique NECT 3D CT (same infant as previous) shows beaked and fused sagittal suture ➘.

## TERMINOLOGY

### Abbreviations and Synonyms
- Craniostenosis, sutural synostosis, craniosynostosis, cranial dysostosis

### Definitions
- Heterogeneous group of disorders with premature fusion (osseous obliteration) of cranial sutures
  - Non-syndromic craniosynostosis (more common)
  - Syndromic (> 150 syndromes)

## IMAGING FINDINGS

### General Features
- Best diagnostic clue: Skull growth is ↓ perpendicular to, & ↑ parallel to fused suture
- Location: Calvarium, ± skeletal anomalies
- Size: Single suture or universal synostosis
- Morphology: Classic imaging appearance: Calvarial (and facial) distortion

### CT Findings
- NECT
  - Fibrous or bony "bridging"; bony sutural "beaking"
  - Scaphocephaly: ↓ Transverse, ↑ AP ⇒ sagittal synostosis
  - Trigonocephaly: "Ax-head"; "pear-shaped" on axial ⇒ metopic
  - Plagiocephaly: Asymmetry ⇒ unilateral single or asymmetric multiple
  - Brachycephaly: ↑ Transverse, ↓ AP ⇒ bicoronal or bilambdoid
  - Turricephaly: "Towering skull" ⇒ bicoronal or bilambdoid
  - Kleebattschadel: Bulging temporal, shallow orbits ⇒ bicoronal **and** bilambdoid
  - Craniofacial dysostoses: "Towering skull", shallow orbits

### MR Findings
- T1WI: Syndromic: See cerebellar tonsillar ectopia, hydrocephalus; agenesis corpus callosum (Apert craniofacial dysostosis)
- T2WI: Non-syndromic, single synostoses: Brain normal

## DDx: Acquired Synostosis

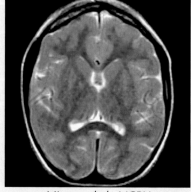

Microcephaly MCPH

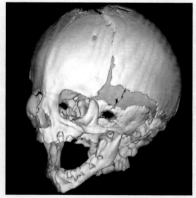

Newborn, MCPH

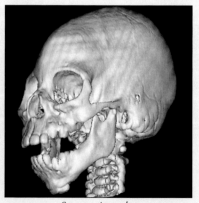

Severe Atrophy

# CRANIOSTENOSES

## Key Facts

### Terminology
- Heterogeneous group of disorders with premature fusion (osseous obliteration) of cranial sutures
- Non-syndromic craniosynostosis (more common)
- Syndromic (> 150 syndromes)

### Imaging Findings
- Best diagnostic clue: Skull growth is ↓ perpendicular to, & ↑ parallel to fused suture
- Size: Single suture or universal synostosis
- Morphology: Classic imaging appearance: Calvarial (and facial) distortion
- Fibrous or bony "bridging"; bony sutural "beaking"
- Scaphocephaly: ↓ Transverse, ↑ AP ⇒ sagittal synostosis
- Trigonocephaly: "Ax-head"; "pear-shaped" on axial ⇒ metopic

- Plagiocephaly: Asymmetry ⇒ unilateral single or asymmetric multiple
- Brachycephaly: ↑ Transverse, ↓ AP ⇒ bicoronal or bilambdoid
- Turricephaly: "Towering skull" ⇒ bicoronal or bilambdoid
- Kleebattschadel: Bulging temporal, shallow orbits ⇒ bicoronal **and** bilambdoid
- Craniofacial dysostoses: "Towering skull", shallow orbits

### Top Differential Diagnoses
- Postural Flattening
- Secondary Craniosynostosis

---

- MRV: Post-operative dural venous occlusions occur

## Radiographic Findings
- Radiography
  - Skull: Dense suture; "bone bridge" on tangential view; digital markings; inner table scalloping
  - Plain films (extremity): Many anomalies described, certain are specific
    - Apert: Hand/foot syndactyly
    - Pfeiffer: Wide, "stub" thumbs
    - Saethre-Chotzen: Duplicated distal phalanx and cone-shaped epiphysis of hallux
    - Muenke-type mutations: Calcaneo-cuboid fusion
    - Crouzon: Hands/feet normal

## Ultrasonographic Findings
- Fetal diagnosis of craniosynostosis defined by calvarial deformities and loss of normal sutural hypoechogenicity

## Nuclear Medicine Findings
- Bone Scan
  - Bone scintigraphy: Less accurate than PF or CT
    - Especially in the very young infant
- Brain scintigraphy: Focal ↓ cerebral blood flow (CBF) subjacent to stenosed suture

## Imaging Recommendations
- Cephalometrics (plain skull radiographs): Optional
- Low dose 3D CT for surgical planning and follow-up
- Common indication for imaging
  - Evaluate whether suture patent or fused
  - Assess brain anomalies, pre-operative ventricle size
  - Surgical planning and routine follow-up
  - Complications: Post-operative dural vein thrombosis, hydrocephalus, infection

## DIFFERENTIAL DIAGNOSIS

### Postural Flattening
- Hypotonic infant ⇒ especially unilateral lambdoid ("sticky" suture)

  - Postural: Parallelogram skull, ipsilateral anterior ear displacement
  - Lambdoid synostosis: Trapezoid skull, ipsilateral posterior ear displacement
- Premature infant ⇒ especially sagittal

### Secondary Craniosynostosis
- Arrest of brain growth ⇒ especially metopic or universal craniosynostosis

## PATHOLOGY

### General Features
- General path comments
  - Embryology-anatomy
    - 13 weeks: Mineralization proceeds outwards from ossification centers
    - 18 weeks: Bone fronts meet ⇒ induce sutures
    - Skull enlarges by appositional growth at suture
    - Bone plates separated by osteogenic stem cell filled space
    - ↑ Cell proliferation in sutures prior to onset of fusion ⇒ ↑ collagenous extracellular matrix ⇒ subsequent ossification
    - Synostosis of one suture ⇒ excessive growth at unfused sutures
    - Growth ↓ perpendicular to fused suture
    - Growth ↑ parallel to fused suture
- Genetics
  - Syndromic synostoses usually autosomal dominant
  - Heterozygous gene mutations (FGFR: 1-3, TWIST and MSX2)
    - Fibroblastic growth factors (FGFs) bind to fibroblastic growth factor receptors (FGFRs) ⇒ signal cell proliferation and differentiation
    - TWIST and MSX2 (transcription factors) determine the expression of target effector genes
- Etiology
  - Up regulation of factors signaling sutural fusion: Transforming growth factor (TGF) and FGFs/FGFRs
  - Intact dura regulates overlying sutural activity

- Acts as internal periosteum with osteogenic/directional role
  - Regional differentiated dura mater induces fusion or allows patency in adjacent suture
  ○ Other craniosynostosis etiologies: Metabolic bone disease: ↑ Thyroid, "↓ PO4-vitamin D-resistant rickets", mucopolysaccharidoses/mucolipidoses
- Epidemiology
  ○ 1:2,500
  ○ Sagittal 60%, coronal 20-30%, metopic 1-2%
- Associated abnormalities: Syndromic synostoses frequently associated with limb anomalies

## Gross Pathologic & Surgical Features
- Fibrous or bony "bridging"; focal synostotic foci or diffuse bony "beaking" along suture

## Microscopic Features
- ↑ Osteoblastic cell differentiation/maturation

## CLINICAL ISSUES

### Presentation
- Most common signs/symptoms: Asymmetric face/cranium or ↓ head growth
- Clinical Profile
  ○ Craniofacial asymmetry, with or without extremity malformations
  ○ Non-syndromic patients have normal cognitive and motor development
  ○ More common in twins, possibly mechanical forces

### Demographics
- Age
  ○ Infancy
  ○ At birth if severe or if extremity malformations
- Gender
  ○ Scaphocephaly M:F = 3.5:1
  ○ Trigonocephaly M:F = 2:1
  ○ Apert M:F = 1:1
- Ethnicity: Apert population-based study: Asian highest prevalence, Hispanic lowest prevalence

### Natural History & Prognosis
- Abnormal skull growth ⇒ ↑ ICP, impaired CBF, airway obstruction
  ○ Craniofacial deformity socially stigmatizing if severe
- Single suture ⇒ 2° mandibular/maxillary deformities
- Multiple suture ⇒ above and ↑ ICP, ↓ CBF; airway/aural/visual compromise
- Syndromic: (±) Midline brain anomalies, (±) developmental delays

### Treatment
- Mild deformity or positional
  ○ Aggressive physiotherapy and head repositioning
  ○ Orthotic head-band or helmet
    ▪ Helmet therapy more effective with posterior plagiocephaly than with brachycephaly
- Moderate to severe: Surgical cranial vault reshaping
  ○ Alternative: Distraction osteogenesis of cranial vault
    ▪ Advantages: Less invasive, shorter operation time, easy care, minimal dural dissection

- Disadvantages: Limited initial reshaping and necessity of a 2nd operation for device removal
- Post-operative CT imaging very important
  ○ Establishes baseline
  ○ Rate of reossification can be assessed in regions where dura is left uncovered
  ○ Focal or generalized "copper-beaten" appearance & sclerotic hyperdense bands represent recurrence
  ○ As pediatric skull grows, evaluates for migration of fixation screws, plates, & wires
    ▪ May end up buried within skull or even intracranially
    ▪ Development of absorbable hardware may eradicate this problem

## DIAGNOSTIC CHECKLIST

### Consider
- Non-syndromic doesn't mean not genetic, single sutural synostoses also governed by genes

### Image Interpretation Pearls
- In positional lambdoid flattening: Long-axis of skull is oblique (forehead to contralateral occiput)
- In unilateral lambdoid synostosis: Long-axis of skull remains unilateral AP (forehead to ipsilateral occiput)

## SELECTED REFERENCES

1. Cho BC et al: Distraction osteogenesis of the cranial vault for the treatment of craniofacial synostosis. J Craniofac Surg. 15(1):135-44, 2004
2. Glass RB et al: The infant skull: a vault of information. Radiographics. 24(2):507-22, 2004
3. Teichgraeber JF et al: Molding helmet therapy in the treatment of brachycephaly and plagiocephaly. J Craniofac Surg. 15(1):118-23, 2004
4. Azimi C et al: Clinical and genetic aspects of trigonocephaly: a study of 25 cases. Am J Med Genet A. 117(2):127-35, 2003
5. Delahaye S et al: Prenatal ultrasound diagnosis of fetal craniosynostosis. Ultrasound Obstet Gynecol. 21(4):347-53, 2003
6. Panthaki ZJ et al: Hand abnormalities associated with craniofacial syndromes. J Craniofac Surg. 14(5):709-12, 2003
7. Rice DP et al: Molecular mechanisms in calvarial bone and suture development, and their relation to craniosynostosis. Eur J Orthod. 25(2):139-48, 2003
8. Trusen A et al: The pattern of skeletal anomalies in the cervical spine, hands and feet in patients with Saethre-Chotzen syndrome and Muenke-type mutation. Pediatr Radiol. 33(3):168-72, 2003
9. Warren SM et al: Regional dura mater differentially regulates osteoblast gene expression. J Craniofac Surg. 14(3):363-70, 2003
10. Greenwald JA et al: Regional differentiation of cranial suture-associated dura mater in vivo and in vitro: implications for suture fusion and patency. J Bone Miner Res. 15(12):2413-30, 2000
11. Nah H: Suture biology: Lessons from molecular genetics of craniosynostosis syndromes. Clin Orthod Res. 3(1):37-45, 2000
12. Tolarova MM et al: Birth prevalence, mutation rate, sex ratio, parents' age, and ethnicity in Apert syndrome. Am J Med Genet. 72(4):394-8, 1997

# CRANIOSTENOSES

## IMAGE GALLERY

### Typical

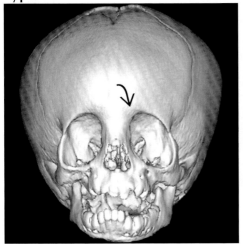

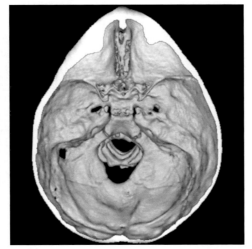

*(Left)* Coronal NECT 3D CT shows "quizzical" orbits, with elevation of the medial aspect ➘ of the superior orbital rim. There is hypotelorism. The metopic suture is ridge-like and fused. *(Right)* Axial NECT 3D reconstruction (same toddler as previous image) shows typical trigonocephaly due to metopic synostosis.

### Typical

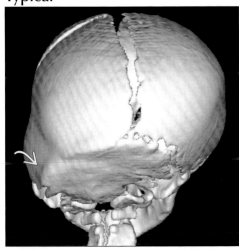

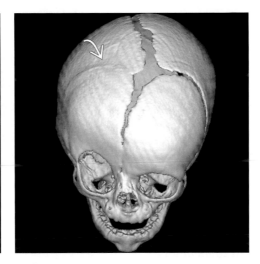

*(Left)* Coronal NECT 3D CT shows fusion of the right lambdoid and petrosquamous suture. Growth along the mastoid fontanel leads to a prominent mastoid "bump" ➘ in the lambdoid synostosis. *(Right)* Coronal oblique NECT 3D reconstruction shows a fused right coronal suture ➘. The sagittal suture is unfused and tilted. The ipsilateral orbital rim is flat and the nasal bone tilted.

### Typical

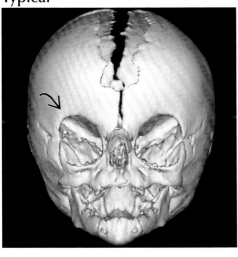

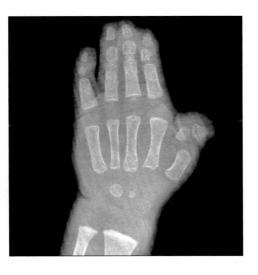

*(Left)* Coronal NECT 3D reconstruction in Apert syndrome shows bilateral coronal synostosis. Coronal synostosis leads to elevation of the lateral orbital rim ➘, resulting in the harlequin orbit. *(Right)* Anteroposterior radiograph shows typical syndactyly in Apert syndrome.

# THICK SKULL

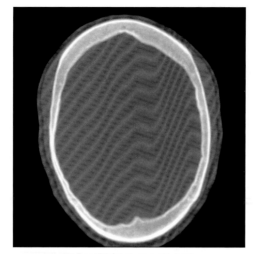

Axial bone CT shows diffuse secondary calvarial thickening, result of acquired asymmetrical loss of brain substance; thickened calvarium (left > right) with preserved normal bone structure.

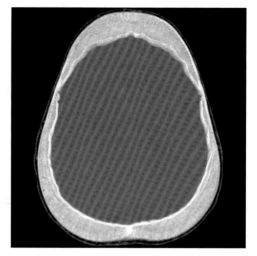

Axial bone CT in thalassemia major shows diffuse primary calvarial thickening (normal underlying brain): Thick diploe; "hair on end" appearance due to blood-forming bone marrow hyperplasia.

## TERMINOLOGY

### Abbreviations and Synonyms
- Skull thickening (ST)

### Definitions
- Diploic space expansion with/without adjacent cortical thickening

## IMAGING FINDINGS

### General Features
- Best diagnostic clue: Widened skull width
- Location
  - Diffuse
  - Localized
    - Can affect any bone of calvarium or skull base
    - Occipital squamae do not contain marrow and are usually spared
- Size
  - Diffuse: Involving nearly entire skull
  - Localized: Small focal/regional involvement at any skull location

- Morphology
  - Thickening of calvarium, or of skull base (including face)
  - When localized
    - Mono- or poly-ostotic
    - Highly dependent on underlying etiology

### CT Findings
- NECT
  - Thickened skull
    - Diffuse or localized
    - Mono- or poly-ostotic
    - Appearance can vary dependent on etiology
    - Inner table, outer table, diploic space involvement varies; dependent on etiology
  - Findings may be classic/pathognomic
    - Dyke-Davidoff-Masson syndrome: Focal cerebral atrophy with ipsilateral compensatory osseous thickening & dilated paranasal sinuses
    - β-thalassemia: "Hair on end" skull
    - Shunted hydrocephalus with cortical atrophy: Shunt presence with atrophy and ST
    - Chronic encephalopathies with secondary atrophy

---

## DDx: Other Pericerebral Calcification, Thickening, Bone Dystrophy

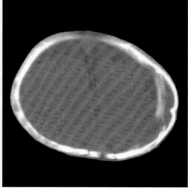

*Calcified SDH*

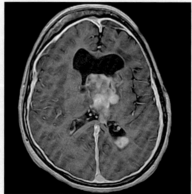

*Subdural Fibrosis*

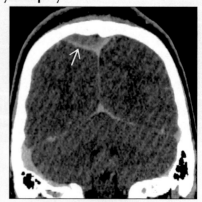

*Transosseous Ewing Sarcoma*

# THICK SKULL

## Key Facts

### Terminology
- Diploic space expansion with/without adjacent cortical thickening

### Imaging Findings
- Best diagnostic clue: Widened skull width
- NECT as the primary approach
- MR + contrast if cellular, aggressive causes (e.g., tumor) are suspected

### Top Differential Diagnoses
- Normal Anatomic Variation
- Other Pericalvarial Calcification & Thickening
- Bone Invasive/Destructive Lesions

### Clinical Issues
- Most often asymptomatic; macrocephaly, dysmorphic features dependent on etiology
- Patients with skull base ST may be symptomatic from foraminal or canal encroachment
- ST of no clinical concern by itself, except if neural, venous involvement
- Usually no specific treatment required
- Skull findings often harbinger of underlying disease

### Diagnostic Checklist
- Risk of neurological compromise
- ST may be only clue to severe causal disease
- CT for bony changes, MR for diploe, nerves, veins

---

- Fibrous dysplasia: Medullary expansion with a "ground glass" appearance
- CECT: Diploic enhancement in some etiologies

### MR Findings
- T1WI: May show alterations in normal diploic space signal → varies with etiology
- T2WI: May show alterations in normal diploic space signal → varies with etiology
- STIR: May show alterations in normal diploic space signal → varies with etiology
- T1 C+: Diploic enhancement in some etiologies
- MRV
  - Focal etiologies may have dural sinus displacement
  - Disease of skull base may result in stenosis/occlusion of venous outlets and collateral channels

### Radiographic Findings
- Radiography
  - Less sensitive for diffuse, although may be apparent when ST is striking
  - Focal more easily appreciated as subtle but definite increased density without defined borders
  - Some etiologies have dramatic and unique findings which can quickly lead to diagnosis
    - Fibrous dysplasia → ground glass appearance
    - β-thalassemia → "hair on end" skull

### Nuclear Medicine Findings
- PET: 18F-fluoro-2-deoxyglucose (FDG) PET: May show uptake in aggressive etiologies
- Bone Scan
  - Variable, dependent on cause of ST
    - May be cold or hot
    - Differences possible in early vascular vs. later bone uptake phases

### Angiographic Findings
- Conventional
  - Focal involvement may have dural sinus displacement
  - Disease of skull base may result in stenosis/occlusion of venous outlets with collateral pathways

### Imaging Recommendations
- Best imaging tool
  - NECT as the primary approach
  - MR + contrast if cellular, aggressive causes (e.g., tumor) are suspected
- Protocol advice
  - Bone reconstruction algorithm
  - Thin-section, high-resolution CT
    - Tri-planar reformats
    - Thoroughly investigate bone structure
    - Evaluate sella, ear, foramina & canals

## DIFFERENTIAL DIAGNOSIS

### Normal Anatomic Variation
- Upper limits of normal
- Normal appearing cortices & diploic space

### Other Pericalvarial Calcification & Thickening
- Calcified SDH
- Subdural fibrosis
- Chronic cephalohematoma

### Dystrophic Macrocephaly without ST
- Craniosynostosis, achondroplasia, mucopolysaccharidoses etc.

### Bone Invasive/Destructive Lesions
- Tumors, proliferative hemopathic processes, infection
- Thickening may occur due to bone sclerosis/reconstruction

## PATHOLOGY

### General Features
- General path comments: Skull thickening
- Genetics: Some etiologies associated with genetic involvement/predisposition
- Etiology

# THICK SKULL

- ○ Etiologies more likely to cause generalized ST
  - Drug therapy e.g., Dilantin (phenytoin)
  - Secondary brain atrophy with inward growth of calvarium
  - Shunted hydrocephalus with brain volume loss
  - Chronic severe anemia: Sickle cell anemia, iron deficiency anemia, β-thalassemia
  - Hormonal: Hyperparathyroidism, acromegaly
  - Hurler: Mucopolysaccharidosis
  - Osteopetrosis
  - Engelmann disease ("sclerosing diaphyseal dysplasia") at skull base
- ○ Etiologies more likely to cause regional or focal ST
  - Hemangioma
  - Langerhans cell histiocytosis
  - Osteoma
  - Calcifying cephalohematoma
  - Dyke-Davidoff-Masson syndrome
- ○ Etiologies causing both focal or generalized ST
  - Fibrous dysplasia: Monostotic (67%), poly-ostotic (30%), McCune-Albright syndrome (3%)
- Epidemiology: Highly variable dependent on etiology
- Associated abnormalities: Many causes are systemic & have a plethora of associated abnormalities

## Gross Pathologic & Surgical Features

- Skull thickening with/without specific diploic changes
  - ○ Cortical bone may be thick but usually spared
- Sinusal equivalent of calvarial overgrowth is dilatation (e.g., Dyke-Davidoff-Masson, acromegaly)

## Microscopic Features

- Inner/outer table cortical thickening with/without diploic space involvement
- Specific histopathology depends on underlying cause

# CLINICAL ISSUES

## Presentation

- Most common signs/symptoms
  - ○ Most often asymptomatic; macrocephaly, dysmorphic features dependent on etiology
  - ○ Without skull base disease: Most symptoms referable to causal disease
  - ○ Patients with skull base ST may be symptomatic from foraminal or canal encroachment
    - Manifests as cranial nerve (CN) deficit(s)
    - Sino-orbital & auditive complications
  - ○ Venous sinuses
    - Displaced/compressed by focal calvarial expansion
    - Narrowed by skull base expansion (possible pseudo-tumor cerebri, hydrocephalus)
- Clinical Profile
  - ○ Features/tests may discriminate between etiologies
    - Dilantin (phenytoin) therapy: Medical history
    - Acromegaly: Global appearance, ↑ growth hormone & IGF-1
    - Dyke-Davidoff-Masson syndrome: Paresis/spasticity contralateral to abnormal calvarium
    - Sickle cell anemia: Hemoglobin electrophoresis & Sickledex test abnormal

- Iron deficiency anemia: ↓ Hematocrit & hemoglobin; small red blood cells; ↓ serum ferritin & iron; high iron binding capacity (TIBC)
- β-thalassemia: Blood smear & hemoglobin electrophoresis abnormal
- Hyperparathyroidism: ↑ Serum calcium, ↑ parathyroid hormone, ↓ serum phosphorus,
- Osteopetrosis: Radiographic skeletal series diagnostic for diffusely dense bones
- Engelmann disease: Radiographic skeletal series show diaphyseal dysplasia

## Demographics

- Age: Depends on etiology
- Gender: May depend on etiology

## Natural History & Prognosis

- ST of no clinical concern by itself, except if neural, venous involvement

## Treatment

- Usually no specific treatment required
  - ○ Skull findings often harbinger of underlying disease
  - ○ Therapy aimed at treating underlying etiology
- Indications for partial or total surgical excision
  - ○ Cosmesis (commonest)
  - ○ Sino-orbital & auditive complications (less common)
  - ○ Peripheral compressive cranial neuropathies (uncommon)
  - ○ Central neurological manifestations (rarest)

# DIAGNOSTIC CHECKLIST

## Consider

- Risk of neurological compromise
- ST may be only clue to severe causal disease

## Image Interpretation Pearls

- CT for bony changes, MR for diploe, nerves, veins

# SELECTED REFERENCES

1. Goisis M et al: Fibrous dysplasia of the orbital region: current clinical perspectives in ophthalmology and cranio-maxillofacial surgery. Ophthal Plast Reconstr Surg. 22(5):383-7, 2006
2. Unal O et al: Left hemisphere and male sex dominance of cerebral hemiatrophy (Dyke-Davidoff-Masson Syndrome). Clin Imaging. 28(3):163-5, 2004
3. Lucey BP et al: Marked calvarial thickening and dural changes following chronic ventricular shunting for shaken baby syndrome. Arch Pathol Lab Med. 127(1):94-7, 2003
4. Sharma RR et al: Symptomatic cranial fibrous dysplasias: clinico-radiological analysis in a series of eight operative cases with follow-up results. J Clin Neurosci. 9(4):381-90, 2002
5. Ikedo D et al: Stimulatory effects of phenytoin on osteoblastic differentiation of fetal rat calvaria cells in culture. Bone. 25(6):653-60, 1999
6. Di Preta JA et al: Hyperostosis cranii ex vacuo: a rare complication of shunting for hydrocephalus. Hum Pathol. 25(5):545-7, 1994
7. Watts RW et al: Computed tomography studies on patients with mucopolysaccharidoses. Neuroradiology. 21(1):9-23, 1981

## IMAGE GALLERY

### Typical

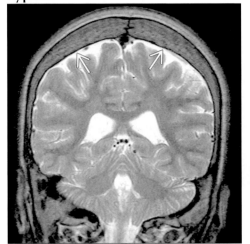 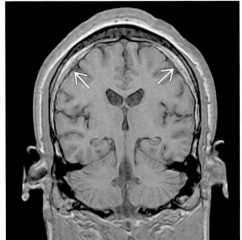

*(Left)* Coronal T2WI MR in sickle cell disease shows diffuse skull thickening ➡️ with diploic widening (from blood-forming bone marrow). Abnormality involves skull base; brain essentially normal. *(Right)* Coronal T1WI MR shows diffuse calvarial thickening in patient with severe epilepsy, likely due to phenytoin treatment. Note thickened inner calvarium ➡️; skull base not involved.

### Typical

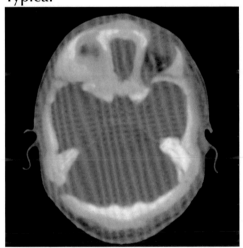 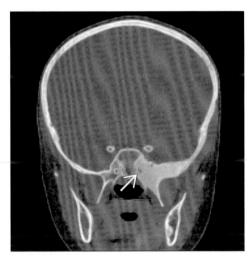

*(Left)* Axial bone CT shows diffuse primary bone dystrophy with loss of normal bone organization specific for osteopetrosis; the whole skull is involved including face and petrous bones. *(Right)* Coronal bone CT shows localized primary bone dysplasia of sphenoid bone (poly-ostotic fibrous dysplasia, frontal involved also); note narrowing of the vidian canal ➡️.

I

6

67

### Typical

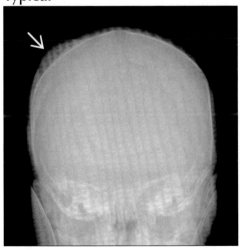 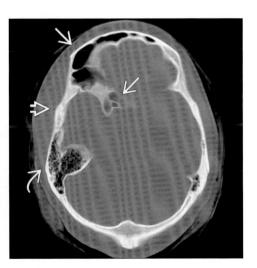

*(Left)* Coronal radiograph shows localized acquired bone thickening with rounded appearance specific for calcifying cephalhematoma (sub-periosteal hematoma) ➡️ in 4 weeks old infant. *(Right)* Axial bone CT shows Dyke-Davidoff-Masson phenomenon: Unilateral dilation of anterior sinuses ➡️ and mastoid air cells ➡️, with thickening of temporal squama ➡️.

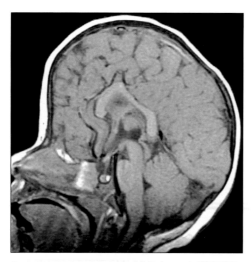

*Sagittal T1WI MR shows typical findings of small clivus, low pituitary gland with long infundibulum, compressed pons. Face is small due to premature closure of facial sutures.*

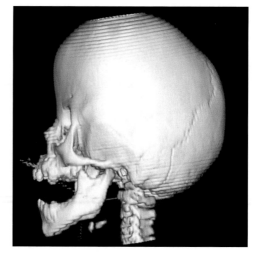

*Lateral NECT 3D reformation shows turricephaly due to bilateral coronal suture synostosis and small face due to premature fusion of facial sutures.*

## TERMINOLOGY

### Definitions
- A constellation of findings leading to increased intracranial pressure and macrocephaly, resulting from a small skull base

## IMAGING FINDINGS

### General Features
- Best diagnostic clue: Small posterior fossa: Small cisterns, short clivus
- Location: Sphenoid, temporal, occipital bones
- Size: Bones, foramina of skull base are too small
- Morphology: Small skull base due to early fusion of sutures

### MR Findings
- T1WI
  - Frontal bossing, sometimes turricephaly or brachycephaly
  - Small posterior fossa
- MRV
  - Venous anomalies common; absent transverse sinuses, persistence of fetal sinuses
    - Emissary veins enlarge to increase intracranial to extracranial venous flow

### Imaging Recommendations
- Best imaging tool: CT for bones, MR for neural structures
- Protocol advice
  - CT with 3D reformations for skull base
  - MR: Sag T1, T2 for crowding of brain stem; axial T2 for compression of craniocervical junction

## DIFFERENTIAL DIAGNOSIS

### Achondroplasia
- Open skull base sutures, ventriculomegaly, congenital spinal stenosis

### Craniosynostosis Syndromes
- Crouzon and Pfeiffer syndromes have earliest, most severe skull base hypoplasia

## DDx: Syndromes with Small Skull Base

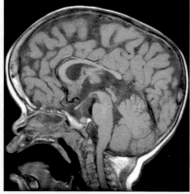

*Achondroplasia*

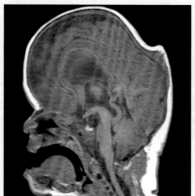

*Crouzon Syndrome*

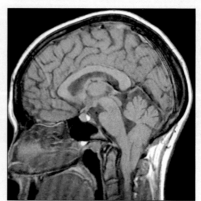

*Chiari I*

# SMALL SKULL BASE

## Key Facts

### Terminology
- A constellation of findings leading to increased intracranial pressure and macrocephaly, resulting from a small skull base

### Imaging Findings
- Best diagnostic clue: Small posterior fossa: Small cisterns, short clivus
- Size: Bones, foramina of skull base are too small

- Frontal bossing, sometimes turricephaly or brachycephaly
- Small posterior fossa
- Venous anomalies common; absent transverse sinuses, persistence of fetal sinuses

### Top Differential Diagnoses
- Achondroplasia
- Craniosynostosis Syndromes
- Chiari I Malformation

## Chiari I Malformation
- Small posterior fossa but no craniosynostoses

## PATHOLOGY

### General Features
- Genetics
  - Variable; most are autosomal dominant
  - When due to sutural synostosis, mutations of fibroblast growth factor receptors (FGFRs), especially FGFR2, are found
    - Many modifying genes may be responsible for differing phenotypes caused by the same mutation
- Etiology: Impaired growth of enchondral bone vs. premature suture closure

### Gross Pathologic & Surgical Features
- Small skull base, narrow skull base foramina lead to clinical features

## CLINICAL ISSUES

### Presentation
- Most common signs/symptoms: Frontal bossing, macrocephaly

### Demographics
- Age: Infancy, early childhood

## Natural History & Prognosis
- Increased intracranial pressure may resolve as emissary veins enlarge
- Small skull base may result in tonsillar herniation, cranial neuropathies, compression of craniocervical junction

## Treatment
- May require shunting for increased intracranial pressure
- Tonsillar herniation may require foramen magnum decompression

## DIAGNOSTIC CHECKLIST

### Consider
- Consider venous anomalies when evaluating small skull base patients for decompression

## SELECTED REFERENCES
1. Aydin S et al: Chiari type I malformations in adults: a morphometric analysis of the posterior cranial fossa. Surg Neurol. 64(3):237-41; discussion 241, 2005
2. Sgouros S: Skull vault growth in craniosynostosis. Childs Nerv Syst. 21(10):861-70, 2005
3. Taylor WJ et al: Enigma of raised intracranial pressure in patients with complex craniosynostosis: the role of abnormal intracranial venous drainage. J Neurosurg. 94(3):377-85, 2001

## IMAGE GALLERY

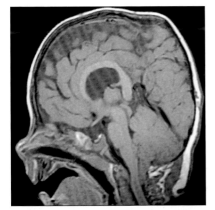
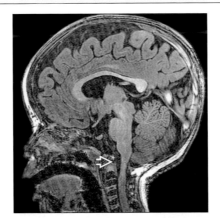
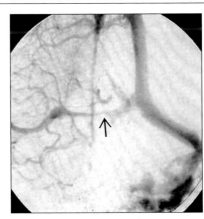

*(Left)* Sagittal T1WI MR shows brachycephaly, suggesting coronal synostosis. In addition clivus is short, infundibulum is long, and tonsils are herniated, signs of small posterior fossa. *(Center)* Sagittal T1WI MR shows compression of the craniocervical junction ➡ due to the small skull base. The clivus is short and the infundibulum is long. *(Right)* Anteroposterior angiography venous phase shows abnormal venous drainage with narrow right transverse sinus ➡ without sigmoid sinus or jugular vein, instead draining through emissary veins.

# CALVARIUM FRACTURE

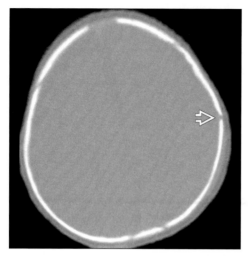

Axial NECT photographed at bone windows shows a linear skull fracture ⊟ in the left parietal bone.

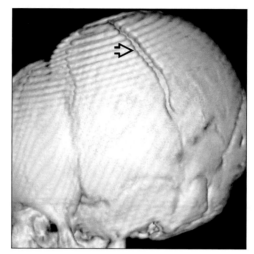

Lateral NECT 3D surface reconstruction (same patient as previous image) shows a linear skull fracture ⊟ in the parietal bone extending from the sagittal suture inferiorly toward the temporal bone.

## TERMINOLOGY

### Abbreviations and Synonyms
- Fracture (Fx)
- Calvarial, skull, skull base, basilar skull

### Definitions
- Fx or break in the cranial (skull) bones

## IMAGING FINDINGS

### General Features
- Best diagnostic clue: Linear calvarial lucency
- Location
  - Fracture at thin squamous temporal/parietal bones, petrous ridge of temporal bone, sphenoid wings
  - Middle cranial fossa is weakest with thin bones & multiple foramina
  - Other sites: Cribriform plate, orbital roof, occipital condyles, region between mastoid & dural sinuses
- Morphology: Fx can be linear, depressed, diastatic, comminuted, overriding, closed or open, growing

### CT Findings
- CTA: Evaluates for associated vascular injury, consider if carotid canal or region of venous sinuses involved
- NECT
  - Intracranial air may be only sign on axial images
  - Linear Fx: Sharply delineated lucent line with overlying soft tissue swelling
  - Depressed Fx: Fragment(s) displaced inwards
  - Diastatic Fx from spreading sutures
    - Cranial "burst fracture" unique in infants: Wide diastasis (> 4 mm) → brain herniates through Fx, extrudes under scalp
  - Skull base Fx
    - Longitudinal, transverse, pneumocephalus common
    - AF level within adjacent air cell(s)
    - Nasal cavity fluid → cerebrospinal fluid (CSF) rhinorrhea
    - Ear cavity fluid from CSF otorrhea or blood density from hemotympanum
    - Air in TMJ glenoid fossa may be only CT sign of an inconspicuous skull base Fx
  - Longitudinal temporal bone Fx

## DDx: Fracture Mimics

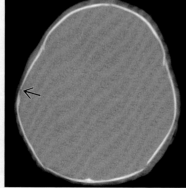

Accessory Suture

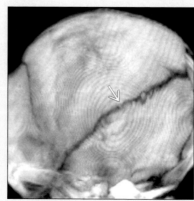

Accessory Suture (NECT MIP)

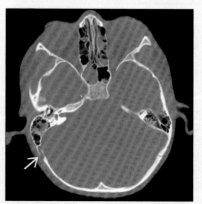

Vascular Channel

# CALVARIUM FRACTURE

## Key Facts

### Imaging Findings
- Intracranial air may be only sign on axial images
- CTA: Evaluates for associated vascular injury, consider if carotid canal or region of venous sinuses involved
- MR if suspect underlying parenchymal injury or to find subtle SDH
- Helical thin section CT, bone algorithm, reformat to minimal slice thickness, get minimum intensity projections (MIPs) or surface rendering

### Top Differential Diagnoses
- Suture Line
- Vascular Groove
- Venous Lake

### Pathology
- Accidental trauma: Parietal linear skull Fx less than 5 cm most common
- Non-accidental trauma: > 5 cm, multiple/complex, depressed, wide, growing fracture, involvement > 1 cranial bone, non-parietal fracture, associated intracranial injury
- Intracranial hemorrhage (ICH) rare in infants; increasing incidence > 2 years
- Skull fracture better predictor of ICH than loss of consciousness (LOC) (unlike adult)

### Clinical Issues
- Linear Fx: Often asymptomatic without LOC
- Clinical Profile: Blunt trauma

---

- Fx line parallel to long axis of petrous bone
- Tympanic membrane disruption
- Ossicular disruption; most commonly incudostapedial joint
- AF levels in mastoid air cells
  - Transverse temporal bone Fx
    - Fx line perpendicular to long axis of petrous bone
    - Inner ear architecture commonly involved
    - Dense hemorrhage in mesotympanum
  - Mixed temporal bone Fx: Imaging elements of both longitudinal & transverse Fx
  - Occipital condylar fracture
  - Growing Fx: Herniation of CSF & soft tissue densities into epidural or subgaleal spaces

## MR Findings
- T1WI FS: Detect dissection if fracture involves carotid canal
- T2WI: Assess for associated parenchymal contusion
- FLAIR: Assess for associated parenchymal contusion, epidural hematoma (EDH), subdural hematoma (SDH), or SAH
- T2* GRE: Best at detecting associated parenchymal hemorrhage
- MRA: May detect associated arterial injury (if fracture involves carotid canal)
- MRV: May detect associated venous injury (if fracture near venous sinuses)

## Radiographic Findings
- Radiography
  - Linear Fx: Sharply defined, linear, lucent line
  - Depressed Fx: Bone-on-bone density
  - Skull base Fx: Insensitive; AF levels
  - Sutural diastasis: Asymmetric widening of suture
  - Growing Fx: Widening Fx lines over time

## Imaging Recommendations
- Best imaging tool
  - NECT
  - MR if suspect underlying parenchymal injury or to find subtle SDH
  - MR or CTA if suspect dissection or venous injury

- Plain films no role
- Protocol advice
  - Helical thin section CT, bone algorithm, reformat to minimal slice thickness, get minimum intensity projections (MIPs) or surface rendering
  - Thin-slice high-resolution NECT for skull base Fx
    - Sagittal/coronal reconstructions
  - Consider lowering kVp to 80 if just looking for bone detail

## DIFFERENTIAL DIAGNOSIS

### Suture Line
- < 2 mm width, fracture (< 2 mm)
- Same width throughout (fracture widest at center)
- Specific anatomic sites
- Less distinct, irregular margins, sclerotic borders (better seen in older children)
- Not straight line

### Vascular Groove
- Corticated margins, non-linear (branches like a tree)
- Typical location (i.e., middle meningeal artery [MMA])

### Arachnoid Granulation
- Corticated margins; typical location (parasagittal, transverse sinus)

### Venous Lake
- Corticated margins; typical location (i.e., parasagittal)

## PATHOLOGY

### General Features
- Etiology
  - Direct trauma: Falls, MVA, bicycle, pedestrian vs. car most common
  - Linear Fx: Low-energy blunt trauma over a wide surface area of skull
  - Depressed Fx: High-energy direct blow to a small surface area with a blunt object (e.g., baseball bat)

# CALVARIUM FRACTURE

○ Occipital condylar fracture: High-energy trauma with axial load, lateral bending, or rotational injury
• Epidemiology
  ○ For < 2 years
    ▪ Accidental trauma: Parietal linear skull Fx less than 5 cm most common
    ▪ Non-accidental trauma: > 5 cm, multiple/complex, depressed, wide, growing fracture, involvement > 1 cranial bone, non-parietal fracture, associated intracranial injury
  ○ Skull Fx present in 75% of fatal injuries at autopsy
  ○ 25-35% with severe brain injury don't have Fx
  ○ Skull base Fx = 19-21% of all skull fractures
    ▪ Sphenoid Fx accounts for 15% of skull base Fx
  ○ 75-90% of depressed Fx are open Fx
• Associated abnormalities
  ○ ~ 30% of linear Fx have intracranial pathology: Epi-/subdural hematoma, contusion
  ○ Intracranial hemorrhage (ICH) rare in infants; increasing incidence > 2 years
  ○ Skull fracture better predictor of ICH than loss of consciousness (LOC) (unlike adult)
  ○ 10-15% with severe head trauma have C1 or C2 Fx

## CLINICAL ISSUES

### Presentation
• Most common signs/symptoms
  ○ Linear Fx: Often asymptomatic without LOC
  ○ Depressed Fx
    ▪ Loss of consciousness (25% none, 25% < 1 hour)
    ▪ Often symptoms referable to epidural hematoma
  ○ Skull base Fx: "Vernet"/"jugular foramen" syndrome
    ▪ Foraminal involvement → CN 9, 10, & 11 deficits
    ▪ Difficulty in phonation, aspiration
    ▪ Ipsilateral paralysis: Vocal cord, soft palate, superior pharyngeal constrictor, sternocleidomastoid, & trapezius
  ○ Longitudinal temporal bone Fx
    ▪ Conductive hearing loss
    ▪ 10-20% CN 7 palsy from facial canal involvement
  ○ Transverse temporal bone Fx
    ▪ Neurosensory hearing loss, vertigo
    ▪ 50% CN 7 palsy from IAC Fx
• Clinical Profile: Blunt trauma

### Demographics
• Age: Infants, adolescents
• Gender: M > F

### Natural History & Prognosis
• Sequelae: CSF leak, delayed CN deficit(s), infarct
• Healing process
  ○ Infants: Usually heals in 3-6 months without a trace
  ○ Children: Heals within 12 months
• Transverse temporal bone Fx
  ○ Permanent neurosensory hearing loss
  ○ Persistent vertigo, unrelenting CN 7 palsy
• Growing Fx ("post-traumatic encephalocele") can be a late complication
  ○ Herniation of CSF, brain, & vessels through lacerated dura/fracture into epidural/subgaleal space

### Treatment
• Most skull Fx, even depressed, do not require surgery
• Contaminated open fractures: Broad spectrum antibiotics & tetanus vaccination
• Type II & III occipital condylar Fx: Treated conservatively with neck stabilization via hard (Philadelphia) collar or halo traction
• Indications for surgery
  ○ Depressed segment > 5 mm below inner table of adjacent bone or cosmesis
  ○ Gross contamination, dural tear with pneumocephalus, underlying hematoma
  ○ Correction of ossicle disarticulation
  ○ Occipital condylar type III Fx (unstable) which requires atlantoaxial arthrodesis
  ○ Persistent CSF leak
• Repeat NECT
  ○ Patient with SDH or small EDH to ensure stability
  ○ Patients with contaminated open depressed skull fractures to check for infection/abscess
  ○ Dictated by complications; seizures, CSF leak

## DIAGNOSTIC CHECKLIST

### Consider
• Non accidental trauma when young and trauma undocumented

### Image Interpretation Pearls
• Sutures curvilinear, irregular; fractures linear, smooth
• Look for adjacent EDH or contralateral SDH

## SELECTED REFERENCES

1. Boran BO et al: Evaluation of mild head injury in a pediatric population. Pediatr Neurosurg. 42(4):203-7, 2006
2. Holmes JF et al: Epidemiology of blunt head injury victims undergoing ED cranial computed tomographic scanning. Am J Emerg Med. 24(2):167-73, 2006
3. Reed MJ et al: Can we abolish skull x rays for head injury? Arch Dis Child. 90(8):859-64, 2005
4. Williamson LM et al: Trends in head injury mortality among 0-14 year olds in Scotland (1986-95). J Epidemiol Community Health. 56(4):285-8, 2002
5. Graham CA et al: Neonatal head injuries. J Accid Emerg Med. 17(5):334-6, 2000
6. Kim KA et al: Analysis of pediatric head injury from falls. Neurosurg Focus. 8(1):e3, 2000
7. Jennett B: Epidemiology of head injury. Arch Dis Child. 78(5):403-6, 1998
8. Chan KH et al: The significance of skull fracture in acute traumatic intracranial hematomas in adolescents: a prospective study. J Neurosurg. 72(2):189-94, 1990
9. Mann KS et al: Skull fractures in children: their assessment in relation to developmental skull changes and acute intracranial hematomas. Childs Nerv Syst. 2(5):258-61, 1986
10. Hobbs CJ: Skull fracture and the diagnosis of abuse. Arch Dis Child. 59(3):246-52, 1984
11. Da Dalt L et al: F, Barbone F. Predictors of intracranial injuries in children after blunt head trauma.
12. Leventhal JM et al: Fractures in young children. Distinguishing child abuse from unintentional injuries.

# CALVARIUM FRACTURE

## IMAGE GALLERY

### Typical

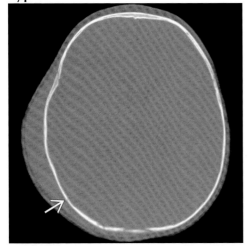
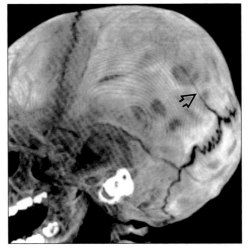

*(Left)* Axial NECT photographed using bone windows shows a subtle linear skull fracture ➡ with overlying soft tissue swelling in the right parietal bone. *(Right)* Lateral NECT MIP (same patient as previous image) makes the linear skull fracture ⇨ more easily seen.

### Typical

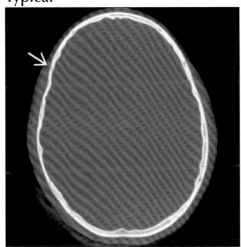
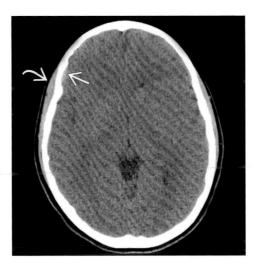

*(Left)* Axial NECT photographed using bone windows shows a linear skull fracture ➡ in the left frontal bone. No parenchymal abnormalities are seen. *(Right)* Axial NECT using brain windows (same patient as previous image) shows a small epidural hematoma ➡ and some overlying soft tissue swelling ➡.

### Typical

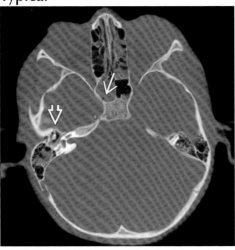
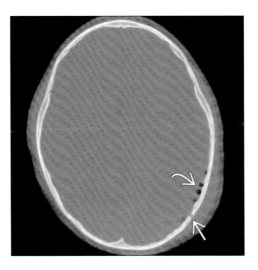

*(Left)* Axial NECT after head trauma shows a small air bubble in fluid-filled sphenoid sinus adjacent to sphenoid wing fracture ➡. Transverse temporal bone fracture ⇨ with fluid in mastoid. *(Right)* Axial NECT shows left parietal bone linear fracture ➡ with overlying soft tissue swelling and adjacent pneumocephalus ➡. The intracranial air suggests a fracture through the temporal bone.

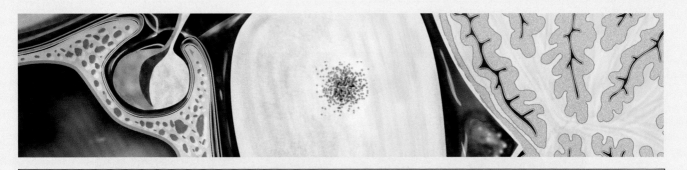

# SECTION 7: Blood Vessels

# PERSISTENT TRIGEMINAL ARTERY

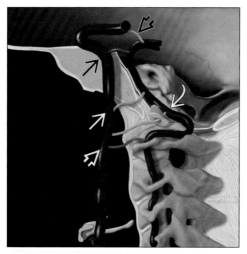

Graphic of persistent vestigial CB anastomoses: Trigeminal ➡, otic ➡, hypoglossal (hypoglossal canal) ➡, proatlantal ➡; final mature CB anastomosis is posterior communicating ➡.

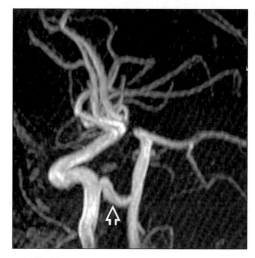

Lateral MRA maximum intensity projection shows large arterial trunk ➡ extending from proximal cavernous ICA to mid-BA in the absence of associated anomalies.

## TERMINOLOGY

### Abbreviations and Synonyms
- Persistent trigeminal artery (PTA)

### Definitions
- Most common of persistent carotid basilar anastomosis (PCBA) between cavernous ICA, basilar artery (BA)

## IMAGING FINDINGS

### General Features
- Best diagnostic clue: Abnormal vessel between proximal cavernous ICA and BA
- Location: Lateral or medial

### CT Findings
- CTA: Delineates vascular anomaly, associated disease
- CECT: Large vessel between BA and cavernous ICA

### MR Findings
- T2WI: Abnormal prepontine arterial channel
- MRA: Depicts channel, possible associated lesions

### Angiographic Findings
- Conventional
  - Saltzman type I: PTA supplies distal BA, PComAs usually absent, proximal BA hypoplastic
  - Saltzman type II: PTA feeds superior cerebellar arteries, patent persistent communicating arteries (PComAs) supply posterior cerebral arteries (PCA)
  - Associated vascular anomalies in 25% of cases (aneurysms: 15%)

### Imaging Recommendations
- Best imaging tool: MR + MRA
- Protocol advice: No DSA unless associated disease

## DIFFERENTIAL DIAGNOSIS

### Carotid ("Fetal") Origin of PCA
- Common (10% right, 10% left, 8% bilateral), from the supracavernous ICA; proximal PCA hypoplastic/absent

### Other PCBAs
- Persistent hypoglossal artery (PHA), 2nd most common (0.03-0.26%)

## DDx: Other ICA-BA Anastomoses

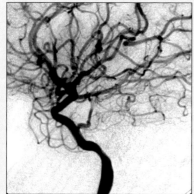

"Fetal" PComA and PTA

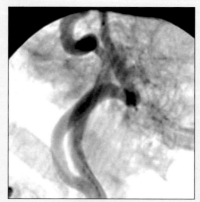

Hypoglossal

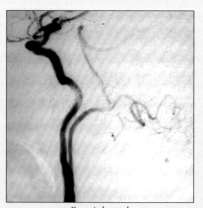

Pro-Atlantal

# PERSISTENT TRIGEMINAL ARTERY

## Key Facts

### Imaging Findings
- Best diagnostic clue: Abnormal vessel between proximal cavernous ICA and BA
- Best imaging tool: MR + MRA

### Pathology
- Epidemiology: Most common PCBA (0.1-0.2%)
- 25% prevalence of other vascular disease (e.g., aneurysm, moyamoya)

### Clinical Issues
- Incidental finding at imaging
- Trigeminal neuralgia, pituitary dysfunction rare
- Benign if no associated disease

### Diagnostic Checklist
- When incidental no further investigation

---

- From cervical ICA at C1/3 (or lower) to BA, along CN12 through hypoglossal canal (caudocranial); PComAs and VAs usually hypoplastic/absent
- Pro-atlantal intersegmental artery (PIA), most caudal
  - From cervical ICA at C2/3 (or lower) (type I), ECA (type II), or CCA rarely, to one VA above C1 through foramen magnum; VAs usually absent or hypoplastic
- Persistent otic artery (POA), rarest (two cases reported)
  - From petrous ICA to caudal BA through internal acoustic meatus; VAs absent or hypoplastic

## PATHOLOGY

### General Features
- General path comments
  - Embryology
    - Before vertebral arteries develop, ICA supplies hindbrain arteries through four transient segmental connections
  - Anatomy
    - PTA arises from cavernous ICA
    - Runs posterolaterally along trigeminal nerve (41%) or medially through dorsum sellae (59%)
    - Small PComAs, VAs, proximal BA
- Etiology: Unknown
- Epidemiology: Most common PCBA (0.1-0.2%)
- Associated abnormalities
  - 25% prevalence of other vascular disease (e.g., aneurysm, moyamoya)

- Rarely: Carotid-cavernous fistula, AVM, fenestration, NF1, abnormal CC/ICA, aorta coarctation

## CLINICAL ISSUES

### Presentation
- Most common signs/symptoms
  - Incidental finding at imaging
  - Trigeminal neuralgia, pituitary dysfunction rare
- Hemorrhage, ischemia from associated arterial disease

### Natural History & Prognosis
- Benign if no associated disease

## DIAGNOSTIC CHECKLIST

### Consider
- When incidental no further investigation

## SELECTED REFERENCES

1. Suttner N et al: Persistent trigeminal artery: a unique anatomic specimen--analysis and therapeutic implications. Neurosurgery. 47(2):428-33; discussion 433-4, 2000
2. Uchino A et al: Persistent trigeminal artery variants detected by MR angiography. Eur Radiol. 10:1801-4, 2000
3. Hirai T et al: MR angiography of the persistent trigeminal artery variant. J Comput Assist Tomogr. 19(3):495-7, 1995
4. Silbergleit R et al: Persistent trigeminal artery detected with standard MRI. J Comput Assist Tomogr. 17(1):22-5, 1993

## IMAGE GALLERY

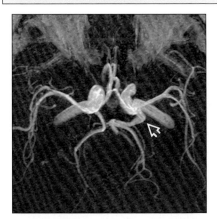 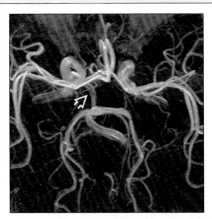 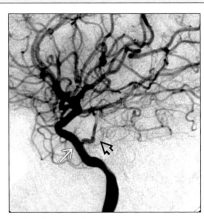

*(Left) Axial MRA collapsed view shows the lateral location of left persisting trigeminal artery ➡. Note the absence of ipsilateral posterior communicating artery. (Center) Axial MRA collapsed view shows medial location of a right persisting trigeminal artery ➡. Ipsilateral posterior communicating artery is absent. (Right) Lateral angiography shows the persistent trigeminal artery ➡ originating from the cavernous portion of the ICA ➡, and coursing posteriorly to supply the terminal portion of the BA.*

# SINUS PERICRANII

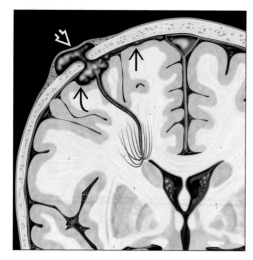

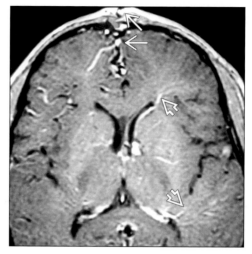

*Coronal graphic shows a complex lateral sinus pericranii (SP). In addition to a scalp varix ⇒, a DVA, intracranial varix ⇒ and cortical vein ⇒ comprise SP.*

*Axial T1 C+ MR shows enlarged cortical and scalp veins in the region of superior sagittal sinus ⇒. This patient with blue rubber-bleb nevus syndrome also has many DVAs ⇒.*

## TERMINOLOGY

### Abbreviations and Synonyms
- Sinus pericranii (SP)

### Definitions
- Abnormal communication between intracranial (IC) and extracranial venous circulation
  - Most common arrangement: Communication of dural venous sinus (DVS) with overlying scalp varix or prominent scalp veins via transcalvarial diploic or emissary vein(s)

## IMAGING FINDINGS

### General Features
- Best diagnostic clue: Scalp lesion with vascular enhancement communicating with underlying DVS
- Location
  - Frontal (40%), parietal (34%), occipital (23%), temporal (4%)
  - Midline or parasagittal
    - Lateral location uncommon

- Superior sagittal sinus most common DVS
  - Transverse sinus, torcular distant second
- Size
  - Scalp lesion: 1-13 cm; most 2-6 cm
  - Transcalvarial bone defect: Single/multiple 1-4 mm holes; rare large defect
- Morphology
  - Extracranial SP morphology
    - Tubular, round, lobular varix or multiple veins
    - Venous malformation (VM) or AVM (rare) less common
  - Intracranial SP morphology
    - DVS
    - Varix or prominent cortical vein(s) less common
    - May be associated with developmental venous anomaly (DVA)

### CT Findings
- NECT
  - Homogeneous (varix) or heterogeneous (VM)
    - Septations, phleboliths if VM
  - Bone algorithm
    - Single/multiple well-defined bone defects
    - Pressure erosion from overlying varix

I

7

4

## DDx: Pediatric Scalp Lesions

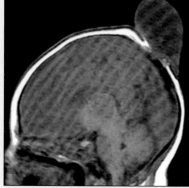

*Atretic Parietal Cephalocele*

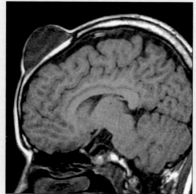

*Dermoid*

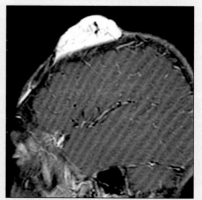

*Infantile Hemangioma*

# SINUS PERICRANII

## Key Facts

### Terminology
- Abnormal communication between intracranial (IC) and extracranial venous circulation

### Imaging Findings
- Best diagnostic clue: Scalp lesion with vascular enhancement communicating with underlying DVS
- Midline or parasagittal

### Top Differential Diagnoses
- Cephalocele
- Dermoid/Epidermoid
- Vascular Anomalies of the Scalp (Isolated)
- Rhabdomyosarcoma, Langerhans Cell Histiocytosis, Neuroblastoma Metastases

### Pathology
- Congenital or acquired, traumatic or spontaneous
- Rare

### Clinical Issues
- Nontender, fluctuant, bluish forehead/scalp mass
- Reduces in upright position
- Distends when prone or with Valsalva
- Age: Children, young adults (range: Newborn to 70 years)
- Stable or slow enlargement
- Prognosis excellent following surgical removal

### Diagnostic Checklist
- Pre-operative evaluation of entire DVS network important, particularly in setting of syndromic craniosynostoses

---

- CECT
  - Varix: Homogeneous, vascular enhancement
    - Heterogeneous if thrombus present or if VM
- CTV: Delineates all vascular components of SP

## MR Findings
- T1WI
  - Variable; most hypo-, isointense or mixed
    - Hyperintense if thrombus present
    - Flow voids in rapidly flowing varix/VM
- T2WI
  - Variable; most hyperintense
    - Mixed signal in large varix/VM 2° turbulent flow
    - Flow voids in rapidly flowing varix/VM
- T1 C+
  - Varix: Homogeneous, vascular enhancement
  - VM: Heterogeneous enhancement
    - Peripheral puddling with delayed "fill in" classic
- MRV: Delineates all vascular components of SP

## Radiographic Findings
- Skull radiograph: Normal or focal bone defect, thinning, erosion

## Ultrasonographic Findings
- Grayscale Ultrasound: Hypoechoic scalp mass
- Color Doppler: Identifies scalp, transcalvarial vein and direction of flow

## Nuclear Medicine Findings
- Bone Scan: ↑ Activity venous and blood pool phases

## Angiographic Findings
- Conventional
  - SP identified during venous phase
  - "Closed" and "drainer" classification based on venous drainage pattern
    - Closed: Blood comes from and drains into DVS
    - Drainer: Blood comes from DVS and drains into scalp veins

## Other Modality Findings
- Percutaneous venography (PV)
  - Visualization of scalp veins
  - Visualization of transcalvarial vein, DVS, intracranial varix/cortical vein inconstant

## Imaging Recommendations
- Best imaging tool
  - MR C+/MRV
    - Scalp veins best separated from cortical veins on MRV source images
    - Transcalvarial vein may not be identified on conventional sequences
- Protocol advice
  - CT/CTV suitable alternative to MR
  - Angiography or PV may be required to accurately demonstrate venous anatomy pre-operatively
  - US emerging as suitable tool for demonstration of scalp and transcalvarial vein and direction of flow

## DIFFERENTIAL DIAGNOSIS

### Cephalocele
- Brain/CSF-filled dural herniation through skull defect
- No enhancement unless vessels/DVS herniate
- Atretic parietal cephalocele (APC): Midline with small bone defect; characteristic persistent falcine sinus

### Dermoid/Epidermoid
- Anterior fontanelle location classic
- Well-defined fluid/fat signal, none to mild rim-enhancement
- Pressure erosion; focal defect in calvarial location uncommon

### Vascular Anomalies of the Scalp (Isolated)
- Infantile hemangioma (IH), AVF, AVM, VM
- MR C+: Solid enhancement (IH), flow voids (AVM, AVF), heterogeneous (VM)
- Pressure erosion without definable IC communication

### Rhabdomyosarcoma, Langerhans Cell Histiocytosis, Neuroblastoma Metastases
- Enhancing, destructive masses
- DVS invasion appears as filling defect

# SINUS PERICRANII

## PATHOLOGY

### General Features
- Etiology
  - Congenital or acquired, traumatic or spontaneous
  - Congenital
    - Incomplete sutural fusion over prominent/abundant diploic or emissary veins
    - In utero DVS thrombosis or DVS/internal jugular vein hypoplasia/atresia; SP forms as alternate venous outlet
    - SP part of VM or other congenital vascular malformation
  - Traumatic
    - Disruption of diploic/emissary veins at outer table
    - Laceration or thrombosis of DVS
  - Spontaneous
    - Likely 2° to remote, "forgotten" trauma
    - Subclinical, post-natal DVS thrombosis
- Epidemiology
  - Rare
  - 11% of patients presenting for treatment of craniofacial VMs
- Associated abnormalities
  - Blue rubber-bleb nevus syndrome
  - Systemic VMs
  - Syndromic (multi-sutural) craniosynostosis
  - Isolated reports of cutis aplasia congenita

### Gross Pathologic & Surgical Features
- Scalp varix/VM: Bluish, blood-filled sac or network of sacs beneath > above periosteum

### Microscopic Features
- Scalp Varix/VM: Non-muscular venous channel(s)
  - Endothelial lining = congenital origin
  - Fibrous lining/capsule = traumatic origin
- +/- Hemosiderin laden macrophages, thrombus

### Staging, Grading or Classification Criteria
- Classification based on venous drainage pattern
  - "Closed": Blood comes from and drains into DVS
  - "Drainer": Blood comes from DVS, drains into scalp veins

## CLINICAL ISSUES

### Presentation
- Most common signs/symptoms
  - Nontender, fluctuant, bluish forehead/scalp mass
    - Reduces in upright position
    - Distends when prone or with Valsalva
  - Rare: Pain, headache, nausea, dizziness
- Clinical Profile: Child with long history of painless, reducible scalp mass

### Demographics
- Age: Children, young adults (range: Newborn to 70 years)
- Gender: M = F (post-traumatic cases M > F)

### Natural History & Prognosis
- Stable or slow enlargement
- Rare spontaneous regression
- Potential lifetime risk hemorrhage or air embolism
- Prognosis excellent following surgical removal
  - Very rare recurrence

### Treatment
- Once medical attention sought, SP usually treated
- Surgery
  - Pre-operative evaluation of entire DVS network necessary to ensure feasibility of SP removal
  - Removal of scalp lesion; closure of bone holes with bone wax, diamond drilling
  - Rare cranioplasty for large bone defects
  - Small risk of significant blood loss
- Endovascular therapy
  - Suitable for single/small drainer SPs
  - Percutaneous injection sclerosant/coils into draining scalp veins
  - Risk of overlying skin necrosis

## DIAGNOSTIC CHECKLIST

### Consider
- Blue rubber-bleb nevus syndrome if SP associated with multiple intracranial DVAs

### Image Interpretation Pearls
- Pre-operative evaluation of entire DVS network important, particularly in setting of syndromic craniosynostoses
  - SP may serve as important venous outflow channel if associated DVS/IJV stenosis/atresia
- Imaging appearance characteristic
  - Unless SP thrombosed, main competing DDx is cephalocele with herniated DVS

## SELECTED REFERENCES

1. Yanik B et al: Sinus pericranii: color Doppler ultrasonographic findings. J Ultrasound Med. 25(5):679-82, 2006
2. Wen CS et al: Sinus pericranii: from gross and neuroimaging findings to different pathophysiological changes. Childs Nerv Syst. 21(6):482-8, 2005
3. Brisman JL et al: Sinus pericranii involving the torcular sinus in a patient with Hunter's syndrome and trigonocephaly: case report and review of the literature. Neurosurgery. 55(2):433, 2004
4. Burry MV et al: Use of gadolinium as an intraarticular contrast agent for pediatric neuroendovascular procedures. J Neurosurg. 100:105-5, 2004
5. Burrows PE et al: Venous variations of the brain and cranial vault. Neuroimaging Clin N Am. 13:13-26, 2003
6. Kurosu A et al: Craniosynostosis in the presence of a sinus pericranii: case report. Neurosurgery. 34:1090-93, 1994
7. Nakasu Y et al: Multiple sinus pericranii with systemic angiomas: case report. Surg Neurol. 39:41-5, 1993
8. Bollar A et al: Sinus pericranii: radiological and etiopathological considerations. J Neurosurg. 77:469-72, 1992
9. Sherry RG et al: Sinus pericranii and venous angioma in the Blue-Rubber bleb nevus syndrome. AJNR. 5:832-34, 1984

# SINUS PERICRANII

## IMAGE GALLERY

### Typical

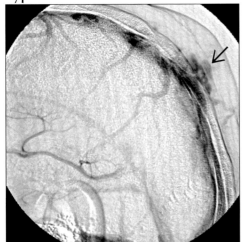

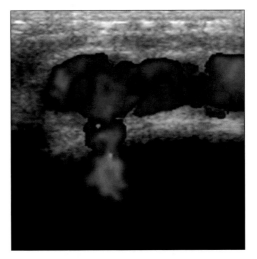

(Left) Lateral angiography venous phase shows typical appearance and location of SP. Several dilated scalp veins ➡ fill from the superior sagittal sinus via a small transosseous feeder. (Right) Transcranial color Doppler shows venous blood within a tubular scalp lesion and a transcalvarial vein. Shadowing from the skull precludes further intracranial evaluation.

### Typical

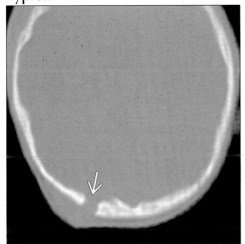

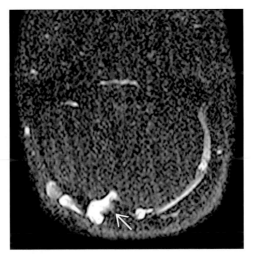

(Left) Axial NECT shows a well-defined bone defect ➡ with overlying scalp swelling. The parasagittal location is typical for SP. Occipital bone location is less common than frontal or parietal. (Right) Source images from axial neck MRV in same patient as previous image show transcalvarial communication ➡ of a scalp varix with the torcular. SPs arising from the torcular/transverse sinus are infrequent.

### Typical

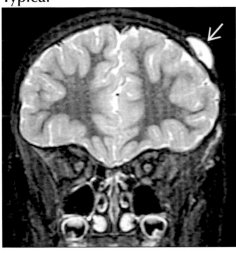

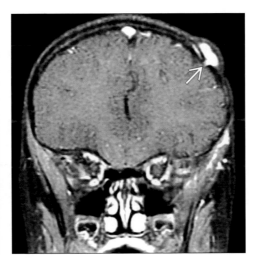

(Left) Coronal T2WI FS MR shows a well-defined, hyperintense scalp lesion ➡ with underlying bone thinning. While the T2 appearance is consistent with SP, the lateral location is unusual. (Right) Coronal T1 C+ FS MR in same patient as previous image shows vascular enhancement of the scalp varix and a small transosseous vein ➡. A cortical vein ultimately bridged the varix with the sagittal DVS.

# CAPILLARY TELANGIECTASIA

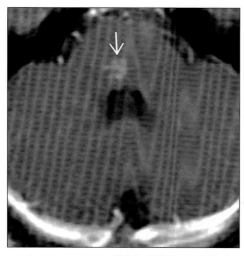

*Axial T1 C+ MR shows brush like contrast enhancement ➡ with no mass effect in the central pons, the most common location for capillary telangiectasias.*

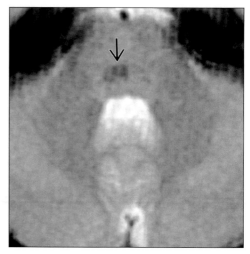

*Axial T2\* GRE MR shows mildly decreased signal intensity ➡ and no mass effect from the telangiectasia.*

## TERMINOLOGY

### Abbreviations and Synonyms
- Brain capillary telangiectasia (BCT)

### Definitions
- Cluster of capillaries interspersed with normal brain

## IMAGING FINDINGS

### General Features
- Best diagnostic clue: Hypointense T2\* lesion, faint "brush-like" enhancement, no mass effect
- Location
  - Midbrain, pons, medulla, spinal cord most common
  - One-third found elsewhere (subcortical WM, etc.)
- Size: Usually < 1 cm
- Morphology: Small, poorly-demarcated lesion; no mass effect or edema

### CT Findings
- NECT: Usually normal (occasionally may have Ca++)
- CECT: Usually normal

### MR Findings
- T1WI: Usually normal
- T2WI: 50% normal; 50% stippled foci of hyperintensity
- FLAIR: Usually normal; may show hyperintense foci
- T2\* GRE
  - Lesion moderately but not profoundly hypointense (deoxyhemoglobin)
  - Less common: Multifocal BCTs ("gray dots")
- DWI: Usually normal
- T1 C+
  - Faint stippled or speckled "brush-like" enhancement
  - May show punctate, linear/branching vessels ± collecting vein if mixed with developmental venous anomaly (DVA)

### Angiographic Findings
- Conventional
  - Usually normal
  - Faint vascular "stain" or draining vein if mixed with DVA

### Imaging Recommendations
- Best imaging tool: MR with T2\*, T1 C+ sequences

---

### DDx: Capillary Telangiectasia Mimics

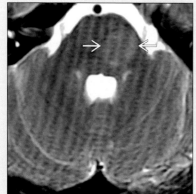

*Demyelinating Lesion*

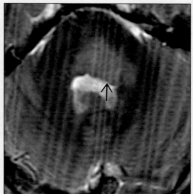

*Brainstem Tumor*

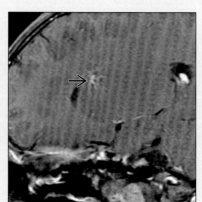

*"Medusa Head" of DVA*

# CAPILLARY TELANGIECTASIA

## Key Facts

### Terminology
- Cluster of capillaries interspersed with normal brain

### Imaging Findings
- Best diagnostic clue: Hypointense T2* lesion, faint "brush-like" enhancement, no mass effect
- Less common: Multifocal BCTs ("gray dots")
- Best imaging tool: MR with T2*, T1 C+ sequences

### Top Differential Diagnoses
- Neoplasm
- Developmental Venous Anomaly (DVA)
- Cavernous Malformation

### Diagnostic Checklist
- Enhancing lesion with no mass effect, minimal T2 abnormality

## DIFFERENTIAL DIAGNOSIS

### Demyelinating Lesion
- T2 lesion without blooming on GRE T2 and peripheral enhancement

### Neoplasm
- Mass effect, more prominent T2 signal abnormality

### Developmental Venous Anomaly (DVA)
- Medusa head and draining vein on T1 C+, mixed with BCT

### Cavernous Malformation
- Blood locules with blood at different stages, hemosiderin rim

## PATHOLOGY

### General Features
- General path comments: Usually incidental finding
- Genetics: None known
- Etiology: Unknown
- Epidemiology: 15-20% of intracranial vascular malformations

### Microscopic Features
- Cluster of dilated but histologically normal capillaries with normal brain in-between
- Uncomplicated CTs have no gliosis, hemorrhage, Ca++

## CLINICAL ISSUES

### Presentation
- Most common signs/symptoms: Asymptomatic; headache, vertigo, tinnitus rare
- Clinical Profile: Incidental finding

### Demographics
- Age: Any age but adult more common

### Natural History & Prognosis
- Clinically benign, quiescent unless histologically mixed
- Case reports of progression if large

### Treatment
- None

## DIAGNOSTIC CHECKLIST

### Image Interpretation Pearls
- Enhancing lesion with no mass effect, minimal T2 abnormality

## SELECTED REFERENCES

1. Castillo M et al: MR imaging and histologic features of capillary telangiectasia of the basal ganglia. AJNR Am J Neuroradiol. 22(8):1553-5, 2001

## IMAGE GALLERY

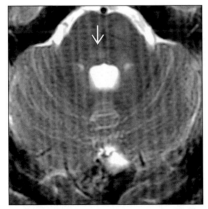 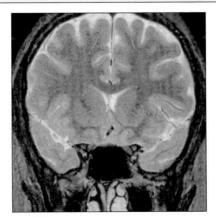 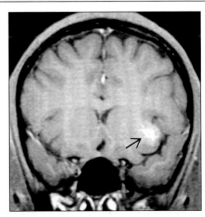

*(Left)* Axial T2WI MR shows subtle increased T2 ➡ but no mass effect, differentiating it from an acute process or a neoplasm. *(Center)* Coronal T2WI MR is normal, showing no mass effect and no T2 abnormality. *(Right)* Coronal T1 C+ MR in same patient as previous image shows a large area of brush-like enhancement ➡ but no mass effect.

# DEVELOPMENTAL VENOUS ANOMALY

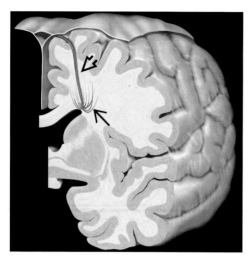

Coronal graphic shows a central enlarged transcerebral collector vein ⇒ draining a crown of dilated periventricular medullary veins ⇒ toward the superior sagittal sinus.

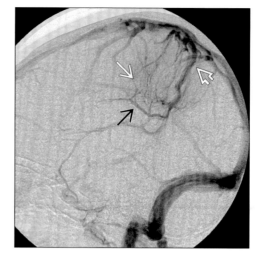

Lateral angiography shows parietal transcerebral vein ⇒ that collects numerous smaller periventricular medullary veins ⇒, and a subependymal vein ⇒, toward superior sagittal sinus.

## TERMINOLOGY

### Abbreviations and Synonyms
- Developmental venous anomaly (DVA); medullary venous malformation (MVM); venous angioma

### Definitions
- Strictly venous malformation with angiogenically mature venous elements
- Sometimes considered a normal anatomic variant of venous drainage, but commonly associated with other pathologies (cavernomas, vascular syndromes)

## IMAGING FINDINGS

### General Features
- Best diagnostic clue: "Medusa head": Crown of dilated medullary veins converging toward an enlarged central vein
- Location
  - Anywhere in the brain, extending between the pial and the ependymal surfaces
    - Cerebral mantle, basal ganglia, brainstem
    - More common: Frontal, parietal, cerebellar
    - May drain to the surface or to the ventricle, or both
- Size: Varies (may be extensive) but usually < 2-3 cm
- Morphology
  - "Caput Medusae" (Medusa head): Appearance of an umbrella, a jellyfish
  - Large trans-parenchymal vein collecting a surrounding field of either superficial or periventricular dilated medullary veins
  - Usually solitary, can be multiple in vascular syndromes, especially blue rubber bleb nevus syndrome (BRBNS)

### CT Findings
- NECT
  - Usually normal
  - Occasional Ca++ if associated cavernous malformation
  - Rarely acute parenchymal hemorrhage (cavernoma, thrombosis of central vein)
- CECT
  - Numerous linear or dot-like enhancing foci

## DDx: Prominent Draining Veins

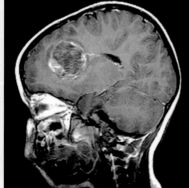

*High Grade Glioma*

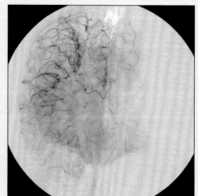

*Ill-Defined AVM*

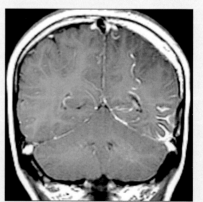

*Sturge-Weber Syndrome*

# DEVELOPMENTAL VENOUS ANOMALY

## Key Facts

### Terminology
- Strictly venous malformation with angiogenically mature venous elements

### Imaging Findings
- Best diagnostic clue: "Medusa head": Crown of dilated medullary veins converging toward an enlarged central vein
- Strong linear transcerebral enhancement
- Protocol advice: Include T2* GRE sequence to look for cavernoma

### Pathology
- Most common cerebral vascular malformation at autopsy

### Clinical Issues
- Usually asymptomatic, incidental
- Hemorrhage with focal neurologic deficit: May occur if associated with cavernoma, or in case of (rare) thrombosis/hemorrhage
- Hemorrhage risk 0.15% per lesion/per year
- Stenosis or thrombosis of draining vein increases hemorrhage risk
- Co-existing cavernous malformation increases hemorrhage risk

### Diagnostic Checklist
- Prominent group of venous channels with a central transcerebral collector
- If a DVA is hemorrhagic, look for associated cavernoma or tiny AVM

---

- In well-defined round/ovoid areas on sequential sections
- Converge on single enlarged tubular draining vein
- Occasionally seen as linear structure in a single slice

### MR Findings
- T1WI
  - Can be normal if DVA is small
  - Variable signal depending on size, flow
    - Flow void, other flow artifacts
  - Hemorrhage if thrombosis of vein or associated cavernoma
- T2WI
  - +/- Flow void
  - +/- Blood products (rare)
  - Flow mismapped into parenchyma
- FLAIR: Usually normal; may show hyperintense region if gliosis, venous ischemia, or hemorrhage if present
- T2* GRE: May bloom if co-existing blood, cavernoma
- DWI
  - Usually normal
  - Rare: Acute venous infarct seen as hyperintense area of reduced diffusion
- T1 C+
  - Strong linear transcerebral enhancement
    - Stellate, tubular vessels converge on collector vein
    - Vein drains into superficial or subependymal vein
- MRA
  - Arterial tree usually normal
  - Contrast-enhanced MRA may demonstrate slow-flow DVA
- MRV: Delineates "Medusa head" and drainage pattern
- MRS: Normal

### Angiographic Findings
- Conventional
  - DSA
    - Arterial phase normal in > 95% of cases
    - Capillary phase usually normal (rare: Prominent "blush" ± A-V shunt)
    - Venous phase: "Medusa head"

- 5% atypical (transitional form of venous-arteriovenous malformation with enlarged feeders, A-V shunting)

### Imaging Recommendations
- Best imaging tool: T1 C+ MR plus MRV
- Protocol advice: Include T2* GRE sequence to look for cavernoma

## DIFFERENTIAL DIAGNOSIS

### Tiny AVM with Single Draining Vein
- Vein fills early, during the arterial phase

### Vascular Neoplasm
- Enlarged medullary veins draining hypervascular tumor
- Mass effect, usually enhances

### Collateral Drainage of Dural Sinus Occlusion
- Typically multiple and disseminated, medullary veins may enlarge as collateral drainage
- Clot in the lumen of the sinus

### Sturge-Weber Syndrome
- May develop strikingly enlarged medullary, subependymal, choroid plexus veins
- Co-existing pial, and facial, angiomas

### Venous Varix (Isolated)
- Prominent vein without hydrodynamic explanation

### Demyelinating Disease
- Rare: Active, aggressive demyelination may have prominent medullary veins, but no caput medusa

## PATHOLOGY

### General Features
- General path comments
  - Embryology: Unknown

# DEVELOPMENTAL VENOUS ANOMALY

- DVA functions as a trans-parenchymal collateral drainage
- Variably considered as resulting from developmental arrest ("persistent" hypothetic large embryonic medullary vein), or from previous occlusion of adjacent collectors, but genetic inheritance common
- Genetics
  - Mutations in chromosome 9p
    - Encodes for surface cell receptors
    - Tie-2 mutation results in missense activation
    - Segregates pedigrees with skin, oral and GI mucosa, brain venous malformations
  - Approximately 50% inherited as autosomal dominant
- Etiology
  - Does not express growth factors
  - Expresses structural proteins of mature angiogenesis
- Epidemiology
  - Most common cerebral vascular malformation at autopsy
  - 60% of cerebral vascular malformations
  - 2.5-9% prevalence on contrast-enhanced MR scans
- Associated abnormalities
  - 15-20% occur with co-existing cavernous malformation
  - Blue rubber bleb nevus syndrome (BRBNS)
  - Sinus pericranii
  - Cervicofacial venous or lymphatic malformation (CAMS-3)
  - Cortical malformations

## Gross Pathologic & Surgical Features
- Radially oriented dilated medullary veins
- Venous roots are embedded in normal brain
- Enlarged transcortical or subependymal draining vein

## Microscopic Features
- Dilated thin-walled vessels diffusely distributed in normal white matter (no gliosis)
- Occasional: Thickened, hyalinized vessel walls
- 20% have mixed histology (cavernoma most common), may hemorrhage
- Variant: "Angiographically occult" DVA with malformed, compactly arranged vessels and partly degenerated walls

# CLINICAL ISSUES

## Presentation
- Most common signs/symptoms
  - Usually asymptomatic, incidental
  - Uncommon
    - Headache
    - Seizures
    - Hemorrhage with focal neurologic deficit: May occur if associated with cavernoma, or in case of (rare) thrombosis/hemorrhage
- Clinical Profile: Asymptomatic patient with DVA found incidentally on MR

## Demographics
- Age: Commonly seen at all ages

- Gender: M = F
- Ethnicity: None known

## Natural History & Prognosis
- Hemorrhage risk 0.15% per lesion/per year
  - Stenosis or thrombosis of draining vein increases hemorrhage risk
  - Co-existing cavernous malformation increases hemorrhage risk
- Seizures may be associated with cavernoma, or cortical malformation

## Treatment
- Incidental DVA: None (attempt at removal may cause venous infarction)
- Histologically mixed DVA: Determined by co-existing lesion
- DVAs provide main venous drainage for intervening normal brain! should not be removed!

# DIAGNOSTIC CHECKLIST

## Image Interpretation Pearls
- Prominent group of venous channels with a central transcerebral collector
- If a DVA is hemorrhagic, look for associated cavernoma or tiny AVM

# SELECTED REFERENCES

1. Campeau NG et al: De novo development of a lesion with the appearance of a cavernous malformation adjacent to an existing developmental venous anomaly. AJNR Am J Neuroradiol. 26(1):156-9, 2005
2. Rollins N et al: MR venography in the pediatric patient. AJNR Am J Neuroradiol. 26(1):50-5, 2005
3. Abe M et al: Histologically classified venous angiomas of the brain: a controversy. Neurol Med Chir (Tokyo). 43(1):1-10; discussion 11, 2003
4. Gabikian P et al: Developmental venous anomalies and sinus pericranii in the blue rubber-bleb nevus syndrome. Case report. J Neurosurg. 99(2):409-11, 2003
5. Wurm G et al: Recurrent cryptic vascular malformation associated with a developmental venous anomaly. Br J Neurosurg. 17(2):188-95, 2003
6. Desai K et al: Developmental deep venous system anomaly associated with congenital malformation of the brain. Pediatr Neurosurg. 36(1):37-9, 2002
7. Hammoud D et al: Ischemic complication of a cerebral developmental venous anomaly: case report and review of the literature. J Comput Assist Tomogr. 26(4):633-6, 2002
8. Agazzi S et al: Developmental venous anomaly with an arteriovenous shunt and a thrombotic complication. Case report. J Neurosurg. 94(3):533-7, 2001
9. Clatterbuck RE et al: The juxtaposition of a capillary telangiectasia, cavernous malformation, and developmental venous anomaly in the brainstem of a single patient: case report. Neurosurgery. 49(5):1246-50, 2001
10. Kilic T et al: Expression of structural proteins and angiogenic factors in cerebrovascular anomalies. Neurosurgery. 46(5):1179-91; discussion 1191-2, 2000
11. Naff NJ et al: A longitudinal study of patients with venous malformations: documentation of a negligible hemorrhage risk and benign natural history. Neurology. 50(6):1709-14, 1998

# DEVELOPMENTAL VENOUS ANOMALY

### Typical

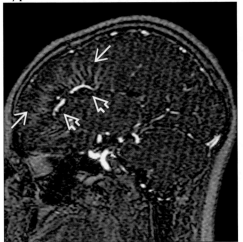
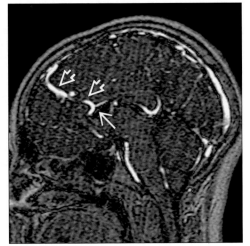

*(Left)* Sagittal MRA source image shows multiple medullary veins ➜ converging toward larger subependymal trunks ⮞ in the frontal horn and body of the lateral ventricle. *(Right)* Sagittal MRA source image (same patient as previous image) shows an enlarged transcerebral collector vein ⮞ draining the subependymal veins ➜ toward the superior sagittal sinus.

### Typical

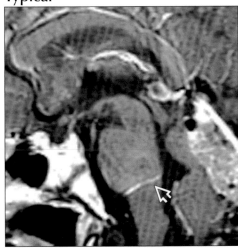
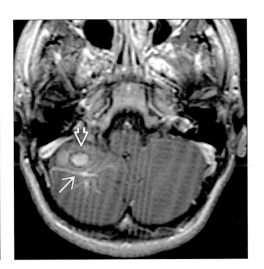

*(Left)* Sagittal T1 C+ MR shows DVA ⮞ crossing upper medulla at pontomedullary sulcus, to drain subependymal veins toward inferior petrosal sinus (incidental finding, MR for medulloblastoma). *(Right)* Axial T1 C+ MR shows typical DVA ➜ in the right cerebellar hemisphere adjacent to a bleeding cavernoma ⮞ and draining to the surface. Child was admitted for acute cerebellar hemorrhage.

### Typical

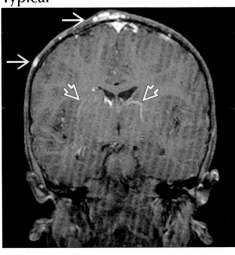
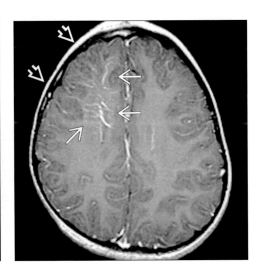

*(Left)* Coronal T1 C+ FS MR shows venous malformations (varices) ➜ in the scalp, together with multiple DVAs ⮞ in the basal ganglia. Patient with blue rubber bleb nevus syndrome (BRBNS). *(Right)* Axial T1 C+ FS MR shows extensive DVA ➜ in the white matter subjacent to a right frontal cortical dysplasia with the appearance of a polymicrogyria ⮞.

# CAVERNOUS MALFORMATION

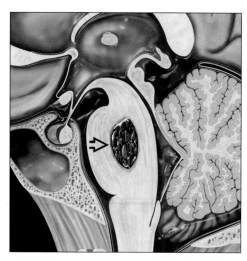
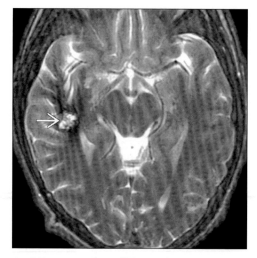

Sagittal graphic shows multiple blood containing locules ⊡ in the central pons. The lesion contains blood of varying ages. This is a common location for infratentorial cavernous malformations.

Axial T2WI MR shows ➡ a multicystic "popcorn" lesion with surrounding hemosiderin.

## TERMINOLOGY

### Abbreviations and Synonyms
- Cavernous malformation (CM); cavernoma; cavernous angioma, cavernous hemangioma, cryptic vascular malformation or cavernous venous malformation (CVM)

### Definitions
- Benign sporadic or familial low pressure vascular lesion with tendency to bleed

## IMAGING FINDINGS

### General Features
- Best diagnostic clue
  - "Popcorn ball", blood in different phases, hemosiderin rim
  - May present as large hemorrhage in children
- Location: Brain CMs: 80% supratentorial (frontal > temporal parietal, cortical > deep, 7% intraventricular, 20% infratentorial (14.7% pons); spinal cord rare
- Size
  - CMs vary from microscopic to giant (> 6 cm)
  - CMs reach larger size in children than adults (6-7 cm vs. 2-3 cm)
- Morphology
  - Locules of variable size contain blood products at different stages of evolution
  - Complete hemosiderin rim surrounds lesion unless recent bleed

### CT Findings
- CTA: Negative but may be adjacent vascular malformation
- NECT
  - Negative in 30-50%
  - Round/ovoid hyperdense lesion, may be large in children
  - 40-60% Ca++
  - Little mass effect relative to size
- CECT: Little/no enhancement unless mixed with other lesion like capillary telangiectasia, developmental venous anomaly (DVA)

### MR Findings
- T1WI

## DDx: Cavernous Malformation

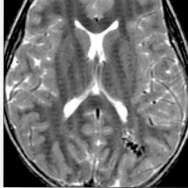
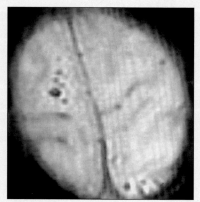
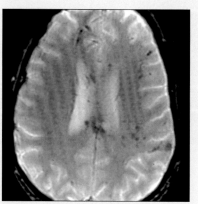

Arteriovenous Malformation | Venous Hemorrhage | Diffuse Axonal Injury

# CAVERNOUS MALFORMATION

## Key Facts

### Imaging Findings
- "Popcorn ball", blood in different phases, hemosiderin rim
- May present as large hemorrhage in children
- T2* most sensitive; susceptibility effect ("blooming")
- May see only punctate hypointense foci, black dots, on T2*
- Include T1 C+ to look for associated DVA if single CM

### Top Differential Diagnoses
- AVM: "Flow voids" ± hemorrhage, usually single phase of blood products
- Hemorrhagic neoplasm: Incomplete hemosiderin rim, mass effect, often enhancement
- Old trauma: Diffuse axonal injury, contusions

### Pathology
- Incidence of familial cases ~ 20%
- Early brain radiation a risk factor
- 75% occur as solitary, sporadic lesion
- 10-30% multiple, familial

### Clinical Issues
- Two peaks: 6 months to 3 yrs and 11 to 16 yrs; fetal and neonatal very rare
- Annual hemorrhage rate 3% (range 0.25-6.4%, larger than adult)

### Diagnostic Checklist
- Number 2 cause of spontaneous ICH in children after AVM; do T2* for additional lesions
- Continued surveillance to monitor change

---

- ○ "Popcorn ball" appearance of mixed hyper-, hypointense blood-containing "locules"
- ○ Can also have uniform increased, isointense or decreased T1 core
- T2WI
  - ○ "Popcorn ball" appearance of mixed hyper-, hypointense blood-containing "locules"
  - ○ Can have uniform increased, isointense or decreased T2 core, ± fluid-fluid levels
  - ○ Uniform and complete thin rim of decreased T2 unless recent hemorrhage
  - ○ No surrounding edema unless recent hemorrhage
- FLAIR: Similar to T2WI
- T2* GRE
  - ○ T2* most sensitive; susceptibility effect ("blooming")
  - ○ May see only punctate hypointense foci, black dots, on T2*
- DWI: Typically low or isointense signal on DWI
- T1 C+
  - ○ No significant enhancement early (may show associated DVA)
  - ○ After delay (1 hr) can show intense enhancement
- MRA: Normal (may show associated DVA)
- Large acute hemorrhage may obscure diagnostic features of CM

## Angiographic Findings
- Conventional
  - ○ DSA
    - Typically normal (angiographically occult)
    - ± Associated DVA
    - Occasionally venous pooling or capillary blush
    - Avascular mass effect if large acute hemorrhage
    - Rare: Venous pooling, contrast "blush"

## Imaging Recommendations
- Best imaging tool
  - ○ MR with T2* GRE
  - ○ Angiography to rule out arteriovenous malformation (AVM) only if MR not diagnostic, CTA inconclusive
- Protocol advice
  - ○ T2* GRE essential: Small lesions may be detected only on this sequence

- ○ T2WI: Look for "popcorn" appearance and thin, complete rim of decreased T2
- ○ Include T1 C+ to look for associated DVA if single CM

## DIFFERENTIAL DIAGNOSIS

### "Popcorn Ball" Hemorrhagic Lesion
- AVM: "Flow voids" ± hemorrhage, usually single phase of blood products
- Hemorrhagic neoplasm: Incomplete hemosiderin rim, mass effect, often enhancement
- Venous hemorrhage: Classically lateral temporal or parasagittal; with venous thrombosis

### Multiple "Black Dots"
- Old trauma: Diffuse axonal injury, contusions
- Hemorrhagic micro-hemorrhages (history of prior cardiac surgery, coagulopathy)
- Hypertensive microbleeds (history of long-standing hypertension; rare in children)

## PATHOLOGY

### General Features
- General path comments
  - ○ Discrete collection of endothelial-lined, hemorrhage-filled vessels without intervening normal brain
  - ○ CMs are angiogenically immature lesions with endothelial proliferation, increased neoangiogenesis
  - ○ VEGF, βFGF, TGFα expressed
  - ○ Receptors (e.g., Flk-1) upregulated
- Genetics
  - ○ Incidence of familial cases ~ 20%
  - ○ At least 3 genes implicated in hereditary form: CCM1, CCM2, CCM3 genes
  - ○ Multiple (familial) CM syndrome is autosomal dominant, variable penetrance
    - Mutation in chromosomes 3.7q (KRIT1 mutation at CCM1 locus)

# CAVERNOUS MALFORMATION

- Nonsense, frame-shift or splice-site mutations consistent with two-hit model for CM
  - Mutations encode a truncated KRIT1 protein
  - KRIT1 interacts with endothelial cell microtubules; loss of function leads to inability of endothelial cells to mature, form capillaries
- Etiology
  - Incompletely understood
  - Genetic forms
  - Sporadic forms
  - Early brain radiation a risk factor
  - Role of DVA in creation of CM topic of debate
- Epidemiology
  - Prevalence 0.37-0.53%
  - 75% occur as solitary, sporadic lesion
  - 10-30% multiple, familial
- Associated abnormalities
  - DVA unusual in pediatric age group
  - Adjacent capillary telangiectasias or dysmorphic vessels common, especially < 3 yrs

## Gross Pathologic & Surgical Features
- Discrete, lobulated, bluish-purple ("mulberry-like") nodule
- Pseudocapsule of gliotic, hemosiderin-stained brain
- Large cysts common in infants

## Microscopic Features
- Thin-walled epithelial-lined spaces
- Embedded in collagenous matrix
- Hemorrhage in different stages of evolution
- ± Ca++
- Does not contain normal brain
- May be histologically mixed (VM most common)

## Staging, Grading or Classification Criteria
- Zabramski classification of CMs
  - Type 1: Subacute hemorrhage (hyperintense on T1WI; hyper- or hypointense on T2WI)
  - Type 2: Mixed signal intensity on T1-, T2WI with degrading hemorrhage of various ages (classic "popcorn ball" lesion)
  - Type 3: Chronic hemorrhage (hypo- to iso on T1-, T2WI)
  - Type 4: Punctate microhemorrhages ("black dots"), poorly seen except on GRE sequences

# CLINICAL ISSUES

## Presentation
- Most common signs/symptoms
  - New onset seizure 25% (less than adult) ± focal deficit
  - 30% hemorrhage (more than adult), infratentorial > supratentorial
  - New onset focal neurological deficit
  - Asymptomatic (less common than adult)
- Clinical Profile: Familial CM = Hispanic-American

## Demographics
- Age
  - Two peaks: 6 months to 3 yrs and 11 to 16 yrs; fetal and neonatal very rare

- Familial CMs tend to present earlier than sporadic lesions
- Gender: M = F
- Ethnicity
  - Multiple (familial) CM syndrome in Hispanic-Americans of Mexican descent
    - Founder mutation in KRIT1 (Q445X)
    - Positive family history = 90% chance of mutation resulting in CM
  - CMs may occur in any ethnic population

## Natural History & Prognosis
- Annual hemorrhage rate 3% (range 0.25-6.4%, larger than adult)
- Broad range of dynamic behavior (may progress, enlarge, regress, occur de novo)
- MR findings not yet correlated with risk of future hemorrhage
- Propensity for growth via repeated intralesional hemorrhages
  - Risk factor for future hemorrhage = previous hemorrhage
  - Rehemorrhage rate high initially, decreases 2-3 years after 1st bleed
- Familial CMs at especially high risk for hemorrhage, forming new lesions

## Treatment
- Total removal via microsurgical resection optimal
  - Caution: If mixed DVA, venous drainage must be preserved
- Stereotaxic XRT limited effectiveness, radiation related complications for CM > AVM

# DIAGNOSTIC CHECKLIST

## Consider
- Number 2 cause of spontaneous ICH in children after AVM; do T2* for additional lesions
- Atypical appearance in setting of recent hemorrhage requires F/U imaging to confirm dx
- DNA testing of family to determine if genetic cause
- Continued surveillance to monitor change

## Image Interpretation Pearls
- Look for popcorn-like lesion in acute hematoma

# SELECTED REFERENCES

1. D'Angelo VA et al: Supratentorial cerebral cavernous malformations: clinical, surgical, and genetic involvement. Neurosurg Focus. 21(1):e9, 2006
2. Duhem R et al: Cavernous malformations after cerebral irradiation during childhood: report of nine cases. Childs Nerv Syst. 21(10):922-5, 2005
3. Thiex R et al: Giant cavernoma of the brain stem: value of delayed MR imaging after contrast injection. Eur Radiol. 13 Suppl 4:L219-25, 2003
4. Mottolese C et al: Central nervous system cavernomas in the pediatric age group. Neurosurg Rev. 24(2-3):55-71; discussion 72-3, 2001

# CAVERNOUS MALFORMATION

## IMAGE GALLERY

Typical

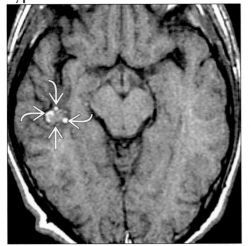
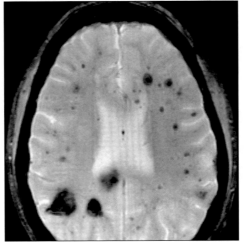

*(Left) Axial T1WI MR shows mixed → isointense and → hyperintense regions within the lesion, representing blood products of various ages. Note the minimal mass effect. (Right) Axial T2\* GRE MR in a patient with familial syndrome of multiple cavernomas shows innumerable foci of "blooming" signal loss caused by ferromagnetic blood products in multiple tiny CMs.*

Typical

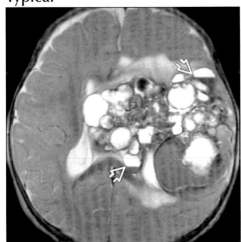
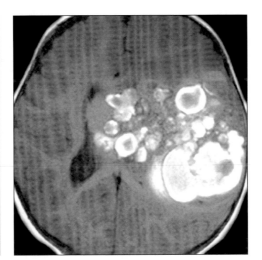

*(Left) Axial T2WI MR shows giant CM crossing the midline with numerous fluid-fluid levels ⇥. Note that most cysts have a complete hypointense hemosiderin rim. (Right) Axial T1WI MR of same patient as previous image shows various signal intensities within the individual collections of blood products. This finding is consistent with blood of various stages.*

Typical

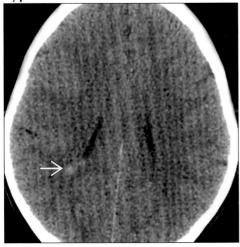
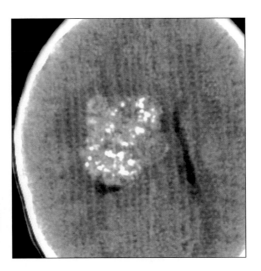

*(Left) Axial NECT shows subtle increased attenuation → from blood products or calcification within the CM. Note lack of surrounding edema. (Right) Axial NECT shows a giant CM with variable attenuation secondary to hemorrhage intermixed with calcification. Mass effect is minimal given size of the lesion.*

# DURAL A-V FISTULA

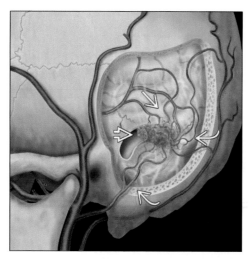

*Lateral graphic shows thrombosed transverse sinus ⊵, and a dense network of dural arterial branches from MMA ➔ and posterior transosseous auricular and occipital arteries ↗.*

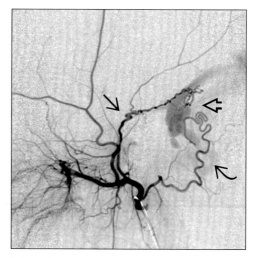

*Lateral angiography shows a partly occluded transverse/sigmoid sinus with a fistula ⊵ fed by branches of the MMA ➔ and occipital artery ↗. This corresponds to the adult type dAVF.*

## TERMINOLOGY

### Abbreviations and Synonyms
- Dural arteriovenous fistula (dAVF)
- Dural arteriovenous (AV) shunt

### Definitions
- dAVF: Direct AV communication in the wall of a dural sinus

## IMAGING FINDINGS

### General Features
- Best diagnostic clue
  - Congenital type
    - Enlarged fistular channels in wall of dural venous sinus, draining into sinus
    - Fed from dural/transosseous arteries
    - Vessels hugely dilated, but normal mature anatomy
  - Adult type: Network of tiny vessels in the wall of dural sinus
- Location: Dural venous sinuses

- Size: Typically large shunts in congenital type
- Morphology
  - Collection of numerous AV channels within dural sinus wall
  - Sinus thrombosed in adult type

### CT Findings
- CTA: May be useful in static depiction of angioarchitecture
- NECT
  - Brain: Normal early
  - Progressive changes later: Loss of volume, hydrocephalus, dystrophic Ca++
- CECT
  - Enlarged dural sinus and related veins (superior ophthalmic vein, cortical veins)
  - Mass effect possible (occipital lobes, midbrain, exophthalmos)
  - Enlarged arterial foramina (foramen spinosum)
  - May be normal

### MR Findings
- T1WI
  - Large dural sinuses with flow artifacts
  - May be normal

## DDx: Non-Dural Extracerebral Vascular Malformations

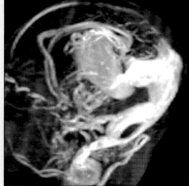

*Vein of Galen Malformation*

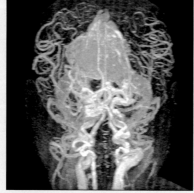

*Vein of Galen Malformation*

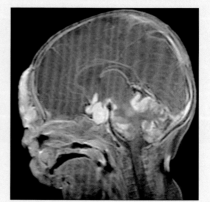

*PHACE(S) Syndrome*

# DURAL A-V FISTULA

## Key Facts

### Terminology
- dAVF: Direct AV communication in the wall of a dural sinus

### Imaging Findings
- Collection of numerous AV channels within dural sinus wall
- Large dural sinuses with flow artifacts
- Most common = torcular AVF
- Best imaging tool: DSA with superselective catheterization of dural and transosseous feeders

### Top Differential Diagnoses
- Vein of Galen Malformation (VOGM)
- Meningeal Angiomatosis
- Carotid-Cavernous Fistula

### Pathology
- Mature arterial and venous configuration
- Most are congenital
- Pathological activation of neoangiogenesis (adult type)
- Epidemiology: Uncommon: 10% of intra-cranial AV shunts in children (against 15-20% in adults)

### Clinical Issues
- Neonate: Congestive heart failure (CHF), prominent venous collateral
- Progressive neurological, ophthalmic deterioration
- Multiplication of fistular sites even after treatment

### Diagnostic Checklist
- If patient has objective pulsatile bruit, angiography necessary to completely exclude dAVF

---

- T2WI
  - Same, signs of chronic brain ischemia
  - Hemorrhage, ischemia uncommon in children dAVF
  - Focal hyperintensity in adjacent brain = retrograde leptomeningeal venous drainage (RLVD), venous perfusion abnormalities
- FLAIR: Same
- T2* GRE: Usually normal (no blooming) in uncomplicated dAVF
- DWI: Normal, rarely venous infarct or ischemia
- T1 C+
  - Enlarged dural sinuses and related veins
  - Chronically thrombosed sinus usually enhances
- MRA
  - MRA useful for gross depiction of angioarchitecture & dynamics
  - However
    - May be negative with small or slow flow shunts
    - May yield incomplete depiction of high flow lesions
- MRV: Depicts occluded parent sinus, collateral flow

## Angiographic Findings
- Conventional
  - Most common = torcular AVF
    - Multiple dural branches from middle meningeal (MMA), internal carotid (ICA), vertebral (VA), transosseous branches from occipital, posterior auricular arteries
    - Arterial inflow into parallel venous channel ("recipient pouch") common; can be embolized with preservation of parent sinus
    - Hugely dilated torcular, transverse sinus, with contrast dilution
    - Adult type: Tortuous engorged pial veins ("pseudophlebitic pattern"), venous congestion/hypertension (clinically aggressive: Ischemia, hemorrhage)
  - Cavernous sinus (CS) = second most common
    - Proximal MMA, ICA feeders
    - Dilated superior ophthalmic vein
  - Superior sagittal sinus, other dural sinuses

## Imaging Recommendations
- Best imaging tool: DSA with superselective catheterization of dural and transosseous feeders
- Protocol advice
  - For screening: CT-CTA, MR-MRA
  - Assessment: DSA to delineate vascular supply, venous drainage, planning treatment

## DIFFERENTIAL DIAGNOSIS

### Vein of Galen Malformation (VOGM)
- Feeders mostly from cerebral, not dural arteries: Anterior cerebral, choroidal, midbrain/tectal, falcine/tentorial branches only accessory
- Dilated venous sac on dorsal midline (velum interpositum, supratectal)
- Fetal arterial/venous configuration with abnormal venous drainage channels (falcine sinuses)
- Stenosed, occluded sinuses common

### Meningeal Angiomatosis
- Syndromic
- Mostly extracerebral vascular malformations

### Carotid-Cavernous Fistula
- Direct opening of the carotid siphon into the CS, usually traumatic in children

## PATHOLOGY

### General Features
- General path comments
  - Numerous large AV fistular channels in wall of enlarged sinuses
  - Mature arterial and venous configuration
- Etiology
  - Most are congenital
    - Assumed to be acquired during early fetal life, cause and mechanism unknown, presumably multifactorial

- No familial incidence, no association with other vascular malformations (no syndromic forms)
- No associated dural sinus thrombosis
- Secondary dural/pial shunts develop commonly after successful transarterial embolization, recruitment of new small arterial feeders
  - Adult type can occur in response to trauma, venous occlusion or venous hypertension
    - Multiple tiny feeders in wall of occluded sinus
  - Pathological activation of neoangiogenesis (adult type)
    - Proliferating capillaries within granulation tissue in dural sinus obliterated by organized thrombi
    - Budding/proliferation of microvascular network in inner dura connects to plexus of thin-walled venous channels, creating microfistulae
    - High bFGF, VEGF expression in dAVFs
- Epidemiology: Uncommon: 10% of intra-cranial AV shunts in children (against 15-20% in adults)
- Associated abnormalities: Cortical drainage associated with edema, chronic ischemic encephalopathy

## Gross Pathologic & Surgical Features
- Network of AV microfistulae in wall of dural sinus

## Microscopic Features
- Arterialized veins with irregular intimal thickening, variable loss of internal elastic lamina

# CLINICAL ISSUES

## Presentation
- Most common signs/symptoms
  - Neonate: Congestive heart failure (CHF), prominent venous collateral
    - Brain typically normal (possible tonsillar prolapse due to intracranial)
  - Older children: Chronic features
    - CSF resorption impaired
    - Arterial steal: Chronic ischemia with progressive neurological deterioration
    - Objective bruit possible, but no subjective tinnitus (AVF present at birth)
    - Proptosis (venous rerouting)
  - Adult type: Uncommon
    - Tinnitus
  - Dural AVF in fetus
    - Not exceptional
    - Detected with routine US: Extracerebral anechoic mass not fitting the usual topography of arachnoid cysts
    - Diagnosed with fetal MR ultrafast single-shot: Dilatation of dural sinus/venous pouch
    - Brain is typically normal
    - May thrombose and regress spontaneously
- Other signs/symptoms: Late: Secondary fistular sites, dural sinus stenosis with possible features of veno-occlusive disease, venous rerouting

## Demographics
- Age
  - Commonly neonate, infant
  - Late presentation possible (then mostly adult type)

## Natural History & Prognosis
- Progressive neurological, ophthalmic deterioration
- Spontaneous closure rare
- Multiplication of fistular sites even after treatment

## Treatment
- To prevent complications: Hydrocephalus, progressive deterioration, acute ischemia/bleed
- Options
  - Endovascular: Multiple sessions common, good immediate results (CHF)
    - Typically transarterial: Hyperselective, multi-arterial embolization
    - May be venous, or combined
  - Surgical resection: Attempts usually fail (extensive, massively hemorrhagic, usually incomplete surgery)
  - Stereotaxic radiosurgery: May help to complement endovascular treatment
  - New fistular sites may develop secondarily

# DIAGNOSTIC CHECKLIST

## Consider
- Venous collateral flow in dural sinus thrombosis can become very prominent, mimic dAVF
- Single pedicle or small dAVF may be missed even with focused CT with CTA, MR with MRA
- If patient has objective pulsatile bruit, angiography necessary to completely exclude dAVF

## Image Interpretation Pearls
- CT-CTA, MR-MRA shows large sinus/veins
- Always examine both ICAs, ECAs, VAs and look for dAVF if enlarged sinuses, veins

# SELECTED REFERENCES

1. Noguchi K et al: Intracranial dural arteriovenous fistulas: evaluation with combined 3D time-of-flight MR angiography and MR digital subtraction angiography. AJR Am J Roentgenol. 182(1):183-90, 2004
2. Burrows PE et al: Venous variations of the brain and cranial vault. Neuroimaging Clin N Am. 13(1):13-26, 2003
3. Kai Y et al: Pre- and post-treatment MR imaging and single photon emission CT in patients with dural arteriovenous fistulas and retrograde leptomeningeal venous drainage. AJNR Am J Neuroradiol. 24(4):619-25, 2003
4. Klisch J et al: Transvenous treatment of carotid cavernous and dural arteriovenous fistulae: results for 31 patients and review of the literature. Neurosurgery. 53(4):836-56; discussion 856-7, 2003
5. Rucker JC et al: Diffuse dural enhancement in cavernous sinus dural arteriovenous fistula. Neuroradiology. 45(2):88-9, 2003
6. van Dijk JM et al: Venous congestive encephalopathy related to cranial dural arteriovenous fistulas. Neuroimaging Clin N Am. 13(1):55-72, 2003
7. Coley SC et al: Dural arteriovenous fistulae: noninvasive diagnosis with dynamic MR digital subtraction angiography. AJNR Am J Neuroradiol. 23(3):404-7, 2002
8. Kincaid PK et al: Dural arteriovenous fistula in children: endovascular treatment and outcomes in seven cases. AJNR Am J Neuroradiol. 22(6):1217-25, 2001

# DURAL A-V FISTULA

## IMAGE GALLERY

### Typical

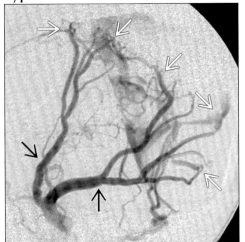
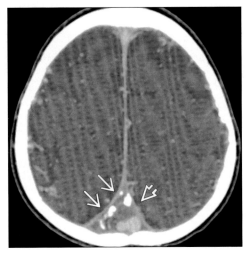

*(Left)* Lateral angiography shows multiple, markedly dilated branches of the MMA ➡ feeding numerous AVF ➡ in the wall of a hugely enlarged torcular, hardly opacified by diluted contrast. *(Right)* Axial CECT shows, months after the embolization, the partly occluded dural ➡ sinus with occlusion material in the fistular channels ➡ contained within the dural wall of the SSS.

### Other

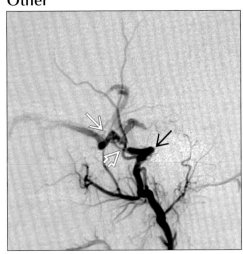
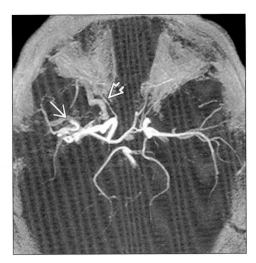

*(Left)* Lateral angiography shows a dilated MMA ➡ feeding an AVF of the wall of the CS ➡ shortly after entering the skull through the foramen spinosum. Prominent superior ophthalmic vein ➡. *(Right)* Axial MIP shows MR appearance in the same case: An enlarged MMA ➡ and a prominent superior ophthalmic vein ➡ in this one month old child investigated for exophthalmos.

### Typical

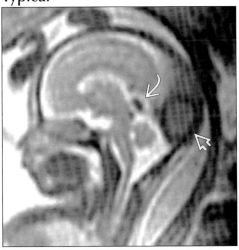
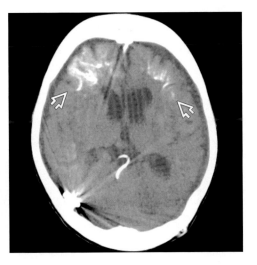

*(Left)* Sagittal T2WI FS MR shows dilated torcular ➡ in a 23 week old fetus, larger than on previous study three weeks before; upstream enlargement of vein of Galen ➡ and other afferent veins. *(Right)* Axial NECT shows a thick skull (from shunted hydrocephalus) with white matter loss and characteristic subcortical dystrophic Ca++ ➡ due to chronic ischemia from vascular steal effect.

# ARTERIOVENOUS MALFORMATION

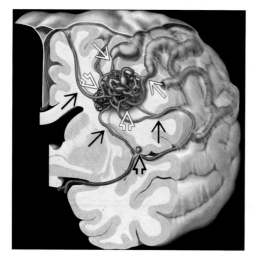

Coronal graphic shows cerebral AVM with centrum semi-ovale nidus ➡ fed from cortical and central arteries ➡, drained by cortical veins ➡ with proximal flow-related aneurysm ➡.

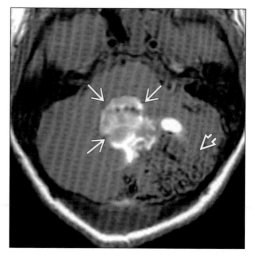

Axial T1WI MR shows a large ventricular and paraventricular hematoma ➡ adjacent to an extensive bed of dilated vessels (AVM ➡) in the left cerebellar hemisphere.

## TERMINOLOGY

### Abbreviations and Synonyms
- Arteriovenous malformation (AVM)

### Definitions
- Vascular malformation with arteriovenous shunting, no intervening capillary bed

## IMAGING FINDINGS

### General Features
- Best diagnostic clue: Brain hemorrhage adjacent to parenchymal conglomeration of dilated vessels (nidus) with enlarged afferent arteries and efferent veins
- Location
  - Anywhere in brain tissue (including choroid plexuses)
  - Respond to vascular organization
  - Typically solitary (sporadic), but also (rarely) multiple (syndromic)
- Size: From tiny/small (common in children) to giant
- Morphology: Tightly packed mass of enlarged vascular channels with flow voids

### CT Findings
- CTA: See enlarged arteries ⇒ nidus ⇒ draining veins
- NECT: Mostly acute brain hemorrhage in a child; if none, the isodense blood in the vessels may be missed; Ca++ occasionally
- CECT: Strong vascular enhancement of dilated vascular bed

### MR Findings
- T1WI: Hemorrhage, flow voids of adjacent nidus, feeding arteries and draining veins
- T2WI: Same as T1, no or little brain tissue in the nidus
- FLAIR: Same as T2, associated gliosis sometimes
- T2* GRE: Hemorrhagic blooming acutely, blood residues later
- DWI: Usually normal
- T1 C+: Strong vascular enhancement of nidus and prominent related arteries and veins
- MRA: Gross depiction of arteries, nidus, veins

### Angiographic Findings
- Conventional

## DDx: Other Hemorrhages and Vascular Malformations

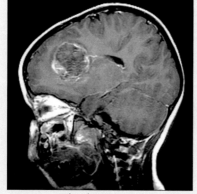

Bleeding Tumor

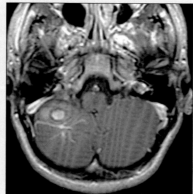

Cavernoma and DVA

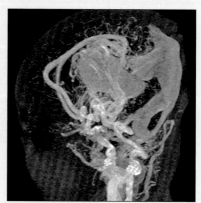

Vein of Galen Malformation

# ARTERIOVENOUS MALFORMATION

## Key Facts

### Terminology
- Vascular malformation with arteriovenous shunting, no intervening capillary bed

### Imaging Findings
- Best diagnostic clue: Brain hemorrhage adjacent to parenchymal conglomeration of dilated vessels (nidus) with enlarged afferent arteries and efferent veins
- T1WI: Hemorrhage, flow voids of adjacent nidus, feeding arteries and draining veins
- Best imaging tool: Conventional angiogram; superselective angiogram if needed for planning treatment

### Pathology
- Bleeding typically is from rupture of draining vein (dilation, kinking, thrombosis); rupture of flow-related aneurysm rare in children

### Clinical Issues
- Annual bleeding risk at 3.2%, spontaneous obliteration exceptional (< 1% of cases)

### Diagnostic Checklist
- AVM is the most common cause for brain hemorrhage in children (perinatal period excluded); cavernomas, tumors, aneurysms are less common
- Dilated vessels, especially if adjacent to hematoma

---

- Always bilateral internal-external carotid (ICA-ECA) and vertebrobasilar (VB) angiograms (multiple feeders)
- Depicts three components of AVMs
  - Enlarged arterial feeders: Number, origin, cortical or perforant, terminal or lateral feeders (risks for normal parenchyma), possible high flow aneurysm
  - Nidus of tightly packed vessels; classically may be hidden if compressed by hematoma
  - Early filling (fast flow), dilated draining veins (cortical and subependymal) that overly arteries; may be partly thrombosed (collaterals)
- Locates AVM
  - Structure, lobe (lateral, medial, inferior aspects), gyrus/sulcus; neighboring eloquent areas
  - Superficial (pial fistula in neonate, infants), deep, central nuclei, choroid plexus, cerebellum
- Evaluates shunt: Size of nidus, size of related vessels, speed of flow

### Imaging Recommendations
- Best imaging tool: Conventional angiogram; superselective angiogram if needed for planning treatment
- Protocol advice: CT or MR (include contrast-enhanced MRA, GRE sequences) followed by conventional angiography

## DIFFERENTIAL DIAGNOSIS

### Tumoral Bleed
- Added mass effect, enhancement, tumor blush, no vascular dilatation; may need later repeat study

### Cavernomas
- Characteristic blooming artifact on T2* GRE, surrounding or adjacent to the hematoma; no nidus, no dilated vessels (but DVA common); may be multiple

### Extracerebral Arteriovenous Fistula
- Vein of Galen malformation (VOGM): Extraparenchymal, dorsal fistula associated with venous sac, fed by anterior cerebral, choroidal, mesencephalic and dural branches
- Dural arteriovenous fistula, with or without cerebral venous drainage; primarily fed by enlarged ECA/dural branches

### Arterial Aneurysm
- No dilated vessels, hematoma extends to cortex, subarachnoid blood common, aneurysm may be seen on CTA/MRA

## PATHOLOGY

### General Features
- General path comments: Tangle of dilated vessels in brain parenchyma, without interposed capillary bed
- Genetics
  - Sporadic AVMs: Multiple up-, down-regulated genes
    - Homeobox genes involved in angiogenesis, such as Hox D3 and B3, may malfunction
  - Syndromic AVMs (2% of cases)
    - Familial multiple AVMs in hereditary hemorrhagic telangiectasia (HHT)
    - Cerebrofacial arteriovenous metameric syndromes (CAMS) involve face and brain
- Etiology
  - Most AVMs are sporadic, even if due to gene dysregulation
    - Vascular endothelial growth factors (VEGFs) receptors mediate endothelial proliferation/migration
    - Cytokine receptors mediate vascular maturation/remodeling
    - Syndromic AVMs may be familial, such as HHT1 (9q34.1), HHT2 (12q11-q14), HHT3 (5q31.3-q32) and JPHT (18q21.1), or not (Wyburn-Mason)

○ Bleeding typically is from rupture of draining vein (dilation, kinking, thrombosis); rupture of flow-related aneurysm rare in children
○ Large AVMs generate arterial steal with progressive neurological deterioration and/or chronic epilepsy, congestive heart failure (CHF) in infants
• Epidemiology
○ Global prevalence of sporadic AVMs = 0.04-0.52%; 20% are diagnosed in children
○ AVMs: Most common cause for brain hemorrhage in children (excluding neonatal period)

## Gross Pathologic & Surgical Features
• Intraparenchymal compact mass of tangled dilated vessels

## Microscopic Features
• Vascular changes
○ Feeding arteries enlarged but mature with some wall thickening
○ Draining veins enlarged, varicose, often kinked, sometimes thrombosed
○ Nidus
  ▪ Conglomeration of numerous AV shunts without interposed brain tissue and no capillary bed
  ▪ Thin-walled dysplastic vessels, no subendothelial support, variable muscularization (loss of normal contractile properties), disorganized collagen
○ Perinidal capillary network (PDCN) may be cause of recurrence of surgically resected AVMs
  ▪ Dilated capillaries (10-25 times larger than normal capillaries) form a ring (1-7 mm) surrounding nidus
  ▪ Connected to nidus, to feeding arteries/draining veins, to surrounding normal brain vessels
○ Adjacent gliosis, atrophy, blood residues

## Staging, Grading or Classification Criteria
• Spetzler-Martin scale: Classification by size, location in relation to eloquent cortex, type of venous drainage
• Multiple brain AVMs: Typically part of HHT (pulmonary AVMs, cutaneous and mucosal telangiectasia, hepatic AVMs)
• Metameric AVMs: Typically Wyburn-Mason syndrome: Diencephalic optic pathway and midbrain/thalamic AVMs
• Other cerebrofacial arteriovenous metameric syndromes (CAMS)
○ CAMS 1 = prosencephalic metameric AVMs (hypothalamus/hypophysis, nose)
○ CAMS 2 = lateral prosencephalic group (occipital lobe, thalamus and maxilla)
○ CAMS 3 = rhombencephalic group (cerebellum, pons, mandible)

## CLINICAL ISSUES

### Presentation
• Most common signs/symptoms
○ Hemorrhage (headaches, neurological deficit, coma) in 80% of children AVMs
○ Epilepsy (10%), progressive neurological deficits (15%) with large lesions

○ CHF in infants (pial AV fistula)

## Demographics
• Age: Exceptional in infants (then almost exclusively pial fistula), but most common cause of brain hemorrhage after 6-7 years
• Gender: M = F
• Ethnicity: Occurs in all ethnic groups

## Natural History & Prognosis
• Recurrent complications
○ Annual bleeding risk at 3.2%, spontaneous obliteration exceptional (< 1% of cases)
○ Vascular steal can only become worse
• Spontaneous prognosis severe

## Treatment
• Surgery often needed acutely to address hemorrhage; also indicated for accessible AVMs or for small, distal AVM (beyond reach of endovascular)
• Endovascular treatment: Fast flow AVMs with accessible feeders
• Radiosurgery on single or adjacent limited volumes (may take years to reach effect; risk of rebleed)
• Combination of the three gives significant results

## DIAGNOSTIC CHECKLIST

### Consider
• AVM is the most common cause for brain hemorrhage in children (perinatal period excluded); cavernomas, tumors, aneurysms are less common

### Image Interpretation Pearls
• Dilated vessels, especially if adjacent to hematoma
• Tiny AVMs common in children; isolated early filling vein may be the only clue to diagnosis

## SELECTED REFERENCES

1.  Cohen-Gadol AA et al: Radiosurgery for arteriovenous malformations in children. J Neurosurg. 104(6 Suppl):388-91, 2006
2.  DeCesare B et al: Spontaneous thrombosis of congenital cerebral arteriovenous malformation complicated by subdural collection: in utero detection with disappearance in infancy. Br J Radiol. 79(946):e140-4, 2006
3.  Sato S et al: Perinidal dilated capillary networks in cerebral arteriovenous malformations. Neurosurgery. 54(1):163-8; discussion 168-70, 2004
4.  Battacharya JJ et al: Wyburn-Mason or Bonnet-Dechaume-Blanc as cerebrofacial arteriovenous metameric syndromes (CAMS): a new concept and classification. Interv Neuroradiol 7:5-17, 2001
5.  Vikkula M et al: Molecular genetics of vascular malformations. Matrix Biol. 20(5-6):327-35, 2001
6.  Di Rocco C et al: Cerebral arteriovenous malformations in children. Acta Neurochir (Wien). 142(2):145-56; discussion 156-8, 2000
7.  Rodesch G et al: Non galenic cerebral arteriovenous malformations in neonates and infants. Review of 26 consecutive cases (1982-1992). Childs Nerv Syst. 11(4):231-41, 1995
8.  Kondziolka D et al: Arteriovenous malformations of the brain in children: a forty year experience. Can J Neurol Sci. 19(1):40-5, 1992

# ARTERIOVENOUS MALFORMATION

## IMAGE GALLERY

### Typical

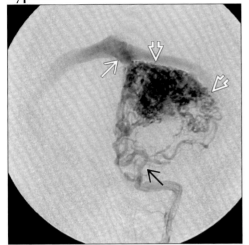
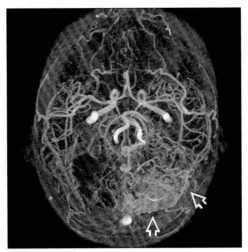

*(Left) Axial oblique angiography shows a large AVM ⟐ of the posterior portion of the left cerebellar hemisphere, fed by the left PICA ➔ with an early filling into the torcular ➔. (Right) Axial MIP (same patient as previous image) shows the extensive vascular bed ⟐ in left cerebellar hemisphere. MR imaging is enough for the diagnosis, but angiography is needed for planning treatment.*

### Typical

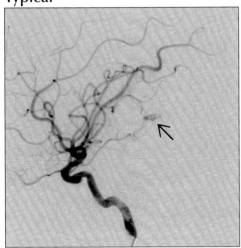
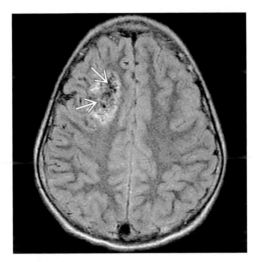

*(Left) Lateral angiography shows a tiny AVM ➔ fed by a distal branch of the anterior choroidal artery. Tiny AVMs are common in children, and most often present with a hemorrhage. (Right) Axial FLAIR MR shows a large, non-hemorrhagic right frontal AVM (flow voids ➔) with gliosis (bright signal) of the surrounding brain tissue. This patient presented with seizures.*

### Variant

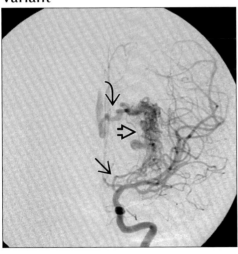
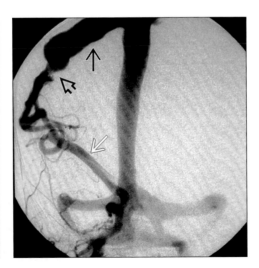

*(Left) Anteroposterior angiography shows a large AVM of the basal ganglia-thalamus ⟐, fed by anterior choroidal ➔ and deep perforators, with early drainage in deep cerebral veins ➔. (Right) Anteroposterior angiography shows a single large, congenital, high-flow pial fistula ⟐ in neonate who presented with CHF. Note markedly enlarged MCA ➔ and cortical draining vein ➔.*

# VEIN OF GALEN ANEURYSMAL MALFORMATION

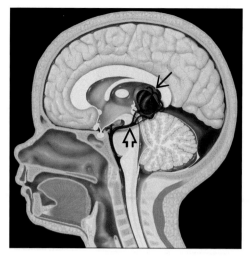

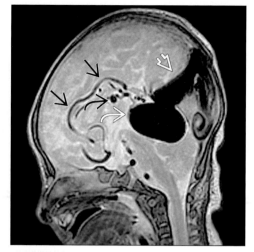

*Sagittal graphic shows a Galenic varix ➔ supplied by posterior choroidal arteries ⟹ and draining to the median vein of Markowski.*

*Sagittal T2WI MR shows typical VGAM. Note dilated pericallosal artery ➔ and choroidal ⟹ feeders. A persistent falcine vein ⟹ drains the Galenic varix ➔.*

## TERMINOLOGY

### Abbreviations and Synonyms
- Vein of Galen malformation (VGAM, VGM), vein of Galen "aneurysm", galenic varix

### Definitions
- Arteriovenous fistula (AVF) between deep choroidal arteries and the median prosencephalic vein (MPV) of Markowski
  - There is no aneurysm of the true vein of Galen, which fails to form because of fistula

## IMAGING FINDINGS

### General Features
- Best diagnostic clue: Large midline varix in neonate/infant
- Location: Quadrigeminal plate cistern
- Size
  - Varix can be several centimeters in diameter
    - Large varix reflects downstream venous stenosis
- Morphology: Spherical or tubular varix

## CT Findings
- NECT
  - Venous pouch mildly hyperdense to brain
  - Hydrocephalus
    - Due to decreased resorption or tectal compression
  - Subcortical white matter (WM) Ca++ from chronic venous ischemia
  - Streak artifact from coils or glue make CT a poor choice for post-treatment imaging
- CECT: Strong enhancement of feeding arteries and varix

## MR Findings
- T1WI
  - Pulsation artifact from varix
  - Varix contents hypointense and heterogeneous (turbulent flow)
  - Compression of tectum
  - Prominent sulci
    - Elevated venous pressures cause decreased resorption of cerebrospinal fluid (CSF)
  - Herniation of cerebellar tonsils
- T2WI
  - Varix homogeneously hypointense

## DDx: Vascular Lesions in Children

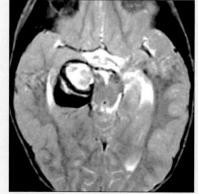

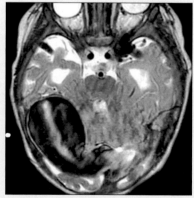

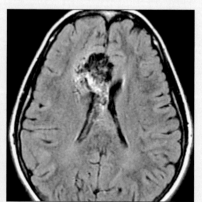

*Giant Aneurysm*

*Dural Arteriovenous Fistula*

*Arteriovenous Malformation*

# VEIN OF GALEN ANEURYSMAL MALFORMATION

## Key Facts

### Terminology
- Arteriovenous fistula (AVF) between deep choroidal arteries and the median prosencephalic vein (MPV) of Markowski

### Imaging Findings
- Pulsation artifact from varix
- Elevated venous pressures cause decreased resorption of cerebrospinal fluid (CSF)
- MRA is key for pre- and post-treatment assessment of feeders to malformation
- MRA is unaffected by coils or acrylic embolic material
- Significant antenatal end-organ injury is a contradiction to aggressive treatment
- Frequent venous abnormalities
- Diagnostic arteriography performed in concert with embolization

### Top Differential Diagnoses
- Arteriovenous malformation (AVM) with drainage into true vein of Galen
- Childhood Dural Arteriovenous Fistula (dAVF)

### Pathology
- Up to 30% of all pediatric vascular malformations
- "Choroidal" or "mural" classification based on angioarchitecture of VGM

### Clinical Issues
- Delay in treatment until 4-6 months, associated with better outcome
- Transcatheter embolization (TCE) at 4-6 months
- May require staged embolizations
- Shunt placement associated with exacerbation of venous ischemia

---

- ○ Prominent flow voids from feeding arteries around varix
- ○ Sharp delineation of malformation
- DWI
  - ○ Reduced diffusion in areas of acute ischemia or infarction
    - ▪ Valuable in immediate post-treatment studies
- MRA
  - ○ MRA is key for pre- and post-treatment assessment of feeders to malformation
    - ▪ MRA is unaffected by coils or acrylic embolic material
- MRV
  - ○ Essential in initial and follow-up evaluation
  - ○ Presence and degree of venous stenosis can have major influence on prognosis
- Fetal MR
  - ○ Can identify presence or absence of brain or other end-organ injury
    - ▪ Significant antenatal end-organ injury is a contradiction to aggressive treatment

### Radiographic Findings
- Radiography: Cardiomegaly and edema from heart failure (CHF) evident on chest X-ray

### Ultrasonographic Findings
- Cardiac dilatation, hydrops fetalis = poor prognosis

### Angiographic Findings
- Conventional
  - ○ Common arterial feeders
    - ▪ Medial and lateral posterior choroidal arteries
    - ▪ Pericallosal arteries
  - ○ Frequent venous abnormalities
    - ▪ Embryonic falcine sinus drains MPV in 50%
    - ▪ Frequent stenoses at sigmoid-jugular junction

### Echocardiographic Findings
- Dilatation of right heart, superior vena cava, ascending aorta and great vessels
- Poor prognostic indicators
  - ○ Descending aorta diastolic flow reversal

- ○ Suprasystemic pulmonary artery hypertension
- ○ Persistent ductus arteriosus with significant right to left shunt

### Imaging Recommendations
- Best imaging tool
  - ○ MR with MRA and MRV
  - ○ Diagnostic arteriography performed in concert with embolization
- Protocol advice
  - ○ Maximize MRA evaluation
    - ▪ 3D reconstruction can provide valuable insight

## DIFFERENTIAL DIAGNOSIS

### Vein of Galen Aneurysmal Dilation (VGAD)
- Arteriovenous malformation (AVM) with drainage into true vein of Galen
- Much less common than VGAM

### Childhood Dural Arteriovenous Fistula (dAVF)
- High-flow fistulas with venous varices
- Massive torcular enlargement may thrombose spontaneously after delivery
  - ○ Especially when supplied exclusively by external carotid artery branches

### Giant Aneurysm
- Not associated with venous abnormalities
- "Onion skin" layers in wall

### Complex Developmental Venous Anomaly (DVA)
- Dilatation of veins draining normal brain parenchyma
- Associated with blue rubber-bleb nevus syndrome

### Pial AVM
- Distinguished by true nidus at transition
- Rarely present before 3 years of age

# VEIN OF GALEN ANEURYSMAL MALFORMATION

## PATHOLOGY

### General Features
- General path comments
  - Embryology
    - Abnormal connection of choroidal arteries to MPV occurs at 6-11 weeks gestation
    - Flow through fistula prevents normal regression of MPV
- Genetics: Sporadic ⇒ no increased risk in sibs
- Epidemiology
  - Rare
    - < 1% cerebral vascular malformations
    - Up to 30% of all pediatric vascular malformations
  - Most common extracardiac cause of high-output heart failure in newborn
- Associated abnormalities
  - Venous occlusion or stenosis
    - Primary atresia vs. occlusion 2° to increased pressure and flow
    - Provides some protection for right heart
  - Cerebral ischemia/atrophy
    - Arterial steal and/or chronic venous hypertension
  - Hydrocephalus
    - ↓ CSF resorption 2° to elevated venous pressure
    - ± Cerebral aqueduct obstruction
  - Sinus venosus atrial septal defects
    - May exacerbate CHF
  - Aortic coarctation

### Gross Pathologic & Surgical Features
- Malformation of structures adjacent to MPV
  - Pineal gland, tela choroidea of 3rd ventricle

### Staging, Grading or Classification Criteria
- "Choroidal" or "mural" classification based on angioarchitecture of VGM
  - Choroidal has multiple feeders from pericallosal, choroidal, and thalamoperforating arteries
  - Mural has single or few feeders from collicular or posterior choroidal arteries

## CLINICAL ISSUES

### Presentation
- Most common signs/symptoms
  - Neonate: High output CHF, cranial bruit
  - Infant: Macrocrania, prominent superficial cranial veins
- Other signs/symptoms: Developmental delay, failure to thrive, hydrocephalus, seizure, headache, hepatic failure

### Demographics
- Age
  - Most commonly diagnosed in neonatal period
  - Rarely diagnosed after 3 years old
  - Occasional older child or adult ⇒ compensated
- Gender: M:F = 2:1

### Natural History & Prognosis
- Prognosis related to volume of shunt and timing/success of treatment
  - High volume shunts requiring treatment in newborn period, have worse prognosis
  - Delay in treatment until 4-6 months, associated with better outcome
- Without treatment ⇒ progression of CHF or brain damage resulting in death
- Chronic venous ischemia and cerebral atrophy without treatment ⇒ "melting brain"
  - Consequence of venous insufficiency
- Up to 60% neurologically normal after treatment
- Incomplete closure of fistula can be associated with good outcome

### Treatment
- Multi-system organ failure or brain damage at presentation are contra-indications to treatment
- Medical therapy for CHF until 4-6 months of age
  - Failure of therapy warrants earlier neuro-intervention
- Transcatheter embolization (TCE) at 4-6 months
  - Permanent occlusion of fistula point from arterial side
    - Acrylic or coils
  - Filling of venous pouch with acrylic or coils
    - May be technically more simple in neonates
    - Risks further injury to already compromised venous system
    - May increase risk of "melting brain"
- May require staged embolizations
- Frequent neurological and MR assessments after TCE
  - Evidence of deterioration warrants further therapy
- Treatment for hydrocephalus controversial
  - Shunt placement associated with exacerbation of venous ischemia
  - Hemorrhage risk from engorged subependymal veins
  - Ideally placed only after all TCEs performed

## DIAGNOSTIC CHECKLIST

### Image Interpretation Pearls
- Meticulous evaluation of MRA can identify essentially all feeders to VGAM
- MRA C+ can show arterial & venous anatomy together

## SELECTED REFERENCES

1.  Gailloud P et al: Diagnosis and management of vein of galen aneurysmal malformations. J Perinatol. 25:542-51, 2005
2.  Foran A et al: Vein of Galen aneurysm malformation (VGAM): closing the management loop. Ir Med J. 97(1):8-10, 2004
3.  Jones BV et al: Vein of Galen aneurysmal malformation: diagnosis and treatment of 13 children with extended clinical follow-up. AJNR Am J Neuroradiol. 23:1717-24, 2002
4.  Mitchell PJ et al: Endovascular management of vein of Galen aneurysmal malformations presenting in the neonatal period. AJNR Am J Neuroradiol. 22:1403-9, 2001
5.  Lasjaunias P et al: Cerebral arteriovenous malformations in children. Management of 179 consecutive cases and review of the literature. Childs Nerv Syst. 11:66-79; discussion 79, 1995

# VEIN OF GALEN ANEURYSMAL MALFORMATION

## IMAGE GALLERY

### Typical

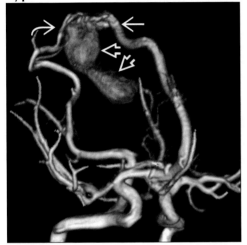

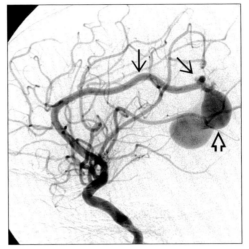

*(Left) Coronal oblique volume rendered MRA shows an elongated VGAM varix ⮞ supplied by an enlarged pericallosal artery ➡ and a distal branch of the right posterior cerebral artery ➡. (Right) Lateral arteriographic image from a left internal carotid artery injection shows supply to a VGAM ⮞ from the pericallosal artery ➡.*

### Variant

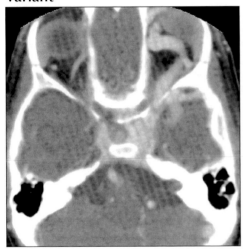

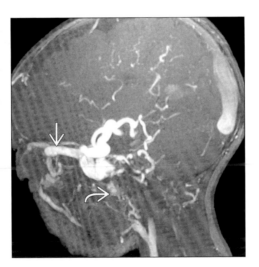

*(Left) Axial CECT shows massive enlargement of the left superior ophthalmic vein (SOV) and pericavernous veins in a 6 month old with a compensated VGAM and bilateral jugular bulb stenosis. (Right) Sagittal MRV (same infant as previous image) shows how cerebral venous drainage has been "captured" by the petrosal sinuses ➡ and SOV ➡ as a consequence of jugular compromise.*

### Variant

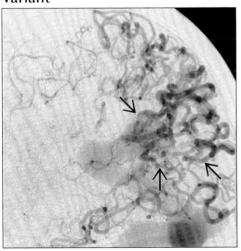

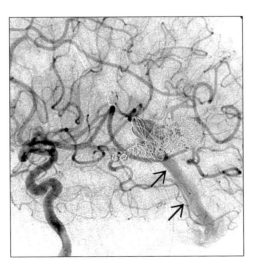

*(Left) Lateral RICA injection from cerebral arteriogram shows multiple cortical MCA branches tracking centrally to supply the fistula at the vein of Galen ➡. (Right) Lateral RICA injection (same child as previous image) 6 months after coil embolization of the varix shows complete resolution of the cortical feeders, with preservation of flow to straight sinus ➡.*

# MOYAMOYA

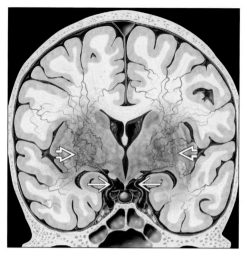
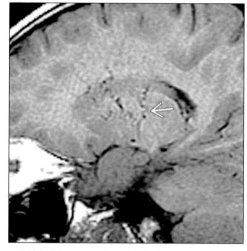

*Coronal graphic shows severe tapering of both distal internal carotid arteries ➡️ and strikingly enlarged lenticulostriate arteries ➡️. This is the "puff of smoke"/moyamoya pattern.*

*Sagittal T1WI MR shows curvilinear flow voids in the basal ganglia and thalami resulting from enlarged and tortuous lenticulostriate arteries ➡️.*

## TERMINOLOGY

### Abbreviations and Synonyms
- Idiopathic progressive arteriopathy of childhood; spontaneous occlusion of the circle of Willis

### Definitions
- Progressive narrowing of distal ICA and proximal circle of Willis (COW) vessels with secondary collateralization
- Moyamoya-like collateralization may occur with ANY progressive vascular occlusion (inherited or acquired)

## IMAGING FINDINGS

### General Features
- Best diagnostic clue: Multiple punctate dots (CECT) & flow-voids (MR) in basal ganglia (BG)
- Location: COW; anterior > > > posterior circulation
- Size: Large vessel occlusion
- Morphology: "Puff or spiral of smoke" (moyamoya in Japanese) = cloud-like lenticulostriate and thalamostriate collaterals on angiography

## CT Findings
- CTA: Abnormal COW & "net-like" collaterals
- NECT
  ○ Children: 50-60% show anterior > posterior atrophy
  ○ Adults: Hemorrhage (esp. intraventricular)
- CECT: Enhancing dots (big lenticulostriates) in BG & abnormal "net-like" vessels at base of brain
- Xe-133 CT: ↓ Cerebral reserve with acetazolamide challenge

## MR Findings
- T1WI: Multiple dot-like or curvilinear flow voids in BG
- T2WI
  ○ ↑ Signal small vessel cortical and white matter infarcts
  ○ Collateral vessels = "net-like" cisternal filling defects
- FLAIR
  ○ Bright sulci = leptomeningeal "ivy sign"
    ▪ Slow-flowing engorged pial vessels, thickened arachnoid membranes
- T2* GRE: Hemosiderin if prior hemorrhage
- DWI: Positive in acute stroke; VERY useful in "acute on chronic" disease
- T1 C+

## DDx: Different Etiologies of Moyamoya

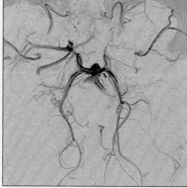
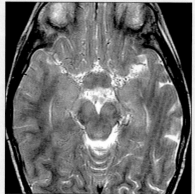
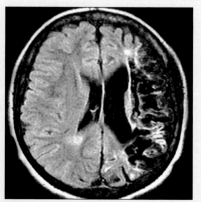

*Progeria*

*NF1 with ONG*

*Sickle Cell Disease*

# MOYAMOYA

## Key Facts

### Terminology
- Idiopathic progressive arteriopathy of childhood; spontaneous occlusion of the circle of Willis
- Progressive narrowing of distal ICA and proximal circle of Willis (COW) vessels with secondary collateralization
- Moyamoya-like collateralization may occur with ANY progressive vascular occlusion (inherited or acquired)

### Imaging Findings
- Best diagnostic clue: Multiple punctate dots (CECT) & flow-voids (MR) in basal ganglia (BG)
- Morphology: "Puff or spiral of smoke" (moyamoya in Japanese) = cloud-like lenticulostriate and thalamostriate collaterals on angiography
- Bright sulci = leptomeningeal "ivy sign"
- Slow-flowing engorged pial vessels, thickened arachnoid membranes
- DWI: Positive in acute stroke; VERY useful in "acute on chronic" disease
- MRA or catheter angiography: Predominantly (not exclusively) anterior circulation
- Dilatation and branch extension of anterior choroidal artery predicts adult hemorrhagic events

### Clinical Issues
- Initially described in Japanese children, but panethnic distribution now known

### Diagnostic Checklist
- Need to seek etiology
- Moyamoya in children typically presents with cerebral ischemia vs. hemorrhage in adults

---

- ○ Lenticulostriate collaterals ⇒ enhancing "dots" in BG and "net-like" thin vessels in cisterns
- ○ Leptomeningeal enhancement (contrast-enhanced "ivy sign") ↓ after "effective bypass surgery"
- MRA: Narrowed distal ICA and proximal COW vessels, ± synangiosis
- MRV: Some vasculopathies leading to moyamoya may also involve veins
- MRS
  - ○ Lactate in acutely infarcted tissue
  - ○ NAA/Cr and Cho/Cr ratios frontal white matter improve/increase after revascularization
- Perfusion-weighted imaging (PWI): ↓ Perfusion deep hemispheric white matter, relative ↑ perfusion posterior circulation
  - ○ PWI may be abnormal when MR still normal
  - ○ Regional cerebral blood volume (rCBV) and time to peak (TTP) correlate with stage of disease

## Ultrasonographic Findings
- Grayscale Ultrasound: Reduction of ICA lumen size
- Pulsed Doppler
  - ○ Doppler spectral waveforms in ICA show no flow (occluded) or high resistance (stenotic) flow pattern
  - ○ ↑ End-diastolic flow velocity and ↓ vascular resistance in ECA collaterals
- Color Doppler: Aliasing suggests stenoses
- Power Doppler: Contrast injection improves visualization of slow flow stenotic vessels and collaterals

## Nuclear Medicine Findings
- PET: ↓ Hemodynamic reserve capacity
- SPECT 123I-Iomazenil: Neuronal density preserved if asymptomatic, ↓ if symptomatic

## Angiographic Findings
- Conventional
  - ○ MRA or catheter angiography: Predominantly (not exclusively) anterior circulation
    - ■ Narrow proximal COW & ICA (earliest)
    - ■ Lenticulostriate & thalamoperforator collaterals (intermediate)
    - ■ Transdural & transosseous EC-IC collaterals (late)
  - ○ Dilatation and branch extension of anterior choroidal artery predicts adult hemorrhagic events

## Imaging Recommendations
- Best imaging tool: MRA
- Protocol advice
  - ○ MRA: COW
  - ○ DWI: Seek "acute on chronic" ischemia
  - ○ MR: FLAIR & T1 C+ illustrate "ivy sign" (reversible if patent bypass)
  - ○ Contrast material improves visualization of synangiosis and collaterals
  - ○ Catheter angiography defines anatomy of occlusions pre-bypass

## DIFFERENTIAL DIAGNOSIS

### "Ivy Sign"
- Leptomeningeal metastases, hemorrhage, meningitis; also seen with high inspired oxygen

### Punctate Foci in Basal Ganglia
- Cribriform lacunar state: No enhancement

### Severely Attenuated Circle of Willis
- Subarachnoid hemorrhage, meningitis, tumor encasement

## PATHOLOGY

### General Features
- General path comments
  - ○ Nearly endless list of etiologies reported
  - ○ Results from any slowly progressive intracranial vascular occlusion
- Genetics
  - ○ Inherited (primary) moyamoya
    - ■ Several gene loci mapped: MYMY1: Chr 3p26-p24.2; MYMY2: 17q25; MYMY3: 8q24
  - ○ Disorders with ↑ association secondary moyamoya

# MOYAMOYA

- Down syndrome, tuberous sclerosis, sickle cell disease, connective tissue disease, progeria
- Midline anomalies (morning glory syndrome); syndromes with aneurysms, cardiac & ocular defects
- NF1, irradiation & suprasellar tumor a disastrous combination
- Inflammatory: CNS angiitis (of childhood), basal meningitis (TB), leptospirosis, atherosclerosis, local infection (tonsillitis/otitis)
- Vasculopathies and prothrombotic states: Kawasaki, anticardiolipin antibody, factor V Leiden, polyarteritis nodosa, Behçet, SLE
- Etiology: Many: Idiopathic, genetic, inflammatory, congenital mesenchymal defects, premature aging syndromes, prothrombotic states
- Epidemiology: 10% of cases are familial
- Associated abnormalities: Depends on primary etiology

## Gross Pathologic & Surgical Features
- Increased perforating (early) and EC-IC (late) collaterals in atrophic brain
- Intracranial hemorrhage (adults)
- Increased saccular aneurysms (esp. basilar in adults)

## Microscopic Features
- Intimal thickening and hyperplasia
- Excessive infolding and thickening of internal elastic lamina
- Increased periventricular pseudoaneurysms (cause of hemorrhage)

## Staging, Grading or Classification Criteria
- Staging criteria (after Suzuki)
  - Stage I: Narrowing of ICA bifurcation
  - Stage II: ACA, MCA, PCA dilated
  - Stage III: Maximal basal moyamoya collaterals; small ACA/MCA
  - Stage IV: Fewer collaterals (vessels); small PCA
  - Stage V: Further reduction in collaterals; absent ACA, MCA, PCA
  - Stage VI: Extensive pial collaterals from ECA

# CLINICAL ISSUES

## Presentation
- Most common signs/symptoms
  - In childhood: TIA, alternating hemiplegia (exacerbated by crying), headache, occasionally just developmental delay and poor feeding
  - In adulthood: SAH and intraventricular hemorrhage
- Clinical Profile
  - Children more likely to have TIA and to progress, adults more likely to infarct (but slower progression)
  - Children more likely to have ipsilateral anterior PLUS posterior circulation involvement

## Demographics
- Age: Bimodal age peaks: 6 years > 35 years
- Gender: M:F = 1:1.8
- Ethnicity

- Initially described in Japanese children, but panethnic distribution now known
- Present in 0.07% of asymptomatic Japanese
- Remains most frequent cause of stroke in Asian children

## Natural History & Prognosis
- Progressive narrowing, collateralization and ischemia
- Prognosis depends on etiology, ability to form collaterals, age/stage at diagnosis
- Pediatric cases usually advance to stage V within 10 years
  - Infantile moyamoya progresses faster
- Hemorrhagic moyamoya has poorer outcome

## Treatment
- Anticoagulation; correct/control prothrombotic states and inflammatory etiologies
- Hypertransfusion regimens for sickle cell related moyamoya
- Encephalo-duro-arterio-synangiosis (EDAS), a method of indirect bypass
  - 5 year risk of ipsilateral stroke post EDAS 15%
- Perivascular sympathectomy or superior cervical ganglionectomy (adult)

# DIAGNOSTIC CHECKLIST

## Consider
- Need to seek etiology

## Image Interpretation Pearls
- Enhance asymmetric atrophy found on childhood CT, look for abnormal vascular pattern
- Moyamoya in children typically presents with cerebral ischemia vs. hemorrhage in adults

# SELECTED REFERENCES

1. Kim DS et al: Surgical results in pediatric moyamoya disease: Angiographic revascularization and the clinical results. Clin Neurol Neurosurg. 2006
2. Lim M et al: New vessel formation in the central nervous system during tumor growth, vascular malformations, and Moyamoya. Curr Neurovasc Res. 3(3):237-45, 2006
3. Seol HJ et al: Familial occurrence of moyamoya disease: a clinical study. Childs Nerv Syst. 22(9):1143-8, 2006
4. Togao O et al: Cerebral hemodynamics in Moyamoya disease: correlation between perfusion-weighted MR imaging and cerebral angiography. AJNR Am J Neuroradiol. 27(2):391-7, 2006
5. Lim SM et al: Localized 1H-MR spectroscopy in moyamoya disease before and after revascularization surgery. Korean J Radiol. 4(2):71-8, 2003
6. Morioka M et al: Angiographic dilatation and branch extension of the anterior choroidal and posterior communicating arteries are predictors of hemorrhage in adult moyamoya patients. Stroke. 34(1):90-5, 2003
7. Wityk RJ et al: Perfusion-weighted magnetic resonance imaging in adult moyamoya syndrome: characteristic patterns and change after surgical intervention: case report. Neurosurgery. 51(6):1499-505; discussion 1506, 2002
8. Yoon HK et al: "Ivy sign" in childhood moyamoya disease: depiction on FLAIR and contrast-enhanced T1-weighted MR images. Radiology. 223(2):384-9, 2002

# MOYAMOYA

## IMAGE GALLERY

### Typical

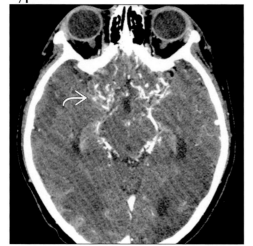

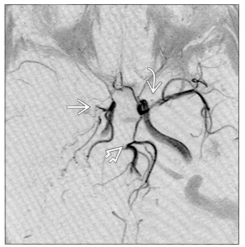

*(Left)* Axial CECT shows dramatic proliferation of "net-like" lenticulostriate collateral arteries ➔ in the basal cisterns. *(Right)* Axial MRA collapsed image shows vascular occlusions of right internal carotid artery ➔, right posterior cerebral artery ➔. Also note stenosis of the left middle cerebral artery ➔.

### Typical

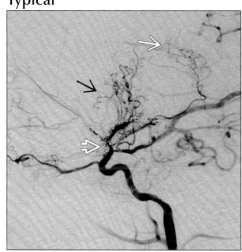

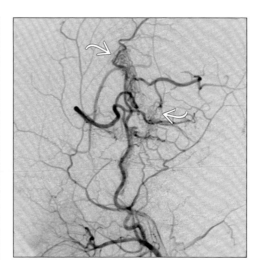

*(Left)* Lateral angiography shows anterior ➔ and posterior ➔ circulation collateral vessels, which are tortuous, dilated. Note tapered occlusion ➔ of the distal internal carotid artery. *(Right)* Lateral angiography of the external carotid artery shows opacification of the synangiosis ➔.

### Variant

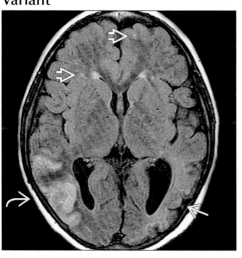

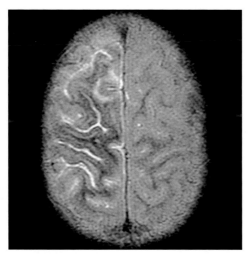

*(Left)* Axial FLAIR MR shows multiple small infarcts ➔, remote left occipital atrophy ➔ and new right occipital infarction with cortical edema ➔ in a child with newly diagnosed moyamoya. *(Right)* Axial FLAIR MR shows asymmetrically bright sulci in moyamoya. This is more severe than the typical "ivy sign" of collaterals.

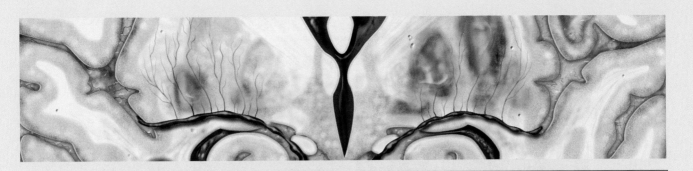

# SECTION 8: Multiple Regions, Brain

# NEUROFIBROMATOSIS TYPE 1

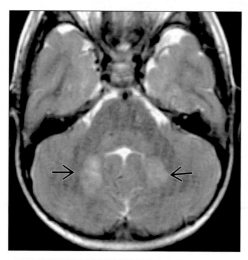

*Axial T2WI MR shows typical signal abnormalities of NF1 ➡ in the deep white matter of the cerebellum. This is the most common location to identify these characteristic lesions.*

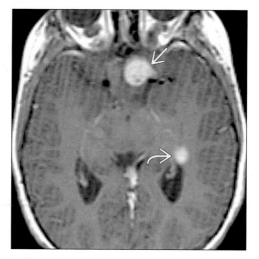

*Axial T1 C+ MR shows enhancing gliomas in the left optic nerve ➡ and the left optic radiations ➡. Multiplicity of gliomas can confound therapeutic strategies in children with NF1.*

## TERMINOLOGY

### Abbreviations and Synonyms
- Synonyms: NF1, Von Recklinghausen disease, peripheral neurofibromatosis

### Definitions
- Neurocutaneous disorder (phakomatosis) characterized by
  - Dynamic reactive/dysplastic white matter (WM) lesions
    - Sometimes called focal areas of signal intensity (FASI), non-specific bright foci (NSBF), unidentified bright objects (UBOs)
  - Astrocytomas, primarily of the visual pathways
    - Visual pathway glioma = optic nerve glioma (ONG)
  - Neurofibromas
  - Vascular dysplasias
  - Skin lesions (cafe-au-lait spots)
  - Dysplastic skeletal lesions

## IMAGING FINDINGS

### General Features
- Best diagnostic clue
  - Hyperintense lesions on T2WI
  - Plexiform neurofibromas
  - Visual pathway gliomas
- Location
  - WM lesions may also involve dentate nuclei of cerebellum, globus pallidus, thalamus, brainstem, pons, midbrain, hippocampus
  - Plexiform lesions are often apparent on brain imaging
    - Scalp lesions over the occiput
    - Skull base lesions extending into retropharynx
    - Orbital lesions extending from cavernous sinus through orbit into periorbital soft tissues
  - Visual pathway gliomas ⇒ intra-orbital optic nerves (ON), chiasm/hypothalamus, optic tracts and radiations
- Size
  - WM lesions: 2-20 mm
  - Visual pathway gliomas: 3-50 mm
  - Plexiform lesions can be massive

## DDx: White Matter Signal Abnormalities

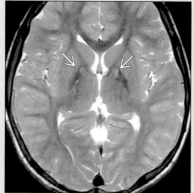

*PKAN*

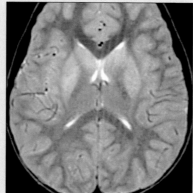

*Ebstein-Barr Virus*

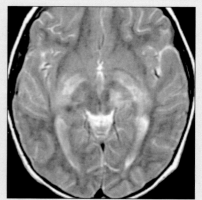

*ADEM*

# NEUROFIBROMATOSIS TYPE 1

## Key Facts

### Terminology
- Synonyms: NF1, Von Recklinghausen disease, peripheral neurofibromatosis

### Imaging Findings
- Hyperintense lesions on T2WI
- Visual pathway gliomas
- WM lesions may also involve dentate nuclei of cerebellum, globus pallidus, thalamus, brainstem, pons, midbrain, hippocampus
- Sphenoid wing and occipital bone dysplasia (absence) are found in association with plexiform tumors
- Visual pathway gliomas have variable enhancement
- Benefit of routine surveillance imaging is questionable

### Pathology
- In children, optic gliomas and WM lesions dominate the clinical picture
- Autosomal dominant; gene locus is chromosome 17q12
- Penetrance = 100%
- ~ 50% new mutations
- Incidence is 1:3,000-5,000
- Most common neurocutaneous syndrome

### Clinical Issues
- Morbidity related to specific manifestations
- Visual pathway glioma ⇒ vision loss, hypothalamic dysfunction

### Diagnostic Checklist
- Absence of visible stigmata does not exclude NF1

---

- Morphology
  - WM lesions: Spherical/ovoid, often amorphous
  - ONG: Conform to and enlarge ON and chiasm, can be spherical in chiasm and hypothalamus

## CT Findings
- CTA: Vascular dysplasias ⇒ moyamoya, aneurysm
- NECT
  - Sphenoid dysplasia
    - Associated enlargement of middle cranial fossa and ipsilateral proptosis
  - Enlarged optic nerves/chiasm
- CECT: Enhancing visual pathway gliomas

## MR Findings
- T1WI
  - WM lesions have variable signal
    - Irregular hyperintensity may reflect myelin clumping or microcalcification
- T2WI
  - WM lesions are hyperintense and typically poorly defined
    - T2WI may be more sensitive than FLAIR for WM lesions in cerebellum
  - ONG are isointense/hyperintense to normal parenchyma
- STIR: Excellent definition of plexiform and paraspinal neurofibromas
- T1 C+
  - WM lesions usually don't enhance
    - Enhancement raises concern for neoplasm, but can be self-limited/reversible
  - Uncommon cases of "wandering" WM enhancement may lead to vascular dysplasia
  - Plexiform lesions have variable enhancement
    - Less well defined than on STIR images
  - Visual pathway gliomas have variable enhancement
    - Significance of ↓ enhancement in response to treatment is uncertain
- T1 C+ FS: Best sequence for evaluation of visual pathway gliomas
- MRA

- Valuable in detection and surveillance of vascular lesions
  - Aneurysms, moyamoya
- MRS
  - May have benefit in evaluation of WM lesions to distinguish from visual pathway glioma
    - WM lesions have relative preservation of NAA
    - Glioma have ↓ NAA with elevated choline

## Radiographic Findings
- Radiography
  - Sphenoid wing and occipital bone dysplasia (absence) are found in association with plexiform tumors
  - Skeletal dysplasias and kyphoscoliosis

## Angiographic Findings
- Conventional
  - Most vascular lesions are non-CNS
    - Renal artery stenosis, aortic stenosis
  - Moyamoya, cerebral aneurysms occasionally encountered

## Imaging Recommendations
- Best imaging tool
  - MR
    - Benefit of routine surveillance imaging is questionable
    - Coronal STIR sequences are essential when imaging spine or head & neck
- Protocol advice
  - Include fat-saturated post-contrast imaging of the orbits
  - Consider MRA if moyamoya suspected

## DIFFERENTIAL DIAGNOSIS

### Demyelinating Disease
- Lesions of acute disseminated encephalomyelitis (ADEM) or multiple sclerosis can mimic WM lesions of NF1

# NEUROFIBROMATOSIS TYPE 1

## Viral Encephalitis
- Ebstein-Barr (EBV), cytomegalovirus (CMV)

## Mitochondrial Encephalopathies
- Pantothenate kinase-associated neurodegeneration (PKAN, Hallervorden-Spatz), Leigh syndrome, glutaric acidurias, Kearns-Sayre syndrome
- Often have lesions in basal ganglia or thalami that resemble WM lesions of NF1

## Krabbe Disease (Globoid Cell Leukodystrophy)
- Can cause optic nerve enlargement mimicking ONG

## Tuberous Sclerosis
- Second most common phakomatosis
- Multiple cortical/subcortical tubers with similar signal to WM lesions of NF1

## PATHOLOGY

### General Features
- General path comments
  - In children, optic gliomas and WM lesions dominate the clinical picture
  - Visual pathway gliomas in NF1 often have a more indolent clinical course than sporadic optic glioma
- Genetics
  - Autosomal dominant; gene locus is chromosome 17q12
    - Penetrance = 100%
  - ~ 50% new mutations
- Etiology
  - NF gene product is neurofibromin
    - Inactivated in NF1 → tissue proliferation, tumor development
  - Oligodendrocyte myelin glycoprotein is embedded in gene
    - This may cause the dysplasia of the WM lesions
- Epidemiology
  - Incidence is 1:3,000-5,000
  - Most common neurocutaneous syndrome
  - Most common inherited tumor syndrome

### Gross Pathologic & Surgical Features
- Gliomas are usually pilocytic astrocytomas
  - Frankly malignant in < 20%
- Slight ↑ incidence of medulloblastoma/ependymoma
- Rare subependymal glial nodules
  - Can result in CSF obstruction

### Microscopic Features
- WM lesions
  - Foci of myelin vacuolization, proliferation of protoplasmic astroglia, microcalcifications, crinkled nuclei
  - No demyelination or inflammation

### Staging, Grading or Classification Criteria
- 2 or more of the following fulfills the diagnostic criteria for NF1
  - 6 + café-au-lait spots measuring ≥ 15 mm in adults or 5 mm in children
  - 2 + neurofibromas or 1 plexiform neurofibroma
  - Axillary/inguinal freckling
  - Visual pathway glioma
  - 2 + Lisch nodules
  - Distinctive bony lesion (sphenoid wing dysplasia, thinning of long bone ± pseudoarthrosis)
  - First-degree relative with NF1

## CLINICAL ISSUES

### Presentation
- Most common signs/symptoms
  - Most children come to attention because of skin lesions
  - ~ 50% have macrocephaly
  - Visual pathway gliomas cause progressive vision loss

### Natural History & Prognosis
- Morbidity related to specific manifestations
  - Visual pathway glioma ⇒ vision loss, hypothalamic dysfunction
  - Plexiform NF ⇒ risk of sarcomatous degeneration
  - Paraspinal NF ⇒ kyphoscoliosis
  - Vascular stenoses ⇒ hypertension (renal artery), stroke
- NF1 related learning disability in 30-60%
  - Associated with WM lesions

### Treatment
- Clinical observation
- Chemotherapy and radiation for visual pathway gliomas

## DIAGNOSTIC CHECKLIST

### Consider
- Absence of visible stigmata does not exclude NF1
- Be aware of potential for vascular lesions

## SELECTED REFERENCES
1. Quigg M et al: Clinical findings of the phakomatoses: neurofibromatosis. Neurology. 66(6):E23-4, 2006
2. Hyman SL et al: The nature and frequency of cognitive deficits in children with neurofibromatosis type 1. Neurology. 65(7):1037-44, 2005
3. Rosser TL et al: Cerebrovascular abnormalities in a population of children with neurofibromatosis type 1. Neurology. 64(3):553-5, 2005
4. Liu GT et al: Optic radiation involvement in optic pathway gliomas in neurofibromatosis. Am J Ophthalmol. 137(3):407-14, 2004
5. Feldmann R et al: Neurofibromatosis type 1: motor and cognitive function and T2-weighted MRI hyperintensities. Neurology. 61(12):1725-8, 2003

# NEUROFIBROMATOSIS TYPE 1

## IMAGE GALLERY

Typical

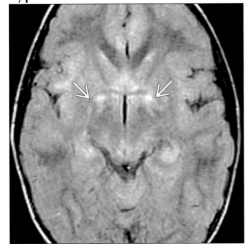
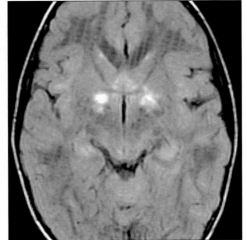

*(Left) Axial FLAIR MR shows relatively subtle signal abnormalities ➡ in the bilateral globus pallidus of a 3 year old with NF1. (Right) Axial FLAIR MR acquired 3 months later (same child as previous image) shows dramatic progression of the white matter lesions. These signal abnormalities typically accelerate in the 1st decade and regress at puberty.*

Typical

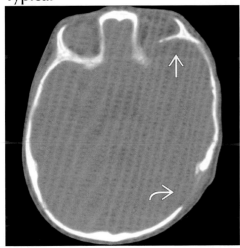
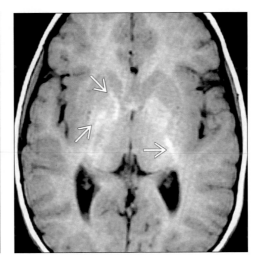

*(Left) Axial bone CT shows a focal defect at the lambdoid suture ➡ and dysplasia of the left sphenoid wing ➡. These bone lesions are associated with plexiform neurofibromas in each location. (Right) Axial T1WI MR shows hyperintense signal abnormalities in thalamic and pallidal lesions ➡. This hyperintensity likely reflects clumping of myelin or the presence of microcalcifications.*

Typical

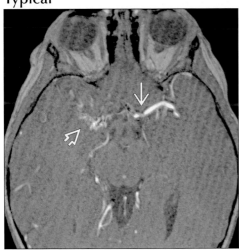
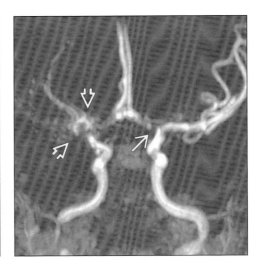

*(Left) Axial MRA shows moyamoya vessels ➡ at site of right middle cerebral artery in a child with NF1. Non-occlusive stenosis ➡ at left carotid terminus has not caused moyamoya changes yet. (Right) Coronal oblique MIP (same child as previous) shows the "puff of smoke" appearance of moyamoya collaterals at right carotid terminus ➡. No collaterals have formed around left sided stenosis ➡.*

# NEUROFIBROMATOSIS TYPE 2

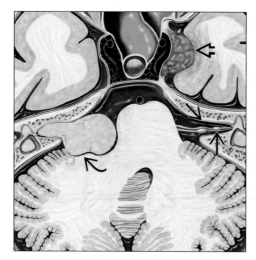

Axial graphic shows a large tumor of right CNs VII-VIII ➘, several small tumors of left CNs VII-VIII ➘, and a meningioma ▷ of the left cavernous sinus and middle cranial fossa.

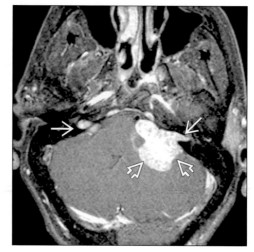

Axial T1 C+ MR shows bilateral schwannomas in the internal auditory canals ➘ and cerebellopontine angle ➘, with significant distortion of the brainstem caused by the left sided tumor.

## TERMINOLOGY

### Abbreviations and Synonyms
- Neurofibromatosis type 2 (NF2)
- MISME
  - Multiple intracranial schwannomas, meningiomas, and ependymomas
- Acoustic neurofibromatosis, central neurofibromatosis, bilateral acoustic neurofibromatosis

### Definitions
- Hereditary syndrome causing multiple cranial nerve schwannomas, meningiomas, and spinal tumors

## IMAGING FINDINGS

### General Features
- Best diagnostic clue: Bilateral vestibular schwannomas
- Location
  - Multiple extra-axial tumors
    - Schwannomas on cranial nerves and spinal nerve roots
    - Meningiomas on dural surfaces

- Intra-axial tumors
  - Ependymomas in spinal cord and brainstem
- Size: Cranial nerve tumors typically symptomatic while still small, but can achieve great size
- Morphology: Tumors grow spherically, but accommodate to bony canals, e.g., internal auditory canal (IAC)
- Multiplicity of lesions
  - Schwannomas of other cranial nerves
  - Schwannoma "tumorlets" of spinal nerves
  - Meningiomas (often multiple)
  - Intramedullary ependymomas (spinal cord)
  - Cerebral calcifications
  - Posterior lens opacities
  - Meningioangiomatosis
  - Glial microhamartomas

### CT Findings
- NECT
  - Vestibular schwannoma
    - Cerebellopontine angle (CPA) mass +/- widened IAC
    - Isodense to hyperdense
    - Rarely cystic/necrotic

## DDx: Cranial Nerve Enhancement

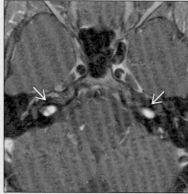

Metastases in IACs

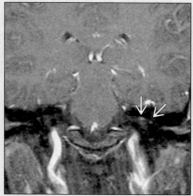

Bell Palsy

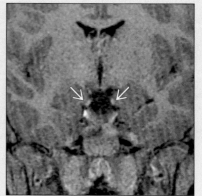

Leukemia (CN III)

# NEUROFIBROMATOSIS TYPE 2

## Key Facts

### Terminology
- Multiple intracranial schwannomas, meningiomas, and ependymomas

### Imaging Findings
- Best diagnostic clue: Bilateral vestibular schwannomas
- Schwannomas on cranial nerves and spinal nerve roots
- Meningiomas on dural surfaces
- Ependymomas in spinal cord and brainstem
- Nonneoplastic cerebral Ca++ (uncommon)
- Use high resolution T1 C+ through basal cisterns with fat-saturation to evaluate cranial nerves
- Evaluation for spinal disease is critical

### Top Differential Diagnoses
- Schwannomatosis
- Multiple Meningiomas
- Metastases

### Pathology
- All NF2 families have chromosome 22q12 abnormalities

### Clinical Issues
- Patients typically become symptomatic in 3rd decade
- Younger age at diagnosis and presence of meningiomas both increase risk of mortality

### Diagnostic Checklist
- Carefully evaluate other cranial nerves in any new diagnosis of vestibular schwannoma

---

- ○ Meningioma
  - ▪ High density dural-based mass(es)
- ○ Nonneoplastic cerebral Ca++ (uncommon)
  - ▪ Extensive choroid plexus Ca++
  - ▪ Cortical surface
  - ▪ Ventricular lining
- CECT
  - ○ Cranial nerve tumor enhancement
  - ○ Meningioma enhancement

## MR Findings
- T1WI
  - ○ Schwannomas
    - ▪ Hypointense to isointense
    - ▪ Rare cystic change
  - ○ Meningiomas
    - ▪ Isointense to hypointense
    - ▪ Occasional hyperintense foci from Ca++
- T2WI
  - ○ Schwannomas
    - ▪ Small intracanalicular lesions can be shown on high resolution T2WI
  - ○ Meningiomas
    - ▪ May incite significant adjacent edema
- T2* GRE: Shows nonneoplastic Ca++ to best advantage
- DWI
  - ○ Some meningiomas have restricted diffusion
    - ▪ Characteristic of atypical or malignant meningioma
- T1 C+
  - ○ Schwannomas
    - ▪ Diffuse enhancement
    - ▪ Usually homogeneous
    - ▪ T1 C+ with fat saturation and thin slice profile essential for identification of small CN tumors
    - ▪ Vestibular schwannomas typically "bulge" into CPA cistern from IAC
  - ○ Meningiomas
    - ▪ Diffuse enhancement of tumor, may be plaque-like
- MRS
  - ○ Meningioma
    - ▪ Absent NAA peak, +/- lactate

- ○ Schwannoma
  - ▪ Absent NAA peak, usually no lactate

## Non-Vascular Interventions
- Myelography
  - ○ Will demonstrate multiple spinal tumorlets
    - ▪ Replaced by contrast-enhanced MR

## Imaging Recommendations
- Best imaging tool: Contrast-enhanced MR
- Protocol advice
  - ○ Use high resolution T1 C+ through basal cisterns with fat-saturation to evaluate cranial nerves
  - ○ Evaluation for spinal disease is critical

## DIFFERENTIAL DIAGNOSIS

### Schwannomatosis
- Multiple schwannomas without vestibular tumors
- No cutaneous stigmata or meningiomas

### Cerebellopontine Angle (CPA) Masses
- Arachnoid cyst
  - ○ Follows CSF on all sequences
- Epidermoid
  - ○ DWI and MRS easily distinguish from arachnoid cyst
- Aneurysm
  - ○ Vertebral or petrous aneurysms may project into CPA
  - ○ Pulsation artifact in phase-encoding direction
- Ependymoma
  - ○ Extends into CPA from fourth ventricle

### Multiple Meningiomas
- Recurrent or metastatic
- Secondary to radiation therapy

### Metastases
- CNS primary
  - ○ Glioblastoma, PNET-MB, germinoma, ependymoma
- Non-CNS primary

# NEUROFIBROMATOSIS TYPE 2

## Inflammatory Disease
- Granulomatous disease: Sarcoidosis, Tuberculosis
- Neuritis: Bell palsy, Lyme disease

# PATHOLOGY

## General Features
- General path comments: Multiple schwannomas, meningiomas, ependymomas
- Genetics
  - Autosomal dominant
  - All NF2 families have chromosome 22q12 abnormalities
  - Germline, somatic NF2 gene mutations
    - NF2 gene functions as tumor suppressor gene
    - Encodes for merlin protein
    - Links cytoskeleton and cell membranes
- Etiology
  - 50% known family history of NF2; 50% new mutations
  - Mutations cause truncated, inactivated merlin protein
  - Loss of both alleles predisposes to tumor formation
- Epidemiology: 1 in 40,000-100,000

## Gross Pathologic & Surgical Features
- Schwannomas are round-ovoid encapsulated masses
- Meningiomas are unencapsulated but sharply circumscribed

## Microscopic Features
- NF2-related schwannomas have higher proliferative activity than sporadic tumors but not necessarily more aggressive course

## Staging, Grading or Classification Criteria
- NF2-associated schwannomas are WHO grade I
- Diagnostic criteria
  - Bilateral vestibular schwannomas; or
  - 1st degree relative with NF2 and 1 vestibular schwannoma; or
  - 1st degree relative with NF2 and 2 of the following
    - Neurofibroma
    - Meningioma
    - Glioma
    - Schwannoma
    - Posterior subcapsular lenticular opacity

# CLINICAL ISSUES

## Presentation
- Most common signs/symptoms
  - 1/3 of children with NF2 present with hearing loss
  - 1/3 present with other cranial nerve symptoms
- Other signs/symptoms: Scoliosis, paraplegia or neck pain from spinal lesions
- Clinical Profile: Young adult with multiple cranial neuropathies, cataracts, and extremity weakness

## Demographics
- Age

- Patients typically become symptomatic in 3rd decade
- Screening of children of NF2 parents can identify asymptomatic tumors

## Natural History & Prognosis
- Younger age at diagnosis and presence of meningiomas both increase risk of mortality
- Diagnosis before age 25 ⇒ 60% survival at 10 yrs
- Diagnosis after age 25 ⇒ 67% survival at 10 yrs

## Treatment
- Complete resection of CN 8 schwannoma if feasible
- Subtotal microsurgical resection with functional cochlear nerve preservation in the last hearing ear

# DIAGNOSTIC CHECKLIST

## Consider
- Carefully evaluate other cranial nerves in any new diagnosis of vestibular schwannoma
  - Be highly suspicious if < 30 yrs
- Study entire neuraxis in suspected cases (multiple small, asymptomatic schwannomas on cauda equina common)

## Image Interpretation Pearls
- Coronal thin slice T1 C+ with fat saturation to assess cranial nerves

# SELECTED REFERENCES

1. Bosch MM et al: Optic nerve sheath meningiomas in patients with neurofibromatosis type 2. Arch Ophthalmol. 124(3):379-85, 2006
2. Omeis I et al: Meningioangiomatosis associated with neurofibromatosis: report of 2 cases in a single family and review of the literature. Surg Neurol. 65(6):595-603, 2006
3. Gelal F et al: Islets of meningioma in an acoustic schwannoma in a patient with neurofibromatosis-2: pathology and magnetic resonance imaging findings. Acta Radiol. 46(5):519-22, 2005
4. Kim JE et al: Neurofibromatosis type 2 in an infant presenting with visual impairment confirmed by genetic mutation analysis. Retina. 25(7):938-40, 2005
5. Ruggieri M et al: Earliest clinical manifestations and natural history of neurofibromatosis type 2 (NF2) in childhood: a study of 24 patients. Neuropediatrics. 36(1):21-34, 2005
6. Rushing EJ et al: Central nervous system meningiomas in the first two decades of life: a clinicopathological analysis of 87 patients. J Neurosurg. 103(6 Suppl):489-95, 2005
7. Nunes F et al: Neurofibromatosis 2 in the pediatric population. J Child Neurol. 18(10):718-24, 2003
8. Otsuka G et al: Age at symptom onset and long-term survival in patients with neurofibromatosis Type 2. J Neurosurg. 99(3):480-3, 2003
9. Baser ME et al: Predictors of the risk of mortality in neurofibromatosis 2. Am J Hum Genet. 71(4):715-23, 2002
10. Shaida AM et al: Schwannomatosis in a child--or early neurofibromatosis type 2. J Laryngol Otol. 116(7):551-5, 2002
11. Mayfrank L et al: Intracranial calcified deposits in neurofibromatosis type 2. A CT study of 11 cases. Neuroradiology. 32(1):33-7, 1990

## IMAGE GALLERY

### Typical

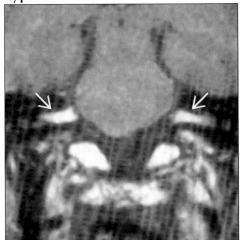

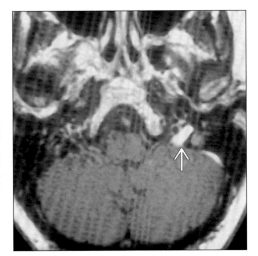

*(Left) Coronal T1 C+ MR shows vestibular schwannomas ➡ filling both internal auditory canals of this teenager. A careful survey of all cranial nerves is required when imaging NF2 patients. (Right) Axial T1 C+ MR shows diffuse enhancement of a twelfth cranial nerve schwannoma ➡ filling the left hypoglossal canal. Atypical cranial nerve involvement is a harbinger of NF2.*

### Typical

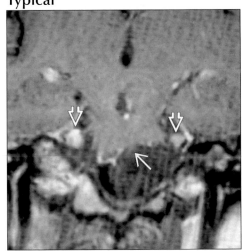

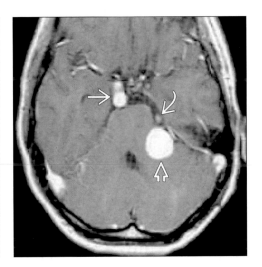

*(Left) Coronal T1 C+ MR shows enlargement and enhancement of cisternal segments of both trigeminal nerves ➡. Note pontine deformity ➡ from previously resected vestibular nerve schwannoma. (Right) Axial T1 C+ MR shows tumors of the right trochlear nerve ➡, left trigeminal nerve ➡, and left vestibular nerve ➡ in this patient with NF2.*

### Typical

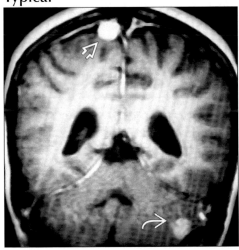

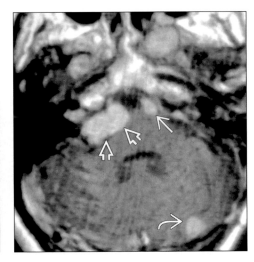

*(Left) Coronal T1 C+ MR shows a parafalcine meningioma over the right parietal lobe ➡ and a similar sized meningioma impinging upon the left cerebellar hemisphere ➡. (Right) Axial T1 C+ MR shows schwannomas of the right 7th/8th nerve complex ➡ and of the left 6th cranial nerve ➡, as well as a meningioma dorsal to the left cerebellar hemisphere ➡.*

# TUBEROUS SCLEROSIS COMPLEX

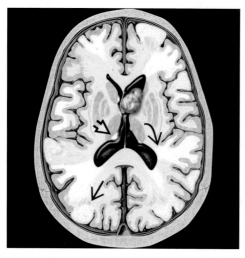

Axial graphic shows a giant cell astrocytoma in the left foramen of Monro, mild left frontal horn obstruction, subependymal nodules ⇒, radial lines ⇒ and many cortical/subcortical tubers ⇒.

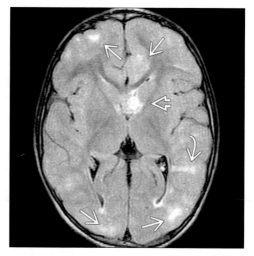

Axial FLAIR MR shows subependymal giant cell astrocytoma ⇒, multiple cortical/subcortical tubers expanding gyri ⇒, and a radial line ⇒ extending to the left trigone.

## TERMINOLOGY

### Abbreviations and Synonyms
- Tuberous sclerosis complex (TSC); Bourneville-Pringle syndrome

### Definitions
- Inherited tumor disorder with multi-organ hamartomas
  - Spectrum of central nervous system (CNS) hamartomas, all contain giant balloon cells

## IMAGING FINDINGS

### General Features
- Best diagnostic clue
  - Calcified (Ca++) subependymal nodules (hamartomas)
    - 98% have subependymal nodules (SENs)
- Location
  - Subependymal giant cell astrocytoma (SGCA) 15%
  - Cortical/subcortical tubers, white matter lesions 70-95%
    - Frontal > parietal > occipital > temporal > cerebellum
    - ↑ Number tubers ⇒ ↑ neurologic symptoms
  - White matter lesions along lines of neuronal migration
  - Cyst-like white matter lesions (cystoid brain degeneration)
- Size: Thickened cortex, enlarged gyri associated with cortical/subcortical tubers
- Morphology
  - Pyramidal-shaped gyral expansion
  - 20% have "eye-of-potato" central depression

### CT Findings
- NECT
  - SENs
    - Along caudothalamic groove > atrial > > temporal
    - 50% Ca++ (progressive after 1 year)
  - Tubers
    - Early: Low density/Ca++ cortical/subcortical mass
    - Later: Isodense/Ca++ (50% by 10 years)
  - Ventriculomegaly common even without SGCA
- CECT: Enhancing/enlarging SEN suspicious for SGCA

## DDx: Tubers and Calcifications

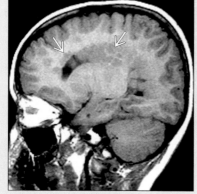

Heterotopia

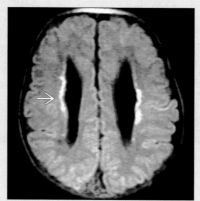

Cytomegalovirus

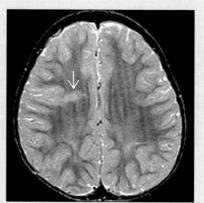

Transmantle GM

# TUBEROUS SCLEROSIS COMPLEX

## Key Facts

### Terminology
- Tuberous sclerosis complex (TSC); Bourneville-Pringle syndrome
- Inherited tumor disorder with multi-organ hamartomas

### Imaging Findings
- Calcified (Ca++) subependymal nodules (hamartomas)
- Subependymal giant cell astrocytoma (SGCA) 15%
- Cortical/subcortical tubers, white matter lesions 70-95%
- White matter lesions along lines of neuronal migration
- Cyst-like white matter lesions (cystoid brain degeneration)
- Cortical/subcortical tubers: Early T1 ↑, but variable after myelin maturation
- SEN enhancement more visible on MR than on CT
- 30-80% enhance (enlarging SEN at foramen of Monro: SGCA)
- Fetal documentation of rhabdomyoma: TSC confirmed in 96%

### Top Differential Diagnoses
- X-Linked Subependymal Heterotopia
- (S)TORCH
- Taylor Type Cortical Dysplasia

### Pathology
- Mutations in TSC tumor suppressor genes cause abnormal cellular differentiation, proliferation

## MR Findings
- T1WI
  - Cortical/subcortical tubers: Early T1 ↑, but variable after myelin maturation
  - Focal lacune-like cysts (vascular etiology)
- T2WI: Variable signal (relative to myelin maturation)
- FLAIR
  - White matter (WM) lesions
    - Streaky linear or wedge-shaped hyperintensities (along radial migration lines from ventricle to cortex)
  - FLAIR becomes more positive with age
- T2* GRE: Ca++ SEN more readily discerned
- DWI: ↑ ADC values in epileptogenic tubers
- T1 C+
  - SEN enhancement more visible on MR than on CT
    - 30-80% enhance (enlarging SEN at foramen of Monro: SGCA)
    - Other enhancing lesions followed [unless growing, or obstructing cerebrospinal fluid (CSF)]
  - 12% cortical/subependymal tubers enhance
- MRA: Rare aneurysms and dysplasias
- MRS: ↓ NAA/Cr, ↑ mI/Cr in subcortical tubers, SENs

## Radiographic Findings
- Radiography
  - Bone islands (skull)
  - Undulating periosteal new bone

## Ultrasonographic Findings
- Grayscale Ultrasound
  - Fetal documentation of rhabdomyoma: TSC confirmed in 96%
    - Rhabdomyomas identifiable as early as 20 weeks gestation

## Nuclear Medicine Findings
- PET: ↓ Glucose metabolism in lateral temporal gyri in TSC plus autism
- Brain SPECT: ↓ Uptake quiescent tubers; ictal SPECT ↑ uptake tubers with active seizure focus
  - Helps localize for surgery

## Angiographic Findings
- Conventional: DSA/MRA: Vascular dysplasia (rare: Moyamoya, aneurysm)

## Imaging Recommendations
- Best imaging tool: MR with contrast
- Protocol advice
  - MR with contrast; +/- NECT (document Ca++ SENs)
  - Yearly surveillance imaging if: Incompletely calcified SGCA or enhancing SGCA
    - Look for rapid growth, +/- ventricular obstruction

# DIFFERENTIAL DIAGNOSIS

## X-Linked Subependymal Heterotopia
- Isointense to gray matter (GM) T1/T2; don't enhance or Ca++

## (S)TORCH
- Cytomegalovirus (CMV)
  - Periventricular Ca++
  - Typical WM lesions
  - Polymicrogyria

## Taylor Type Cortical Dysplasia
- Considered forme fruste TSC (single cortical lesion can mimic neoplasm)

# PATHOLOGY

## General Features
- General path comments: Inherited tumor disorder with multi-organ hamartomas
- Genetics
  - Approximately 50% of TSC cases inherited
    - De novo: Spontaneous mutation/germ-line mosaicism
    - Autosomal dominant, high but variable penetrance
  - Mutations in TSC tumor suppressor genes cause abnormal cellular differentiation, proliferation

- Two distinct loci: TSC1 (9q34.3) encodes "hamartin"; TSC2 (16p13.3) encodes "tuberin"
- Etiology
  - Abnormal differentiation/proliferation of germinal matrix cells
  - Migrational arrest of dysgenetic neurons
- Epidemiology: 1:10,000-20,000
- Associated abnormalities
  - Renal: Angiomyolipoma and cysts 40-80%
  - Cardiac: Rhabdomyomas 50-65%; majority involute over time
  - Lung: Cystic lymphangiomyomatosis/fibrosis
  - Solid organs: Adenomas; leiomyomas
  - Skin: Ash-leaf spots (majority) including scalp/hair; facial angiofibromas; shagreen patches 20-35% post pubertal
  - Extremities: Subungual fibromas 15-20%; cystic bone lesions; undulating periosteal new bone formation
  - Ocular: "Giant drusen" (50%); retinal astrocytomas (which may regress)
  - Dental pitting permanent teeth in most adults with TSC

## Gross Pathologic & Surgical Features
- Firm cortical masses ("tubers") with dimpling ("potato eye")

## Microscopic Features
- Cortical dysplasia with balloon cells, ectopic neurons
- Myelin loss, vacuolation and gliosis

## Staging, Grading or Classification Criteria
- SGCA: WHO grade I

## CLINICAL ISSUES

### Presentation
- Most common signs/symptoms
  - Classic clinical triad
    - Facial angiofibromas 90%; mental retardation (MR) 50-80%; seizures (Sz) 80-90%
    - All three ("epiloia"): 30%
- Clinical Profile
  - Sz (infantile type spasms in very young), facial angiofibroma, hypopigmented skin lesions, MR
  - Infant/toddler: Infantile spasms (65%), autism (50%) ⇒ bad prognosis
    - Infantile spasms occur before development of facial lesions, shagreen patches
  - Diagnostic criteria: Two major or one major + one minor
    - Major: Facial angiofibroma/forehead plaque, sub-/periungual fibroma, ≥ 3 hypomelanotic macules, shagreen patch, multiple retinal nodular hamartomas, cortical tuber, SEN, SGCA, cardiac rhabdomyoma, lymphangioleiomyomatosis, renal angiomyolipoma
    - Minor: Dental enamel pits, hamartomatous rectal polyps, bone cysts, cerebral WM radial migration lines (> 3 = major sign), gingival fibromas, non-renal hamartoma, retinal achromic patch, confetti skin lesions, multiple renal cysts

## Demographics
- Age
  - Diagnosed at any age
    - First year of life if: Infantile spasms or surveillance for positive family history
    - Child: Autistic-like behavior, mental retardation, seizures, or skin lesions
    - Adult diagnoses reported with demonstration of symptomatic SGCA on brain imaging

## Natural History & Prognosis
- CNS: SGCAs 10-15%

## Treatment
- Treat seizures, infantile spasms respond to Vigabatrin
- Resect isolated tubers if seizure focus or if able to identify seizure focus among many tubers
- SGCAs resected if obstructing foramen of Monro
- Oral rapamycin reported to cause regression of SGCA (may also spontaneously regress)

## DIAGNOSTIC CHECKLIST

### Consider
- Systemic involvement common

### Image Interpretation Pearls
- T1WI readily documents early white matter abnormalities (pre-myelin maturation)

## SELECTED REFERENCES

1. Chong-Kopera H et al: TSC1 stabilizes TSC2 by inhibiting the interaction between TSC2 and the HERC1 ubiquitin ligase. J Biol Chem. 2006
2. Franz DN et al: Rapamycin causes regression of astrocytomas in tuberous sclerosis complex. Ann Neurol. 59(3):490-8, 2006
3. Pinto Gama HP et al: Comparative analysis of MR sequences to detect structural brain lesions in tuberous sclerosis. Pediatr Radiol. 36(2):119-25, 2006
4. Bader RS et al: Fetal rhabdomyoma: Prenatal diagnosis, clinical outcome, and incidence of associated tuberous sclerosis complex. J Pediatr 143(5):620-4, 2003
5. Jansen FE et al: Diffusion-weighted MRI and identification of the epileptogenic tuber in patients with tuberous sclerosis. Arch Neurol 60(11):1580-4, 2003
6. Rott HD et al: Cyst-like cerebral lesions in tuberous sclerosis. Am J Med Genet 111(4):435-9, 2002
7. Cristophe C et al: MRI spectrum of cortical malformations in tuberous sclerosis complex. Brain Dev 22(8):487-493, 2000
8. Baron Y et al: MR imaging of tuberous sclerosis in neonates and young infants. AJNR 20(5):907-16, 1999
9. Griffiths PD et al: White matter abnormalities in tuberous sclerosis complex. Acta Radiol 39(5):482-6, 1998
10. Jay V et al: Cerebellar pathology in tuberous sclerosis. Ultrastruct Pathol 22(4):331-9, 1998
11. Roach ES et al: Tuberous sclerosis complex consensus conference: Revised clinical diagnostic criteria. J Child Neurol 13:624-28, 1998

# TUBEROUS SCLEROSIS COMPLEX

## IMAGE GALLERY

### Typical

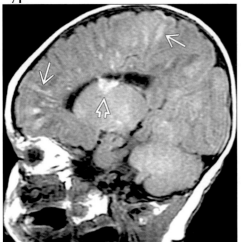 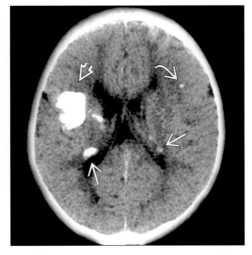

*(Left) Sagittal T1WI MR shows radial white matter lines ➡, well seen on unenhanced T1WI prior to myelin maturation and FLAIR after myelin maturation. Subependymal hamartomas ➡ show increased signal. (Right) Axial NECT shows multiple calcified subependymal nodules ➡. These undergo progressive calcification after infancy. Small ➡ and unusually large ➡ calcified tubers are also present.*

### Typical

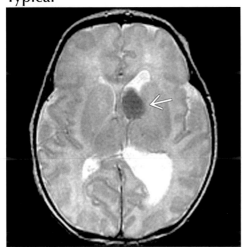 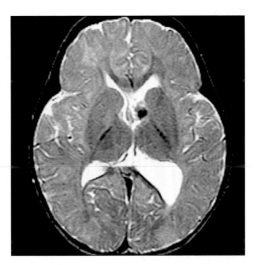

*(Left) Axial T2WI MR shows neonate with very large and obstructing left giant cell astrocytoma ➡. Lesion is quite low signal on T2WI and was markedly increased in signal on T1WI image (not shown). (Right) Axial T2WI MR shows marked reduction in size of the left foramen of Monro lesion in the same infant as previous image, 10 months later. No treatment was given. The left lateral ventricle is less obstructed.*

### Variant

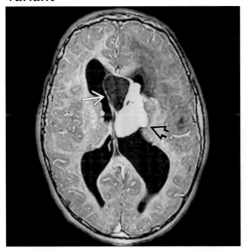 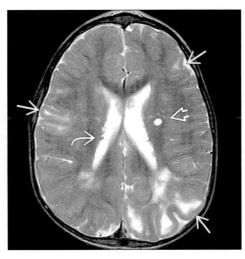

*(Left) Axial T1 C+ MR shows large subependymal giant cell astrocytoma with cystic ➡ and solid ➡ components, left frontal lobe edema and lateral ventricular obstruction. (Right) Axial T2WI MR shows multiple cortical/subcortical tubers ➡ expanding gyri. Small dimples mark the gyral crest in several. Subependymal hamartomas ➡ and oval cystic lesion ➡ are present.*

# STURGE-WEBER SYNDROME

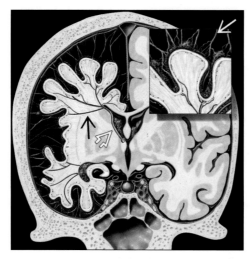

Coronal graphic shows extensive pial angiomatosis ➡, prominent medullary collaterals ➡, enlarged ipsilateral choroid plexus ⇨, and atrophy of the right hemisphere.

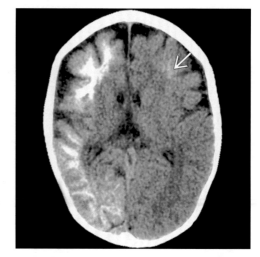

Axial NECT shows extensive right hemispheric calcification and atrophy, both of which have developed rapidly in the first year of life. Note subtle left frontal calcification ➡.

## TERMINOLOGY

### Abbreviations and Synonyms
- Sturge-Weber syndrome (SWS); Sturge-Weber-Dimitri; encephalotrigeminal angiomatosis

### Definitions
- Usually a sporadic congenital (but not inherited) malformation in which fetal cortical veins fail to develop normally
  - Imaging features are sequelae of progressive venous occlusion and chronic venous ischemia

## IMAGING FINDINGS

### General Features
- Best diagnostic clue: Cortical Ca++, atrophy, and enlarged ipsilateral choroid plexus
- Location
  - Pial angiomatosis unilateral 80%, bilateral 20%
  - Occipital > parietal > frontal/temporal lobes > diencephalon/midbrain > cerebellum
- Size: Small focal or bilateral multi-lobar involvement

### CT Findings
- NECT
  - Gyral/subcortical white matter (WM) Ca++
    - Ca++ not in leptomeningeal angioma
    - Progressive, generally posterior to anterior
  - Late
    - Atrophy
    - Hyperpneumatization of paranasal sinuses
    - Thick diploe
- CECT
  - Serpentine leptomeningeal enhancement
  - Ipsilateral choroid plexus enlargement usual
    - Choroidal fissure if frontal involvement
    - Trigonal glomus if posterior involvement (common)

### MR Findings
- T1WI: ↑ WM volume subjacent to pial angiomatosis (early); atrophy of WM and gray matter (late)
- T2WI
  - Early: Transient hyperperfusion ⇒ "accelerated" myelin maturation
  - Late: ↑ Signal in region of gliosis & ↓ cortical signal in regions of calcification

## DDx: Abnormal Enhancement

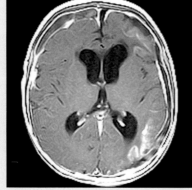

Bilateral Empyema

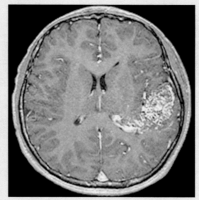

Arteriovenous Malformation

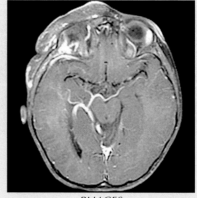

PHACES

# STURGE-WEBER SYNDROME

## Key Facts

### Terminology

- Sturge-Weber syndrome (SWS); Sturge-Weber-Dimitri; encephalotrigeminal angiomatosis
- Usually a sporadic congenital (but not inherited) malformation in which fetal cortical veins fail to develop normally
- Imaging features are sequelae of progressive venous occlusion and chronic venous ischemia

### Imaging Findings

- Best diagnostic clue: Cortical Ca++, atrophy, and enlarged ipsilateral choroid plexus
- Pial angiomatosis unilateral 80%, bilateral 20%
- Radiography: Tram-track calcification
- Early: Transient hyperperfusion ⇒ "accelerated" myelin maturation
- Late: ↑ Signal in region of gliosis & ↓ cortical signal in regions of calcification
- Early: Serpentine leptomeningeal enhancement, pial angiomatosis of subarachnoid space
- Late: "Burnt-out" ⇒ ↓ pial enhancement, ↑ cortical/subcortical Ca++; atrophy
- Progressive sinovenous occlusion

### Pathology

- Epidemiology: Rare: 1:50,000

### Clinical Issues

- Clinical Profile: "Port-wine stain", seizures, hemiparesis
- ↑ Extent of lobar involvement and atrophy ⇒ ↑ likelihood Sz

---

- FLAIR
  - Late: Gliosis in involved lobes
  - FLAIR C+: Improved visualization of enhancement
- T2* GRE: Tram-track gyral calcifications
- DWI: Restricted diffusion in acute ischemia
- T1 C+
  - Early: Serpentine leptomeningeal enhancement, pial angiomatosis of subarachnoid space
  - Late: "Burnt-out" ⇒ ↓ pial enhancement, ↑ cortical/subcortical Ca++; atrophy
  - Engorged, enhancing choroid plexus
- MRA: Rare high-flow arteriovenous malformations
- MRV
  - Progressive sinovenous occlusion
    - Lack of superficial cortical veins
    - ↓ Flow transverse sinuses/jugular veins
    - ↑↑ Prominence deep collateral (medullary/subependymal) veins
- MRS: ↑ Choline; ↓ NAA in affected areas
- Fat-saturation: Orbital enhancement > 50%, best seen with T1 C+ fat-saturation
  - Choroidal angioma, periorbital soft tissues, bony orbit and frontal bone

## Radiographic Findings

- Radiography: Tram-track calcification

## Ultrasonographic Findings

- Pulsed Doppler: ↓ Middle cerebral artery velocity

## Nuclear Medicine Findings

- PET: Progressive hypoperfusion; progressive glucose hypometabolism
- Bone Scan
  - Hypertrophied ipsilateral cortex, diploe
  - Intracranial dystrophic gyral calcification
- SPECT: Transient hyperperfusion (early); hypoperfusion (late)
  - Pattern inconsistent, may be smaller or larger than abnormality detected on CT/MR

## Angiographic Findings

- Conventional
  - Pial blush, rare arteriovenous malformation
  - Findings mostly venous: Paucity of normal cortical veins, extensive medullary and deep collaterals

## Imaging Recommendations

- Best imaging tool: Enhanced MR
- Protocol advice
  - NECT to evaluate for calcification (may be more extensive than recognized on MR)
  - MR with contrast (assess extent, uni-/bilaterality, orbital involvement)
    - FLAIR + contrast improves conspicuity of leptomeningeal angiomatosis
    - Perfusion may predict progression

## DIFFERENTIAL DIAGNOSIS

### Other Vascular Phakomatoses (Neurocutaneous Syndromes)

- Blue-rubber-bleb nevus syndrome
  - Multiple small cutaneous venous malformations plus intracranial developmental venous anomalies
- Wyburn-Mason syndrome
  - Facial vascular nevus; visual pathway and/or brain arteriovenous malformation (AVM)
- Klippel-Trenaunay-Weber syndrome
  - Osseous/soft tissue hypertrophy, extremity vascular malformations
  - May be combined with some features of SWS
- PHACES
  - Posterior fossa malformations, hemangiomas, arterial anomalies, coarctation of the aorta, cardiac, eye and sternal anomalies
- Meningioangiomatosis
  - Ca++ common; variable leptomeningeal enhancement; atrophy usually absent
  - May invade brain through Virchow-Robin perivascular spaces

### Celiac Disease

- Bilateral occipital Ca++; no brain/face involvement

# STURGE-WEBER SYNDROME

## Leptomeningeal Enhancement
- Meningitis; leptomeningeal metastases, & leukemia

## PATHOLOGY

### General Features
- General path comments
  - Cutaneous nevus flammeus CN V1 & V2; ± visceral angiomatosis
  - Embryology
    - 4-8 weeks: Embryonic cortical veins fail to coalesce & develop ⇒ persistent primordial vessels
    - Visual cortex adjacent to optic vesicle and upper fetal face
- Genetics
  - Usually sporadic: Probable somatic mutation or cutaneous mosaicism
    - Fibronectin (found in SWS port-wine-derived fibroblasts and SWS surgical brain samples) regulates angiogenesis and vasculogenesis
  - Very rarely familial, but occasionally with other vascular phakomatosis
- Etiology: Persistent fetal vasculature ⇒ deep venous occlusion/stasis ⇒ anoxic cortex
- Epidemiology: Rare: 1:50,000
- Associated abnormalities: 50% have extracranial port-wine stains (torso or extremities), so evaluate for other vascular phakomatoses

### Gross Pathologic & Surgical Features
- Meningeal hypervascularity & angiomatosis
- Subjacent cortical & subcortical Ca++

### Microscopic Features
- Pial angioma = multiple thin-walled vessels in enlarged sulci
- Cortical atrophy, Ca++
- Occasional underlying cortical dysplasia

### Staging, Grading or Classification Criteria
- Roach scale
  - Type I: Leptomeningeal plus facial; ± glaucoma
  - Type 2: Facial only; ± glaucoma
  - Type 3: Leptomeningeal only

## CLINICAL ISSUES

### Presentation
- Most common signs/symptoms
  - CN V1 facial nevus flammeus ("port-wine stain") 98%; (± V2, V3)
    - Check mucous membranes for occult lesions
  - Eye findings especially with upper and lower lid nevus flammeus
    - Choroidal angioma 70% ⇒ ↑ intraocular pressure/congenital glaucoma ⇒ buphthalmos
    - Retinal telangiectatic vessels; scleral angioma; iris heterochromia
  - Seizures 90%; hemiparesis 30-66%
  - Stroke-like episodes; neurological deficit; migraines
- Clinical Profile: "Port-wine stain", seizures, hemiparesis

## Demographics
- Age
  - Facial lesion visible at birth
    - Pial angiomatosis may be occult if no facial lesion and no seizures to prompt imaging
  - Seizures (Sz) develop first year of life
    - Infantile spasms ⇒ tonic/clonic, myoclonic
- Gender: M = F
- Ethnicity: No ethnic predilection

### Natural History & Prognosis
- ↑ Extent of lobar involvement and atrophy ⇒ ↑ likelihood Sz
- If Sz ⇒ developmental delay 43%, emotional/behavioral problems 85%, special education 70%, employability 46%
- Progressive hemiparesis 30%, homonymous hemianopsia 2%

### Treatment
- Treat seizures; ± resect affected lobes (hemisphere)

## DIAGNOSTIC CHECKLIST

### Consider
- In "Sturge-Weber-like" syndromes, look for extracranial manifestations

### Image Interpretation Pearls
- Ipsilateral choroid plexus engorgement
  - May be only finding in first 6 months of life
  - If both sides enlarged, look for bilateral involvement (may be subtle)

## SELECTED REFERENCES

1. Evans AL et al: Cerebral perfusion abnormalities in children with Sturge-Weber syndrome shown by dynamic contrast bolus magnetic resonance perfusion imaging. Pediatrics. 117(6):2119-25, 2006
2. Comi AM et al: Increased fibronectin expression in sturge-weber syndrome fibroblasts and brain tissue. Pediatr Res. 53(5):762-9, 2003
3. Lin DD et al: Early characteristics of Sturge-Weber syndrome shown by perfusion MR imaging and proton MR spectroscopic imaging. AJNR Am J Neuroradiol. 24(9):1912-5, 2003
4. Pfund Z et al: Quantitative analysis of gray- and white-matter volumes and glucose metabolism in Sturge-Weber syndrome. J Child Neurol. 18:119-26, 2003
5. Portilla P et al: Sturge-Weber disease with repercussion on the prenatal development of the cerebral hemisphere. AJNR Am J Neuroradiol. 23(3):490-2, 2002
6. Cohen MM Jr: Asymmetry: molecular, biologic, embryopathic, and clinical perspectives. Am J Med Genet. 101(4):292-314, 2001
7. Griffiths PD et al: 99mTechnetium HMPAO imaging in children with the Sturge-Weber syndrome: a study of nine cases with CT and MRI correlation. Neuroradiology. 39(3):219-24, 1997

# STURGE-WEBER SYNDROME

## IMAGE GALLERY

### Typical

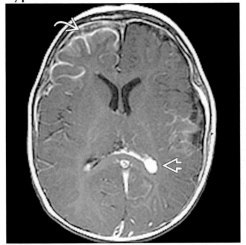 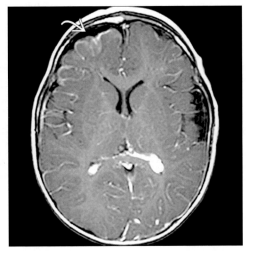

*(Left)* Axial T1 C+ MR at 3 months of age shows right frontal pial angiomatosis ⟶ and contralateral Sylvian atrophy and angiomatosis. Note associated engorgement of the choroid plexus ⟹. *(Right)* Axial T1 C+ MR at follow-up shows decrease in the degree of enhancement of right frontal pial angiomatosis and cortical volume loss over time ⟶.

### Typical

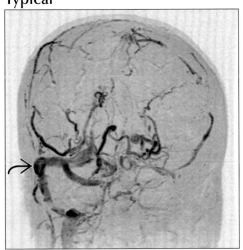 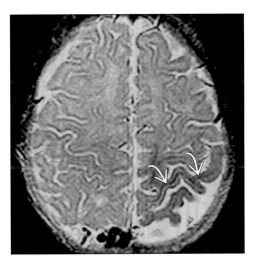

*(Left)* Coronal MRV shows extensive diminution of normal venous structures. Only the right transverse, sigmoid and jugular system ⟶ remain patent. *(Right)* Axial T2WI MR in a young infant shows white matter hypointensity, possibly due to accelerated myelin maturation of atrophied left Rolandic cortex and subcortical white matter ⟶.

### Variant

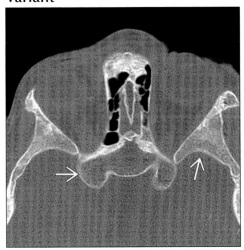 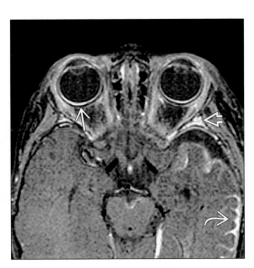

*(Left)* Axial bone CT shows irregular thickening and distortion of bone ⟶ in extensive bilateral Sturge-Weber syndrome. Involvement is much more severe than usual. *(Right)* Axial T1 C+ FS MR shows bilateral choroidal angiomas ⟶, marrow enhancement ⟹ and left temporal atrophy with pial angiomatosis ⟶.

# VON HIPPEL LINDAU

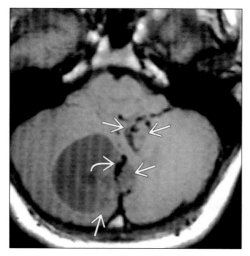

Axial T1WI MR shows two masses ➡ in the cerebellum with multiple curvilinear signal voids ➡, representing arteries, within them.

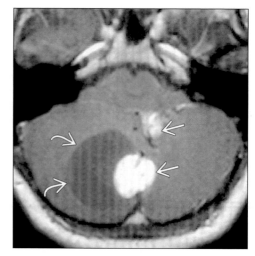

Axial T1 C+ MR shows that the masses are composed of a uniformly enhancing solid portion ➡. The larger mass, in the midline and right hemisphere, has a larger cystic component ➡.

## TERMINOLOGY

### Abbreviations and Synonyms
- von Hippel Lindau (VHL) syndrome (OMIM 19330)

### Definitions
- Autosomal dominant familial syndrome with hemangioblastomas (HGBLs), clear cell renal carcinoma, cystadenomas, pheochromocytomas
  - Affects six different organ systems, including eye, ear, central nervous system (CNS)
  - Involved tissues often have multiple lesions
  - Lesions ⇒ benign cysts, vascular tumors, carcinomas

## IMAGING FINDINGS

### General Features
- Best diagnostic clue: 2 or more CNS HGBL or 1 HGBL + retinal hemorrhage
- Location
  - HGBLs in VHL
    - Typically multiple
    - 50% in spinal cord (posterior half)

- 35-40% cerebellum
- 10% brainstem (posterior medulla)
- 1% supratentorial (along optic pathways, in cerebral hemispheres)
  - Ocular angiomas
    - Found in 75% of VHL gene carriers
    - Cause retinal detachment, hemorrhage
  - Cystadenoma of endolymphatic sac (ELS)
    - Large, located posterior to internal auditory canal
- Size: HGBLs vary from tiny mass to very large with even larger associated cysts
- Morphology: Symptomatic HGBLs more often cystic with mural nodule than solid

### CT Findings
- NECT
  - HGBL: 2/3 ⇒ well-delineated cerebellar cyst + nodule
    - Nodule typically abuts pial surface
    - 1/3 solid, without cyst
  - Cystadenoma of ELS ⇒ destructive changes in petrous bone
- CECT: Intense enhancement of tumor nodule

## DDx: Cerebellar Tumors Mimicking VHL

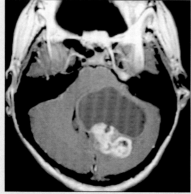

*Pilocytic Astrocytoma*

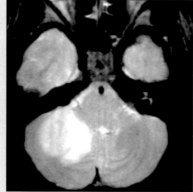

*Hemispheric Medulloblastoma*

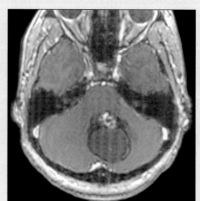

*Solitary Hemangioblastoma*

# VON HIPPEL LINDAU

## Key Facts

### Terminology
- Autosomal dominant familial syndrome with hemangioblastomas (HGBLs), clear cell renal carcinoma, cystadenomas, pheochromocytomas

### Imaging Findings
- Best diagnostic clue: 2 or more CNS HGBL or 1 HGBL + retinal hemorrhage
- Size: HGBLs vary from tiny mass to very large with even larger associated cysts

### Top Differential Diagnoses
- Solitary Hemangioblastoma
- Pilocytic Astrocytoma
- Hemispheric Medulloblastoma in Teen/Young Adult
- Multiple AVMs in Vascular Neurocutaneous Syndrome

### Pathology
- Etiology: Both alleles of VHL tumor suppressor gene on chromosome 3 inactivated

### Clinical Issues
- Earliest symptom in VHL often visual
- Phenotypes based on absence or presence of pheochromocytoma
- HGBLs ⇒ multiple periods of tumor growth (usually associated with increasing cyst size) separated by periods of arrested growth
- On average, new lesion develops every 2 years in VHL

### Diagnostic Checklist
- Solitary HGBL in a young patient may indicate VHL

## MR Findings
- T1WI
  - HGBL: Mixed iso ⇒ hypointense nodule, +/- "flow voids"
  - Associated cyst slightly hyperintense to cerebrospinal fluid (CSF)
  - Cystadenoma of ELS: Heterogeneous hyper/hypointense
- T2WI
  - HGBL: Hyperintense nodule, cyst
  - Cystadenoma of ELS: Hyperintense mass
- FLAIR
  - HGBL: Hyperintense cyst with variable edema
  - Cystadenoma of ELS: Hyperintense mass
- T2* GRE: HGBL: Blooms if hemorrhage present
- T1 C+
  - HGBL: Tumor nodule enhances strongly; cyst wall does not enhance
  - May detect tiny asymptomatic enhancing nodules
  - Cystadenoma of ELS: Heterogeneous enhancement

## Angiographic Findings
- Conventional
  - HGBL: DSA shows intensely vascular mass, prolonged stain
  - A-V shunting (early draining vein) common

## Imaging Recommendations
- Best imaging tool: Brain: MR without & with contrast
- Protocol advice: Scan entire brain and spine
- NIH recommendations
  - Contrast-enhanced MR of brain/spinal cord from age 11 years, every 2 years
  - US of abdomen from 11 years, yearly
  - Abdominal CT from 20 years, yearly or every other year
  - MR of temporal bone if hearing loss, tinnitus/vertigo

## DIFFERENTIAL DIAGNOSIS

### Solitary Hemangioblastoma
- 25-40% of HGBLs occur in VHL
- No VHL mutations, family history, other tumors or cysts

### Pilocytic Astrocytoma
- Usually younger than VHL patients
- No family history, lacks retinal angioma/hemorrhages
- Tumor nodule lacks vascular flow voids (more characteristic of HGBL)
- Tumor nodule often does not abut pial or ependymal surface

### Hemispheric Medulloblastoma in Teen/Young Adult
- Rare; occur in peripheral cerebellar hemisphere
- May appear extraparenchymal
- Solid, gray matter intensity on T2WI

### Multiple AVMs in Vascular Neurocutaneous Syndrome
- Osler-Weber-Rendu, Wyburn-Mason, etc.
- Small AVMs may resemble HGBL at angiography

## PATHOLOGY

### General Features
- General path comments
  - VHL characterized by development of
    - Capillary hemangioblastomas of the CNS and retina
    - ELS tumors
    - Cysts, renal clear cell carcinoma
    - Pancreatic cysts, islet cell tumors
    - Pheochromocytoma
    - Epididymal cysts, cystadenomas
- Genetics
  - Autosomal dominant inheritance with high penetrance, variable expression

# VON HIPPEL LINDAU

- ○ Germline mutations of VHL tumor suppressor gene
  - Chromosome 3p25-26
  - Involved in cell cycle regulation, angiogenesis
  - Disease features vary depending on specific VHL mutations
- Etiology: Both alleles of VHL tumor suppressor gene on chromosome 3 inactivated
- Epidemiology: 1:35-50,000

## Gross Pathologic & Surgical Features
- HGBL seen as well-circumscribed, very vascular, reddish nodule
  - ○ 75% at least partially cystic, contain amber-colored fluid

## Microscopic Features
- Two components in HGBL
  - ○ Rich capillary network
  - ○ Large vacuolated stromal cells with clear cytoplasm

## Staging, Grading or Classification Criteria
- Capillary hemangioblastoma: WHO grade I

## CLINICAL ISSUES

### Presentation
- Most common signs/symptoms
  - ○ VHL is clinically very heterogeneous; phenotypic penetrance: 97% at 65 years
  - ○ Retinal angiomas
    - Earliest symptom in VHL often visual
    - Retinal detachment, vitreous hemorrhages
  - ○ Cerebellar HGBLs
    - Headache (obstructive hydrocephalus)
    - Nearly 75% of symptom-producing tumors have associated cyst
  - ○ Spinal cord HGBLs
    - Progressive myelopathy
    - 95% associated syrinx
- Clinical Profile
  - ○ Phenotypes based on absence or presence of pheochromocytoma
    - Type 1: Without pheochromocytoma
    - Type 2A: With both pheochromocytoma, renal cell carcinoma
    - Type 2B: With pheochromocytoma, without renal cell carcinoma
  - ○ Diagnosis of VHL: Capillary hemangioblastoma in CNS/retina and one of typical VHL-associated tumors or previous family history

### Demographics
- Age
  - ○ VHL presents in young adults; uncommon in children
    - Retinal angioma: Mean age: 25 years
    - Cerebellar: Mean age: 30 years
  - ○ Mean age of presentation with other VHL-associated tumors
    - Pheochromocytoma (30 years)
    - Renal carcinoma (33 years)
    - Endolymphatic sac tumor
- Gender: M = F

## Natural History & Prognosis
- Renal carcinoma proximal cause of death in 15-50%
- HGBLs ⇒ multiple periods of tumor growth (usually associated with increasing cyst size) separated by periods of arrested growth
- On average, new lesion develops every 2 years in VHL

## Treatment
- Ophthalmoscopy yearly from infancy
- Physical/neurological examination, from 2 years, then yearly
- Surgical resection of symptomatic cerebellar/spinal hemangioblastoma
- Stereotactic radiosurgery may control smaller lesions
- Laser treatment of retinal angiomata

## DIAGNOSTIC CHECKLIST

### Consider
- Follow NIH screening rules
- Look for ELS tumors in VHL patients with dysequilibrium, hearing loss or aural fullness

### Image Interpretation Pearls
- Solitary HGBL in a young patient may indicate VHL

## SELECTED REFERENCES

1. Choo D et al: Endolymphatic sac tumors in von Hippel-Lindau disease. J Neurosurg 100:480-7, 2004
2. Wanebo JE et al: The natural history of hemangioblastomas of the central nervous system in patients with von Hippel-Lindau disease. J Neurosurg. 98(1):82-94, 2003
3. Weil RJ et al: Surgical management of brainstem hemangioblastomas in patients with von Hippel-Lindau disease. J Neurosurg. 98(1):95-105, 2003
4. Weil RJ et al: Clinical and molecular analysis of disseminated hemangioblastomatosis of the central nervous system in patients without von Hippel-Lindau disease. Report of four cases. J Neurosurg. 96(4):775-87, 2002
5. Allen RC et al: Molecular characterization and ophthalmic investigation of a large family with type 2A Von Hippel-Lindau Disease. Arch Ophthalmol. 119(11):1659-65, 2001
6. Conway JE et al: Hemangioblastomas of the central nervous system in von Hippel-Lindau syndrome and sporadic disease. Neurosurg 48:55-63, 2001
7. Friedrich CA: Genotype-phenotype correlation in von Hippel-Lindau syndrome. Hum Mol Genet. 10(7):763-7, 2001
8. Sims KB: Von Hippel-Lindau disease: gene to bedside. Curr Opin Neurol. 14(6):695-703, 2001
9. Sora S et al: Incidence of von Hippel-Lindau disease in hemangioblastoma patients: the University of Tokyo Hospital experience from 1954-1998. Acta Neurochir (Wien). 143(9):893-6, 2001
10. Bohling T et al: Von Hippel-Lindau disease and capillary hemangioblastoma. In Kleihues P, Cavanee WK (eds): Tumours of the Central Nervous System, 223-6, IARC Press, 2000
11. North PE et al: GLUT1 immunoreaction patterns reliably distinguish hemangioblastoma from metastatic renal cell carcinoma. Clin Neuropathol. 19(3):131-7, 2000

# VON HIPPEL LINDAU

## IMAGE GALLERY

### Typical

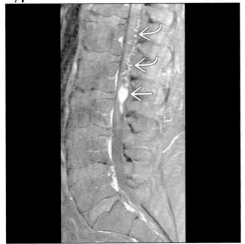 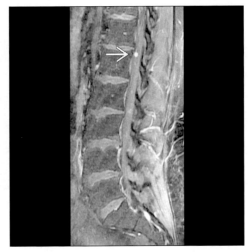

*(Left)* Sagittal T1 C+ FS MR shows an enhancing mass ➡ at the level of the L2-L3 intervertebral disc, representing a hemangioblastoma. Note the multiple enlarged, enhancing veins ➡ coursing rostrally. *(Right)* Sagittal T1 C+ FS MR shows an adjacent parasagittal image (same patient as previous image) with a second, smaller, hemangioblastoma ➡ at the level of the L1 vertebral body.

### Typical

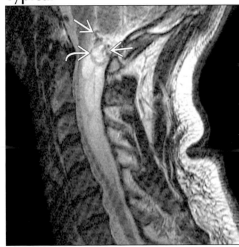 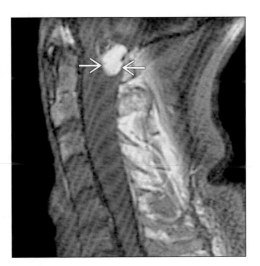

*(Left)* Sagittal T2WI MR shows an ovoid hyperintense mass ➡ with multiple curvilinear flow voids ➡ surrounding it at the dorsal cervicomedullary junction. Syrinx is developing below tumor. *(Right)* Sagittal T1 C+ MR shows that the mass ➡ uniformly and intensely enhances after administration of paramagnetic contrast. The developing syrinx is hypointense.

### Typical

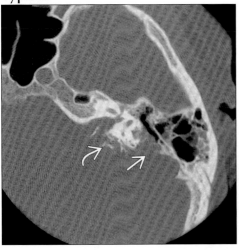 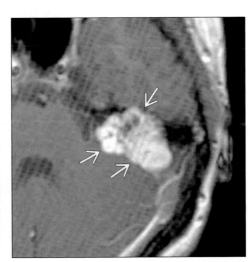

*(Left)* Axial NECT shows erosive changes ➡ involving the posteromedial aspect of the petrous pyramid, including spicules of bone ➡. These are centered in the region of the endolymphatic sac. *(Right)* Axial T1 C+ MR (same patient as previous image) shows a large enhancing mass ➡ that is centered in the region of the endolymphatic sac, and was an endolymphatic sac cystadenoma at surgery.

# BASAL CELL NEVUS SYNDROME

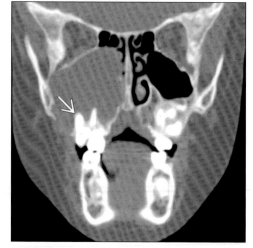

Axial NECT shows a large unilocular odontogenic keratocyst filling the right maxillary sinus. An unerupted tooth ➡ is evident posteriorly. The sinus walls ➡ are eroded.

Coronal NECT (reformatted images) in the same patient as previous image shows the root of a molar tooth ➡ within the wall of the mass. The mass distorts the nasal cavity and the floor of the orbit.

## TERMINOLOGY

### Abbreviations and Synonyms
- Basal cell nevus syndrome (BCNS), Nevoid basal cell carcinoma syndrome (NBCCS), Gorlin syndrome, Gorlin-Goltz syndrome

### Definitions
- BCNS: Hereditary tumor syndrome characterized by multiple basal cell epitheliomas (BCE)/basal cell carcinomas (BCC), odontogenic keratocysts, palmoplantar pits, dural Ca++, +/- medulloblastoma

## IMAGING FINDINGS

### General Features
- Best diagnostic clue
  - Multiple jaw cysts, prominent dural Ca++, macrocephaly
  - Other skeletal features: Hyperaerated paranasal sinuses, splayed/fused/bifid ribs, kyphoscoliosis, platybasia, Sprengel deformity of scapulae
- Location
  - Cysts: Mandible, maxilla
  - Ca++: Intracranial dura
- Size: Variable enlargement of mandible, maxilla

### CT Findings
- NECT
  - Odontogenic keratocysts (OKC) in 80-90%
    - Large, uni- or multilocular sharply marginated cysts, containing unerupted teeth
    - Mandible > maxilla
  - Early Ca++ of falx cerebri, tentorium, peri-clinoid ligaments (dural bridging), dura, pia, choroid plexus & basal ganglia
  - +/- Ventriculomegaly
  - +/- Callosal dysgenesis
  - Cysts of all kinds common
- CECT
  - Look for
    - Desmoplastic medulloblastoma
    - Meningioma
    - Colloid cyst

### MR Findings
- T1WI
  - Macrocephaly with increased cranio-facial ratio

## DDx: Mandibular/Maxillary Masses

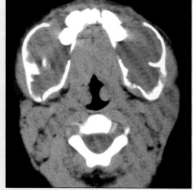

Cherubism

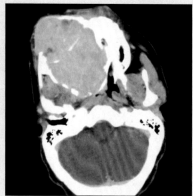

Giant Cell Granuloma

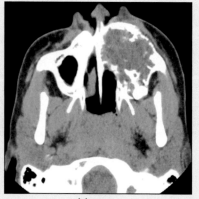

Myxoma

# BASAL CELL NEVUS SYNDROME

## Key Facts

### Terminology

- Basal cell nevus syndrome (BCNS), Nevoid basal cell carcinoma syndrome (NBCCS), Gorlin syndrome, Gorlin-Goltz syndrome
- BCNS: Hereditary tumor syndrome characterized by multiple basal cell epitheliomas (BCE)/basal cell carcinomas (BCC), odontogenic keratocysts, palmoplantar pits, dural Ca++, +/- medulloblastoma

### Imaging Findings

- Multiple jaw cysts, prominent dural Ca++, macrocephaly
- Odontogenic keratocysts (OKC) in 80-90%
- Large, uni- or multilocular sharply marginated cysts, containing unerupted teeth

- Early Ca++ of falx cerebri, tentorium, peri-clinoid ligaments (dural bridging), dura, pia, choroid plexus & basal ganglia

### Top Differential Diagnoses

- Ameloblastoma
- Dentigerous Cyst
- Cherubism
- Aneurysmal Bone Cyst
- Giant Reparative Granuloma
- Odontogenic Myxoma

### Clinical Issues

- Usually diagnosed during the 1st decade of life

---

- ○ OKC are hypointense to isointense, contain a hypointensity representing the unerupted tooth
- ○ Dural Ca++ difficult to observe on MR
- T2WI: OKC are hyperintense, contain a hypointensity representing the unerupted tooth
- T1 C+
  - ○ Cysts may show thin peripheral enhancing rim
  - ○ Look for perineural spread of head and neck BCC using fat-saturated images

## Radiographic Findings

- Radiography
  - ○ Diffuse, tiny, lytic (kerato) cysts of bones (35%), especially jaws
  - ○ Other
    - ▪ Thick calvarium with platybasia
    - ▪ Rib anomalies (bifid ribs; splayed, fused or misshapen)
    - ▪ Short 4th metacarpals
    - ▪ Spina bifida occulta; vertebral segmentation anomalies

## Nuclear Medicine Findings

- Bone Scan: May show ↑ uptake

## Imaging Recommendations

- Best imaging tool
  - ○ MR to screen for medulloblastoma, cystic jaw lesions
  - ○ CT of face for oral surgery planning
- Protocol advice
  - ○ Low mA 2-3 mm axial CT of the face including mandible, coronal reformats
  - ○ Fat-saturated T2's and T1 C+ to diagnose jaw cysts, perineural BCC spread

## DIFFERENTIAL DIAGNOSIS

### Ameloblastoma

- Bubbly-appearing, solitary lesion may contain unerupted tooth
- When large, associated enhancing soft tissue mass nearly always present

- May have enhancing solid mural nodule

### Dentigerous Cyst

- Unilocular cyst surrounding tooth crown
- No enhancing intra- or extra-cyst soft tissue

### Cherubism

- Symmetrical cystic fibrous dysplasia of mandible

### Aneurysmal Bone Cyst

- Multilocular, multi-septated mass in mandible
- Enhancing soft tissues inside and outside of bony rim

### Giant Reparative Granuloma

- Solitary mass, generally solid, does not contain unerupted tooth

### Odontogenic Myxoma

- Radiolucent areas with bony trabeculations
- Well or poorly defined margins, aggressive growth. Benign histology

### Miscellaneous Maxillary Masses

- Maxillary sinus mucocele: Contains no cyst or septae, smooth expansion of sinus walls
- Incisor canal cyst: Found in midline anterior maxilla, posterior to incisors, water density/intensity, small
- Globulomaxillary cyst: Located between lateral incisor and canine, small

## PATHOLOGY

### General Features

- General path comments
  - ○ 3x more common in mandible than in maxilla
    - ▪ Mainly in premolar and retromolar triangle area
  - ○ Usually, multiple, small or large, unilocular or multilocular
  - ○ May cross the midline
- Genetics
  - ○ Autosomal dominant: Complete penetrance, variable expression
  - ○ New mutations ↑ with advanced paternal age

# BASAL CELL NEVUS SYNDROME

- o Mutation inactivated tumor suppressor genes PTCH1&2 (9q22.3-q31)
- Etiology: The PATCHED (PTCH) gene encodes a Sonic hedgehog (SHH) receptor and a tumor suppressor protein that is defective in BCNS
- Epidemiology
  - o 1 in 57,000 (1 in 200 with BCC have syndrome, 1 in 5 if < 19 yrs)
  - o Most BCNS have OKC; 5% of patients with OKC have BCNS
- Associated abnormalities
  - o Associated neoplasms (mutation inactivated tumor suppressor genes)
    - ▪ Rare ameloblastoma & squamous cell cancer
    - ▪ Desmoplastic medulloblastoma: Seen in 4-20% (1-2% medulloblastoma have BCNS)
    - ▪ Cardiac, abdominal and pelvic mesenchymal tumors

## Gross Pathologic & Surgical Features
- OKC: Expansile mandible and/or maxillary cysts with unerupted tooth
  - o Satellite cyst formation is common; may involve coronoid process
  - o Maxillary canine/premolar area > retromolar

## Microscopic Features
- OKC: Parakeratinized lining and ↑ epithelial growth factor receptor

## Staging, Grading or Classification Criteria
- Need 2 major or 1 major and 2 minor criteria for diagnosis
- Major criteria: > 2 (or 1 under 30 yrs) basal cell carcinomas; > 10 basal cell nevi; odontogenic keratocyst or polyostotic bone cyst; ≥ 3 palmar/plantar pits; lamellar or (under 20 yrs) falx Ca++; family history
- Minor criteria: Rib or vertebral anomalies, macrocrania/frontal bossing; cardiac or ovarian fibromas; mesenteric cysts; facial clefting (5-13%), hand (long fingers, short 4th metacarpal, polydactyly) or ocular anomalies

# CLINICAL ISSUES

## Presentation
- Most common signs/symptoms: Jaw and maxilla deformity with pain
- Clinical Profile: Desmoplastic medulloblastoma in boys 2 years and younger (before syndrome apparent), beware, irradiation induced ↑↑ number BCC
- BCE (75%) onset puberty, resemble nevi or skin tags; BCC by 40 years
- Skin (other): Epidermal (kerato) cysts (55%), milia, fibromas, lipomas
- Palmar and plantar pits (> 85%): Usually noticed after childhood
- Multiple OKC that may fracture or become infected
- Dysmorphic facies; large head/large brow, everted mandibular angle, hypertelorism, lip clefts common, macrosomia, tall stature

- Cognition normal if no malformations/tumors and no prior irradiation

## Demographics
- Age
  - o Usually diagnosed during the 1st decade of life
    - ▪ OKC usually form before 7 years of age
- Gender: No predilection
- Ethnicity: No predilection

## Natural History & Prognosis
- Develop enormous numbers BCCs
  - o Especially fair skin, sun exposure, irradiation
  - o Darkly pigmented skin protective, has smaller numbers BCC

## Treatment
- Options, risks, complications: After surgery, recurrence is very high (up to 60%)
- Skin lesions: Lifelong monitoring; topical tretinoin/5-fluorouracil, photodynamic therapy; early surgical removal
- Surgery/chemotherapy, avoid radiotherapy for medulloblastoma

# DIAGNOSTIC CHECKLIST

## Consider
- BCNS when precocious dural Ca++ and OKC are detected

## Image Interpretation Pearls
- Multiple mandibular cysts containing teeth or parts of teeth

# SELECTED REFERENCES

1. Kimonis VE et al: Radiological features in 82 patients with nevoid basal cell carcinoma (NBCC or Gorlin) syndrome. Genet Med. 6(6):495-502, 2004
2. Kahn JL et al: [Imaging of mandibular malformations and deformities] J Radiol. 84(9):975-81, 2003
3. Ozturk A et al: Neuroradiological findings in a mother and daughter with Gorlin syndrome. Clin Dysmorphol. 12(2):145-6, 2003
4. Leonardi R et al: Bilateral hyperplasia of the mandibular coronoid processes in patients with nevoid basal cell carcinoma syndrome: an undescribed sign. Am J Med Genet 110:400-403. Am J Med Genet. 120A(3):446, 2002
5. Rozylo-Kalinowska I et al: Odontogenic keratocyst in Gorlin-Goltz syndrome. Ann Univ Mariae Curie Sklodowska [Med]. 57(2):79-85, 2002
6. Stavrou T et al: Intracranial calcifications in childhood medulloblastoma: relation to nevoid basal cell carcinoma syndrome. AJNR Am J Neuroradiol. 21(4):790-4, 2000
7. Iwanaga S et al: Gorlin syndrome: unusual manifestations in the sella turcica and the sphenoidal sinus. AJNR. 19:956-8, 1998
8. Wicking C et al: De novo mutations of the PATCHED gene in nevoid BCC syndrome help to define the clinical phenotype. Am J Med Genet. 73(3):304-7, 1997
9. Mosskin M et al: Nevoid basal cell carcinoma syndrome. Int J Neuroradiol. 2(5):480-8, 1996

# BASAL CELL NEVUS SYNDROME

## IMAGE GALLERY

Typical

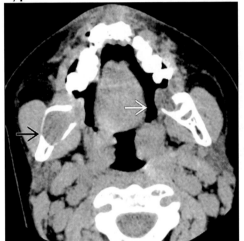
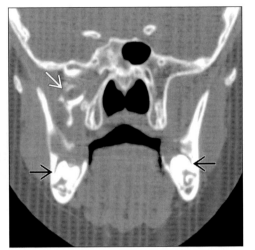

*(Left)* Axial NECT shows a small well marginated mass ➡ in the right posterior mandible. A smaller lesion ➡ is seen in the left posterior mandible. *(Right)* Coronal NECT in the same patient as previous image shows the unerupted teeth ➡ at the base of the mandibular odontogenic cysts. A maxillary tooth ➡ with a cyst is evident in the right maxilla.

Typical

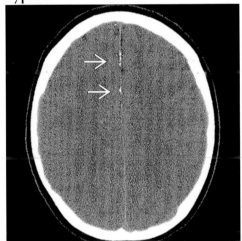
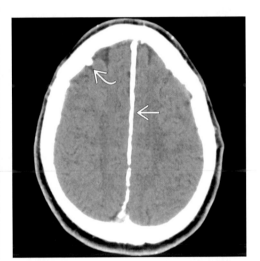

*(Left)* Axial NECT shows early, small calcifications of the falx cerebri ➡ in a 10 year old boy. Dural calcifications are seen in childhood in Gorlin syndrome. *(Right)* Axial NECT shows more extensive falcine calcification ➡ in an older patient. Calcification of the dura over the convexities ➡ is also present.

Typical

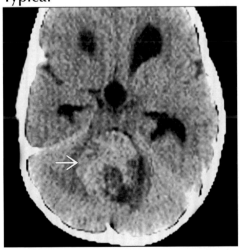
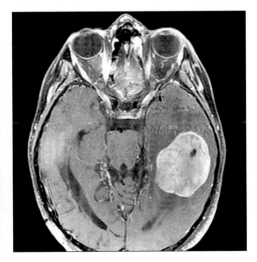

*(Left)* Axial NECT shows a hyperdense heterogeneous mass ➡ in the 4th ventricle and midline cerebellum, typical of medulloblastoma. Ventricles are enlarged from obstructive hydrocephalus. *(Right)* Axial T1WI FS MR shows an enhancing mass in the left middle cranial fossa/temporal lobe. A meningioma was resected in this adolescent previously irradiated for a medulloblastoma.

I
8
25

# HHT

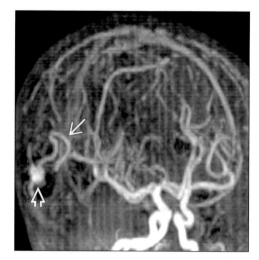

Coronal angiography by selective catheterization of bronchial arteries shows pulmonary AVM → with early venous return →. Pulmonary AVMs are a common feature of HHT in children.

Sagittal oblique MRA (same patient as previous image) shows posterior tangle of vessels ⇒ with dilated feeding artery → indicating associated brain AVM, an uncommon finding in children with HHT.

## TERMINOLOGY

### Abbreviations and Synonyms
- Hereditary hemorrhagic telangiectasia (HHT); Rendu-Osler-Weber syndrome (ROW)

### Definitions
- Autosomal dominant disorder with widely distributed, multisystem angiodysplastic lesions
  - Mucocutaneous, visceral telangiectasias
  - Arteriovenous malformations/fistulae (AVM/AVF) of lungs, brain, GI tract, liver

## IMAGING FINDINGS

### General Features
- Best diagnostic clue: Multiple pulmonary (pAVM) or cerebral (cAVM) AVM in patient with recurrent epistaxis
- Location
  - Capillary telangiectasias in scalp, nasopharynx, orbit
  - Intracranial vascular malformations may occur anywhere; less common in children
- Size: cAVMs in HHT are usually small, often incidental
- Morphology: Mottled, purplish skin, scalp, mucosal lesions

### CT Findings
- CTA: May demonstrate visceral, CNS high-flow AVMs, AVFs
- NECT
  - Brain: AVM = isodense serpentine vessels; abscess = low density with iso- to hyperdense rim
  - Lung: Well-delineated vascular mass(es) on high-resolution **noncontrast** multislice CT, usually in lower lobes
- CECT
  - Brain: Strong, uniform, well-delineated enhancement of cAVMs; ring-enhancement of abscesses (late cerebritis, early capsule stage)
    - Developmental venous anomalies (DVA) not rare (8%)
  - Liver: Multi-detector contrast-enhanced CT demonstrates abnormalities in 75% of HHT patients
    - Arterioportal, arteriosystemic shunts (100%)
    - Intraparenchymal telangiectases (60-65%)
    - Large confluent vascular masses (25%)

## DDx: Other Multiple Vascular Malformations

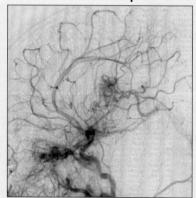

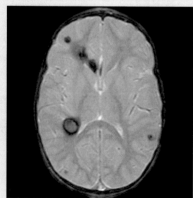

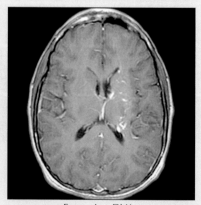

*Wyburn-Mason*  *Multiple Cavernomas*  *Extensive DVAs*

# HHT

## Terminology
- Hereditary hemorrhagic telangiectasia (HHT); Rendu-Osler-Weber syndrome (ROW)
- Autosomal dominant disorder with widely distributed, multisystem angiodysplastic lesions

## Imaging Findings
- Best diagnostic clue: Multiple pulmonary (pAVM) or cerebral (cAVM) AVM in patient with recurrent epistaxis
- Capillary telangiectasias in scalp, nasopharynx, orbit
- Intracranial vascular malformations may occur anywhere; less common in children
- Liver: Multi-detector contrast-enhanced CT demonstrates abnormalities in 75% of HHT patients

- Baseline screening of brain in all patients with HHT highly recommended (cAVMs can have devastating neurologic sequelae)

## Top Differential Diagnoses
- Nasal Mucosal "Blush"
- Multiple Intracranial AVMs without HHT

## Pathology
- Autosomal dominant; four known mutations, all affecting the transforming growth factor β (TGF-β) transduction pathway

## Clinical Issues
- Epistaxis typically begins by age 10, most HHT patients are symptomatic by age 21 years

## MR Findings
- T1WI: cAVM: "Flow voids" common, ± hemorrhage; telangiectasias typically not visualized
- T2WI: cAVM: "Flow voids", without/with hemorrhage, mass effect, edema, gliosis
- FLAIR: Nest of flow voids, adjacent brain changes
- T2* GRE: Useful in detecting micro-hemorrhages; may show flow in cAVMs; capillary telangiectasias become mildly hypointense
- T1 C+: AVMs, DVAs, slow-flow vascular telangiectasias enhance
- MRA: Demonstrates intermediate to large cAVMs; small AVMs may not be visualized without contrast-enhanced MRA
- MRV: May demonstrate DVAs

## Angiographic Findings
- Conventional
  - Demonstrates vascular malformations in the brain (AVM, AVF, DVA), as well as on the nasopharyngeal mucosa
  - AVMs in HHT can be micro-, small, or macro-AVM, but only 10-12% are > 10 mm

## Imaging Recommendations
- Best imaging tool
  - Brain: MR with contrast
    - Baseline screening of brain in all patients with HHT highly recommended (cAVMs can have devastating neurologic sequelae)
  - Lungs, liver: Multislice CT/CTA
- Protocol advice: Brain: Contrast, T2* GRE, MRA

## DIFFERENTIAL DIAGNOSIS

### Nasal Mucosal "Blush"
- Prominent but normal nasal mucosal blush can mimic capillary telangiectasia

### Multiple Intracranial AVMs without HHT
- Rare in absence of vascular neurocutaneous syndrome

- 50% of the cases associated with other disorders (Wyburn-Mason, etc.)

### Multiple Intracranial DVAs
- Association with HHT less common than with blue rubber bleb nevus syndrome

### Multiple Capillary Telangiectasias
- Can be found incidentally without HHT
- Capillary telangiectasias in HHT much more common outside the brain than in it!

### Multiple Cavernous Malformations
- Typically uncommon in HHT

## PATHOLOGY

### General Features
- General path comments: Abnormalities of vascular structures account for all recognized phenotypic manifestations of HHT
- Genetics
  - Autosomal dominant; four known mutations, all affecting the transforming growth factor β (TGF-β) transduction pathway
    - HHT1: Endoglin gene mutation (9q34.1): Telangiectasias, early onset of epistaxis; pAVMs
    - HHT2: Activin receptor like kinase 1 (ALK-1) gene mutation (12q11-q14): Lower penetrance, milder disease, gastrointestinal bleeds
    - HHT3: Unidentified gene mutation on 5q31.3-q32
    - JP/HHT: MADH4 gene mutation on 18q21.1 (predisposition to gastrointestinal malignancy but also involved in TGF-β signaling pathway); families associate features of HHT with colon polyp/cancer
  - AVMs, AVFs appear in certain forms of HHT only
- Etiology: Abnormalities of TGF-β transduction pathway affect vasculogenesis, angiogenesis, and properties of endothelial cells
- Epidemiology: Rare: 1-2/10,000
- Associated abnormalities

# HHT

- 70% of patients with pAVMs have HHT
- > 50% of patients with multiple cAVMs have HHT
- 5-15% of patients with HHT have pAVMs
- 5-13% of patients with HHT have cAVMs
- 2-17% have hepatic AVMs (depends on kindred)

## Gross Pathologic & Surgical Features

- Multiple telangiectasias of mucosa, dermis, viscera
- Most pAVMs are actually AVFs (direct connection between pulmonary artery and vein through thin-walled aneurysm)
- Hepatic AV shunts less common, often numerous

## Microscopic Features

- Smallest telangiectasias are focal dilatations of post-capillary venules that enlarge and extend through capillaries toward arterioles, resulting in direct AVF/AVM

## Staging, Grading or Classification Criteria

- Most cAVMs are of low grade (Spetzler-Martin I or II)

## CLINICAL ISSUES

### Presentation

- Most common signs/symptoms: Recurrent epistaxis from nasal mucosal telangiectasias; can be severe, exsanguinating
- Other signs/symptoms
  - Telangiectasias lips, mouth, tongue, fingers, around nails
  - Gastrointestinal bleeding
- Clinical Profile
  - HHT diagnosis based on combination of findings
    - Mucocutaneous telangiectasias
    - Spontaneous/recurrent episodes of epistaxis
    - Visceral AVMs (lungs, brain, liver)
    - Family history
- Neurologic symptoms common
  - Intracranial bleed from cAVM; TIA/stroke/abscess complicate pulmonary AVMs
- Pulmonary AVMs cause
  - R/L shunts
  - Dyspnea, cyanosis, fatigue
  - Polycythemia
  - Serious complication = cerebral emboli/abscess

### Demographics

- Age
  - Epistaxis typically begins by age 10, most HHT patients are symptomatic by age 21 years
  - Skin lesions appear later (most by 40 years)
- Gender: M = F

### Natural History & Prognosis

- Epistaxis increases in frequency, severity
- cAVMs in HHT have lower bleeding risk than sporadic AVMs; rare cases may regress spontaneously
- Significant lifetime risk of brain abscess or stroke if pAVM present
- Heart failure: Poor prognosis in patients with hepatic AVM
- Gastrointestinal bleeding limits lifespan when under age 50; many require multiple transfusions and endoscopies

### Treatment

- PAVMs: Surgery no longer indicated, excellent results of embolization
- CAVMs: Embolization and radiosurgery, depending on size, location
- Mucosal telangiectasias (nose, GI tract): Laser coagulation
- Prophylactic antibiotics prior to all dental work if pAVM present
- IV iron administration if oral iron fails to maintain satisfactory level

## DIAGNOSTIC CHECKLIST

### Consider

- Screening family members with brain MR

### Image Interpretation Pearls

- cAVM, not capillary telangiectasia is the most common intracranial vascular malformation in HHT patients
- Brain ischemia and abscess are uncommon but a serious risk in HHT patients with pAVMs

## SELECTED REFERENCES

1. Ianora AA et al: Hereditary hemorrhagic telangiectasia: multi-detector row helical CT assessment of hepatic involvement. Radiology. 230(1):250-9, 2004
2. Abdalla SA et al: Visceral manifestations in hereditary haemorrhagic telangiectasia type 2. J Med Genet. 40(7):494-502, 2003
3. Berg J et al: Hereditary haemorrhagic telangiectasia: a questionnaire based study to delineate the different phenotypes caused by endoglin and ALK1 mutations. J Med Genet. 40(8):585-90, 2003
4. Kuwayama K et al: Central nervous system lesions associated with hereditary hemorrhagic telangiectasia--three case reports. Neurol Med Chir (Tokyo). 43(9):447-51, 2003
5. Larson AM: Liver disease in hereditary hemorrhagic telangiectasia. J Clin Gastroenterol. 36(2):149-58, 2003
6. Marchuk DA et al: Vascular morphogenesis: tales of two syndromes. Hum Mol Genet. 12 Spec No 1:R97-112, 2003
7. Sabba C et al: Hereditary hemorrhagic teleangiectasia (Rendu-Osler-Weber disease). Minerva Cardioangiol. 50(3):221-38, 2002
8. Shah RK et al: Hereditary hemorrhagic telangiectasia: a review of 76 cases. Laryngoscope. 112(5):767-73, 2002
9. Arnold SM et al: Acute hepatic encephalopathy with diffuse cortical lesions. Neuroradiology. 43(7):551-4, 2001
10. Byard RW et al: Osler-Weber-Rendu syndrome--pathological manifestations and autopsy considerations. J Forensic Sci. 46(3):698-701, 2001
11. Dong SL et al: Brain abscess in patients with hereditary hemorrhagic telangiectasia: case report and literature review. J Emerg Med. 20(3):247-51, 2001
12. Willemse RB et al: Bleeding risk of cerebrovascular malformations in hereditary hemorrhagic telangiectasia. J Neurosurg. 92(5):779-84, 2000

## IMAGE GALLERY

### Typical

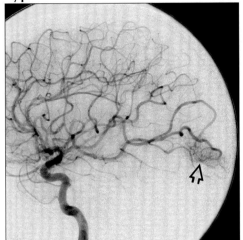

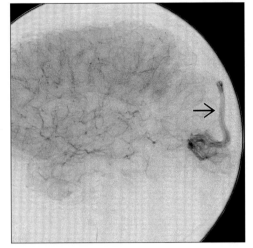

*(Left)* Lateral angiography shows faintly opacified occipital telangiectatic network ⊳ fed by posterior branch of temporo-occipital artery. Study requested to evaluate bleeding risk of lesion. *(Right)* Lateral angiography shows early filling vein → indicating behavior like an AVM, with significant risk of bleeding. Such lesion are typically found in adolescent/young adult.

### Typical

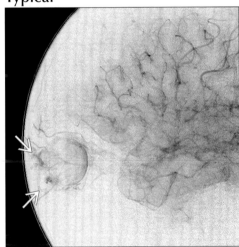

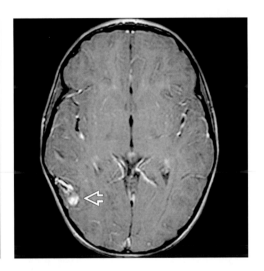

*(Left)* Lateral angiography shows multiple mucosal telangiectasias → in the territory of ethmoidal branches of ICA, indicating significant risk of massive epistaxis. *(Right)* Axial T1 C+ MR shows cavernous pouch of blood in posterior right temporal region ⊳. This is the location of the telangiectatic network demonstrated at conventional angiography.

### Typical

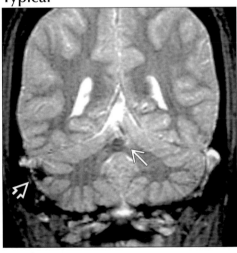

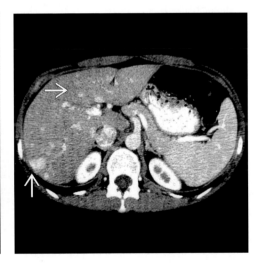

*(Left)* Coronal T2* GRE MR shows cavernoma-like telangiectasia ⊳ with hemosiderin deposit in lateral right cerebellum in another child with HHT. Note similar, fainter abnormality in vermis →. *(Right)* Axial CECT shows multiples angiomas disseminated across the liver → in still another child with HHT. (Courtesy A. Burdette, MD).

I

8

29

# ENCEPHALOCRANIOCUTANEOUS LIPOMATOSIS

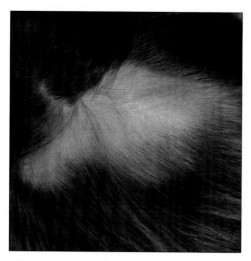

*Clinical photograph shows "nevus psiloliparus", the hallmark of encephalocraniocutaneous lipomatosis (ECCL). A well-circumscribed area of alopecia overlies a scalp lipoma.*

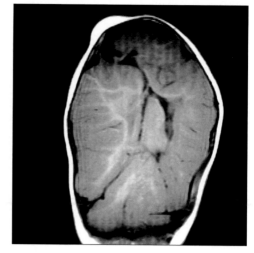

*Coronal T1WI MR shows a right scalp lipoma and CNS dysgenesis in this patient with nevus psiloliparus. Although both hemispheres are abnormal, the right is mildly atrophic compared to left.*

## TERMINOLOGY

### Abbreviations and Synonyms
- Encephalocraniocutaneous lipomatosis (ECCL)
- Haberland syndrome, Fishman syndrome

### Definitions
- Rare congenital neurocutaneous syndrome characterized by ipsilateral scalp, eye and brain abnormalities
- First described in 1970 by Catherine Haberland

## IMAGING FINDINGS

### General Features
- Best diagnostic clue
  - Unilateral cerebral hemispheric atrophy ipsilateral to scalp lipoma
  - Other frequent ipsilateral CNS abnormalities
    - Middle cranial fossa arachnoid cyst
    - Cortical dysplasia
    - Cortical Ca⁺⁺
  - Intracranial (IC) lipomas occur inconsistently

- Spinal lipomas in 15%; cervicothoracic > lumbar
  - Rarely, CNS abnormalities limited to IC lipoma
- Location
  - IC lipomas
    - CP angle, Meckel cave, foramen magnum
    - Usually ipsilateral to scalp lipoma; occasionally contra- or bilateral
  - All other CNS anomalies ipsilateral to scalp lipoma
- Morphology: Focal occipital lobe atrophy and occipital horn enlargement characteristic

### CT Findings
- CTA: Arterial ectasias, pouches, and aneurysms described in older patients
- NECT
  - Hemispheric atrophy, ventriculomegaly
    - Ventriculomegaly primarily due to volume loss although hydrocephalus occasionally present
  - Low density scalp lipoma (may be difficult to identify, particularly if at vertex)
  - ± Cortical Ca⁺⁺
    - Identified as early as first month of life, progressive
  - ± Focal calvarial enlargement

8

30

## DDx: Neurocutaneous Syndromes with Unilateral Hemispheric Abnormalities

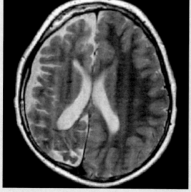

*Sturge-Weber*

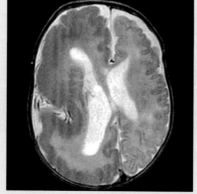

*Epidermal Nevus*

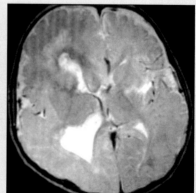

*Proteus*

# ENCEPHALOCRANIOCUTANEOUS LIPOMATOSIS

## Key Facts

### Terminology
- Rare congenital neurocutaneous syndrome characterized by ipsilateral scalp, eye and brain abnormalities

### Imaging Findings
- Unilateral cerebral hemispheric atrophy ipsilateral to scalp lipoma
- Intracranial (IC) lipomas occur inconsistently

### Top Differential Diagnoses
- Sturge-Weber Syndrome (SWS)
- Oculocerebrocutaneous Syndrome (OCCS)
- Epidermal Nevus Syndrome (ENS)
- Proteus Syndrome

### Pathology
- Epidemiology: Rare; ~ 40 reported cases (likely under-reported)

### Clinical Issues
- Nevus psiloliparus: Sharply demarcated focus of scalp alopecia overlying scalp lipoma
- Hallmark of ECCL
- Newborn with nevus psiloliparus, scleral mass, and periocular papules
- Majority with variable degrees of psychomotor impairment and dependency

### Diagnostic Checklist
- Considerable imaging overlap with SWS ⇒ search for scalp lipoma

---

- ▪ Usually underlies scalp lipoma
- CECT: ± Diffuse, ipsilateral leptomeningeal (LM) enhancement

### MR Findings
- T1WI
  - ○ Scalp/intracranial lipomas
  - ○ Polymicrogyria of temporal, parietal, and/or occipital lobes
  - ○ Scleral choristoma occasionally visible: Heterogeneous with focal areas of hyperintensity
- T2WI
  - ○ Cortical Ca++ hypointense
  - ○ Lipomas hyperintense on FSE T2
  - ○ Arachnoid cysts isointense to CSF
- FLAIR: Nulling of signal from arachnoid cyst
- T2* GRE: Blooming of cortical Ca++
- DWI: Arachnoid cyst isointense to CSF
- T1 C+: ± Diffuse, ipsilateral leptomeningeal enhancement
- MRA: Arterial ectasias, pouches, and aneurysms described in older patients

### Ultrasonographic Findings
- Prenatal US: Ventriculomegaly reported on 3rd trimester US

### Angiographic Findings
- Conventional: Arterial ectasias, pouches, and aneurysms described in older patients

### Imaging Recommendations
- Best imaging tool: Contrast-enhanced MR
- Protocol advice
  - ○ Multiplanar MR with fat-saturation for identification of scalp lipoma (may be missed on CT)
  - ○ MRA may disclose vascular abnormalities

## DIFFERENTIAL DIAGNOSIS

### Sturge-Weber Syndrome (SWS)
- Unilateral hemispheric cerebral atrophy, cortical Ca++, LM enhancement ipsilateral to forehead port wine nevus
  - ○ CNS findings frequently posterior

### Oculocerebrocutaneous Syndrome (OCCS)
- Characterized by unique cutaneous striated muscle hamartoma, cystic microphthalmia, and giant tectum absent vermis malformation
- Cortical dysplasia, agnesis of the corpus callosum, and Dandy Walker malformation frequently present
- Cutaneous, eye, and CNS anomalies usually ipsilateral but less consistently than ECCL

### Epidermal Nevus Syndrome (ENS)
- Ipsilateral epidermal nevus, hemimeganencephaly, facial lipoma, and hemi-hypertrophy
- Occasional scleral choristoma

### Proteus Syndrome
- Progressive asymmetric, bilateral trunk/limb hypertrophy
- Osteomas, lipomas, and pigmented nevi common
- CNS anomalies uncommon; hemimeganencephaly most common

## PATHOLOGY

### General Features
- General path comments
  - ○ ECCL considered distinct entity; however, some clinical/imaging overlap with SWS, OCCS, ENS, and Proteus syndrome
  - ○ Few reports heart, limb involvement, café-au-lait spots, maxillary/mandibular odontomas
  - ○ Embryology-anatomy
    - ▪ 3rd week gestation: Embryonic disc consists of ectoderm, mesoderm, entoderm

# ENCEPHALOCRANIOCUTANEOUS LIPOMATOSIS

- Neural tube develops from ectoderm during 3rd week gestation
- 4th & 5th week gestation: Mesoderm forms mesenchymal sheath over brain and spinal cord ⇒ precursor blood vessels, bone, cartilage and fat
- Genetics
  - Sporadic
  - Best theory: Survival autosomal lethal gene by somatic mosaicism
- Etiology
  - Theory: Primary mesodermal dysgenesis of unknown etiology
    - Neuroectoderm secondarily involved
- Epidemiology: Rare; ~ 40 reported cases (likely under-reported)

## Gross Pathologic & Surgical Features
- Brain: Cortical atrophy, white matter hypoplasia, ventriculomegaly, polymicrogyria, Wallerian degeneration brainstem
  - Arterial ectasias, pouches, aneurysms described in older patients
- Leptomeninges: Thick, gray, gelatinous with excess underlying arteries, veins, and varicose capillaries
- Skull: Macrocranium with focal hyperostosis
- Scalp: Focal lipomatous thickening with overlying circumscribed alopecia
- Face: Multiple tiny white/purple/yellow periocular > perinasal papules
- Eye: Yellowish scleral/limbal mass

## Microscopic Features
- Brain: Abnormal, four-layered cytoarchitecture; mineral concretions outer cortical lamina; scattered glial nodules
- Leptomeninges: Lipoangiomatosis
- Skull: Diploic replacement with mature fat cells
- Scalp: Benign lipoma > fibrolipoma expanding into dermis; absent hair follicles with preserved erector pili muscles
- Skin: Subcutaneous angiofibroma, fibrolipoma, or lipoma
- Eye: Corneal limbus/scleral choristoma
  - Other ocular abnormalities: Persistent hyaloid vasculature, coloboma, cloudy cornea, lens dislocation, ectopic pupils

## CLINICAL ISSUES

### Presentation
- Most common signs/symptoms
  - Nevus psiloliparus: Sharply demarcated focus of scalp alopecia overlying scalp lipoma
    - Hallmark of ECCL
- Other signs/symptoms
  - Ipsilateral ocular choristomas and periocular > perinasal papules
  - Macrocranium (unrelated to hydrocephalus)
  - Seizures, psychomotor delay, spastic hemiparesis
  - Infrequent scoliosis, foot deformities, sensorimotor deficits (2° to spinal lipoma)
- Clinical Profile

---

- Newborn with nevus psiloliparus, scleral mass, and periocular papules
- Infant with seizures, nevus psiloliparus, scleral mass, and periocular papules

### Demographics
- Age
  - Newborn > infant presentation
  - Rare presentation teen/adult with cutaneous, ocular lesions
- Gender: M = F
- Ethnicity: No racial or geographic predilection

### Natural History & Prognosis
- Natural history
  - Reported growth lipomas and ocular choristomas; remaining congenital abnormalities static
  - Reports of abnormal vasculature, aneurysms later in life
- Prognosis
  - Majority with variable degrees of psychomotor impairment and dependency
  - Few reports neurologically normal patients with nevus psiloliparus: Non-syndromic nevus psiloliparus vs. ECCL with minimal CNS involvement

### Treatment
- Anti-epileptics
- Shunt placement for hydrocephalus

## DIAGNOSTIC CHECKLIST

### Image Interpretation Pearls
- Considerable imaging overlap with SWS ⇒ search for scalp lipoma
- Low density IC lipoma may be difficult to distinguish from CSF on CT

## SELECTED REFERENCES

1. Hunter AG. Related Articles et al: Oculocerebrocutaneous and encephalocraniocutaneous lipomatosis syndromes: blind men and an elephant or separate syndromes? Am J Med Genet A. 2006
2. Sofiatti A et al: Encephalocraniocutaneous lipomatosis: clinical spectrum of systemic involvement. Pediatr Dermatol. 2006
3. Happle R et al: Nevus psiloliparus: report of two nonsyndromic cases. Eur J Dermatol. 14(5):314-6, 2004
4. Gawel J et al: Encephalocraniocutaneous lipomatosis. J Cutan Med Surg. 7(1):61-5, 2003
5. Parazzini C et al: Encephalocraniocutaneous lipomatosis: complete neuroradiologic evaluation and follow-up of two cases. AJNR Am J Neuroradiol. 20(1):173-6, 1999
6. Rizzo R et al: Encephalocraniocutaneous lipomatosis, Proteus syndrome, and somatic mosaicism. Am J Med Genet. 47(5):653-5, 1993
7. Fishman MA. Related Articles et al: Encephalocraniocutaneous lipomatosis. J Child Neurol. 2(3):186-93, 1987
8. Haberland C et al: Encephalocraniocutaneous lipomatosis. A new example of ectomesodermal dysgenesis. Arch Neurol. 22(2):144-55, 1970

# ENCEPHALOCRANIOCUTANEOUS LIPOMATOSIS

## IMAGE GALLERY

### Typical

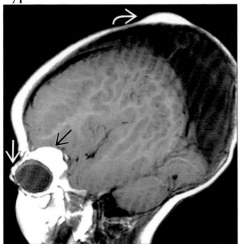

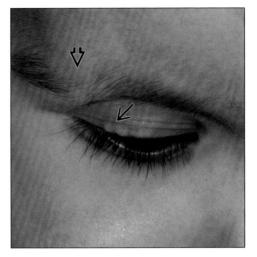

*(Left)* Sagittal T1WI MR shows typical findings of ECCL: Scalp lipoma ➡ ipsilateral to hemispheric abnormalities, and scleral choristoma ➡. Also note orbital lipoma ➡ and buphthalmos. *(Right)* Clinical photograph of the eye shows typical periocular findings: Small eyebrow nevus psiloliparus ➤ and eyelid papules ➡. The findings are ipsilateral to the scalp nevus psiloliparus.

### Typical

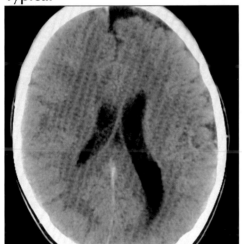

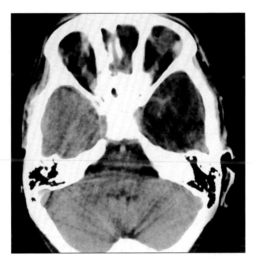

*(Left)* Axial NECT shows left hemispheric atrophy and ventriculomegaly in a patient with ECCL. Cortical Ca$^{++}$ are absent. The scalp lipoma (nevus psiloliparus) is more obvious clinically than by CT. *(Right)* Axial NECT shows a middle cranial fossa arachnoid cyst in a patient with ECCL. The cyst is ipsilateral to hemispheric atrophy and a scalp lipoma.

### Variant

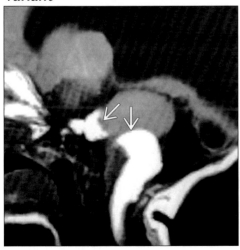

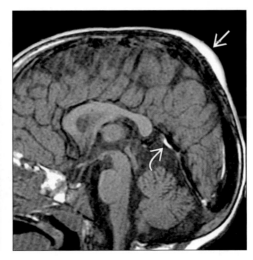

*(Left)* Sagittal T1WI MR shows craniocervical and cerebellopontine angle ➡ lipomas. Severe ventriculomegaly is likely secondary to CSF obstruction at foramen magnum and cerebral atrophy. *(Right)* Sagittal T1WI MR shows a tentorial ➡ and scalp ➡ lipoma. There is no other intracranial abnormality. The patient is clinically normal. The findings represent a forme fruste of ECCL.

# MISSILE AND PENETRATING INJURY

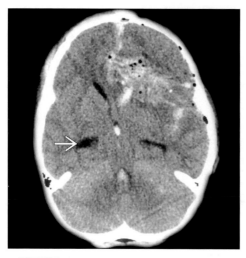

*Axial NECT shows GSW in 3 y/o. Bullet entered through left temporal squamosa, traveled anteriorly/superiorly. Parenchymal, SAH and IVH are evident. Big temporal horn ➡ early hydrocephalus.*

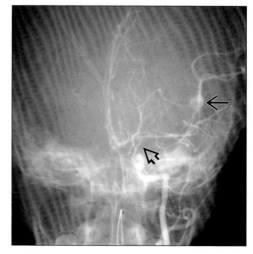

*Anteroposterior angiography following selective injection of the left CCA. A pseudoaneurysm ➡ in an anterior branch of the left MCA is seen. Severe vasospasm affects the ICA ➡ and MCA.*

## TERMINOLOGY

### Abbreviations and Synonyms
- Gun shot wound (GSW)

### Definitions
- Cranial trauma from high-velocity projectile (typically GSW)

## IMAGING FINDINGS

### General Features
- Best diagnostic clue: Single or multiple intracranial foreign bodies, missile tract, pneumocephalus, entry ± exit wound
- Morphology
  - Extremely variable depending on
    - Size, shape & number of projectiles
    - Projectile velocities
    - Entry/exit site(s) & course through brain
  - Skull fracture(s)
    - Entry site → embedded bullet & bone fragments
    - Pneumocephalus

- Intracranial hemorrhage
  - Epidural, subdural, subarachnoid hemorrhage
  - Hemorrhagic tract through brain
  - Intracerebral, intraventricular hemorrhage
- Secondary effects
  - Ischemia & infarction
  - Brain herniation

### CT Findings
- NECT
  - Best assessment of extent of soft tissue injury
  - Identify entrance & exit wounds

### MR Findings
- T1WI: Variable signal from hemorrhage, foreign bodies & air
- T2WI: Edema from pressure wave
- T2* GRE: Hemosiderin deposition as well as susceptibility artifact from foreign bodies
- MRV
  - Venous injury or thrombosis if missile tract crosses or tears interdural veins or lacerates sinus
  - Dural sinus thrombosis → reported incidence < 5% with penetrating trauma

---

## DDx: Stick-like Objects Penetrating Cranial Cavity through Posterior Orbit

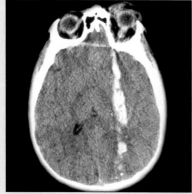

*Metal Rod through Orbit*

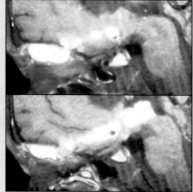

*Wooden Flagpole through Orbit*

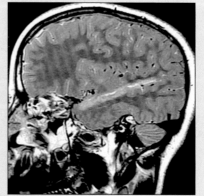

*Metal Skewer through Nose, Orbit*

# MISSILE AND PENETRATING INJURY

## Key Facts

### Terminology
- Gun shot wound (GSW)

### Imaging Findings
- Best diagnostic clue: Single or multiple intracranial foreign bodies, missile tract, pneumocephalus, entry ± exit wound
- Entry site → embedded bullet & bone fragments
- Epidural, subdural, subarachnoid hemorrhage
- Hemorrhagic tract through brain

- Intracerebral, intraventricular hemorrhage
- Ischemia & infarction
- Brain herniation
- Initial study ⇒ NECT ± CTA
- Conventional cerebral angiography depending on type of trauma & degree of injury

### Diagnostic Checklist
- Post-traumatic pseudoaneurysm may be overlooked on CT → often obscured by hemorrhagic contusion

---

## Angiographic Findings
- Conventional
  - Traumatic intracranial aneurysms occur in atypical locations → proximal to/beyond circle of Willis & major arterial bifurcations
  - Vascular spasm from projectile velocity or SAH
  - Extracranial pseudoaneurysms vary from small saccular lesions & fusiform dilatations to large collections with huge cavitating hematomas
  - Also: Direct CCFs, dural AVFs involving meningeal vessels, extracranial AVFs, arterial dissection

## Imaging Recommendations
- Protocol advice
  - Initial study ⇒ NECT ± CTA
  - Conventional cerebral angiography depending on type of trauma & degree of injury
  - MR/MRA if retained bullet fragment non-ferromagnetic

## PATHOLOGY

### General Features
- Etiology: Pressure wave in front of missile crushes/stretches/disintegrates tissue, creates temporary cavitation

### Microscopic Features
- Highly variable ranging from axonal transection to axonal edema

- Vessels: Transection to luminal injury

## CLINICAL ISSUES

### Natural History & Prognosis
- Transventricular or bihemispheric central type of trajectory ⇒ predictive of high morbidity/mortality

## DIAGNOSTIC CHECKLIST

### Consider
- Could there be a vascular injury/aneurysm?
- Post-traumatic pseudoaneurysm may be overlooked on CT → often obscured by hemorrhagic contusion

## SELECTED REFERENCES

1. Coughlan MD et al: Craniocerebral gunshot injuries in children. Childs Nerv Syst. 19(5-6):348-52, 2003
2. Martins RS et al: Prognostic factors and treatment of penetrating gunshot wounds to the head. Surg Neurol. 60(2):98-104; discussion 104, 2003
3. Cruz J et al: Cerebral extraction of oxygen and intracranial hypertension in severe, acute, pediatric brain trauma: preliminary novel management strategies. Neurosurgery. 50(4):774-9; discussion 779-80, 2002
4. Di Roio C et al: Craniocerebral injury resulting from transorbital stick penetration in children. Childs Nerv Syst. 16(8):503-6; discussion 507, 2000

## IMAGE GALLERY

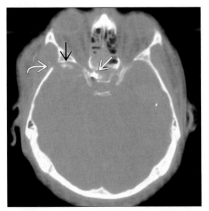 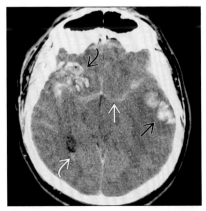 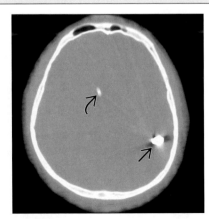

*(Left)* Axial bone CT shows the entrance of a bullet through the right pterion ➡. Inward displacement of bone fragments ➡. A large bullet fragment is lodged in the optic canal ➡. *(Center)* Axial NECT shows extensive bihemispheric damage from GSW. Hemorrhagic contusions in the right anterior sylvian ➡ and the left mid sylvian ➡ regions. SAH ➡, IVH ➡ are evident. *(Right)* Axial bone CT in same patient as prior shows the largest bullet fragment in the left posterior sylvian region ➡. A ventricular drain ➡ has been inserted.

# CHILD ABUSE, BRAIN

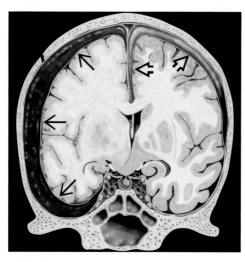

Coronal graphic shows a large subdural hematoma over the right hemisphere ➡ and a smaller collection over the left hemisphere ➡; differences in color imply different ages of blood.

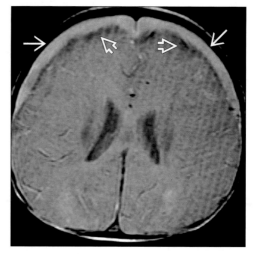

Axial FLAIR MR in an infant shows hyperintense subdural collections over both frontal lobes ➡; note darker CSF signal in the SAS ➡ under the collections, matching ventricular CSF.

## TERMINOLOGY

### Abbreviations and Synonyms
- Nonaccidental trauma (NAT); nonaccidental injury (NAI), shaken-baby syndrome (SBS), battered child syndrome, Caffey-Kempe syndrome
- Rule out parental abuse (ROPA), whiplash shaken infant syndrome, nonaccidental head injury (NAHI), trauma-X
- Multiple alternate titles have been suggested in attempts to minimize accusatory labeling in clinical settings

### Definitions
- Traumatic injury deliberately inflicted on infants and children by adults

## IMAGING FINDINGS

### General Features
- Best diagnostic clue
  - Multiple brain injuries disproportionally severe relative to proffered history

- Can be divided into two major groupings
  - Direct impact injury ⇒ result of direct blow to cranium or impact of skull on object
  - Shaking injury ⇒ result of violent to-and-fro motion of head
  - Groups not exclusive: Shaking injury often compounded by impact
- Direct impact injury characterized by skull fractures and injury to immediately underlying brain
  - Superficial injury (scalp laceration, swelling) strongly associated
  - High association with other organ injury
- Shaking injury characterized by diffusely distributed subdural hematomas
  - Imaging characteristics often suggest injuries of differing ages
  - High association with "ischemic" parenchymal injury

### CT Findings
- CTA
  - Detectable vascular injury relatively uncommon in child abuse

## DDx: Extra-axial Collections in Children

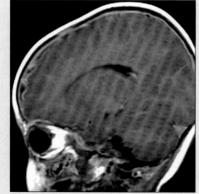

Empyema

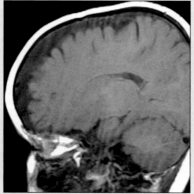

Glutaric Aciduria

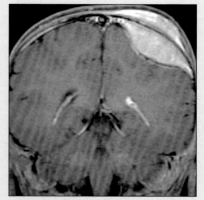

Neuroblastoma

# CHILD ABUSE, BRAIN

## Key Facts

### Terminology
- Traumatic injury deliberately inflicted on infants and children by adults

### Imaging Findings
- Multiple brain injuries disproportionally severe relative to proffered history
- Direct impact injury ⇒ result of direct blow to cranium or impact of skull on object
- Shaking injury ⇒ result of violent to-and-fro motion of head
- Groups not exclusive: Shaking injury often compounded by impact
- CT is the primary imaging tool in initial evaluation of child abuse
- Parenchymal injury often accompanies shaking injury

### Pathology
- 85% of fatal child abuse victims have evidence of impact head injury at postmortem examination
- #1 cause of brain injury death in children < 2 yrs

### Clinical Issues
- "Killer couch" ⇒ injuries commonly blamed on infant rolling off couch onto floor
- Retinal hemorrhage can be missed on cursory exam
- Retinal hemorrhage can be seen in glutaric acidurias
- High mortality ⇒ 15-38% (60% if coma at presentation)

### Diagnostic Checklist
- Avoid use of vague, oblique, obscuring language in reports
- Avoid temptation to precisely time ICH

---

- Post-traumatic aneurysm, dissection can be demonstrated by CTA
- NECT
  - CT is the primary imaging tool in initial evaluation of child abuse
  - Sensitive in detection and characterization of fractures
    - Fractures oriented in axial plane may be missed!
  - Very sensitive in the detection and characterization of intracranial hemorrhage (ICH)
  - Subarachnoid hemorrhage (SAH) is common (> 50%)
  - Subdural hemorrhage (SDH) is very common
    - Over cerebral convexities, in interhemispheric fissure, overlying tentorium
    - Normal density of subarachnoid space (SAS) stands out next to increased density of SDH
  - Great caution should be exercised if attempting to estimate "age" of ICH
    - Blood loses density based upon multiple factors ⇒ cerebrospinal fluid (CSF) dilution, hematocrit, coagulation status
    - SDHs of same age can have significantly different density
    - Chronic SDHs tend to be uniform in density, slightly greater than CSF in SAH and ventricles
    - Acute SDHs are more likely to be hyperdense
    - However, acute SDH can be hypodense, and focal clots and membranes can cause hyperdensity in chronic SDH
  - Parenchymal injury often accompanies shaking injury
    - Initial CT ⇒ loss of gray-white differentiation, decreased density of supratentorial brain relative to cerebellum
    - Subsequent studies show multiple regions of decreased attenuation, not corresponding to arterial territories
  - Subdural hygromas can develop at 12-26 hours after injury
    - CSF density subdural collections of CSF that leak from SAS

### MR Findings
- T1WI
  - Hyperintense hemorrhagic staining of injured cortex
  - Subdurals in posterior fossa clearly shown on sagittal T1WI
- T2WI: Shows loss of cortical ribbon and deep nuclei in neonates
- PD/Intermediate: Possibly most sensitive sequence for detection of small SDH
- T2* GRE: Sensitive for hemorrhagic staining, remote hemorrhage
- DWI: Key sequence for identification of parenchymal insult in shaking injury in acute/subacute stage
- MRA: Proximal vascular correlate (dissection, spasm) rarely shown in association with parenchymal injury
- MRS: Will show ↓ NAA, ↑ lactate in regions of parenchymal injury

### Radiographic Findings
- Radiography
  - More sensitive in the detection of skull fractures than standard CT
    - CT is more sensitive and specific for depression and complications of fractures
  - Detection of fractures, a key component in forensic evaluation of suspected child abuse
  - Some fracture patterns are considered more suspicious for child abuse
    - Analysis of abuse and accidental injuries does not support this
  - Multiple, compound, diastatic fractures, and fractures crossing sutures imply significant trauma
    - Discordance with suggested history best indicator for child abuse

### Nuclear Medicine Findings
- Bone Scan
  - Can be used to document associated skeletal injury
    - Can miss skull fractures, metaphyseal injuries

### Imaging Recommendations
- Best imaging tool

- NECT to evaluate brain initially
  - MR of greater benefit at 48-72 hours
- Radiographs to detect skull fractures (as part of skeletal survey)
- Protocol advice
  - Use PD/Intermediate sequence to detect subtle SDH on MR
  - Use DWI to assess parenchymal injury
  - Consider concomitant spine injury
  - Use MRA or CTA to evaluate suspected pseudoaneurysm

## DIFFERENTIAL DIAGNOSIS

### Accidental Trauma
- Appropriate history for degree of injury

### Benign Macrocrania
- Self-limited communicating hydrocephalus
- Prominence of extra-axial spaces ⇒ isodense to CSF

### Mitochondrial Encephalopathies
- Several mitochondrial encephalopathies cause atrophy with subdural collections
- Glutaric acidurias (types I & II), Menkes syndrome
- Rare diseases with pre-existing neurologic symptoms

### Overshunting
- "Passive" subdurals can develop from decreased volume associated with CSF shunting

### Subdural Empyema
- Febrile, sinusitis, meningitis

### Dural Based Tumor
- Neuroblastoma, leukemia

## PATHOLOGY

### General Features
- General path comments
  - 85% of fatal child abuse victims have evidence of impact head injury at postmortem examination
  - Cause of death in 80% of fatalities is brain swelling
    - Severe hypoxic ischemic encephalopathy > diffuse axonal injury (DAI)
  - Retinal hemorrhage 70-96% (usually bilateral, always with SDH)
- Etiology
  - Increased vulnerability in infants due to
    - Large head/body ratio + weak neck muscles
    - Developing brain ⇒ less structural integrity prior to myelination, greater susceptibility to injury
- Epidemiology
  - 17-25:100,000 annual incidence
    - Almost certainly under-reported
  - #1 cause of brain injury death in children < 2 yrs

## CLINICAL ISSUES

### Presentation
- Most common signs/symptoms

- Discordance between stated history & degree of injury
  - Attempt by perpetrator to minimize suspicion
- "Killer couch" ⇒ injuries commonly blamed on infant rolling off couch onto floor
  - Frequently in infants too young to roll over at all
- Difficulty breathing, unresponsive
- Other signs/symptoms
  - Poor feeding, vomiting, irritability, seizures, lethargy, coma, apnea
  - Retinal hemorrhage can be missed on cursory exam
  - Retinal hemorrhage can be seen in glutaric acidurias
- Clinical Profile
  - Perpetrators are most often direct caretakers ⇒ parents, baby-sitters, mother's boyfriend
  - Developmentally delayed, "colicky", premature or low birth weight infants at higher risk
  - Psychosocial stressors and poor coping mechanisms in family environment

### Demographics
- Age
  - Majority < 1 year
  - Most common 2-6 months
- Gender: Male > female

### Natural History & Prognosis
- High mortality ⇒ 15-38% (60% if coma at presentation)

### Treatment
- Notification of local Child Protection Agency mandated in US/Canada/Australia/some European countries
- Multidisciplinary child abuse & neglect team intervention

## DIAGNOSTIC CHECKLIST

### Consider
- Avoid use of vague, oblique, obscuring language in reports
  - Can hamper care of child and legal investigation
  - May increase likelihood of interpretation being challenged

### Image Interpretation Pearls
- Avoid temptation to precisely time ICH
  - Impossible to precisely state age of bleeding in the absence of "before and after" imaging
  - Reasonable estimates and conclusions are more defensible in court

## SELECTED REFERENCES

1. Kleinman PK: Diagnostic Imaging of Child Abuse, 2nd ed. Mosby. 285-342, 1998
2. Caffey J: The parent-infant traumatic stress syndrome; (Caffey-Kempe syndrome), (battered babe syndrome). Am J Roentgenol Radium Ther Nucl Med. 114(2):218-29, 1972
3. Silverman FN: Unrecognized trauma in infants, the battered child syndrome, and the syndrome of Ambroise Tardieu. Rigler Lecture. Radiology. 104(2):337-53, 1972

## IMAGE GALLERY

### Typical

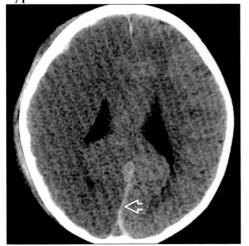 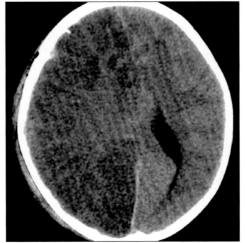

*(Left)* Axial NECT shows subdural blood along the posterior falx ➤ and loss of gray-white differentiation in the right cerebral hemisphere, with effacement of sulci and right to left shift. *(Right)* Axial NECT (same child as previous image) 24 hours later shows the "reversal sign"; white matter is denser than gray matter on the injured right side, contrasting with a normal appearance on the left.

### Typical

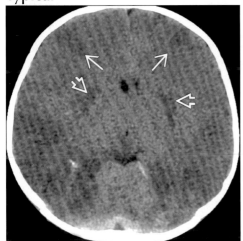 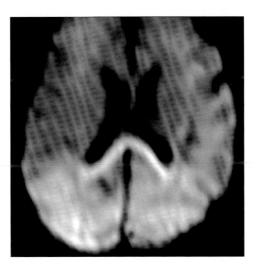

*(Left)* Axial NECT shows parenchymal injury as patchy regions of decreased attenuation at the temporal-parietal lobe junctions, in the lenticular nuclei ➤, and frontal lobes ➤. *(Right)* Axial DWI MR (same infant as previous image) shows bright signal caused by restricted diffusion throughout the occipital and inferior parietal lobes.

### Typical

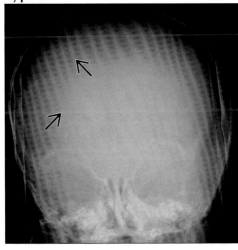 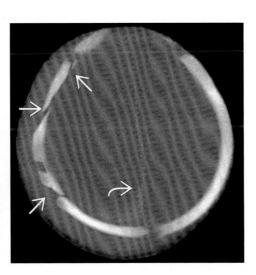

*(Left)* Anteroposterior radiograph shows diastatic and complex fractures ➤ of the right hemicranium in this child who was reported to have rolled off the couch onto the floor. *(Right)* Axial NECT (same child as previous image) shows the same fractures ➤ extending across the coronal suture. Note the subdural hematoma extending into the interhemispheric fissure ➤.

# LIPOMA

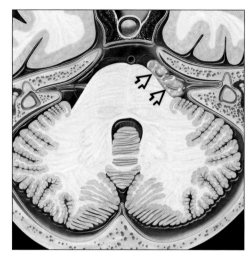

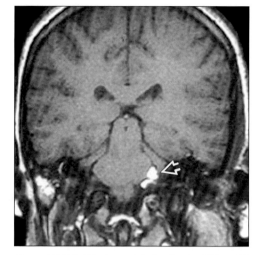

Axial graphic shows fatty mass ⇒ in left cerebellopontine angle. Note the nerves and blood vessels coursing through and around the mass because lipomas are maldeveloped subarachnoid space.

Coronal T1WI MR shows lobulated mass ⇒ in left cerebellopontine angle. This was an incidental finding, as lipomas are rarely symptomatic.

## TERMINOLOGY

### Abbreviations and Synonyms

- Intracranial lipoma (ICL); lipomatous hamartoma

### Definitions

- Mass of mature non-neoplastic adipose tissue
  - CNS lipomas are congenital malformations, not true neoplasm
  - Lipoma variants in the central nervous system (CNS) include: Angiolipoma, hibernoma, osteolipoma

## IMAGING FINDINGS

### General Features

- Best diagnostic clue: Well-delineated lobulated extra-axial mass with fat attenuation/intensity
- Location
  - Midline location common
  - 80% supratentorial
    - 30-40% interhemispheric fissure superior (sometimes posterior) to corpus callosum; may extend into lateral ventricles, choroid plexus

  - 20-25% pineal region (usually attached to tectum)
  - 15-20% suprasellar (attached to tuber cinereum)
  - Small lipomas common in cavernous sinuses
  - Uncommon: Sylvian fissures, middle cranial fossa
  - 20% infratentorial
    - Cerebellopontine angle (may extend into internal auditory canal (IAC), vestibule)
    - Uncommon: Jugular foramen, foramen magnum
- Size: Varies from tiny to very large
- Morphology
  - Lobulated pial-based fatty mass that may encase vessels & cranial nerves
  - Two kinds of interhemispheric lipoma
    - Curvilinear type (thin ICL curves around corpus callosum (CC) body, splenium)
    - Tubulonodular type (bulky mass; frequent Ca++, usually associated with CC agenesis)

### CT Findings

- CTA: Aberrant anterior cerebral artery (ACA) course in interhemispheric CC lipoma associated with callosal dysgenesis
- NECT
  - -50 to -100 H (fat density)

## DDx: Intracranial Lipoma

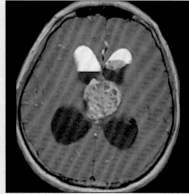

Dermoid Tumor

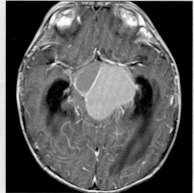

Craniopharyngioma

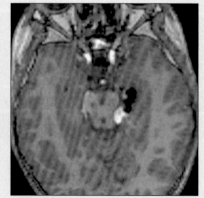

Thrombosed Aneurysm

# LIPOMA

## Key Facts

### Terminology
- Mass of mature non-neoplastic adipose tissue
- CNS lipomas are congenital malformations, not true neoplasm

### Imaging Findings
- Best diagnostic clue: Well-delineated lobulated extra-axial mass with fat attenuation/intensity
- 30-40% interhemispheric fissure superior (sometimes posterior) to corpus callosum; may extend into lateral ventricles, choroid plexus
- -50 to -100 H (fat density)
- Ca++ varies from none to extensive
- Standard SE: Hyperintense on T1WI
- Becomes hypointense with fat suppression
- Standard SE: Hypointense with striking chemical shift artifact (CSA) on T2WI

### Top Differential Diagnoses
- Dermoid
- Teratoma
- Lipomatous Differentiation/Transformation of Neoplasm
- Craniopharyngioma
- Subacute Hemorrhage

### Pathology
- Cranial, spinal intradural fat is a congenital anomaly (not a true neoplasm)
- Identical to adipose tissue elsewhere

### Diagnostic Checklist
- When in doubt, use fat-saturation sequence

---

- Ca++ varies from none to extensive
  - Present in 65% of bulky tubulonodular CC lipomas
- CECT: Doesn't enhance

## MR Findings
- T1WI
  - Standard SE: Hyperintense on T1WI
  - Becomes hypointense with fat suppression
- T2WI
  - Standard SE: Hypointense with striking chemical shift artifact (CSA) on T2WI
    - Round/linear "filling defects" present where vessels, cranial nerves pass through lipoma
    - May show low signal intensity foci (Ca++)
  - FSE: Iso- to hyperintense (j-coupling)
- PD/Intermediate
  - Standard SE: Iso- to hyperintense [depending on repetition time/echo time (TR/TE)]
    - Striking CSA
- STIR: Hypointense
- FLAIR: Hyperintense

## Ultrasonographic Findings
- Grayscale Ultrasound
  - Generally hyperechoic
  - Look for other fetal anomalies (CC agenesis, etc.)
- Color Doppler: See normal flow in vessels coursing through lipoma

## Angiographic Findings
- Conventional
  - ACA courses directly superiorly if CC agenesis present
  - Arteries & veins often embedded within lipoma

## Imaging Recommendations
- Best imaging tool: MR
- Protocol advice: Add fat suppression sequence for confirmation

---

## DIFFERENTIAL DIAGNOSIS

### Dermoid
- Density usually 20-40 H (lipoma -50 to -100 H)
- Signal intensity usually more heterogeneous than lipoma
- Rupture with cisternal fat droplets common
- Usually no associated malformations (common with lipoma)
- Dermoids often calcify, lipomas in locations other than interhemispheric don't

### Teratoma
- Locations similar to lipoma
- Tissue from all 3 embryonic germ layers ⇒ fat often present
  - Look for: Mucous cysts, chondroid nodules, bony spicules
- Imaging appearance usually more heterogeneous
  - May show foci of contrast-enhancement

### Lipomatous Differentiation/Transformation of Neoplasm
- May occur occasionally in neuroectodermal tumors (PNETs, ependymoma, gliomas)
- Cerebellar liponeurocytoma
  - Mixed mesenchymal/neuroectodermal posterior fossa neoplasm
  - Primarily hypointense on T1WI, mixed with hyperintense foci
  - Patchy, irregular enhancement
- Meningioma (lipomatous transformation uncommon)

### Craniopharyngioma
- T1 shortening, Ca++ (CT) can be confused with lipoma
- Look for enhancement of cyst rim, fluid-fluid levels

### Subacute Hemorrhage
- In aneurysm or subarachnoid hematoma
- Look for susceptibility effects on gradient echo images

# LIPOMA

## PATHOLOGY

### General Features
- General path comments
  - Fat not normally present in CNS
  - Cranial, spinal intradural fat is a congenital anomaly (not a true neoplasm)
  - Cortical dysplasia may be found next to sylvian fissure lipomas
- Genetics
  - No known defects in sporadic ICL
  - Occurs in encephalocraniocutaneous lipomatosis, a congenital neurocutaneous syndrome
- Etiology
  - Persistence, maldevelopment of embryonic meninx primitiva
    - Normally differentiates into leptomeninges, cisterns
    - Maldifferentiates into fat instead
  - Developing pia-arachnoid invaginates through embryonic choroid fissure
    - Explains frequent intraventricular extension of interhemispheric lipomas
- Epidemiology: < 0.5% of all intracranial tumors (not true neoplasm)
- Associated abnormalities
  - Most common: Interhemispheric lipoma + corpus callosum anomalies
  - Other congenital malformations
    - Cephaloceles
    - Closed spinal dysraphism
  - Encephalocraniocutaneous lipomatosis ⇒ Fishman syndrome
  - Pai syndrome ⇒ facial clefts, skin lipomas; occasional ICLs, usually interhemispheric

### Gross Pathologic & Surgical Features
- Yellow lobulated fatty mass attached to leptomeninges, sometimes adherent to brain
- Cranial nerves, arteries/veins pass through lipoma

### Microscopic Features
- Identical to adipose tissue elsewhere
- Cells vary slightly in shape/size, measure up to 200 microns
- Occasional nuclear hyperchromasia
- Mitoses rare/absent
- Liposarcoma: Extremely rare malignant intracranial adipose tumor

## CLINICAL ISSUES

### Presentation
- Most common signs/symptoms
  - Usually found incidentally at imaging, autopsy
  - Rare: Cranial neuropathy (vestibulocochlear dysfunction, facial pain), seizures (associated with other congenital anomalies)

### Demographics
- Age: Any age
- Gender: M = F

## Natural History & Prognosis
- Fat cells grow during first year of life
  - Enlarging lipoma in infant does not imply aggressive nature
- Benign, usually stable in children, adults
- May expand with corticosteroids
  - High dose, long term administration may result in neural compressive symptoms

## Treatment
- Generally not a surgical lesion; high morbidity/mortality
- Reduce/eliminate steroids

## DIAGNOSTIC CHECKLIST

### Consider
- Could high signal on T1WI be due to other substances with short T1 (e.g., subacute hemorrhage)?

### Image Interpretation Pearls
- When in doubt, use fat-saturation sequence

## SELECTED REFERENCES

1. Yildiz H et al: Intracranial lipomas: importance of localization. Neuroradiology. 48(1):1-7, 2006
2. Given CA et al: Interhemispheric lipoma connected to subcutaneous lipoma via lipomatous stalk. Pediatr Radiol. 35(11):1110-2, 2005
3. Kakita A et al: Cerebral lipoma and the underlying cortex of the temporal lobe: pathological features associated with the malformation. Acta Neuropathol (Berl). 109(3):339-45, 2005
4. Yilmazlar S et al: Quadrigeminal cistern lipoma. J Clin Neurosci. 12(5):596-9, 2005
5. Gaskin CM et al: Lipomas, lipoma variants, and well-differentiated liposarcomas (atypical lipomas). AJR 182: 733-9, 2004
6. Spallone A et al: Lipomas of the pineal region. Surg Neurol. 62(1):52-8; discussion 58-9, 2004
7. Fitoz S et al: Intracranial lipoma with extracranial extension through foramen ovale in a patient with encephalocraniocutaneous lipomatosis syndrome. Neuroradiol 44: 175-8, 2002
8. Tankere F et al: Cerebellopontine angle lipomas: report of four cases and review of the literature. Neurosurg 50: 626-31, 2002
9. Feldman RP et al: Intracranial lipoma of the sylvian fissure. Case report and review of the literature. J Neurosurg. 94(3):515-9, 2001
10. Ickowitz V et al: Prenatal diagnosis and postnatal follow-up of pericallosal lipoma: Report of seven new cases. AJNR 22: 767-72, 2001
11. Amor DJ et al: Encephalocraniocutaneous lipomatosis (Fishman syndrome): a rare neurocutaneous syndrome. J Paediatr Child Health. 36(6):603-5, 2000
12. Ichikawa T et al: Intracranial lipomas: demonstration by computed tomography and magnetic resonance imaging. J Nippon Med Sch. 67(5):388-91, 2000
13. Kieslich M et al: Midline developmental anomalies with lipomas in the corpus callosum region. J Child Neurol. 15(2):85-9, 2000

# LIPOMA

### Typical

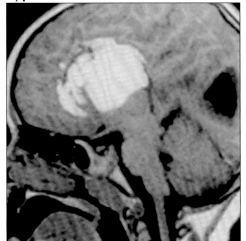
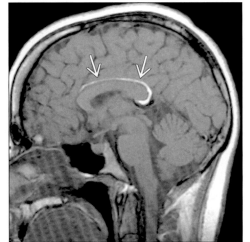

*(Left)* Sagittal T1WI MR shows large tubulonodular interhemispheric lipoma that extended laterally into the lateral ventricles through the choroidal fissure and inferiorly into the third ventricle. *(Right)* Sagittal T1WI MR shows curvilinear interhemispheric lipoma ➡ dorsal to callosal body and wrapping around splenium. Do not mistake for thrombosed vein (use fat suppression)!

### Typical

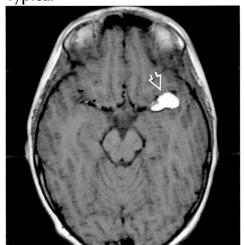
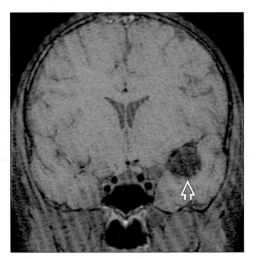

*(Left)* Axial T1WI MR shows left sylvian fissure lipoma ➡. This was initially thought to represent a thrombosed middle cerebral artery aneurysm. *(Right)* Coronal T1WI FS MR shows that the hyperintensity disappears after application of a fat suppression pulse, confirming a diagnosis of lipoma. The lipoma ➡ lies adjacent to the middle cerebral artery (MCA).

### Typical

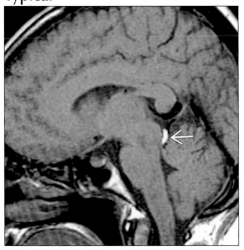
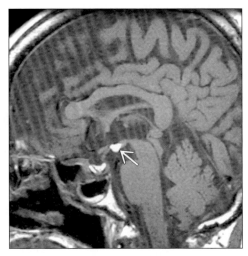

*(Left)* Sagittal T1WI MR shows collicular/supravermian lipoma ➡ in typical location, adjacent to the inferior colliculus and the superior surface of the cerebellar vermis. *(Right)* Sagittal T1WI MR shows typical hypothalamic lipoma ➡, extending into the suprasellar cistern from the tuber cinereum, between the median eminence and the mamillary bodies.

I

8

43

# CONGENITAL MUSCULAR DYSTROPHY

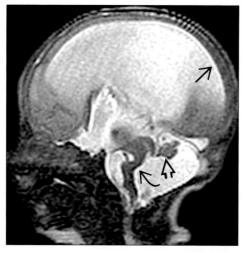

Sagittal T2WI MR in WWS shows a Z-shaped brain stem ➔ with kinking of the pons-midbrain junction. The cerebellum is small, dysplastic ➔ and rotated. Note thin cortex ➔ and hydrocephalus.

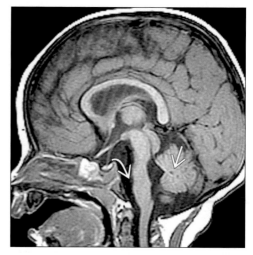

Sagittal T1WI MR in another child with congenital muscular dystrophy (MEB phenotype) shows a notched pons ➔ and small cysts ➔ within the fastigial white matter of the vermis.

## TERMINOLOGY

### Abbreviations and Synonyms
- Congenital muscular dystrophy (CMD)
- Cobblestone lissencephaly (LIS); type 2 lissencephaly
- Walker-Warburg syndrome (WWS), muscle-eye-brain disease (MEB), Fukuyama congenital muscular dystrophy (FCMD)

### Definitions
- CMDs = heterogeneous group of autosomal recessive myopathies presenting at birth with hypotonia
- CMDs without major brain malformations are either merosin positive or merosin negative
  - Merosin (-): Significant dys-/hypomyelination of white matter (WM)
  - Merosin (+): Normal/very mild imaging findings [cerebellar (CBLL) hypoplasia, nonspecific WM changes, focal polymicrogyria (PMG)]
- ~ 50% of children with CMD have major brain abnormalities with a spectrum of overlapping findings including abnormal signal of WM & ocular, cortical (cobblestone cortex), brainstem & CBLL anomalies

## IMAGING FINDINGS

### General Features
- Best diagnostic clue: "Z-shaped", kinked or notched brainstem in a hypotonic infant
- Morphology
  - CMDs with brain malformations (WWS most severe)
    - Cortical dysplasia, cobblestone LIS or pachygyria
    - Varying degrees agenesis or hypogenesis of corpus callosum, septum pellucidum, vermis
    - Flat or "Z-shaped" brainstem or "notched" pons
    - ± Hydrocephalus or encephalocele

### CT Findings
- NECT
  - All imaging findings most severe in WWS
    - ↓ Attenuation WM, vermian dysgenesis (resembles Dandy Walker spectrum)
    - ± Occipital cephalocele, ± hydrocephalus, shallow or absent sulci

### MR Findings
- T1WI

## DDx: Kinked Brainstem

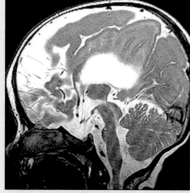

Aneuploidy

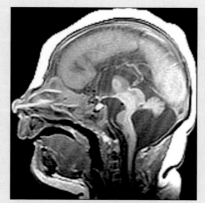

Microlissencephaly

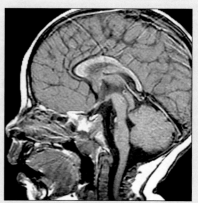

Cleft Pons

# CONGENITAL MUSCULAR DYSTROPHY

## Key Facts

### Terminology
- CMDs = heterogeneous group of autosomal recessive myopathies presenting at birth with hypotonia
- CMDs without major brain malformations are either merosin positive or merosin negative
- ~ 50% of children with CMD have major brain abnormalities with a spectrum of overlapping findings including abnormal signal of WM & ocular, cortical (cobblestone cortex), brainstem & CBLL anomalies

### Imaging Findings
- Best diagnostic clue: "Z-shaped", kinked or notched brainstem in a hypotonic infant
- All imaging findings most severe in WWS

### Pathology
- Marked phenotypic overlap amongst FCMD, Walker-Warburg, and MEB
- Muscle biopsy: Mild to moderate dystrophic changes, ± inflammatory infiltrate, ± absent staining laminin-α2
- CMDs with brain anomalies have hypoglycosylation of α-dystroglycan allowing neuronal overmigration through gaps in external lamina ⇒ "pebbled" surface of brain

### Clinical Issues
- Most common signs/symptoms: Hypotonia, cognitive and motor delay, poor vision, ↑ serum creatine kinase
- Clinical Profile: Floppy newborn
- Supportive: Respiratory & cardiovascular concerns

---

- Thin, dysplastic, PMG or "pebbled" supratentorial cortex, ± hydrocephalus
- ± Callosal, vermian, or septal hypogenesis
- Flat, deeply clefted, notched or "Z-shaped" brainstem
- T2WI
  - Polymicrogyria of cerebellar cortex, ± cysts
  - CMD merosin (-): Dysmyelination of centrum semiovale, ± subcortical U-fibers, but normal corpus callosum signal
  - FCMD, MEB: WM abnormalities in half
  - WWS: Severe WM hypomyelination
- MRS: Laminin-α2 deficiency: ↓ Metabolites (NAA, creatine, choline) suggest edema, astrocytosis & reduced cellular white matter density

## Imaging Recommendations
- Best imaging tool: MR
- Protocol advice: Multiplanar T2/FLAIR of posterior fossa to define CBLL cysts & kinked brainstem

## DIFFERENTIAL DIAGNOSIS

### Dandy Walker Malformation
- Small vermian remnant rotated superiorly by cyst, pons usually normal in size and not clefted or notched

### Microlissencephaly
- Microcephaly, Z-shaped brainstem, hypoplastic CBLL, smooth cerebrum (**not** cobblestone)

### Congenital Cytomegalovirus Infection
- Delayed myelination, polymicrogyria, small CBLL

### Horizontal Gaze Palsy Associated with Progressive Scoliosis (HGPS): Chr 11q23
- Horizontal gaze palsy, progressive scoliosis, brainstem hypoplasia/clefting, mild CBLL volume loss

## PATHOLOGY

### General Features
- General path comments
  - Marked phenotypic overlap amongst FCMD, Walker-Warburg, and MEB
  - Muscle biopsy: Mild to moderate dystrophic changes, ± inflammatory infiltrate, ± absent staining laminin-α2
  - CMDs with brain anomalies have hypoglycosylation of α-dystroglycan allowing neuronal overmigration through gaps in external lamina ⇒ "pebbled" surface of brain
- Genetics
  - At least 12 gene mutations known
  - Abnormal extracellular matrix proteins
    - CMD type 1A (MDC1A): LAMA2
    - CMD type 1B Ullrich CMD (UCMD)
  - Abnormal membrane receptors for extracellular matrix involving O-glycosylation of α-dystroglycan; these cause gaps in external limiting membrane & overmigration of neurons/glia into subpial & subarachnoid spaces
    - FCMD: Mutation in gene encoding fukutin (FCMD at 9q31)
    - MEB: O-Mannoside N-acetyl-glucosaminyl-transversae (POMGnT1), FKRP
    - WWS: O-Mannosyltransferase gene (POMT1, POMT2); occasionally LARGE, FCMD or FKRP
    - CMD type 1C: (MDC1C) FKRP gene
    - CMD type 1D: (MDC1D) LARGE gene
    - CMD with integrin-α7 deficiency, ITGA7 gene
    - NOTE: Phenotype depends more on severity of mutation than on gene involved
  - Abnormal endoplasmic reticulum protein
    - CMD w/spine rigidity type 1 (RSMD1) SEPN1 gene
  - Other CMD variants with known defects
    - CMD with familial junctional epidermolysis bullosa (plectin gene on Chr 8)
  - Mixed patterns and intermediate forms occur

- CMD merosin (-) with brain anomalies, cerebellar cysts, vermis hypoplasia, mental retardation
- Etiology: Mutations in molecules with roles in cell migration and connection
- Epidemiology: 7-12 per 100,000 children in Japan; incidence elsewhere uncertain
- Associated abnormalities: CMD variants with "not yet found" mutations: Occipito-temporal polymicrogyria, occipital agyria, calf-hypertrophy, arthrogryposis, ptosis, adducted thumbs

## Gross Pathologic & Surgical Features

- CMDs with brain malformations
  - Supratentorial: Cobblestone cortex, abnormal myelination, ± hydrocephalus
  - Brainstem: Variable degrees of pontine hypoplasia and fused colliculi ⇒ flat, cleft or "Z-shaped"
  - Infratentorial: CBLL hypoplasia, PMG & cysts related to defects in limiting membrane, ± encephalocele
  - Ocular anomalies: Retinal/optic nerve dysplasias, microphthalmia, buphthalmos, glaucoma, anterior chamber dysplasias, cataracts

## Microscopic Features

- Cerebral and CBLL PMG
- Overmigration of neurons/glia into subpial/subarachnoid space
- Hypoplasia of many WM tracts

## Staging, Grading or Classification Criteria

- Various phenotypes from least severe to most severe
  - Mutations of genes → different phenotypes depending on severity of mutation
- CMD 1A-D
- FCMD
  - Frontal polymicrogyria, occipital cobblestone cortex, delayed myelin with "peripheral first" pattern, CBLL involved
- MEB
  - Hydrocephalus, vermian hypogenesis, dysplastic cortex, patchy abnormal WM, ± callosal dysgenesis
- WWS (most severe)
  - Hydrocephalus, vermian hypogenesis, kinked pons-midbrain, cobblestone cortex, no myelin, ± cephalocele, ± callosal dysgenesis

# CLINICAL ISSUES

## Presentation

- Most common signs/symptoms: Hypotonia, cognitive and motor delay, poor vision, ↑ serum creatine kinase
- Clinical Profile: Floppy newborn

## Demographics

- Age
  - CMD with brain malformations can be diagnosed in utero via US and MR, otherwise in early infancy
  - FCMD: High percentage spontaneous abortions
- Gender: Autosomal recessive: M = F usual
- Ethnicity
  - FCMD most common in Japan (carrier state 1:88)
  - MEB more prevalent in Finland
  - WWS has worldwide distribution

- Other country and population-isolate specific variants are known

## Natural History & Prognosis

- Varies with mutation: CMD 1 least severe (decreased fetal movement, hypotonia, proximal weakness, contractures, mild or nonprogressive course, most sit, some walk, intellect usually normal); WWS most severe (death within first year)

## Treatment

- Supportive: Respiratory & cardiovascular concerns

# DIAGNOSTIC CHECKLIST

## Consider

- Typical brainstem and cerebellar findings should prompt the diagnosis of CMD, even if eyes and supratentorial cortex radiographically normal

## Image Interpretation Pearls

- Not all "Z-shaped" brainstems are CMD
- Not all CMD have "Z-shaped" brainstems, remember merosin (-) CMD

# SELECTED REFERENCES

1. Brockmann K et al: Quantitative proton MRS of cerebral metabolites in laminin alpha2 chain deficiency. Brain Dev. 2006
2. Martin PT: Mechanisms of Disease: congenital muscular dystrophies-glycosylation takes center stage. Nat Clin Pract Neurol. 2(4):222-230, 2006
3. Mendell JR et al: The congenital muscular dystrophies: recent advances and molecular insights. Pediatr Dev Pathol. 9(6):427-43, 2006
4. Leite CC et al: Merosin-deficient congenital muscular dystrophy (CMD): a study of 25 Brazilian patients using MRI. Pediatr Radiol. 35(6):572-9, 2005
5. Van Reeuwijk J et al: POMT2 mutations cause alpha-dystroglycan hypoglycosylation & Walker-Warburg syndrome. J Med Genet. 42(12):907-12, 2005
6. Beltran-Valero de Bernabe D et al: Mutations in the FKRP gene can cause muscle-eye-brain disease and Walker-Warburg syndrome. J Med Genet. 41(5):e61, 2004
7. Triki C et at: Merosin-deficient congenital muscular dystrophy with mental retardation & cerebellar cysts, unlinked to the LAMA2, FCMD, MEB and CMD1B loci, in 3 Tunisian patients. Neuromuscul Disord. 13(1):4-12, 2003
8. Zolkipli Z et al: Occipito-temporal polymicrogyria and subclinical muscular dystrophy. Neuropediatrics. 34(2):92-5, 2003
9. Mercuri E et al: Early white matter changes on brain magnetic resonance imaging in a newborn affected by merosin-deficient congenital muscular dystrophy. Neuromuscul Disord. 11(3):297-9, 2001
10. Philpot J et al: Brain magnetic resonance imaging abnormalities in merosin-positive congenital muscular dystrophy. Eur J Paediatr Neurol. 4(3):109-14, 2000
11. Barkovich AJ: Neuroimaging manifestations and classification of congenital muscular dystrophies. AJNR Am J Neuroradiol. 19(8):1389-96, 1998
12. van der Knaap MS et al: Magnetic resonance imaging in classification of congenital muscular dystrophies with brain abnormalities. Ann Neurol. 42(1):50-9, 1997

# CONGENITAL MUSCULAR DYSTROPHY

## IMAGE GALLERY

Typical

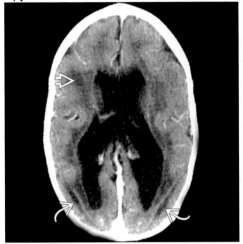

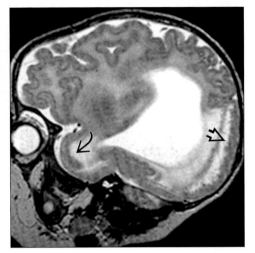

*(Left) Axial CECT shows diffuse pachygyria, abnormally low density of white matter ⇨ and bilateral focal cobblestone cortex of the posterior occipital cortex ⇨. (Right) Sagittal T2WI MR (same patient as previous image) shows FCMD phenotype with cobblestone cortex of the occipital ⇨ and temporal ⇨ lobes. The frontal cortex is dysplastic with microgyri.*

Typical

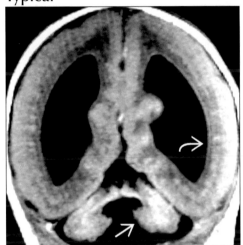

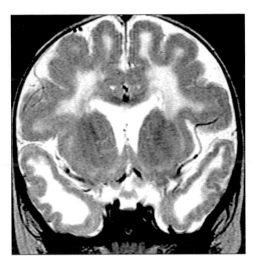

*(Left) Coronal T1WI MR (WWS phenotype) shows diffuse, symmetric cobblestone cortex of parietal and occipital ⇨ lobes. The cerebellum is small, vermis deficient and hemispheres ⇨ dysplastic. (Right) Coronal T2WI MR shows diffuse abnormally increased signal white matter and fronto-temporal cortical dysplasia typical of CMDs.*

Typical

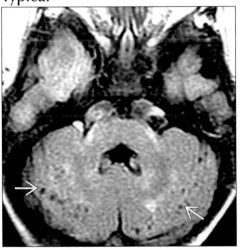

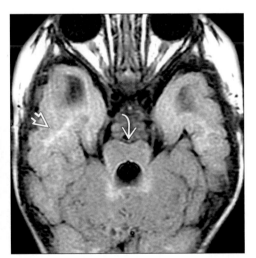

*(Left) Axial FLAIR MR shows multiple tiny cysts ⇨ throughout the cerebellar hemispheres. (Right) Axial FLAIR MR shows additional cysts, white matter hypersignal ⇨ and a notched pons ⇨.*

# NEURENTERIC CYST, INTRACRANIAL

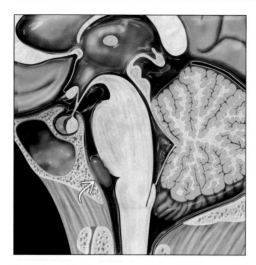

Sagittal graphic shows neurenteric cyst ➘, an ovoid mass situated anterior to the pontomedullary junction in the prepontine cistern.

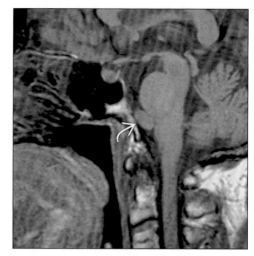

Sagittal T1WI MR shows an isointense ovoid mass ➘ situated anterior to the pontomedullary junction. The clivus immediately anterior to the mass has an unusual configuration.

## TERMINOLOGY

### Abbreviations and Synonyms
- Neurenteric cyst (NEC); enterogenous cyst

### Definitions
- Benign malformative endodermal CNS cyst

## IMAGING FINDINGS

### General Features
- Best diagnostic clue: Round/lobulated nonenhancing, slightly hyperintense [to cerebrospinal fluid (CSF)] mass in front of medulla, near pontomedullary junction
- Location
  - Spine > > brain
  - Most intracranial NECs found in posterior fossa
    - Common: Anterior to brainstem, cerebellopontine angle (CPA), clivus
    - Rare: Suprasellar, quadrigeminal cisterns; anterior fossa
- Size: Variable; usually < 2 cm

- Morphology: Smooth, lobulated, well-demarcated

### CT Findings
- CECT: Nonenhancing ventral iso- to slightly hyperdense mass

### MR Findings
- T1WI: Iso-/slightly hyperintense to CSF
- T2WI: Hyperintense to CSF
- PD/Intermediate: Hyperintense to CSF
- FLAIR: Hyperintense to CSF
- T1 C+: No enhancement

### Imaging Recommendations
- Best imaging tool: MR without, with contrast
- Protocol advice: FLAIR useful in distinguishing intracranial cysts

## DIFFERENTIAL DIAGNOSIS

### Epidermoid or Dermoid
- CPA most common site for epidermoid
- "White" epidermoid (rare) is hyperintense on T1WI, can be difficult to distinguish if midline

### DDx: Parapontine Masses

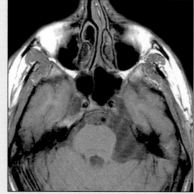

Arachnoid Cyst

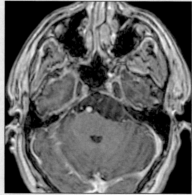

Epidermoid

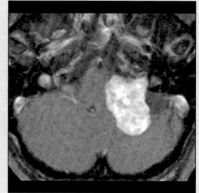

Schwannoma

# NEURENTERIC CYST, INTRACRANIAL

## Key Facts

### Terminology
- Benign malformative endodermal CNS cyst

### Imaging Findings
- Best diagnostic clue: Round/lobulated nonenhancing, slightly hyperintense [to cerebrospinal fluid (CSF)] mass in front of medulla, near pontomedullary junction
- Most intracranial NECs found in posterior fossa
- T1WI: Iso-/slightly hyperintense to CSF

- T2WI: Hyperintense to CSF
- FLAIR: Hyperintense to CSF
- T1 C+: No enhancement
- Protocol advice: FLAIR useful in distinguishing intracranial cysts

### Top Differential Diagnoses
- Epidermoid or Dermoid
- Arachnoid Cyst
- Schwannoma

---

### Arachnoid Cyst
- Like CSF on all sequences

### Schwannoma
- Enhances strongly; usually not midline

## PATHOLOGY

### General Features
- Etiology: Part of split spinal cord malformation spectrum; persistent neurenteric canal
- Epidemiology: Intracranial cases are very rare
- Associated abnormalities: Vertebral segmentation anomalies in 50% of spinal NECs

### Gross Pathologic & Surgical Features
- Transparent, thin-walled smooth round/lobulated cyst
- Contents vary from clear, colorless fluid (like CSF) to thicker, more viscous/mucoid

### Microscopic Features
- Contains mucin-secreting goblet cells

## CLINICAL ISSUES

### Presentation
- Most common signs/symptoms
  - Spine: Cord compression, myelopathy
  - Brain: Asymptomatic or headache

### Demographics
- Gender: M = F

### Natural History & Prognosis
- Stable or slowly enlarging

### Treatment
- Total surgical excision

## DIAGNOSTIC CHECKLIST

### Consider
- Nonenhancing midline mass ventral to brainstem, slightly hyperdense/intense to CSF may be NEC

### Image Interpretation Pearls
- Not all NECs associated with bony defects

## SELECTED REFERENCES

1. Tubbs RS et al: Neurenteric cyst: Case report and a review of the potential dysembryology. Clin Anat. 2005
2. Christov C et al: Giant supratentorial enterogenous cyst: Report of a case, literature review, and discussion of pathogenesis. Neurosurg 54:759-63, 2004
3. Agrawal D et al: Intramedullary neurenteric cyst presenting as infantile paraplegia: a case and review. Pediatr Neurosurg. 37(2):93-6, 2002
4. Gao P-Y et al: Neurenteric cysts: Pathology, imaging spectrum, differential diagnosis. INR 1: 17-27, 1995

I
8
49

## IMAGE GALLERY

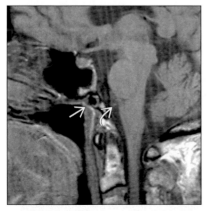
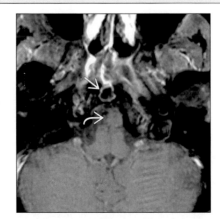
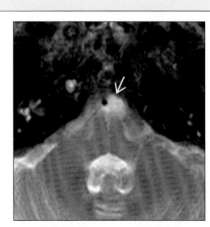

*(Left)* Sagittal T1WI MR shows the defect ➡ better in the clivus immediately anterior to the neurenteric cyst ➡. *(Center)* Axial T1 C+ MR shows the mass ➡ to be nonenhancing, remaining isointense to the brain stem. The defect in the clivus ➡ is better seen in this plane. *(Right)* Axial T2WI MR shows that the mass ➡ is hyperintense compared to brain tissue, contrasted by the hypointensity of the rapidly moving CSF surrounding it.

# ENCEPHALITIS (MISCELLANEOUS)

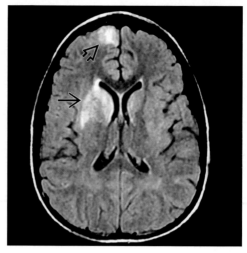

Axial T2WI MR shows typical findings of EBV encephalitis: Bilateral symmetric involvement of the caudate ➡; multifocal cortical swelling ➡; and periatrial hyperintensities.

Axial FLAIR MR in a patient with viral encephalitis shows asymmetric involvement, primarily in the right corpus striatum ➡ and in the right frontal pole ➡.

## TERMINOLOGY

### Definitions
- Diffuse brain parenchymal inflammation caused by a variety of pathogens, most commonly viruses
- Meningoencephalitis: Diffuse inflammation of the brain parenchyma and the meninges

## IMAGING FINDINGS

### General Features
- Best diagnostic clue
  - Abnormal T2 hyperintensity of gray matter (GM) ± white matter (WM), or deep gray nuclei
  - Large, poorly-delineated areas of involvement common, ± patchy hemorrhage
- Location
  - Cytomegalovirus (CMV): Periventricular WM
  - Epstein-Barr virus (EBV): Symmetric basal ganglia (BG), thalami, cortex or brainstem
  - Varicella-zoster virus (VZV)
    - Varicella: May affect multifocal areas of cortex; cerebellitis
    - Zoster: Brainstem/cortical GM, cranial nerves
  - Cerebellitis: Bilateral cerebellar hemispheres
  - Eastern equine encephalitis (EEE): BG, thalami, WM
  - Enteroviral encephalomyelitis (EV71)
    - EV71: Posterior medulla, pons, midbrain, dentate nuclei, spinal cord
    - Polio, coxsackie: Midbrain, anterior spinal cord
  - Hantavirus: Pituitary gland hemorrhage
  - Japanese encephalitis (influenza): Bilateral thalami, brainstem, cerebellum, spinal cord, cerebral cortex
  - Murray valley encephalitis (MVE): Bilateral thalami; may affect midbrain, cervical spinal cord
  - Rabies encephalitis: Brainstem, hippocampi, hypothalamus, WM, GM
  - Rhombencephalitis: Brainstem and cerebellum
  - St. Louis encephalitis: Substantia nigra
  - West Nile virus (WNV) (like polio): Cerebral white matter, brainstem, substantia nigra, anterior horn (cord), cerebellum

### CT Findings
- NECT: Initial CT negative or mild swelling in most patients

## DDx: Multifocal/Infiltrative Cerebral Processes

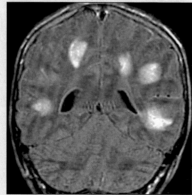

ADEM

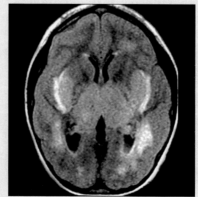

Leigh Disease

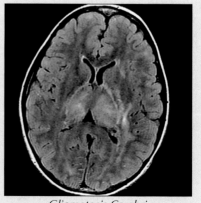

Gliomatosis Cerebri

# ENCEPHALITIS (MISCELLANEOUS)

## Key Facts

### Terminology
- Diffuse brain parenchymal inflammation caused by a variety of pathogens, most commonly viruses

### Imaging Findings
- Abnormal T2 hyperintensity of gray matter (GM) ± white matter (WM), or deep gray nuclei
- Large, poorly-delineated areas of involvement common, ± patchy hemorrhage
- NECT: Initial CT negative or mild swelling in most patients
- Best imaging tool: MR is most sensitive

### Top Differential Diagnoses
- Acute Disseminated Encephalomyelitis (ADEM)
- Ischemia
- Infiltrating Neoplasm

- Herpes Encephalitis
- Status Epilepticus
- Toxic/Metabolic Lesions

### Clinical Issues
- Varies widely: Slight meningeal to severe encephalitic symptoms, ± fever, prodrome
- Many encephalitides have high morbidity, mortality
- Rapid diagnosis, early treatment with antiviral or antibacterial agents can decrease mortality, may improve outcome

### Diagnostic Checklist
- Imaging often nonspecific
- Use MR for early diagnosis, differentiate from ADEM, toxic/metabolic disorders

## MR Findings
- T1WI
  - Japanese encephalitis: Low signal foci in WM, brainstem, BG, thalami bilaterally
  - Rabies encephalitis: Hyperintense bilateral BG, rare
- T2WI
  - CMV: Patchy increased signal in periventricular WM
  - EBV: Hyperintensity in BG, thalamus, cortex
  - Varicella: Multifocal increased cortical signal
  - Zoster: Increased signal in brainstem, cortex
  - Cerebellitis: Hyperintense cerebellar signal
  - EEE: Increased signal in BG & thalami; may involve brainstem, cortex, periventricular WM
  - EV71: Hyperintense lesions in posterior medulla, pons, midbrain, dentate nuclei of cerebellum
    - Less common: Cervical spinal cord, thalamus and putamen
  - Japanese encephalitis (influenza): High signal foci in WM, brainstem, BG, thalami bilaterally
  - MVE: Hyperintensity in bilateral thalami; may involve midbrain, cerebral peduncles
  - Rabies encephalitis: Ill-defined mild hyperintensity in brainstem, hippocampi, thalami, WM, BG
    - Paralytic rabies: Medulla and spinal cord hyperintensity
  - Rhombencephalitis: Patchy hyperintensity in pons, medulla, midbrain, ± cerebellum
  - St. Louis encephalitis: May see hyperintensity of substantia nigra; often normal
- T2* GRE: Japanese encephalitis: Thalamic hemorrhage
- DWI: Diffusion restriction is seen early in course of disease; not as prominent as seen in ischemia
- T1 C+
  - Variable enhancement: None to intense
  - Meningeal enhancement can be seen
  - Herpes zoster oticus (Ramsay Hunt syndrome): Enhancing CNs 7, 8, membranous labyrinth
- MRS: May help differentiate encephalitis from infarct

## Imaging Recommendations
- Best imaging tool: MR is most sensitive

- Protocol advice: Multiplanar MR with T1, T2, FLAIR, DWI and contrast

## DIFFERENTIAL DIAGNOSIS

### Acute Disseminated Encephalomyelitis (ADEM)
- Post infectious demyelination, 1-2 week latency
- WM > GM involvement, patchy or confluent; contrast enhancement unusual

### Ischemia
- Typical vascular distribution, DWI positive

### Infiltrating Neoplasm
- Typically unilateral disease
- Subacute onset

### Herpes Encephalitis
- Limbic system and temporal lobe involvement

### Status Epilepticus
- Active seizures with cerebral hyperperfusion, transient BBB disruption may cause abnormal signal, cortical swelling, enhancement

### Toxic/Metabolic Lesions
- Symmetric BG involvement common

## PATHOLOGY

### General Features
- General path comments
  - Herpes viruses include: HSV-1, HSV-2, CMV, EBV, VZV, B virus, HSV-6, HSV-7
  - Flaviviruses include: West Nile virus, Japanese encephalitis, St. Louis encephalitis virus, Murray valley encephalitis, Kunjin virus
  - Varicella: Meningoencephalitis, cerebellar ataxia, and aseptic meningitis (< 1% of patients)
  - Zoster infection: Encephalitis, neuritis, myelitis, or herpes ophthalmicus

# ENCEPHALITIS (MISCELLANEOUS)

- Immunocompetent patients: Cranial and peripheral nerve palsies
- Immunosuppressed patients: Diffuse encephalitis
○ Varicella-mediated angiitis: Delayed onset cerebral infarction (post-herpes zoster ophthalmicus, chickenpox)
○ EBV is the agent in infectious mononucleosis
- Diffuse encephalitis seen in < 1% of patients
- Associated with meningoencephalitis, Guillain-Barre syndrome, transverse myelitis
○ Enteroviruses include: Coxsackie viruses A & B, poliovirus, echoviruses, enteroviruses 68-71
○ Arboviruses (arthropod-borne viruses) include: Eastern, Western, & Venezuelan equine encephalitis, St. Louis encephalitis, Japanese B encephalitis, California encephalitis, tick-borne encephalitis
○ Nipah encephalitis: Paramyxovirus related to close contact with infected pigs
○ Cerebellitis: Most cases caused by a virus of the herpes family
○ Rhombencephalitis: Enteroviruses most commonly
- Etiology
○ Most (but not all) are caused by viruses
○ Viruses are obligate intracellular parasites
○ Replicate in skin or mucous membranes of respiratory, GI tracts
○ Spread of virus to CNS is hematogenous or neural
○ Some invade along CNs (i.e., HSV-1 via lingual nerve to trigeminal ganglia)
○ Latent infections may reactivate, spread along meningeal branches
○ Zoster: Latent virus in ganglia of CNs (often 5 & 7) can reactivate, spread to brainstem
○ Rabies: Reaches CNS by retrograde axoplasmic flow
○ Arboviruses are transmitted by mosquitoes and ticks
- Epidemiology
○ Viral nonseasonal: Herpes (most common), varicella-zoster, EBV, CMV, adenovirus, enterovirus, rabies
○ Viral seasonal: St. Louis, Western/Eastern equine; Japanese, Venezuelan

## Gross Pathologic & Surgical Features
- Vascular congestion, generalized or local edema, ± hemorrhage, necrosis

## Microscopic Features
- Infiltration by polymorphonuclear cells (PMNs), lymphocytes, plasma cells, and mononuclear cells
- Perivascular cuffing characteristic
- May see inclusion bodies (i.e., Negri bodies in rabies)

## CLINICAL ISSUES

### Presentation
- Most common signs/symptoms
○ Varies widely: Slight meningeal to severe encephalitic symptoms, ± fever, prodrome
○ Varicella and herpes zoster: Different clinical manifestations of infection by same virus (VZV)
○ Varicella encephalitis: Fever, headache, vomiting, seizures, altered mental status days-weeks after onset of (chicken-pox) rash

○ Zoster: Immunocompetent; CN & peripheral nerve palsies in dermatomes involved by skin lesions
- CN 5, Ophthalmic branch most affected (herpes zoster ophthalmicus)
- Rare complication: Contralateral hemiplegia related to cerebral angiitis and mycotic aneurysms
○ Zoster: Immunosuppressed patient with fever, meningismus, altered mental status
○ Cerebellitis: Sudden onset of limb and/or gait ataxia after infectious prodrome
○ Enterovirus encephalitis (EV71)
- Hand-foot-and-mouth disease (HFMD): Fever, vesicles on hands, feet, elbows, knees, lips
- Herpangina: Ulcers of palate and pharynx
- Cranial neuropathies, ocular disturbance, dyspnea, tachycardia if brainstem involved
○ MVE: Fever, headache, confusion, tremors; may progress to paralysis, coma, respiratory failure
○ Rabies
- Encephalitic: Fever, malaise, altered mental status, limbic dysfunction, autonomic stimulation signs
- Paralytic: Weakness of all extremities
○ Rhombencephalitis: Areflexia, ataxia, ophthalmoplegia
○ St. Louis encephalitis: Tremors, fevers
○ WNV: Can cause WN fever, or WN neuroinvasive disease (includes encephalitis, meningitis and acute flaccid paralysis)
- Clinical Profile
○ Variable
○ CSF studies often abnormal

## Natural History & Prognosis
- Many encephalitides have high morbidity, mortality
- Rapid diagnosis, early treatment with antiviral or antibacterial agents can decrease mortality, may improve outcome

## Treatment
- Dependent on etiology

## DIAGNOSTIC CHECKLIST

### Consider
- Imaging often nonspecific
- Use MR for early diagnosis, differentiate from ADEM, toxic/metabolic disorders

### Image Interpretation Pearls
- DWI may detect lesions earlier than conventional MR
- Post contrast FLAIR images best to detect superficial cortical inflammation

## SELECTED REFERENCES

1. Silvia MT et al: Pediatric central nervous system infections and inflammatory white matter disease. Pediatr Clin North Am. 52(4):1107-26, ix, 2005
2. Kennedy PG: Viral encephalitis: causes, differential diagnosis, and management. J Neurol Neurosurg Psychiatry. 75 Suppl 1:i10-5, 2004
3. Kleinschmidt-DeMasters BK et al: The expanding spectrum of herpesvirus infections of the nervous system. Brain Pathol. 11(4):440-51, 2001

# ENCEPHALITIS (MISCELLANEOUS)

## IMAGE GALLERY

Typical

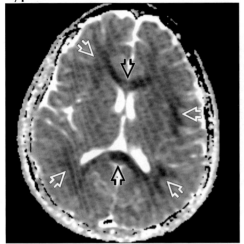 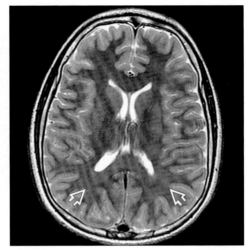

*(Left)* Axial ADC shows reduced diffusivity (low signal on ADC) in the corpus callosum ⇨ and asymmetrically in the subcortical white matter of the cerebral hemispheres ⇨. *(Right)* Axial T2WI MR (same patient as previous) shows subtle hyperintensity in the callosal splenium and the posterior white matter ⇨, but not anteriorly. MR study was performed within a day of admission.

Typical

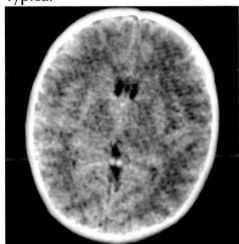 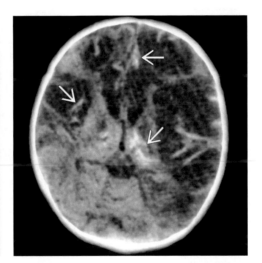

*(Left)* Axial NECT in a 3 week-old infant shows low attenuation throughout the cerebrum, including the basal ganglia and the thalami. Patient presented with 3 days of fever and new focal seizures. *(Right)* Axial NECT (same patient as previous) 3 weeks later shows diffuse, asymmetric liquefaction of cerebral mantle. Basal ganglia are atrophic. Foci of high attenuation ➔ likely represent calcification, ± hemorrhage.

Typical

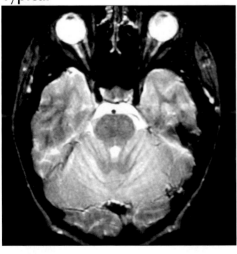 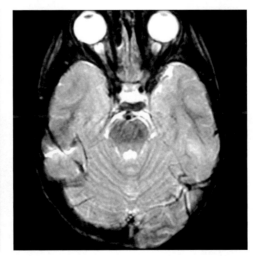

*(Left)* Axial T2WI MR shows diffuse cerebellar edema in a 15 year-old with viral cerebellitis. Cerebellar folia are obliterated. Cerebellar cortex is blurry, mildly hyperintense compared to cerebral cortex. *(Right)* Axial T2WI MR (same patient as previous) 3 years later shows resolution of the cerebellar swelling. Cerebellar folia are normally appreciated.

# TUBERCULOSIS

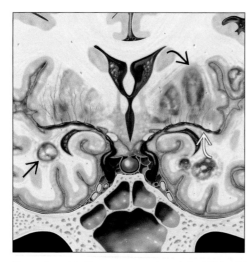

Coronal graphic illustrates narrowing of the MCAs ➘ from basilar meningitis, and resulting basal ganglia infarction ➔. Multiple granulomas ➔ are pictured.

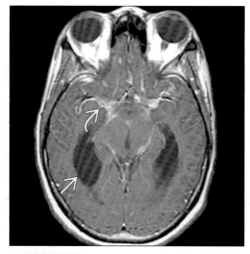

Axial T1 C+ MR shows diffuse meningeal enhancement with typical predilection for the basal cisterns ➘. Hydrocephalus is evident, with marked dilatation ➔ of the temporal horns.

## TERMINOLOGY

### Definitions
- Infection by Mycobacterium tuberculosis (TB), an acid-fast bacillus
- Typically causes tuberculous meningitis (TBM) and/or localized CNS infection, tuberculoma

## IMAGING FINDINGS

### General Features
- Best diagnostic clue
  - Basilar meningitis + extracerebral TB (pulmonary)
  - Meningitis + parenchymal lesions highly suggestive
- Location
  - TBM: Basal meningitis
  - Tuberculomas: Typically parenchymal
    - Infratentorial lesions are less common, can involve brainstem (up to 8%)
    - Dural tuberculomas may occur
- Size: Tuberculomas range from 1 mm to 6 cm (usually < 2 cm)
- Morphology

  - TBM: Thick basilar exudate
  - Tuberculoma: Round or oval mass
    - Solitary or multiple (more common)
- Associated findings
  - TB spondylitis (Pott disease)
    - Spine is most frequent osseous site
  - Less common sites: Calvarium (± dura), otomastoid
  - TB cervical adenitis: Child/young adult with pulmonary disease, conglomerate nodal neck mass

### CT Findings
- NECT
  - TBM: May be normal early (10-15%)
    - Isodense to hyperdense exudate effaces CSF spaces, fills basal cisterns, sulci
  - Tuberculoma
    - Hypodense to hyperdense round or lobulated nodule/mass with moderate to marked edema
    - Ca++ uncommon (approximately 20%)
- CECT
  - TBM: Intense basilar meningeal enhancement
  - Tuberculomas: Solid or ring-enhancing

## DDx: Disseminated CNS Lesions (Intra-/Extra-Axial)

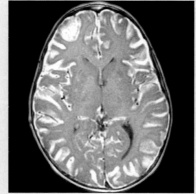

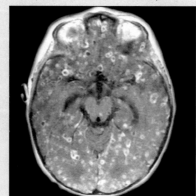

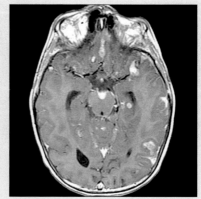

Disseminated Medulloblastoma | Profuse Cysticercosis | Metastatic Retinoblastoma

# TUBERCULOSIS

## Key Facts

### Terminology
- Typically causes tuberculous meningitis (TBM) and/or localized CNS infection, tuberculoma

### Imaging Findings
- Basilar meningitis + extracerebral TB (pulmonary)
- Meningitis + parenchymal lesions highly suggestive
- Tuberculomas: Typically parenchymal
- Tuberculomas: Solid or ring-enhancing

### Top Differential Diagnoses
- Meningitis
- Neurocysticercosis
- Abscess
- Neoplasm
- Neurosarcoidosis

### Pathology
- Childhood TB is typically a primary infection
- Most TB CNS infections accompany generalized miliary TB
- Meningitis is most frequent manifestation of CNS TB
- Reemerging disease (immigration from endemic areas, AIDS, drug resistant strains)
- In some countries, TB represents 10-30% of intracranial masses

### Clinical Issues
- Varies from mild meningitis with no neurologic deficit to comatose
- Long term morbidity up to 80%: Mental retardation, paralysis, seizures, rigidity, speech or visual deficits

---

- "Target sign": Central Ca++ or enhancement surrounded by enhancing rim (not pathognomonic for TB)

## MR Findings
- T1WI
  - TBM: Exudate isointense or hyperintense to CSF
  - Tuberculoma
    - Noncaseating granuloma: Hypointense to brain
    - Caseating granuloma with solid center: Hypointense or isointense to brain
    - Caseating granuloma with necrotic center: Hypointense or isointense to brain with central hypointensity
    - Caseating granulomas may have hyperintense rim (paramagnetic material)
- T2WI
  - TBM: Exudate is isointense or hyperintense to CSF; may see low signal nodules (rare)
  - Tuberculoma (noncaseating/caseating granulomas)
    - Noncaseating granuloma: Hyperintense to brain
    - Caseating granuloma with solid center: Iso- to hypointense with hypointense rim (hypointensity due to free radicals, solid caseation or increased cellular density)
    - Caseating granuloma with necrotic center: Central hyperintensity with hypointense rim
    - Hypointense rim + surrounding edema common
- FLAIR
  - TBM: Increased intensity in basal cisterns, sulci related to proteinaceous exudate
  - Tuberculoma: Similar to T2 characteristics
- DWI
  - May show hyperintense center of tuberculoma
  - Helpful for detecting complications (stroke, cerebritis)
- T1 C+
  - TBM: Marked meningeal enhancement, basilar prominence; may be nodular
    - Punctate/linear basal ganglia enhancement = vasculitis
    - Rare: Ventriculitis, choroid plexitis

- Rare: Pachymeningitis with dural thickening, enhancement (may mimic meningioma)
  - Tuberculomas
    - Noncaseating granuloma: Nodular, homogeneous enhancement
    - Caseating granuloma with solid center: Peripheral rim-enhancement
    - Caseating granuloma with necrotic center: Peripheral rim-enhancement, central low signal
- MRA: May see vessel narrowing, irregularity, occlusion
- MRS
  - TB abscess has prominent lipid, lactate but no amino acid resonances
    - Lipids at 0.9 ppm, 1.3 ppm, 2.0 ppm, 2.8 ppm
    - Mimics neoplasm, treated bacterial abscess
- Complications: Hydrocephalus, ischemia common
- Chronic changes: Atrophy, Ca++, chronic ischemia

## Angiographic Findings
- Conventional
  - Narrowing of major arteries at base of brain (supraclinoid ICA, M1, A1)
  - Narrowing and occlusion of small and/or medium sized arteries

## Imaging Recommendations
- Best imaging tool: MR is most sensitive to delineate extent and complications
- Protocol advice: Contrast-enhanced MR with FLAIR, DWI, ± MRA

# DIFFERENTIAL DIAGNOSIS

## Meningitis
- Infectious meningitis (bacterial, fungal, viral, parasitic)
  - Coccidioidomycosis, cryptococcus often basilar
- Carcinomatous meningitis (CNS or systemic primary)
  - Disseminated PNET, glioma most common

## Neurocysticercosis
- Single/multiple cystic lesions, ± ring-enhancement
- Look for scolex: Usually no basal meningitis

# TUBERCULOSIS

## Abscess
- Other granuloma, parasite, bacteria
- Pyogenic abscess often has more edema
- Classically T2 hypointense rim & DWI positive

## Neoplasm
- Single lesion, thick, nodular enhancing wall
- Typically more indolent onset, history may help

## Neurosarcoidosis
- Typically leptomeningeal and/or dural enhancement
- Rarely causes parenchymal nodules

## PATHOLOGY

### General Features
- General path comments
  - Childhood TB is typically a primary infection
  - Most TB CNS infections accompany generalized miliary TB
  - Meningitis is most frequent manifestation of CNS TB
- Etiology
  - TBM pathophysiology
    - Penetration of meningeal vessel walls by hematogenous spread
    - Rupture of subependymal or subpial granulomata into the CSF
  - Tuberculoma pathophysiology
    - Hematogenous spread (GM-WM junction lesions)
    - Extension of meningitis into parenchyma via cortical veins or small penetrating arteries
  - Arteries directly involved by basilar exudate or indirectly by reactive arteritis
    - Infection causes arterial spasm resulting in thrombosis and infarct
    - Lenticulostriate arteries, middle cerebral arteries (MCA), thalamoperforators most often affected
    - Infarcts most common in basal ganglia, thalami, cerebral cortex, pons, cerebellum
- Epidemiology
  - Incidence of TB in USA falling since 1993
  - Reemerging disease (immigration from endemic areas, AIDS, drug resistant strains)
  - In some countries, TB represents 10-30% of intracranial masses

### Gross Pathologic & Surgical Features
- TBM: Thick, gelatinous cisternal exudate
- Tuberculoma: Noncaseating, caseating with solid center, or caseating with necrotic center
  - Rarely progresses to TB abscess
  - Lobulated mass with thick rim, occurs in parenchyma, subarachnoid space, dura

### Microscopic Features
- TBM: Inflammatory cells, fragile neocapillaries
  - Caseous necrosis, chronic granulomas, endarteritis, perivascular inflammatory changes
- Tuberculoma
  - Early capsule: Peripheral fibroblasts, epithelioid cells, Langerhans giant cells, lymphocytes
  - Late capsule: Thick collagen layer; central liquefied caseating material in mature tuberculoma

## CLINICAL ISSUES

### Presentation
- Most common signs/symptoms
  - Varies from mild meningitis with no neurologic deficit to comatose
  - TBM: Fevers, confusion, headache, lethargy, meningismus
  - Tuberculoma: Seizures, increased intracranial pressure, papilledema
- Clinical Profile
  - LP: Increased protein, pleocytosis (lymphocytes), low glucose, negative for organisms
    - CSF positive on initial LP in < 40%
    - Mycobacteria grow slowly, culture 4-8 weeks
    - PCR for TB may help confirm diagnosis earlier
  - TB skin test may be negative, particularly early
  - Elevated erythrocyte sedimentation rate common

### Natural History & Prognosis
- Long term morbidity up to 80%: Mental retardation, paralysis, seizures, rigidity, speech or visual deficits
- Complications: Hydrocephalus (70%), stroke (up to 40%), cranial neuropathies (3, 4, 6 common), syrinx
- Tuberculomas may take months to years to resolve
  - Size of lesion determines healing time

### Treatment
- Untreated TBM can be fatal in as little as 3 weeks
- Multidrug therapy required: Isoniazid, rifampin, pyrazinamide, ± ethambutol or streptomycin
- Despite therapy, lesions may develop or increase
- Hydrocephalus typically requires CSF diversion

## DIAGNOSTIC CHECKLIST

### Consider
- TB often mimics other diseases like neoplasm

### Image Interpretation Pearls
- Combination of meningitis and parenchymal lesions suggests TB!

## SELECTED REFERENCES
1. Ranjan P et al: Serial study of clinical and CT changes in tuberculous meningitis. Neuroradiology. 45(5):277-82, 2003
2. Wasay M et al: Brain CT and MRI findings in 100 consecutive patients with intracranial tuberculoma. J Neuroimaging. 13(3):240-7, 2003
3. Pui MH et al: Magnetic resonance imaging findings in tuberculous meningoencephalitis. Can Assoc Radiol J. 52(1):43-9, 2001
4. Uysal G et al: Magnetic resonance imaging in diagnosis of childhood central nervous system tuberculosis. Infection. 29(3):148-53, 2001
5. Wallace RC et al: Intracranial tuberculosis in children: CT appearance and clinical outcome. Pediatr Radiol. 21(4):241-6, 1991

# TUBERCULOSIS

## IMAGE GALLERY

### Typical

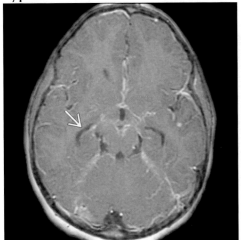
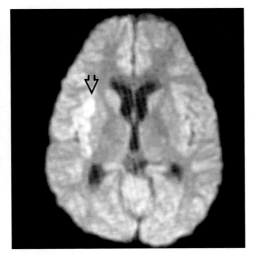

*(Left)* Axial T1 C+ MR shows meningeal enhancement in the cisterns around the mesencephalon. The temporal horns ➡ are dilated. *(Right)* Axial DWI MR in the same patient as previous image shows acute ischemic change in the right sylvian cortex ▷ secondary to the spasm/arteritis of the right MCA. Lateral and third ventricles are mildly dilated.

### Typical

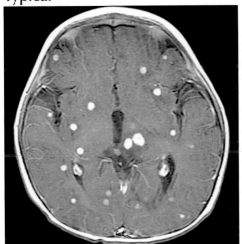
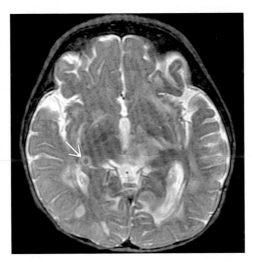

*(Left)* Axial T1 C+ MR in a 9 month old with disseminated miliary TB. Multiple enhancing granulomas are evident throughout the cerebral hemispheres, thalami. The meninges are normal. *(Right)* Axial T2WI MR in the same patient as previous image shows predominantly iso- to hypointense ➡ T2 signal within the center of the granulomas. A moderate amount of edema surrounds the granulomas.

### Typical

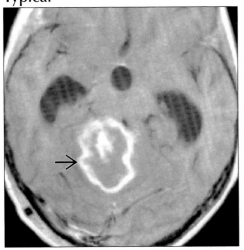
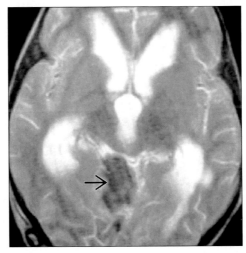

*(Left)* Axial T1 C+ MR of a caseating granuloma in the superior right cerebellum shows irregular rim-enhancement ➡ with central enhancing nodule ("target sign"). The mass causes obstructive hydrocephalus. *(Right)* Axial T2WI MR in the same patient as previous image shows marked hypointensity ➡ within the center of the mass, highly suggestive of a caseating tuberculoma.

# NEUROCYSTICERCOSIS

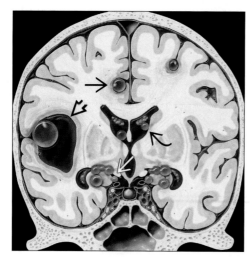

*Coronal graphic shows multiple cysts of NCC in various locations: Parenchymal ➔, intraventricular ➔, sylvian ➔ and parasellar/choroidal fissure ➔.*

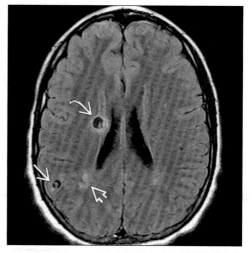

*Axial FLAIR MR shows a vesicular cyst with viable scolex ➔ and a cyst with early degeneration ➔. Ill-defined WM hyperintensities ➔ represent residual edema (late granular stage).*

## TERMINOLOGY

### Abbreviations and Synonyms
- Neurocysticercosis (NCC), cysticercosis

### Definitions
- Intracranial parasitic infection caused by the pork tapeworm, Taenia solium
- Four pathologic stages: Vesicular, colloidal vesicular, granular nodular, nodular calcified

## IMAGING FINDINGS

### General Features
- Best diagnostic clue: Cyst with "dot" inside
- Location
  - Convexity subarachnoid spaces most common
  - May involve cisterns > parenchyma > ventricles
  - Parenchymal cysts often hemispheric, at gray-white junction
  - Intraventricular cysts are often isolated
  - Basal cistern cysts may be racemose (multiple, grape-like)
  - Rare CNS locations: Sella, orbit, spinal cord
- Size
  - Cysts variable, typically 1 cm, range from 5-20 mm and contain a (1-4 mm) scolex
  - Parenchymal cysts 1 cm or less
  - Racemose subarachnoid cysts may be larger, up to 9 cm
- Morphology
  - Rounded or ovoid cyst, solitary in 20-50%
  - When multiple, usually small number of cysts
  - Disseminated form ("miliary" NCC) rare
  - Imaging varies with development stage, host response
  - Lesions may be at different stages in same patient
  - Inflammatory response around cyst may seal sulcus, make lesions appear intra-axial

### CT Findings
- NECT
  - Vesicular stage (viable larva): Smooth, thin-walled cyst, isodense to CSF, no edema
    - Hyperdense "dot" within cyst = protoscolex
  - Colloidal stage (degenerating larva): Hyperdense cyst fluid with surrounding edema

I
8

58

## DDx: Cystic Pediatric CNS Lesions

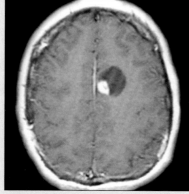

*Pilocytic Astrocytoma*

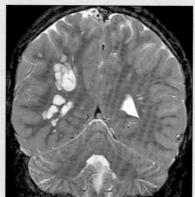

*Enlarged Virchow Robin Spaces*

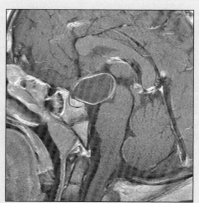

*Craniopharyngioma*

# NEUROCYSTICERCOSIS

## Key Facts

### Terminology
- Intracranial parasitic infection caused by the pork tapeworm, Taenia solium
- Four pathologic stages: Vesicular, colloidal vesicular, granular nodular, nodular calcified

### Imaging Findings
- Best diagnostic clue: Cyst with "dot" inside
- Convexity subarachnoid spaces most common
- May involve cisterns > parenchyma > ventricles
- Intraventricular cysts are often isolated
- Imaging varies with development stage, host response

### Top Differential Diagnoses
- Abscess
- Tuberculosis
- Neoplasm
- Arachnoid Cyst
- Enlarged Perivascular Spaces
- Other Parasitic Infection

### Pathology
- Cysticercosis is most common, most widely disseminated parasitic infection in the world
- CNS infection found in 60-90% of cysticercosis cases

### Clinical Issues
- Seizure, headaches, intracranial hypertension, hydrocephalus, learning disabilities
- Diagnosis confirmed by ELISA of serum or CSF
- Most common cause of epilepsy in endemic areas
- Oral albendazole (reduces parasitic burden, seizures) indicated in patients with viable NCC

---

- Granular (healing) stage: Mild edema
- Nodular calcified (healed) stage: Small, Ca++ nodule
- CECT
  - Vesicular stage: No (or mild) wall enhancement
  - Colloidal stage: Thicker ring-enhancing fibrous capsule
  - Granular stage: Involuting enhancing nodule
  - Nodular calcified stage: Shrunken, calcified nodule
- Subarachnoid lesions: Multiple isodense cysts without scolex, may cause meningitis
- Intraventricular cysts not well seen on CT, may see hydrocephalus

### MR Findings
- T1WI
  - Vesicular stage: Cystic lesion isointense to CSF
    - May see discrete, eccentric scolex (hyperintense)
  - Colloidal stage: Cyst is mildly hyperintense to CSF
  - Granular stage: Thickened, retracted cyst wall; edema decreases
  - Nodular calcified stage: Difficult to detect
- T2WI
  - Vesicular stage: Cystic lesion isointense to CSF
    - May see discrete, eccentric scolex
    - No surrounding edema
  - Colloidal stage: Cyst is hyperintense to CSF
    - Surrounding edema, mild to marked
  - Granular stage: Thickened, retracted cyst wall; edema decreases
  - Nodular calcified stage: Shrunken, Ca++ lesion
- FLAIR
  - Vesicular stage: Cystic lesion isointense to CSF
    - May see discrete, eccentric scolex (hyperintense to CSF); no edema
  - Colloidal stage: Cyst is hyperintense to CSF
    - Surrounding edema, mild to marked
  - Useful to detect intraventricular cysts (hyperintense)
  - 100% inspired oxygen increases conspicuity
- T2* GRE: Will often miss small calcified nodules
- DWI: Cystic lesion typically isointense to CSF
- T1 C+
  - Vesicular stage: No enhancement typical, may see mild enhancement

- May see discrete, eccentric scolex enhancement
  - Colloidal stage: Thick cyst wall enhances
    - Enhancing marginal nodule (scolex)
  - Granular stage: Thickened, retracted cyst wall; may have nodular or ring-enhancement
  - Nodular calcified stage: Rare minimal enhancement
- MRS: Few reports show elevated lactate, alanine, succinate, choline; decreased NAA and Cr
- May see "encephalitic cysticercosis" with multiple small enhancing lesions and diffuse edema: More common in children than in adults
- Intraventricular cysts may cause ventriculitis and/or hydrocephalus
- Cisternal NCC may appear racemose (multilobulated, grape-like): Lacks scolex
  - Complications: Meningitis, hydrocephalus, vasculitis

### Imaging Recommendations
- Best imaging tool
  - MR >> CT in identification of extraparenchymal NCC (intraventricular, basal subarachnoid)
  - CT >> MR in detections of calcified nodules
- Protocol advice
  - MR with T1, T2, FLAIR, GRE, contrast
  - Thin (< 3 mm) slices to identify scolex

## DIFFERENTIAL DIAGNOSIS

### Abscess
- Typically T2 hypointense rim and reduced diffusion
- Multiple lesions may occur related to septic emboli

### Tuberculosis
- Tuberculomas often occur with meningitis
- Typically not cystic
- Lipid peak may be seen with MRS

### Neoplasm
- Juvenile pilocytic astrocytoma: Cystic mass with mural nodule

# NEUROCYSTICERCOSIS

- Craniopharyngioma: Can present as primarily cystic suprasellar mass
- Hemangioblastoma: Rare in absence of von Hippel Lindau

## Arachnoid Cyst
- Solitary lesion with CSF density/intensity
- No enhancement

## Enlarged Perivascular Spaces
- Follow CSF on all MR sequences
- No enhancement

## Other Parasitic Infection
- May be cystic, but no scolex seen

## PATHOLOGY

### General Features
- General path comments
  - Four pathologic stages
    - Vesicular, colloidal, granular, nodular calcified
  - Vesicular stage: Larva is a small marginal nodule projecting into small cyst with clear fluid
    - Viable parasite with little or no inflammation
    - May remain in this stage for years or degenerate
  - Colloidal stage: Larva begins to degenerate
    - Scolex shows hyaline degeneration, slowly shrinks
    - Cyst fluid becomes turbid and capsule thickens
    - Surrounding edema and inflammation
  - Granular stage: Cyst wall thickens and scolex is transformed into coarse mineralized granules
    - Surrounding edema regresses
  - Nodular calcified stage: Lesion is completely mineralized and small; no edema
  - Racemose cysts: Multilocular, nonviable cysts; no scolex
    - Can be several cms in size
    - CP angle, suprasellar region, sylvian fissure, basilar cisterns
- Etiology
  - Caused by larval form of pig tapeworm, T solium
  - Man is intermediate host in life cycle of tapeworm
    - Ingestion of eggs from contaminated water, food
    - From GI tract, primary larvae (oncospheres) disseminate into CNS and skeletal muscle
    - Once intracranial, primary develop into secondary larvae, cysticerci
  - Man can also be the definitive host (infected with tapeworm)
    - Typically from uncooked pork that contain larval cysts
    - Larval cysts develop into adult worms in human intestine
    - Creates a symptom-free (most commonly) tapeworm carrier in the household
- Epidemiology
  - Cysticercosis is most common, most widely disseminated parasitic infection in the world
  - CNS infection found in 60-90% of cysticercosis cases
  - Endemic in many countries (Latin America, parts of Asia, India, Africa, Eastern Europe)

- Increased migration and travel have spread disease to high-income countries

## CLINICAL ISSUES

### Presentation
- Most common signs/symptoms
  - Seizure, headaches, intracranial hypertension, hydrocephalus, learning disabilities
  - Varies with organism, development stage, host immune response
  - NCC asymptomatic until larvae degenerate
- Clinical Profile
  - Most common parasitic infection worldwide
  - Diagnosis confirmed by ELISA of serum or CSF

### Demographics
- Ethnicity: In US, Latin American patients most commonly seen

### Natural History & Prognosis
- Most common cause of epilepsy in endemic areas
- Variable time from initial infection until symptoms, 6 months to 30 years, typically 2-5 years
- Variable time to progress through pathologic stages, 1-9 years, mean 5 years
- Subarachnoid disease may be complicated by meningitis, vasculitis and hydrocephalus
- Intraventricular NCC has increased morbidity and mortality
  - Increased morbidity related to acute obstructive hydrocephalus

### Treatment
- Oral albendazole (reduces parasitic burden, seizures) indicated in patients with viable NCC
- Steroids often required to decrease edema during medical therapy
- Surgical excision or drainage of parenchymal lesions may be required
- Endoscopic resection of intraventricular lesions in selected cases

## DIAGNOSTIC CHECKLIST

### Consider
- Complex parasitic cysts may mimic brain tumor

### Image Interpretation Pearls
- FLAIR and T1WI helpful to identify scolex and intraventricular lesions

## SELECTED REFERENCES

1. Garcia HH et al: Neurocysticercosis: updated concepts about an old disease. Lancet Neurol. 4(10):653-61, 2005
2. Jayakumar PN et al: MRI and in vivo proton MR spectroscopy in a racemose cysticercal cyst of the brain. Neuroradiology. 46:72-4, 2004
3. Zee CS et al: Imaging of neurocysticercosis. Neuroimaging Clin N Am. 10(2):391-407, 2000

## IMAGE GALLERY

### Typical

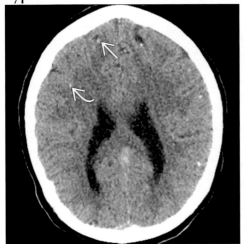
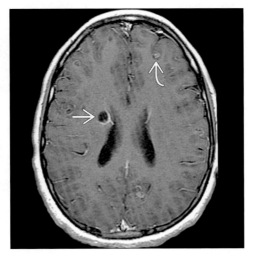

*(Left)* Axial NECT shows multiple small calcifications ➨, located primarily in the cortex/depths of sulci, typical of the nodular stage. A calcified granular lesion ➨ is also present. *(Right)* Axial T1 C+ MR in the same patient as previous image at the same level (different angulation), shows NCC in the vesicular ➨ and granular ➨ stages. The calcifications seen on CT are not appreciated.

### Typical

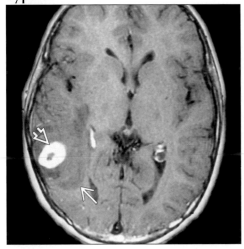
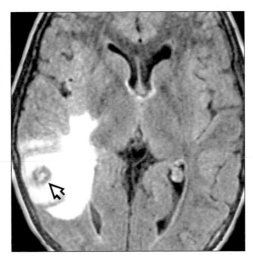

*(Left)* Axial T1 C+ MR shows a large, thick rimmed, enhancing lesion ➨ with surrounding vasogenic edema ➨. Unless the scolex is observed, this mass is not easily differentiated from a tuberculoma. *(Right)* Axial FLAIR MR in the same patient as previous image better demonstrates the extensive vasogenic edema surrounding the lesion. No scolex can be seen in this degenerating colloidal cysticercosis ➨.

### Typical

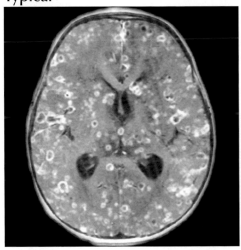
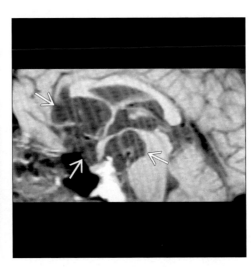

*(Left)* Axial T1 C+ MR in a one year old shows innumerable small ring and dot-size enhancing lesions typical of profuse NCC. This one year old presented with macrocephaly and encephalopathy. *(Right)* Sagittal T1WI MR shows multiple cysts ➨ with marked mass effect filling the basal cisterns, typical of racemose (grape-like) neurocysticercosis. No scolex is identifiable.

# PARASITES, MISCELLANEOUS

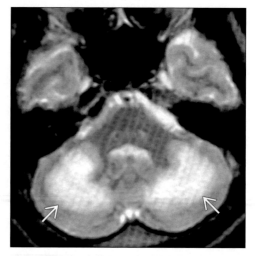

Axial CECT shows typical involvement of the thalami ➡ by malaria. Symmetric, bilateral thalamic hypodensity is evident, with mass effect. There is no contrast enhancement.

Axial T2WI MR shows typical involvement of the cerebellum by malaria. Symmetric, bilateral hemispheric ➡ T2 bright abnormalities are seen, extending into the middle cerebellar peduncles.

## TERMINOLOGY

### Definitions
- Parasitic infection affecting the CNS

## IMAGING FINDINGS

### General Features
- Best diagnostic clue: Enhancing supratentorial mass, may be multiloculated
- Location
  - Majority of parasitic infections are supratentorial
  - Malaria: Predilection for basal ganglia, cortex
  - Echinococcus: Parietal lobe common; MCA territory
  - Amebic encephalitis: Supratentorial, frontal lobes and basal ganglia
  - Paragonimiasis: Hemispheric, commonly posterior
- Morphology
  - Malaria: Punctate and ring hemorrhages, infarcts, cerebral edema
  - Echinococcosis: Large uni- or multilocular cyst ± detached germinal membrane, daughter cysts, no edema

- Amebic encephalitis: Meningoencephalitis; single or multiple focal, nodular or ring-enhancing masses
- Paragonimiasis: Acutely may cause hemorrhage or infarct, followed later by granuloma formation
  - In chronic stage, round and ovoid Ca++ in mass
- Schistosomiasis: Granulomatous encephalitis, hyperintense mass, enhancing dots along linear area
- Sparganosis: Conglomerate, multicystic mass with surrounding edema
- Trichinosis: Eosinophilic meningoencephalitis, vascular thrombi, infarcts
- Trypanosomiasis: Meningoencephalitis ⇒ brain edema, congestion, petechial hemorrhages

### CT Findings
- NECT
  - Malaria: 4 patterns, correlate with disease severity
    - Normal
    - Diffuse cerebral edema
    - Focal infarct: Cortex, basal ganglia, thalamus, pons, cerebellum; ± hemorrhage
    - Bilateral thalamic and cerebellar hypodensity
  - Echinococcus: Unilocular or multilocular cyst, isodense to CSF, no edema; Ca++ rare, < 1%

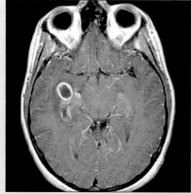
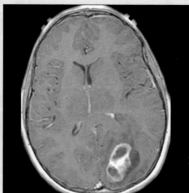
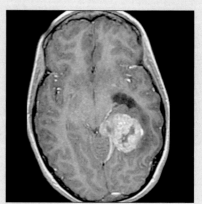

## DDx: Enhancing Cerebral Masses

*Pyogenic Abscess*  *Pilocytic Astrocytoma*  *Ependymoma*

# PARASITES, MISCELLANEOUS

## Key Facts

### Imaging Findings
- Majority of parasitic infections are supratentorial
- Malaria: Punctate and ring hemorrhages, infarcts, cerebral edema
- Echinococcosis: Large uni- or multilocular cyst ± detached germinal membrane, daughter cysts, no edema
- Amebic encephalitis: Meningoencephalitis; single or multiple focal, nodular or ring-enhancing masses
- Paragonimiasis: Acutely may cause hemorrhage or infarct, followed later by granuloma formation
- Schistosomiasis: Granulomatous encephalitis, hyperintense mass, enhancing dots along linear area
- Trichinosis: Eosinophilic meningoencephalitis, vascular thrombi, infarcts

- Trypanosomiasis: Meningoencephalitis ⇒ brain edema, congestion, petechial hemorrhages

### Top Differential Diagnoses
- Neoplasm
- Abscess
- Neurocysticercosis
- Porencephalic Cyst
- Arachnoid Cyst

### Diagnostic Checklist
- Complex conglomerated parasitic cysts of any etiology may mimic brain tumor!
- Patient's travel history is often key to diagnosis

---

- ○ Amebic encephalitis: Diffuse edema
- ○ Paragonimiasis: Multiple conglomerated granulomas, ± hemorrhage
  - ■ Multiple round or oval calcifications ("soap bubble" appearance), surrounding low density, cortical atrophy, ventriculomegaly
- ○ Schistosomiasis: Single or multiple hyperdense lesions with edema, mass effect
- ○ Sparganosis: Conglomerate, multicystic mass with surrounding edema; ± Ca++
  - ■ Atrophy, ventricular dilatation in chronic cases
- ○ Trichinosis: Hypodense white matter lesions, cortical infarcts
- ○ Trypanosomiasis: Edema with scattered petechial hemorrhage
- CECT
  - ○ Echinococcus: No enhancement typical
  - ○ Amebic encephalitis: Single or multiple focal, punctate, nodular or ring-enhancing masses
  - ○ Paragonimiasis: Ring-enhancement
  - ○ Trichinosis: Ring-enhancing lesions
  - ○ Sparganosis: Irregular/multilocular enhancing mass with surrounding edema

## MR Findings
- T1WI
  - ○ Amebic encephalitis: Centrally hypointense mass
  - ○ Echinococcus: Cyst isointense to CSF
- T2WI
  - ○ Malaria: Cortical and white matter ischemia, hyperintense
    - ■ Deep gray nuclei and cerebellar hyperintensity
  - ○ Echinococcus: Cyst isointense to CSF with hypointense rim; no perilesional edema
  - ○ Amebic encephalitis: Hyperintense lesions, ± hemorrhage
    - ■ May have hypointense rim
  - ○ Paragonimiasis: Heterogeneous mass with surrounding edema, ± hemorrhage
    - ■ May have isointense or hypointense rim
  - ○ Schistosomiasis: Hyperintense mass with surrounding edema

- ○ Sparganosis: Conglomerate, multicystic mass with surrounding edema, ± hemorrhage
  - ■ May see mixed signal lesion, central low signal and peripheral high signal
  - ■ Unilateral white matter degeneration, cortical atrophy in chronic cases
- T1 C+
  - ○ Echinococcus: No enhancement typical; may see fine peripheral enhancement
  - ○ Amebic encephalitis: Heterogeneous or ring-enhancement
  - ○ Paragonimiasis: Conglomerated, multiple ring-enhancing lesions
    - ■ Chronic: Atrophy and calcification
  - ○ Schistosomiasis: Central linear enhancement surrounded by multiple punctate nodules, arborized appearance
  - ○ Sparganosis: Variable; pattern may change on follow-up related to worm migration

## Imaging Recommendations
- Best imaging tool
  - ○ Contrast MR is most sensitive for detection
  - ○ CT may be helpful to identify associated Ca++
- Protocol advice: Contrast-enhanced MR

## DIFFERENTIAL DIAGNOSIS

### Neoplasm
- Primary CNS, rarely metastatic
- Cyst with mural nodule vs. solid mass

### Abscess
- T2 hypointense rim and ↓ diffusion typical
- Ring-enhancement, thinner on ventricular margin

### Neurocysticercosis
- Cyst with marginal scolex
- Multiple lesions common

### Porencephalic Cyst
- Encephalomalacia ± surrounding gliosis
- Often communicates with ventricle

# PARASITES, MISCELLANEOUS

## Arachnoid Cyst
- Nonenhancing solitary lesion with CSF density/intensity

# PATHOLOGY

## General Features
- General path comments: Findings depend on number, size, stage of infection
- Etiology
  - Malaria: Infection of erythrocytes by P. falciparum
    - Vascular occlusion of capillaries by infected erythrocytes
  - Echinococcus (hydatid disease) is caused by E. granulosis most commonly and E. multilocularis
    - Dogs or other carnivores are definitive hosts
    - Sheep or cattle are intermediate hosts
    - Humans are secondarily infected by ingestion of food or water contaminated with parasite eggs
    - Parasite from GI tract to portal system, lymphatics
    - Infection usually occurs in liver and lungs
  - Amebic encephalitis: Entamoeba histolytica, Naegleria fowleri, Acanthamoeba most common
    - Infection from swimming in contaminated freshwater lake or inhaling dust or soil with amebic cysts
    - Ascends along olfactory tract to brain or hematogenous spread
  - Paragonimiasis: Ingestion of undercooked fresh water crabs or crayfish contaminated with Westermani flukes (lung fluke)
    - Worms penetrate skull base foramina and meninges and directly invade brain parenchyma
  - Schistosomiasis: Infestation from trematode (fluke) worms
    - Host is freshwater snail
    - Humans affected through skin
    - Migrates to lungs and liver, reach venous system
  - Sparganosis: Ingestion of contaminated water or food (snake, frogs)
  - Trichinosis: Ingestion of uncooked meat containing infective encysted larvae
  - Trypanosomiasis: African (sleeping sickness) and American (Chaga disease)
    - African: Transmitted to humans by tsetse fly; invades meninges, subarachnoid space
    - American: Transmitted by reduviid bugs
- Epidemiology: Increased travel, immigration have spread diseases

## Gross Pathologic & Surgical Features
- Malaria: Ischemia, edema, petechial hemorrhage
- Echinococcus: Cysts (4-10 cm) with thick, smooth wall
  - Cyst wall composed of 3 layers: Host forms outer fibrous layer (pericyst), middle laminated membrane layer, inner germinal layer (produces scolex)
- Amebic encephalitis: Cerebral edema, hemorrhage, necrosis, meningeal exudate
- Paragonimiasis: Cystic lesions elaborate toxins that result in infarction, meningitis, adhesions
- Sparganosis: Live worm or degenerated worm with surrounding granuloma found at surgery

- Trichinosis: Eosinophilic meningoencephalitis, ischemic lesions, petechial hemorrhage, necrosis
- Trypanosomiasis: Edema, congestion, hemorrhage

# CLINICAL ISSUES

## Presentation
- Most common signs/symptoms
  - Malaria: Altered consciousness, seizures
  - Echinococcus: Mass effect related to lesion location
- Clinical Profile
  - Varies with organism, development stage, host immune response
  - ELISA studies can be helpful in some diseases

## Demographics
- Age
  - Children between 6 months and 5 years particularly susceptible to CNS malaria
  - Peak incidence of CNS hydatid disease: 5-10 years
  - CNS paragonimiasis especially common in adolescent males

## Natural History & Prognosis
- Some parasitic infections (e.g., echinococcosis) develop slowly over many years
- Malaria: Most common cause of death from parasites
  - 15-25% mortality despite appropriate therapy
  - Neurocognitive impairments common in children who survive
- Echinococcus complicated by rupture, hemorrhage, secondary infection
- Amebiasis: Second cause of death from parasites
- Trichinosis: Mortality in 5-10% of affected individuals
- Trypanosomiasis, American: Mortality 2-10% if meningoencephalitis

## Treatment
- Variable, ranges from oral therapy to lesion resection

# DIAGNOSTIC CHECKLIST

## Consider
- Complex conglomerated parasitic cysts of any etiology may mimic brain tumor!
- Patient's travel history is often key to diagnosis

# SELECTED REFERENCES

1. Idro R et al: Pathogenesis, clinical features, and neurological outcome of cerebral malaria. Lancet Neurol. 4(12):827-40, 2005
2. Klion AD et al: The role of eosinophils in host defense against helminth parasites. J Allergy Clin Immunol. 113(1):30-7, 2004
3. Polat P et al: Hydatid disease from head to toe. Radiographics. 23(2):475-94; quiz 536-7, 2003
4. Lowichik A et al: Parasitic infections of the central nervous system in children. Part II: Disseminated infections. J Child Neurol. 10(2):77-87, 1995
5. Lowichik A et al: Parasitic infections of the central nervous system in children. Part III: Space-occupying lesions. J Child Neurol. 10(3):177-90, 1995

# PARASITES, MISCELLANEOUS

## IMAGE GALLERY

### Typical

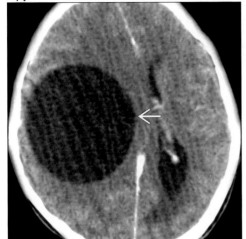

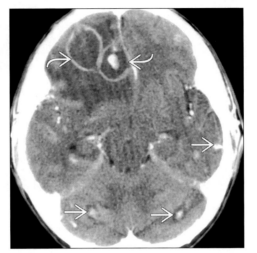

*(Left)* Axial CECT of echinococcus. A unilocular cyst ➡ is present in the right cerebral hemisphere, with no surrounding edema or enhancement. The mass causes subfalcine herniation to the left. *(Right)* Axial CECT of amebic encephalitis. Multiple punctate ➡ and ring-enhancing lesions ➡ are seen in the cerebellum and cerebrum. Edema and mass effect accompany multiple lesions.

### Typical

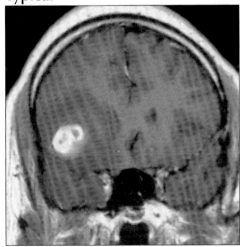

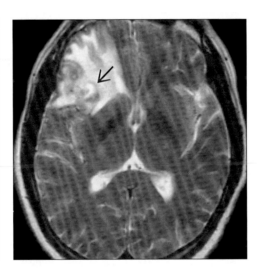

*(Left)* Coronal T1 C+ MR in a patient from East Asia with paragonimiasis. The right frontal mass displays conglomerated, ring-enhancement and surrounding edema. It mimics a neoplasm. *(Right)* Axial T2WI MR in the same patient as previous image shows the heterogeneous lesion with mass effect and marked surrounding edema. The hypointense rim ➡ is typical of paragonimiasis.

### Typical

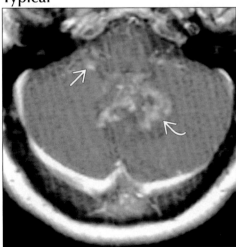

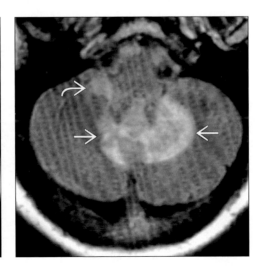

*(Left)* Axial T1 C+ MR in a patient with schistosomiasis. Irregular punctate enhancement is evident in the inferior cerebellum ➡ and in the right flocculus ➡. *(Right)* Axial FLAIR MR (same patient as previous image) shows edema surrounding a hyperintense inflammatory mass ➡. The lesion extends towards the flocculus where a smaller nodular mass ➡ is identified.

I
8

65

# LEIGH SYNDROME

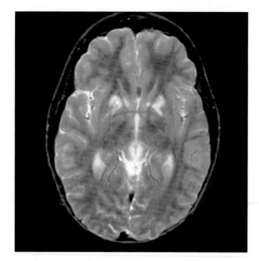

Axial T2WI MR shows abnormal T2 prolongation in the caudate heads, putamina, and the periaqueductal gray matter, classic foci of involvement for Leigh syndrome due to pyruvate dehydrogenase deficiency.

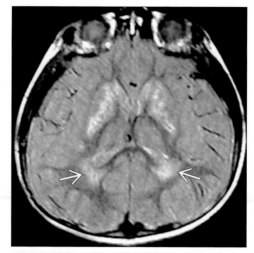

Axial FLAIR MR shows abnormal hyperintensity in the peritrigonal white matter ➡ as well as the basal ganglia, another common pattern in Leigh syndrome due to pyruvate dehydrogenase deficiency.

## TERMINOLOGY

### Abbreviations and Synonyms
- Leigh syndrome (LS)
- Subacute necrotizing encephalomyelopathy

### Definitions
- Genetically heterogeneous mitochondrial disorder characterized by progressive neurodegeneration

## IMAGING FINDINGS

### General Features
- Best diagnostic clue: Bilateral, symmetric ↑ T2/FLAIR putamina and peri-aqueductal gray matter (PAG)
- Location
  - Common
    - Basal ganglia (BG): Corpora striata (putamina > caudate heads) > globi pallidi (GP)
    - Brain stem (BS): PAG, substantia nigra/subthalamic nuclei, central tegmental tract
    - Thalami, cerebellar dentate nuclei
  - Infrequent: White matter (WM, cerebral > cerebellar), spine, cortical gray matter
- Size
  - BS: Small, discrete foci (< 1 cm), central tegmental tracts
  - BG: Caudate/putamina involvement classic but variable
  - Thalami: Focal involvement dorsomedial nuclei classic but variable
- Morphology
  - Except WM, lesions are bilaterally symmetric
  - Edema characteristic of early disease; volume loss characteristic of late disease
    - PAG edema may cause hydrocephalus
  - Involvement of lower BS (pons, medulla) and lack of BG involvement characteristic of LS 2° to complex IV involvement
  - Uncommon appearances
    - Mass-like BS involvement (especially PAG)
    - Predominant WM disease (simulates leukodystrophy)

### CT Findings
- NECT: Hypodense; occasionally normal

## DDx: Basal Ganglia Lesions

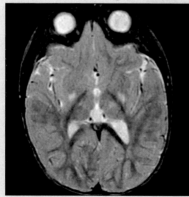

Neonatal HIE

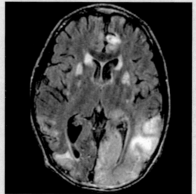

MELAS

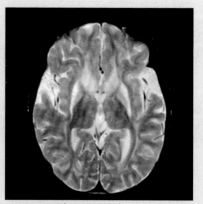

Glutaric Aciduria I

# LEIGH SYNDROME

## Key Facts

### Terminology
- Genetically heterogeneous mitochondrial disorder characterized by progressive neurodegeneration

### Imaging Findings
- Best diagnostic clue: Bilateral, symmetric ↑ T2/FLAIR putamina and peri-aqueductal gray matter (PAG)

### Top Differential Diagnoses
- Profound Perinatal Asphyxia: Request Birth History
- Mitochondrial Encephalopathy, Lactic Acidosis, Stroke-Like Episodes (MELAS)
- Glutaric Aciduria Type I (GA-1)
- Wilson Disease

### Pathology
- LS characterized by extreme genetic heterogeneity

- Autosomal recessive (AR), X-linked, and maternal inheritance of mutated proteins involved in mitochondrial energy production underlie LS
- Bioenergetic failure (ATP loss) and production reactive oxygen species likely key factors
- LS in children < 6 years of age: 1:32,000 (most common mitochondrial disease in this age group)

### Clinical Issues
- Presentation: Psychomotor delay/regression, hypotonia
- Majority present by age 2
- Childhood & adult presentations uncommon
- Natural history: Progressive neurodegeneration leading to respiratory failure and death in childhood
- No curative treatment

---

- CECT: Enhancement uncommon

## MR Findings
- T1WI
  - Hypointense
    - Hyperintensity suggests blood or myelin degradation products
- T2WI: Hyperintense
- FLAIR
  - Hyperintense
    - Resolution of signal abnormality or cystic necrosis (hypointense) may be seen in chronic disease
- DWI: Reduced diffusivity in acutely affected areas
- T1 C+: Enhancement uncommon
- MRS: ↑ Choline, ↓ NAA, (+) lactate

## Ultrasonographic Findings
- Hyperechoic deep gray structures, WM

## Imaging Recommendations
- Best imaging tool: MR with DWI/MRS
- Protocol advice: MRS obtained in BG

## DIFFERENTIAL DIAGNOSIS

### Profound Perinatal Asphyxia: Request Birth History
- ↑ T2 & T1 dorsolateral putamina, lateral thalami, dorsal BS, peri-Rolandic cortex
  - T1 hyperintensity seen in first week

### Mitochondrial Encephalopathy, Lactic Acidosis, Stroke-Like Episodes (MELAS)
- ↑ T2/FLAIR putamina: May be asymmetric/unilateral
- Stroke-like signal abnormality parietal-occipital lobes
  - Non-vascular distribution and (-) DWI typical

### Glutaric Aciduria Type I (GA-1)
- ↑ T2/FLAIR corpora striata, GP, +/- WM disease
- Characteristic widening of sylvian fissures

### Wilson Disease
- ↑ T2/FLAIR putamina, GP, midbrain, thalami
  - T2 changes evident older children, teens
- ↑ T1 GP 2° to hepatic failure in younger children

### Other Organic Acidopathies: Propionic Acidemia, 3-Methylglutaconic Aciduria, etc.
- Differentiate by clinical, laboratory features

## PATHOLOGY

### General Features
- General path comments
  - 50-75% patients with LS have detectable biochemical or molecular abnormality
  - Embryology-anatomy
    - Main role mitochondria: Production ATP via oxidative phosphorylation
    - Hundreds to thousands mitochondria/cell (↑ where ↑ energy requirements)
    - Mitochondria contain own DNA (mtDNA, average of 5 mtDNA per mitochondrion)
    - mtDNA contribution to zygote exclusively from oocyte (maternal inheritance)
    - Mitochondria/mtDNA randomly distributed among daughter cells
    - MtDNA and nuclear DNA (nDNA) encode subunits of electron transport chain (ETC) complexes (COs) I, III-V (nuclear DNA encodes all subunits of CO II)
  - Brain & striated muscle highly dependent on oxidative phosphorylation ⇒ most severely affected in mitochondrial disorders
  - Variable number of mitochondria/cell, and random distribution mitochondria/mtDNA into daughter cells account for phenotypic heterogeneity typical of all mitochondrial disorders
- Genetics
  - LS characterized by extreme genetic heterogeneity

# LEIGH SYNDROME

○ Autosomal recessive (AR), X-linked, and maternal inheritance of mutated proteins involved in mitochondrial energy production underlie LS

- Mutations frequently involve ETC COs I-V leading to CO deficiencies
- AR: Mutation SURF1 gene (9q34) is most frequent cause of LS due to CO IV (cytochrome C oxidase, COX) deficiency
- Other AR mutations: NDUFV1/NDUFS8 (11q13), NDUFS4 (5q11.1) NDUFS7 genes ⇒ CO I deficiency; NDUFS3 gene ⇒ NADH dehydrogenase deficiency; SDHA gene (5p15) ⇒ CO II deficiency; BCS1L gene (2q33) ⇒ CO III deficiency, and non-SURF1 mutations ⇒ COX deficiency
- X-linked: PDHA1 gene (Xp22.2-p22.1) ⇒ pyruvate dehydrogenase CO deficiency
- Maternally inherited (mtDNA mutations): MTATP6 gene ⇒ CO V deficiency (causes LS if mutation load > 90%, NARP {neuropathy, ataxia, retinitis pigmentosa} if load 70-90%); MTND5, MTND6 genes ⇒ CO I deficiency; MTCO3 gene ⇒ COX deficiency; MTTK, MTTV tRNA genes

- Etiology
  ○ Exact mechanistic relationship between mitochondrial dysfunction and neurodegeneration unknown
  ○ Bioenergetic failure (ATP loss) and production reactive oxygen species likely key factors
- Epidemiology
  ○ Mitochondrial disorders: 1:8,500
  ○ LS in children < 6 years of age: 1:32,000 (most common mitochondrial disease in this age group)

## Gross Pathologic & Surgical Features

- Brownish-gray, gelatinous or cavitary foci in corpora striata, GP, BS, dentate nuclei, thalami, spinal cord, WM

## Microscopic Features

- Spongiform degeneration, gliosis, neuronal loss, demyelination, capillary proliferation

# CLINICAL ISSUES

## Presentation

- Most common signs/symptoms
  ○ Presentation: Psychomotor delay/regression, hypotonia
  ○ Other signs/symptoms
    - Progressive BS & BG dysfunction ⇒ ataxia, ophthalmoplegia, ptosis, vomiting, swallowing and respiratory difficulties, dystonia
    - Variable seizures (generalized, focal, myoclonic and rarely infantile spasms), peripheral neuropathy
  ○ CO IV deficiency 2° SURF1 mutation ⇒ early presentation, BS dysfunction, peripheral neuropathy, rapid neurologic deterioration
  ○ Metabolic stressors (e.g., infection) may unmask disease or cause deterioration
  ○ Elevated CSF, serum, urine lactate classic but not invariable

○ Biochemical defect identified by mitochondrial analysis of muscle biopsy or cultured skin fibroblasts
○ Prenatal diagnosis: Chorionic villus sampling (mutations and biochemical defects)

- Clinical Profile: Progressive neurodegeneration; signs/symptoms of BS & BG dysfunction; ↑ lactate in blood, CSF

## Demographics

- Age
  ○ Majority present by age 2
  ○ Childhood & adult presentations uncommon
- Gender: No gender predilection
- Ethnicity: No ethnic predilection

## Natural History & Prognosis

- Natural history: Progressive neurodegeneration leading to respiratory failure and death in childhood
- Prognosis: Dismal (particularly SURF1); childhood/adult LS more slowly progressive

## Treatment

- No curative treatment
- Variable improvement with quinone derivatives, vitamins, dichloroacetate

# DIAGNOSTIC CHECKLIST

## Image Interpretation Pearls

- Putaminal involvement classic but variable
- Thalamic and PAG involvement simulates Wernicke encephalopathy; however, mamillary bodies spared in LS
- Involvement of corpus callosum suggests CO I or CO II involvement

# SELECTED REFERENCES

1. O'Brien TW et al: Nuclear MRP genes and mitochondrial disease. Gene. 354:147-51, 2005
2. Benit P et al: Mutant NDUFS3 subunit of mitochondrial complex I causes Leigh syndrome. J Med Genet. 41(1):14-7, 2004
3. Rossi A et al: Leigh Syndrome with COX deficiency and SURF1 gene mutations: MR imaging findings. AJNR Am J Neuroradiol. 24(6):1188-91, 2003
4. Schon EA et al: Neuronal degeneration and mitochondrial dysfunction. J Clin Invest. 111:303-12, 2003
5. Farina L et al: MR Findings in Leigh Syndrome with COX Deficiency and SURF-1 Mutations. AJNR Am J Neuroradiol. 23:1095-100, 2002
6. Munich et al: Clinical Spectrum and Diagnosis of Mitochondrial Disorders. Am J Med Genet. 106:4-17, 2001
7. Tanji K et al: Neuropathological features of mitochondrial disorders. Semin Cell Dev Biol. 12(6):429-39, 2001
8. Arii J et al: Leigh syndrome: serial MR imaging and clinical follow-up. AJNR Am J Neuroradiol. 21(8):1502-9, 2000
9. Medina L et al: MR findings in patients with subacute necrotizing encephalomyelopathy (Leigh syndrome): correlation with biochemical defect. AJR Am J Roentgenol. 154(6):1269-74, 1990

# LEIGH SYNDROME

## IMAGE GALLERY

### Typical

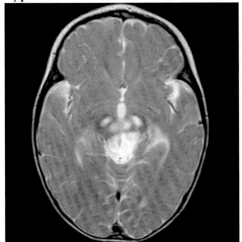 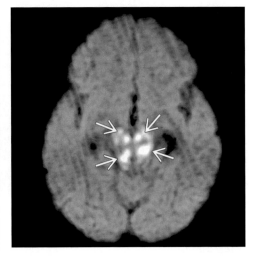

*(Left)* Axial T2WI MR shows abnormal hyperintensity in the dorsal midbrain, substantia nigra, and subthalamic nuclei. This is a common pattern for Leigh syndrome due to cytochrome oxidase (CO IV) deficiency. *(Right)* Axial DWI MR shows areas of reduced diffusivity ⇥ in the substantia nigra and in a portion of the dorsal mid brain. The reduced diffusivity is in areas of acute involvement.

### Variant

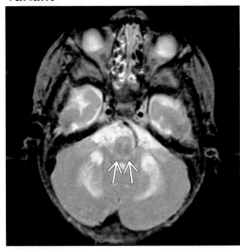 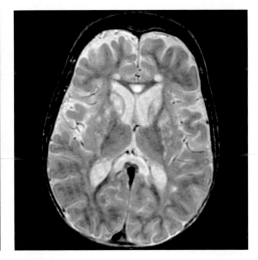

*(Left)* Axial T2WI MR shows involvement of dorsal brain stem tracts ⇥ and cerebellar white matter; cerebellum is less commonly involved than cerebrum. *(Right)* Axial T2WI MR shows involvement of periventricular white matter, basal ganglia, and corpus callosum, common areas of involvement in Leigh syndrome due to electron transport chain complexes I and II.

### Typical

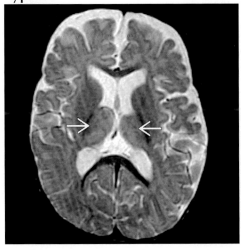 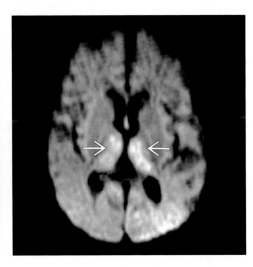

*(Left)* Axial T2WI MR shows subtle thalamic ⇥ involvement in this infant with Leigh syndrome. Initially thalamic involvement may be isolated when patients become symptomatic in infancy. *(Right)* Axial DWI MR shows reduced diffusivity ⇥ in the thalami. The abnormality is more easily seen on this diffusion weighted image than on the T2 weighted image from the same study (previous image).

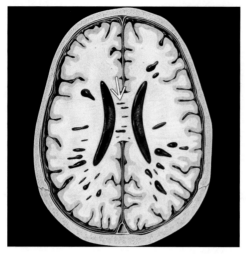

*Axial graphic shows dilated Virchow-Robin spaces (VRS) radially oriented in the white matter. They are predominantly posterior with the typical involvement of the corpus callosum →.*

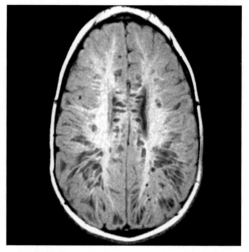

*Axial T1WI MR shows severe white matter involvement by dilated VRS in toddler with MPS 1H and minimal neurological symptoms. Peritrigonal and callosal involvement is pronounced.*

## TERMINOLOGY

### Abbreviations and Synonyms

- Mucopolysaccharidoses (MPS); old term "gargoylism"
  - Prototype: MPS 1H (Hurler)

### Definitions

- Inherited disorder of metabolism characterized by enzyme deficiency and inability to break down glycosaminoglycan (GAG)
  - Failure to break down GAG ⇒ accumulation of toxic intracellular substrate

## IMAGING FINDINGS

### General Features

- Best diagnostic clue: Perivascular spaces (PVS), also known as Virchow-Robin spaces (VRS), dilated by accumulated GAG
- Location: Favored sites of dilated VRS in MPS = corpus callosum (CC), peritrigonal white matter (WM), but can occur in other lobes
- Size

  - Variably-sized dilated VRS; one to many; usually under 5 mm
    - Occasional large obstructed VRS occur
- Morphology: Round, oval, spindle, parallel to veins

### CT Findings

- NECT
  - Metopic beaking despite macrocrania
  - Macrocrania, ↓ density WM, dilated VRS are rarely visible on CT
  - Progressive hydrocephalus and atrophy
- CECT: Enhancing pannus associated with ligaments and dura at craniovertebral junction (CVJ)

### MR Findings

- T1WI
  - Cribriform appearance WM, CC, basal ganglia (BG)
    - Dilated VRS filled with GAG: "Hurler holes"
    - Especially in severe MPS (MPS 1H, 2 > other types)
    - Exception MPS 4 (Morquio): CNS spared
  - Occasional arachnoid cysts (meningeal GAG deposition)
- T2WI
  - ↑ Signal of WM surrounding dilated VRS: Gliosis, edema, de- or dysmyelination

## DDx: Perivascular Spaces in White Matter

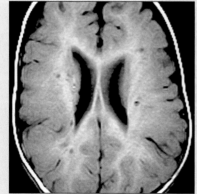

*Macrocephaly*

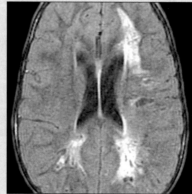

*Hypomelanosis of Ito*

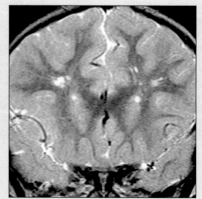

*Velocardiofacial*

# MUCOPOLYSACCHARIDOSES, SKULL AND BRAIN

## Key Facts

### Terminology
- Prototype: MPS 1H (Hurler)
- Inherited disorder of metabolism characterized by enzyme deficiency and inability to break down glycosaminoglycan (GAG)
- Failure to break down GAG ⇒ accumulation of toxic intracellular substrate

### Imaging Findings
- Best diagnostic clue: Perivascular spaces (PVS), also known as Virchow-Robin spaces (VRS), dilated by accumulated GAG
- Cribriform appearance WM, CC, basal ganglia (BG)
- Exception MPS 4 (Morquio): CNS spared
- Occasional arachnoid cysts (meningeal GAG deposition)

- Compression craniovertebral junction in majority MPS
- Always visualize foramen magnum on any CNS study to seek CVJ compression

### Top Differential Diagnoses
- Velocardiofacial Syndrome (Microdeletion Chr 22)
- Macrocephaly with Dilated VRS
- Hypomelanosis of Ito
- Normal VR Spaces

### Pathology
- Thick meninges
- Cribriform (honeycomb) appearance cut surface of brain

### Diagnostic Checklist
- Airway: Major sedation and anesthesia risk

---

- ○ ± Additional patchy WM signal
- ○ Hypomyelination and severe atrophy in MPS 3B
- FLAIR
  - ○ VRS isointense with CSF
  - ○ ↑ Signal surrounds VRS
- DWI
  - ○ Slightly hyperintense WM due to T2 shine-through
  - ○ Diffusivity of cysts similar to CSF
- MRS
  - ○ ↓ NAA, ↑ Cho/Cr ratio; ↑ peak at 3.7 ppm contains signals from MPS
    - Reduction of presumptive MPS peaks following bone marrow transplant (BMT)
- Spinal MR
  - ○ Compression craniovertebral junction in majority MPS
    - C2 meningeal hypertrophy
    - Progressive odontoid dysplasia ⇒ risk atlantoaxial subluxation if no BMT; some correction reported following BMT
    - Short C1 posterior arch
  - ○ Upper lumbar gibbus
    - MPS 1H (Hurler): Inferior beaking
    - MPS 4 (Morquio): Middle beaking

### Radiographic Findings
- Radiography: Dysostosis multiplex, broad ribs, trident hands, J-shaped sella, "rosette" formation of multiple impacted teeth in a single follicle

### Nuclear Medicine Findings
- 123I-IMP: ↓ Perfusion

### Imaging Recommendations
- Best imaging tool: MR brain
- Protocol advice
  - ○ Baseline MR/MRS
  - ○ F/U: Complications (CVJ compression, hydrocephalus); therapeutic response to BMT
  - ○ Always visualize foramen magnum on any CNS study to seek CVJ compression

## DIFFERENTIAL DIAGNOSIS

### Velocardiofacial Syndrome (Microdeletion Chr 22)
- Dilated VRS and plaques, typical frontal predominance; deviated upper cervical carotid arteries

### Macrocephaly with Dilated VRS
- Lacks typical beaked metopic suture and foramen magnum compression

### Hypomelanosis of Ito
- Periventricular signal change (brighter and more persistent than MPS) with large VRS
- ± Hemimegalencephaly
- Typical whorled skin lesions
- Lack "beaked" metopic suture present in MPS

### Perinatal Hypoxic Ischemic Encephalopathy
- Transient cystic phase occasionally follows hypoxic ischemic encephalopathy ⇒ atrophy

### Normal VR Spaces
- Vary in number and prominence

## PATHOLOGY

### General Features
- General path comments
  - ○ GAG accumulates in most organs/ligaments
    - Hepatosplenomegaly (HSM), umbilical hernia
    - Skeletal dysostosis multiplex, joint contractures
    - Arterial wall (mid-aortic stenosis) and cardiac valve thickening
    - Dural thickening (cord compression at foramen magnum)
    - Coarse facies (formerly "gargoylism")
    - Upper airway obstruction (38%): Submucosal deposition ⇒ small, abnormal shape trachea (difficult intubation) and vocal cords
  - ○ Embryology-anatomy
    - Dilated VRS may be seen in utero

# MUCOPOLYSACCHARIDOSES, SKULL AND BRAIN

- Genetics: MPS: Autosomal recessive (exception: X-linked MPS 2)
- Etiology: MPS: Ganglioside accumulation (toxic to neurons)
- Epidemiology
  - 1:29,000 live births (series from Australia)
    - MPS 1H: 1 in 107,000 live births
    - MPS 2: 1 in 165,000 male live births
    - MPS 3: 1 in 58,000 live births
    - MPS 4A: 1 in 640,000 live births
    - MPS 6: 1 in 320,000 live births
- Associated abnormalities
  - Dermal melanocytosis (mongolian-like spots)
    - Extensive, blue skin pigmentation differs from typical mongolian spots in persistence, progression

## Gross Pathologic & Surgical Features
- Thick meninges
- Cribriform (honeycomb) appearance cut surface of brain

## Microscopic Features
- MPS: Glycosaminoglycans accumulate in leptomeninges + VRS

## Staging, Grading or Classification Criteria
- MPS 1-9, depends upon specific enzyme deficiency
  - MPS 1H, 1HS (Hurler/Hurler-Scheie): α-L-iduronidase (4p16.3)
  - MPS 2 (Hunter): Iduronate 2-sulfatase (Xq28)
  - MPS 3A (Sanfilippo): Heparin N-sulfatase (17q25.3)
  - MPS 4A (Morquio): Galactose 6-sulfatase (16q24.3)
  - MPS 6 (Maroteaux-Lamy): Arylsulfatase B (5q11-q13)

# CLINICAL ISSUES

## Presentation
- Most common signs/symptoms
  - Typical coarse facies develop (mild in MPS 3,6,7)
    - Macroglossia, bushy eyebrows, flat nasal bridge
- Clinical Profile
  - Prototype MPS 1H, appear normal at birth
    - Corneal clouding (except MPS 2): Proteoglycans in keratocytes
    - Mental retardation (significant except MPS 2b, 4, 1HS)
    - Joint contractures, dysostosis multiplex, short stubby fingers, carpal tunnel syndrome
    - Loses walking skills: Spinal claudication/myelopathy C1-2 and vascular claudication from mid-aortic stenosis
    - Recurrent upper respiratory infection, nasal discharge, ear infections, sleep apnea, sensorineural deafness
    - Middle ear effusions (73%), otolaryngologist notes this pre-diagnosis MPS
  - MPS 7 may present with fetal nuchal translucency, hydrops fetalis or isolated ascites

## Demographics
- Age: Differs in different syndromes; MPS 1H presents in infancy

- Gender: MPS 2 (Hunter) is X-linked: Male
- Ethnicity: Prevalence of specific MPS disorders varies with country

## Natural History & Prognosis
- Progressive deterioration without therapy, rate depends upon specific deficiency
- Severe white matter changes more likely to be associated with mental retardation

## Treatment
- BMT or IV recombinant human enzyme (e.g., MPS 1H: α-L-iduronidase)
  - ↓ Visceral accumulation MPS; ameliorate some manifestations
- Murine embryonic stem cell models under evaluation for gene therapy

# DIAGNOSTIC CHECKLIST

## Consider
- Airway: Major sedation and anesthesia risk

## Image Interpretation Pearls
- Not all MPS have typical facial features, dilated VRS may still signal one of the less common MPS
- Not all dilated VRS are MPS
- Always look for CVJ compression as treatable cause of morbidity

# SELECTED REFERENCES

1. Beck M. Related Articles et al: New therapeutic options for lysosomal storage disorders: enzyme replacement, small molecules and gene therapy. Hum Genet. 2006
2. Van der Knaap MS et al: Magnetic Resonance of Myelin, Myelination, and Myelin Disorders. 3rd ed. Springer-Verlag, Berlin. 123-32, 2005
3. Gabrielli O et al: Correlation between cerebral MRI abnormalities and mental retardation in patients with MPS. Am J Med Genet. 125A(3):224-31, 2004
4. Hanson M et al: Association of dermal melanocytosis with lysosomal storage disease: clinical features and hypotheses regarding pathogenesis. Arch Dermatol. 139(7):916-20, 2003
5. Nelson J et al: Incidence of the mucopolysaccharidoses in Western Australia. Am J Med Genet A. 123(3):310-3, 2003
6. Brooks DA: Alpha-L-iduronidase and enzyme replacement therapy for mucopolysaccharidosis I. Expert Opin Biol Ther. 2(8):967-76, 2002
7. Geipel A et al: Mucopolysaccharidosis VII (Sly disease) as a cause of increased nuchal translucency and non-immune fetal hydrops: study of a family and technical approach to prenatal diagnosis in early and late pregnancy. Prenat Diagn. 22(6):493-5, 2002
8. Takahashi Y et al: Evaluation of accumulated mucopolysaccharides in the brain of patients with mucopolysaccharidoses by (1)H-magnetic resonance spectroscopy before and after bone marrow transplantation. Pediatr Res. 49(3):349-55, 2001
9. Zafeiriou DI et al: Serial magnetic resonance imaging findings in mucopolysaccharidosis IIIB (Sanfilippo's syndrome B). Brain Dev. 23(6):385-9, 2001
10. Nakamura T et al: Rosette formation of impacted molar teeth in mucopolysaccharidoses and related disorders. Dentomaxillofac Radiol. 21(1):45-9, 1992

# MUCOPOLYSACCHARIDOSES, SKULL AND BRAIN

## IMAGE GALLERY

### Typical

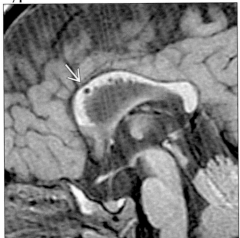
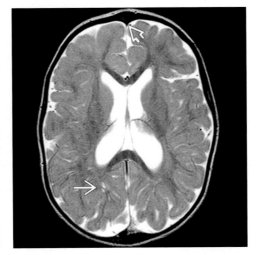

*(Left)* Sagittal T1WI MR shows VRS ➡ throughout the corpus callosum in a toddler with MPS 1H. Callosal involvement by these dilated perivascular spaces is typical. *(Right)* Axial T2WI MR in same toddler as previous image shows only a few ➡ peritrigonal VRS. Metopic "beak" ➡ in the presence of frontal bossing and macrocrania is a typical feature of MPS.

### Typical

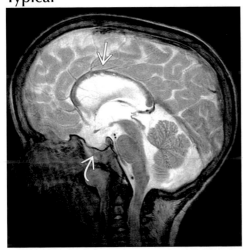
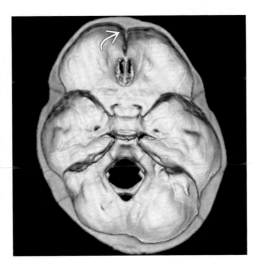

*(Left)* Sagittal T2WI MR in child with MPS 2 shows a few callosal VRS ➡, scaphocephaly with frontal bossing, ventriculomegaly and a large J-shaped sella turcica ➡. *(Right)* Axial bone CT with 3D reconstruction shows typical metopic beak ➡ in MPS. Metopic beak is rare in macrocrania unless there is concomitant MPS.

### Typical

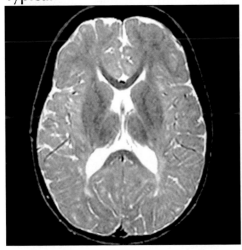
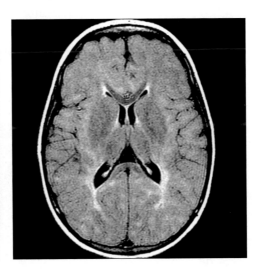

*(Left)* Axial T2WI MR in MPS 3B shows prominent ventricles and sulci in addition to the common finding of delayed myelin maturation. *(Right)* Axial FLAIR MR in same patient as previous image shows abnormal increased signal in the peritrigonal white matter. The presence of VRS in MPS 3B is variable. Progressive atrophy is typical.

# OSMOTIC DEMYELINATION SYNDROME

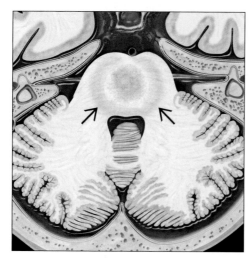

Axial graphic shows acute osmotic demyelination affecting the central pons ➡. The pons is slightly swollen with mild mass effect on the 4th ventricle.

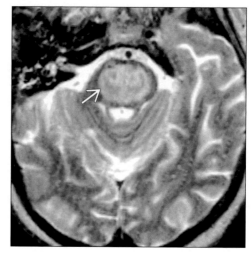

Axial T2WI MR shows a confluent, symmetric hyperintensity ➡ in the central pons. The periphery of the pons is spared. There is little associated mass effect.

## TERMINOLOGY

### Abbreviations and Synonyms
- Osmotic demyelination syndrome (ODMS); formerly called "central pontine myelinolysis" (CPM) and/or "extrapontine myelinolysis" (EPM)

### Definitions
- Acute demyelination caused by rapid shifts in serum osmolality
- Classic setting: Rapid correction of hyponatremia
  - ODMS may occur in normonatremic patients

## IMAGING FINDINGS

### General Features
- Best diagnostic clue: Central pons T2 hyperintensity with sparing of periphery
- Location
  - 50% in pons (CPM)
    - Central fibers involved; peripheral fibers spared
  - 50% extra-pontine sites (EPM)
    - Basal ganglia (BG)

- Cerebral white matter (WM)
- Uncommon: Cerebral cortex, middle cerebellar peduncles
  - CPM + EPM: Almost pathognomonic for ODMS
- Size: Variable extent
- Morphology
  - Imaging findings in children similar to adult presentation
  - Round or triangular-shaped (pons)
  - Regardless of site, demyelination often bilateral/symmetric
  - Gyriform (cortical involvement)

### CT Findings
- NECT
  - Low density in affected areas (pons, BG, etc.)
  - No hemorrhage
- CECT
  - Classic: No enhancement
  - Early, acute/severe demyelination may enhance moderately strongly

### MR Findings
- T1WI
  - Acute

## DDx: Pontine Lesions in Children

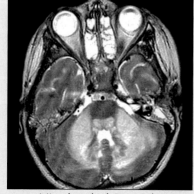

Mitochondrial Cytopathy

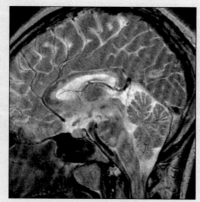

Multiple Sclerosis

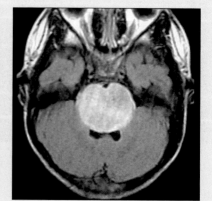

Infiltrative Pontine Glioma

# OSMOTIC DEMYELINATION SYNDROME

## Key Facts

### Terminology
- Osmotic demyelination syndrome (ODMS); formerly called "central pontine myelinolysis" (CPM) and/or "extrapontine myelinolysis" (EPM)
- Acute demyelination caused by rapid shifts in serum osmolality
- Classic setting: Rapid correction of hyponatremia
- ODMS may occur in normonatremic patients

### Imaging Findings
- Best diagnostic clue: Central pons T2 hyperintensity with sparing of periphery
- 50% in pons (CPM)
- 50% extra-pontine sites (EPM)
- Basal ganglia (BG)
- Cerebral white matter (WM)
- CPM + EPM: Almost pathognomonic for ODMS

- Acute: Confluent hyperintensity in central pons with sparing of periphery and corticospinal tracts
- Symmetric hyperintensity in BG, WM or GM (EPM)
- Subacute: Hyperintensity often normalizes, may resolve completely
- ADC: Variable; normal to mildly hyperintense
- Usually does not enhance
- Best imaging tool: MR > > CT

### Top Differential Diagnoses
- Demyelinating Disease
- Rhombencephalitis
- Pontine Neoplasm (Astrocytoma)
- Leigh Syndrome
- Hypertensive Encephalopathy
- Wilson Disease
- Pontine Ischemia/Infarction

---

- Classic: Mildly/moderately hypointense
- Less common: Can be isointense with surrounding normal brain
- Findings may be transitory, resolve completely
- Initial study may be normal
  - Subacute
    - May resolve completely
    - Less common: Hyperintensity at 1-4 months (coagulative necrosis)
- T2WI
  - Acute: Confluent hyperintensity in central pons with sparing of periphery and corticospinal tracts
    - Symmetric hyperintensity in BG, WM or GM (EPM)
  - Subacute: Hyperintensity often normalizes, may resolve completely
- PD/Intermediate: Hyperintense
- FLAIR: Hyperintense
- T2* GRE: Hemorrhage, "blooming" rare
- DWI
  - Restricted (mildly hyperintense)
  - ADC: Variable; normal to mildly hyperintense
- T1 C+
  - Usually does not enhance
  - Less common: Moderate confluent enhancement

### Nuclear Medicine Findings
- PET
  - Early metabolic stress = variable hypermetabolism
  - Late = hypometabolic areas in affected sites

### Imaging Recommendations
- Best imaging tool: MR > > CT
- Protocol advice
  - MR
    - Include FLAIR, T1 C+, DWI
    - Repeat imaging

## DIFFERENTIAL DIAGNOSIS

### Demyelinating Disease
- Look for typical lesions elsewhere

- "Horseshoe" (incomplete ring) enhancement pattern in acute MS common

### Rhombencephalitis
- Enterovirus common agent
- Look for cerebellar, cranial nerve involvement

### Pontine Neoplasm (Astrocytoma)
- Infiltrative (diffuse) neoplasm; mass effect
- Usually little/no contrast-enhanced at presentation

### Leigh Syndrome
- Pyruvate dehydrogenase complex defects: Caudate + putamen, delayed myelination
- Cytochrome oxydase deficiency: Subthalamic nuclei, medulla, dorsal pons
- Complex V deficiency: Anterior putamen, dorsal mesencephalon + pons

### Hypertensive Encephalopathy
- Parieto-occipital lobes = most common site in hypertensive encephalopathy
- Pontine hypertensive encephalopathy: Typically does not spare peripheral fibers

### Wilson Disease
- Basal ganglia, thalamus > pons

### Pontine Ischemia/Infarction
- Often asymmetric
- Usually involves both central, peripheral pontine fibers
- Caution: Perforating BA infarct(s) may involve central pons, mimic CPM (including DWI)

## PATHOLOGY

### General Features
- General path comments
  - Demyelination without associated inflammation
    - Nonspecific (pattern, distribution suggests ODMS)
- Etiology

# OSMOTIC DEMYELINATION SYNDROME

- ○ Heterogeneous disorder with common etiology = osmotic stress
- ○ Osmotic stress = any change in osmotic gradient
- ○ Most common = iatrogenic correction of hyponatremia
- ○ Less common = osmotic derangement with azotemia, hyperglycemia, hypokalemia, ketoacidosis
- ○ Precise mechanism of osmotic stress-related myelinolysis unknown
  - ▪ Osmotic insult = change in serum osmolality
  - ▪ Relative intracellular hypotonicity
  - ▪ Serum osmolality change causes endothelial damage
  - ▪ Organic osmolyte deficiency predisposes to endothelial breakdown
  - ▪ Endothelial cells shrink, causing breakdown of blood brain barrier
  - ▪ Accumulation of hypertonic sodium-rich fluid in extracerebral fluid (ECF)
  - ▪ Hypertonic ECF, release of myelin toxins damages WM
  - ▪ Cell death ensues
- ○ "Co-morbid" conditions that may exacerbate ODMS
  - ▪ Hepatic, renal, adrenal, pituitary, paraneoplastic disease
  - ▪ Nutritional (alcohol, malnutrition, vomiting)
  - ▪ Burn, transplantation, other surgical patients
- Epidemiology: Reported with various pediatric disorders: Fulminant hepatitis, liver transplantation, chronic debilitation, malnutrition, diabetes

## Gross Pathologic & Surgical Features
- Bilateral/symmetrical, soft, gray-tan discoloration

## Microscopic Features
- Extensive demyelination, gliosis
- Macrophages contain engulfed myelin bits and fragments
- Axis cylinders, nerve cells preserved
- No inflammation

# CLINICAL ISSUES

## Presentation
- Most common signs/symptoms
  - ○ Seizures, altered mental status
  - ○ Often biphasic when hyponatremia present
    - ▪ ODMS symptoms emerge 2-4 days (occasionally weeks) after correction of hyponatremia
    - ▪ Changing level of consciousness, disorientation
    - ▪ Pseudobulbar palsy, dysarthria, dysphagia (CPM)
    - ▪ Movement disorder (EPM)
  - ○ Symptoms may resolve with serum osmolality increase
- Clinical Profile: Sick, hyponatremic child with rapid correction of serum sodium

## Natural History & Prognosis
- Spectrum of outcomes
  - ○ Complete recovery may occur
  - ○ Minimal residual deficits
    - ▪ Memory, cognitive impairment
    - ▪ Ataxia, spasticity, diplopia

- ○ May progress to
  - ▪ Spastic quadriparesis
  - ▪ "Locked in"; may progress to coma, death
- "Co-morbid" conditions common, poorer prognosis

## Treatment
- No consensus; no "optimal" correction rate for hyponatremia
- Self-correction (fluid restriction, discontinue diuretics) if possible
- Plasmapheresis, steroids, glucose infusions being studied

# DIAGNOSTIC CHECKLIST

## Image Interpretation Pearls
- Classic CPM spares peripheral pontine fibers
- EPM can occur without CPM
- Repeat MR may be necessary as initial study may be normal

# SELECTED REFERENCES
1. Rizek KA et al: Early diagnosis of central pontine myelinolysis with diffusion-weighted imaging. AJNR. 25:210-3, 2004
2. Bonkowsky JL et al: Extrapontine myelinolysis in a pediatric case of diabetic ketoacidosis and cerebral edema. J Child Neurol. 18(2): 144-7, 2003
3. Kim JS et al: Decreased striatal dopamine transporter binding in a patient with extrapontine myelinolysis. Mov Disord. 18(3): 342-5, 2003
4. Mochizuki H et al: Benign type of central pontine myelinolysis in alcoholism--clinical, neuroradiological and electrophysiological findings. J Neurol. 250(9): 1077-83, 2003
5. Chua GC et al: MRI findings in osmotic myelinolysis. Clin Radiol. 57(9): 800-6, 2002
6. Lampl C et al: Central pontine myelinolysis. Eur Neurol. 47(1): 3-10, 2002
7. Lin SH et al: Osmotic demyelination syndrome after correction of chronic hyponatremia with normal saline. Am J Med Sci. 323(5): 259-62, 2002
8. Agildere AM et al: MRI of neurologic complications in end-stage renal failure patients on hemodialysis: pictorial review. Eur Radiol. 11(6):1063-9, 2001
9. Ashrafian H et al: A review of the causes of central pontine myelinosis: yet another apoptotic illness? Eur J Neurol. 8(2): 103-9, 2001
10. Cramer SC et al: Decreased diffusion in central pontine myelinolysis. AJNR. 22:1476-9, 2001
11. Niehaus L et al: Reversible central pontine and extrapontine myelinolysis in a 16-year-old girl. Childs Nerv Syst. 17(4-5): 294-6, 2001
12. Brown WD: Osmotic demyelination disorders: central pontine and extrapontine myelinolysis. Curr Opin Neurol. 13(6): 691-7, 2000
13. Calakos N et al: Cortical MRI findings associated with rapid correction of hyponatremia. Neurology. 55(7): 1048-51, 2000
14. Chan CY et al: Clinics in diagnostic imaging (45). Osmotic myelinolysis ( central potine myelinolysis). Singapore Med J. 41(1): 45-8, 2000
15. Waragai M: Serial MRI of extrapontine myelinolysis of the basal ganglia: a case report. J Neurol Sci. 161:173-5, 1998

# OSMOTIC DEMYELINATION SYNDROME

## IMAGE GALLERY

### Typical

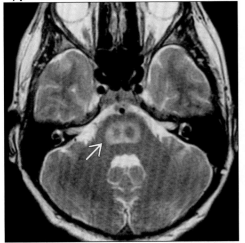 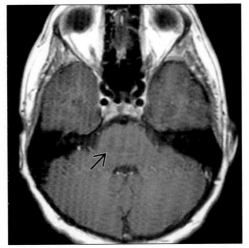

*(Left)* Axial T2WI MR shows central, confluent symmetric osmotic demyelination within the pons of a sick, diabetic teenager. The lesion ➡ is T2 bright with central sparing (of the corticospinal tracts). *(Right)* Axial T1 C+ MR (same patient as previous image) at the same level shows mild hypointensity ➡ in the portions of the lesion that are T2 hyperintense. The lesion does not enhance.

### Typical

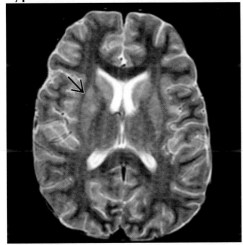 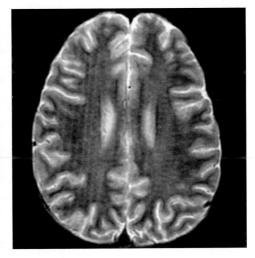

*(Left)* Axial T2WI MR in a 7year old s/p severe hyponatremia demonstrates EPM with patchy hyperintensities in the basal ganglia ➡ and thalami. The white matter also shows patchy demyelination. *(Right)* Axial T2WI MR (same patient as previous image) at the upper lateral ventricular level demonstrates the patchy, "tigroid" pattern of demyelination throughout the cerebral WM. The cortex is spared.

### Typical

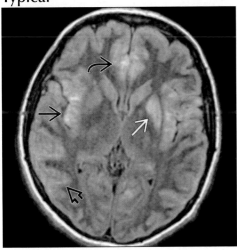 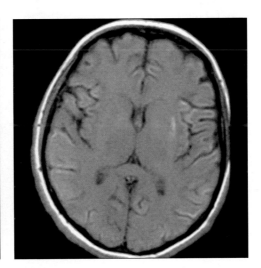

*(Left)* Axial FLAIR MR shows asymmetric involvement of the left putamen ➡. Patchy cortical swelling is most evident in the cingulate gyri ➡, insular cortex ➡, parietal lobes ➡. *(Right)* Axial T1WI MR at the same level shows T1 bright signal changes indicative of cortical laminar necrosis: An unusual manifestation of ODMS. The distribution of T1 abnormalities is similar to the T2 findings.

# LANGERHANS CELL HISTIOCYTOSIS, SKULL & BRAIN

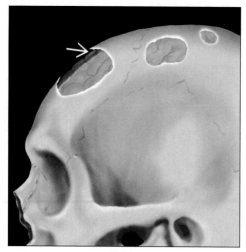

Lateral graphic shows multiple well defined lytic skull lesions characteristic of LCH. Prior to treatment the lesions lack marginal sclerosis and show beveled edges ➡.

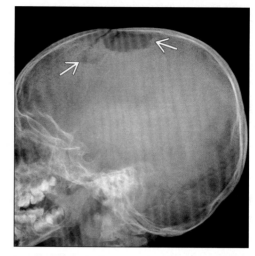

Lateral radiograph shows two lytic LCH lesions of the calvarium ➡. The larger lesion shows a characteristic geographic sharp border, lacking sclerosis. With healing, sclerosis occurs.

## TERMINOLOGY

### Abbreviations and Synonyms
- Langerhans cell histiocytosis (LCH)
- Eosinophilic granuloma
- Formerly called histiocytosis X

### Definitions
- Proliferation of Langerhans cell histiocytes forming granulomas within any organ system

## IMAGING FINDINGS

### General Features
- Best diagnostic clue
  - Skull ⇒ sharply marginated lytic skull defect with beveled margins
  - Mastoid ⇒ geographic destruction, soft tissue mass
  - Brain ⇒ thick enhancing infundibulum, absent posterior pituitary bright spot
- Location
  - Skull

- Calvarium is most common bony site involved, especially prevalent in frontal, parietal bones
- Also mastoid portion of temporal bone, mandible, orbit, facial bones
  - Brain ⇒ pituitary infundibulum, hypothalamus
    - Rare: Choroid plexus, leptomeninges, basal ganglia, cerebellar white matter (WM), and brain parenchyma
- Size
  - Skull and facial bones: Lesions grow fast, moderate soft tissue mass common
  - Pituitary infundibulum: Small lesions due to early endocrine dysfunction; diabetes insipidus (DI)
- Morphology
  - Variable patterns of bony lysis
  - Soft tissue masses vary from discrete to infiltrative

### CT Findings
- NECT
  - Calvarium ⇒ lytic defect, beveled (inner table > outer table), small soft tissue mass
  - Mastoid ⇒ bone destruction, often bilateral, soft tissue mass
  - Brain ⇒ thickened pituitary stalk

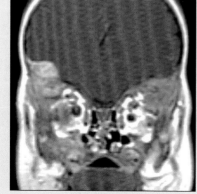

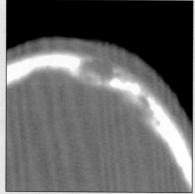

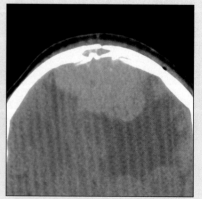

## DDx: Calvarial Mimics of LCH

Neuroblastoma

Osteomyelitis

Leukemia

# LANGERHANS CELL HISTIOCYTOSIS, SKULL & BRAIN

## Key Facts

### Terminology
- Proliferation of Langerhans cell histiocytes forming granulomas within any organ system

### Imaging Findings
- Skull ⇒ sharply marginated lytic skull defect with beveled margins
- Mastoid ⇒ geographic destruction, soft tissue mass
- Brain ⇒ thick enhancing infundibulum, absent posterior pituitary bright spot
- Rare ⇒ enhancing: Choroid plexus masses, nodules of the leptomeninges, and basal ganglia
- PET: 18-FDG: ↑ Uptake in proliferating lesions, ↓ uptake for "burned-out" lesions

### Top Differential Diagnoses
- Lytic Calvarial Lesions

- Temporal Bone Destructive Processes
- Pituitary Infundibular/Hypothalamic Thickening or Masses

### Pathology
- Etiology: Uncertain: Inflammatory ↔ neoplastic
- Affects 4:1 million
- Peak age at onset 1 year (isolated), 2-5 years (multifocal disease)
- Inverse relation between severity of involvement and age
- Monostotic involvement 50-75%

### Diagnostic Checklist
- Skull is most frequent bony site involved by LCH
- Thick enhancing pituitary stalk is the most common CNS manifestation of LCH

---

- CECT
  - Calvarium ⇒ enhancing soft tissue in lytic defect
  - Mastoid ⇒ soft tissue mass variably enhances
  - Brain ⇒ enhancing, thick pituitary stalk, ± hypothalamic mass or enhancement

## MR Findings
- T1WI
  - Soft tissue mass at site of bony lysis
    - Variable, T1 shortening if LCH lesion is proliferative (lipid-laden macrophages)
  - Brain
    - Infundibulum: Hypointense or isointense to GM
    - Absence of posterior pituitary bright spot
- T2WI
  - Skull, mastoid, orbital/facial lesions: Soft tissue masses show slight hyperintensity
  - Brain
    - Infundibulum/hypothalamus: Slightly hyperintense
    - ± Cerebellar white matter hyperintensity (autoimmune mediated demyelination)
    - Dural and choroid plexus masses very hypointense
- FLAIR: Hyperintensity of the rare cerebellar white matter demyelination
- DWI: Cerebellar demyelination with central nervous system (CNS) LCH may show restricted diffusion
- T1 C+
  - Skull, mastoid, orbital/facial: Strongly enhancing soft tissue masses (defined or infiltrating)
  - Brain
    - Infundibulum: Vivid enhancement and stalk thickening
    - Rare ⇒ enhancing: Choroid plexus masses, nodules of the leptomeninges, and basal ganglia

## Radiographic Findings
- Radiography
  - Calvarium: Well defined lytic lesion, beveled edge, lack of marginal sclerosis
    - ± Button sequestra or sclerotic margins when healing

- Mastoid: Geographic destruction, often bilateral, little regional adenopathy,
- Facial/orbital: More variable patterns of bony lysis, discrete ↔ permeative

## Nuclear Medicine Findings
- PET: 18-FDG: ↑ Uptake in proliferating lesions, ↓ uptake for "burned-out" lesions
- Bone Scan
  - Tc-Bone scan: Variable (cold ↔ warm)
    - Calvarium: ↓ Central uptake with halo of ↑ activity

## Imaging Recommendations
- Best imaging tool
  - Skull: NECT
  - Mastoid disease: CECT
  - Brain: MR with contrast
- Protocol advice
  - Suspected mastoid LCH: CECT, axial and coronal
  - Brain MR: Patient with diabetes insipidus
    - Pituitary: Small FOV, thin-section, no gap, sagittal and coronal T1 imaging with contrast
    - If initial study is normal, repeat in 2-3 months

## DIFFERENTIAL DIAGNOSIS

### Lytic Calvarial Lesions
- Surgical (burr hole, shunt, surgical defect)
- Epidermoid, dermoid, leptomeningeal cyst
- Osteomyelitis, TB, syphilis, sarcoid
- Leukemia, lymphoma, metastases (neuroblastoma),

### Temporal Bone Destructive Processes
- Severe mastoiditis: Infection usually spares bony labyrinth
- Fibrous dysplasia: Skull base lesions may be lytic
- Rhabdomyosarcoma: Often with large ipsilateral cervical nodes

## Pituitary Infundibular/Hypothalamic Thickening or Masses
- Germinoma, glioma, PNET, lymphoma, metastasis
- Lymphocytic hypophysitis, sarcoidosis, meningitis

## PATHOLOGY

### General Features
- General path comments: Masses of proliferating: Histiocytes, plasma cells, and eosinophilic inflammatory cells forming granulomas
- Genetics
  - Familial cases documented
  - Monoclonality of pathologic Langerhans cell
  - T (7;12) translocation, involvement of the tel gene on chromosome 12
- Etiology: Uncertain: Inflammatory ↔ neoplastic
- Epidemiology
  - Affects 4:1 million
  - Peak age at onset 1 year (isolated), 2-5 years (multifocal disease)
  - Inverse relation between severity of involvement and age
  - Monostotic involvement 50-75%
  - Familial LCH < 2%
  - Bone lesions are most common manifestations of LCH ⇒ 80-95% of children with LCH
- Associated abnormalities: ↑ Risk of LCH: Family history of thyroid disease, underimmunization, penicillin use, solvent exposure

### Gross Pathologic & Surgical Features
- Yellow, gray, or brown tumor mass

### Microscopic Features
- Monoclonality of Langerhans cells
  - Presence of CD1a and Birbeck granules needed to establish diagnosis

### Staging, Grading or Classification Criteria
- Formerly classified into one of 3 overlapping forms
  - Eosinophilic granuloma: Localized, calvarium most common, 70%
  - Hand Schueller Christian: Chronic disseminated form, multifocal, 20%
  - Letterer-Siwe: Acute disseminated form, onset < 2 years of age, ± skeletal involvement, 10%
- Now classified according to risk factors
  - Young age, multifocal involvement, multiorgan dysfunction, relapse

## CLINICAL ISSUES

### Presentation
- Most common signs/symptoms
  - Calvarial: Pain, subscalp mass, bony defect
  - Mastoid destruction: Pain, chronic otitis externa, retroauricular subscalp mass
  - Retroorbital mass: Exophthalmos, ± painful ophthalmoplegia

- Pituitary infundibular involvement: DI, ± visual disturbance, ± hypothalamic dysfunction
- Clinical Profile: Child < 2 years with diabetes insipidus, ± lytic calvarial lesion

### Demographics
- Age: LCH typically presents under 2 years of age
- Gender: M:F = 2:1
- Ethnicity: More common among Caucasians

### Natural History & Prognosis
- Variable depending on age of onset and extent of involvement
  - Spontaneous regression within 3 months up to 2 years
  - Behavior of LCH may change with time, and assume aggressive form
  - Multifocal and systemic LCH: Mortality may approach 18%
- Rarely, may spontaneously hemorrhage ⇒ epidural hematoma

### Treatment
- Therapeutic options depend upon symptoms, location, and extent of disease
  - Observation, excision/curettage, sclerotherapy/injection, radiation/chemotherapy
- Solitary eosinophilic granuloma has best prognosis with spontaneous remission common
  - Curettage if painful, observe asymptomatic
- LCH patients with DI: Oral or nasal vasopressin, ± chemotherapy and radiation

## DIAGNOSTIC CHECKLIST

### Consider
- CNS LCH for ataxic patient with choroid plexus masses and cerebellar WM demyelination

### Image Interpretation Pearls
- Skull is most frequent bony site involved by LCH
- Thick enhancing pituitary stalk is the most common CNS manifestation of LCH

## SELECTED REFERENCES

1. Grois N et al: Neuropathology of CNS disease in Langerhans cell histiocytosis. Brain. 128(Pt 4):829-38, 2005
2. Jubran RF et al: Predictors of outcome in children with Langerhans cell histiocytosis. Pediatr Blood Cancer. 45(1):37-42, 2005
3. Steiner M et al: Modern imaging methods for the assessment of Langerhans' cell histiocytosis-associated neurodegenerative syndrome: case report. J Child Neurol. 20(3):253-7, 2005
4. Prayer D et al: MR imaging presentation of intracranial disease associated with Langerhans cell histiocytosis. AJNR Am J Neuroradiol. 25(5):880-91, 2004
5. Prosch H et al: Central diabetes insipidus as presenting symptom of Langerhans cell histiocytosis. Pediatr Blood Cancer. 43(5):594-9, 2004
6. Kleinjung T et al: Langerhans' cell histiocytosis with bilateral temporal bone involvement. Am J Otolaryngol. 24(4):265-70, 2003

## IMAGE GALLERY

### Typical

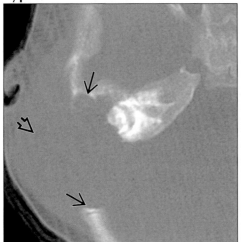
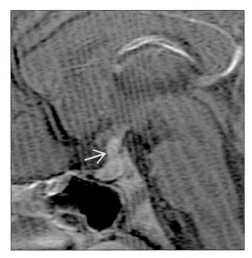

*(Left)* Axial NECT shows a destructive lesion of the mastoid segment of the temporal bone. Note the "cookie-cutter" sharp borders ➡ and accompanying large postauricular soft tissue mass ⇨. *(Right)* Sagittal T1 C+ MR shows thickening and enhancement ➡ of the pituitary stalk (infundibulum) in a patient with acquired diabetes insipidus.

### Typical

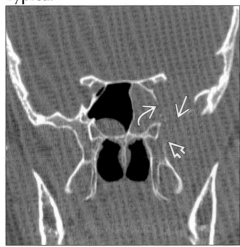
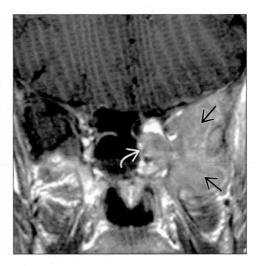

*(Left)* Coronal NECT shows a destructive left skull base lesion. LCH bone lysis involves the floor of the middle cranial fossa ➡, lateral sphenoid sinus ➡, and lateral pterygoid bone ⇨. *(Right)* Coronal T1 C+ MR shows a heterogeneously enhancing mass involving the masticator space and anterior middle cranial fossa ➡. The tumor invades the sphenoid sinus ➡.

### Variant

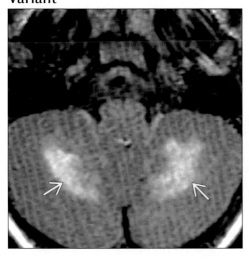
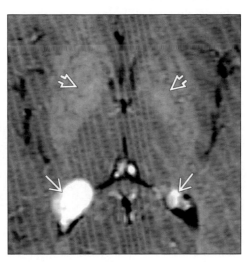

*(Left)* Axial FLAIR MR shows bilateral cerebellar white matter hyperintensity ⬛ due to demyelination, which is believed to be autoimmune in etiology. *(Right)* Axial T1 C+ MR shows robustly enhancing eosinophilic granulomas ➡ in the choroid plexus. The mosaic pattern of basal ganglia enhancement ➡ results from perivascular spread of LCH.

# ATYPICAL TERATOID-RHABDOID TUMOR

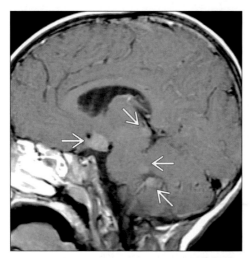

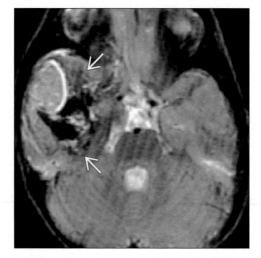

*Sagittal T1 C+ MR shows multiple foci of enhancing tumor in an infant with AT/RhT ➡. Diffuse spread of tumor at presentation may make the primary site of origin impossible to determine.*

*Axial T2WI MR shows a markedly aggressive AT/RhT ➡ centered over the right middle cerebral artery. Extensive hypointense signal reflects calcification and hemorrhagic staining.*

## TERMINOLOGY

### Abbreviations and Synonyms
- Atypical teratoid-rhabdoid tumor (AT/RhT), AT/RT
- Malignant rhabdoid tumor of brain, cranial rhabdoid tumor

### Definitions
- Rare aggressive tumor of early childhood composed of rhabdoid cells, areas resembling pineal region primitive neuroectodermal tumor (PNET), and malignant mesenchymal or epithelial tissue

## IMAGING FINDINGS

### General Features
- Best diagnostic clue
  - Heterogeneous intracranial mass in an infant
  - Think of AT/RhT when medulloblastoma (PNET-MB) is considered
- Location
  - 50% infratentorial (most off-midline)
    - Cerebello-pontine angle (CPA)

- Cerebellum and/or brainstem
  - 40% supratentorial
    - Hemispheric or suprasellar
  - 15-20% present with disseminated tumor
- Size: Most = 1-3 cm at presentation (can be very large)
- Morphology: Roughly spherical, irregular

### CT Findings
- NECT
  - Hyperattenuating mass
  - Commonly contains cysts or hemorrhage
  - May contain Ca++
  - Obstructive hydrocephalus common
- CECT: Heterogeneous enhancement

### MR Findings
- T1WI
  - Heterogeneous
    - Isointense to brain with foci of hyperintensity corresponding to hemorrhage
    - Cysts slightly hyperintense to CSF
- T2WI
  - Heterogeneous
    - Regions of marked hypointense signal from hemorrhage

## DDx: Disseminated Tumor in Infants

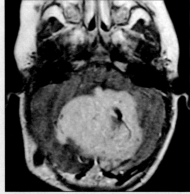

*Medulloblastoma*

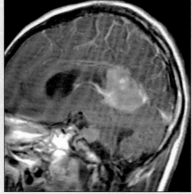

*Pineoblastoma*

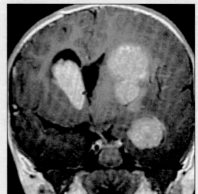

*Choroid Plexus Carcinoma*

# ATYPICAL TERATOID-RHABDOID TUMOR

## Key Facts

### Terminology
- Rare aggressive tumor of early childhood composed of rhabdoid cells, areas resembling pineal region primitive neuroectodermal tumor (PNET), and malignant mesenchymal or epithelial tissue

### Imaging Findings
- Heterogeneous intracranial mass in an infant
- 50% infratentorial (most off-midline)
- 15-20% present with disseminated tumor
- Commonly contains cysts or hemorrhage
- May contain Ca++
- Decreased diffusivity
- Heterogeneous enhancement
- Entire CNS must be imaged at presentation to identify subarachnoid spread of tumor

### Top Differential Diagnoses
- Medulloblastoma (PNET-MB)
- Ependymoma

### Pathology
- Rhabdoid cells resemble those in malignant rhabdoid tumor of kidney
- Divergent differentiation accounts for "teratoid" label

### Clinical Issues
- Clinical Profile: Child under 3 with increasing head size, vomiting, and lethargy
- Median survival = 6 months

### Diagnostic Checklist
- Always consider AT/RhT when large tumor found in child < 3 years

---

- Hyperintense cystic foci
- FLAIR
  - Cysts hyperintense to CSF
  - Solid tumor isointense to hyperintense
  - Interstitial edema
- T2* GRE: Hypointense "blooming" of hemorrhagic foci
- DWI
  - Hyperintense
  - Decreased diffusivity
- T1 C+
  - Heterogeneous enhancement
  - Leptomeningeal spread
    - Diffuse linear
    - Multiple nodular
- MRA: May show narrowing of encased vessels
- MRS
  - Aggressive metabolite pattern
    - Elevated choline
    - Low or absent NAA and creatine
    - Lipid/lactate peak

### Imaging Recommendations
- Best imaging tool: MR with contrast
- Protocol advice
  - MRA may be of benefit for identifying vascular compromise
  - Entire CNS must be imaged at presentation to identify subarachnoid spread of tumor

## DIFFERENTIAL DIAGNOSIS

### Medulloblastoma (PNET-MB)
- Posterior fossa tumor
- AT/RhT more likely to have cysts than PNET-MB

### Ependymoma
- "Plastic" tumor, extends out 4th ventricle foramina
- Ca++, cysts, hemorrhage common; heterogeneous enhancement

### Pilocytic Astrocytoma (PA)
- More commonly contains large cyst

- Older children (5-15 years)

### Pineoblastoma
- PNET
- May present with widespread metastases

### Choroid Plexus Tumors
- Choroid plexus papilloma (CPP) or carcinoma (CP carcinoma)
- Intraventricular mass that can have dissemination

### Gliosarcoma
- High grade glioma
- Exophytic from brainstem

### Teratoma
- More often pineal or parasellar in location
- Heterogeneous on imaging due to Ca++, hemorrhage

### Hemangioblastoma
- Large cyst with small enhancing mural nodule
- Adult tumor!
- Often associated with von Hippel Lindau disease

## PATHOLOGY

### General Features
- General path comments
  - Defined as distinct lesion in 1987
  - Combination of primitive neuroectodermal, peripheral epithelial, and mesenchymal elements
  - Divergent differentiation
- Genetics
  - Monosomy of chromosome 22 or deletion of band 22q11
    - Band 22q11 is site of hSNF5/INI1 gene
    - INI1 is part of an ATP-dependent chromatin-remodeling complex
    - Inactivation of INI1 protein expression may result in altered transcriptional regulation of downstream target genes
  - Chromosome 22 abnormalities are also found in other CNS tumors

# ATYPICAL TERATOID-RHABDOID TUMOR

- Etiology
  - Unknown
  - Rhabdoid cells resemble those in malignant rhabdoid tumor of kidney
  - Divergent differentiation accounts for "teratoid" label
    - Diverse immunohistological staining suggests multiple cell lines
    - Cells do not develop beyond primitive stage, unlike teratoma
- Epidemiology
  - Rare over 3 years of age
  - Up to 20% of primitive CNS tumors in children under 3
  - No gender predominance

## Gross Pathologic & Surgical Features
- Frequently unresectable at presentation
- Poorly defined tumor margins
- Infiltration into parenchyma

## Microscopic Features
- Sheets of nonspecific cells interrupted by fibrovascular septa
- Rhabdoid cells
  - Large, pale, bland cells with moderate eosinophilic cytoplasm
- Embracing cells
  - Sickle-shaped cells that "embrace" rhabdoid cells
- Frequent positive immunoreactivity
  - Vimentin (VIM)
  - Glial fibrillary acidic protein (GFAP)
  - Synaptophysin
  - Smooth muscle actin
  - Cytokeratin
  - Chromogranin
  - Neuron specific enolase (NSE)
  - Epithelial membrane antigen (EMA)

## Staging, Grading or Classification Criteria
- WHO grade IV

# CLINICAL ISSUES

## Presentation
- Most common signs/symptoms
  - Signs of increased intracranial pressure
    - Lethargy
    - Vomiting
    - Increased head circumference
  - Other signs/symptoms
    - Torticollis
    - Seizure
    - Regression of skills
- Clinical Profile: Child under 3 with increasing head size, vomiting, and lethargy

## Demographics
- Age: < 3 years
- Gender: M = F

## Natural History & Prognosis
- Median survival = 6 months

- Overall 2 year survival of less than 15% for children < 3 years at diagnosis

## Treatment
- Some question benefit of gross total resection
- Radiation rarely an option due to young age
- Chemotherapy regimens designed for PNET-MB largely ineffectual

# DIAGNOSTIC CHECKLIST

## Consider
- Always consider AT/RhT when large tumor found in child < 3 years

## Image Interpretation Pearls
- Imaging appearance is nonspecific
- More likely to be heterogeneous or supratentorial than PNET

# SELECTED REFERENCES

1. El Kababri M et al: Atypical teratoid rhabdoid tumor in a child with neurofibromatosis 1. Pediatr Blood Cancer. 46(2):267-8, 2006
2. Fujisawa H et al: Cyclin D1 is overexpressed in atypical teratoid/rhabdoid tumor with hSNF5/INI1 gene inactivation. J Neurooncol. 73(2):117-24, 2005
3. Janson K et al: Predisposition to atypical teratoid/rhabdoid tumor due to an inherited INI1 mutation. Pediatr Blood Cancer. 2005
4. Reddy AT: Atypical teratoid/rhabdoid tumors of the central nervous system. J Neurooncol. 75(3):309-13, 2005
5. Strother D: Atypical teratoid rhabdoid tumors of childhood: diagnosis, treatment and challenges. Expert Rev Anticancer Ther. 5(5):907-15, 2005
6. Arslanoglu A et al: Imaging findings of CNS atypical teratoid/rhabdoid tumors. AJNR. 25:476-80, 2004
7. Lee YK et al: Atypical teratoma/rhabdoid tumor of the cerebellum: Report of two infantile cases. AJNR. 25:481-3, 2004
8. Fenton LZ et al: Atypical teratoid/rhabdoid tumor of the central nervous system in children: an atypical series and review. Pediatr Radiol. 33(8):554-8, 2003
9. Bambakidis NC et al: Atypical teratoid/rhabdoid tumors of the central nervous system: clinical, radiographic and pathologic features. Pediatr Neurosurg. 37(2):64-70, 2002
10. Lee MC et al: Atypical teratoid/rhabdoid tumor of the central nervous system: clinico-pathological study. Neuropathology. 22(4):252-60, 2002
11. Guler E et al: Extraneural metastasis in a child with atypical teratoid rhabdoid tumor of the central nervous system. J Neurooncol. 54(1):53-6, 2001
12. Hauser P et al: Atypical teratoid/rhabdoid tumor or medulloblastoma? Med Pediatr Oncol. 36(6):644-8, 2001
13. Zuccoli G et al: Central nervous system atypical teratoid/rhabdoid tumour of infancy. CT and mr findings. Clin Imaging. 23(6):356-60, 1999

# ATYPICAL TERATOID-RHABDOID TUMOR

## IMAGE GALLERY

### Typical

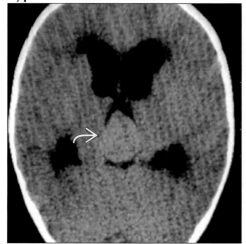

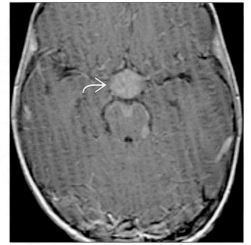

*(Left) Axial NECT shows slightly hyperattenuating pineal region AT/RhT ➔. Like PNETs and ependymomas, these tumors tend to be slightly more dense than brain parenchyma. (Right) Axial T1 C+ MR shows a dominant primary suprasellar tumor ➔ with widespread subarachnoid metastatic disease filling sulci and the interpeduncular and perimesencephalic cisterns.*

### Typical

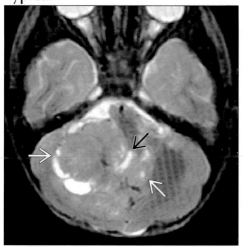

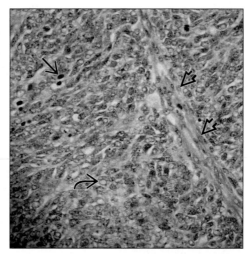

*(Left) Axial T2WI MR shows mass ➔ isointense to gray matter, centered in the vermis and right cerebellar hemisphere, with marked displacement and compression of the 4th ventricle ➔. (Right) Micropathology, low power, H&E shows fibrovascular septa ➔, dense nucleoli ➔, and a small number of "rhabdoid" cells ➔. The latter do not necessarily dominate the histology of AT/RhT.*

### Typical

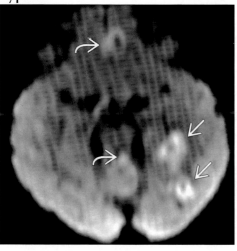

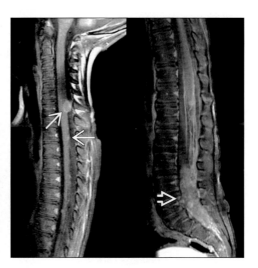

*(Left) Axial DWI MR shows reduced diffusivity of AT/RhT at primary site in the left temporal lobe ➔ and at metastases ➔ in superior cerebellar peduncle and in frontal lobe. (Right) Sagittal T1 C+ FS MR of the spinal column shows nodular tumor foci ➔ in the cervical and thoracic spine, with a large mass of tumor in the lumbar canal ➔.*

# LEUKEMIA

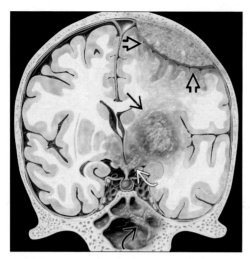

*Coronal graphic shows leukemic infiltrates in the sphenoid bone ⤷, infundibulum and hypothalamus ⤷, basal ganglia ⤷, and epidural space ⤷.*

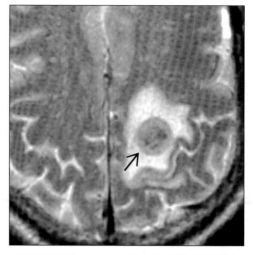

*Axial T2WI MR shows a well defined left parietal lobe leukemic metastasis ⤷ with moderate surrounding edema.*

## TERMINOLOGY

### Abbreviations and Synonyms
- Granulocytic sarcoma, chloroma, extramedullary leukemic tumors (EML)
- Extramedullary myeloblastoma, extramedullary myeloid cell tumors (EmMCT)

### Definitions
- Solid tumor of myeloblasts, myelocytes, and promyelocytes occurring in patients with myeloproliferative disorders
- There are multiple intracranial manifestations or complications of leukemia and its treatment
  - Posterior reversible encephalopathy syndrome (PRES)
  - Invasive aspergillus infection
  - Late development of cavernous angiomas after radiation therapy
  - Post-transplantation lymphoproliferative disease (PTLD) after bone marrow transplantation
  - Venous thrombosis associated with chemotherapy (L-asparaginase)
  - Vasculitis

- Primary manifestation of leukemia
- Secondary to treatment (trans-retinoic acid)
- Secondary to infection (aspergillus)

## IMAGING FINDINGS

### General Features
- Best diagnostic clue
  - Homogeneous enhancing tumor(s) in patient with known or suspected myeloproliferative disorder
  - Most often a complication of acute myelogenous leukemia (AML)
- Location: May be dural-based or less commonly intraparenchymal
- Morphology: Variable

### CT Findings
- NECT
  - Isodense or hyperdense to brain
    - Parenchymal lesions often hyperdense
  - May present with or mimic hematoma
  - May rapidly become hypodense related to necrosis or liquefaction
- CECT

## DDx: Multiple Hemorrhagic Parenchymal Lesions

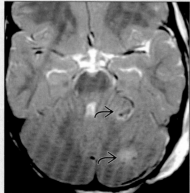

*Shear Injury*

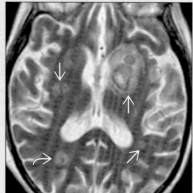

*Aspergillus*

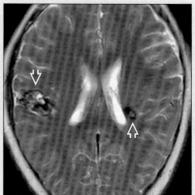

*Cavernomas*

# LEUKEMIA

## Key Facts

### Imaging Findings
- Homogeneous enhancing tumor(s) in patient with known or suspected myeloproliferative disorder
- Most often a complication of acute myelogenous leukemia (AML)
- Location: May be dural-based or less commonly intraparenchymal
- Homogeneous enhancement
- Use fat-saturation techniques for contrast MR

### Top Differential Diagnoses
- Metastatic Neuroblastoma (NBL)
- Meningioma
- Extramedullary Hematopoiesis
- Fungal Infection

### Pathology
- "Chloroma" (from green color) coined in 1853
- Re-named granulocytic sarcoma in 1966
- Epidemiology: 11% of patients with AML

### Clinical Issues
- May precede marrow diagnosis of leukemia
- 50% of cases diagnosed only at autopsy

### Diagnostic Checklist
- Hemorrhagic lesions in children with AML can be manifestation of chloroma or complication of therapy
- Remember that chloromas can rarely mimic abscess with enhancing rim

---

- ○ Homogeneous enhancement
  - ■ Hyperdensity or presence of hemorrhage may mask enhancement
- ○ May have rim-enhancement mimicking abscess

## MR Findings
- T1WI
  - ○ Hypointense or isointense to brain
    - ■ Hemorrhagic parenchymal lesions can be hyperintense
  - ○ Can distinguish between acute hematoma and non-hemorrhagic mass
- T2WI
  - ○ Heterogeneous and hyperintense to isointense
    - ■ Hemorrhagic parenchymal lesions will be hypointense
  - ○ Leptomeningeal disease in perivascular spaces may appear as patchy bright signal in white matter
- FLAIR: More sensitive than T2WI for leptomeningeal disease
- T2* GRE
  - ○ Sensitive for hemorrhagic lesions
    - ■ Helpful for identifying cavernous angiomas as very late complication of leukemia treatment
- DWI: Can distinguish ischemic lesions from posterior reversible encephalopathy syndrome (PRES)
- T1 C+
  - ○ Homogeneous enhancement
    - ■ May become heterogeneous with necrosis/liquefaction
  - ○ Leptomeningeal or perivascular space enhancement
  - ○ Fat-saturation technique essential for assessment of skull base disease
  - ○ Subtraction techniques may help identify enhancement, separate from hyperintense hemorrhagic components
- MRA
  - ○ May show vasospasm in cases of PRES
  - ○ May identify medium vessel vasculitis
- MRV
  - ○ Essential in evaluation of hemorrhagic lesions
  - ○ Identify presence or extent of venous thrombosis

## Nuclear Medicine Findings
- PET: Avid uptake on FDG-PET exams
- Bone Scan
  - ○ Tc-99m MDP commonly used for bone disease in leukemia
  - ○ Soft tissue uptake typically reflects hypercalcemia, not chloroma

## Imaging Recommendations
- Best imaging tool: MR with contrast and T2* GRE
- Protocol advice
  - ○ Use fat-saturation techniques for contrast MR
  - ○ Consider extramedullary hematopoiesis in differential diagnosis

## DIFFERENTIAL DIAGNOSIS

### Metastatic Neuroblastoma (NBL)
- Rarely occurs without extracranial disease
- Characteristic "raccoon eyes" clinical presentation
- Spiculated periostitis

### Meningioma
- May be very difficult to distinguish
- Dural "tail" may be more common in meningioma

### Extra-Axial Hematoma
- Extracranial soft tissue swelling or skull fracture
- If no appropriate history, consider possibility of child abuse

### Extramedullary Hematopoiesis
- Markedly hypointense on T2WI
- Same at-risk patient population

### Langerhans Cell Histiocytosis (LCH)
- Destruction of adjacent bone without periosteal reaction
- Diabetes insipidus

# LEUKEMIA

## Fungal Infection
- Multiple hemorrhagic parenchymal lesions are characteristic of aspergillus infection in the immunocompromised patient
- Children with leukemia treated with bone marrow transplant are at high risk for these infections

## Multiple Cavernous Angiomas
- Multiple hemorrhagic/hemosiderin-stained parenchymal lesions

## Shear Injury
- Multiple hemorrhagic/hemosiderin-stained parenchymal lesions

## PATHOLOGY

### General Features
- General path comments
  - CNS leukemia presents in three forms
    - Meningeal disease, usually with acute lymphoblastic leukemia (ALL)
    - Intravascular aggregates (leukostasis) that can rupture in patients with markedly high leukocyte counts
    - Tumor masses (chloroma)
  - Leukemic masses first described in 1811
    - "Chloroma" (from green color) coined in 1853
    - Re-named granulocytic sarcoma in 1966
- Genetics
  - Children with CNS leukemic infiltrates in AML have higher rate of chromosome 11 abnormalities than those without CNS disease
  - Chromosomal 8 and 21 translocations reported in cases of AML with chloroma
- Etiology
  - Some association with exposures
    - Ionizing radiation, hydrocarbons, benzene, alkylating agents
- Epidemiology: 11% of patients with AML
- Associated abnormalities
  - AML has higher incidence in some genetic syndromes
    - Fanconi anemia, Down syndrome, Bloom syndrome
  - Less commonly seen in other myeloproliferative disorders

### Gross Pathologic & Surgical Features
- Green color of chloroma (in 70% of cases) caused by high levels of myeloperoxidase

### Microscopic Features
- Moderate to large cells with pleomorphic nuclei
- Multiple mitoses give "starry sky" appearance

### Staging, Grading or Classification Criteria
- French-American-British (FAB) classification divides AML into 8 subtypes
- Chloroma is additional variant presentation, not separate subtype

## CLINICAL ISSUES

### Presentation
- Most common signs/symptoms
  - May precede marrow diagnosis of leukemia
  - 50% of cases diagnosed only at autopsy
- Clinical Profile
  - Child with AML develops new neurological signs or symptoms
    - Focal signs from local mass effect
    - Headache from hemorrhage

### Demographics
- Age: 60% of patients are < 15 yrs
- Gender: M:F = 1.4:1
- Ethnicity: Hispanic children < 19 yrs have highest rates of leukemia

### Natural History & Prognosis
- Overall survival rates for AML are around 40-50%
- Chloroma in setting of other myeloproliferative syndrome is a poor prognostic sign

### Treatment
- Options, risks, complications
  - Bone marrow transplant for consolidation
  - Chemotherapy for induction
    - Cytarabine (Ara-C), anthracycline

## DIAGNOSTIC CHECKLIST

### Consider
- Hemorrhagic lesions in children with AML can be manifestation of chloroma or complication of therapy

### Image Interpretation Pearls
- Multiple lesions at multiple sites are suggestive of diagnosis
- Remember that chloromas can rarely mimic abscess with enhancing rim

## SELECTED REFERENCES

1. Barredo JC et al: Isolated CNS relapse of acute lymphoblastic leukemia treated with intensive systemic chemotherapy and delayed CNS radiation: a pediatric oncology group study. J Clin Oncol. 24(19):3142-9, 2006
2. Chan MS et al: MR imaging of the brain in patients cured of acute lymphoblastic leukemia--the value of gradient echo imaging. AJNR Am J Neuroradiol. 27(3):548-52, 2006
3. Guermazi A et al: The dural tail sign--beyond meningioma. Clin Radiol. 60(2):171-88, 2005
4. Porto L et al: Central nervous system imaging in childhood leukaemia. Eur J Cancer. 40(14):2082-90, 2004
5. Nikolic B et al: CT changes of an intracranial granulocytic sarcoma on short-term follow-up. AJR Am J Roentgenol. 180(1):78-80, 2003
6. Okafuji T et al: CT and MR findings of brain aspergillosis. Comput Med Imaging Graph. 27(6):489-92, 2003
7. Ahn JY et al: Meningeal chloroma (granulocytic sarcoma) in acute lymphoblastic leukemia mimicking a falx meningioma. J Neurooncol. 60(1):31-5, 2002
8. Guermazi A et al: Granulocytic sarcoma (chloroma): imaging findings in adults and children. AJR Am J Roentgenol. 178(2):319-25, 2002

# LEUKEMIA

## IMAGE GALLERY

### Typical

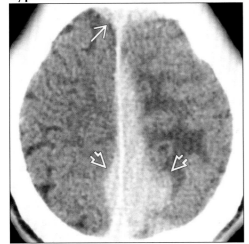 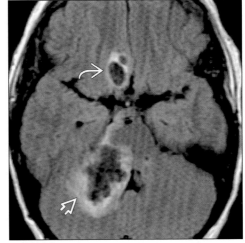

*(Left)* Axial CECT shows enhancing dural based leukemic infiltrates on both sides of the falx ➡. Note additional extra-axial disease along anterior dural margin ➡. *(Right)* Axial FLAIR MR in a child with ALL shows hemorrhagic tumors in the middle cerebellar peduncle ➡ and in the posterior aspect of the right gyrus rectus ➡.

### Typical

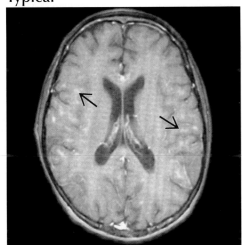 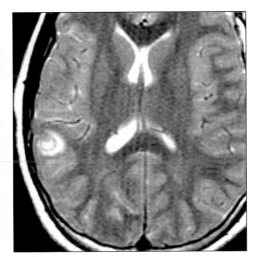

*(Left)* Axial T1 C+ MR shows multiple foci of enhancement filling perivascular spaces throughout the brain ➡. The imaging appearance of this manifestation mimics granulomatous disease. *(Right)* Axial T2WI MR in the same child shows the significant edema around the neoplasm and the ring-like hypointense signal at the margin, mimicking a small abscess.

### Variant

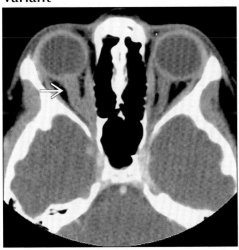 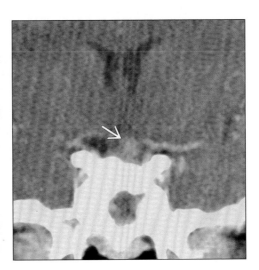

*(Left)* Axial CECT of the orbits in a child with ALL shows abnormal enhancement and thickening of the right optic nerve ➡ due to leukemic infiltration. *(Right)* Coronal CECT shows a rounded, thickened infundibulum ➡. This results from leukemic infiltration of the infundibulum, which is a rare complication of systemic leukemia.

# PART II
**Head & Neck**

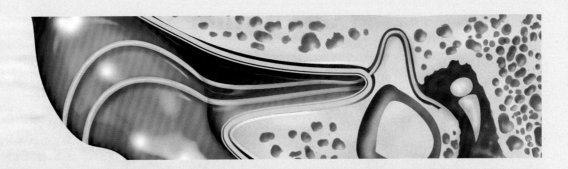

# SECTION 1: Temporal Bone & Skull Base

# LABYRINTHINE APLASIA

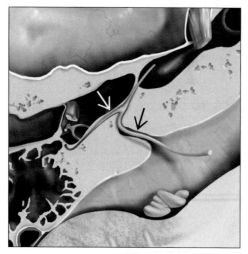

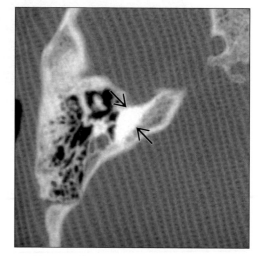

*Axial graphic depicts labyrinthine aplasia. Note complete absence all inner ear structures with the exception of small IAC ➡ with only CN7. Lateral wall of inner ear ➡ is flattened.*

*Axial bone CT shows complete labyrinthine aplasia with absence of inner ear structures ➡: Cochlea, vestibule and semicircular canals.*

## TERMINOLOGY

### Abbreviations and Synonyms
• Old synonym: Michel deformity

### Definitions
• Complete absence of cochlea

## IMAGING FINDINGS

### General Features
• Best diagnostic clue: Absent cochlea, vestibule, and semicircular canals (SCCs)

### CT Findings
• NECT
  ○ Mild form of labyrinthine aplasia
    ▪ Petrous bone lacks cochlea, vestibule & SCCs
    ▪ Small internal auditory canal (IAC) and petrous apex, middle ear normal
  ○ More severe form of labyrinthine aplasia
    ▪ Absent IAC, petrous apex and ossicles (or fused)
  ○ Lateral wall of inner ear is FLAT

  ○ Facial nerve bony canal prominent, geniculate ganglion more posterior than normal

### MR Findings
• T2WI
  ○ No normal high signal intensity fluid in membranous labyrinth on high-resolution T2WI
  ○ Sagittal T2WI through IAC show normal CN7 but absent cochlear-vestibular complex

### Imaging Recommendations
• Best imaging tool
  ○ High resolution temporal bone CT
  ○ Thin section T2WI MRI

## DIFFERENTIAL DIAGNOSIS

### Cochlear Aplasia: Late 3rd Week Arrest
• Absent cochlea, dysmorphic vestibule and SCCs

### Common Cavity Deformity: 4th Week Arrest
• Ovoid single inner ear cavity

---

### DDx: Inner Ear Abnormalities

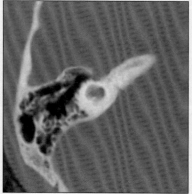

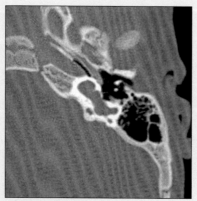

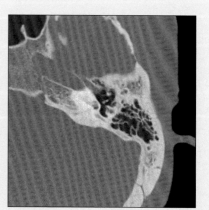

*Common Cavity*

*Cystic Cochleovestibular Anomaly*

*Labyrinthine Ossification*

# LABYRINTHINE APLASIA

## Key Facts

### Terminology
- Old synonym: Michel deformity

### Imaging Findings
- Best diagnostic clue: Absent cochlea, vestibule, and semicircular canals (SCCs)
- No normal high signal intensity fluid in membranous labyrinth on high-resolution T2WI

### Top Differential Diagnoses
- Cochlear Aplasia: Late 3rd Week Arrest
- Common Cavity Deformity: 4th Week Arrest
- Cystic Cochleovestibular Anomaly (CCVA) (Incomplete Partition, Type 1)
- Large Endolymphatic Sac Anomaly (LESA) (Incomplete Partition, Type 2)
- Labyrinthine Ossification, Obliterative Type

## Cystic Cochleovestibular Anomaly (CCVA) (Incomplete Partition, Type 1)
- 5th week arrest with "figure 8" cystic cochlea & vestibule with dysplastic SCCs

## Large Endolymphatic Sac Anomaly (LESA) (Incomplete Partition, Type 2)
- 7th week arrest with large vestibular aqueduct, endolymphatic sac and duct, and cochlear dysplasia

## Labyrinthine Ossification, Obliterative Type
- Post-meningitis ossification, normal lateral bulge of promontory

## PATHOLOGY

### General Features
- General path comments
  - Embryology
    - Arrest of otic placode development at 3rd gestational week
- Genetics: Autosomal dominant inheritance
- Etiology: usually unknown, rarely Thalidomide exposure
- Epidemiology: Extremely rare, < 1% of inner ear malformations
- Associated abnormalities: Klippel-Feil syndrome

## CLINICAL ISSUES

### Presentation
- Most common signs/symptoms: Congenital SNHL

### Natural History & Prognosis
- Affected ear will never hear

### Treatment
- Unilateral - no treatment
- Bilateral - profound deafness
  - Not a cochlear implant candidate

## DIAGNOSTIC CHECKLIST

### Consider
- Labyrinthine aplasia if bony labyrinth is featureless, with no cochlea, vestibule or SCCs
- Lateral wall of otic capsule FLAT, not convex

## SELECTED REFERENCES

1. Sennaroglu L et al: A new classification for cochleovestibular malformations. Laryngoscope. 112:2230-41, 2002
2. Schuknecht HF: Pathology of the Ear, 2nd ed. Philadelphia: Lea and Febiger, Vol. 180-1, 1993
3. Jackler R et al: Congenital malformation of the inner ear. Laryngoscope. 97:2-14, 1987

## IMAGE GALLERY

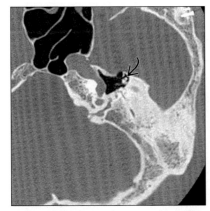 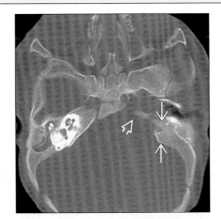 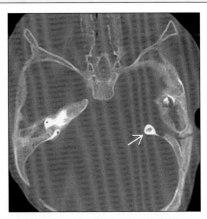

*(Left)* Axial bone CT shows a severe case of labyrinthine aplasia without definable cochlea, vestibule or SCCs with dysmorphic ossicles ⟋ fused to the small lateral epitympanic cavity. *(Center)* Axial bone CT shows severe labyrinthine aplasia and skull base deformity. The left petrous apex is absent ⇨ and the left cochlea and semicircular canals ⇨ are not formed. *(Right)* Axial bone CT in the same patient as previous image shows a small dysmorphic hypodense structure ⇨ that may represent an early otocyst.

# AURAL ATRESIA

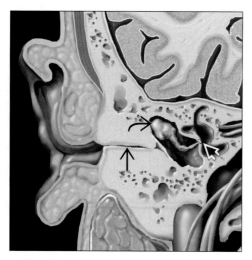

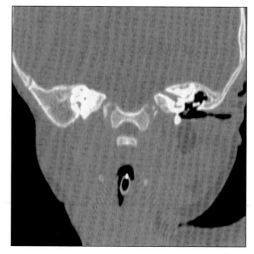

*Coronal graphic of EAC shows deformed auricle & bony EAC atresia →. Ossicular fusion & rotation ⟶ with oval window atresia ▷ are also present.*

*Coronal bone CT shows absence of right external auditory canal, lack of aerated middle ear cavity and mastoid air cells, and absent middle ear ossicles in a child with Goldenhar syndrome.*

## TERMINOLOGY

### Abbreviations and Synonyms
- External auditory canal (EAC) atresia
- Congenital aural dysplasia (CAD)

### Definitions
- Dysplasia of the outer ear (auricle and EAC)
  - Stenosis or atresia of EAC

## IMAGING FINDINGS

### General Features
- Best diagnostic clue: Soft tissue or bony atretic plate occluding the EAC where tympanic membrane (TM) should be
- Location
  - EAC, middle ear & mastoid complex
  - Inner ear spared in most cases
- Size: Stenosis usually extends from external opening of canal to tympanic membrane
- Morphology
  - Dysplastic auricle (microtia)

- Mildest form has narrowed EAC
- More severe has no identifiable EAC
- Hypoplasia or underpneumatization of middle ear cavity (MEC) & mastoid complex
- Dysmorphic ossicular chain, especially malleus & incus
  - Hypoplastic, absent, abnormal joint or fusion to attic wall

### CT Findings
- NECT
  - External ear & EAC
    - Small, dysmorphic pinna
    - Bony, soft tissue, or mixed stenosis/atresia of membranous and bony portions of EAC
    - Variable thickness of atretic plate
  - Middle ear findings depend on severity of atresia
    - Small middle ear cavity (especially hypotympanum)
    - Fusion, abnormal rotation, hypoplasia or absence of malleus & incus
    - Abnormal malleoincudal or incudostapedial articulation
    - Oval window atresia may be associated

## DDx: External Auditory Canal Occlusion

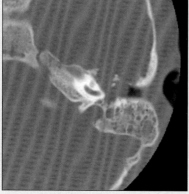

*Rhabdomyosarcoma*

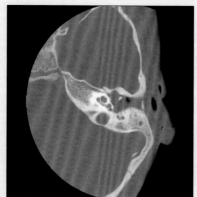

*Cholesteatoma*

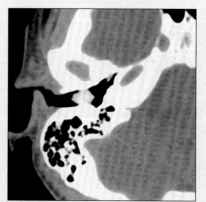

*Foreign Body: Silicone Ear Plug*

# AURAL ATRESIA

## Key Facts

### Terminology
- External auditory canal (EAC) atresia
- Congenital aural dysplasia (CAD)
- Dysplasia of the outer ear (auricle and EAC)

### Imaging Findings
- Small, dysmorphic pinna
- Bony, soft tissue, or mixed stenosis/atresia of membranous and bony portions of EAC
- Small middle ear cavity (especially hypotympanum)
- Fusion, abnormal rotation, hypoplasia or absence of malleus & incus
- Congenital or acquired cholesteatoma in EAC or behind atresia plate (< 10%)
- Aberrant course of tympanic & mastoid portions of facial nerve common

### Top Differential Diagnoses
- Rhabdomyosarcoma
- EAC Osteoma or Exostosis
- EAC Cholesteatoma
- Foreign Body (FB)

### Pathology
- Failure of canalization leads to EAC atresia
- Inner ear forms earlier during gestation, so anomalies of labyrinth & IAC rarely associated with EAC atresia

### Diagnostic Checklist
- Severity of auricular dysplasia parallels degree of deformity of middle ear & ossicles

---

- Normal morphology & location of stapes important for surgical reconstruction of ossicular function
- Congenital or acquired cholesteatoma in EAC or behind atresia plate (< 10%)
- Facial nerve canal findings
  - Aberrant course of tympanic & mastoid portions of facial nerve common
  - Tympanic segment may be dehiscent and or caudally displaced, overlying oval or round windows
  - Mastoid segment usually anteriorly and laterally displaced
  - May exit skull base into glenoid fossa, between glenoid fossa and styloid process or lateral to styloid process
- Inner ear findings
  - Inner ear & inner auditory canal (IAC) normal in most cases
  - 12% abnormal: Hypoplastic cochlea, hypoplastic or large lateral semicircular canal, large vestibule or large vestibular aqueduct

### MR Findings
- Unnecessary for initial imaging
- Helpful if associated cholesteatoma

### Imaging Recommendations
- Best imaging tool: High-resolution axial & coronal plane bone CT

## DIFFERENTIAL DIAGNOSIS

### Rhabdomyosarcoma
- Enhancing soft tissue mass, usually with associated osseous erosion

### EAC Osteoma or Exostosis
- Usually unilateral
- Benign bony growth obliterating EAC

### EAC Cholesteatoma
- Unilateral with normal auricle

- Soft tissue mass protrudes into EAC
- Underlying bony EAC scalloping
- May have bone fragments in soft tissue mass

### Foreign Body (FB)
- May see surgical packing in adults
- Small toys, beans & beads in children

## PATHOLOGY

### General Features
- General path comments
  - Non-syndromal EAC atresia usually unilateral
  - Bilateral atresia common when EAC atresia syndromal
  - Atresia is membranous, bony or mixed
  - Embryology-anatomy
    - 1st & 2nd branchial arches & 1st pharyngeal pouch develop at same time during embryogenesis
    - Associated middle ear & mastoid anomalies are common with EAC atresia
    - Branchial groove & 1st pharyngeal pouch give rise to EAC
    - Initially, core of epithelial cells solid in future EAC location, 3rd trimester core canalizes to form EAC
    - Failure of canalization leads to EAC atresia
    - 1st branchial arch forms malleus head, incus body & short process & tensor tympani tendon
    - 2nd branchial arch forms manubrium of malleus, long process of incus, stapes (except footplate) & stapedial muscle and tendon
    - Inner ear forms earlier during gestation, so anomalies of labyrinth & IAC rarely associated with EAC atresia
- Genetics
  - 14% have family history
  - May be associated with inherited syndromes
    - Crouzon, Goldenhar or Pierre Robin syndromes
- Etiology: Presumed to be in utero insult, epithelial cells of 1st branchial groove fail to split & canalize
- Epidemiology
  - 1 in 10,000 births

# AURAL ATRESIA

- 1 in 900 births in the era of thalidomide embryopathy
  - Bony > > membranous atresia
- Associated abnormalities
  - Inner ear anomaly occurs in up to 12%
  - May be isolated malformation, or part of craniofacial syndrome

## Gross Pathologic & Surgical Features
- Pinna is malformed & abnormally positioned
- Atresia plate can be membranous or bony and of variable thickness

## Microscopic Features
- Cholesteatoma may occur in rudimentary MEC

## Staging, Grading or Classification Criteria
- Mild anomaly may have normal pinna, minimal deformity of malleus & incus, hypoplastic MEC
- Moderate malformation has rudimentary auricle, more severe ossicular anomalies & aberrant facial nerve course
- Severe anomaly may have no pinna, rudimentary middle ear cleft, absent ossicles & inner ear malformations

# CLINICAL ISSUES

## Presentation
- Most common signs/symptoms
  - Conductive hearing loss
  - Physical exam
    - Dysplastic auricle, EAC absent or stenotic

## Demographics
- Age: Congenital lesion
- Gender: Occurs more commonly in males

## Natural History & Prognosis
- Status at birth remains unchanged through life, unless there is associated middle ear cholesteatoma
- In unilateral atresia, other ear has normal hearing
- Bilateral atresia may present as bilateral conductive hearing loss
  - Surgical success depends on degree of associated middle and inner ear anomalies
- Auricle reconstruction may require 4-5 staged surgeries

## Treatment
- Unilateral atresia usually treated with auricle reconstruction and bone anchored hearing aid if other ear is normal
- Course of facial nerve, status of oval and round window, ossicles, inner ear structures, and IAC should be established by CT prior to surgery
- Bilateral atresia is treated at 5-8 years of age, when mastoid development is complete
  - Reconstruction of auricle precedes surgical treatment of middle ear & ossicular deformities
  - Surgical reconstruction on side with mildest EAC atresia if bilateral
  - Both auricles are repaired for cosmetic reasons

# DIAGNOSTIC CHECKLIST

## Consider
- EAC atresia = clinical diagnosis
  - CT provides pre-operative roadmap
- Severity of auricular dysplasia parallels degree of deformity of middle ear & ossicles
- Temporal bone CT later in life to exclude associated cholesteatoma

## Image Interpretation Pearls
- Pre-operative T-bone CT checklist essential for surgical planning
  - Type (bony or membranous) & thickness of atresia plate
  - Size of mastoid complex & middle ear cavity helps determine surgical approach
  - Status of ossicular chain, including presence, morphology, & fusion to lateral MEC wall
  - Carefully assess malleoincudal and incudostapedial articulations
  - Status of oval window & stapes inspected for oval window atresia
  - Trace course of facial nerve, as aberrant and/or dehiscent nerve may be at risk during surgery
  - Hypoplastic or aplastic IAC with deficient cochlear nerve, and hypoplastic cochlea may be a surgical contraindication

# SELECTED REFERENCES

1. Blevins NH et al: External auditory canal duplication anomalies associated with congenital aural atresia. J Laryngol Otol. 117(1):32-8, 2003
2. Klingebiel R et al: Multislice computed tomographic imaging in temporal bone dysplasia. Otol Neurotol. 23(5):715-22, 2002
3. Benton C et al: Imaging of congenital anomalies of the temporal bone. Neuroimaging Clin N Am. 10(1):35-53, vii-viii, 2000
4. Calzolari F et al: Clinical and radiological evaluation in children with microtia. Br J Audiol. 33(5):303-12, 1999
5. Declau F et al: Diagnosis and management strategies in congenital atresia of the external auditory canal. Study Group on Otological Malformations and Hearing Impairment. Br J Audiol. 33(5):313-27, 1999
6. Selesnick S et al: Surgical treatment of acquired external auditory canal atresia. Am J Otol. 19(2):123-30, 1998
7. Mayer TE et al: High-resolution CT of the temporal bone in dysplasia of the auricle and external auditory canal. AJNR Am J Neuroradiol. 18(1):53-65, 1997
8. Nishizaki K et al: A computer-assisted operation for congenital aural malformations. Int J Pediatr Otorhinolaryngol. 36(1):31-7, 1996
9. Yeakley JW et al: CT evaluation of congenital aural atresia: what the radiologist and surgeon need to know. J Comput Assist Tomogr. 20(5):724-31, 1996
10. Chandrasekhar SS et al: Surgery of congenital aural atresia. Am J Otol. 16(6):713-7, 1995
11. Andrews JC et al: Three-dimensional CT scan reconstruction for the assessment of congenital aural atresia. Am J Otol. 13(3):236-40, 1992
12. Jahrsdoerfer RA et al: Grading system for the selection of patients with congenital aural atresia. Am J Otol. 13(1):6-12, 1992

## IMAGE GALLERY

### Typical

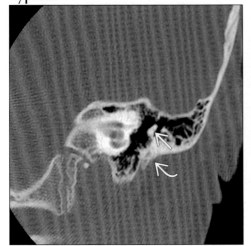
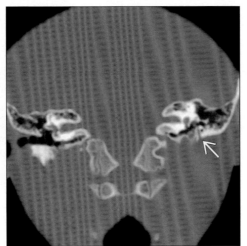

*(Left)* Coronal bone CT shows left external auditory canal atresia ➔ with a moderate sized left middle ear cavity. Small dysmorphic ossicles ➔ are fused to the lateral epitympanic wall. *(Right)* Coronal bone CT in same patient as previous image shows comparison with normal contralateral right temporal bone and anomalous position of the left descending facial nerve canal ➔.

### Typical

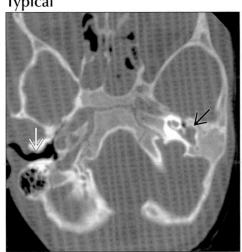
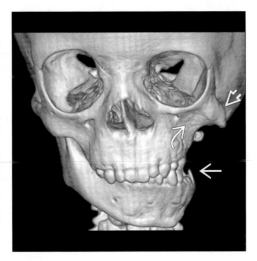

*(Left)* Axial bone CT shows complete absence of the left EAC, absent mastoid air cells and small, opacified left middle ear cavity ➔. Note normal right EAC ➔ for comparison. *(Right)* Frontal 3D face CT in a patient with Goldenhar syndrome shows hypoplasia of the left mandible ➔, malar eminence ➔ and zygomatic arch ➔.

### Typical

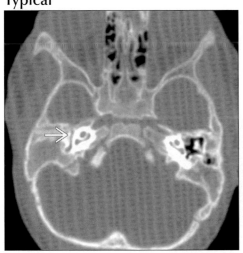
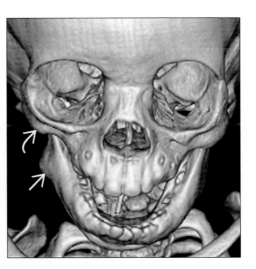

*(Left)* Axial bone CT shows complete absence of the right EAC, middle ear cavity, mastoid air cells and middle ear ossicles with inferiorly displaced tympanic segment of facial nerve canal ➔. *(Right)* Frontal 3D face CT in a patient with Goldenhar syndrome shows small ipsilateral right hemimandible ➔ and malar eminence ➔.

# COCHLEAR APLASIA, INNER EAR

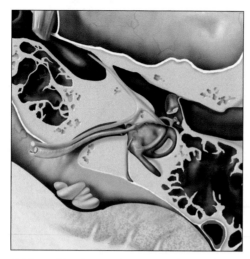

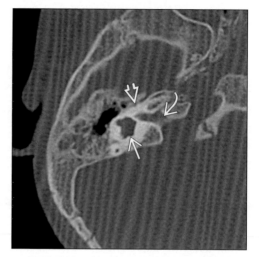

*Axial graphic depicts classic example of cochlear aplasia. The drawing shows an absence of both the cochlea and the cochlear nerve. Note the enlarged vestibule.*

*Axial bone CT shows cochlear aplasia ⊟ with associated vestibular dysplasia ⊟ and small internal auditory canal ⊅. Lateral semicircular canal is small, dysplastic.*

## TERMINOLOGY

### Abbreviations and Synonyms
- Absent cochlea

### Definitions
- Absent cochlea; vestibule, semicircular canals (SCCs) & internal auditory canal (IAC) present

## IMAGING FINDINGS

### General Features
- Best diagnostic clue: Absent cochlea, usually associated with dysmorphic vestibule & SCCs
- Location: Anterior membranous labyrinth, unilateral or bilateral

### CT Findings
- NECT
  - Complete absence of cochlea
    - Vestibule, SCCs & IAC normal, hypoplastic or dilated (cystic)

- Cochlear promontory flat, instead of normal lateral convexity when cochlea present
- Labyrinthine, geniculate ganglion & anterior tympanic portions of facial nerve occupy site where cochlea should be
- EAC, middle ear, ossicular chain, bony vestibular aqueduct & endolymphatic duct have normal size

### MR Findings
- T2WI
  - Absence of cochlea
  - Oblique sag ⇒ small IAC, absent cochlear nerve
  - Bone signal intensity replaces cochlea site
  - Vestibule, SCCs & IAC variably affected

### Imaging Recommendations
- Best imaging tool
  - High resolution temporal bone CT
  - High resolution oblique sag T2 for cochlear nerve

## DIFFERENTIAL DIAGNOSIS

### Labyrinthine Aplasia: 3rd Week Arrest
- Otic capsule development arrest at 3rd week gestation

### DDx: Absent Cochlea

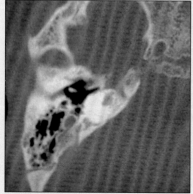
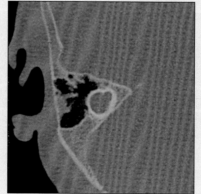
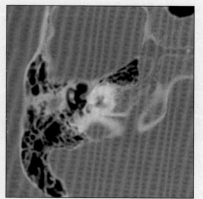

*Labyrinthine Aplasia*  *Common Cavity Deformity*  *Labyrinthine Ossification*

# COCHLEAR APLASIA, INNER EAR

## Key Facts

### Terminology
- Absent cochlea; vestibule, semicircular canals (SCCs) & internal auditory canal (IAC) present

### Imaging Findings
- Complete absence of cochlea

### Top Differential Diagnoses
- Labyrinthine Aplasia: 3rd Week Arrest
- Common Cavity Deformity: 4th Week Arrest

- Cystic Cochleovestibular Anomaly (CCVA) (Incomplete Partition, Type 1)
- Labyrinthine Ossification, Obliterative Type

### Pathology
- Arrest of otic placode development at late 3rd gestational week

### Clinical Issues
- Congenital sensorineural hearing loss

---

- Cochlea, vestibule & SCCs absent

## Common Cavity Deformity: 4th Week Arrest
- Ovoid single inner ear cavity

## Cystic Cochleovestibular Anomaly (CCVA) (Incomplete Partition, Type 1)
- 5th week arrest with "figure 8" cystic cochlea & vestibule with dysplastic SCCs

## Labyrinthine Ossification, Obliterative Type
- Post-meningitis ossification, normal lateral bulge of cochlear promontory

## PATHOLOGY

### General Features
- General path comments
  - Embryology
    - Arrest of otic placode development at late 3rd gestational week
- Etiology: Unknown
- Epidemiology: Extremely rare, < 1% of inner ear anomalies
- Associated abnormalities: Dysmorphic vestibule and SCCs

## CLINICAL ISSUES

### Presentation
- Congenital sensorineural hearing loss

### Demographics
- Age: Congenital, present at birth

### Natural History & Prognosis
- Affected ear will never hear

## DIAGNOSTIC CHECKLIST

### Consider
- Cochlear aplasia if no cochlea is seen on CT or T2 MR, but rest of membranous labyrinth present
- Be sure to distinguish from obliterative labyrinthine ossification

## SELECTED REFERENCES

1. Sennaroglu L et al: A new classification for cochleovestibular malformations. Laryngoscope. 112(12):2230-41, 2002
2. Schuknecht HF: Pathology of the Ear. 2nd ed. Philadelphia, Lea and Febiger. 180-1, 1993
3. Jackler RK et al: Congenital malformations of the inner ear: a classification based on embryogenesis. Laryngoscope. 97(3 Pt 2 Suppl 40):2-14, 1987

## IMAGE GALLERY

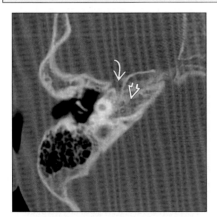 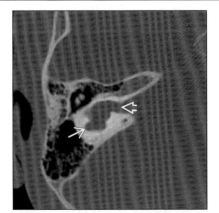 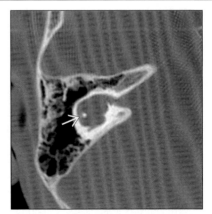

*(Left)* Axial bone CT shows no anterior labyrinth ➡ and low-lying geniculate fossa ➡. *(Center)* Axial bone CT (same patient as previous) shows a dysplastic vestibule ➡ that communicates with a small IAC ➡. There is no cochlea anterior to the dysplastic vestibule. *(Right)* Axial bone CT (same patient as previous) shows dilated dysplastic lateral semicircular canal containing a small central bone island ➡ inside the canal.

# COMMON CAVITY, INNER EAR

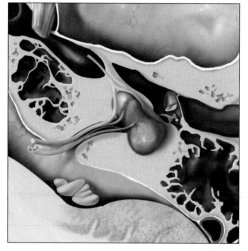

Axial graphic shows features of common cavity malformation. Note cochlea and vestibule are melded into one common cyst. Semicircular canals are not distinct from cystic vestibular component.

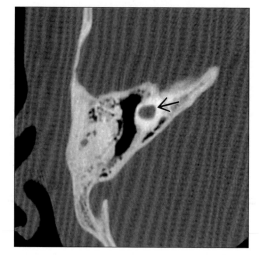

Axial bone CT shows small, featureless common cavity → without differentiation into cochlea and vestibule.

## TERMINOLOGY

### Abbreviations and Synonyms
- Cystic common cavity

### Definitions
- Common cavity: Rudimentary cochlea & vestibule

## IMAGING FINDINGS

### General Features
- Best diagnostic clue: Featureless common cavity: Rudimentary cochlea, vestibule & semicircular canals (SCCs)
- Size: Small or large

### CT Findings
- NECT
  - Cochlea, vestibule & SCCs form common cavity
  - SCCs usually absent
    - May be normal or dysplastic

- Internal auditory canal (IAC) always abnormal: Large with large common cavity, small with small common cavity, frequently enters center of cavity with defective fundus
- Middle ear structures, including ossicles, & vestibular aqueduct are normal

### MR Findings
- T2WI
  - High signal intensity fluid within featureless cystic cochlea & vestibule & absent modiolus
  - SCCs usually absent but may be normal or dysplastic
  - IAC small - hypoplastic or absent CN8 components, normal CN7

### Imaging Recommendations
- Best imaging tool
  - High resolution temporal bone CT
  - High resolution oblique sag T2 - for cochlear nerve

## DIFFERENTIAL DIAGNOSIS

### Cochlear Aplasia: Late 3rd Week Arrest
- Absent cochlea, dysmorphic vestibule and SCCs

## DDx: Inner Ear Anomalies (Cochlea)

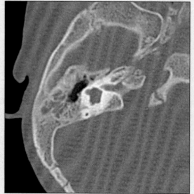

Cochlear Aplasia

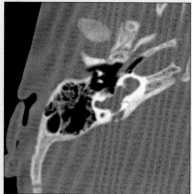

Cystic Cochleovestibular Anomaly

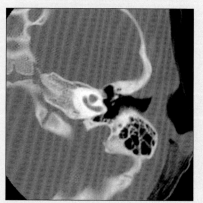

IP Type 2

# COMMON CAVITY, INNER EAR

## Key Facts

### Terminology
- Common cavity: Rudimentary cochlea & vestibule

### Imaging Findings
- Cochlea, vestibule & SCCs form common cavity
- SCCs usually absent

### Top Differential Diagnoses
- Cochlear Aplasia: Late 3rd Week Arrest

- Cystic Cochleovestibular Anomaly (CCVA) (Incomplete Partition, Type 1)
- Large Endolymphatic Sac Anomaly (LESA) (Incomplete Partition, Type 2)

### Pathology
- Rare, < 1% of all congenital inner ear malformations

### Clinical Issues
- Most common signs/symptoms: Congenital SNHL

---

## Cystic Cochleovestibular Anomaly (CCVA) (Incomplete Partition, Type 1)
- 5th week arrest with "figure 8" cystic cochlea and vestibule with dysplastic SCCs

## Large Endolymphatic Sac Anomaly (LESA) (Incomplete Partition, Type 2)
- 7th week arrest with large vestibular aqueduct, endolymphatic sac and duct, and cochlear dysplasia

## PATHOLOGY

### General Features
- General path comments
  - Embryology
    - Arrest of development at 4th gestational week, after differentiation of otic (auditory) placode into otocyst
- Etiology: Unknown
- Epidemiology
  - Rare, < 1% of all congenital inner ear malformations
  - 25% of all cochlear malformations

### Microscopic Features
- May be some differentiation of organ of Corti, but neural populations absent or low

## CLINICAL ISSUES

### Presentation
- Most common signs/symptoms: Congenital SNHL

### Treatment
- Successful cochlear implantation (CI) has been performed in common cavity deformity, suggesting some cochlear nerve fibers present

## DIAGNOSTIC CHECKLIST

### Consider
- Common cavity when cochlea & vestibule form single cavity without differentiation

### Image Interpretation Pearls
- T2 sagittal MR images through IAC necessary to determine presence of cochlear nerve if CI planned

## SELECTED REFERENCES

1. Sennaroglu L et al: A new classification for cochleovestibular malformations. Laryngoscope. 112(12):2230-41, 2002
2. Schuknecht HF: Pathology of the Ear. 2nd ed. Philadelphia, Lea and Febiger. 180-1, 1993
3. Jackler RK et al: Congenital malformations of the inner ear: a classification based on embryogenesis. Laryngoscope. 97(3 Pt 2 Suppl 40):2-14, 1987

## IMAGE GALLERY

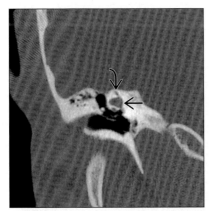 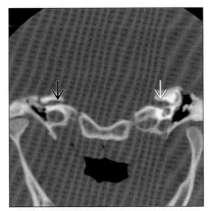 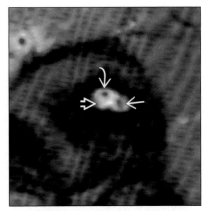

*(Left)* Coronal bone CT shows featureless common cavity ➡ with rudimentary superior semicircular canal ➡. The middle ear appears normal. *(Center)* Coronal bone CT in the same patient shows ipsilateral small right IAC ➡, compared to contralateral normal IAC ➡. *(Right)* Sagittal oblique T2WI MR shows the facial nerve ➡ and vestibular nerves ➡ present but the cochlear nerve absent ➡, in a patient with common cavity deformity.

# CYSTIC COCHLEOVESTIBULAR ANOMALY

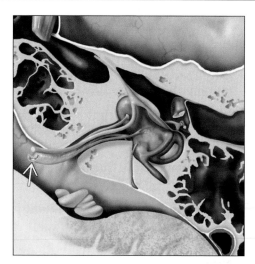

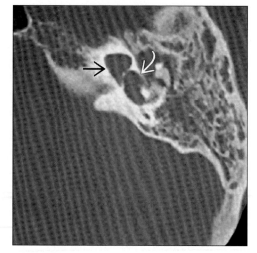

*Axial graphic depicts "figure 8" confluent cystic cochlea and vestibule. Modiolus is absent with all components of CN8 small →. IAC is ~ 75% of normal size. CN7 is normal in position.*

*Axial bone CT shows classic cystic cochleovestibular anomaly with dilated featureless cochlea → and vestibule →, resulting in a "figure 8" configuration. The modiolus is absent.*

## TERMINOLOGY

### Abbreviations and Synonyms
- Cystic cochleovestibular anomaly (CCVA)
- Incomplete partition (IP) type 1
- Cystic cochleovestibular malformation

### Definitions
- Malformation due to arrest of inner ear development at 5th gestational week

## IMAGING FINDINGS

### General Features
- Best diagnostic clue: "Snowman" shaped inner ear with cystic featureless cochlea and dilated cystic vestibule
- Location: Membranous labyrinth
- Morphology: Cochlea & vestibule have "figure 8" contour with no internal features

### CT Findings
- NECT
  - Cystic, featureless cochlea lacks modiolus

- Vestibule dilated & cystic
- Semicircular canals present, variable shape & degree of dilatation
- IAC may be dilated with defective fundus
- EAC, middle ear & ossicular chain, bony vestibular aqueduct & endolymphatic sac normal
- CN7 canal normal size, near normal in location

### MR Findings
- T2WI
  - Fluid-filled dilated, featureless cochlea & vestibule
    - Results in "figure 8" contour
  - Cochlea is cystic
    - No turns or modiolus
  - IAC small or normal size, deficient or absent cochleovestibular nerves, normal CN7

### Imaging Recommendations
- Best imaging tool
  - High-resolution T2WI MR
  - High-resolution temporal bone CT also helpful

## DDx: Inner Ear Anomalies

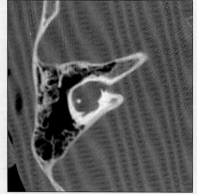

*Cochlear Aplasia*

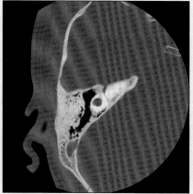

*Common Cavity*

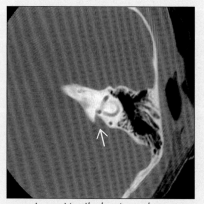

*Large Vestibular Aqueduct*

# CYSTIC COCHLEOVESTIBULAR ANOMALY

## Key Facts

### Terminology
- Malformation due to arrest of inner ear development at 5th gestational week

### Imaging Findings
- Morphology: Cochlea & vestibule have "figure 8" contour with no internal features
- IAC small or normal size, deficient or absent cochleovestibular nerves, normal CN7

### Top Differential Diagnoses
- Cochlear Aplasia: Late 3rd Week Arrest
- Common Cavity Deformity: 4th Week Arrest
- Large Endolymphatic Sac Anomaly (LESA) (Incomplete Partition, Type 2)

### Clinical Issues
- Most common signs/symptoms: Congenital SNHL
- May be relative contraindication to cochlear implant

## DIFFERENTIAL DIAGNOSIS

### Cochlear Aplasia: Late 3rd Week Arrest
- Absent cochlea, dysmorphic vestibule and semicircular canals

### Common Cavity Deformity: 4th Week Arrest
- Ovoid single inner ear cavity

### Large Endolymphatic Sac Anomaly (LESA) (Incomplete Partition, Type 2)
- 7th week arrest with large vestibular aqueduct (VA), endolymphatic sac and duct and cochlear dysplasia
- Clinical presentation: Cascading bilateral SNHL in 1st years of life

## PATHOLOGY

### General Features
- General path comments
  - Embryology
    - Arrest of otic placode development at ~ 5th gestational week
- Epidemiology: Rare inner ear anomaly, < 2% of all congenital labyrinthine lesions

### Microscopic Features
- Cochleovestibular nerves deficient
- Internal architecture of cochlea & vestibule lack normal structures

## CLINICAL ISSUES

### Presentation
- Most common signs/symptoms: Congenital SNHL

### Treatment
- May be relative contraindication to cochlear implant

## DIAGNOSTIC CHECKLIST

### Consider
- CCVA if cochlea & vestibule have rudimentary contours, but no internal architecture

### Image Interpretation Pearls
- T2WI MR shows full extent of lesion, including status of CN7 & CN8 in IAC

## SELECTED REFERENCES

1. Sennaroglu L et al: A new classification for cochleovestibular malformations. Laryngoscope. 112:2230-41, 2002
2. Schuknecht HF: Pathology of the ear, 2nd ed. Philadelphia, Lea and Febiger. 180-1, 1993
3. Jackler R et al: Congenital malformations of the inner ear. Laryngoscope. 97:2-14, 1987

## IMAGE GALLERY

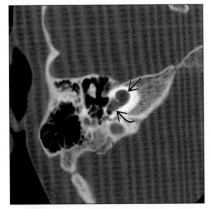 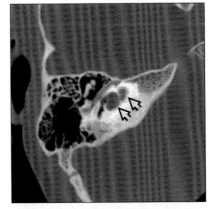 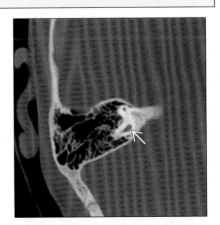

*(Left)* Axial bone CT image shows featureless cochlea ➡, absent modiolus and dilated inferior vestibule ➡. *(Center)* Axial bone CT 1 mm more superior, in the same patient as previous image, shows a "figure 8" configuration of the cystic cochleovestibular anomaly ➡. *(Right)* Axial bone CT 6 mm more superior, in the same patient as previous image, shows dilated, dysplastic posterior semicircular canal ➡.

# SEMICIRCULAR CANAL DYSPLASIA

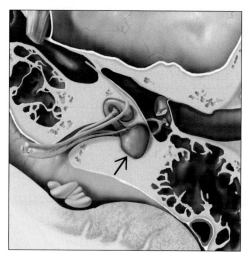

Axial graphic depicts severe, syndromic type of semicircular canal dysplasia with complete absence of all semicircular canals, cochlear dysplasia & dysmorphic vestibule ➡.

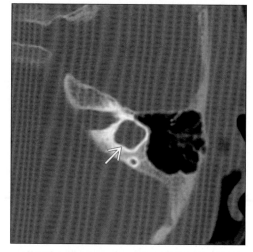

Axial bone CT shows homogeneous, nearly square, dysmorphic vestibule/lateral semicircular canal forming a single cavity ➡. Note absence of the normal central bone island.

## TERMINOLOGY

### Abbreviations and Synonyms
- Semicircular canal dysplasia (SCCD)
- Semicircular canal-vestibule dysplasia

### Definitions
- SCCD: Malformation, hypoplasia or aplasia of one or all of semicircular canals (SCC)

## IMAGING FINDINGS

### General Features
- Best diagnostic clue: Spectrum of anomalies, most common appearance is short, dilated lateral SCC & vestibule forming single cavity
- Location: Posterior membranous labyrinth
- Size: Varies from aplasia of SCCs to dysmorphic small SCCs to enlarged & dilated vestibule-lateral SCC
- Morphology: SCCs may be short & dilated, wide or aplastic

### CT Findings
- NECT
  - Most common, least severe appearance of SCCD is dilated lateral SCC forming single cavity with vestibule
    - Posterior & superior SCC may be normal, dilated or hypoplastic
    - Cochlea can be normal or incompletely partitioned (apical & middle turn)
    - Middle ear & mastoids variable, ranging from normal to ossicular anomalies
    - Oval window atresia commonly associated
  - Next most common is SCCD associated with CHARGE syndrome
    - All SCCs absent in both ears
    - Vestibule small & dysmorphic
    - Oval window atresia always present
    - Tympanic segment of facial nerve may be found overlying atretic oval window
    - Cochlear anomalies usually associated
    - Most common cochlear anomaly: "Isolated cochlea" with lack of cochlear nerve aperture

## DDx: Inner Ear Abnormalities

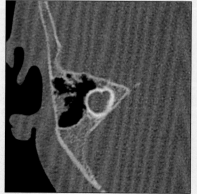

Common Cavity Deformity

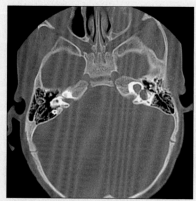

Cystic Cochleovestibular Anomaly

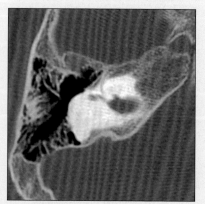

Labyrinthine Ossification

# SEMICIRCULAR CANAL DYSPLASIA

## Key Facts

### Terminology
- SCCD: Malformation, hypoplasia or aplasia of one or all of semicircular canals (SCC)

### Imaging Findings
- Most common, least severe appearance of SCCD is dilated lateral SCC forming single cavity with vestibule
- Next most common is SCCD associated with CHARGE syndrome

### Top Differential Diagnoses
- Common Cavity Deformity
- Cystic Cochleovestibular Anomaly (CCVA) (Incomplete Partition Type I)
- Large Endolymphatic Sac Anomaly (LESA) (Incomplete Partition Type II)

- Labyrinthine Ossification

### Pathology
- SCC aplasia or hypoplasia may be part of genetic syndromes
- Etiology: 6-8 week gestational arrest or insult

### Clinical Issues
- Sensorineural hearing loss (SNHL) common
- Conductive hearing loss often present due to oval window atresia & ossicular chain anomalies
- Bilateral syndromic SCCD may benefit from cochlear implantation
- High-resolution oblique sagittal T2 MR through internal auditory canal (IAC) recommended prior to cochlear implantation to confirm presence of cochlear nerve

---

○ SCC dysplasia or aplasia may be associated with labyrinthine aplasia, cochlear hypoplasia, common cavity deformity or other more mild forms of cochlear dysplasia

### MR Findings
- T1WI: Labyrinthine structures poorly visualized
- T2WI
  ○ Sporadic SCCD
    ▪ Common sac formed by dilated vestibule & short, wide, dysmorphic lateral SCC
    ▪ Posterior & lateral SCCs normal or mildly dysplastic
  ○ Syndromic SCCD
    ▪ High signal from lateral, posterior & superior SCCs absent in both ears
    ▪ Small, dysmorphic high signal vestibule apparent
    ▪ "Isolated cochlea" with aplastic cochlear nerve aperture (black bony bar across cochlear aperture), cochlear nerve absent

### Imaging Recommendations
- Best imaging tool: Temporal bone CT best study to delineate dysplastic or aplastic SCC components
- Protocol advice
  ○ Axial images best show lateral & posterior SCC
  ○ Coronal images (direct or reformatted) best show superior SCC
  ○ Combination of 2 planes needed to confirm oval window atresia

## DIFFERENTIAL DIAGNOSIS

### Common Cavity Deformity
- Cochlea & vestibule fused into single cavity
- SCCs may be normal or absent

### Cystic Cochleovestibular Anomaly (CCVA) (Incomplete Partition Type I)
- Cochlea & vestibule separate but featureless, with a "figure 8" appearance

- SCCs variable; normal, dilated & dysmorphic, or absent

### Large Endolymphatic Sac Anomaly (LESA) (Incomplete Partition Type II)
- Vestibular aqueduct greater than 1.5 mm on T-bone CT (new literature greater than 1.1 mm at the midpoint or greater than 2.1 mm at the operculum is abnormal)
- Endolymphatic duct & sac dilated on T2 MR
- Middle & apical cochlear turns form common cavity & associated dilated vestibule
- SCCs usually normal

### Labyrinthine Ossification
- Bony replacement of any portion of membranous labyrinth
- When affects SCCs, may mimic SCCD
- History of profound sensorineural hearing loss after episode of meningitis

## PATHOLOGY

### General Features
- General path comments
  ○ SCC dysplasia without congenital syndrome
    ▪ Lateral SCC most often involved
    ▪ +/- Abnormal vestibule
- Genetics
  ○ Embryology
    ▪ Membranous labyrinth - pars superior & inferior
    ▪ Pars superior, phylogenetically older structure, gives rise to SCCs & utricle
    ▪ Because lateral SCC last to form, more susceptible to developmental anomalies
    ▪ Pars inferior gives rise to cochlea & saccule
  ○ JAG 1 gene mutation linked to SCC anomalies in mice
    ▪ JAG1 gene mutation causes Alagille syndrome in humans
  ○ SCC aplasia or hypoplasia may be part of genetic syndromes

# SEMICIRCULAR CANAL DYSPLASIA

- CHARGE association (coloboma, heart disease, atresia of nasal choana, mental or growth retardation, genital hypoplasia, ear anomalies): Complete SCC aplasia or isolated lateral canal aplasia usually seen
  - Alagille syndrome (arteriohepatic dysplasia): Posterior SCC hypoplasia seen
  - Waardenburg syndrome (hypertelorism, iris heterochromia, white forelock): Posterior SCC aplasia seen
  - Crouzon syndrome (craniofacial dysostosis): Large vestibule & short lateral SCC
  - Apert syndrome (acrocephalosyndactylism type I): Large vestibule & short lateral SCC
- Etiology: 6-8 week gestational arrest or insult
- Epidemiology
  - Rare inner ear anomaly
  - Lateral SCC dysplasia more common than other SCC dysplasia variants
- Associated abnormalities: Common & varied with syndromic SCC dysplasia

## Gross Pathologic & Surgical Features

- SCCs either completely absent, rudimentary or dilated & dysmorphic
- Tympanic portion of facial nerve canal often dehiscent & inferiorly displaced
- Oval window atresia commonly associated
- Cochlea, endolymphatic duct & sac variable

## CLINICAL ISSUES

### Presentation

- Most common signs/symptoms
  - Sensorineural hearing loss (SNHL) common
    - Cochlea may appear normal on imaging
  - Conductive hearing loss often present due to oval window atresia & ossicular chain anomalies
  - Other signs/symptoms
    - Vestibular function variable, even with SCC aplasia
    - Caloric responses may be absent
- Clinical Profile
  - Sporadic SCCD: Range from mild to profound SNHL
  - Syndromic SCCD: Usually profound SNHL with other associated anomalies

### Demographics

- Age: Congenital; present at birth

### Natural History & Prognosis

- Mild, sporadic SCCD may have minimal clinical impact
- In syndromic SCCD affected ear severe hearing loss

### Treatment

- Unilateral sporadic SCCD requires no treatment
- Bilateral syndromic SCCD may benefit from cochlear implantation
- High-resolution oblique sagittal T2 MR through internal auditory canal (IAC) recommended prior to cochlear implantation to confirm presence of cochlear nerve

## DIAGNOSTIC CHECKLIST

### Consider

- If one or all of SCCs are dysplastic or missing, SCCD is present
- If child has CHARGE syndrome, look for T-bone CT findings of severe SCCD

### Image Interpretation Pearls

- Both axial & coronal T-bone CT planes recommended to assess ossicular chain & oval window

## SELECTED REFERENCES

1. Kiernan AE et al: The Notch ligand JAG1 is required for sensory progenitor development in the mammalian inner ear. PLoS Genet. 2(1):e4, 2006
2. Koch B et al: Partial absence of the posterior semicircular canal in Alagille syndrome: CT findings. Pediatr Radiol. 36(9):977-979, 2006
3. Morimoto AK et al: Absent semicircular canals in CHARGE syndrome: radiologic spectrum of findings. AJNR Am J Neuroradiol. 27(8):1663-71, 2006
4. Vore AP et al: Deletion of and novel missense mutation in POU3F4 in 2 families segregating X-linked nonsyndromic deafness. Arch Otolaryngol Head Neck Surg. 131(12):1057-63, 2005
5. Satar B et al: Congenital aplasia of the semicircular canals. Otol Neurotol. 24(3):437-46, 2003
6. Yu KK et al: Molecular genetic advances in semicircular canal abnormalities and sensorineural hearing loss: a report of 16 cases. Otolaryngol Head Neck Surg. 129(6):637-46, 2003
7. Sennaroglu L et al: A new classification for cochleovestibular malformations. Laryngoscope. 112(12):2230-41, 2002
8. Scholtz AW et al: Goldenhar's syndrome: congenital hearing deficit of conductive or sensorineural origin? Temporal bone histopathologic study. Otol Neurotol. 22(4):501-5, 2001
9. Benton C et al: Imaging of congenital anomalies of the temporal bone. Neuroimaging Clin N Am. 10(1):35-53, vii-viii, 2000
10. Lemmerling MM et al: Unilateral semicircular canal aplasia in Goldenhar's syndrome. AJNR Am J Neuroradiol. 21(7):1334-6, 2000
11. Bamiou DE et al: Unilateral sensorineural hearing loss and its aetiology in childhood: the contribution of computerised tomography in aetiological diagnosis and management. Int J Pediatr Otorhinolaryngol. 51(2):91-9, 1999
12. Wiener-Vacher SR et al: Vestibular function in children with the CHARGE association. Arch Otolaryngol Head Neck Surg. 125(3):342-7, 1999
13. Higashi K et al: Aplasia of posterior semicircular canal in Waardenburg syndrome type II. J Otolaryngol. 21(4):262-4, 1992
14. Mizuno M et al: Labyrinthine anomalies with normal cochlear function. ORL J Otorhinolaryngol Relat Spec. 54(5):278-81, 1992
15. Parnes L et al: Bilateral semicircular canal aplasia with near-normal cochlear development. Ann Otol Rhinol Laryngol. 99:957-59, 1990

# SEMICIRCULAR CANAL DYSPLASIA

## IMAGE GALLERY

### Typical

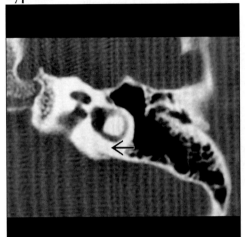 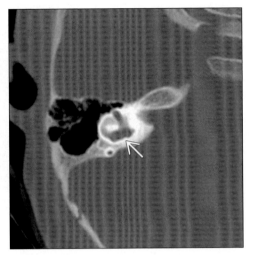

*(Left)* Axial bone CT shows absence of the normally seen left posterior SCC (it should be at site marked by ➡) in this child with Alagille syndrome. *(Right)* Axial bone CT shows a mildly enlarged posterior limb of the right lateral semicircular canal ➡ in another patient with nonsyndromic SCCD.

### Typical

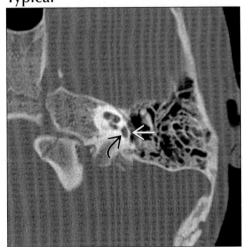 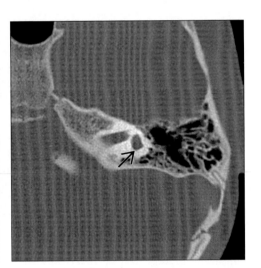

*(Left)* Axial bone CT shows rudimentary vestibule ➡ and atretic oval window ➡ in a patient with CHARGE syndrome. *(Right)* Axial bone CT in the same patient shows a single dysmorphic, featureless SCC ➡.

### Typical

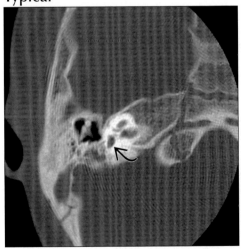 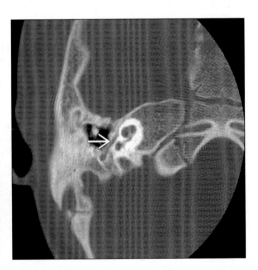

*(Left)* Axial bone CT shows dysplastic rudimentary vestibule ➡ and oval window atresia in a patient with CHARGE syndrome. The SCCs were absent and the anomalies were bilateral. *(Right)* Axial bone CT in the same patient shows low-lying tympanic segment of facial nerve canal ➡.

# LARGE ENDOLYMPHATIC SAC ANOMALY

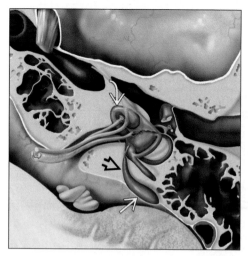

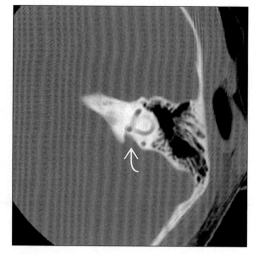

*Axial graphic of left inner ear shows intradural ➜ & intraosseous ➤ components of the enlarged endolymphatic sac. Notice also the cochlea ➜ is mildly dysplastic.*

*Axial bone CT shows an enlarged vestibular aqueduct ➜ in a child with impaired hearing in the left ear. The semicircular canals appear normal.*

## TERMINOLOGY

### Abbreviations and Synonyms

- Large endolymphatic sac anomaly (LESA); term used for T2 MR
- Large vestibular aqueduct syndrome (LVAS); term used for CT
- Incomplete partition (IP) type 2
- Mondini malformation: Obsolete term with multiple confusing definitions
  - Probably should no longer be used

### Definitions

- LESA/LVAS: Arrested development of inner ear at 7th week gestation with large endolymphatic sac and cochlear dysplasia
- Incomplete partition (IP) type 2
  - Sennaroglu et al proposed this term in 2002
    - Defined as "cochlea with 1.5 turns (middle & apical turns coalesce to form a cystic apex) accompanied by dilated vestibule & enlarged vestibular aqueduct"
  - This newest term awaits widespread acceptance

## IMAGING FINDINGS

### General Features

- Best diagnostic clue
  - Bone CT: Large bony vestibular aqueduct (VA)
  - T2 MR: Large endolymphatic sac and duct
- Location: Posterior temporal bone
- Size
  - Axial bone CT: Bony VA transverse dimension at midpoint > 1.5 mm
    - Newer data suggests abnormal ≥ 1 mm at midpoint and ≥ 2 mm at operculum
  - High resolution axial T2 MR: Obvious sac in fovea is abnormal, normal sac barely visible
- Morphology
  - Axial bone CT: "V-shaped" enlarged bony VA
  - Axial T2 MR: Elongated sac

### CT Findings

- NECT
  - Enlarged bony VA > 1.5 mm at midpoint
  - Newer data suggests abnormal ≥ 1 mm at midpoint and ≥ 2 mm at operculum

## DDx: Inner Ear Anomalies

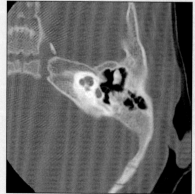

*Cochlear Hypoplasia*

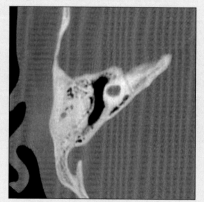

*Common Cavity*

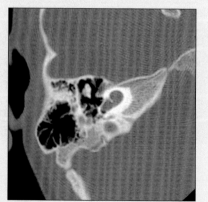

*CCV Anomaly*

# LARGE ENDOLYMPHATIC SAC ANOMALY

## Key Facts

### Terminology
- Large endolymphatic sac anomaly (LESA); term used for T2 MR
- Large vestibular aqueduct syndrome (LVAS); term used for CT
- LESA/LVAS: Arrested development of inner ear at 7th week gestation with large endolymphatic sac and cochlear dysplasia

### Imaging Findings
- Bone CT: Large bony vestibular aqueduct (VA)
- T2 MR: Large endolymphatic sac and duct
- Axial bone CT: Bony VA transverse dimension at midpoint > 1.5 mm
- Newer data suggests abnormal ≥ 1 mm at midpoint and ≥ 2 mm at operculum

### Top Differential Diagnoses
- Cochlea Aplasia
- Common Cavity
- Cystic Cochleovestibular (CCV) Anomaly
- Cochlear Hypoplasia

### Pathology
- Best hypothesis SNHL: Cochlea is "fragile" & susceptible to injury from mild trauma as a result of microscopic infrastructural deficiencies
- LESA/LVA: Most common congenital anomaly of inner ear found by imaging

### Clinical Issues
- Cochlear implantation (CI) for bilateral profound SNHL

---

- ○ Bony VA diameter > posterior semicircular canal (SCC) diameter
- ○ Cochlear dysplasia with apical turn dysmorphism & modiolar deficiency

### MR Findings
- T1WI: Low to intermediate signal sac visible along posterior wall of T-bone
- T2WI
  - ○ High signal enlarged endolymphatic sac obvious
  - ○ Associated cochlear dysplasia findings usually subtle, may be obvious
  - ○ Cochlear turn dysmorphism seen as bulbous apical turn (more severe dysmorphism sometimes present)
  - ○ Modiolar deficiency common (may also be normal or absent)
  - ○ Scalar chamber asymmetry with more anterior scala vestibuli larger than more posterior scala tympani

### Imaging Recommendations
- Thin-section T-bone CT (0.625 or 1 mm)
  - ○ Must look for & find large bony vestibular aqueduct
  - ○ Diagnosis easily missed if specific search not completed
  - ○ CT less sensitive for associated cochlear anomalies
- Thin-section high-resolution T2 MR (0.8-1 mm slice thickness) best imaging tool in experienced hands
  - ○ Better identifies large endolymphatic sac & cochlear dysplasia

## DIFFERENTIAL DIAGNOSIS

### Cochlea Aplasia
- Absent cochlea with vestigial vestibule & SCCs

### Common Cavity
- Cochlea, vestibule & SCCs = single cyst

### Cystic Cochleovestibular (CCV) Anomaly
- Bilobed cystic cochlea & cystic vestibule

### Cochlear Hypoplasia
- Modiolar deficiency, cochlear aperture large

## PATHOLOGY

### General Features
- General path comments
  - ○ Anatomic comments
    - ■ Endolymphatic sac has intradural portion (larger part) & intraosseous portion
    - ■ Delineation between intradural & intraosseous portions is by histopathology in sac wall
    - ■ Endolymphatic duct is short connection between utriculosaccular duct & intraosseous sac
    - ■ Normal endolymphatic sac & duct usually not identified, but may be barely visible on thin-section high-resolution T2 MR
- Genetics
  - ○ 15% of patients with LVAS have Pendred syndrome
    - ■ SLC26A4 Pendrin gene mutation, severe sensorineural hearing loss (SNHL)
    - ■ 50% have goiter/hypothyroidism
- Etiology
  - ○ LESA/LVAS: Result of arrested development of inner ear at approximately 7th week of fetal development
  - ○ Etiology of SNHL
    - ■ Best hypothesis SNHL: Cochlea is "fragile" & susceptible to injury from mild trauma as a result of microscopic infrastructural deficiencies
    - ■ Other hypothesis: Protein-rich endolymph refluxes into cochlea & vestibule
- Epidemiology
  - ○ LESA/LVA: Most common congenital anomaly of inner ear found by imaging
    - ■ LVA present in 32% of patients with SNHL
  - ○ Bilateral anomaly in up to 90%
- Associated abnormalities
  - ○ Associated cochlear dysplasia (≥ 75%)
  - ○ Associated vestibule and/or SCC anomaly (50%)
  - ○ Distal renal tubular acidosis rarely associated
    - ■ Characterized by a defect in urinary acidification with various degrees of metabolic acidosis
  - ○ Brachio-oto-renal syndrome rarely associated

# LARGE ENDOLYMPHATIC SAC ANOMALY

## Gross Pathologic & Surgical Features
- Enlarged endolymphatic sac is found in dural sleeve in fovea in posterior wall of T-bone

## Staging, Grading or Classification Criteria
- Inner ear anomalies (grading from severe to mild)
  - Labyrinthine aplasia (Michel deformity): 3rd week arrest
  - Cochlear aplasia: Late 3rd week arrest
  - Common cavity: 4th week arrest
  - CCV malformation (IP type 1): 5th week arrest
  - Cochlear hypoplasia: 6th week arrest
  - LESA (IP type 2): 7th week arrest

## CLINICAL ISSUES

### Presentation
- Most common signs/symptoms
  - SNHL in a child who hears at birth but hearing deteriorates over early years of life
    - Fluctuating or "cascading" SNHL often with post-traumatic potentiation

### Demographics
- Age
  - Pediatric onset most common
  - Most present < 10 years of age
- Gender: 2:1, M:F

### Natural History & Prognosis
- If bilateral, inevitably leads to profound SNHL
- SNHL develops with variable speed
  - Hearing loss may not be present until early adult life
- Prognosis is best when SNHL is unilateral or early adult onset

### Treatment
- Avoidance of contact sports or other activities that may lead to head trauma is essential
- Cochlear implantation (CI) for bilateral profound SNHL
  - Postlingual deafness group does best with CI
  - Initial fears regarding LESA/LVAS and CI dispelled
  - No increase in cochlear implant complications
  - Significant improvement in quality of life reported

## DIAGNOSTIC CHECKLIST

### Consider
- Use high-resolution T2 MR as modality of choice to make & refine diagnosis
- No relationship between size of endolymphatic sac & severity of SNHL

### Image Interpretation Pearls
- When LESA/LVAS diagnosed, remember to quantify severity of cochlear dysplasia
  - Cochlear implant surgeon may want to implant least affected side when bilateral

## SELECTED REFERENCES

1. Vijayasekaran S et al: When is the vestibular aqueduct enlarged? A statistical analysis of the normative distribution of vestibular aqueduct size. AJNR in press, 2007
2. Kim LS et al: Cochlear implantation in children with inner ear malformations. Ann Otol Rhinol Laryngol. 115(3):205-14, 2006
3. Simons JP et al: Computed tomography and magnetic resonance imaging in pediatric unilateral and asymmetric sensorineural hearing loss. Arch Otolaryngol Head Neck Surg. 132(2):186-92, 2006
4. Berrettini S et al: Distal renal tubular acidosis associated with isolated large vestibular aqueduct and sensorineural hearing loss. Ann Otol Rhinol Laryngol. 111(5 Pt 1):385-91, 2002
5. Bichey BG et al: Changes in quality of life and the cost-utility associated with cochlear implantation in patients with large vestibular aqueduct syndrome. Otol Neurotol. 23(3):323-7, 2002
6. Mafong DD et al: Use of laboratory evaluation and radiologic imaging in the diagnostic evaluation of children with sensorineural hearing loss. Laryngoscope. 112(1):1-7, 2002
7. Miyamoto RT et al: Cochlear implantation with large vestibular aqueduct syndrome. Laryngoscope. 112(7 Pt 1):1178-82, 2002
8. Naganawa S et al: Serial MR imaging studies in enlarged endolymphatic duct and sac syndrome. Eur Radiol. 12 Suppl 3:S114-7, 2002
9. Sennaroglu L et al: A new classification for cochleovestibular malformations. Laryngoscope. 112(12):2230-41, 2002
10. Pyle GM: Embryological development and large vestibular aqueduct syndrome. Laryngoscope. 110(11):1837-42, 2000
11. Davidson HC et al: MR evaluation of vestibulocochlear anomalies associated with large endolymphatic duct and sac. AJNR Am J Neuroradiol. 20(8):1435-41, 1999
12. Naganawa S et al: MR imaging of the cochlear modiolus: area measurement in healthy subjects and in patients with a large endolymphatic duct and sac. Radiology. 213(3):819-23, 1999
13. Phelps PD et al: Radiological malformations of the ear in Pendred syndrome. Clin Radiol. 53(4):268-73, 1998
14. Dahlen RT et al: Overlapping thin-section fast spin-echo MR of the large vestibular aqueduct syndrome. AJNR Am J Neuroradiol. 18(1):67-75, 1997
15. Tong KA et al: Large vestibular aqueduct syndrome: a genetic disease? AJR Am J Roentgenol. 168(4):1097-101, 1997
16. Okumura T et al: Magnetic resonance imaging of patients with large vestibular aqueducts. Eur Arch Otorhinolaryngol. 253(7):425-8, 1996
17. Weissman JL: Hearing loss. Radiology. 199(3):593-611, 1996
18. Harnsberger HR et al: Advanced techniques in magnetic resonance imaging in the evaluation of the large endolymphatic duct and sac syndrome. Laryngoscope. 105(10):1037-42, 1995
19. Zalzal GH et al: Enlarged vestibular aqueduct and sensorineural hearing loss in childhood. Arch Otolaryngol Head Neck Surg. 121(1):23-8, 1995
20. Bagger-Sjoback D: Surgical anatomy of the endolymphatic sac. Am J Otol. 14(6):576-9, 1993
21. Jackler RK et al: The large vestibular aqueduct syndrome. Laryngoscope. 99(12):1238-42; discussion 1242-3, 1989
22. Valvassori GE et al: The large vestibular aqueduct syndrome. Laryngoscope. 88(5):723-8, 1978

# LARGE ENDOLYMPHATIC SAC ANOMALY

## IMAGE GALLERY

### Typical

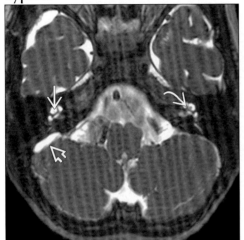 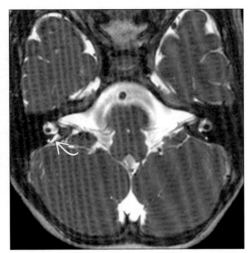

*(Left)* Axial 3D T2 TSE T2WI shows large right endolymphatic sac ➡. The right modiolus ➡ is also smaller than the left ➡, a common association showing extensive dysgenesis. *(Right)* Axial 3D T2 TSE High resolution axial T2WI shows enlarged right endolymphatic sac/duct ➡ in a patient with Pendred syndrome.

### Typical

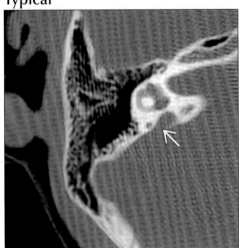 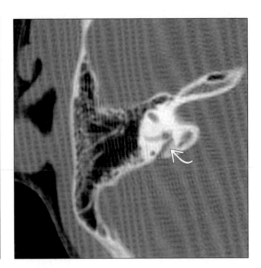

*(Left)* Axial bone CT in a 5 year old with hearing loss shows enlargement of the right vestibular aqueduct, at the operculum ➡. The lateral semicircular canal is dysplastic. *(Right)* Axial bone CT (same patient as previous image) 1 mm more superior, shows that the midpoint ➡ of the vestibular aqueduct is also enlarged.

### Typical

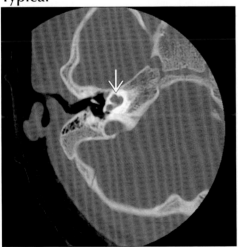 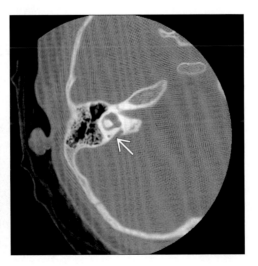

*(Left)* Axial bone CT shows incomplete partitioning of the cochlea ➡ in a patient with severe SNHL and Pendrin gene mutation (Pendred syndrome). *(Right)* Axial bone CT at a more superior level in the same patient as previous image shows that the vestibular aqueduct ➡ is abnormally enlarged.

# EPIDERMOID CYST, CPA-IAC

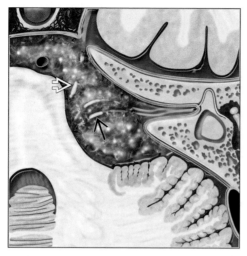

*Axial graphic shows large CPA epidermoid with typical "bed of pearls" appearance. Notice 5th ⇨ and 7th & 8th cranial nerves ➡ are characteristically engulfed.*

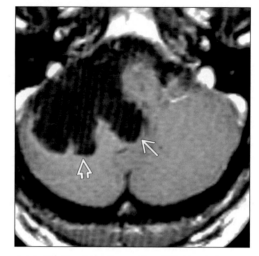

*Axial T1 C+ MR shows the CSF signal intensity epidermoid in the right CPA, insinuating into the foramen of Luschka ➡ and right cerebellar hemisphere ⇨.*

## TERMINOLOGY

### Abbreviations and Synonyms
- Epidermoid of cerebellopontine angel (CPA) cistern (Ep-CPA)
- Epidermoid tumor, epidermoid cyst, primary cholesteatoma or epithelial inclusion cyst

### Definitions
- Congenital intradural mass 2° inclusion of ectodermal epithelial elements during neural tube closure
- "White epidermoid" - rare variant
  - Epidermoid with high protein content causing high signal on T1, lower signal on T2 MR sequences

## IMAGING FINDINGS

### General Features
- Best diagnostic clue
  - CPA cisternal mass with high signal on diffusion MR (DWI)
    - Engulfs cranial nerves (7th & 8th), vessels (AICA, vertebral artery)

- Location
  - Posterior fossa most common site
    - CPA 75%, 4th ventricle 25%
  - May extend cephalad → medial middle cranial fossa
  - Rarely intramedullary in brain stem
- Size
  - Variable, may be large at presentation
  - Usually larger than acoustic schwannoma at presentation
- Morphology
  - Mass insinuates into cisterns, engulfs cranial nerves & vessels
  - Margins scalloped, irregular or cauliflower-like
  - When large may distort adjacent brainstem ± cerebellum

### CT Findings
- NECT
  - Low attenuation like cerebral spinal fluid (CSF)
  - Calcification in 20%, usually along margins
  - Pressure erosion of adjacent bone may occur
- CECT
  - No enhancement is rule
    - Sometimes margin of cyst minimally enhances

## DDx: Cystic CPA Mass

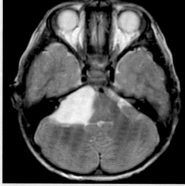

*Arachnoid Cyst*

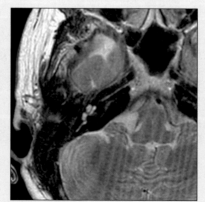

*Neurenteric Cyst*

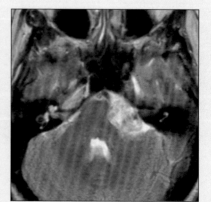

*Schwannoma*

# EPIDERMOID CYST, CPA-IAC

## Key Facts

### Terminology
- Epidermoid tumor, epidermoid cyst, primary cholesteatoma or epithelial inclusion cyst
- Congenital intradural mass 2° inclusion of ectodermal epithelial elements during neural tube closure

### Imaging Findings
- CPA cisternal mass with high signal on diffusion MR (DWI)
- Engulfs cranial nerves (7th & 8th), vessels (AICA, vertebral artery)

### Top Differential Diagnoses
- Arachnoid Cyst
- Neurenteric Cyst
- Cystic Neoplasm

### Pathology
- 3rd most common CPA mass
- 1% of all intracranial masses
- Pearly white mass in CPA

### Clinical Issues
- Clinical Profile: Young adult with minor symptoms has mass discovered in CPA cistern on MR

### Diagnostic Checklist
- Insinuating CPA mass has low signal on T1, high on T2 (similar to, but not identical to CSF)
- Mixed signal on FLAIR
- Reduced diffusion (high signal) on DWI
- DWI is key to correct diagnosis of initial lesion & recurrence

---

- If nodular enhancement seen, consider rare squamous cell carcinoma arising from Ep-CPA
  - "Dense" epidermoid
    - Rare high attenuation Ep-CPA variant

### MR Findings
- T1WI
  - Isointense or slightly hyperintense to CSF signal
  - Usually slightly heterogeneous
  - "White epidermoid": High T1 signal
- T2WI
  - Isointense to hyperintense compared to CSF
  - "White epidermoid": Low T2 signal
- FLAIR
  - Mixed signal, partly hyperintense to CSF
    - Part of lesion isointense to CSF, part hyperintense
- DWI
  - High signal intensity of T2 hyperintense lesion establishes diagnosis
    - High signal intensity indicates reduced diffusivity compared to CSF
  - High signal intensity foci in surgical bed post-op indicates recurrence
- T1 C+
  - No enhancement is rule
  - Mild peripheral enhancement occurs in approximately 25% of cases
- MRA
  - Vessels of CPA may be displaced or engulfed by EpC-CPA
  - Artery wall dimension not affected

### Imaging Recommendations
- Best imaging tool: Brain MR with FLAIR, DWI & post-contrast T1 sequences
- Protocol advice
  - Begin with routine enhanced MR imaging
  - FLAIR & diffusion sequences added to confirm diagnosis
  - Follow-up study looking for recurrence must include FLAIR & diffusion sequences

## DIFFERENTIAL DIAGNOSIS

### Arachnoid Cyst
- Displaces, does not engulf adjacent structures
- Does not insinuate
- T1 & T2 signal follows CSF signal
  - May be higher signal on T2 (lacks CSF pulsations)
- Low signal on FLAIR sequence
- Low signal (high diffusivity) on DWI

### Neurenteric Cyst
- Most common location pre-pontine cistern
- May have high T1 signal (can mimic "white epidermoid")
- T2 signal often low

### Cystic Neoplasm
- All contain areas of contrast-enhancement
  - Cystic schwannoma rare; intramural cysts more common in larger lesions
  - Cystic ependymoma originates in 4th ventricle, extends out foramen of Luschka to CPA cisterna
  - Cystic astrocytoma: Pedunculated lesion extending from brainstem
  - Cystic meningioma rare, dural tail common

## PATHOLOGY

### General Features
- Etiology
  - Inclusion of ectodermal elements during neural tube closure, results in migration abnormalities of epiblastic cells
  - 3rd-5th week of embryogenesis
- Epidemiology
  - 3rd most common CPA mass
  - 1% of all intracranial masses

### Gross Pathologic & Surgical Features
- Pearly white mass in CPA
- Surgeons refer to it as "the beautiful tumor"
- Lobulated, cauliflower-shaped surface features

# EPIDERMOID CYST, CPA-IAC

- Insinuating growth pattern in cisterns
  - Engulfs cisternal vessels & nerves
    - May become adherent
    - May cause hyperactive dysfunction of cranial nerve (CN) 5 or 7

## Microscopic Features

- Cyst wall: Simple stratified cuboidal squamous epithelium
- Cyst contents: Solid crystalline cholesterol, keratinaceous debris
  - Does not contain hair follicles, sebaceous glands or fat (in contrast to dermoid)
- Grows in successive layers by desquamation from cyst wall

## CLINICAL ISSUES

### Presentation

- Most common signs/symptoms
  - Principal presenting symptom: Dizziness
  - Other symptoms: Depend on location, growth pattern
    - Trigeminal neuralgia (tic douloureux)
    - Sensorineural hearing loss
    - Facial neuralgia (hemifacial spasm)
    - Headache
  - Symptoms usually present for > 4 years before Ep-CPA is diagnosed
- Clinical Profile: Young adult with minor symptoms has mass discovered in CPA cistern on MR

### Demographics

- Age
  - Although congenital, most often presents in adult life
  - Broad presentation from 1st to 6th decades
    - Peak age = 40 years

### Natural History & Prognosis

- Slow growing congenital lesions that remain clinically silent for many years
- Smaller cisternal lesions are readily cured with surgery
- Larger lesions where upward supratentorial herniation has occurred are more difficult to completely remove
  - Larger lesions tend to have more significant surgical complications

### Treatment

- Complete surgical removal is goal
  - Total removal possible in < 50%
  - Near-total removal often better surgical choice
    - Aggressive total removal may cause significant cranial neuropathy
    - Used when Ep-CPA capsule is adherent to brainstem & cranial nerves
- If brain stem involved, resection is typically subtotal
- If recurs, takes many years to grow
  - DWI is the key in assessing for recurrence

## DIAGNOSTIC CHECKLIST

### Consider

- MR diagnosis Ep-CPA when
  - Insinuating CPA mass has low signal on T1, high on T2 (similar to, but not identical to CSF)
  - Mixed signal on FLAIR
  - Reduced diffusion (high signal) on DWI

### Image Interpretation Pearls

- DWI is key to correct diagnosis of initial lesion & recurrence

## SELECTED REFERENCES

1. Ziyal IM et al: Epidermoid cyst of the brain stem symptomatic in childhood. Childs Nerv Syst. 21(12):1025-9, 2005
2. Nguyen JB et al: Magnetic resonance imaging and proton magnetic resonance spectroscopy of intracranial epidermoid tumors. Crit Rev Comput Tomogr. 45(5-6):389-427, 2004
3. Hamlat A et al: Malignant transformation of intracranial epidermoid cyst with leptomeningeal carcinomatosis: case report. Acta Neurol Belg. 103(4):221-4, 2003
4. Dutt SN et al: Radiologic differentiation of intracranial epidermoids from arachnoid cysts. Otol Neurotol. 23(1):84-92, 2002
5. Kobata H et al: Cerebellopontine angle epidermoids presenting with cranial nerve hyperactive dysfunction: pathogenesis and long-term surgical results in 30 patients. Neurosurgery. 50(2):276-85; discussion 285-6, 2002
6. Dechambre S et al: Diffusion-weighted MRI postoperative assessment of an epidermoid tumour in the cerebellopontine angle. Neuroradiology. 41:829-31, 1999
7. Ochi M et al: Unusual CT and MR appearance of an epidermoid tumor of the cerebellopontine angle. AJNR Am J Neuroradiol. 19(6):1113-5, 1998
8. Talacchi A et al: Assessment and surgical management of posterior fossa epidermoid tumors: report of 28 cases. Neurosurgery. 42(2):242-51; discussion 251-2, 1998
9. Timmer FA et al: Chemical analysis of an epidermoid cyst with unusual CT and MR characteristics. AJNR Am J Neuroradiol. 19(6):1111-2, 1998
10. Ikushima I et al: MR of epidermoids with a variety of pulse sequences. AJNR Am J Neuroradiol. 18(7):1359-63, 1997
11. Kallmes DF et al: Typical and atypical MR imaging features of intracranial epidermoid tumors. AJR Am J Roentgenol. 169(3):883-7, 1997
12. Kuzma BB et al: Epidermoid or arachnoid cyst? Surg Neurol. 47(4):395-6, 1997
13. Mohanty A et al: Experience with cerebellopontine angle epidermoids. Neurosurgery. 40:24-30, 1997
14. Tien RD et al: Variable bandwidth steady-state free-precession MR imaging: a technique for improving characterization of epidermoid tumor and arachnoid cyst. AJR Am J Roentgenol. 164(3):689-92, 1995
15. Gao PY et al: Radiologic-pathologic correlation. Epidermoid tumor of the cerebellopontine angle. AJNR Am J Neuroradiol. 13(3):863-72, 1992
16. Altschuler EM et al: Operative treatment of intracranial epidermoid cysts and cholesterol granulomas: report of 21 cases. Neurosurgery. 26(4):606-13; discussion 614, 1990
17. deSouza CE et al: Cerebellopontine angle epidermoid cysts: a report on 30 cases. J Neurol Neurosurg Psychiatry. 52(8):986-90, 1989
18. Tampieri D et al: MR imaging of epidermoid cysts. AJNR Am J Neuroradiol. 10(2):351-6, 1989

## IMAGE GALLERY

### Typical

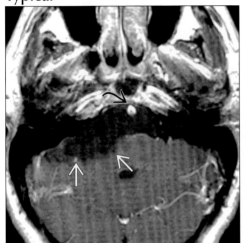
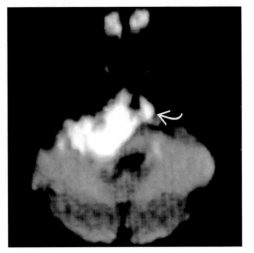

*(Left)* Axial T1 C+ MR shows a cystic appearing prepontine and right CPA mass ➡, nearly isointense to CSF, without contrast-enhancement. Basilar artery ➡ is engulfed. *(Right)* Axial DWI MR in the same patient as previous image shows reduced diffusion, confirming the diagnosis of epidermoid and better defining the margins of the lesion, extending into the left CPA cistern ➡.

### Typical

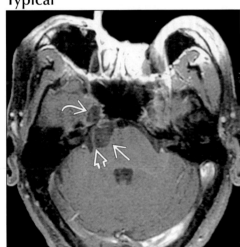
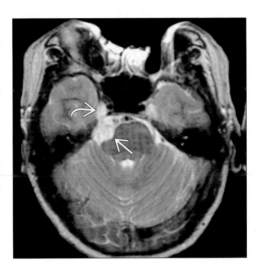

*(Left)* Axial T1 C+ MR shows nonenhancing cystic mass in right CPA cistern ➡, extending into the right trigeminal cistern ➡ and deflecting cisternal segment of right trigeminal nerve ➡. *(Right)* Axial T2WI MR in the same patient as previous image shows hyperintense signal of the right CPA cistern mass ➡ and extension into the ipsilateral trigeminal cistern ➡.

### Typical

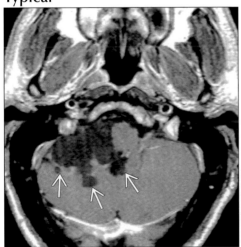
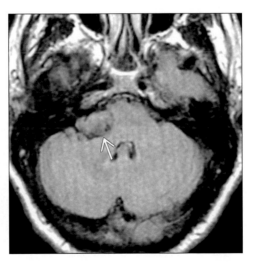

*(Left)* Axial T1 C+ MR shows nonenhancing, irregular irregular hypointense right CPA mass ➡, typical of epidermoid. The irregularity and absence of enhancement strongly suggest this diagnosis. *(Right)* Axial FLAIR MR shows incomplete fluid attenuation of right CPA cistern mass ➡, resulting in a mixed signal intensity that is typical of epidermoid tumors.

# ARACHNOID CYST, CPA-IAC

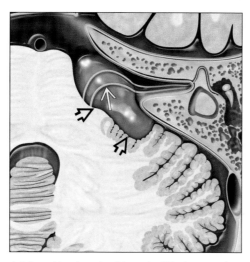

Axial graphic of arachnoid cyst in CPA shows its thin, translucent wall. Notice the displacement of the 7th & 8th cranial nerves ➡ and mass effect upon the brainstem-cerebellum ⟫.

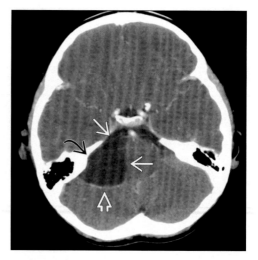

Axial CECT shows a nonenhancing right CPA arachnoid cyst ➡. Note imperceptible walls, mass effect on medulla and cerebellar hemisphere ⟫ and scalloping of dorsal petrous bone ↗.

## TERMINOLOGY

### Abbreviations and Synonyms
- Abbreviation: Arachnoid cyst (AC)
- Synonyms: Primary AC or congenital AC

### Definitions
- Definition: Arachnoid or collagen-lined cavities that do not communicate directly with ventricular system or subarachnoid space

## IMAGING FINDINGS

### General Features
- Best diagnostic clue
  - Cystic cisternal mass with imperceptible walls
  - Isointense to CSF on all MR sequences
    - Complete fluid attenuation on FLAIR MR imaging
    - Diffusivity similar to CSF on DWI MR imaging
  - Isodense to CSF on CT
- Location
  - 33% of all AC occur in posterior fossa
    - Cerebellopontine angle (CPA) = most common infratentorial site
  - Patterns of extension
    - Most remain confined to CPA (60%)
    - May extend dorsal to brainstem (25%)
    - May extend into internal auditory canal (IAC) (15%)
- Size
  - Variable, may be large but asymptomatic
  - When large, will exert mass effect on adjacent brainstem & cerebellum
- Morphology
  - Sharply demarcated lesion with broad arching margins
  - Displaces, does not engulf surrounding structures

### CT Findings
- NECT
  - Attenuation usually same as CSF
  - Rare high attenuation from hemorrhage or proteinaceous fluid
  - Bone changes: May cause pressure erosion/scalloping of adjacent bone
- CECT: No enhancement of cavity or wall

## DDx: Cystic CPA Mass

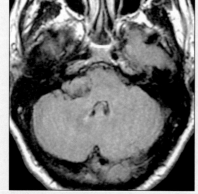

Epidermoid

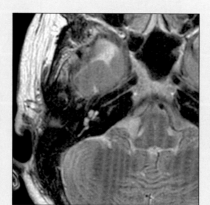

Neurenteric Cyst

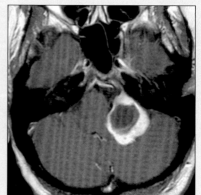

Schwannoma

# ARACHNOID CYST, CPA-IAC

## Key Facts

### Terminology
- Abbreviation: Arachnoid cyst (AC)
- Synonyms: Primary AC or congenital AC
- Definition: Arachnoid or collagen-lined cavities that do not communicate directly with ventricular system or subarachnoid space

### Imaging Findings
- Cystic cisternal mass with imperceptible walls
- Isointense to CSF on all MR sequences
- Isodense to CSF on CT
- 33% of all AC occur in posterior fossa
- Cerebellopontine angle (CPA) = most common infratentorial site

### Top Differential Diagnoses
- Epidermoid
- Neurenteric Cyst
- Cystic Neoplasm

### Pathology
- Embryonic meninges fail to merge
- Noncommunicating CSF-containing fluid compartment surrounded by arachnoid

### Clinical Issues
- Clinical Profile: Child or adult undergoing brain MR for unrelated symptoms
- Most cases require no treatment

### Diagnostic Checklist
- Differentiate AC from epidermoid cyst
- AC has low signal on DWI = best clue
- FLAIR MR sequence will show AC as a low signal (fluid attenuated) lesion

## MR Findings
- T1WI
  - Low signal lesion isointense to CSF
  - Well-circumscribed, pushing lesion compresses adjacent brainstem & cerebellum when large
  - Rarely associated with hydrocephalus when large
- T2WI
  - High signal lesion isointense to CSF
  - May have brighter signal than CSF if fluid within cyst which lacks CSF pulsations that normally decreases CSF signal intensity
- FLAIR: Signal intensity similar to CSF
- DWI: Diffusivity similar to CSF
- T1 C+
  - No contrast-enhancement
  - Imperceptible wall

## Imaging Recommendations
- Best imaging tool: Whole brain MR imaging
- Protocol advice
  - If suspect AC on brain MR, add following sequences
    - FLAIR: Low signal intensity
    - DWI: Low signal intensity
    - Post-contrast T1WI: No enhancement with imperceptible cyst wall

## DIFFERENTIAL DIAGNOSIS

### Epidermoid
- Lesion most similar to arachnoid cyst
- FLAIR MR: Mixed hypo- and hyperintense signal
- DWI: Increased (similar to CSF) signal
- Morphology: Insinuates into adjacent CSF spaces & surrounds vessels-cranial nerves

### Neurenteric Cyst
- Most common location pre-pontine cistern
- May contain T1 high signal (may mimic "white epidermoid")
- T2 signal often low

### Cystic Neoplasm
- All contain areas of contrast-enhancement
  - Cystic schwannoma rare: Intramural cysts more common in larger lesions
  - Cystic ependymoma: Originates in 4th ventricle, extends out foramen of Luschka to CPA cistern
  - Cystic astrocytoma: Pedunculated lesion extending from brainstem
  - Cystic meningioma rare: Dural tail common

## PATHOLOGY

### General Features
- General path comments
  - Soft, thin-walled mass that contains CSF
  - Intracranial AC
    - Most common location is middle cranial fossa (50%)
    - Second most common location is posterior fossa (33%): CP angle, retrocerebellar, supravermian
    - Suprasellar (10%) and other sporadic intracranial locations (7%)
- Etiology
  - Embryonic meninges fail to merge
  - Cyst lies between split in arachnoid membrane
  - Noncommunicating CSF-containing fluid compartment surrounded by arachnoid
- Epidemiology: Accounts for 1% of intracranial masses
- Associated abnormalities
  - Extraparenchymal tumors may have adjacent AC
    - Meningiomas, schwannomas most common
  - Acoustic schwannoma has associated AC in 0.5%

### Gross Pathologic & Surgical Features
- Fluid-containing cyst with translucent membrane
- May surround or displace but does not engulf adjacent vessels or cranial nerves

### Microscopic Features
- Thin wall of flattened but normal arachnoid cells

# ARACHNOID CYST, CPA-IAC

- No glial limiting membrane or epithelial lining is present in AC wall
- No inflammation or neoplastic change

## CLINICAL ISSUES

### Presentation
- Most common signs/symptoms
  - Small AC: Asymptomatic
    - Incidental finding on MR
  - Large AC: May have clinical manifestations
    - Symptoms from direct compression &/or raised intracranial pressure
    - May compress/block foramina of Luschka or Magendie
- Clinical Profile: Child or adult undergoing brain MR for unrelated symptoms
- Other symptoms: Defined by location & size
  - Vague, nonspecific symptoms common
  - Headache
  - Dizziness, tinnitus and/or sensorineural hearing loss (SNHL)
  - Hemifacial spasm or trigeminal neuralgia

### Demographics
- Age
  - May be diagnosed at any age
    - 75% of AC found in children
- Gender: M:F = 3:1

### Natural History & Prognosis
- Most AC do not enlarge over time
  - Infrequently enlarge via CSF pulsation through ball-valve opening into AC
  - Hemorrhage with subsequent decrease in size has been reported
- If surgery is limited to AC where symptoms are clearly related, prognosis is excellent
- Radical cyst removal may result in cranial neuropathy and/or vascular compromise

### Treatment
- Most cases require no treatment
- Surgical intervention is highly selective process
  - Reserved for cases where clear symptoms can be directly linked to AC anatomic location
  - Endoscopic cyst decompression via fenestration
    - Least invasive initial approach
    - Suboccipital retrosigmoid approach preferred

## DIAGNOSTIC CHECKLIST

### Consider
- Differentiate AC from epidermoid cyst
  - AC has low signal on DWI = best clue
- Determine if symptoms match location of AC before considering surgical treatment
- Progressively less surgical treatment is trend

### Image Interpretation Pearls
- AC signal parallels CSF on all MR sequences = key to radiologic diagnosis

- Remember T2 signal may be higher than CSF from lack of CSF pulsation
- DWI MR sequence will show AC as low signal lesion
- FLAIR MR sequence will show AC as a low signal (fluid attenuated) lesion
- No enhancement of AC, including wall
- If any nodular enhancement, consider alternative diagnosis

## SELECTED REFERENCES

1. Alaani A et al: Cerebellopontine angle arachnoid cysts in adult patients: what is the appropriate management? J Laryngol Otol. 119(5):337-41, 2005
2. Chernov MF et al: Double-endoscopic approach for management of convexity arachnoid cyst: case report. Surg Neurol. 61(5):483-6; discussion 486-7, 2004
3. Nguyen JB et al: Magnetic resonance imaging and proton magnetic resonance spectroscopy of intracranial epidermoid tumors. Crit Rev Comput Tomogr. 45(5-6):389-427, 2004
4. Sinha S et al: Familial posterior fossa arachnoid cyst. Childs Nerv Syst. 20(2):100-3, 2004
5. McBride LA et al: Cystoventricular shunting of intracranial arachnoid cysts. Pediatr Neurosurg. 39(6):323-9, 2003
6. O'reilly RC et al: Posterior fossa arachnoid cysts can mimic Meniere's disease. Am J Otolaryngol. 24(6):420-5, 2003
7. Boltshauser E et al: Outcome in children with space-occupying posterior fossa arachnoid cysts. Neuropediatrics. 33(3):118-21, 2002
8. Dutt SN et al: Radiologic differentiation of intracranial epidermoids from arachnoid cysts. Otol Neurotol. 23(1):84-92, 2002
9. Ottaviani F et al: Arachnoid cyst of the cranial posterior fossa causing sensorineural hearing loss and tinnitus: a case report. Eur Arch Otorhinolaryngol. 259(6):306-8, 2002
10. Bonneville F et al: Unusual lesions of the cerebellopontine angle: a segmental approach. Radiographics. 21(2):419-38, 2001
11. Gangemi M et al: Endoscopic surgery for large posterior fossa arachnoid cysts. Minim Invasive Neurosurg. 44(1):21-4, 2001
12. Ucar T et al: Bilateral cerebellopontine angle arachnoid cysts: case report. Neurosurgery. 47(4):966-8, 2000
13. Samii M et al: Arachnoid cysts of the posterior fossa. Surg Neurol. 51(4):376-82, 1999
14. Choi JU et al: Pathogenesis of arachnoid cyst: congenital or traumatic? Pediatr Neurosurg. 29(5):260-6, 1998
15. Shukla R et al: Posterior fossa arachnoid cyst presenting as high cervical cord compression. Br J Neurosurg. 12(3):271-3, 1998
16. Takano S et al: Facial spasm and paroxysmal tinnitus associated with an arachnoid cyst of the cerebellopontine angle--case report. Neurol Med Chir (Tokyo). 38(2):100-3, 1998
17. Jallo GI et al: Arachnoid cysts of the cerebellopontine angle: diagnosis and surgery. Neurosurgery. 40(1):31-7; discussion 37-8, 1997
18. Higashi S et al: Hemifacial spasm associated with a cerebellopontine angle arachnoid cyst in a young adult. Surg Neurol. 37(4):289-92, 1992
19. Babu R et al: Arachnoid cyst of the cerebellopontine angle manifesting as contralateral trigeminal neuralgia: case report. Neurosurgery. 28(6):886-7, 1991
20. Wiener SN et al: MR imaging of intracranial arachnoid cysts. J Comput Assist Tomogr. 11(2):236-41, 1987
21. Flodmark O: Neuroradiology of selected disorders of the meninges, calvarium, and venous sinuses.

## IMAGE GALLERY

### Typical

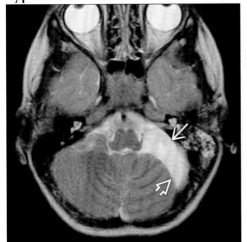 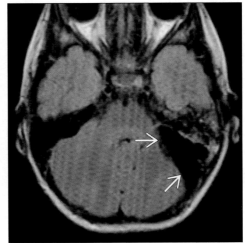

*(Left) Axial T2WI MR shows a hyperintense, sharply marginated left CPA cyst causing scalloping ⮕ of petrous pyramid and mass effect on the left cerebellar hemisphere ⮕. (Right) Axial FLAIR MR of the same patient as previous image shows complete attenuation of the hyperintense T2 signal in this CPA cistern cyst ⮕, distinguishing it from an epidermoid.*

### Typical

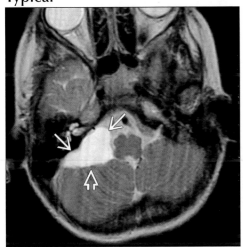 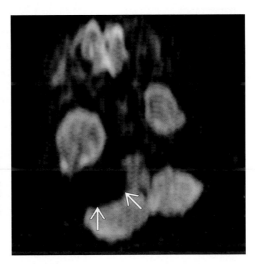

*(Left) Axial T2WI MR shows a hyperintense right CPA cyst ⮕ causing mild mass effect on the right cerebellar hemisphere ⮕. Cyst fluid is hyperintense to CSF in surrounding cisterns. (Right) Axial DWI MR in the same patient as previous image shows hypointensity ⮕ within the cyst, proving high diffusivity and thus confirming suspicion of arachnoid cyst.*

### Typical

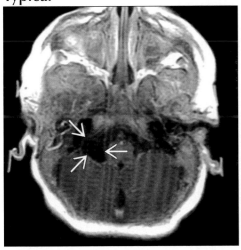 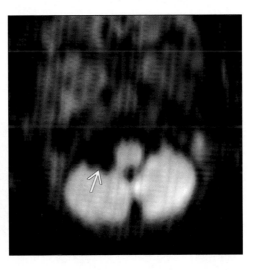

*(Left) Axial T1 C+ MR shows a small, sharply-marginated CSF signal intensity right CPA cyst ⮕, causing minimal flattening of the adjacent medulla and right cerebellar hemisphere. (Right) Axial DWI MR in the same patient as previous image shows hypointensity ⮕, confirming high diffusivity of fluid and suggesting the diagnosis of arachnoid cyst rather than epidermoid or other solid mass.*

# CONGENITAL CHOLESTEATOMA

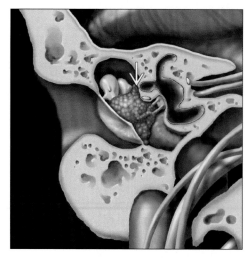

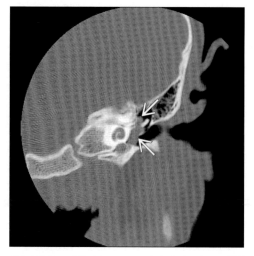

*Coronal graphic shows congenital cholesteatoma involving the middle ear. The lesion has extended medial to the ossicles ➡ as it engulfs the entire ossicular chain. The tympanic membrane is intact.*

*Coronal bone CT shows congenital cholesteatoma ➡ in the mesotympanum and hypotympanum, medial to the ossicles.*

## TERMINOLOGY

### Abbreviations and Synonyms
- Congenital cholesteatoma (CCh)
- Primary cholesteatoma, epidermoid, "skin in the wrong place"

### Definitions
- Aberrant rest of epithelial cells

## IMAGING FINDINGS

### General Features
- Best diagnostic clue: Smooth, well-circumscribed middle ear mass ± ossicular erosions
- Location
  - Majority middle ear (CCh-ME)
    - Anterosuperior tympanic cavity near eustachian tube or stapes: Most common
    - Posterior epitympanum at tympanic isthmus (area between middle ear cavity & attic)
  - Other locations: External auditory canal (EAC), middle ear-mastoid, petrous apex, CP angle, geniculate ganglion
- Size
  - Usually small, identified on otoscopic exam
  - Rarely fills entire middle ear cavity
- Morphology: Lobular, discrete middle ear (ME) mass

### CT Findings
- Bone CT
  - Appearance depends on size of lesion and location
  - Small CCh-ME: Detected early, appears as well-circumscribed ME lesion
  - Large CCh-ME: Larger mass may erode ossicles, middle ear wall, lateral semicircular canal or tegmen tympani
    - Bone erosion less common than in acquired cholesteatoma
    - Bone erosion occurs late in disease
    - Ossicular erosion unusual with anterior mesotympanum involvement
    - Long process of incus & stapes superstructure most commonly destroyed ossicles

## DDx: Middle Ear Masses

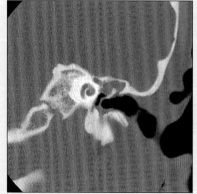

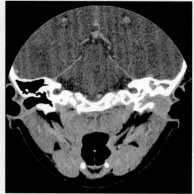

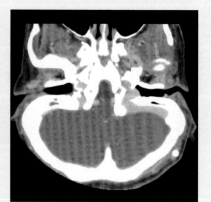

*Acquired Cholesteatoma*   *Rhabdomyosarcoma*   *Dehiscent Jugular Bulb*

# CONGENITAL CHOLESTEATOMA

II

1

31

## Key Facts

### Terminology
- Primary cholesteatoma, epidermoid, "skin in the wrong place"

### Imaging Findings
- Best diagnostic clue: Smooth, well-circumscribed middle ear mass ± ossicular erosions
- Other locations: External auditory canal (EAC), middle ear-mastoid, petrous apex, CP angle, geniculate ganglion

### Top Differential Diagnoses
- Acquired Cholesteatoma
- Rhabdomyosarcoma, Middle Ear
- Dehiscent Jugular Bulb
- Facial Nerve Schwannoma, Middle Ear

### Pathology
- Congenital abnormal ectodermal rest
- Epidemiology: 2-5% of cholesteatomas are congenital
- Early or "closed" CCh
- Small, encapsulated focal anterior tympanic cavity mass
- Late or "open" CCh
- Large ME mass, extends throughout cavity & mastoid complex

### Clinical Issues
- Avascular ME mass behind intact TM
- No prior history of inflammation or trauma
- Unilateral conductive hearing loss (CHL) 60% in one series

---

- Labyrinthine extension may occur but only late in disease process
- If aditus ad antrum occluded, mastoid air cells opacify with retained secretions
- Common locations of CCh-ME
  - Anterosuperior middle ear, adjacent to eustachian tube & anterior tympanic ring, medial to ossicular structures
  - Inferior but adjacent to tensor tympani muscle, mimics pars tensa acquired middle ear cholesteatoma that also often ends up medial to ossicles
  - Near stapes
  - Posterior epitympanum, at tympanic isthmus

### MR Findings
- T1WI: Iso- to hypointense ME mass
- T2WI
  - Intermediate intensity ME mass
  - With larger lesions, aditus ad antrum obstruction seen as high signal retained secretions in mastoid air cells
- T1 C+
  - Peripherally-enhancing ME mass
    - CCh-ME is nonenhancing material surrounded by thin subtle rim-enhancement
  - If lesion is long-standing, associated scar may be seen as thickened area of enhancement adjacent to CCh-ME

### Imaging Recommendations
- Temporal bone CT is examination of choice
- T1 C+ MR is complimentary exam in certain circumstances, recommended if
  - Recurrent or large CCh-ME
  - Diagnosis uncertain

## DIFFERENTIAL DIAGNOSIS

### Acquired Cholesteatoma
- Otoscopy reveals retraction pocket, pars flaccida or pars tensa tympanic membrane (TM) perforation

- Imaging: Pars flaccida cholesteatoma, acquired
  - Scutum erosion with lesion in Prussak space of lateral epitympanum
  - Ossicular chain & lateral semicircular canal more likely eroded
  - Chronic inflammatory changes present
- Imaging: Pars tensa cholesteatoma, acquired
  - Lesion enlarges medial to ossicles
  - Ossicular erosion common

### Rhabdomyosarcoma, Middle Ear
- Aggressive, destructive mass in middle ear and mastoid
- Lateral extension into EAC
- Medial extension into internal auditory canal
- Cephalad extension into middle cranial fossa
- Posterior extension into posterior cranial fossa
- Inferior extension into nasopharyngeal, temporal mandibular joint, masticator or parotid space

### Dehiscent Jugular Bulb
- Usually asymptomatic, incidental finding in imaging studies
  - May present with blue mass behind intact tympanic membrane on otoscopic exam
- Superior and lateral extension of jugular bulb into middle ear cavity via dehiscent jugular plate of sigmoid sinus

### Facial Nerve Schwannoma, Middle Ear
- Otoscopy shows avascular mass behind intact TM; rare in children
- Tubular mass emanating from tympanic facial nerve canal, enhancing on T1 C+ MR
  - Enlarged bony facial nerve canal and geniculate fossa
  - Extends from geniculate ganglion along tympanic segment of facial nerve

## PATHOLOGY

### General Features
- Etiology

# CONGENITAL CHOLESTEATOMA

- ○ Congenital abnormal ectodermal rest
  - In middle ear: Abnormal migration of external canal ectoderm beyond tympanic ring
  - Becomes a mass-like middle ear accumulation of stratified epithelial squamous cells
- Epidemiology: 2-5% of cholesteatomas are congenital
- Associated abnormalities
  - ○ EAC atresia can present with associated CCh
  - ○ Rarely associated with 1st branchial cleft remnant

## Gross Pathologic & Surgical Features
- Circumscribed, pearly-white mass with capsular sheen
- When detected early, no associated inflammatory changes

## Microscopic Features
- Identical to epidermoid inclusion cyst
- Stratified squamous epithelium, with progressive exfoliation of keratinous material
- Contents rich in cholesterol crystals

## Staging, Grading or Classification Criteria
- Early or "closed" CCh
  - ○ Small, encapsulated focal anterior tympanic cavity mass
- Late or "open" CCh
  - ○ Large ME mass, extends throughout cavity & mastoid complex

# CLINICAL ISSUES

## Presentation
- Most common signs/symptoms
  - ○ Avascular ME mass behind intact TM
  - ○ No prior history of inflammation or trauma
- Other symptoms
  - ○ Unilateral conductive hearing loss (CHL) 60% in one series
  - ○ Large lesions can obstruct eustachian tube with resultant ME effusion & infection
  - ○ May be discovered surgically after chronic ME effusion unresponsive to tympanostomy tubes

## Demographics
- Age
  - ○ Average age of presentation or detection
    - Anterior or anterosuperior: 4 years
    - Posterosuperior & mesotympanum: 12 years
    - Attic & mastoid antrum involvement: 20 years
- Gender: M:F = 3:1

## Natural History & Prognosis
- CCh-ME: Smaller, anterior lesions have better outcome, with complete surgical resection
- If untreated, keratin debris accumulates over time, with resultant larger lesion
  - ○ Enlarging, cyst-like CCh may rupture, extending throughout ME
  - ○ If eustachian tube obstructed, ME effusions & otitis occur
  - ○ Larger lesions with infection may be difficult to differentiate from acquired cholesteatoma

- Large lesions or posterior epitympanic CCh have recurrence rates as high as 20%
  - ○ Staged surgical resection often used for large lesions
- Temporal bone CT to assess for recurrence

## Treatment
- Complete surgical extirpation = treatment of choice
- Ossicular chain reconstruction may be necessary

# DIAGNOSTIC CHECKLIST

## Consider
- CCh-ME mass is seen behind intact TM
- No history of prior TM perforation
- ME is opacified with wall erosion in patient with external auditory canal atresia

# SELECTED REFERENCES

1. Kojima H et al: Congenital cholesteatoma clinical features and surgical results. Am J Otolaryngol. 27(5):299-305, 2006
2. Thakkar KH et al: Congenital cholesteatoma isolated to the mastoid. Otol Neurotol. 27(2):282-3, 2006
3. El-Bitar MA et al: Congenital middle ear cholesteatoma: need for early recognition--role of computed tomography scan. Int J Pediatr Otorhinolaryngol. 67(3):231-5, 2003
4. Darrouzet V et al: Congenital middle ear cholesteatomas in children: our experience in 34 cases. Otolaryngol Head Neck Surg. 126(1):34-40, 2002
5. El-Bitar MA et al: Bilateral occurrence of congenital middle ear cholesteatoma. Otolaryngol Head Neck Surg. 127(5):480-2, 2002
6. Koltai PJ et al: The natural history of congenital cholesteatoma. Arch Otolaryngol Head Neck Surg. 128(7):804-9, 2002
7. Nelson M et al: Congenital cholesteatoma: classification, management, and outcome. Arch Otolaryngol Head Neck Surg. 128(7):810-4, 2002
8. Potsic WP et al: A staging system for congenital cholesteatoma. Arch Otolaryngol Head Neck Surg. 128(9):1009-12, 2002
9. Potsic WP et al: Congenital cholesteatoma: 20 years' experience at The Children's Hospital of Philadelphia. Otolaryngol Head Neck Surg. 126(4):409-14, 2002
10. Shohet JA et al: The management of pediatric cholesteatoma. Otolaryngol Clin North Am. 35(4):841-51, 2002
11. Yammine FG et al: Anterior and posterior middle ear congenital cholesteatomas in children. J Otolaryngol. 30(1):29-33, 2001
12. Yeo SW et al: The clinical evaluations of pathophysiology for congenital middle ear cholesteatoma. Am J Otolaryngol. 22(3):184-9, 2001
13. Liu JH et al: Congenital cholesteatoma of the middle ear. Clin Pediatr (Phila). 39(9):549-51, 2000
14. Melero GA et al: Facial paralysis: An unusual presentation of congenital cholesteatoma. Otolaryngol Head Neck Surg. 122(4):615-6, 2000
15. Tos M: A new pathogenesis of mesotympanic (congenital) cholesteatoma. Laryngoscope. 110(11):1890-7, 2000
16. De la Cruz A et al: Detection and management of childhood cholesteatoma. Pediatr Ann. 28(6):370-3, 1999
17. Friedberg J: Congenital cholesteatoma. Laryngoscope. 104(3 Pt 2):1-24, 1994

# CONGENITAL CHOLESTEATOMA

## IMAGE GALLERY

### Typical

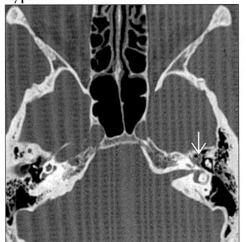
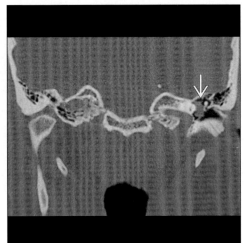

*(Left)* Axial bone CT shows a small CCh in the left middle ear cavity ➡, anteromedial to the intact middle ear ossicles. *(Right)* Coronal bone CT (same patient as previous image) shows the soft tissue mass ➡, medial to the uninvolved ossicles, abutting the cochlear promontory.

### Typical

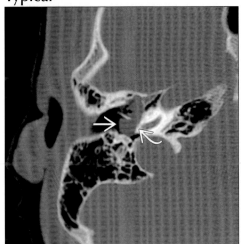
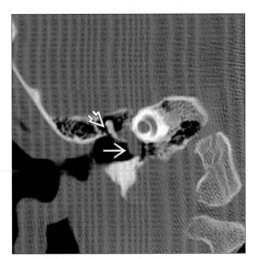

*(Left)* Axial bone CT shows a lobulated CCh in the right middle ear cavity ➡, abutting the cochlear promontory ➡ in a patient without a prior history of infection. *(Right)* Coronal bone CT (same patient as previous image) shows the middle ear mass ➡, medial to the ossicles, without involvement of Prussak space ➡.

### Typical

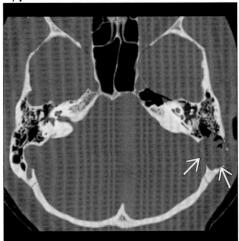
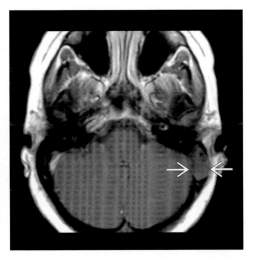

*(Left)* Axial bone CT shows a large CCh filling the left posterior mastoid air cells and destroying the adjacent inner and outer tables of the calvarium ➡. *(Right)* Axial T1 C+ MR (same patient as previous image) shows no significant enhancement of the lesion ➡. The patient presented in adulthood without a prior history of ear infections or trauma.

# ACQUIRED CHOLESTEATOMA

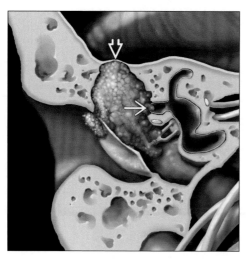

Coronal graphic shows large pars flaccida acquired cholesteatoma. Complications include erosion of ossicles and lateral semicircular canal ⇨ with thinning of tegmen tympani ⇨.

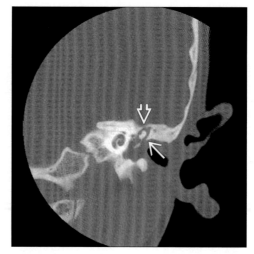

Coronal bone CT shows left pars flaccida ACh filling the left middle ear cavity. Note truncation of the scutum ⇨ and focal thinning of the tegmen tympani ⇨.

## TERMINOLOGY

### Abbreviations and Synonyms

- Secondary or acquired cholesteatoma (ACh)
  - "Attic" or "Prussak space" cholesteatoma = pars flaccida cholesteatoma (PFC)
  - Pars tensa cholesteatoma (PTC): "Sinus" cholesteatoma = PTC involving sinus tympani

### Definitions

- Stratified squamous epithelium-lined sac filled with exfoliated keratin debris

## IMAGING FINDINGS

### General Features

- Best diagnostic clue
  - PFC: Nonenhancing soft tissue mass in Prussak space with scutum erosion
    - ± Tegmen tympani, lateral semicircular canal (SCC), facial nerve canal or sigmoid sinus plate dehiscence

  - PTC: Nonenhancing mass in posterior tympanum medial to ossicles
- Location
  - Pars flaccida ACh: 82% of all cholesteatomas
    - Secondary to tympanic membrane (TM) perforation or retraction pocket involving anterior superior pars flaccida portion of the TM (Shrapnell membrane)
  - Pars tensa ACh: 18% of all cholesteatomas
    - Secondary to TM perforation or retraction pocket in the inferior pars tensa portion of TM
  - Mural = automastoidectomy, atypical ACh shell
    - Residual ACh rind left behind after middle ear (ME)-mastoid ACh extrudes central matrix through TM or external auditory canal (EAC) bony wall
  - Other: Petrous apex, cerebellopontine angle
- Size: Few mm to several cm

### CT Findings

- CECT
  - No enhancement of cholesteatoma
  - Surrounding granulation tissue may enhance
- Bone CT

## DDx: ME-Mastoid Disease with Bone Destruction

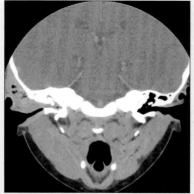

*Otomastoiditis*

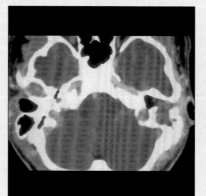

*Langerhans Cell Histiocytosis*

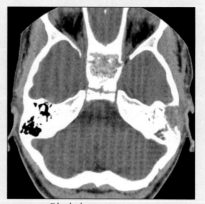

*Rhabdomyosarcoma*

## Key Facts

### Terminology
- Secondary or acquired cholesteatoma (ACh)
- "Attic" or "Prussak space" cholesteatoma = pars flaccida cholesteatoma (PFC)
- Pars tensa cholesteatoma (PTC): "Sinus" cholesteatoma = PTC involving sinus tympani

### Imaging Findings
- PFC: Nonenhancing soft tissue mass in Prussak space with scutum erosion
- PTC: Nonenhancing mass in posterior tympanum medial to ossicles

### Top Differential Diagnoses
- Acute Coalescent Otomastoiditis with Abscess
- Langerhans Cell Histiocytosis (LCH)
- Rhabdomyosarcoma

- Congenital Cholesteatoma

### Pathology
- TM retraction or TM perforation results in accumulation of stratified squamous epithelial cells in ME cavity, produces mass-like ball of keratin
- Continually enlarges, ± erosion of adjacent bone
- Associated chronic inflammation may cause further bone erosion

### Diagnostic Checklist
- When ME and mastoid opacified, difficult to differentiate effusion from cholesteatoma
- Presence of ossicular erosion supports diagnosis of cholesteatoma but may also occur in non-cholesteatomatous chronic otitis media

---

- ○ Pars flaccida ACh
  - Soft tissue mass in Prussak space, **lateral** to malleus head, scutum erosion characteristic
  - Ossicles displaced medially
  - Ossicular erosion in 70%: Incus long process most common, incus body & malleus head less common
  - May extend posterolateral to aditus ad antrum and mastoid antrum or inferiorly to posterior ME recesses
  - May also erode lateral SCC, facial nerve canal, tegmen tympani and/or sigmoid sinus plate
- ○ Pars tensa ACh
  - Erosive mass in posterior tympanum **medial** to ossicles
  - May involve sinus tympani, facial recess, aditus ad antrum and/or mastoid
  - Ossicular erosion common (90%), especially medial aspect of incus long process, stapes suprastructure and malleus manubrium
  - ± Posterior tegmen tympani dehiscence
- ○ Mural ACh
  - "Hollowed out" ME-mastoid with residual cholesteatoma rind along walls of cavity
- ○ Radiologists search pattern and report should include
  - Location of mass, relationship to ossicles
  - Integrity of ossicles, scutum, lateral SCC, tegmen tympani, facial nerve canal and sigmoid sinus plate
  - Extension into mastoid antrum
  - Assessment of mastoid air cells: Aerated or opaque, coalescent or non-coalescent, may be small and underpneumatized with sclerotic septations secondary to chronic infection

### MR Findings
- T1WI: ME mass hypointense
- T2WI: Mildly hyperintense, usually less than trapped secretions
- DWI: Hyperintense
- T1 C+
  - ○ PFC or PTC does not enhance

- ○ Associated granulation tissue or scar may enhance
- ○ If tegmen tympani dehiscent, coronal may show dural enhancement adjacent to bony defect

### Imaging Recommendations
- Best imaging tool
  - ○ Noncontrast bone CT: Axial and coronal
    - Prussak space mass, scutum and tegmen tympani best evaluated on coronal images
    - Ossicular erosion, lateral SCC and facial nerve canal erosion: Need to view axial and coronal images
    - Sigmoid plate erosion best evaluated on axial images
  - ○ Coronal T1 C+ MR useful adjunct when cephalocele, intracranial extension or intracranial infection suspected

---

## DIFFERENTIAL DIAGNOSIS

### Acute Coalescent Otomastoiditis with Abscess
- Clinical presentation: Fever, periauricular erythema, pain, fluctuance
- Rim-enhancing fluid collection adjacent to opacified mastoid air cells = abscess, may be intracranial or extracranial
- Variable trabecular & cortical erosions
- Regional complications: Subperiosteal abscess, meningitis, brain abscess, epidural abscess, sigmoid sinus thrombosis secondary to thrombophlebitis, Bezold abscess around sternocleidomastoid muscle, labyrinthitis, petrous apicitis, communicating hydrocephalus secondary to sinus thrombosis or obstruction of arachnoid granulations

### Langerhans Cell Histiocytosis (LCH)
- Enhancing soft tissue mass with bone destruction
- Locations in head and neck: Orbit, maxilla, mandible, temporal bone, cervical spine, skull

# ACQUIRED CHOLESTEATOMA

## Rhabdomyosarcoma
- Parameningeal in ME, paranasal sinus, nasopharynx
- Soft tissue mass with variable contrast-enhancement
- Aggressive osseous destruction common

## Congenital Cholesteatoma
- 2% of all cholesteatomas
- Well-defined ME mass behind intact TM
- Osseous erosion similar to ACh if large
- Usually lacks history of recurrent infection or TM perforation

## Chronic Otitis Media with Ossicular Erosion
- Non-cholesteatomatous ossicular erosion: Distal incus most common, TM often retracted
- May lack surrounding inflammatory debris, mastoid may be sclerotic secondary to chronic otitis media during mastoid formation
- May be indistinguishable from ACh on CT

# PATHOLOGY

## General Features
- Etiology
  - TM retraction or TM perforation results in accumulation of stratified squamous epithelial cells in ME cavity, produces mass-like ball of keratin
  - Continually enlarges, ± erosion of adjacent bone
  - Associated chronic inflammation may cause further bone erosion
- Associated abnormalities: Increased risk in patients with cleft palate

## Gross Pathologic & Surgical Features
- Pearly white mass

## Microscopic Features
- Mass of stratified squamous epithelium filled with exfoliated keratin debris, rich in cholesterol crystals
- Chronic inflammatory changes usually present

# CLINICAL ISSUES

## Presentation
- Most common signs/symptoms
  - Conductive hearing loss (CHL)
  - Recurrent or chronic ME infections with TM perforation or retraction pocket, foul smelling aural discharge
  - ME mass with TM perforation on examination
- Other signs/symptoms: Painless otorrhea, vertigo, otalgia, facial nerve paralysis

## Demographics
- Age
  - Occurs in children and adults
  - Unusual in children less than 4 years of age

## Natural History & Prognosis
- Natural history

- Small ACh forms within retraction pocket, progressive increase in size, destruction of adjacent structures (ossicles, SSCs, tegmen tympani, facial nerve canal, transverse sinus invasion)
- If untreated: CN 7 involvement, venous sinus thrombosis and intracranial extension = late complications
- Prognosis
  - Excellent if complete removal of small lesions
  - Residual CHL, sensorineural hearing loss and peripheral facial nerve paralysis possible
  - Sinus tympani extension associated with high post-surgical recurrence rate

## Treatment
- Surgical excision, mastoidectomy and ossicular chain reconstruction if needed

# DIAGNOSTIC CHECKLIST

## Image Interpretation Pearls
- When ME and mastoid opacified, difficult to differentiate effusion from cholesteatoma
- Presence of ossicular erosion supports diagnosis of cholesteatoma but may also occur in non-cholesteatomatous chronic otitis media

# SELECTED REFERENCES

1. De Foer B et al: Single-shot, turbo spin-echo, diffusion-weighted imaging versus spin-echo-planar, diffusion-weighted imaging in the detection of acquired middle ear cholesteatoma. AJNR Am J Neuroradiol. 27(7):1480-2, 2006
2. Dubrulle F et al: Diffusion-weighted MR imaging sequence in the detection of postoperative recurrent cholesteatoma. Radiology. 238(2):604-10, 2006
3. Schraff SA et al: Pediatric cholesteatoma: a retrospective review. Int J Pediatr Otorhinolaryngol. 70(3):385-93, 2006
4. Shohet JA et al: The management of pediatric cholesteatoma. Otolaryngol Clin North Am. 35(4):841-51, 2002
5. Watts S et al: A systematic approach to interpretation of computed tomography scans prior to surgery of middle ear cholesteatoma. J Laryngol Otol. 114(4):248-53, 2000
6. Fageeh NA et al: Surgical treatment of cholesteatoma in children. J Otolaryngol. 28(6):309-12, 1999
7. Mafee MF: MRI and CT in the evaluation of acquired and congenital cholesteatomas of the temporal bone. J Otolaryngol. 22(4):239-48, 1993
8. Vartiainen E et al: Long-term results of surgical treatment in different cholesteatoma types. Am J Otol. 14(5):507-11, 1993
9. Schuring AG et al: Staging for cholesteatoma in the child, adolescent, and adult. Ann Otol Rhinol Laryngol. 99(4 Pt 1):256-60, 1990
10. Michaels L: Biology of cholesteatoma. Otolaryngol Clin North Am. 22(5):869-81, 1989
11. Mafee MF et al: Cholesteatoma of the middle ear and mastoid. A comparison of CT scan and operative findings. Otolaryngol Clin North Am. 21(2):265-93, 1988
12. Nardis PF et al: Unusual cholesteatoma shell: CT findings. J Comput Assist Tomogr. 12(6):1084-5, 1988
13. Swartz JD: Cholesteatomas of the middle ear. Diagnosis, etiology, and complications. Radiol Clin North Am. 22(1):15-35, 1984

## IMAGE GALLERY

### Typical

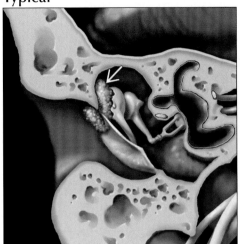

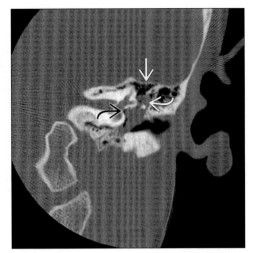

*(Left)* Coronal graphic shows small ACh originating at pars flaccida portion of the tympanic membrane. The mass ➡ fills Prussak space with slight medial displacement of the ossicles. *(Right)* Coronal bone CT shows ACh filling Prussak space ➡, partially filling the middle ear cavity and extending into the oval window ➘. The tegmen tympani ➡ is intact.

### Typical

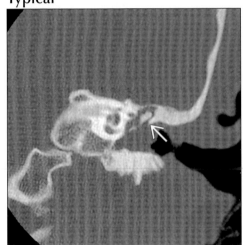

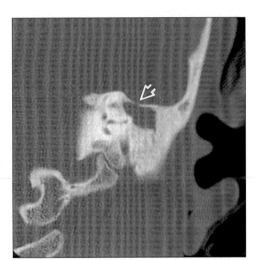

*(Left)* Coronal bone CT shows ACh filling the middle ear cavity and Prussak space and engulfing the ossicles. Note also the mild truncation of the scutum ➡. *(Right)* Coronal bone CT (same patient as previous image) shows filling of the epitympanum and thinning of the overlying tegmen tympani ➡ secondary to ACh.

### Typical

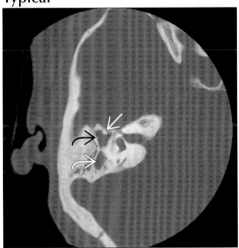

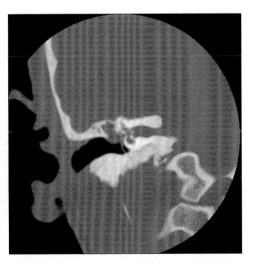

*(Left)* Axial bone CT shows complete opacification of the epitympanum ➚ and mastoid antrum ➚, truncated malleus head ➡ and nonvisualization/erosion of incus long process. *(Right)* Coronal bone CT (same patient as previous image) shows absence of the incus short process and the stapes in this patient with ACh.

# CHONDROSARCOMA

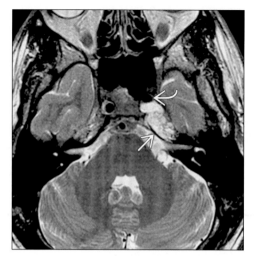

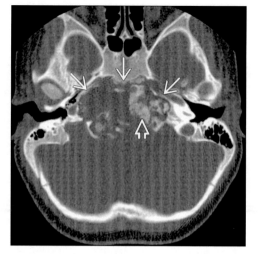

*Axial T2WI MR shows mildly heterogeneous hyperintense mass ➡ centered at the left petrooccipital synchondrosis. The the left petrous internal carotid artery ➡ is anteriorly displaced.*

*Axial bone CT shows a large skull base mass ➡ involving clivus and both petrous apices, expanding posteriorly to compress the brain stem. Note chondroid calcification ➡ within tumor.*

## TERMINOLOGY

### Abbreviations and Synonyms
- Chondrosarcoma, skull base (CSa-SB)

### Definitions
- CSa-SB: Chondroid malignancy of the skull base

## IMAGING FINDINGS

### General Features
- Best diagnostic clue: Chondroid matrix in a tumor centered on the petrooccipital synchondrosis
- Location
  - Base of skull
    - Typically centered on the petrooccipital synchondrosis
    - Rarely arise in basisphenoid or dural surface of clivus
  - Other locations: Maxillary sinus, mandible, nasal cavity, neck, nasopharynx, orbit
- Size: Variable, usually > 3 cm
- Morphology

- Lobulated margins
- Usually solitary but may be multiple

### CT Findings
- NECT
  - 50% have chondroid matrix calcification (arc or ring-like)
  - Sharp, narrow, nonsclerotic transition zone
  - > 50% have associated bone destruction
  - Soft tissue component relatively dense
- CECT: Variable enhancement

### MR Findings
- T1WI
  - Low to intermediate signal intensity relative to gray matter
    - Low signal foci within tumor may suggest underlying coarse matrix mineralization or fibrocartilaginous elements
- T2WI
  - High often heterogeneous T2 signal
  - Hypointense foci (calcifications) less conspicuous than on CT
- T2WI FS: Preferred over T2WI without FS as margins better defined

## DDx: Clival Lesions

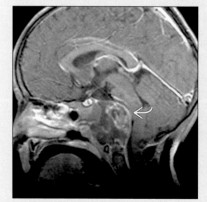

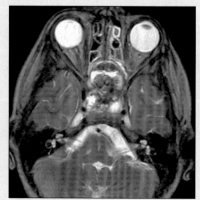

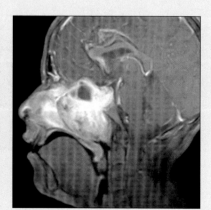

*Chordoma*

*Craniopharyngioma*

*Juvenile Angiofibroma*

# CHONDROSARCOMA

## Key Facts

### Terminology
- Chondrosarcoma, skull base (CSa-SB)
- CSa-SB: Chondroid malignancy of the skull base

### Imaging Findings
- Best diagnostic clue: Chondroid matrix in a tumor centered on the petrooccipital synchondrosis
- 50% have chondroid matrix calcification (arc or ring-like)
- Sharp, narrow, nonsclerotic transition zone
- High often heterogeneous T2 signal
- Heterogeneous or homogeneous enhancement

### Top Differential Diagnoses
- Chordoma
- Craniopharyngioma
- Rathke Pouch Cyst

- Juvenile Angiofibroma
- Pituitary Adenoma
- Nerve Sheath Tumors

### Clinical Issues
- Most common signs/symptoms: Abducens (CN6) palsy
- Rare in pediatric age group, consider Ollier disease or Maffucci syndrome

### Diagnostic Checklist
- Classic: T1 C+ MR heterogeneously-enhancing tumor at petrooccipital synchondrosis with high T2 signal
- CT: Chondroid mineralization (50%)
- Invasive bone changes in petrooccipital fissure strongly favors diagnosis of CSa

---

- T1 C+
  - Heterogeneous or homogeneous enhancement
    - Whorls of enhancing lines within tumor matrix often seen
- T1 C+ FS: Preferred over T1 C+ without FS as margins better defined

### Angiographic Findings
- Conventional
  - Avascular or hypovascular mass
  - Internal carotid artery displacement & encasement

### Imaging Recommendations
- Best imaging tool: CT and MR
- Protocol advice
  - Thin section CT with bone algorithm and coronal reformats
  - Focused C+ MR of skull base
    - Multiplanar T2 FS and T1 C+ FS
    - Consider MRA & MRV
  - In selected cases pre-operative angiography with test occlusion

## DIFFERENTIAL DIAGNOSIS

### Chordoma
- Key tumor to differentiate from CSa
- Bone CT: Destructive midline clival lesion; bone fragments within matrix
- MR: Low T1, high T2, enhancing mass
- Midline > lateral location

### Craniopharyngioma
- Bone CT: Often calcification within mass
- MR: Cystic and solid, may have intrinsic T1 shortening

### Rathke Pouch Cyst
- Cystic mass in sella, no solid component

### Juvenile Angiofibroma
- Adolescent boy, intense enhancement, flow voids

### Pituitary Adenoma
- Well-marginated, homogeneously enhancing

### Nerve Sheath Tumors
- Well marginated, dumbbell shape, ± cystic components

### Cholesteatoma, Petrous Apex
- Bone CT: Expansile, smooth petrous apex lesion
- MR: Low T1, high T2 lesion without enhancement

### Esthesioneuroblastoma
- Intermediate T1, T2 ± peripheral tumor cysts

### Osteogenic Sarcoma
- Bone CT: Indefinite margins, sclerosis or mixed, ± "sunburst" spicules of mineralized tumor

### Chondromyxoid (CM) Fibroma
- Bone CT: Expansile, non-infiltrating skull base mass, ± ground-glass

## PATHOLOGY

### General Features
- General path comments: CSa-SB arises from remnants of embryonal cartilage or metaplasia of meningeal fibroblasts
- Genetics: May complicate Ollier disease, Maffucci syndrome
- Etiology: Arises from cartilage, endochondral bone or from primitive mesenchymal cells in meninges
- Epidemiology
  - 6% of all skull base tumors
  - 75% of all cranial CSa in skull base

### Gross Pathologic & Surgical Features
- Smooth, lobulated mass welling up from petrooccipital fissure
- Cut surface shows a gray-white, glistening tumor parenchyma

# CHONDROSARCOMA

## Microscopic Features

- Hypercellular tumor composed of chondrocytes with hyperchromatic, pleomorphic nuclei & prominent nucleoli
- Binucleate or multinucleate cells are rule
- Hyaline matrix may calcify in "ringlets"
- Intercellular matrix is solid in hyaline type compared to mucinous/gelatinous matrix in myxoid or mixed types
- Histology may overlap with, be confused with that of chordomas
  - Especially chondroid chordoma, myxoid chondrosarcoma
  - Differentiation facilitated by immunohistochemical staining

## Staging, Grading or Classification Criteria

- Classification
  - Conventional CSa: Hyaline (7%), myxoid (30% of cases) or mixed (63% of cases)
  - Dedifferentiated, clear cell or mesenchymal
- Grading from low grade to high grade
  - Based on degree of cellularity, pleomorphism, mitoses & multinucleated cells

# CLINICAL ISSUES

## Presentation

- Most common signs/symptoms: Abducens (CN6) palsy
- Other signs/symptoms: Headaches, decreased hearing, dizziness, tinnitus, nasal stuffiness or discharge, sinusitis, other cranial nerve palsies (CN 3, 5, 7, 8)
- Clinical Profile
  - Rare in pediatric age group, consider Ollier disease or Maffucci syndrome
  - Typically middle age patient with insidious onset of headaches & cranial nerve palsies
    - Mean duration of symptoms at diagnosis = 27 months

## Demographics

- Age: 10-80 years, mean 40 years
- Gender: M > F

## Natural History & Prognosis

- Prognosis depends on extent at diagnosis, histologic grade & completeness of resection
- Most skull base CSa well to moderately differentiated
- Most slow-growing, locally invasive, rarely metastasize
  - High grade CSa metastasizes to bones & lung more frequently
- 10 year survival rates of 99% recently reported
  - Radical resection & proton beam irradiation

## Treatment

- Combined radical resection & high dose, fractionated conformal radiation or proton beam therapy
- Basal subfrontal approach used for tumor that invades clivus & extends anteriorly into sphenoid & ethmoid sinuses
- Subtemporal & preauricular infratemporal approach when extends laterally beyond petrous internal carotid artery

# DIAGNOSTIC CHECKLIST

## Consider

- Is lesion in midline (chordoma) or off-midline (CSa)?
- Do calcifications represent arc-whorl intralesional calcifications (CSa) or fragmented destroyed bone (chordoma)?

## Image Interpretation Pearls

- Classic: T1 C+ MR heterogeneously-enhancing tumor at petrooccipital synchondrosis with high T2 signal
  - CT: Chondroid mineralization (50%)
  - Invasive bone changes in petrooccipital fissure strongly favors diagnosis of CSa

# SELECTED REFERENCES

1. Hug EB et al: Proton radiotherapy in management of pediatric base of skull tumors. Int J Radiat Oncol Biol Phys. 52(4):1017-24, 2002
2. Neff B et al: Chondrosarcoma of the skull base. Laryngoscope. 112(1):134-9, 2002
3. Schmidinger A et al: Natural history of chondroid skull base lesions--case report and review. Neuroradiology. 44(3):268-71, 2002
4. Tsai EC et al: Tumors of the skull base in children: review of tumor types and management strategies. Neurosurg Focus. 12(5):e1, 2002
5. Crockard HA et al: A multidisciplinary team approach to skull base chondrosarcomas. J Neurosurg. 95(2):184-9, 2001
6. Richardson MS: Pathology of skull base tumors. Otolaryngol Clin North Am. 34(6):1025-42, vii, 2001
7. Hug EB et al: Proton radiation therapy for chordomas and chondrosarcomas of the skull base. J Neurosurg. 91(3):432-9, 1999
8. Rosenberg AE et al: Chondrosarcoma of the base of the skull: a clinicopathologic study of 200 cases with emphasis on its distinction from chordoma. Am J Surg Pathol. 23(11):1370-8, 1999
9. Korten AG et al: Intracranial chondrosarcoma: review of the literature and report of 15 cases. J Neurol Neurosurg Psychiatry. 65(1):88-92, 1998
10. Keel SB et al: Chondromyxoid fibroma of the skull base: a tumor which may be confused with chordoma and chondrosarcoma. A report of three cases and review of the literature. Am J Surg Pathol. 21(5):577-82, 1997
11. Ramina R et al: Maffucci's syndrome associated with a cranial base chondrosarcoma: case report and literature review. Neurosurgery. 41(1):269-72, 1997
12. Rapidis AD et al: Chondrosarcomas of the skull base: review of the literature and report of two cases. J Craniomaxillofac Surg. 25(6):322-7, 1997
13. Geirnaerdt MJ et al: Calcified meningioma of the skull base simulating chondrosarcoma. Eur J Radiol. 21(2):148-51, 1995
14. Weber AL et al: Cartilaginous tumors and chordomas of the cranial base. Otolaryngol Clin North Am. 28(3):453-71, 1995
15. Brown E et al: Chondrosarcoma of the skull base. Neuroimaging Clin N Am. 4(3):529-41, 1994
16. Meyers SP et al: Chondrosarcomas of the skull base: MR imaging features. Radiology. 184(1):103-8, 1992

# CHONDROSARCOMA

## IMAGE GALLERY

### Typical

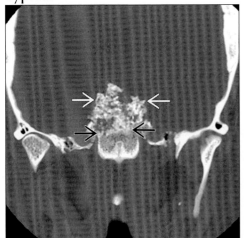
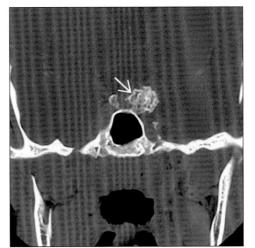

*(Left)* Coronal bone CT shows better the rings, arcs, and stipples ➡ of the chondroid matrix calcification and the sharp, narrow, nonsclerotic transition zone ➡ in this clival chondrosarcoma. *(Right)* Coronal bone CT shows the calcified chondroid mass ➡ arising from the left anterior clinoid process and compressing the superior aspect of the cavernous sinus.

### Typical

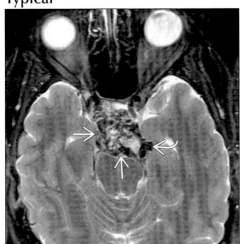
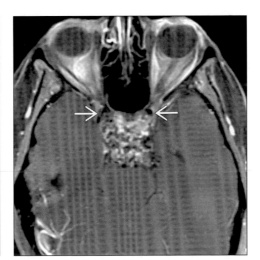

*(Left)* Axial T2WI FS MR shows heterogeneous clival mass ➡ extending into the prepontine cistern. Notice the multiple low signal foci ➡ due to matrix calcification. *(Right)* Axial T1 C+ FS MR in the same patient as previous image shows heterogeneously enhancing mass that expands the clivus and compresses the cavernous segments of the internal carotid arteries ➡.

### Typical

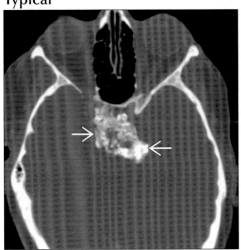
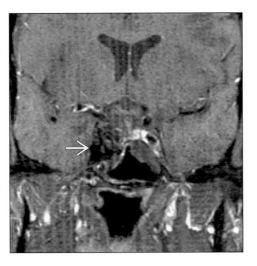

*(Left)* Axial bone CT in same patient as previous image shows the mass is heterogeneous with rings and arcs of high density consistent with chondroid matrix calcification ➡. *(Right)* Coronal T1 C+ FS MR shows ➡ a low signal mass centered on the right petrooccipital synchondrosis with no enhancement. Chondrosarcomas typically enhance.

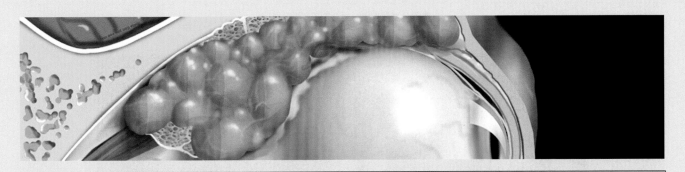

# SECTION 2: Orbit, Nose and Sinuses

# NASAL GLIOMA

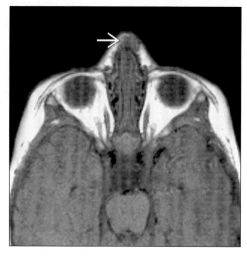

Axial T1WI MR in a child presenting with a subcutaneous nasal mass ➜ shows a low signal intensity extranasal glioma just to the left of midline at the nasal dorsum.

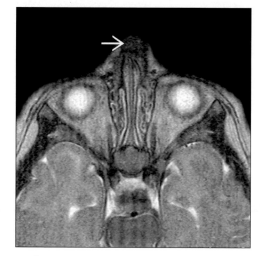

Axial T2WI FS MR in the same patient as previous image shows a low signal intensity extranasal glioma ➜ to the left of midline at nasal dorsum.

## TERMINOLOGY

### Abbreviations and Synonyms
- Nasal glioma (NG)
  - Extranasal glioma (ENG); intranasal glioma (ING)
- Nasal cerebral heterotopia, glial heterotopia

### Definitions
- Rare, developmental mass of dysplastic neurogenic tissue sequestered & isolated from subarachnoid space
- "Glioma" is a misnomer as this is non-neoplastic tissue
- Best thought of as encephalocele that has lost its intracranial connection

## IMAGING FINDINGS

### General Features
- Best diagnostic clue: Well-circumscribed, solid soft tissue mass off midline at nasal dorsum or within nasal cavity in infant with **no** CSF connection to brain
- Location
  - ENG (60%): Mass along nasal dorsum
    - Glabella most frequent location

- Also medial canthus, nasopharynx, mouth, pterygopalatine fossa (very rare)
  - ING (30%): Nasal cavity mass
    - May be attached to concha of middle turbinate, nasal septum or lateral nasal wall
    - Nasal or nasopharyngeal cavity, mouth or rarely pterygopalatine fossa
  - Mixed extra-intranasal (10%)
    - Components communicate through defect in or lateral edge of nasal bone or rarely through defect in orbital plate of frontal bone or sinus
  - Both ENG & ING usually off midline; right > left
- Size: 1-3 cm in diameter
- Morphology: Well-circumscribed round, ovoid or polypoid mass

### CT Findings
- NECT
  - ENG: Well-circumscribed soft tissue attenuation mass (isodense to brain) located over nasal bones
    - Nasal bones may be thinned
  - ING: Soft tissue attenuation mass within nasal cavity
    - Typically high in nasal vault

## DDx: Nasal Region Masses

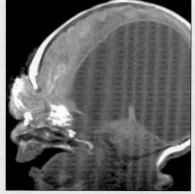

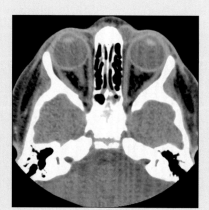

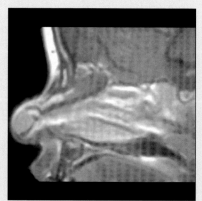

Nasofrontal Encephalocele     Nasal Dermoid     Nasal Dermal Sinus

# NASAL GLIOMA

## Key Facts

### Terminology
- Nasal glioma (NG)
- Rare, developmental mass of dysplastic neurogenic tissue sequestered & isolated from subarachnoid space
- "Glioma" is a misnomer as this is non-neoplastic tissue

### Imaging Findings
- Best diagnostic clue: Well-circumscribed, solid soft tissue mass off midline at nasal dorsum or within nasal cavity in infant with **no** CSF connection to brain

### Top Differential Diagnoses
- Frontoethmoidal Cephalocele
- Dermoid-Epidermoid, Isolated
- Nasal Dermal Sinus

- Nasal Polyp

### Pathology
- NG in similar spectrum of congenital anomalies as frontoethmoidal cephaloceles
- Epidemiology: Very rare lesion
- Fibrous or gemistocytic astrocytes & neuroglial fibers

### Clinical Issues
- Clinical Profile: Off-midline intranasal (ING) or dorsum of nose (ENG) mass in newborn

### Diagnostic Checklist
- Most important to differentiate NG from cephalocele
- Document lack of connecting brain tissue and/or contiguous CSF space

---

- ■ Fibrous pedicle connecting lesion intracranially may not be well seen on CT
- ■ Defect in cribriform plate (10-30%)
- ○ Calcification rare
- CECT
  - ○ Lesion does not enhance significantly
  - ○ If intrathecal contrast used
    - ■ Fails to document connection of lesion to subarachnoid space

### MR Findings
- T1WI
  - ○ Predominantly mixed-to-low signal intensity mass
  - ○ Gyral structure of gray matter rarely visible
- T2WI
  - ○ Iso to hyperintense
  - ○ No CSF-space connection
- T1 C+
  - ○ Dysplastic tissue typically does not enhance
  - ○ Rare lesion where enhancement is "perceived"
    - ■ "Perceived" enhancement at periphery of intranasal lesions may actually represent adjacent nasal mucosa

### Imaging Recommendations
- Best imaging tool
  - ○ Multiplanar MR
    - ■ Sagittal T2 may show pedicle of fibrous tissue (not brain parenchyma) between ING & intracranial cavity
    - ■ Sagittal T1 & T2 images also differentiate NG from cephalocele or dermoid
- Protocol advice
  - ○ Thin-section sagittal T1 and T2 MR important
  - ○ Thin-section axial bone noncontrast CT may help construct surgical plan

## DIFFERENTIAL DIAGNOSIS

### Frontoethmoidal Cephalocele
- Frontonasal (FN) & nasoethmoidal (NE) cephalocele types

- Clinical: Congenital mass on or around bridge of nose
- Imaging: MR imaging shows connection to intracranial brain parenchyma

### Dermoid-Epidermoid, Isolated
- Clinical: Focal mass on bridge of nose or in medial orbit without associated tract
- Imaging
  - ○ Dermoid: Fat density/signal intensity
  - ○ Epidermoid: Fluid density/signal

### Nasal Dermal Sinus
- Clinical: Pit on tip or bridge of nose
- Imaging
  - ○ Dermoid or epidermoid along anterior neuropore tract from tip of nose to intracranial site anterior to crista galli
  - ○ Single or multiple
  - ○ Possible intracranial connection via sinus tract

### Nasal Polyp
- Clinical: Polyp is less firm, more translucent that ING
  - ○ Polyps unusual under the age of 5 years
- Imaging
  - ○ Typically inferolateral to middle turbinate (ING medial)
  - ○ Thin enhancement of peripheral mucosa on MR

## PATHOLOGY

### General Features
- General path comments
  - ○ Dysplastic, heterotopic neuroglial & fibrous tissue separated from brain during development of anterior skull or anterior skull base
  - ○ Does not contain CSF and not contiguous with subarachnoid or intraventricular spaces
  - ○ 15% remain connected with intracranial structures usually through a defect in or near cribriform plate
  - ○ Not locally invasive
- Etiology

# NASAL GLIOMA

- ○ NG in similar spectrum of congenital anomalies as frontoethmoidal cephaloceles
- ○ ENG: Fonticulus frontalis (potential space prior to fusion of frontal & nasal bones) fuses prior to regression of dural diverticulum
  - ▪ Dysplastic parenchyma is sequestered over nasal bones
- ○ ING: Dysplastic neural tissue is trapped in developing prenasal space, through foramen cecum, prior to fusion of nasal bones with cartilaginous nasal capsule
- Epidemiology: Very rare lesion
- Associated abnormalities: Rarely associated with other brain or systemic anomalies

## Gross Pathologic & Surgical Features
- Firm, smooth mass
- Rarely recognized as brain tissue at surgery
- 10-30% attached to brain by a stalk of fibrous tissue through defect in or near cribriform plate
- Mixed extra-intranasal lesions connect through defect in nasal bone

## Microscopic Features
- Fibrous or gemistocytic astrocytes & neuroglial fibers
- Fibrous, vascularized connective tissue & sparse neurons
- Glial fibrillary acidic protein (GFAP) & S-100 protein positive
- No mitotic features or bizarre nuclear forms
- Only 10% contain neurons

## CLINICAL ISSUES

### Presentation
- Most common signs/symptoms
  - ○ Extranasal glioma
    - ▪ Congenital subcutaneous blue or red mass along nasal dorsum
    - ▪ May be covered by capillary telangiectasia
  - ○ Intranasal glioma
    - ▪ Firm, polypoid submucosal nasal cavity mass
    - ▪ Nasal obstruction & septal deviation may be present
    - ▪ May be confused clinically with nasal polyp
    - ▪ May protrude through nostril
  - ○ Other signs/symptoms
    - ▪ No change in size with crying, Valsalva, or pressure on jugular vein (vs. frontoethmoidal cephalocele)
    - ▪ ENG: Capillary telangiectasia may cover
    - ▪ ING: Respiratory distress, epiphora
- Clinical Profile: Off-midline intranasal (ING) or dorsum of nose (ENG) mass in newborn

### Demographics
- Age: Usually identified at birth or within first few years of life

### Natural History & Prognosis
- Grows slowly in proportion to adjacent tissue
  - ○ May deform nasal skeleton, maxilla or orbit

- ING: Pedicle attaches brain & lesion may grow at same rate as brain, may become infected resulting in meningitis
- Complete resection results in cure
  - ○ 10% recurrence rate with incomplete resection

### Treatment
- Surgical resection is treatment of choice
- ENG without intracranial connection removed via external incision with stalk dissection
- ING without intracranial connection may be removed endoscopically
  - ○ Less post-operative deformity than with craniotomy
- Rare gliomas with intracranial extension best treated with combined intra- and extracranial approach

## DIAGNOSTIC CHECKLIST

### Consider
- Most important to differentiate NG from cephalocele
- Document lack of connecting brain tissue and/or contiguous CSF space

### Image Interpretation Pearls
- Must evaluate images for connection to intracranial cavity through skull base defect (encephalocele)
- Combined use of thin-section MR & bone CT accomplishes this task
  - ○ Focus imaging to fronto-ethmoid area only

## SELECTED REFERENCES

1. Al-Ammar AY et al: A midline nasopharyngeal heterotopic neuroglial tissue. J Laryngol Otol. 120(7):E25, 2006
2. Cannady SB et al: PHACE syndrome: report of a case with a glioma of the anterior skull base and ocular malformations. Int J Pediatr Otorhinolaryngol. 70(3):561-4, 2006
3. De Biasio P et al: Prenatal diagnosis of a nasal glioma in the mid trimester. Ultrasound Obstet Gynecol. 27(5):571-3, 2006
4. Hedlund G: Congenital frontonasal masses: developmental anatomy, malformations, and MR imaging. Pediatr Radiol. 36(7):647-62; quiz 726-7, 2006
5. Khanna G et al: Causes of facial swelling in pediatric patients: correlation of clinical and radiologic findings. Radiographics. 26(1):157-71, 2006
6. Ma KH et al: Nasal glioma. Hong Kong Med J. 12(6):477-9, 2006
7. Chau HN et al: A rare case of nasal glioma in the sphenoid sinus of an adult presenting with meningoencephalitis. Eur Arch Otorhinolaryngol. 262(7):592-4, 2005
8. Agirdir BV et al: Endoscopic management of the intranasal glioma. J Pediatr Surg. 39(10):1571-3, 2004
9. Penner CR et al: Nasal glial heterotopia: a clinicopathologic and immunophenotypic analysis of 10 cases with a review of the literature. Ann Diagn Pathol. 7(6):354-9, 2003
10. Rahbar R et al: Nasal glioma and encephalocele: diagnosis and management. Laryngoscope. 113(12):2069-77, 2003
11. Hoeger PH et al: Nasal glioma presenting as capillary haemangioma. Eur J Pediatr. 160(2):84-7, 2001
12. Shah J et al: Pedunculated nasal glioma: MRI features and review of the literature. J Postgrad Med. 45(1):15-7, 1999
13. Barkovich AJ et al: Congenital nasal masses: CT and MR imaging features in 16 cases. AJNR Am J Neuroradiol. 12(1):105-16, 1991

# NASAL GLIOMA

## IMAGE GALLERY

### Typical

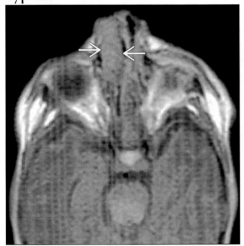
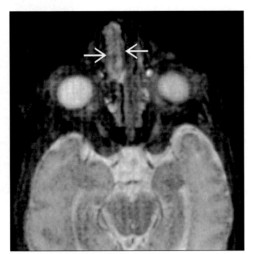

*(Left) Axial T1WI MR shows an off-midline, slightly heterogeneous, well-circumscribed, gray matter-intensity intranasal glioma ➡ within the right nasal cavity. (Right) Axial T2WI MR in the same patient as previous image shows the off-midline, slightly heterogeneous well-circumscribed intranasal glioma ➡ to have low signal intensity.*

### Variant

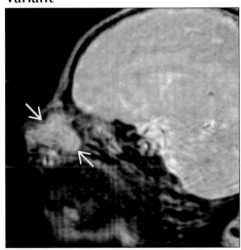
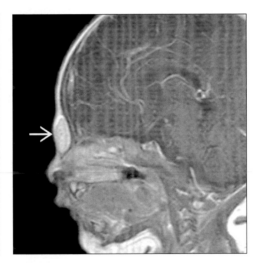

*(Left) Sagittal T2WI MR shows a slightly heterogeneous, well-circumscribed intranasal glioma ➡. No connection to the intracranial cavity was detected by imaging or at surgery. (Right) Sagittal T1 C+ MR shows an atypical extranasal glioma ➡ with diffuse enhancement. A benign mesenchymal neoplasm, such as a hemangioma, could have a similar appearance.*

### Typical

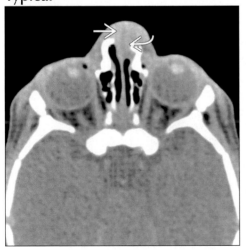
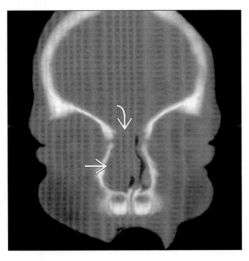

*(Left) Axial NECT shows a mixed extra- and intranasal glioma ➡ at the dorsum of the nose. Note the associated defect in the nasal bone ➡ and associated intranasal extension. (Right) Coronal bone CT shows a large soft tissue mass ➡ in the right nasal cavity in an infant. Note absence of ossification in cribriform plate ➡; this cannot be differentiated from cephalocele by CT.*

# SINCIPITAL CEPHALOCELE

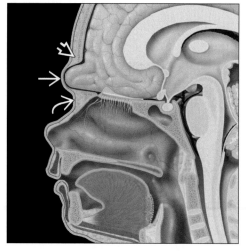

Sagittal graphic of a nasofrontal cephalocele shows herniation of brain through a patent fonticulus frontalis ➡ between the frontal ➡ and nasal ➡ bones.

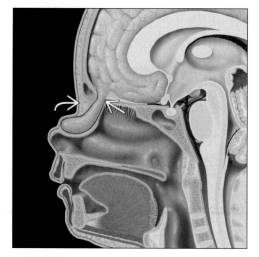

Sagittal graphic of a nasoethmoidal cephalocele shows herniation of brain through a patent foramen cecum ➡ behind the nasal bone ➡.

## TERMINOLOGY

### Abbreviations and Synonyms
- Frontoethmoidal cephalocele (FECeph)
  - Nasofrontal cephalocele (NFCeph) or frontonasal cephalocele
  - Nasoethmoidal cephalocele (NECeph)
  - Naso-orbital cephalocele (NOCeph)

### Definitions
- Congenital herniation of meninges, CSF ± brain through defect in anterior skull causing visible mass
- 3 types: NFCeph, NECeph & NOCeph

## IMAGING FINDINGS

### General Features
- Best diagnostic clue: Frontal, nasal or medial orbital soft tissue mass contiguous with intracranial brain parenchyma extending through bony defect
- Location
  - NFCeph: Between nasal and frontal bones through embryonic fonticulus frontalis

- NECeph: Between nasal bone and nasal cartilage through foramen cecum
- NOCeph: Between the maxilla and lacrimal bones
- Size: Variable (1-2 cm to larger than infant's head)
- Morphology
  - Well-circumscribed, round, globular
  - 90% of FECeph terminate intracranially at single midline defect
  - 10% terminate intracranially at paired openings in anterior cribriform plates

### CT Findings
- NECT
  - NFCeph: Frontal bones displaced superiorly while nasal bones, frontal processes of maxillae & nasal cartilage pushed inferiorly
  - NECeph: Nasal bone bowed with tract through anterior ethmoid area
    - Crista galli may be bifid or absent
    - Deficient or absent cribriform plate, frontal bone, lacrimal bone
  - NOCeph: Uni- or bilateral naso-orbital bony defects
  - **Note**: Nasal process of frontal bone, nasal bone and ethmoid bones incompletely ossified until > 1 yr

## DDx: Skull Base and Nasal Region Lesions

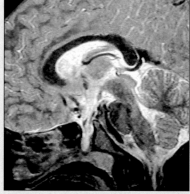

*Basal Cephalocele*

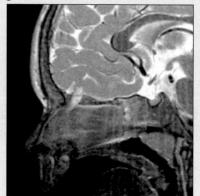

*Nasal Dermoid with Sinus Tract*

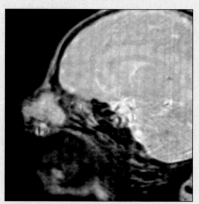

*Nasal Glioma*

# SINCIPITAL CEPHALOCELE

## Key Facts

### Terminology
- Frontoethmoidal cephalocele (FECeph)
- 3 types: NFCeph, NECeph & NOCeph

### Imaging Findings
- Best diagnostic clue: Frontal, nasal or medial orbital soft tissue mass contiguous with intracranial brain parenchyma extending through bony defect
- NFCeph: Between nasal and frontal bones through embryonic fonticulus frontalis
- NECeph: Between nasal bone and nasal cartilage through foramen cecum
- NOCeph: Between the maxilla and lacrimal bones
- **Note:** Nasal process of frontal bone, nasal bone and ethmoid bones incompletely ossified until > 1 yr
- MR superior to CT < 1 yr to avoid misinterpreting cartilaginous unossified bones as defects on CT

- Thin (2 mm) T2 FS sagittal and coronal optimal for visualizing parenchyma through defects

### Top Differential Diagnoses
- Basal Cephalocele
- Nasal Glioma
- Nasal Dermal Sinus
- Dermoid-Epidermoid, Isolated
- Dacryocystocele

### Pathology
- FECeph most common type in Southeast Asia

### Clinical Issues
- Newborn with externally visible, firm nasal or medial orbital mass

## MR Findings
- T1WI: Soft tissue mass with isointense signal to gray matter showing contiguity with intracranial parenchyma extending through bony defect
- T2WI
  - Hyperintense CSF surrounds herniated soft tissue parenchyma
  - Tissue may show ↑ signal due to gliosis
- T1 C+
  - No abnormal enhancement noted within soft tissue
  - Meninges may enhance if infection/inflammation of meninges present

## Ultrasonographic Findings
- OB US: Frontal or nasal soft tissue mass; widened interorbital distance

## Imaging Recommendations
- Best imaging tool
  - MR superior to CT < 1 yr to avoid misinterpreting cartilaginous unossified bones as defects on CT
  - MR shows cephalocele extension through bony defect
  - MR superior for showing other associated brain anomalies
- Protocol advice
  - Thin (2 mm) T2 FS sagittal and coronal optimal for visualizing parenchyma through defects
  - DWI to rule out epidermoids
  - Thin section (1.5 mm) CT bone algorithm

## DIFFERENTIAL DIAGNOSIS

### Basal Cephalocele
- Unlike sincipital not visible externally

### Nasal Glioma
- Clinical: Soft tissue mass along dorsum of nose (extranasal type) or under nasal bones (intranasal type)
- MR imaging shows no connection between mass in intracranial contents

### Nasal Dermal Sinus
- Clinical: Pit on tip or bridge of nose
- Dermoid or epidermoid along anterior neuropore tract from tip of nose to intracranial site anterior to crista galli
- Single or multiple
- Possible intracranial connection via sinus tract

### Dermoid-Epidermoid, Isolated
- Clinical: Focal mass on bridge of nose or in medial orbit without associated tract
- Fat density/intensity if dermoid
- Fluid density/intensity if epidermoid

### Dacryocystocele
- Well-circumscribed, cystic mass at medial canthus
- No connection to skull base or brain parenchyma
- Dilated nasolacrimal duct, cystic mass at inferior meatus

## PATHOLOGY

### General Features
- General path comments: FECeph is congenital herniation of intracranial contents through defects in anterior skull base
- Genetics
  - Sporadic occurrence
  - Unlike occipital cephaloceles not linked to neural tube defects
  - Siblings have 6% incidence of congenital CNS abnormalities
- Etiology
  - Prior to 8th week of gestation 2 potential spaces present
    - Fonticulus frontalis: Between frontal, nasal bones
    - Prenasal space: Between nasal bones, developing cartilaginous nasal septum
    - Anterior neuropore runs in prenasal space, communicating with anterior cranial fossa via foramen cecum

- ○ Dural diverticulum protruding through defects may fail to regress
  - ▪ NFCeph: Protrudes through unobliterated fonticulus frontalis
  - ▪ NECeph: Protrudes through foramen cecum into prenasal space
  - ▪ NOCeph: Protrudes through lacrimal bone into medial orbit
- Epidemiology
  - ○ Anterior encephaloceles rare in West (1:35,000) but up to 1:5,000 live births in Thailand
  - ○ FECeph most common type in Southeast Asia
  - ○ FECeph account for 15% of all cephaloceles
  - ○ NFCeph (50-61%); NECeph (30-33%); NOCeph (6-10%)
- Associated abnormalities
  - ○ Callosal hypogenesis, interhemispheric lipomas, malformations of cortical development, colloid cysts, midline craniofacial dysraphisms, hypertelorism, microcephaly, microphthalmos, hydrocephalus
  - ○ Hypothalamopituitary insufficiency

## Gross Pathologic & Surgical Features

- Well-defined meningeal-lined mass containing CSF ± brain tissue

## Microscopic Features

- Meningoencephalocele: CSF, brain tissue & meninges
- Meningocele: Meninges & CSF only
- Atretic cephalocele: Forme fruste of cephalocele with dura, fibrous tissue & degenerated brain tissue
- Gliocele: Glial-lined CSF-filled cyst

# CLINICAL ISSUES

## Presentation

- Most common signs/symptoms
  - ○ Newborn with externally visible, firm nasal or medial orbital mass
    - ▪ NFCeph: Soft tissue mass at glabella
    - ▪ NECeph: Nasal root or intranasal soft tissue mass
    - ▪ NOCeph: Soft tissue mass in or near medial canthus
- Other signs/symptoms
  - ○ Nasal stuffiness, rhinorrhea
  - ○ Change in size with crying, Valsalva, jugular compression (Furstenberg sign)
- Clinical Profile: Newborn with mass along nose, forehead, or orbital margin with associated broadening of nasal bridge & hypertelorism

## Demographics

- Age: Congenital lesion detected on prenatal ultrasound or presenting at birth
- Gender: M > F
- Ethnicity: FECeph most common in Southeast Asians

## Natural History & Prognosis

- Present at birth; require surgical repair
- If untreated, may grow with child
- Prone to rupture, CSF leak & infection
- When CSF filled, may increase rapidly in size

- Majority have normal neurological development

## Treatment

- Biopsy contraindicated: CSF leak, seizures, meningitis
- Complete surgical resection
  - ○ Herniated brain tissue is dysfunctional: No neuro deficit results
- Meningeal & skull base defect repaired or CSF leak, meningitis or recurrent herniation may result

# DIAGNOSTIC CHECKLIST

## Consider

- Sagittal T1 & T2 MR images are optimal for showing contiguity of mass with intracranial contents
- Bone CT used to evaluate size & location of bony defect prior to surgical repair
- Screening brain for rare associated malformations

## Image Interpretation Pearls

- Determine location of lesion relative to nasal bones
  - ○ Above is NFCeph, below is NECeph

# SELECTED REFERENCES

1. Hedlund G: Congenital frontonasal masses: developmental anatomy, malformations, and MR imaging. Pediatr Radiol. 36(7):647-62; quiz 726-7, 2006
2. Khanna G et al: Causes of facial swelling in pediatric patients: correlation of clinical and radiologic findings. Radiographics. 26(1):157-71, 2006
3. Mahapatra AK et al: Anterior encephaloceles: a series of 103 cases over 32 years. J Clin Neurosci. 13(5):536-9, 2006
4. Rojas L et al: Anterior encephalocele associated with subependymal nodular heterotopia, cortical dysplasia and epilepsy: Case report and review of the literature. Eur J Paediatr Neurol. 10(5-6):227-9, 2006
5. Mahatumarat C et al: Frontoethmoidal encephalomeningocele: surgical correction by the Chula technique. Plast Reconstr Surg. 111(2):556-65; discussion 566-7, 2003
6. Rojvachiranonda N et al: Frontoethmoidal encephalomeningocele: new morphological findings and a new classification. J Craniofac Surg. 14(6):847-58, 2003
7. Mahapatra AK et al: Anterior encephaloceles: a study of 92 cases. Pediatr Neurosurg. 36(3):113-8, 2002
8. Holmes AD et al: Frontoethmoidal encephaloceles: reconstruction and refinements. J Craniofac Surg. 12(1):6-18, 2001
9. De Ponte FS et al: Surgical treatment of frontoethmoidal encephalocele: a case report. J Craniofac Surg. 11(4):342-5, 2000
10. Lowe LH et al: Midface anomalies in children. Radiographics. 20(4):907-22; quiz 1106-7, 1112, 2000
11. Songur E et al: Management of frontoethmoidal (sincipital) encephalocele. J Craniofac Surg. 10(2):135-9, 1999
12. Boonvisut S et al: Morphologic study of 120 skull base defects in frontoethmoidal encephalomeningoceles. Plast Reconstr Surg. 101(7):1784-95, 1998
13. Fitzpatrick E et al: Congenital midline nasal masses: dermoids, gliomas, and encephaloceles. J La State Med Soc. 148(3):93-6, 1996
14. Turgut M et al: Congenital nasal encephalocele: a review of 35 cases. J Craniomaxillofac Surg. 23(1):1-5, 1995
15. Barkovich AJ et al: Congenital nasal masses: CT and MR imaging features in 16 cases. AJNR Am J Neuroradiol. 12(1):105-16, 1991

# SINCIPITAL CEPHALOCELE

## IMAGE GALLERY

### Typical

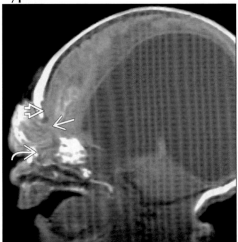

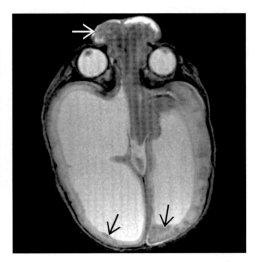

*(Left)* Sagittal T1WI MR of a nasofrontal cephalocele with brain herniating through a patent fonticulus frontalis ➡ between the frontal ⧨ and nasal ⧨ bones. Hydrocephalus is also present. *(Right)* Axial T2WI MR of a nasofrontal cephalocele ➡ with dysplastic frontal lobe tissue herniating through the calvarial defect; associated hydrocephalus and periventricular nodular heterotopia ➡.

### Typical

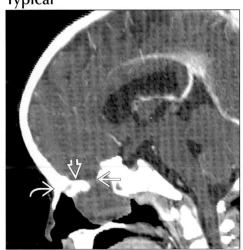

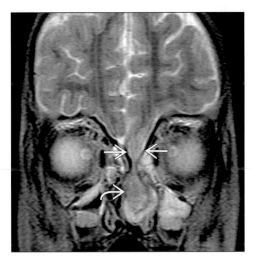

*(Left)* Sagittal bone CT of a nasoethmoidal cephalocele. Inferior frontal lobe herniates through a defect ➡ in the cribriform plate behind the nasal bone ⧨ and crista galli ⧨. *(Right)* Coronal T2WI FS MR of a nasoethmoidal cephalocele with CSF and brain ⧨ herniating into the nasal cavity through a defect ⧨ in the cribriform plate.

### Typical

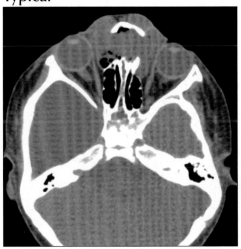

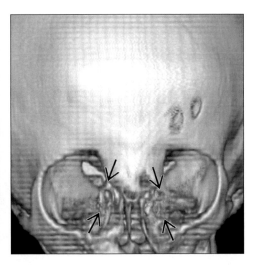

*(Left)* Axial NECT shows a naso-orbital cephalocele with intracranial contents herniating into the bilateral medial orbits through defects between lacrimal bones and maxilla. *(Right)* Anteroposterior bone CT surface reconstruction of the same patient as previous image shows hypertelorism and defects ➡ in the bilateral medial orbital walls.

# NASAL DERMAL SINUS

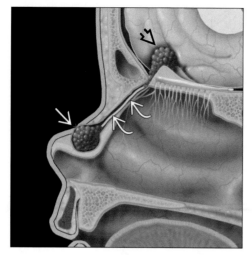

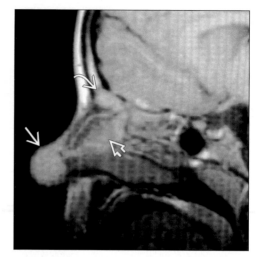

Lateral graphic shows nasal dermal sinus → with 2 dermoids. Extracranial dermoid is just below nasal pit →. Intracranial dermoid ⊳ enters foramen cecum, splits bifid crista galli.

Sagittal T1WI MR shows a "tri-lobed" dermoid with distinct masses at the nasal tip →, in the mid nasal septum ⊟ and at the frontonasal junction →.

## TERMINOLOGY

### Abbreviations and Synonyms
- Nasal dermal sinus (NDS)
- Nasal dermoid sinus; nasal dermoid sinus cyst; anterior neuropore anomaly

### Definitions
- Defective embryogenesis of anterior neuropore resulting in dermoid or epidermoid ± sinus tract in frontonasal region

## IMAGING FINDINGS

### General Features
- Best diagnostic clue
  - Bone CT: Bifid crista galli with large foramen cecum
  - Sagittal T1 MR: Focal low signal (epidermoid or dermoid) or high signal (dermoid) mass found between tip of nose & apex of crista galli
- Location: Epidermoid or dermoid seen from nose tip to apex of crista galli
- Size: 5 mm to 2 cm dermoid or epidermoid

- Morphology: Ovoid mass ± tubular sinus tract

### CT Findings
- NECT
  - Bone CT indirect signs suggestive of intracranial extension
    - Large foramen cecum with bifid or deformed crista galli
    - Cribriform plate deformity
  - NECT findings of epidermoid/dermoid
    - Focal mass within or deep to nasal bridge or along sinus tract to crista galli
    - Fluid density mass = epidermoid/dermoid
    - Fat density mass = dermoid

### MR Findings
- T1WI
  - Sagittal may show epidermoid or dermoid as focal mass from tip of nose to apex of crista galli
    - Fluid intensity mass = epidermoid (or dermoid)
    - Fat intensity mass = dermoid
    - Intracranial mass is seen in region of foramen cecum in a minority of patients
- T2WI
  - Focal high signal if epidermoid/dermoid present

## DDx: Anterior Neuropore Area Lesions

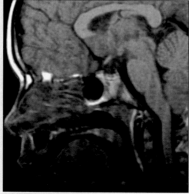

Fatty Marrow CG

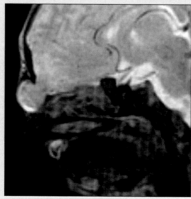

Cephalocele

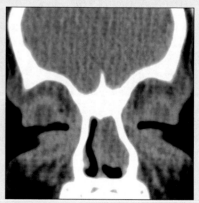

Nasal Glioma

# NASAL DERMAL SINUS

## Key Facts

### Terminology
- Nasal dermoid sinus; nasal dermoid sinus cyst; anterior neuropore anomaly
- Defective embryogenesis of anterior neuropore resulting in dermoid or epidermoid ± sinus tract in frontonasal region

### Imaging Findings
- Bone CT: Bifid crista galli with large foramen cecum
- Thin-section MR imaging focused to frontonasal area best delineates underlying pathology

### Top Differential Diagnoses
- Fatty Marrow in Crista Galli (CG)
- Non-Ossified Foramen Cecum (FC)
- Nasofrontal or Nasoethmoidal Cephalocele
- Nasal Glioma

### Pathology
- Failure of neuropore involution in 4th gestational week; neuroectoderm herniates/migrates along tract of dural stalk
- Dermoid or epidermoid ± nasal dermal tract
- 80% have no intracranial extension

### Clinical Issues
- Child (mean age = 32 months) with nasal pit ± nasoglabellar mass

### Diagnostic Checklist
- Nasoglabellar mass or pit on nose sends clinician in search of NDS with intracranial extension
- Beware! Foramen cecum closes postnatally in first 5 years of life

---

  - ± Sinus tract from tip of nose through enlarged foramen cecum on sagittal MR
- DWI
  - Focal area of diffusion restriction (high signal) if epidermoid
  - Susceptibility artifacts at skull base may obscure signal from epidermoid

### Imaging Recommendations
- Imaging "sweet spot" is small & anterior
  - Focus imaging from tip of nose to back of crista galli
  - Inferior end of axial imaging is hard palate
- Thin-section MR imaging focused to frontonasal area best delineates underlying pathology
  - Sagittal plane important
  - Axial & coronal 3 mm thick T1 & T2 sequences
  - Contrast does not help make diagnosis
  - DWI imaging important additional sequence
- If intracranial extension, add NECT
  - Thin-section (1-2 mm) bone & soft tissue axial & coronal CT nasofrontal region

## DIFFERENTIAL DIAGNOSIS

### Fatty Marrow in Crista Galli (CG)
- No nasoglabellar mass or pit on nose
- CT & MR otherwise normal

### Non-Ossified Foramen Cecum (FC)
- Closes postnatally in first 5 years of life
- Crista galli not deformed or bifid
- If nasal dermoid present, may mistakenly suggest intracranial extension

### Nasofrontal or Nasoethmoidal Cephalocele
- Bone dehiscence is larger, involving a broader area of midline cribriform plate or frontal bone
- Direct extension of meninges, subarachnoid space ± brain projecting into cephalocele on sagittal MR

### Nasal Glioma
- Solid mass of glial tissue separated from brain by subarachnoid space & meninges

- Most commonly found projecting extranasally into paramedian bridge of nose
- Less commonly in anterior nasal septum

### Sutural Dermoid
- Dermoid arising from osseous suture
- Most commonly from suture between nasal process of frontal bone, nasal bone

## PATHOLOGY

### General Features
- General path comments
  - Embryology-anatomy: Normal development
    - Dural stalk passes from floor of anterior cranial fossa, through area of future foramen cecum, into area of osteocartilaginous nasal junction, then regresses completely
    - Failure of involution creates "anterior neuropore anomalies"
  - Anterior neuropore anomaly = general term for anomalous anterior neuropore regression; 3 main types
    - Type 1: Nasal dermal sinus: Epithelium-lined tract from skin to meninges
    - Type 2: Anterior cephalocele: Leptomeninges ± brain tissue herniate through foramen cecum
    - Type 3: Nasal glioma: Brain tissue herniates through foramen cecum; remains in nose/nasal septum
- Genetics: Familial clustering
- Etiology
  - Failure of neuropore involution in 4th gestational week; neuroectoderm herniates/migrates along tract of dural stalk
  - Dermoid or epidermoid ± nasal dermal tract
- Epidemiology
  - 80% have no intracranial extension
  - Intracranial extension associated with dermoid or epidermoid in up to 50%
- Associated abnormalities: Craniofacial anomalies (15%)

## Gross Pathologic & Surgical Features
- If sinus tract is present, tube of tissue can be followed through bones

## Microscopic Features
- Nasal dermal sinus tract is a midline, epithelial-lined
- Often associated with dermoid/epidermoid
  - Dermoid contains epithelium, keratin debris, skin adnexa
  - Epidermoid contains desquamated epithelium

## CLINICAL ISSUES

### Presentation
- Most common signs/symptoms
  - Nasoglabellar mass (30%)
  - Other signs/symptoms
    - Pit on skin of nasal bridge at osteocartilaginous nasal junction ± protruding hair
    - Intermittent sebaceous material discharge from pit
    - < 50% have broadening nasal root & bridge
    - Recurrent meningitis, rare complication of NDS
  - Rarely presents in adult population
    - Patient has congenital pit on nose
    - Meningitis episode followed by imaging analysis
    - NDS with intracranial dermoid or epidermoid found
- Clinical Profile
  - Child (mean age = 32 months) with nasal pit ± nasoglabellar mass
  - Rarely found after work-up for recurrent meningitis or localized infection

### Demographics
- Age: Newborn to 5 years old

### Natural History & Prognosis
- Untreated patients have nasal bridge broadening ± recurrent meningitis
- Curable when surgical correction is successful

### Treatment
- 80% extracranial excision only
  - Local procedure to remove pit
  - Any associated dermoid or epidermoid also simultaneously removed from nasal bridge
- 20% undergo combined extracranial & intracranial resection
  - Biorbitofrontal nasal craniotomy one approach
    - Dermoid or epidermoid along with involved dura-crista galli removed
    - Primary closure of surgical margins of dura completed

## DIAGNOSTIC CHECKLIST

### Consider
- Nasoglabellar mass or pit on nose sends clinician in search of NDS with intracranial extension
- Focused thin-section MR imaging key to diagnosis
  - Key imaging area
    - Anterior to tip of nose

- Posterior to crista galli
- Superior to cephalad margin of crista galli
- Inferior to level of hard palate
- Add bone CT if NDS with intracranial extension found on MR

## Image Interpretation Pearls
- Pearl: If dermal sinus tract is present & reaches dura of anterior cranial fossa, crista galli will be bifid & foramen cecum will be large
  - If foramen cecum is large but the crista galli is not bifid and tract is not seen, foramen cecum may be normal, just not yet closed
    - Do not overcall a "large foramen cecum" or unnecessary craniotomy may result
    - Beware! Foramen cecum closes postnatally in first 5 years of life
    - Repeat imaging in 6-12 months to confirm decrease in size of foramen cecum: Good approach in difficult cases

## SELECTED REFERENCES

1. Hedlund G: Congenital frontonasal masses: developmental anatomy, malformations, and MR imaging. Pediatr Radiol. 36(7):647-62; quiz 726-7, 2006
2. Huisman TA et al: Developmental nasal midline masses in children: neuroradiological evaluation. Eur Radiol. 14(2):243-9, 2004
3. Rahbar R et al: The presentation and management of nasal dermoid: a 30-year experience. Arch Otolaryngol Head Neck Surg. 129(4):464-71, 2003
4. Bloom DC et al: Imaging and surgical approach of nasal dermoids. Int J Pediatr Otorhinolaryngol. 62(2):111-22, 2002
5. Zerris VA et al: Nasofrontal dermoid sinus cyst: report of two cases. Neurosurgery. 51(3):811-4; discussion 814, 2002
6. Lowe LH et al: Midface anomalies in children. Radiographics. 20(4):907-22; quiz 1106-7, 1112, 2000
7. Mankarious LA et al: External rhinoplasty approach for extirpation and immediate reconstruction of congenital midline nasal dermoids. Ann Otol Rhinol Laryngol. 107(9 Pt 1):786-9, 1998
8. Weiss DD et al: Transnasal endoscopic excision of midline nasal dermoid from the anterior cranial base. Plast Reconstr Surg. 102(6):2119-23, 1998
9. Denoyelle F et al: Nasal dermoid sinus cysts in children. Laryngoscope. 107(6):795-800, 1997
10. Fitzpatrick E et al: Congenital midline nasal masses: dermoids, gliomas, and encephaloceles. J La State Med Soc. 148(3):93-6, 1996
11. Castillo M: Congenital abnormalities of the nose: CT and MR findings. AJR Am J Roentgenol. 162(5):1211-7, 1994
12. MacGregor FB et al: Nasal dermoids: the significance of a midline punctum. Arch Dis Child. 68(3):418-9, 1993
13. Barkovich AJ et al: Congenital nasal masses: CT and MR imaging features in 16 cases. AJNR Am J Neuroradiol. 12(1):105-16, 1991
14. Paller AS et al: Nasal midline masses in infants and children. Dermoids, encephaloceles, and gliomas. Arch Dermatol. 127(3):362-6, 1991
15. Wardinsky TD et al: Nasal dermoid sinus cysts: association with intracranial extension and multiple malformations. Cleft Palate Craniofac J. 28(1):87-95, 1991
16. Vibe P et al: Congenital nasal dermoid cysts and fistulas. Scand J Plast Reconstr Surg. 19(1):105-7, 1985
17. Bradley PJ: The complex nasal dermoid. Head Neck Surg. 5(6):469-73, 1983

# NASAL DERMAL SINUS

## IMAGE GALLERY

### Typical

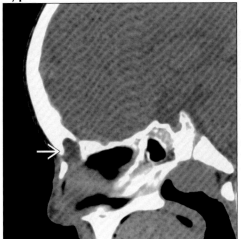

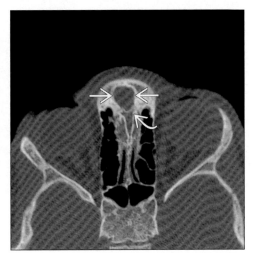

*(Left)* Sagittal NECT shows a well-defined midline dermoid ➡ eroding and enlarging the foramen cecum, a small foramen in front of the crista galli at the frontonasal junction. *(Right)* Axial bone CT in the same patient as previous image shows the enlarged foramen cecum ➡, and mild deformity of the anterior aspect of the crista galli ➡.

### Typical

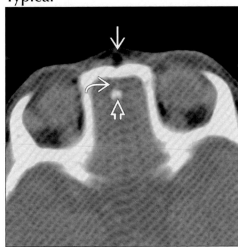

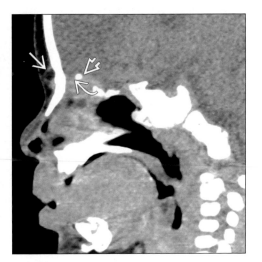

*(Left)* Axial NECT shows a small midline subcutaneous dermoid ➡, normal ossification of the crista galli ➡ and a normal appearance of the foramen cecum for a child of this age ➡. *(Right)* Sagittal NECT in the same patient as previous image shows the sutural dermoid ➡, normal ossification of the crista galli ➡, and a normal size of the foramen cecum ➡.

### Typical

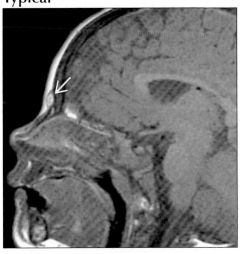

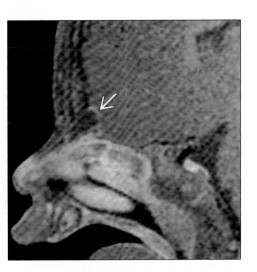

*(Left)* Sagittal T1WI MR in a different patient shows a small hyperintense dermoid ➡ at the glabella in this infant with an asymptomatic glabellar mass, without intracranial extension. *(Right)* Sagittal T1 C+ FS MR shows midline mass ➡ positioned just above, and entering, the foramen cecum. These masses are extradural and often split the layers of the falx cerebri.

# CHOANAL ATRESIA

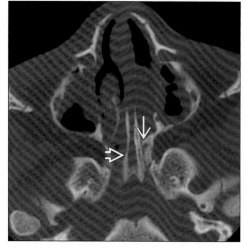

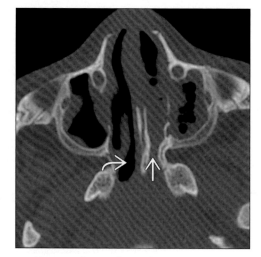

*Axial bone CT shows typical CT appearance of choanal atresia, with bony atresia at superior aspect of choana ➡, thickening of the posterior wall of nasal cavity and enlargement of vomer ➡.*

*Axial bone CT shows soft tissue bridging area of stenosis in the mid choana. This is an area of membranous atresia ➡. Notice the patent right choana ➡.*

## TERMINOLOGY

### Abbreviations and Synonyms
- Choanal atresia (CA), choanal stenosis (CS)

### Definitions
- Atresia or narrowing (stenosis) of the posterior nasal cavity (choana)

## IMAGING FINDINGS

### General Features
- Best diagnostic clue: Narrow posterior nasal cavity, medial bowing and thickening of the lateral wall of the nasal cavity and enlargement of the posterior vomer
- Location
  - Posterior nasal cavity (choana)
  - 50-60% unilateral, 40-50% bilateral (BL)
- Size
  - Choanal atresia
    - Choanal airspace < 0.34 cm in newborn
    - Vomer > 0.34 cm in children less than 8 years

  - Normal mean width of posterior choanal air space
    - Newborns 0.67 cm (± 2 SD = 0.34 - 1.01 cm)
    - 6 years is 0.86 cm (± 2 SD = 0.53 - 1.19 cm)
    - 16 years 1.13 cm (± 2 SD = 0.79 - 1.46 cm)
  - Normal vomer width
    - Children less than 8 years of age usually less than 0.23 cm, should not exceed 0.34 cm
    - Children over 8 years of age 0.28 cm, should not exceed 0.55 cm
- Morphology
  - Purely bony atresia in 29%
  - Mixed bony-membranous malformation in 71%
  - Purely membranous rare
  - Older literature bony 90%, membranous 10%

### CT Findings
- NECT
  - Thin-section axial bone CT
    - Narrowing of posterior choanae < 0.34 cm in newborn
    - Medial bowing and thickening of posterior medial maxilla, may be fused to lateral margin of vomer
    - Thickening of vomer
    - Membranes may be thin or thick

## DDx: Congenital Nasal Obstruction

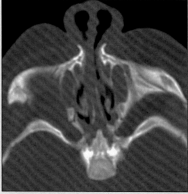

*CNPAS*

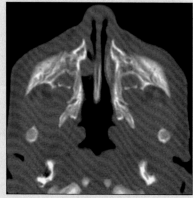

*NLD Mucocele*

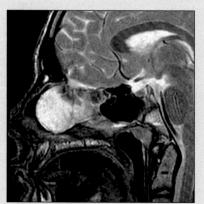

*Cephalocele*

# CHOANAL ATRESIA

## Key Facts

### Terminology
- Atresia or narrowing (stenosis) of the posterior nasal cavity (choana)

### Imaging Findings
- Best diagnostic clue: Narrow posterior nasal cavity, medial bowing and thickening of the lateral wall of the nasal cavity and enlargement of the posterior vomer
- 50-60% unilateral, 40-50% bilateral (BL)
- Choanal airspace < 0.34 cm in newborn
- Vomer > 0.34 cm in children less than 8 years
- Purely bony atresia in 29%
- Mixed bony-membranous malformation in 71%
- Best imaging tool: High-resolution bone CT
- Multiplanar reformations as needed; sagittal plane most useful

### Top Differential Diagnoses
- Congenital Nasal Pyriform Aperture Stenosis (CNPAS)
- Nasolacrimal Duct (NLD) Mucocele
- Cephalocele
- Nasal Dermoid

### Pathology
- Most common congenital abnormality of nasal cavity
- 75% with bilateral atresia have other congenital anomalies

### Clinical Issues
- Bilateral: Severe respiratory distress in newborn
- Unilateral: Chronic purulent rhinorrhea, mild airway symptoms in older child

---

- Retained fluid in nasal cavity
  - False positives can result from imaging in oblique planes
    - Sagittal reformations useful to ensure true stenosis/atresia

### MR Findings
- Not generally needed or useful for choanal atresia itself
- Mainly used to detect associated intracranial anomalies

### Imaging Recommendations
- Best imaging tool: High-resolution bone CT
- Protocol advice
  - Suction secretions and apply topical nasal vasoconstriction agents prior to scan
  - Supine 1-1.5 mm axial images through nasopharynx
  - Imaging plane parallel or 5-10 degrees cephalad to hard palate
  - High-resolution, edge-enhancement bone filters
  - Multiplanar reformations as needed; sagittal plane most useful
  - 3D volume rendering may be helpful

## DIFFERENTIAL DIAGNOSIS

### Congenital Nasal Pyriform Aperture Stenosis (CNPAS)
- Thickened anteromedial maxilla
- Narrow anterior & inferior nasal passage (nasal inlet = pyriform aperture)
- Small triangular-shaped hard palate
- Isolated or in association with other anomalies; solitary central maxillary incisor, holoprosencephaly, hypopituitarism, chromosomal deletion short arm chromosome 18

### Nasolacrimal Duct (NLD) Mucocele
- Round, cystic mass in inferior meatus
- Enlargement of nasolacrimal canal which contains the nasolacrimal duct

- Cystic enlargement of lacrimal sac
- Unilateral or bilateral

### Cephalocele
- Frontonasal or nasoethmoid type
- Meninges ± dysplastic brain extends through bony defect

### Nasal Dermoid
- Epithelium-lined tract from skin to/through meninges
- (Epi)dermoid along tract in ~ 50%
- Bifid crista galli, large foramen cecum

## PATHOLOGY

### General Features
- General path comments
  - 50-60% unilateral
  - Two types
    - Bony atresia (30%)
    - Bony stenosis with membranous atresia (70%)
- Genetics: Sporadic or familial
- Etiology
  - Proposed theories
    - Persistence of buccopharyngeal membrane or failure of bucconasal membrane to perforate
    - Mesodermal defect caused by faulty neural crest cell migration-best explains association with other craniofacial malformation
  - Recently recognized association with antenatal carbimazole exposure (carbimazole embryopathy)
- Epidemiology
  - Most common congenital abnormality of nasal cavity
  - 1:5,000 to 10,000 live births
- Associated abnormalities
  - 75% with bilateral atresia have other congenital anomalies
  - CHARGE syndrome
    - Coloboma
    - Heart/cardiovascular anomalies
    - Atresia of choana

# CHOANAL ATRESIA

- ■ Retarded growth and development
- ■ Genital hypoplasia
- ■ Ear anomalies
- ○ Associations with CA
  - ■ Apert, Crouzon, deLange, fetal alcohol, Di George, Treacher-Collins syndromes
  - ■ Chromosome 12, 18, 22, mutations; XO abnormalities

## Gross Pathologic & Surgical Features
- Membranous soft tissue or bony plate occludes choanal opening

## CLINICAL ISSUES

### Presentation
- Most common signs/symptoms
  - ○ Bilateral: Severe respiratory distress in newborn
    - ■ Aggravated by feeding
    - ■ Relieved by crying
    - ■ Infants are obligate nasal breathers up to 6 months of age
  - ○ Unilateral: Chronic purulent rhinorrhea, mild airway symptoms in older child
    - ■ Less than one year of age: Less severe airway and feeding issues than bilateral involvement
- Other signs/symptoms
  - ○ Inability to pass nasoenteric tube through nasal cavity or absence of nasal mirror misting
  - ○ Nasal stuffiness
  - ○ Grunting, snorting, low-pitched stridor
- Clinical Profile
  - ○ Bilateral: Infant with severe respiratory distress
  - ○ Unilateral: Child with unilateral purulent rhinorrhea

### Demographics
- Age
  - ○ Bilateral atresia presents at birth
  - ○ Unilateral choanal atresia may present in older child

### Natural History & Prognosis
- Bilateral choanal atresia
  - ○ Diagnosed and treated in newborn period
- Unilateral choanal atresia/stenosis
  - ○ May present later in childhood
  - ○ Prognosis is excellent after surgical therapy
- Some patients prone to re-stenosis

### Treatment
- Establish oral airway immediately
- Membranous atresias may be perforated upon passage of nasoenteric tube
- Surgical correction of bilateral atresia performed as soon as possible after diagnosis
- Transnasal endoscopic approaches frequently used for simple membranous & bony atresias
  - ○ May be combined with laser or stenting
- Bilateral bony atresias require transpalatal resection of vomer with choanal reconstruction
- Post-operative scar & incomplete resection of atresia plate best evaluated with bone CT

## DIAGNOSTIC CHECKLIST

### Consider
- Respiratory distress & nasal obstruction in newborn; establish patency of airway
- Thin-section axial bone CT with reformations is imaging modality of choice

### Image Interpretation Pearls
- Determine unilateral or bilateral
- Describe as mixed bony-membranous, purely bony or rarely purely membranous
- Comment on thickness of bony atresia plate
- Look for associated anomalies in head & neck

## SELECTED REFERENCES

1.  Hedlund G: Congenital frontonasal masses: developmental anatomy, malformations, and MR imaging. Pediatr Radiol. 36(7):647-62; quiz 726-7, 2006
2.  Schraff SA et al: Management of choanal atresia in CHARGE association patients: a retrospective review. Int J Pediatr Otorhinolaryngol. 70(7):1291-7, 2006
3.  Wolf D et al: Antenatal carbimazole and choanal atresia: a new embryopathy. Arch Otolaryngol Head Neck Surg. 132(9):1009-11, 2006
4.  Koch BL: Case 73: Nasolacrimal duct mucocele. Radiology. 232(2):370-2, 2004
5.  Samadi DS et al: Choanal atresia: a twenty-year review of medical comorbidities and surgical outcomes. Laryngoscope. 113(2):254-8, 2003
6.  Triglia JM et al: [Choanal atresia: therapeutic management and results in a series of 58 children] Rev Laryngol Otol Rhinol (Bord). 124(3):139-43, 2003
7.  Holzmann D et al: Unilateral choanal atresia: surgical technique and long-term results. J Laryngol Otol. 116(8):601-4, 2002
8.  Sanlaville D et al: A CGH study of 27 patients with CHARGE association. Clin Genet. 61(2):135-8, 2002
9.  Van Den Abbeele T et al: Transnasal endoscopic treatment of choanal atresia without prolonged stenting. Arch Otolaryngol Head Neck Surg. 128(8):936-40, 2002
10. Vanzieleghem BD et al: Imaging studies in the diagnostic workup of neonatal nasal obstruction. J Comput Assist Tomogr. 25(4):540-9, 2001
11. Behar PM et al: Paranasal sinus development and choanal atresia. Arch Otolaryngol Head Neck Surg. 126(2):155-7, 2000
12. Keller JL et al: Choanal atresia, CHARGE association, and congenital nasal stenosis. Otolaryngol Clin North Am. 33(6):1343-51, viii, 2000
13. Black CM et al: Potential pitfalls in the work-up and diagnosis of choanal atresia. AJNR Am J Neuroradiol. 19(2):326-9, 1998
14. Brown OE et al: Choanal atresia: a new anatomic classification and clinical management applications. Laryngoscope. 106(1 Pt 1):97-101, 1996
15. Ey EH et al: Bony inlet stenosis as a cause of nasal airway obstruction. Radiology. 168(2):477-9, 1988
16. Slovis TL et al: Choanal atresia: precise CT evaluation. Radiology. 155(2):345-8, 1985
17. Hengerer AS et al: Choanal atresia: a new embryologic theory and its influence on surgical management. Laryngoscope. 92(8 Pt 1):913-21, 1982
18. Pagon RA et al: Coloboma, congenital heart disease, and choanal atresia with multiple anomalies: CHARGE association. J Pediatr. 99(2):223-7, 1981

# CHOANAL ATRESIA

## IMAGE GALLERY

### Typical

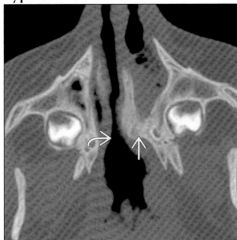
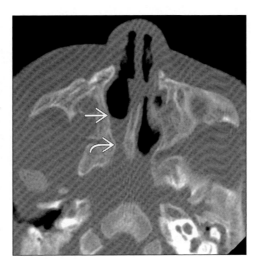

*(Left)* Axial bone CT shows bony choanal atresia at the inferior aspect of the left choana ➡. Notice the patent right choana ➡ in this patient affected unilaterally. *(Right)* Axial bone CT shows narrowing of the right posterior choana ➡, without bony atresia. There are retained secretions causing air-fluid level ➡ in the right nasal cavity.

### Typical

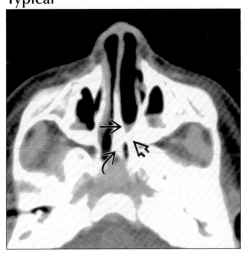
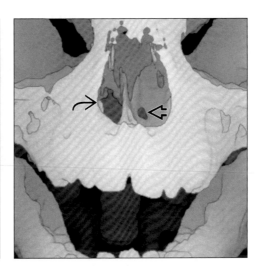

*(Left)* Axial NECT shows unilateral bony choanal atresia ➡ with fluid layering in the posterior nasal cavity ➡ and thickening of the vomer ➡. *(Right)* Anteroposterior volume rendered bone CT shows the bony narrowing of the choana ➡, as compared to the normal right side ➡.

### Typical

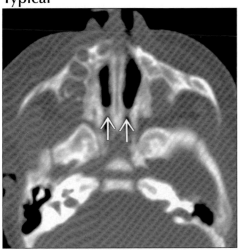
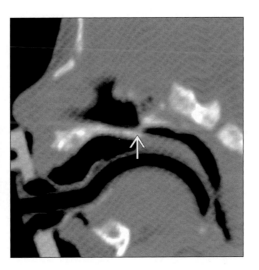

*(Left)* Axial bone CT shows narrow bilateral choana at their inferior aspects ➡ secondary to mixed membranous and osseous atresia. *(Right)* Sagittal bone CT reformation in the same patient as previous image shows the atresia ➡ as a discontinuity of the air passage at the choana in the posterior nasal cavity.

# JUVENILE NASOPHARYNGEAL ANGIOFIBROMA

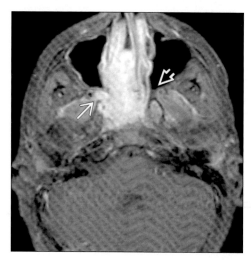

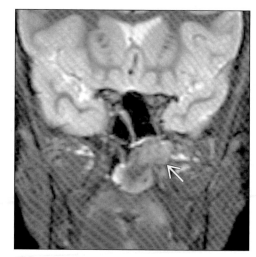

*Axial T1 C+ FS MR shows an avidly enhancing right sided nasopharyngeal angiofibroma with clearly defined tumor in the right PPF ➡. Left PPF ➡ appears normal.*

*Coronal T2WI FS MR shows a small angiofibroma extending from the left PPF ➡ into the posterior nasopharynx. T2WI sequences can help distinguish secretions from tumor.*

## TERMINOLOGY

### Abbreviations and Synonyms
- Juvenile nasal angiofibroma (JNA), juvenile angiofibroma (JAF), angiofibromatous hamartoma

### Definitions
- Benign but aggressive hypervascular mass arising from sphenopalatine foramen (SPF) on lateral nasopharyngeal wall

## IMAGING FINDINGS

### General Features
- Best diagnostic clue: Enhancing mass arising from SPF in an adolescent male
- Location
  ○ Characteristic origin at SPF
  ○ Extends laterally into pterygopalatine fossa (PPF, pterygomaxillary fossa) in 90% of cases
  ○ Extends posteromedially into nasopharynx
  ○ Extends anteriorly into nasal cavity
  ○ Extends superiorly into sphenoid sinus, orbit, skull base and middle cranial fossa
- Size: Usually > 1 cm at diagnosis, can be very large
- Morphology: Usually appears well-defined at imaging

### CT Findings
- CTA
  ○ Can show enlargement of ipsilateral external carotid artery (ECA) feeders to tumor
  ○ Can identify internal carotid artery (ICA) supply
  ○ Helpful in pre-angiographic planning
- NECT
  ○ Soft tissue mass at SPF
  ○ Erosion/destruction of pterygoid plate
  ○ Displacement/destruction of posterior wall of maxillary sinus
  ○ Obliteration of normal fat attenuation in PPF
    ■ Enlargement of PPF
- CECT: Avid and diffuse enhancement of mass

### MR Findings
- T1WI
  ○ Generally isointense to muscle/brain
  ○ Contains foci of hypointensity ⇒ flow voids
- T2WI

## DDx: Nasopharyngeal Masses

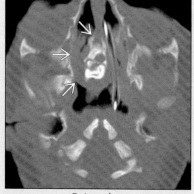

*Epignathus*

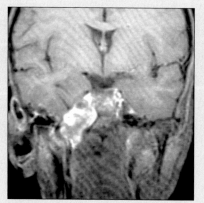

*Rhabdomyosarcoma*

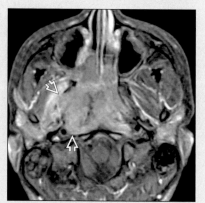

*Nasopharyngeal Carcinoma*

# JUVENILE NASOPHARYNGEAL ANGIOFIBROMA

## Key Facts

### Terminology
- Benign but aggressive hypervascular mass arising from sphenopalatine foramen (SPF) on lateral nasopharyngeal wall

### Imaging Findings
- Extends laterally into pterygopalatine fossa (PPF, pterygomaxillary fossa) in 90% of cases
- Obliteration of normal fat attenuation in PPF
- Enlarged ECA branches supply tumor that has dense capillary blush and delayed wash out
- Distal branches of internal maxillary artery invariably involved
- MR with contrast and fat-saturation essential for identifying intracranial invasion
- Multiplanar reformatting and volume rendering can help in surgical planning

### Top Differential Diagnoses
- Hypervascular Polyp
- Rhabdomyosarcoma

### Pathology
- Pathologic characteristics indicate it may be a vascular malformation rather than a tumor

### Clinical Issues
- Nasal stuffiness: 90%
- Epistaxis: 60%
- Nearly exclusive male incidence ⇒ 75% have androgen receptors
- Local recurrence after surgery in up to 25%
- Surgical resection with pre-operative embolization
- Particles or liquid embolics to reduce blood loss
- Surgery in 24-72 hours

II

2

19

---

- ○ Heterogeneous with flow voids more prominent than on T1WI
- ○ Ideal sequence to distinguish sinus secretions and mucosal thickening from tumor
- T1 C+ FS
  - ○ Best sequence for defining extent of tumor
    - Use of fat-saturation key in post-contrast imaging of head and neck
    - Multiplanar imaging essential to identify intracranial extension
- MRA
  - ○ Can identify ECA and ICA supply to tumor
  - ○ Helpful in pre-angiographic planning

### Radiographic Findings
- Anterior displacement (bowing) of posterior wall of maxillary sinus evident on lateral radiographs
  - ○ Posterior wall may merely appear indistinct
- Soft tissue mass in nasal cavity or nasopharynx
- Erosion of medial pterygoid plate

### Angiographic Findings
- Enlarged ECA branches supply tumor that has dense capillary blush and delayed wash out
  - ○ Distal branches of internal maxillary artery invariably involved
  - ○ Ascending pharyngeal artery, facial artery
- Tumor vessels are tortuous and sometimes irregular
- Important to identify any supply from contralateral ECA
- Essential to identify any supply from ICA
  - ○ Ethmoidal branches of ophthalmic artery, vidian artery
  - ○ Almost invariably present when tumor invades the skull base

### Imaging Recommendations
- Best imaging tool
  - ○ MR with contrast and fat-saturation essential for identifying intracranial invasion
    - Extension through skull base foramina (foramen ovale, foramen rotundum) and dural enhancement best shown on coronal T1 C+ FS

- ○ CT not always essential, but often first exam obtained
    - Defines bone erosion and remodeling best
    - Multiplanar reformatting and volume rendering can help in surgical planning
- Protocol advice
  - ○ All JNA should be evaluated with MR
  - ○ Catheter angiography with bilateral ECA injection and at least ipsilateral ICA injection
  - ○ Endovascular therapy (embolization) as pre-operative adjunct
    - Decrease intra-operative blood loss
    - May allow endoscopic removal of smaller tumors
    - Particles (polyvinyl alcohol), liquid embolic agents

## DIFFERENTIAL DIAGNOSIS

### Hypervascular Polyp
- Angiomatous polyp ⇒ nasopharyngeal polyp that becomes hypervascular due to repeated injury
- Does not involve SPF, PPF
- Not as vascular as JNA, easier to resect

### Rhabdomyosarcoma
- Most common primary malignant head and neck tumor in children
- Does not typically involve SPF, PPF

### Germ Cell Tumors
- Nasopharyngeal teratoma ⇒ epignathus
- More primitive germ cell tumors can arise from same location

### Nasopharyngeal Carcinoma
- Associated with Epstein-Barr virus infection
- Higher incidence in south-east Asia

### Encephalocele
- Congenital herniation of intracranial contents into posterior nasopharynx
- Not hypervascular

# JUVENILE NASOPHARYNGEAL ANGIOFIBROMA

## Fibrous Dysplasia
- Can mimic more aggressive lesions on MR
- Ground-glass appearance on CT diagnostic

## PATHOLOGY

### General Features
- Genetics
  - Increased incidence of JNA has been reported among patients with familial adenomatous polyposis
    - High rate of beta-catenin gene mutations found in sporadic JNAs
    - Nuclear accumulation of beta-catenin found in stromal component
  - Loss of genomic imprinting of IGF II (insulin-like growth factor II) and H19 genes occur in JNA
  - Some cases have failure of expression of the glutathione S transferase M1 (GSTM1) gene
- Etiology
  - Unknown
    - Arise from embryonic fibrocartilage at skull base?
    - Arise from paraganglionic cells from internal maxillary artery branches?
    - Pathologic characteristics indicate it may be a vascular malformation rather than a tumor
- Epidemiology: Rare ⇒ 1:5,000-50,000
- Associated abnormalities: Gardner syndrome (familial adenomatous polyposis) ⇒ 25x increased incidence

### Gross Pathologic & Surgical Features
- Hypervascular mucosa-covered nodular mass

### Microscopic Features
- Vessels and stromal cells
  - Absent elastic laminae in vessels
  - Frequently express vascular endothelial growth factor ⇒ associated with higher vessel density
  - Vimentin-positive stromal cells ⇒ fibroblasts, not myofibroblasts

### Staging, Grading or Classification Criteria
- Fisch classification
  - Stage I: Tumors limited to nasal cavity and nasopharynx; no bony destruction
  - Stage II: Tumors invading PPF, sinuses with bony destruction
  - Stage III: Tumors invading infratemporal fossa, orbit, or parasellar region lateral to cavernous sinus
  - Stage IV: Tumors invading cavernous sinus, optic chiasm, or pituitary
- Sessions classification
  - IA: Tumor limited to posterior nares or nasopharyngeal vault
  - IB: Involvement of at least 1 paranasal sinus
  - IIA: Minimal lateral extension into PPF
  - IIB: Full occupation of PPF with or without superior erosion of orbital bones
  - IIIA: Erosion of skull base, minimal intracranial extension
  - IIIB: Extensive intracranial extension

## CLINICAL ISSUES

### Presentation
- Most common signs/symptoms
  - Nasal stuffiness: 90%
  - Epistaxis: 60%
- Other signs/symptoms
  - Pain, proptosis
  - Swelling of cheek/face
  - Anosmia
  - Otitis media

### Demographics
- Age: Nearly exclusively adolescent ⇒ very unusual before 8 or after 25
- Gender
  - Nearly exclusive male incidence ⇒ 75% have androgen receptors
  - Very small number of cases diagnosed in females ⇒ should prompt genetic testing

### Natural History & Prognosis
- Rare spontaneous regression
- Local recurrence after surgery in up to 25%

### Treatment
- Surgical resection with pre-operative embolization
- Particles or liquid embolics to reduce blood loss
  - Ideal embolization achieves distal distribution of embolic agent
  - Surgery in 24-72 hours
- Radiation therapy
  - Used alone for cure: Up to 80% success
  - Adjuvant for unresectable lesions (intracranial spread)
- Hormonal therapy
  - Generally considered undesirable for adolescent males
  - Can reduce tumor

## SELECTED REFERENCES

1. McAfee WJ et al: Definitive radiotherapy for juvenile nasopharyngeal angiofibroma. Am J Clin Oncol. 29(2):168-70, 2006
2. Uslu C et al: 99mTc-labelled red blood cell single-photon emission computed tomography for the diagnosis and follow-up of juvenile nasopharyngeal angiofibroma. Nucl Med Commun. 27(6):489-94, 2006
3. Baguley C et al: Consumptive coagulopathy complicating juvenile angiofibroma. J Laryngol Otol. 118(11):835-9, 2004
4. Brieger J et al: Vessel density, proliferation, and immunolocalization of vascular endothelial growth factor in juvenile nasopharyngeal angiofibromas. Arch Otolaryngol Head Neck Surg. 130(6):727-31, 2004
5. Beham A et al: Nasopharyngeal angiofibroma: true neoplasm or vascular malformation? Adv Anat Pathol. 7(1):36-46, 2000
6. Hwang HC et al: Expression of androgen receptors in nasopharyngeal angiofibroma: an immunohistochemical study of 24 cases. Mod Pathol. 11(11):1122-6, 1998
7. Endoscopic resection of juvenile angiofibromas--long term results: Rhinology. 2005 Dec;43(4):282-9.

# JUVENILE NASOPHARYNGEAL ANGIOFIBROMA

## IMAGE GALLERY

### Typical

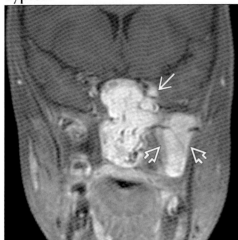 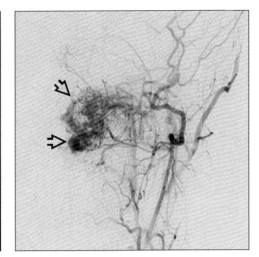

*(Left)* Coronal T1 C+ FS MR shows a JNA that extends superiorly into the cavernous sinus ⇒ and laterally into the infratemporal fossa ⇒. *(Right)* Anteroposterior angiography of the same tumor as previous image shows extensive tumor vascularity ⇒ in the nasopharyngeal component. The full vascularity is often only appreciated with super-selective injections.

### Typical

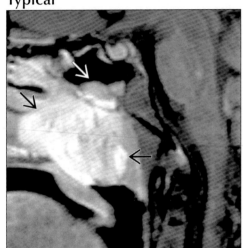 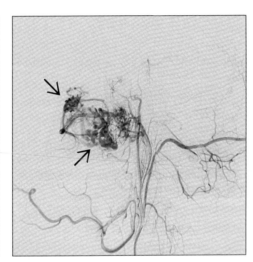

*(Left)* Sagittal T1 C+ MR shows avid enhancement of a nasal angiofibroma that has infiltrated the adenoids ⇒. The tumor has breached the floor of the sphenoid ⇒ but does not enter the calvarium. *(Right)* Lateral view of ECA angiogram (same patient as previous image) shows extensive tumor vascularity ⇒ in the tumor-filled adenoids.

### Typical

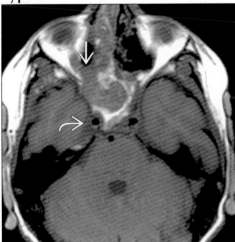 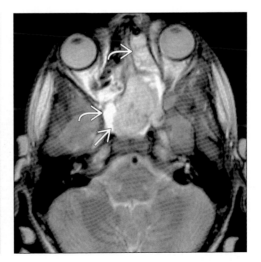

*(Left)* Axial T1WI MR shows a JNA eroding the right orbital apex ⇒ and extending posteriorly through the clivus. Note asymmetric enlargement of the right cavernous sinus ⇒. *(Right)* Axial T2WI MR shows a large angiofibroma ⇒ extended from the posterior nasopharynx into the sphenoid sinus. Note multiple areas of retained secretions ⇒ in nasal cavity and sinuses.

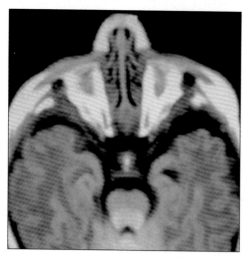

*Axial T1WI MR shows bilateral anophthalmos and resulting small orbits. This is usually autosomal recessive. This patient also had a dysplastic hypothalamus.*

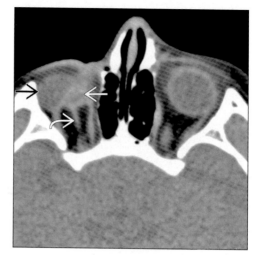

*Axial NECT shows microphthalmia ➡ and optic nerve hypoplasia ➤ with associated cyst ➡ in a 7 year old boy. The etiology was unknown.*

## TERMINOLOGY

### Abbreviations and Synonyms
- Microphthalmos = microphthalmia
- Anophthalmos = anophthalmia

### Definitions
- Microphthalmia: Globe with total axial length (TAL) < 2 standard deviations below mean for age
  - < 19 mm in 1 year old or < 21 mm in adult
- Nanophthalmos: Type of simple microphthalmia with microcornea, bilateral TAL < 18 mm, hyperopia
- Anophthalmia: Complete absence of globe in presence of ocular adnexa

## IMAGING FINDINGS

### General Features
- Location: Unilateral or bilateral
- Embryology
  - During the 4th week of gestation the optic vesicle begins to invaginate and form the optic cup

- During the 5th week mesenchyme invades the open choroidal fissure contributing to formation of the hyaloid artery
- During the 6th week closure of the optic vesicle (globe) occurs
- By term the hyaloid artery within the globe is normally atrophied
- Incomplete regression of hyaloid artery may be associated with remnant vessels in the persistent primary vitreous of the posterior chamber
- Face develops between ~ 4th and 8th weeks
- Anlage of corpus callosum also forms at a similar time (between 3 and ~ 8 weeks)
- Therefore abnormalities involving closure of the midface (medial cleft syndromes) or the corpus callosum may be accompanied by coloboma, microphthalmos or anophthalmos
- Anophthalmia
  - Primary anophthalmia very rare
  - 1. Primary due to failure of optic vesicle development (during weeks 1-3 of gestation)
  - 2. Secondary as part of a general abnormality of forebrain development

## DDx: Mimics of Microphthalmia

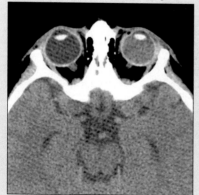

*Coats Disease*

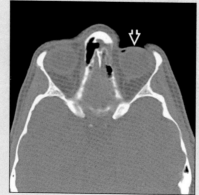

*Enophthalmos*

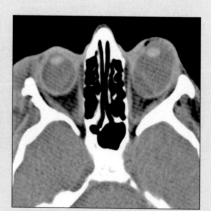

*Left Macrophthalmia*

# ANOPTHALMIA/MICROPHTHALMIA

## Key Facts

### Terminology
- Microphthalmia: Globe with total axial length (TAL) < 2 standard deviations below mean for age
- < 19 mm in 1 year old or < 21 mm in adult
- Nanophthalmos: Type of simple microphthalmia with microcornea, bilateral TAL < 18 mm, hyperopia
- Anophthalmia: Complete absence of globe in presence of ocular adnexa

### Imaging Findings
- Primary anophthalmia very rare
- Isolated; anophthalmos most autosomal recessive (AR), microphthalmos ~ 10% AR
- Phthisis bulbi = inflammation or other process that causes globe destruction

### Top Differential Diagnoses
- Coats Disease
- Ocular Toxocariasis (Sclerosing Endophthalmitis)
- Enophthalmos

### Pathology
- Prevalence of M/A 1.0-1.9 per 10,000
- Associated abnormalities: 1/3 have associated malformations
- Severe: Globe with corneal diameter < 4 mm and TAL < 10 mm at birth or < 12 mm after 1 yr
- Simple: Globe intact but typically mild decrease in TAL
- Complex: Globe with anterior and/or posterior segment dysgenesis and mild, moderate or severe decrease in TAL

---

- ○ 3. Degenerative due to regression or involution of previously formed optic vesicle
- ○ Unilateral associated with severe craniofacial anomalies
- ○ Bilateral associated with absence of optic chiasm, diminished posterior optic pathways, agenesis/dysgenesis corpus callosum
- Microphthalmia
  - ○ More common than true anophthalmos
  - ○ 1. Congenital underdevelopment of globe
    - ■ Sporadic, autosomal dominant, recessive and X-line forms
  - ○ 2. Acquired diminution in size of globe
  - ○ When extreme mimics anophthalmos
- Anophthalmia/microphthalmia (A/M)
  - ○ Hereditary (incomplete list)
    - ■ Isolated; anophthalmos most autosomal recessive (AR), microphthalmos ~ 10% AR
    - ■ Aneuploidy: Trisomy 13 (Patau syndrome), mosaic trisomy 19
    - ■ Deletions (involving chromosomes 4, 7, 14 or X)
    - ■ Chromosomal rearrangements
    - ■ SOX2 related eye disorders; including anophthalmia esophageal-genital (AEG) syndrome
    - ■ PAX6 mutations
    - ■ Waardenburg anophthalmia syndrome
    - ■ Oculocerebrocutaneous syndrome (Delleman syndrome)
    - ■ Anophthalmia-plus syndrome (multiple congenital malformations)
    - ■ Microphthalmia with linear skin defects (MLS) or microphthalmia, dermal aplasia, sclerocornea (MIDAS)
    - ■ Cerebro-oculo-facial-skeletal syndrome (COFS)
    - ■ Nance-Horan syndrome
    - ■ Micro syndrome (mental retardation, microcephaly, congenital cataract, microcornea, microphthalmia, agenesis/hypoplasia corpus callosum, hypogenitalism)

- ■ CHARGE syndrome (coloboma, heart detects, choanal atresia, retarded growth and development and/or CNS abnormalities, genital anomalies in males and ear anomalies/deafness)
- ■ Papillorenal (renal coloboma) syndrome
- ■ Lenz microphthalmia syndrome (X-linked recessive, ANOP1 and ANOP2)
- ■ Branchio-oculo-facial syndrome (BOF)
- ■ Goltz syndrome
- ■ Aicardi syndrome (infantile spasm, corpus callosum agenesis, chorioretinal lacunae)
- ■ Walker-Warburg (WWS), muscle-eye-brain (MEB) syndromes
- ■ Meckel-Gruber syndrome
- ■ Norrie disease
- ■ Incontinentia pigmenti (IP)
- ■ SIX6
- ■ RAX
- ■ Microphthalmia brain atrophy (autosomal recessive)
- ■ Lowe syndrome (oculocerebral renal disease); also cerebral white matter lesions
  - ○ Acquired
    - ■ Congenital infection: Congenital rubella (also cataracts), CMV, syphilis
    - ■ Maternal exposure to alcohol (fetal alcohol syndrome), toxins such as benomyl (fungicide), thalidomide, retinoic acid, LSD, hydantoin
    - ■ Retinopathy of prematurity (ROP or retrolental fibroplasia); also cataracts
    - ■ Trauma
    - ■ Surgery
    - ■ Phthisis bulbi = inflammation or other process that causes globe destruction
  - ○ Unknown
    - ■ Persistent fetal vasculature (previously called persistent hyperplastic primary vitreous or PHPV); also cataracts
    - ■ Associated with coloboma
    - ■ Oculo-auriculo-vertebral spectrum (Goldenhar syndrome)

- Associated with CNS anomalies such as encephaloceles, heterotopia, agenesis corpus callosum, midface abnormalities
- Associated with GU, heart, ear, vertebral abnormalities

## Imaging Recommendations
- Best imaging tool: MR for internal structure of globe, ocular contents and brain

## DIFFERENTIAL DIAGNOSIS

### Coats Disease
- Exudate and retinal detachment with normal sized globe and no calcification

### Ocular Toxocariasis (Sclerosing Endophthalmitis)
- Anterior segment may be uninvolved, retinal detachment, normal sized globe, no calcification

### Enophthalmos
- Globe normal in size but sunken

### Surgical Enucleation
- Up to age 20 years may rarely lead to decreased orbital volume

### Large Contralateral Globe
- Macrophthalmia

### Microcornea with Normal Globe
- TAL within normal limits

## PATHOLOGY

### General Features
- Genetics: Many chromosomal abnormalities, syndromic and nonsyndromic single gene disorders
- Etiology
  - Heterogeneous with many etiologies
  - Environmental, heritable, unknown
- Epidemiology
  - Prevalence of M/A 1.0-1.9 per 10,000
    - Isolated in ~ 5%, chromosomal abnormality in ~ 25%
- Associated abnormalities: 1/3 have associated malformations

### Gross Pathologic & Surgical Features
- Anophthalmos: Structures not derived from neuroectoderm (extra-ocular muscles, eyelids, conjunctiva, lacrimal apparatus) remain
  - May have small cystic structure in orbit that is not a small globe

### Microscopic Features
- Anophthalmos: Almost complete absence of neuroectodermal tissue in orbit

### Staging, Grading or Classification Criteria
- Severe: Globe with corneal diameter < 4 mm and TAL < 10 mm at birth or < 12 mm after 1 yr

- Simple: Globe intact but typically mild decrease in TAL
- Complex: Globe with anterior and/or posterior segment dysgenesis and mild, moderate or severe decrease in TAL
  - Anterior segment dysgenesis; developmental abnormalities of cornea, iris, iridocorneal angle, ciliary body
  - Posterior segment dysgenesis; developmental abnormalities of globe posterior to lens

## CLINICAL ISSUES

### Presentation
- Most common signs/symptoms: Small globe, decreased vision
- Other signs/symptoms: Depends on whether isolated or part of a syndrome

### Demographics
- Age: Typically within first few years
- Gender: Variable depending on cause

### Natural History & Prognosis
- Variable depending on severity and associated abnormalities

### Treatment
- Oculoplastic surgeon: Prosthesis, surgery
- Early intervention and therapy
- If residual sight, good eye patched to strengthen vision in microphthalmic eye
- Surveillance by geneticist to detect emerging features of syndromic causes

## DIAGNOSTIC CHECKLIST

### Consider
- Genetic counseling
- Chromosomal studies to look for evidence of aneuploidy, chromosomal duplication, deletion or rearrangement as well as TORCH titers for congenital infection
- Molecular genetic testing available for mutations in SIX3, HESX1, BCOR, SHH, PAX6, CHD7 (CHARGE syndrome), IKBKG (incontinentia pigmenti), NDP (Norrie disease), SOX2 (SOX2 related eye disorders), POMT1 (Walker-Warburg syndrome), SIX6

## SELECTED REFERENCES

1. Blazer S et al: Early and late onset fetal microphthalmia. Am J Obstet Gynecol. 194(5):1354-9, 2006
2. Forrester MB et al: Descriptive epidemiology of anophthalmia and microphthalmia, Hawaii, 1986-2001. Birth Defects Res A Clin Mol Teratol. 76(3):187-92, 2006
3. Albernaz VS et al: Imaging findings in patients with clinical anophthalmos. AJNR Am J Neuroradiol. 18(3):555-61, 1997
4. Bremond-Gignac DS et al: In utero eyeball development study by magnetic resonance imaging. Surg Radiol Anat. 19(5):319-22, 1997

## IMAGE GALLERY

### Typical

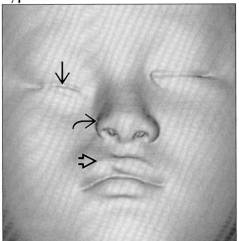 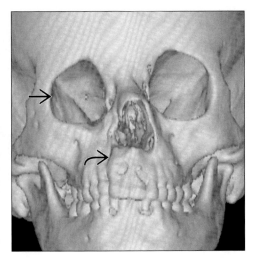

*(Left)* Anteroposterior NECT surface rendering (same patient as previous image) shows small and inferiorly located eyelids ➡, upturned flared nasal ala ➡ and upturned right labia ➡ with rightward deviated philtrum. *(Right)* Anteroposterior NECT bone surface rendering (same patient as previous image) shows a small right orbit ➡ and a Tessier 3 cleft ➡ of the right maxilla.

### Typical

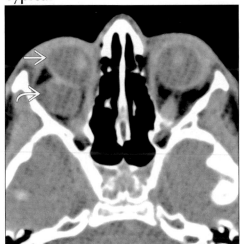 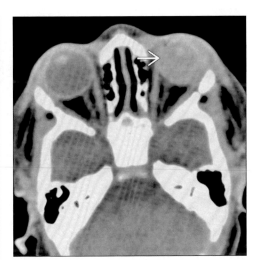

*(Left)* Axial NECT shows a small right globe ➡ and an associated cyst ➡. A coloboma was present in the left eye (not seen on this image). *(Right)* Axial NECT shows left microphthalmia/hyperdense globe ➡ in a 1 month old concerning for hemorrhage due persistent fetal vasculature (persistent hyperplastic primary vitreous).

### Typical

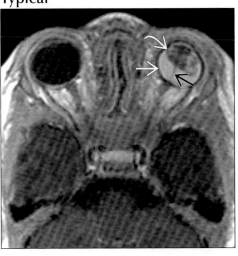 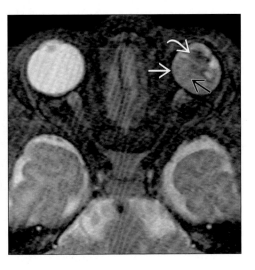

*(Left)* Axial T1 C+ MR in the same patient as previous image shows a retrolental mass ➡ and increased signal ➡ in the vitreous as well as a congenital non-attached retina or Cloquet canal ➡. *(Right)* Axial T2WI MR in the same patient shows as previous image shows the retrolental mass ➡ as hypointense, reduced vitreous signal ➡ due to hemorrhage/exudate and Cloquet canal ➡ as hypointense.

# MACROPHTHALMIA

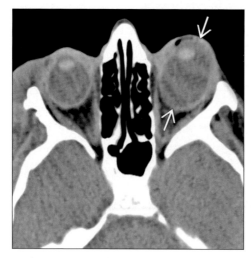

*Axial NECT in a child with neurofibromatosis type 1 with a large left globe ➡ or buphthalmos (congenital glaucoma) and mild left sphenoid wing dysplasia.*

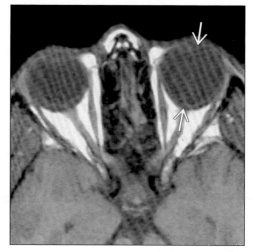

*Axial T1WI MR shows left macrophthalmia ➡ of unknown cause in a 16 year old girl with strabismus and esotropia. Possibly due to dysplastic sclera or due to congenital glaucoma.*

## TERMINOLOGY

### Definitions
- Enlarged globe
- Buphthalmos ("ox eye") is macrophthalmia due to congenital glaucoma or glaucoma in child < 3 years

## IMAGING FINDINGS

### General Features
- Best diagnostic clue: Enlarged globe
- Location: Unilateral > bilateral
- Size
  ○ Globe larger than normal for age
    ▪ Normal mature globe is 24 mm anterior-posterior, 23 mm superior-inferior, 23.5 mm horizontal
    ▪ Normal infant globe is 10-10.5 mm, > 12 mm concerning for macrophthalmia
- Morphology: Generalized or focal

### Imaging Recommendations
- Best imaging tool
  ○ CT for calcified mass in retinoblastoma
  ○ MR for associated orbital or intracranial pathology
  ○ US for intraocular assessment

## DIFFERENTIAL DIAGNOSIS

### Proptosis
- Intraorbital extra-ocular tumor (hemangioma, lymphangioma, optic nerve glioma, lymphoma, NF1, Histiocytosis, venous varix, metastasis, etc.)
- Other causes: Coloboma with retro-ocular cyst, thyroid ophthalmopathy (often bilateral), pseudotumor (bilateral in 1/3)

### Small Contralateral Eye
- Contralateral microphthalmia

## PATHOLOGY

### General Features
- Etiology
  ○ Primary congenital/infantile glaucoma
    ▪ Birth to 3 years
    ▪ No other systemic illness

---

## DDx: Protruding Globes

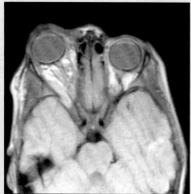

*Proptosis, Lymphangioma*

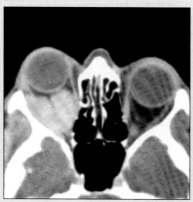

*Proptosis, Hemangioma*

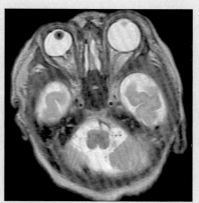

*Small Right Eye (Coloboma)*

# MACROPHTHALMIA

## Key Facts

### Terminology
- Buphthalmos ("ox eye") is macrophthalmia due to congenital glaucoma or glaucoma in child < 3 years

### Imaging Findings
- Globe larger than normal for age
- Normal mature globe is 24 mm anterior-posterior, 23 mm superior-inferior, 23.5 mm horizontal
- Normal infant globe is 10-10.5 mm, > 12 mm concerning for macrophthalmia

### Top Differential Diagnoses
- Proptosis
- Small Contralateral Eye

### Clinical Issues
- Blindness may occur if not treated early
- Congenital glaucoma requires surgical treatment

### Diagnostic Checklist
- Retinoblastoma, melanoma if intraocular mass

---

- Sporadic > autosomal recessive, chromosome 1p36 and 2p21
- Cause not completely understood but significant research to suggest the trabecular meshwork is immature and compressed
- Normal posterior migration of embryonic neural crest cells destined to become the trabecular meshwork is abnormally halted
- 65% male
- Classic triad: Photophobia, epiphora, blepharospasm
- Corneal clouding
- 75% bilateral
- Surgical treatment
- Vision prognosis fair with early treatment
- Other causes of Buphthalmos
  - NF1 (thought to be due to plexiform neurofibroma infiltrating the angle or involving the ciliary body; occurs in up to 50%)
  - Sturge Weber disease (thought to be due to angiomatous change in ciliary body or in the angle of the anterior chamber)
  - Peter anomaly (congenital corneal opacity)
  - Aniridia
  - Axial myopia (most common cause of macrophthalmia, +/- staphyloma, +/- thinning of posterior scleral uveal rim)
  - Proteus syndrome
  - Collagen disorder
  - Staphyloma (focal enlargement, usually idiopathic, bilateral or unilateral)

- Colobomatous macrophthalmia (less common than microphthalmia, autosomal dominant syndrome of macrophthalmia, coloboma and microcornea)
- Secondary to intraocular mass (retinoblastoma, melanoma)

## CLINICAL ISSUES

### Natural History & Prognosis
- Blindness may occur if not treated early

### Treatment
- Congenital glaucoma requires surgical treatment

## DIAGNOSTIC CHECKLIST

### Consider
- Retinoblastoma, melanoma if intraocular mass

## SELECTED REFERENCES

1. Mafee MF et al: Anatomy and pathology of the eye: role of MR imaging and CT. Neuroimaging Clin N Am. 15(1):23-47, 2005
2. Smith M et al: Imaging and differential diagnosis of the large eye. Radiographics. 14(4):721-8, 1994
3. Osborne DR et al: Computed tomographic analysis of deformity and dimensional changes in the eyeball. Radiology. 153(3):669-74, 1984

## IMAGE GALLERY

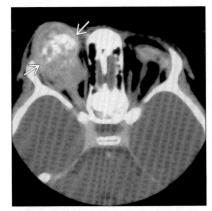 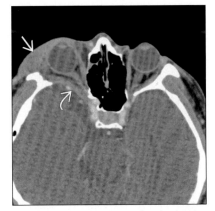 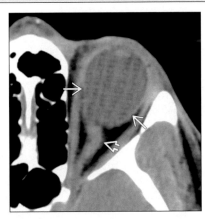

*(Left)* Axial CECT shows right macrophthalmia ➡ due to a large calcified retinoblastoma with retrobulbar extension. Note absent left globe. *(Center)* Axial NECT shows right macrophthalmia in a child with plexiform neurofibroma ➡ and absent sphenoid wing ➡ due to NF1. *(Right)* Axial NECT shows a broad-based coloboma ➡ of the left globe resulting in macrophthalmia. The optic nerve is kinked ➡ as a result of being displaced posteriorly.

# COLOBOMA

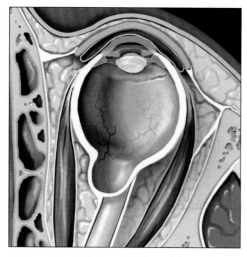

*Axial graphic of classic optic disc coloboma shows a focal defect in the posterior globe at the site of the optic nerve head insertion.*

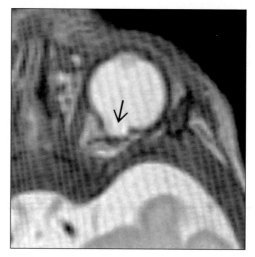

*Axial T2WI MR shows typical optic disc coloboma as a defect in the posterior globe ➡. The high T2 signal in the vitreous is the same as the signal in the coloboma itself.*

## TERMINOLOGY

### Abbreviations and Synonyms
- Optic disc coloboma (ODC)
- Choroidoretinal coloboma (CRC)
- Morning glory disc anomaly (MGDA)
- Peripapillary staphyloma (PPS)

### Definitions
- Coloboma = gap or defect of ocular tissue
  - May involve any or all structures of embryonic cleft
- Primary types of posterior coloboma
  - ODC (isolated): Excavation confined to optic disc
  - CRC: Separate from or extends beyond disc
- Related anomalies
  - MGDA: Congenital disc defect distinct from ODC
  - PPS: Congenital scleral defect at optic nerve head
- Other colobomatous lesions
  - Fuchs coloboma: Inferiorly tilted disc with crescent-shaped defect along inferonasal margin
  - Coloboma of iris, ciliary body, lens or eyelid

## IMAGING FINDINGS

### General Features
- Best diagnostic clue: Focal defect of posterior globe with outpouching of vitreous
- Location
  - Posterior globe at optic nerve head insertion
  - Bilateral ≥ unilateral
- Size: Usually small (few to several mm) unless associated with retrobulbar cyst
- Morphology
  - Crater- or funnel-shaped excavation oriented posteriorly with long axis of globe
  - Retrobulbar colobomatous cyst that communicates with globe may be present
- Associated findings
  - Optic tract & chiasm atrophy; microphthalmia
- Enhancement
  - Sclera enhances; glial tuft in MGDA may enhance
  - Otherwise no abnormal enhancement within defect

### CT Findings
- NECT
  - Defect & retrobulbar cyst fluid isodense to vitreous

## DDx: Abnormal Globe Contour

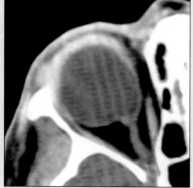

*Staphyloma*

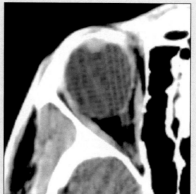

*Buphthalmos*

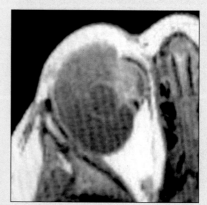

*Microphthalmic Cyst*

# COLOBOMA

## Key Facts

### Terminology
- Coloboma = gap or defect of ocular tissue
- May involve any or all structures of embryonic cleft
- ODC (isolated): Excavation confined to optic disc
- CRC: Separate from or extends beyond disc
- MGDA: Congenital disc defect distinct from ODC

### Imaging Findings
- Best diagnostic clue: Focal defect of posterior globe with outpouching of vitreous
- Crater- or funnel-shaped excavation oriented posteriorly with long axis of globe
- CT diagnoses coloboma easily without sedation

### Top Differential Diagnoses
- Peripapillary Staphyloma (PPS)
- Buphthalmos ("Ox Eye")

- Microphthalmic Cyst
- Morning Glory Disc Anomaly (MGDA)
- Scleral banding (buckling)

### Pathology
- Coloboma: Failure of fusion, superior aspect of embryonic fissure
- Retinal detachment, 25-40% (OCD, MGDA)

### Clinical Issues
- Most common signs/symptoms: ↓ Visual acuity (VA)
- Strabismus and nystagmus secondary to poor VA

### Diagnostic Checklist
- Many known syndromic and systemic associations

---

- ○ Dystrophic Ca++ rarely seen at margins of longstanding defects
- ○ Subretinal high density if hemorrhage

## MR Findings
- T1WI and T2WI
  - ○ Isointense to vitreous; blood products if hemorrhage, signal depends on acuity
  - ○ Glial tuft of MGDA isointense to white matter

## Ultrasonographic Findings
- Outpouching of posterior globe at optic nerve head
- Hypoechoic retrobulbar mass, if cyst present

## Imaging Recommendations
- Best imaging tool
  - ○ CT diagnoses coloboma easily without sedation
  - ○ Key when ocular defects prevent direct visualization

## DIFFERENTIAL DIAGNOSIS

### Peripapillary Staphyloma (PPS)
- Broad excavation defect, encircles disc
- No glial tuft; optic disc sunken but otherwise normal
- Usually unilateral (coloboma frequently bilateral)

### Posterior (Acquired) Staphyloma
- Degenerative ectasia of and thinning of posterior sclera-uveal rim
- Enlarged globe, associated with myopia

### Buphthalmos ("Ox Eye")
- Diffusely enlarged globe from ↑ intraocular pressure
- Seen in neurofibromatosis type 1, infantile glaucoma, aniridia, Sturge-Weber syndrome, Lowe syndrome, homocystinuria

### Microphthalmic Cyst
- Congenital severe ocular derangement
- Deformed small globe with adjacent cyst

### Morning Glory Disc Anomaly (MGDA)
- Funnel-shaped excavation, larger than simple ODC

- Central tuft of glial tissue within defect
- Usually unilateral (coloboma frequently bilateral)

### Other Considerations
- Scleral banding (buckling)
- Globe trauma

## PATHOLOGY

### General Features
- General path comments: Etiology of MGDA and PPS, and relationship with ODC/CRC, are controversial
- Genetics
  - ○ Non-syndromic coloboma
    - Typically autosomal dominant (AD)
    - Mutations: Sonic hedgehog (SHH), PAX2, PAX6, CHX10, MAF, others
  - ○ Syndromic coloboma
    - Usually autosomal recessive (AR)
    - Dozens of syndromes: CHARGE, papillorenal, Aicardi, COACH, Meckel, Warburg, Lenz, others
    - Typically bilateral; especially CRC
  - ○ Sporadic coloboma: Non-inherited
    - Unilateral; especially isolated ODC
  - ○ MGDA: Typically sporadic; rare familial cases
    - Unilateral, except familial often bilateral
  - ○ PPS: Sporadic
    - Unilateral, isolated anomaly
- Etiology
  - ○ Embryology background
    - Embryonic fissure extends along inferonasal aspect optic cup and stalk
    - Fissure fusion (5th-7th week) required for normal globe and nerve formation
  - ○ Coloboma: Failure of fusion, superior aspect of embryonic fissure
  - ○ MGDA: Faulty scleral closure (4th week) vs. mesoectodermal dysgenesis of optic nerve head
  - ○ PPS: Incomplete differentiation of sclera (posterior neural crest cells), diminished peripapillary support
- Epidemiology
  - ○ Coloboma (non-syndromic): 1:12,000

- ○ MGDA and PPS: Rare
- Associated abnormalities
  - ○ Coloboma: CNS, renal, and many other systemic associations; syndromic anomalies (if present)
  - ○ MGDA: Basal cephaloceles, moyamoya, agenesis corpus callosum
  - ○ PPS: Usually isolated; rare associated facial lesions
- Other associated ocular abnormalities
  - ○ Retinal detachment, 25-40% (OCD, MGDA)
  - ○ Congenital optic pit (ODC, MGDA)
  - ○ Cataract; hyaloid artery (ODC, MGDA)
  - ○ Iris coloboma (ODC)
  - ○ PHPV, aniridia (MGDA)

## Gross Pathologic & Surgical Features

- Coloboma (ODC/CRC): Funnel-shaped depression at fundus incorporating optic nerve head
- MGDA: Tuft of whitish tissue overlying enlarged disc
- PPS: Excavation that incorporates sunken optic disk

## Microscopic Features

- Coloboma (ODC/CRC)
  - ○ Invagination of gliotic retina into defect overlying atrophic optic nerve
  - ○ Abrupt termination of choroid and pigmented epithelium at defect margin
- MGDA
  - ○ Central core of vascular connective and glial tissue
  - ○ Peripapillary annulus of subretinal glial tissue and hyperplastic pigmented epithelium
- PPS
  - ○ Large peripapillary defect, thinned sclera, atrophic pigmented epithelium along defect margin

## Staging, Grading or Classification Criteria

- Simple coloboma (normal globe and cornea)
  - ○ Best prognosis; ~ 15%
- Coloboma with microcornea (< 30 mm)
  - ○ Better prognosis; ~ 40%
- Coloboma with microcornea and microphthalmos
  - ○ Worse prognosis; ~ 40%
- Coloboma with microphthalmos cyst
  - ○ Worst prognosis; ~ 5%

## CLINICAL ISSUES

### Presentation

- Most common signs/symptoms: ↓ Visual acuity (VA)
- Clinical Profile
  - ○ VA depends on extent of optic disc involvement and retinal detachment
  - ○ Strabismus and nystagmus secondary to poor VA
  - ○ Reduced visual evoked potentials (VEP)
  - ○ ODC: Visual field deficit, especially superior
  - ○ CRC: VA worse when nerve and macula involved
  - ○ MGDA: May present with leukocoria
  - ○ PPS: Visual loss in children or adults; rare entity
- Funduscopic examination
  - ○ ODC: Enlarged disc with excavation; may resemble glaucomatous cupping
  - ○ CRC: White with pigmented margins; extends inferiorly from or inferior to disc

- ○ MGDA: Enlarged, excavated disc; central core of tissue
  - ■ Central tuft of tissue, surrounding ring of pigmentary disruption; resembles morning glory
  - ■ Retinal vessels abnormally straight and numerous
- ○ PPS: Central crater with recessed optic nerve
  - ■ Normal appearing nerve head, atrophy of surrounding pigment epithelium

## Demographics

- Age: Present at birth
- Gender: MGDA: M < F; also right > left

## Natural History & Prognosis

- Coloboma/MGDA: Visual acuity correlates with retinal status; detachment leads to precipitous vision loss
- Coloboma: Nerve atrophy and cataracts may lead to more insidious vision loss
- PPS: Often poor vision, but usually benign non-progressive course

## Treatment

- Address refractive errors, strabismus, amblyopia
- Retinal detachment
  - ○ Laser treatment, photocoagulation
  - ○ Vitrectomy, air-fluid exchange, scleral buckle
  - ○ Optic nerve sheath fenestration

## DIAGNOSTIC CHECKLIST

### Consider

- Many known syndromic and systemic associations

### Image Interpretation Pearls

- Coloboma is ophthalmoscopic diagnosis
- CT confirms diagnosis & sees coexistent anomalies

## SELECTED REFERENCES

1. Chalouhi C et al: Olfactory evaluation in children: application to the CHARGE syndrome. Pediatrics. 116(1):e81-8, 2005
2. Islam N et al: Optic disc duplication or coloboma? Br J Ophthalmol. 89(1):26-9, 2005
3. Chan RT et al: Morning Glory Syndrome. Clin Exp Optometry. 85(6):383-388, 2002
4. Morrison D et al: National study of microphthalmia, anophthalmia, and coloboma (MAC) in Scotland: investigation of genetic aetiology. J Med Genet. 39(1):16-22, 2002
5. Hornby SJ et al: Regional variation in blindness in children due to microphthalmos, anophthalmos and coloboma. Ophthalmic Epidemiol. 7(2):127-38, 2000
6. Hornby SJ et al: Visual acuity in children with coloboma: clinical features and a new phenotypic classification system. Ophthalmology. 107(3):511-20, 2000
7. Onwochei BC et al: Ocular Colobomata. Surv Ophthalmol. 45:175-94, 2000
8. Gottlieb JL et al: Peripapillary staphyloma. Am J Ophthalmol. 124(2):249-51, 1997
9. Mafee MF et al: Computed tomography of optic nerve colobomas, morning glory anomaly, and colobomatous cyst. Radiol Clin North Am. 25(4):693-9, 1987

# COLOBOMA

## IMAGE GALLERY

### Typical

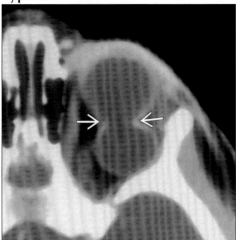
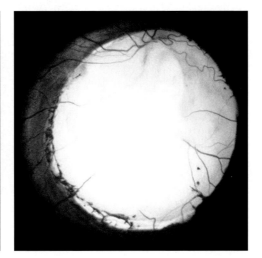

*(Left) Axial CECT shows typical optic disc coloboma with dehiscence of posterior globe through defect ➡ centered on upper optic disc margin. Density in retrobulbar cyst is same as vitreous. (Right) Funduscopy in a patient with coloboma shows large posterior protrusion, centered at the optic nerve head, with marginal pigmentation suggesting chorioretinal involvement. (Courtesy Moran Eye Center).*

### Variant

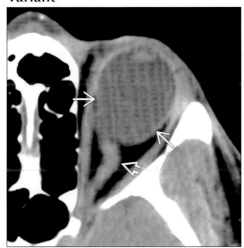
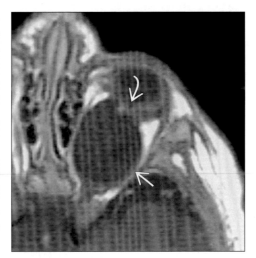

*(Left) Axial NECT shows variant CT case of a broad-based coloboma of the left globe. Defect in posterior globe is broader ➡ than typical coloboma. Optic nerve is kinked ➡ secondarily. (Right) Axial T1 C+ MR reveals an optic disc area defect ➡ with an associated large intraconal retro-ocular cyst ➡ in a patient with Aicardi syndrome. The globe itself in this case is small.*

### Variant

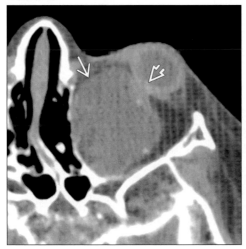
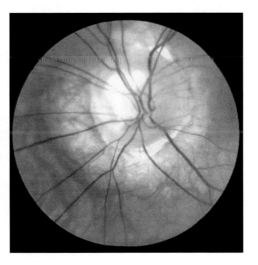

*(Left) Axial CECT of left orbit shows a large retro-ocular cyst ➡ associated with a small globe. The cleft is barely visible along the posterior globe margin as a focal irregular area ➡. (Right) Funduscopy shows an enlarged funnel-shaped optic disc with central glial tissue and annular pigmentation, resulting in appearance that resembles a morning glory flower. (Courtesy Moran Eye Center).*

# NASOLACRIMAL DUCT DACROCYSTOCELE

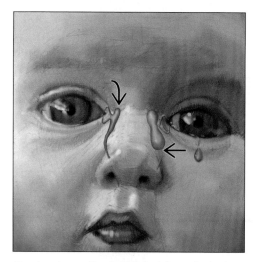

*Drawing shows dilatation of the left nasolacrimal sac secondary to obstruction at the level of the mid nasolacrimal duct ➡. The right nasolacrimal apparatus shows normal structures ➡.*

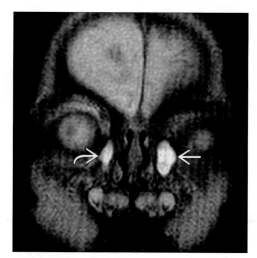

*Coronal T2WI MR shows smooth bulbous dilatation of the left nasolacrimal sac and proximal duct ➡. The right nasolacrimal sac ➡ is also mildly dilated.*

## TERMINOLOGY

### Abbreviations and Synonyms
- Anatomic structures
  - Nasolacrimal apparatus (NLA)
    - Nasolacrimal sac (NLS)
    - Nasolacrimal duct (NLD)
- Synonyms and variations
  - Nasolacrimal duct mucocele
  - Dacrocystocele
  - Congenital dacrocystocele
  - Dacryocele
  - Amniotocele/amniocele
  - Lacrimal sac mucocele
  - Nasolacrimal mucocele

### Definitions
- Two subtypes
  - Proximal
    - Obstruction with dilation of NLS
  - Distal
    - Obstruction at inferior meatus or nasal cavity, with dilatation of NLS and NLD
    - More common than isolated proximal obstruction

## IMAGING FINDINGS

### General Features
- Best diagnostic clue: Well-defined, cystic medial canthal mass in contiguity with NLD in infant
- Location
  - From lacrimal sac to inferior aspect of NLD
  - Proximal lesions located at medial canthus
  - Distal lesions located at inferior meatus
  - Congenital lesions associated with intranasal cysts
- Morphology: Round-ovoid mass at medial canthus extending along NLD course to inferior meatus

### CT Findings
- NECT
  - Hypodense, thin-walled cyst medial canthus
  - Smoothly enlarged NLD to inferior meatus if obstruction is distal
    - Deviated inferior turbinate, nasal septum if large
- CECT
  - Thin rim, minimal or no wall enhancement
  - Thick rim-enhancement ± fluid/debris level if infected (dacryocystitis)

## DDx: Nasolacrimal Region Cystic Mass in a Child

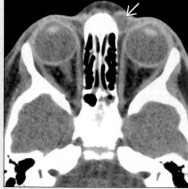

*Epidermoid*

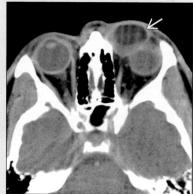

*Dermoid*

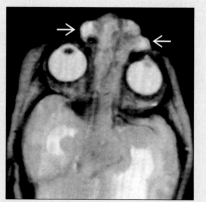

*Frontonasal Cephalocele*

# NASOLACRIMAL DUCT DACROCYSTOCELE

## Key Facts

### Terminology
- Dacryocele
- Amniotocele/amniocele
- Nasolacrimal mucocele

### Imaging Findings
- Best diagnostic clue: Well-defined, cystic medial canthal mass in contiguity with NLD in infant
- Hypodense, thin-walled cyst medial canthus
- Smoothly enlarged NLD to inferior meatus if obstruction is distal
- Thin rim, minimal or no wall enhancement
- Thick rim-enhancement ± fluid/debris level if infected (dacryocystitis)
- Signal intensity varies with protein content of fluid or presence of infection

### Top Differential Diagnoses
- Dermoid/Epidermoid
- Nasoorbital Cephalocele

### Pathology
- Most common abnormality of infant lacrimal apparatus

### Clinical Issues
- Small, round, bluish, medial canthal mass identified at birth or shortly thereafter
- Nasal airway obstruction if bilateral; submucosal nasal cavity mass at inferior meatus

### Diagnostic Checklist
- Imaging useful to exclude other nasoorbital causes of respiratory distress or medial orbital mass in newborn

## MR Findings
- T1WI
  - Hypointense, well-circumscribed mass at medial canthus ± inferior meatus
  - Signal intensity varies with protein content of fluid or presence of infection
- T2WI: Hyperintense typically due to fluid content
- STIR: Intermediate to hyperintense contents within cyst
- FLAIR: Fluid typically appears hypointense, but varies with protein content
- T1 C+
  - Minimal or no wall enhancement around the cyst
  - Thick rim of enhancement with surrounding strandy soft tissue enhancement if inflamed or infected

## Ultrasonographic Findings
- Hypoechoic, rounded lesion with thin wall & increased through transmission

## Imaging Recommendations
- Best imaging tool
  - Thin section axial CECT
    - Excludes (posterior) choanal atresia as cause airway obstruction
- Protocol advice
  - Axial and coronal acquisition or reformation
    - Coronal plane displays contiguity between cysts at lacrimal sac & inferior meatus
  - MR surface coils may improve spatial resolution

## DIFFERENTIAL DIAGNOSIS

### Dermoid/Epidermoid
- Lateral > medial canthus
- 50% fat density/intensity with thin rim-enhancement
- 15% calcification
- Clinical: Childhood presentation common

### Nasoorbital Cephalocele
- Congential herniation through anterior skull and orbital wall defect
- Contains CSF ± brain
- Clinical: Congenital hypertelorism with mass

### Acquired Dacrocystocele
- Medial canthus cyst ± inflammatory changes
- Clinical: Presents in adults
  - Post-inflammatory or neoplastic stenosis
  - NLD injury during sinus surgery
  - LeFort 2 & nasoorbital/nasoethmoid complex fractures

## PATHOLOGY

### General Features
- General path comments
  - Embryology
    - Infolding surface ectoderm into nasoorbital groove 6th week gestation
    - Canalization of ectodermal cord into NLA 3rd month gestation
    - Last area to canalize: Membrane (or valve) of Hasner at opening of NLD into inferior meatus
  - Anatomy
    - Proximal opening: Upper & lower lid lacrimal puncta
    - Canaliculi: Continuation of puncta, converge into common canaliculus prior to entry into NLS
    - Sinus of Maier: Variable bulbous dilatation of distal common canaliculus
    - Valve of Rosenmüller: Oblique angle at junction of common canaliculus & NLS
    - Krause valve: Junction NLS and NLD
  - Physiology
    - Normal breathing, crying ⇒ ↑ intraluminal pressure, stretches mucosa, opens duct
- Genetics
  - Vast majority sporadic
  - Rare familial cases

# NASOLACRIMAL DUCT DACROCYSTOCELE

- Etiology
  - Proximal obstruction
    - Anatomic variation of proximal NLA
    - Distention NLS compresses valve of Rosenmüller, encysting NLA
  - Distal obstruction
    - Imperforate Hasner membrane
    - Tears & mucus accumulate in NLA
- Epidemiology
  - Most common abnormality of infant lacrimal apparatus
  - Imperforate Hasner membrane 6-84% newborns
  - 3rd most common cause neonatal nasal obstruction
    - 1st = mucosal edema, 2nd = choanal atresia
  - Unilateral > bilateral
  - Increase incidence stillborn & premature
    - Failure of normal breathing, crying

## Gross Pathologic & Surgical Features
- Endonasal cyst: Smooth, glistening, thin-walled cyst with mucous or fluid

## Microscopic Features
- Respiratory & squamous epithelium-lined cyst with sero-mucous glands
- Variable inflammatory cells

## CLINICAL ISSUES

### Presentation
- Most common signs/symptoms
  - Proximal
    - Small, round, bluish, medial canthal mass identified at birth or shortly thereafter
  - Distal
    - Nasal airway obstruction if bilateral; submucosal nasal cavity mass at inferior meatus
- Clinical Profile
  - Infant with medial canthal mass ± inflammatory changes
  - Physical examination of eye & nasal cavity
  - Cross-sectional imaging, CT or MR, to evaluate extent of lesion along lacrimal apparatus
- Other symptoms
  - Epiphora, eyelid crusting, anisometropic amblyopia
  - Respiratory distress (with bilateral endonasal cysts)
  - Dacryocystitis: 0.5-6%
    - ↑ Incidence if endonasal component
  - Edema, erythema of eyelid and cyst
  - Preseptal cellulitis; abscess may occur

### Demographics
- Age: Infancy; 4 days to 10 weeks typically
- Gender: M < F = 1:3

### Natural History & Prognosis
- 90% of congenital simple distal obstructions resolve spontaneously by age 1
- Initially unilateral lesion may develop contralateral
- Intervention recommended before infection occurs to prevent dacryocystitis & permanent sequelae
- If persistent and untreated, nasal airway obstruction & mucocele infection may result

### Treatment
- Graded
  - Daily manual massage ± prophylactic systemic or topical antibiotics
  - 10% require probing with irrigation ± silastic stent placement
  - If endonasal component & no response to above
    - ⇒ Endoscopic resection with marsupialization
- Manual massage inappropriate if infected or airway obstruction
- Theoretical risk of NLA scarring, amblyopia, and permanent canthal asymmetry if left untreated
- Occasional recurrence as adult

## DIAGNOSTIC CHECKLIST

### Consider
- Imaging useful to exclude other nasoorbital causes of respiratory distress or medial orbital mass in newborn
  - Choanal stenosis & choanal atresia
  - Nasoorbital cephalocele

### Image Interpretation Pearls
- Comment on full extent of lesion from medial canthus to inferior meatus
- Evaluate for extent of disease in cases complicated by infection, particularly presence of abscess
- Exclude contralateral lesion

## SELECTED REFERENCES

1. Brachlow A et al: Intranasal mucocele of the nasolacrimal duct: an important cause of neonatal nasal obstruction. Clin Pediatr (Phila). 43(5):479-81, 2004
2. Teymoortash A et al: Bilateral congenital dacryocystocele as a cause of respiratory distress in a newborn. Rhinology. 42(1):41-4, 2004
3. DeAngelis D et al: The pathogenesis and treatment of lacrimal obstruction: The value of lacrimal sac and bone analysis. Orbit. 20(3):163-172, 2001
4. Edison BJ et al: Nasolacrimal duct obstruction and dacryocystocele associated with a concha bullosa mucocele. Ophthalmology. 107(7):1393-6, 2000
5. Paysse EA et al: Management and complications of congenital dacryocele with concurrent intranasal mucocele. J AAPOS. 4(1):46-53, 2000
6. Rubin PA et al: Magnetic resonance imaging of the lacrimal drainage system. Ophthalmology. 101(2):235-43, 1994
7. Castillo M et al: Bilateral nasolacrimal duct mucocele, a rare cause of respiratory distress: CT findings in two newborns. AJNR Am J Neuroradiol. 14(4):1011-3, 1993
8. Lavrich JB et al: Disorders of the lacrimal system apparatus. Pediatr Clin North Am. 40(4):767-76, 1993
9. Meyer JR et al: Infected congenital mucocele of the nasolacrimal duct. AJNR Am J Neuroradiol. 14(4):1008-10, 1993
10. Mansour AM et al: Congenital dacryocele. A collaborative review. Ophthalmology. 98(11):1744-51, 1991
11. Rand PK et al: Congenital nasolacrimal mucoceles: CT evaluation. Radiology. 173(3):691-4, 1989
12. Russell EJ et al: CT of the inferomedial orbit and the lacrimal drainage apparatus: normal and pathologic anatomy. AJR Am J Roentgenol. 145(6):1147-54, 1985
13. Harris GJ et al: Congenital dacryocystocele. Arch Ophthalmol. 100(11):1763-5, 1982

# NASOLACRIMAL DUCT DACROCYSTOCELE

## IMAGE GALLERY

### Typical

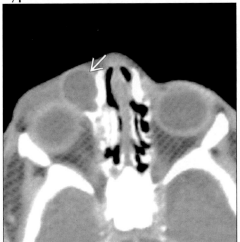

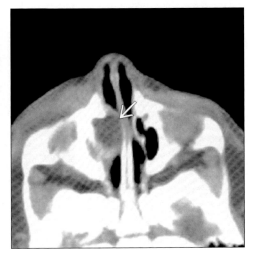

*(Left)* Axial CECT shows a large cystic mass ➡ in the right lacrimal fossa, representing the obstructed lacrimal sac. Note the associated remodeling of the adjacent lacrimal and nasal bones. *(Right)* Axial CECT further inferiorly in the same patient as previous image shows a contiguous cystic mass in the inferior meatus ➡, corresponding to the markedly enlarged distal nasolacrimal duct.

### Typical

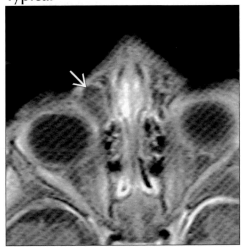

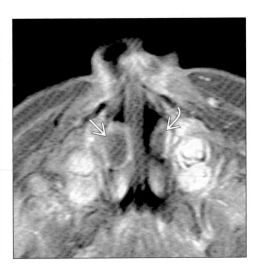

*(Left)* Axial T1 C+ FS MR shows a lobular mass ➡ in the inferomedial right orbit, with rim-enhancement and internal signal slightly higher than simple fluid. *(Right)* Axial T1 C+ FS MR further inferiorly in the same patient as previous image shows a contiguous cystic mass ➡ extending into the right inferior meatus. The left nasolacrimal duct ➡ is also mildly dilated.

### Variant

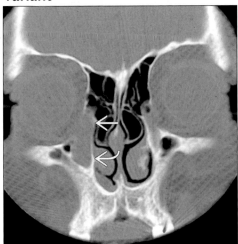

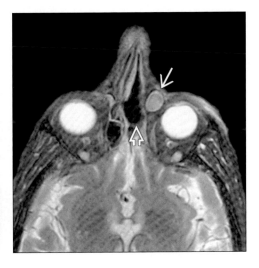

*(Left)* Coronal bone CT in a 20 year old with tearing since birth shows bony remodeling due to nasolacrimal obstruction, with marked enlargement of the lacrimal fossa ➡ and nasolacrimal duct ➡. *(Right)* Axial T2WI MR shows a post-operative dacrocystocele ➡ in an adult, noting changes related to ethmoidectomy ➡. The low internal signal suggests presence of protein or blood products.

# DERMOID AND EPIDERMOID, ORBIT

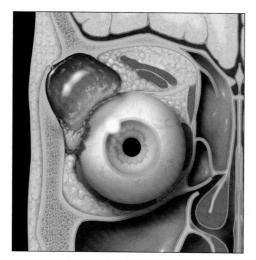
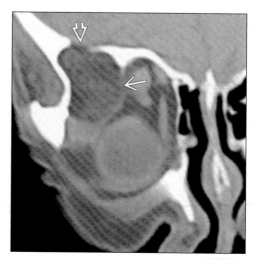

*Coronal graphic depicts a superotemporal dermoid cyst located at the frontozygomatic suture of the right orbit. The dermoid causes mass effect on the globe and remodels the bony orbit.*

*Coronal NECT displayed at wide window reveals an superolateral extraconal dermoid ➡ that has fat density and is associated with congenital focal dehiscence of the orbital roof ➡.*

## TERMINOLOGY

### Abbreviations and Synonyms
- Developmental orbital cyst
- Orbital ectodermal inclusion cyst

### Definitions
- Cyst-like, choristomatous mass lesion of orbit resulting from congenital epithelial inclusion
  - Choristoma: Tumor composed of normal tissue located in abnormal site
- Variations
  - **Dermoid**: Epithelial elements plus dermal substructure including dermal appendages
  - **Epidermoid**: Epithelial elements only

## IMAGING FINDINGS

### General Features
- Best diagnostic clue: Well-demarcated, anterior extraconal mass with fatty, fluid or mixed contents
- Location
  - Tethered to orbital periosteum, near suture lines

- Majority **extraconal** in superolateral orbit, at frontozygomatic suture (65-75%)
- Remainder mostly in superonasal aspect, at frontolacrimal suture
- Can occur anywhere
- Size
  - Less than 2 cm in superficial lesions
  - Larger in deep, complicated lesions
- Morphology
  - Ovoid, well-demarcated cystic mass
  - Most show thin definable wall (75%)
  - No nodular soft tissue outside cyst (80%)
- Contents
  - Internal fat or fluid features; may be mixed or contain debris
  - Lipid components evident in 40-50% of lesions
  - Fluid-fluid levels uncommon (5% of lesions)
  - Dermoids: Typically contain fat & appear more heterogeneous
  - Epidermoids: Typically have features similar to fluid; appear more homogeneous
- Subtypes
  - **Superficial dermoid** (simple, exophytic)
    - Typically smaller, discrete, rounded

## DDx: Superior Orbital Mass

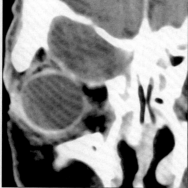
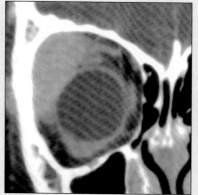
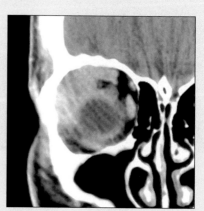

*Frontal Mucocele*     *Idiopathic OID*     *Adenoid Cystic Carcinoma*

# DERMOID AND EPIDERMOID, ORBIT

## Key Facts

### Terminology
- Cyst-like, choristomatous mass lesion of orbit resulting from congenital epithelial inclusion
- **Dermoid**: Epithelial elements plus dermal substructure including dermal appendages
- **Epidermoid**: Epithelial elements only

### Imaging Findings
- Best diagnostic clue: Well-demarcated, anterior extraconal mass with fatty, fluid or mixed contents
- Majority **extraconal** in superolateral orbit, at frontozygomatic suture (65-75%)
- Lipid components evident in 40-50% of lesions
- Osseous remodeling (85%)
- Best imaging tool: CT without contrast frequently adequate for diagnosis

### Clinical Issues
- Most common signs/symptoms: Painless subcutaneous mass (85-90%)
- May present with rupture (10-15%)
- Most frequently presents in childhood and teenage
- Simple, superficial lesions often present in infancy
- Very slow growth, usually dormant for years
- Sudden growth or change following rupture
- Surgical resection is curative
- Steroids used if inflammation in ruptured lesions

### Diagnostic Checklist
- Fat density or signal is essentially pathognomonic
- Posterior extent of complex lesions may not be clinically apparent, therefore imaging is warranted

---

- Present in early childhood
  - **Deep dermoid** (complicated, endophytic)
    - More insidious, frequent bony changes
    - May extend into sinuses, high deep masticator space, or intracranially

## CT Findings
- NECT
  - Hypodense fat (50%)
    - Density -30 to -80 HU
  - Calcification (15%)
    - Fine or punctate, in cyst wall
  - Osseous remodeling (85%)
    - Pressure excavation; smooth, scalloped margins
    - Thinning of bone, may cause focal dehiscence
    - Bony tunnel, cleft, or pit in up to one-third, leading to "dumbbell" appearance
    - Irregular margins indicate rupture and inflammatory reaction
    - Bony changes less common in superficial lesions
- CECT
  - Mild, thin, rim-enhancement
  - Irregular inflammatory enhancement if ruptured

## MR Findings
- T1WI
  - Strongly hyperintense (cf vitreous) if fatty contents
  - Isointense or slightly hyperintense otherwise
- T2WI
  - Isointense or mildly hypointense (cf vitreous)
  - Heterogeneous debris
- T1 C+
  - Thin rim-enhancement
  - More extensive inflammation if ruptured
- Diffusion and FLAIR
  - Epidermoids are hyperintense (cf vitreous)

## Radiographic Findings
- Radiography: Scalloped bony lucency with sclerotic margins

## Ultrasonographic Findings
- Useful for simple superficial lesions

- High internal reflectivity, variable attenuation
- Debris may impair determination of cystic nature

## Imaging Recommendations
- Best imaging tool: CT without contrast frequently adequate for diagnosis
- Protocol advice: Pursue contrast exam and MR if imaging features not characteristic

# DIFFERENTIAL DIAGNOSIS

## Mucocele, Sinonasal
- Associated with chronic inflammatory sinus disease, e.g., polyposis and noninvasive fungal sinusitis
- Expansile mass arising within frontal sinus

## Idiopathic Orbital Inflammatory Disease (IOID)
- Acute onset pain, edema, and proptosis
- Infiltrating mass involving any area of orbit

## Lacrimal Gland Malignancy
- Minor salivary: Adenoid cystic, mucoepidermoid
- Destructive bony changes in malignant lesions

## Lymphoproliferative Lesions, Orbit
- Predilection for lacrimal gland, can involve any area
- Benign (hyperplasia) or malignant (NHL)

## Other Systemic Malignancy
- Langerhans histiocytosis, leukemia, neuroblastoma

## Rhabdomyosarcoma
- Malignancy of children and young adults
- Invasive mass arising anywhere in orbit

## Vascular Lesions
- Venolymphatic lesion, orbit
- Capillary hemangioma, orbit

## Sebaceous Cyst
- Ovoid; fat density and signal
- Mobile, attached to the skin

# DERMOID AND EPIDERMOID, ORBIT

## PATHOLOGY

### General Features
- General path comments
  - Developmental mass, non-neoplastic contents
    - **Epidermoid**: Desquamated keratinaceous debris, cholesterol; thin capsule
    - **Dermoid**: Keratin, sebaceous secretions, lipid metabolites, hair; fibrous capsule
- Etiology
  - Congenital inclusion of dermal elements at site of embryonic suture closure
  - Sequestration of trapped surface ectoderm
- Epidemiology
  - Present from birth; spontaneous occurrence
  - 10% of head and neck dermoid and epidermoid cysts are periorbital
  - 2% of all orbital masses
  - 40% all orbital lesions in childhood

### Gross Pathologic & Surgical Features
- Whitish, well-delineated mass
- Fibrovascular connection to orbital periosteum
- Oily or cheesy material that is tan, yellow, or white

### Microscopic Features
- **Dermoid**
  - Contains dermal structures, including sebaceous glands & hair follicles, blood vessels, fat & collagen within a fibrous capsule
  - Sweat glands in minority (20%)
  - Lined by keratinizing squamous epithelium
- **Epidermoid**
  - Inner surface of thin capsule lined by keratinizing, stratified epithelium
- Inflammatory changes in 40%
- Granulomatous reaction, particularly in deep, complicated lesions

## CLINICAL ISSUES

### Presentation
- Most common signs/symptoms: Painless subcutaneous mass (85-90%)
- Clinical Profile
  - Nontender, firm; painless in 90%
  - Fixed to underlying bone (cf sebaceous cyst)
- May present with rupture (10-15%)
  - Secondary to trauma or spontaneously
  - Acute inflammation mimics cellulitis or inflammatory rhabdomyosarcoma
- Mass effect if very large
  - Diplopia due to restricted movement
- Childhood presentation
  - More common than adult
  - Subcutaneous nodule near orbital rim
  - Smaller, little globe displacement
- Adult presentation
  - More commonly arises deep to orbital rim
  - Often near lacrimal gland in extraconal orbit
  - Less easily palpated; larger, globe displacement

- Less well-defined borders, more likely to erode into adjacent structures

### Demographics
- Age
  - Most frequently presents in childhood and teenage
  - Mean age in late teens to twenties
  - Simple, superficial lesions often present in infancy
  - May present or grow at any age
- Gender: Equal or slight male predominance

### Natural History & Prognosis
- Benign lesion, usually cosmetic considerations
- Very slow growth, usually dormant for years
  - Present during childhood but small and dormant
  - Becomes symptomatic during rapid growth phase in young adult
- Sudden growth or change following rupture
  - Significant inflammation and increased size

### Treatment
- Surgical resection is curative
  - Entire cyst must be removed to prevent recurrence, including growth center at periosteal interface
  - Approach depends on location in orbit
  - Lesions evident in early childhood should be removed to avoid traumatic rupture
- Steroids used if inflammation in ruptured lesions

## DIAGNOSTIC CHECKLIST

### Consider
- Features of typical lesions are distinctive, but deep or inflamed lesions may present diagnostic challenge

### Image Interpretation Pearls
- Fat density or signal is essentially pathognomonic
- Posterior extent of complex lesions may not be clinically apparent, therefore imaging is warranted

## SELECTED REFERENCES

1. Ohtsuka K et al: A review of 244 orbital tumors in Japanese patients during a 21-year period: origins and locations. Jpn J Ophthalmol. 49(1):49-55, 2005
2. Pryor SG et al: Pediatric dermoid cysts of the head and neck. Otolaryngol Head Neck Surg. 132(6):938-42, 2005
3. Shields JA et al: Orbital cysts of childhood--classification, clinical features, and management. Surv Ophthalmol. 49(3):281-99, 2004
4. Shields JA et al: Survey of 1264 patients with orbital tumors and simulating lesions: The 2002 Montgomery Lecture, part 1. Ophthalmology. 111(5):997-1008, 2004
5. Chawda SJ et al: Computed tomography of orbital dermoids: a 20-year review. Clin Radiol. 54(12):821-5, 1999
6. Meyer DR et al: Primary temporal fossa dermoid cysts. Characterization and surgical management. Ophthalmology. 106(2):342-9, 1999
7. Bartlett SP et al: The surgical management of orbitofacial dermoids in the pediatric patient. Plast Reconstr Surg. 91(7):1208-15, 1993
8. Lane CM et al: Orbital dermoid cyst. Eye. 1 ( Pt 4):504-11, 1987
9. Nugent RA et al: Orbital dermoids: features on CT. Radiology. 165(2):475-8, 1987

# DERMOID AND EPIDERMOID, ORBIT

## IMAGE GALLERY

### Typical

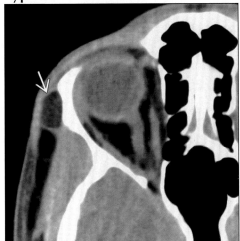

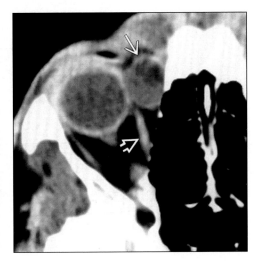

*(Left)* Axial NECT shows a well-circumscribed, oval lesion ➡ within the subcutaneous tissues near the fronto-zygomatic suture of the right orbit. The fat density allows diagnosis of dermoid. *(Right)* Axial CECT demonstrates an oval, well-circumscribed, extraconal, medial orbital dermoid ➡ with mixed fatty & soft tissue density. Note the lateral rectus muscle ➡.

### Variant

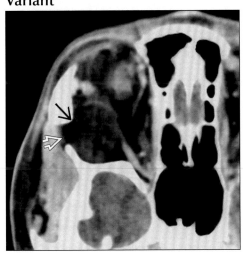

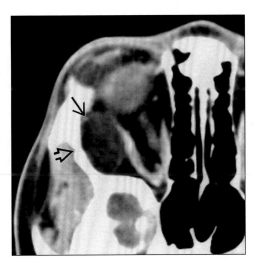

*(Left)* Axial CECT shows large fat-density dermoid ➡, centered in the sphenozygomatic suture. The dermoid extends laterally through a defect ➡ in the lateral orbital wall. *(Right)* Axial CECT of dermoid reveals an ovoid fat-density mass ➡ centered at the sphenozygomatic suture ➡. Frontozygomatic suture association is more common.

### Typical

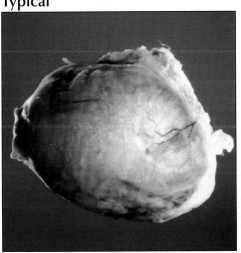

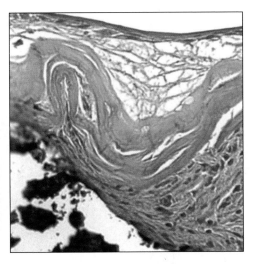

*(Left)* Gross pathology of an unruptured orbital dermoid cyst demonstrates a whitish-yellow, relatively thick fibrous capsule. *(Courtesy Moran Eye Center).* *(Right)* Micropathology reveals the lining of a dermoid, with features of normal epidermal structures, keratinized, stratified squamous epithelium, and underlying glandular structures.

# ORBITAL CELLULITIS

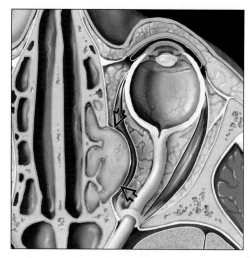

Axial graphic shows the spread of infection ⇒ from the ethmoid sinuses through the lamina papyracea into the medial orbit. Subperiosteal abscess results, putting the optic nerve at risk.

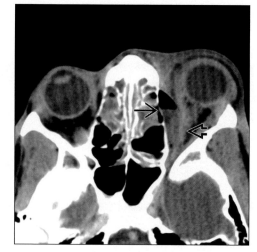

Axial CECT shows bilateral ethmoid disease, a focal left extraconal fluid collection with gas-fluid level ⇒, deviation of the medial rectus muscle ⇒ and mild proptosis.

## TERMINOLOGY

### Abbreviations and Synonyms
- Postseptal cellulitis, preseptal cellulitis = periorbital cellulitis

### Definitions
- Orbital septum
  - Periosteal reflection from bony orbit to tarsal plates of eyelids

## IMAGING FINDINGS

### General Features
- Best diagnostic clue
  - Thickening and edema of orbital soft tissues = cellulitis and/or phlegmon
  - Low-attenuation rim-enhancing subperiosteal collection
    - Majority are drainable subperiosteal abscess (SPA)
    - 20% phlegmon without drainable abscess
- Location
  - Preseptal: Disease anterior to orbital septum
  - Postseptal: Disease posterior to orbital septum
    - Intraconal: Within cone formed by extra-ocular muscles (EOMs)
    - Extraconal: Post-septal disease between bony orbit and EOMs
    - Subperiosteal: Between bony orbit and orbital periosteum
  - Associated myositis
    - Swollen EOMs, may have abnormal contrast-enhancement
  - Beware of associated extra-orbital complications of sinusitis
    - Frontal osteomyelitis, meningitis, empyema, cerebritis, parenchymal abscess

### Imaging Recommendations
- Best imaging tool
  - CECT: Axial and direct coronal or coronal reformatted images (multidetector CT)
  - MR: Best for evaluation of intracranial complications of sinusitis

## DDx: Extra-Orbital Complications of Sinusitis

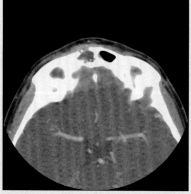

*Pott Puffy Tumor*

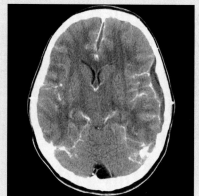

*Empyema*

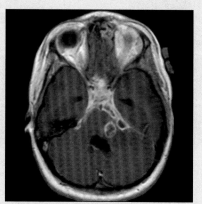

*Abscess & Empyema*

# ORBITAL CELLULITIS

## Key Facts

### Imaging Findings
- Thickening and edema of orbital soft tissues = cellulitis and/or phlegmon
- Low-attenuation rim-enhancing subperiosteal collection
- Preseptal: Disease anterior to orbital septum
- Postseptal: Disease posterior to orbital septum
- Associated myositis
- CECT: Axial and direct coronal or coronal reformatted images (multidetector CT)
- MR: Best for evaluation of intracranial complications of sinusitis

### Top Differential Diagnoses
- Frontal Osteomyelitis - Pott Puffy Tumor (PPT)
- Meningitis
- Empyema

- Cerebritis
- Orbital Myositis

### Pathology
- Sinusitis: Most common cause of orbital cellulitis
- Look for underlying cause of sinusitis
- Potential intracranial spread of infection via diploic veins

### Diagnostic Checklist
- May be difficult to distinguish subperiosteal abscess from phlegmon
- Cavernous sinus thrombosis may be subtle: Compare size, shape and enhancement to contralateral side if unilateral
- Beware of extraorbital complications, sinusitis
- MR indicated if suspect intracranial complication

## DIFFERENTIAL DIAGNOSIS

### Frontal Osteomyelitis - Pott Puffy Tumor (PPT)
- Forehead cellulitis, phlegmon and/or subgaleal abscess
- Frontal bone lytic lesion may be difficult to detect acutely

### Meningitis
- Abnormal meningeal contrast-enhancement

### Empyema
- Epidural (lenticular) or subdural (crescent) extra-axial collection of pus
- Restricted diffusion DWI (increased signal intensity)
- Usually with peripheral dural contrast-enhancement
- Nonenhancing collections may be sterile, i.e. effusions rather than pus

### Cerebritis
- Amorphous intra-axial edema without rim-enhancement

### Orbital Myositis
- Inflammation/infection of EOMs
- EOMs enlarged, markedly enhancing
- Edematous fat surrounds EOMs

## PATHOLOGY

### General Features
- Etiology
  - Sinusitis: Most common cause of orbital cellulitis
    - Other causes: Trauma, foreign body, skin infection, rarely retinoblastoma may present as orbital cellulitis
  - Look for underlying cause of sinusitis
    - Nasolacrimal duct mucocele
    - Antrochoanal polyp
    - Sinonasal foreign body
    - Odontogenic sinusitis

  - Orbital cellulitis: Most common complication of sinusitis
    - Up to 3% of patients with sinusitis
    - May precede signs and symptoms of sinusitis
    - Usually secondary to ethmoiditis
  - Spread of sinus infection to the orbit
    - Direct extension via thin, acquired dehiscence, and/or normal foramina in the lamina papyracea
    - Valveless venous system (diploic veins of Breschet) connects orbital circulation with ethmoid, frontal and maxillary sinus circulation
    - Lymphatic seeding unlikely: No lymph vessels in the orbit
- Associated abnormalities
  - Potential intracranial spread of infection via diploic veins
    - Meningitis
    - Subdural or epidural effusion or empyema
    - Cerebritis
    - Brain abscess

### Microscopic Features
- Microbiology
  - Under 10 years; usually single aerobe
    - Majority Streptococcus pneumoniae, Haemophilus influenza, Moraxella catarrhalis, Streptococcus pyogenes
  - 10-15; years mixed, mostly aerobes
  - Over 15 years; mixed, aerobes and anaerobes

### Staging, Grading or Classification Criteria
- Chandler classification: Orbital complications of sinusitis
  - Preseptal cellulitis
    - Inflammation anterior to the orbital septum
    - Eyelid edema
    - Without tenderness, visual loss or ophthalmoplegia
  - Orbital cellulitis without abscess
    - Diffuse postseptal edema of orbital fat
  - Orbital cellulitis with SPA
    - +/- Proptosis
    - +/- Decreased vision

# ORBITAL CELLULITIS

- +/- Limited EOM motility
  - ○ Orbital cellulitis with abscess in orbital fat
    - Usually severe proptosis
    - Decreased vision
    - Limited EOM motility
  - ○ Cavernous sinus thrombosis secondary to orbital phlebitis
    - Unilateral or bilateral

## CLINICAL ISSUES

### Presentation
- Most common signs/symptoms
  - ○ Depends on degree of inflammation
    - Eyelid swelling, erythema, tenderness
    - Proptosis
    - Ophthalmoplegia results in diplopia
    - Decreased visual acuity
    - Relative afferent pupillary defect (Marcus Gunn pupil) if pressure on optic nerve, dural sheath or vascular supply
- Other signs/symptoms
  - ○ Cranial nerve palsies (CN III, IV, V, VI) with cavernous sinus thrombosis
  - ○ Seizures, mental status change if associated with intracranial complications

### Demographics
- Age: 50% of children are less than 4 years of age

### Natural History & Prognosis
- Good with appropriate treatment
- Rare cause of blindness if untreated

### Treatment
- Imaging indications
  - ○ Significant impairment in visual acuity or ophthalmoplegia: Contrast-enhanced orbit CT
  - ○ No improvement or worsening of symptoms on appropriate antibiotics
  - ○ Suspect subperiosteal or orbital abscess in a patient with severe eyelid edema that prohibits evaluation of vision and EOM motility
- Medical management = intravenous antibiotics
  - ○ Broad spectrum polymicrobial coverage: 2nd or 3rd generation cephalosporins, B-lactamase resistant penicillin combinations, carbapenems
  - ○ Add clindamycin for anaerobic coverage particularly if 10-15 years of age
- Surgical management indications
  - ○ Subperiosteal abscess (not absolute indication)
    - Younger children may only require antibiotics
    - More aggressive surgical drainage in older children
    - Emergent if visual disturbance from optic nerve or retinal compromise
  - ○ Orbital abscess
  - ○ Frontal sinus drainage in osteomyelitis
  - ○ Rarely intracranial drainage of empyemas: Majority resolve with antibiotic therapy

## DIAGNOSTIC CHECKLIST

### Image Interpretation Pearls
- May be difficult to distinguish subperiosteal abscess from phlegmon
- Cavernous sinus thrombosis may be subtle: Compare size, shape and enhancement to contralateral side if unilateral
- Look for potential underlying cause of sinusitis
- Beware of extraorbital complications, sinusitis
- MR indicated if suspect intracranial complication

## SELECTED REFERENCES

1.  Givner LB: Periorbital versus orbital cellulitis. Pediatr Infect Dis J. 21(12):1157-8, 2002
2.  Sobol SE et al: Orbital complications of sinusitis in children. J Otolaryngol. 31(3):131-6, 2002
3.  Younis RT et al: Orbital infection as a complication of sinusitis: are diagnostic and treatment trends changing? Ear Nose Throat J. 81(11):771-5, 2002
4.  Rahbar R et al: Management of orbital subperiosteal abscess in children: Arch Otolaryngol Head Neck Surg. 127(3):281-6, 2001
5.  Starkey CR et al: Medical management of orbital cellulitis. Pediatr Infect Dis J. 20(10):1002-5, 2001
6.  Ambati BK et al: Periorbital and orbital cellulitis before and after the advent of Haemophilus influenzae type B vaccination. Ophthalmology. 107(8):1450-3, 2000
7.  Garcia GH et al: Criteria for nonsurgical management of subperiosteal abscess of the orbit: analysis of outcomes 1988-1998. Ophthalmology. 107(8):1454-6; discussion 1457-8, 2000
8.  Mehra P et al: Odontogenic sinusitis causing orbital cellulitis. J Am Dent Assoc. 130(7):1086-92, 1999
9.  Donahue SP et al: Preseptal and orbital cellulitis in childhood. A changing microbiologic spectrum. Ophthalmology. 105(10):1902-5; discussion 1905-6, 1998
10. Nelson LB et al: Managing orbital cellulitis. J Pediatr Ophthalmol Strabismus. 35(2):68, 1998
11. Pereira KD et al: Management of medial subperiosteal abscess of the orbit in children--a 5 year experience. Int J Pediatr Otorhinolaryngol. 38(3):247-54, 1997
12. Harris GJ: Subperiosteal abscess of the orbit: computed tomography and the clinical course. Ophthal Plast Reconstr Surg. 12(1):1-8, 1996
13. Harris GJ: Subperiosteal abscess of the orbit. Age as a factor in the bacteriology and response to treatment. Ophthalmology. 101(3):585-95, 1994
14. Arjmand EM et al: Pediatric sinusitis and subperiosteal orbital abscess formation: diagnosis and treatment. Otolaryngol Head Neck Surg. 109(5):886-94, 1993
15. Andrews TM et al: The role of computed tomography in the diagnosis of subperiosteal abscess of the orbit. Clin Pediatr (Phila). 31(1):37-43, 1992
16. Handler LC et al: The acute orbit: differentiation of orbital cellulitis from subperiosteal abscess by computerized tomography. Neuroradiology. 33(1):15-8, 1991
17. Patt BS et al: Blindness resulting from orbital complications of sinusitis. Otolaryngol Head Neck Surg. 104(6):789-95, 1991
18. Chandler JR et al: The pathogenesis of orbital complications in acute sinusitis. Laryngoscope. 80(9):1414-28, 1970

# ORBITAL CELLULITIS

## IMAGE GALLERY

### Typical

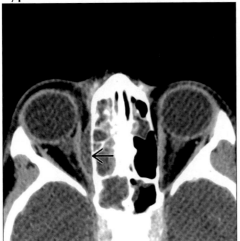

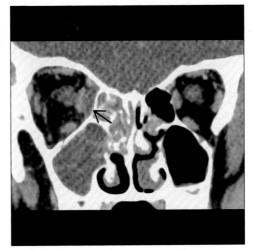

*(Left)* Axial CECT shows a small subperiosteal fluid collection ➡ in the medial right postseptal orbit, deviating the medial rectus muscle laterally, with primarily right sided sinusitis. *(Right)* Coronal CECT shows the same subperiosteal collection ➡, better demonstrates a thin rim of contrast-enhancement, without a definable bony dehiscence.

### Typical

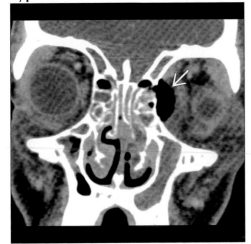

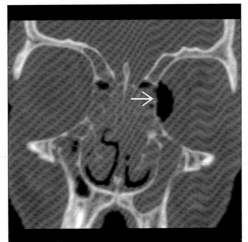

*(Left)* Coronal CECT shows an extraconal gas collection in the left orbit ➡, deviation of the left medial rectus muscle and left globe, and pansinus opacification. *(Right)* Coronal oblique bone CT shows the same gas collection and better demonstrates a focal area of osseous dehiscence in the left lamina papyracea ➡.

### Variant

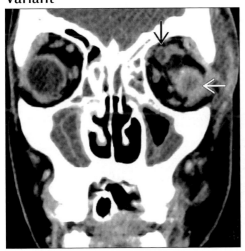

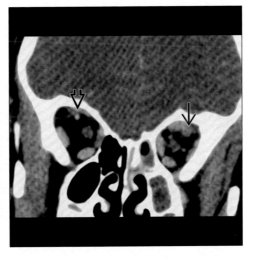

*(Left)* Coronal CECT shows pansinus disease, enlargement and lack of central enhancement in the thrombosed left superior ophthalmic vein ➡, and inferolateral displacement of the left globe ➡. *(Right)* Coronal CECT shows the enlarged left superior ophthalmic vein ➡ more posterior in the left orbit. Notice the normal size and enhancement of the right superior ophthalmic vein ➡.

# LYMPHATIC MALFORMATION, ORBIT

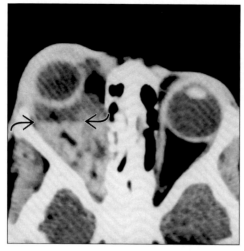

Axial CECT shows a large, trans-spatial orbital lymphangioma, with characteristic blood-fluid levels ➔ with hyperdense blood layering dependently.

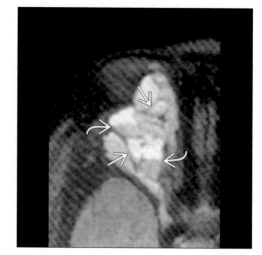

Axial STIR MR shows a complex mass with heterogeneous T2 hyperintensity with fluid-fluid levels ➔. The multiple loculations are separated by thin septations ➔.

## TERMINOLOGY

### Abbreviations and Synonyms
- Lymphangioma, cystic hygroma

### Definitions
- Congenital hamartomatous lymphatic malformation
  - Hemodynamically isolated from systemic drainage

## IMAGING FINDINGS

### General Features
- Best diagnostic clue: Multicystic mass, fluid-fluid levels
- Location
  - Lymphatic malformations (LM) may be superficial or deep
  - Extraconal > intraconal, but often trans-spatial
- Size: Few mm to several cm
- Morphology: Multilocular cystic lesions

### CT Findings
- NECT
  - Multicystic hypodense mass; hyperdense blood products layer dependently
  - Remodeling of bony orbit with large lesions
  - Punctate calcification or phleboliths rare
- CECT: Cystic structures with variable enhancement

### MR Findings
- T1WI
  - Lobulated, poorly circumscribed; variable signal
  - Fluid-fluid levels resulting from hemorrhage into cystic regions
  - Different ages of blood products; subacute blood hyperintense
- T2WI
  - Lobulated, very hyperintense fluid signal
  - Fluid-fluid levels show signal corresponding to age of blood products
  - No flow voids (unlike capillary hemangioma)
- T1 C+: Typically none to minimal peripheral
- MRA: Isolated vasculature, not visible on MRA

### Radiographic Findings
- Radiography: Remodeling of bone with large lesions

---

### DDx: Orbital Masses

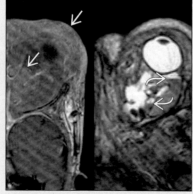

Venolymphatic Malformation

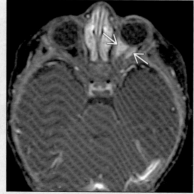

Hemangioma

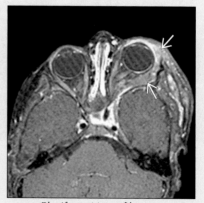

Plexiform Neurofibroma

# LYMPHATIC MALFORMATION, ORBIT

## Key Facts

### Terminology
- Lymphangioma, cystic hygroma
- Congenital hamartomatous lymphatic malformation

### Imaging Findings
- Best diagnostic clue: Multicystic mass, fluid-fluid levels
- Punctate calcification or phleboliths rare
- Fluid-fluid levels show signal corresponding to age of blood products
- T1 C+: Typically none to minimal peripheral

### Top Differential Diagnoses
- Venolymphatic Malformation
- Capillary Hemangioma
- Plexiform Neurofibroma (NF1)
- Orbital Varix

- Cavernous Hemangioma

### Pathology
- Congenital, benign, lymphatic malformation that gradually enlarges
- Mulliken classification of vascular anomalies based on endothelial cell characteristics

### Clinical Issues
- Most common signs/symptoms: Progressive painless proptosis with intermittent worsening
- Most common vascular orbital mass in childhood
- Progressive slow growth during childhood, through puberty and into early adulthood
- Lesions may rapidly ↑ in size with acute hemorrhage
- Observation preferred if vision is not threatened
- Recurrence after surgery common (~ 50%)

## Ultrasonographic Findings
- B-mode: Heterogeneous internal echoes; low echo blood-filled and very low echo lymph-filled cystic spaces
- A-mode: Low reflective blood-filled and lymph-filled spaces; spikes at endothelial walls

## Imaging Recommendations
- Best imaging tool: MR C+
- Protocol advice
  - Fat-sat axial and coronal post-contrast
  - Include brain imaging for associated intracranial abnormalities
  - Does not increase in size with Valsalva maneuver

## DIFFERENTIAL DIAGNOSIS

### Venolymphatic Malformation
- Venous component enhances, lymphatic has fluid-fluid levels

### Capillary Hemangioma
- Lesion of infancy with cutaneous manifestations
- Poorly-marginated, diffusely-enhancing orbital mass

### Plexiform Neurofibroma (NF1)
- Associated with sphenoid and orbit dysplasia
- Infiltrative, trans-spatial mass

### Orbital Varix
- Increases in size with Valsalva
- Rarely can have fluid-fluid levels

### Cavernous Hemangioma
- Well-circumscribed

### Rhabdomyosarcoma
- Most common childhood primary orbital malignancy
- Solid mass with little bone destruction

### Hematologic Malignancy
- Lymphoma, leukemia, Langerhans cell histiocytosis

## PATHOLOGY

### General Features
- General path comments
  - Congenital, benign, lymphatic malformation that gradually enlarges
  - Lymphatic tissue not normally found in the orbit
  - Nonencapsulated infiltrating lesions
- Etiology: Hamartoma from vascular mesenchymal anlage that develops with no systemic vascular or lymphatic connection
- Epidemiology
  - Incidence 3:100,000
  - Less common than capillary and cavernous hemangiomas
  - 8% of all expanding orbital tumors
  - 5% of childhood orbital tumors
- Associated abnormalities
  - LM in other regions of head and neck
  - Venolymphatic malformations associated with intracranial vascular anomalies that can bleed
    - Lesions with this association more likely posterior, diffuse, infiltrative, with poor visual outcome

### Gross Pathologic & Surgical Features
- Thin-walled multilocular mass
- Cysts contain clear fluid or chocolate-colored blood products
- Not well-encapsulated, allowing invasion of surrounding tissues

### Microscopic Features
- Unencapsulated mass of irregularly-shaped sinuses; infiltrates into adjacent stroma
- Dysplastic lymphatic and vascular channels lined with flattened endothelial cells
- Interstitium of smooth muscle fibers and loose connective tissue, with lymphoid follicles and lymphocytic infiltration
- Cystic spaces with lymphatic fluid or chronic blood products

- Positive lymphatic immunohistochemical markers confirm lymphatic origin

## Staging, Grading or Classification Criteria
- Mulliken classification of vascular anomalies based on endothelial cell characteristics
  - Official nomenclature for the International Society for the Study of Vascular Anomalies in 1996
  - Differentiates proliferating tumors (primarily hemangiomas) from vascular malformations, which are structural anomalies involving capillaries, venules, veins, lymphatic channels, and combinations of these structures
  - Low flow malformations include venous, lymphatic, venolymphatic and capillary or venular malformations
- WHO classification of LM
  - Capillary: Capillary-sized lymphatic channels
  - Cavernous: Dilated microscopic channels
  - Cystic: Macroscopic cystic regions of varying size
- Classification of LM based on location
  - Superficial: Conjunctiva or lid (most common)
  - Deep: Retrobulbar orbit
  - Combined: Superficial and deep components
  - Complex: Trans-spatial orbit and face

## CLINICAL ISSUES

### Presentation
- Most common signs/symptoms: Progressive painless proptosis with intermittent worsening
- Clinical Profile: Diplopia, ptosis, restricted EOM movement, compressive optic nerve findings and periorbital ecchymosis

### Demographics
- Age
  - Younger patients: Infants to young adults
  - Usually presents in 1st decade
  - Most common vascular orbital mass in childhood
- Gender: Slight female predominance

### Natural History & Prognosis
- Continues to expand in size; does not involute (unlike capillary hemangioma)
- Progressive slow growth during childhood, through puberty and into early adulthood
- Lesions may intermittently ↑ and ↓ in size in conjunction with upper respiratory infection
  - Due to presence of lymphatic tissue
- Lesions may rapidly ↑ in size with acute hemorrhage
  - Recurrent hemorrhages in 50%
  - Associated with higher lesion recurrence
- Optic nerve compromise late complication of large lesions
- Infiltrating nature results in frequent recurrence
- Refractory visual problems and disfigurement common
- Poor visual acuity associated with multiple surgical resections

### Treatment
- Options, risks, complications

- Conservative therapy
  - Observation preferred if vision is not threatened
- Systemic steroids
  - May ↓ pain, swelling, proptosis, especially in kids
- Surgery
  - Difficult, interdigitation with normal structures
  - Recurrence after surgery common (~ 50%)
  - Multiple surgeries cause visual impairment
  - Acute mass effect due to hemorrhage may require emergent decompression

## DIAGNOSTIC CHECKLIST

### Consider
- Distinction between LM and varix controversial
  - LM is hemodynamically isolated
  - Varix has systemic drainage and therefore pressure-depended distensibility
  - Caveat: Some varices have lymphatic components

### Image Interpretation Pearls
- Blood products + fluid-fluid levels highly suggestive

## SELECTED REFERENCES

1. Gunduz K et al: Correlation of surgical outcome with neuroimaging findings in periocular lymphangiomas. Ophthalmology. 113(7):1236, 2006
2. Bilaniuk LT: Vascular lesions of the orbit in children. Neuroimaging Clin N Am. 15(1):107-20, 2005
3. Boulos PR et al: Intralesional injection of Tisseel fibrin glue for resection of lymphangiomas and other thin-walled orbital cysts. Ophthal Plast Reconstr Surg. 21(3):171-6, 2005
4. Greene AK et al: Periorbital lymphatic malformation: clinical course and management in 42 patients. Plast Reconstr Surg. 115(1):22-30, 2005
5. Shields JA et al: Orbital cysts of childhood--classification, clinical features, and management. Surv Ophthalmol. 49(3):281-99, 2004
6. Gold L et al: Characterization of maxillofacial soft tissue vascular anomalies by ultrasound and color Doppler imaging: an adjuvant to computed tomography and magnetic resonance imaging. J Oral Maxillofac Surg. 61(1):19-31, 2003
7. Vachharajani A et al: Orbital lymphangioma with non-contiguous cerebral arteriovenous malformation, manifesting with thrombocytopenia (Kasabach-Merritt syndrome) and intracerebral hemorrhage. Acta Paediatr. 91(1):98-9, 2002
8. Cursiefen C et al: Orbital lymphangioma with positive immunohistochemistry of lymphatic endothelial markers (vascular endothelial growth factor receptor 3 and podoplanin). Graefes Arch Clin Exp Ophthalmol. 239(8):628-32, 2001
9. Bilaniuk LT: Orbital vascular lesions. Role of imaging. Radiol Clin North Am. 37(1):169-83, xi, 1999
10. Harris GJ: Orbital vascular malformations: a consensus statement on terminology and its clinical implications. Orbital Society. Am J Ophthalmol. 127(4):453-5, 1999
11. Barnes PD et al: Hemangiomas and vascular malformations of the head and neck: MR characterization. AJNR Am J Neuroradiol. 15(1):193-5, 1994
12. Mulliken JB et al: Hemangiomas and vascular malformations in infants and children: a classification based on endothelial characteristics. Plast Reconstr Surg. 69(3):412-22, 1982

# LYMPHATIC MALFORMATION, ORBIT

## IMAGE GALLERY

### Typical

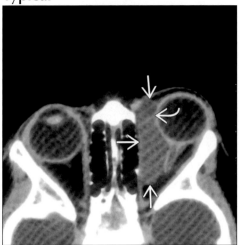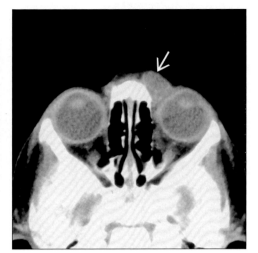

*(Left)* Axial CECT shows a trans-spatial unilocular cystic mass ➡ slightly more dense than vitreous, indicating proteinaceous material or old blood products. Note subtle fluid-fluid level ➡. *(Right)* Axial CECT shows small fluid-density preseptal orbital lymphangioma ➡ lying between the globe and nasal bone no significant enhancement.

### Typical

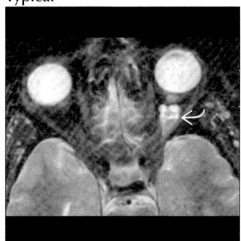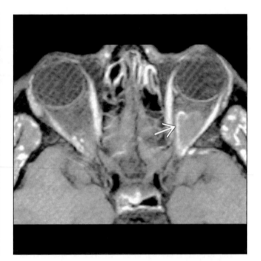

*(Left)* Axial STIR MR shows ➡ layering of blood products within the multiloculated heterogeneous signal retrobulbar lesion. Note minimal proptosis on the affected side. *(Right)* Axial T1 C+ FS MR in the same patient as previous image shows the lesion to be isodense with orbital fat on this fat-suppressed image, with mild irregular marginal enhancement ➡.

### Typical

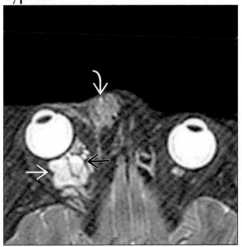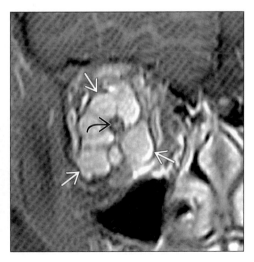

*(Left)* Axial T2WI FS MR shows deep macrocystic hyperintense retrobulbar mass ➡ with a subtle fluid-fluid level ➡ and a superficial microcystic component ➡. Note mild proptosis. *(Right)* Coronal T1 C+ FS MR shows a large retrobulbar multicystic mass ➡ surrounding the optic nerve ➡. The mass is intrinsically bright on T1 likely due to high protein contents.

# VENOLYMPHATIC MALFORMATION, ORBIT

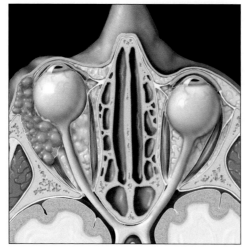

*Axial graphic shows typical example of orbital venolymphatic malformation. Lesions have vascular spaces with venous flow, with varying amounts of lymphangiomatous components with no flow.*

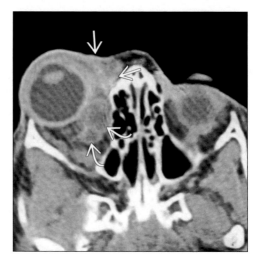

*Axial T1 C+ FS MR shows a heterogeneously enhancing mass with mixed venous ➡ and lymphangiomatous ➡ components. Proptosis with preseptal and intraorbital involvement is evident.*

## TERMINOLOGY

### Abbreviations and Synonyms
- Three subtypes of lesions
  - Lymphatic malformation (LM)
    - Synonyms: Cystic hygroma; lymphangioma
  - Venous malformation (VM)
    - Synonyms: Cavernous malformation
  - Venolymphatic malformation (VLM)
    - Synonyms: Mixed malformation

### Definitions
- Congenital vascular malformations (nonproliferative)
  - Distinct from capillary & cavernous hemangioma
- Hemodynamic classification of malformations
  - No flow
    - No systemic vascular connection
    - Includes LM & isolated (nonconnected) VLM
  - Venous flow
    - Systemic vascular connection
    - Includes systemically connected VLM & VM
    - Distensible channels result in orbital varix
  - Arterial flow
    - Arterial flow through malformation (AVM)

## IMAGING FINDINGS

### General Features
- Best diagnostic clue: Lobulated, irregular, trans-spatial variably enhancing mass
- Location
  - May be superficial (preseptal) or deep (orbit)
  - Extraconal > intraconal; often trans-spatial
- Morphology: Irregular margins, multilocular

### CT Findings
- NECT
  - Hypodense or cystic mass; ± dense hemorrhage
  - Remodeling of bony orbit with large lesions

### MR Findings
- T1WI: Variable signal; fluid-fluid levels if hemorrhage
- T2WI: Lobulated, very hyperintense fluid signal
- T1 C+: Variable enhancement, depending on proportion of venous channels in mixed lesions

### Imaging Recommendations
- Best imaging tool: Enhanced MR with fat suppression
- Protocol advice: CT with Valsalva if varix suspected

## DDx: Enhancing Orbital Mass in a Child

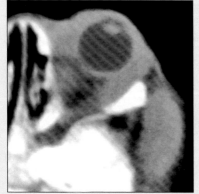

*Capillary Hemangioma*

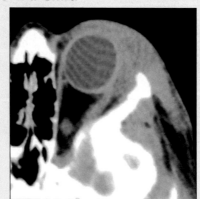

*Plexiform Neurofibroma*

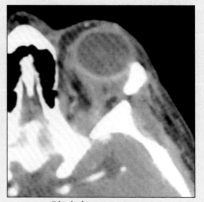

*Rhabdomyosarcoma*

# VENOLYMPHATIC MALFORMATION, ORBIT

## Key Facts

### Terminology
- Congenital vascular malformations (nonproliferative)

### Imaging Findings
- Best diagnostic clue: Lobulated, irregular, trans-spatial variably enhancing mass
- T1 C+: Variable enhancement, depending on proportion of venous channels in mixed lesions
- Protocol advice: CT with Valsalva if varix suspected

### Pathology
- General path comments: Congenital, benign, vascular malformation consisting of dilated vascular channels

### Clinical Issues
- Most common signs/symptoms: Progressive painless mass with proptosis
- Other signs/symptoms: When varix is present, transiently enlarges with Valsalva
- Lesions may rapidly ↑ in size with acute hemorrhage

## DIFFERENTIAL DIAGNOSIS

### Capillary Hemangioma
- Proliferative orbitofacial vascular mass in an infant

### Plexiform Neurofibroma (NF1)
- Infiltrative progressive enhancing masses in a child

### Rhabdomyosarcoma
- Rapidly growing orbital malignancy in a child

## PATHOLOGY

### General Features
- General path comments: Congenital, benign, vascular malformation consisting of dilated vascular channels
- Associated abnormalities: Noncontiguous intracranial vascular malformations

### Gross Pathologic & Surgical Features
- Thin-walled multilocular mass
- Distensible lesions have systemic venous connection

### Microscopic Features
- Unencapsulated mass of irregularly-shaped sinuses
- Infiltrates into adjacent stroma
- Dysplastic venous channels lined with flattened endothelial cells
- Interstitium of smooth muscle fibers and loose connective tissue, with lymphocytic infiltration

## CLINICAL ISSUES

### Presentation
- Most common signs/symptoms: Progressive painless mass with proptosis
- Other signs/symptoms: When varix is present, transiently enlarges with Valsalva

### Demographics
- Age: Younger patients (infants to young adults)

### Natural History & Prognosis
- Progressive growth during and beyond childhood
- Lesions may rapidly ↑ in size with acute hemorrhage
- Infiltrating nature results in frequent recurrence

### Treatment
- Conservative: Observation if vision not threatened
- Systemic steroids: May ↓ pain, swelling, and proptosis
- Surgery: Difficult resection, recurrence common

## DIAGNOSTIC CHECKLIST

### Image Interpretation Pearls
- Varix may be decompressed at rest; transiently enlarges with Valsalva provocation

## SELECTED REFERENCES

1. Orbital vascular malformations: A consensus statement. Am J Ophthalmol. 127(4):453-5, 1999

## IMAGE GALLERY

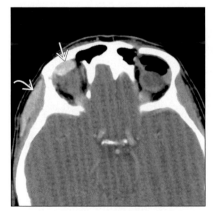
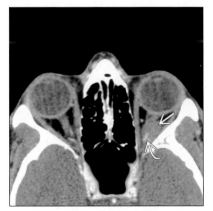
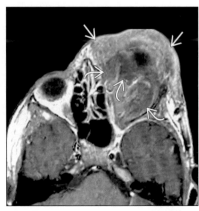

*(Left)* Axial CECT shows an enhancing venous malformation in the superior orbit ➡, with trans-spatial extension into the temporal fossa ➡. *(Center)* Axial CECT shows a low density retrobulbar venolymphatic malformation, with primarily cystic appearance ➡, and a small enhancing venous component ➡. *(Right)* Axial T1 C+ FS MR shows a large, heterogeneous mixed venolymphatic malformation. The mass traverses spatial boundaries, and demonstrates enhancing ➡ and nonenhancing ➡ components.

# HEMANGIOMA, ORBIT

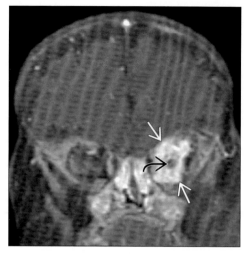

Coronal T1 C+ FS MR shows a left retrobulbar intensely enhancing, lobular mass ➡ surrounding and engulfing the optic nerve ↗.

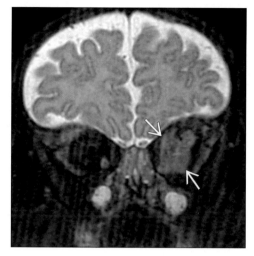

Coronal T2WI FS MR (same patient as previous image) shows the mass ➡ to be irregular and minimally hyperintense. Note the difficulty in differentiating the optic nerve and extraocular muscles.

## TERMINOLOGY

### Abbreviations and Synonyms
- Orbital capillary hemangioma (OCH)
- Benign hemangioendothelioma; infantile periocular hemangioma

### Definitions
- Benign infantile orbital endothelial cell neoplasm
- Distinct lesion from adult or childhood cavernous hemangioma

## IMAGING FINDINGS

### General Features
- Best diagnostic clue: Lobulated, irregular, intensely enhancing mass involving any area of orbit in infant
- Location
  - May involve multiple contiguous areas
  - Predilection for superior orbit, eyelids, supranasal periorbita
  - Sites of orbital involvement
    - Most commonly superomedial extraconal location
    - May extend intraconal, into superior orbital fissure
    - Exclusively retrobulbar in 10%
  - Rarely involved bone or extends intracranially
- Size
  - Typically 2-8 cm size range
  - Superficial lesions detected when smaller
- Morphology
  - Lobulated, irregular contours
  - Margins vary from well-circumscribed to infiltrative

### CT Findings
- NECT
  - Slightly hyperdense, relatively homogeneous
  - No gross calcification
- CECT: Intense enhancement, usually homogeneous

### MR Findings
- T1WI: Iso or hypointense, heterogeneous
- T2WI
  - Hyperintense, heterogeneous
  - Flow voids frequently visible
  - ± Thrombosis or stagnant blood
- T1 C+
  - Diffuse, intense enhancement

## DDx: Orbital Masses

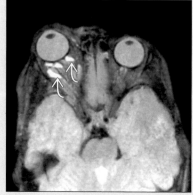

Lymphangioma

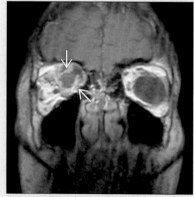

Rhabdomyosarcoma

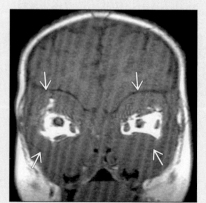

Chloroma (Leukemia)

# HEMANGIOMA, ORBIT

## Key Facts

### Terminology
- Benign hemangioendothelioma; infantile periocular hemangioma

### Imaging Findings
- Best diagnostic clue: Lobulated, irregular, intensely enhancing mass involving any area of orbit in infant
- May be heterogeneous in involuting lesions

### Top Differential Diagnoses
- Lymphangioma
- Orbital Cellulitis
- Rhabdomyosarcoma
- Metastatic Neuroblastoma
- Hematopoietic Malignancy

### Pathology
- Most common benign orbital tumor of infancy

### Clinical Issues
- Bluish discoloration of skin or conjunctiva in 80%
- Enlarge with Valsalva or crying in 50%
- 30% present at birth, most present within first 6 months
- Female predominance 3:1 to 5:1
- Expectant observation unless complications

### Diagnostic Checklist
- Differential diagnosis for rapidly growing mass in infant includes malignancy
- Ultrasound can provide easy bedside confirmation of suspected lesion

○ May be heterogeneous in involuting lesions
- MRA: Often normal since vascular component is primarily at capillary level, small arteries not visible

## Ultrasonographic Findings
- B-scan
  ○ Smooth or irregular mass, homogeneous or heterogeneous, high echogenicity
- Doppler
  ○ High flow supply and drainage

## Angiographic Findings
- Enlarged feeding branches from external carotid, ophthalmic arteries
- Dense parenchymal stain, early draining veins

## Imaging Recommendations
- Best imaging tool
  ○ Ultrasound for rapid bedside confirmation
  ○ Enhanced MR in axial and coronal planes for larger lesions to assess critical structure involvement
- Protocol advice: Use fat-suppression for T2WI and T1 C+ images

# DIFFERENTIAL DIAGNOSIS

## Lymphangioma
- Multilocular, trans-spatial mass with characteristic blood-fluid levels

## Orbital Cellulitis
- Inflammatory changes ± abscess formation

## Rhabdomyosarcoma
- Invasive orbital mass ± bone destruction

## Metastatic Neuroblastoma
- Rapidly progressive orbital metastatic mass
- Frequently involves skull base

## Hematopoietic Malignancy
- Leukemia, lymphoma
- Langerhans cell histiocytosis

# PATHOLOGY

## General Features
- General path comments
  ○ Proliferative vascular mass
  ○ May be considered hamartoma or neoplasm
- Genetics
  ○ Most cases sporadic
  ○ Some associated with pleiotropic genetic syndromes
  ○ Small percent autosomal dominant
    ▪ Gene map locus 5q35.3, 5q31-q33
- Etiology: Hamartomatous proliferation of vascular endothelium
- Epidemiology
  ○ Most common benign orbital tumor of infancy
    ▪ 8-12% term neonates of Western descent, rare in Asians
    ▪ Up to 22% preterm neonates < 1000 g
  ○ 40% hemangiomas present at birth, 80% single
  ○ 50% infant capillary hemangiomas occur in head and neck
- Associated abnormalities
  ○ PHACES syndrome
    ▪ Neurocutaneous syndrome with posterior fossa malformations, hemangiomas, arterial anomalies, coarctation of aorta, eye abnormalities, sternal clefting
  ○ Kasabach-Merritt syndrome
    ▪ Rare condition, seen in patients with extensive hemangiomas
    ▪ Hemorrhagic complications due to thrombocytopenia and coagulopathy

## Gross Pathologic & Surgical Features
- Bluish hue of overlying skin
- May have external or internal carotid arterial supply
- Capable of profuse bleeding

## Microscopic Features
- Unencapsulated cellular neoplasm, lobulated growth
- Thin-walled capillary-sized vascular spaces in lobules with thin fibrous septae

# HEMANGIOMA, ORBIT

- Proliferative phase: Rapidly dividing endothelial cells with different luminal diameter, pericytes, multilaminated basement membranes
- Involutional phase: Mitotic activity decreases, mast cells transiently appear, endothelial cells replaced by perivascular, intralobular fibrous + adipose tissue

## Staging, Grading or Classification Criteria
- Classification by location
  o Deep: Within deep tissues of lid and anterior orbit, or entirely retrobulbar
  o Superficial: Confined to dermis
  o Combined: Both dermal and deep components

## CLINICAL ISSUES

### Presentation
- Most common signs/symptoms
  o Unilateral eyelid, brow or nasal vascular lesion
  o With or without proptosis or decreased vision
- Clinical Profile
  o Rubbery, soft mass
  o Bluish discoloration of skin or conjunctiva in 80%
  o Blanches with pressure (unlike port-wine stain)
  o Enlarge with Valsalva or crying in 50%
  o Loss of visual acuity (noted by parents)
  o Ptosis if eyelid involved
  o Proptosis if retroseptal, especially if intraconal

### Demographics
- Age
  o Tumor of infants
  o 30% present at birth, most present within first 6 months
- Gender
  o Female predominance 3:1 to 5:1
  o Even higher F:M in genetic syndromes

### Natural History & Prognosis
- Proliferative phase
  o Period of rapid growth occurs during first 6 to 18 months of life
- Involutional phase
  o Spontaneous regression usually begins after 1st year
  o May take 5-10 yrs to involute
- Ophthalmic sequelae include deprivation amblyopia (60%, usually if > 1 cm), astigmatism, and corneal exposure
- Cutaneous involvement leaves scar, treat like skin burn

### Treatment
- Expectant observation unless complications
- 20% require treatment
- Indications for treatment
  o Ophthalmic: Visual disturbance, nerve compromise, proptosis, deformity
  o Systemic: Congestive failure, coagulopathy, anemia, airway obstruction
  o Dermatologic: Ulceration, infection, cosmetic disfigurement
- Corticosteroid treatment very effective
  o Intralesional, systemic or topical administration

- Intratumoral laser therapy in larger lesions
- Interferon treatment, surgical ligation or laser ablation options for recalcitrant lesions
- Intravascular embolization contraindicated for intraorbital lesions
- Radiation therapy reserved for advanced lesions

## DIAGNOSTIC CHECKLIST

### Consider
- Differential diagnosis for rapidly growing mass in infant includes malignancy

### Image Interpretation Pearls
- Ultrasound can provide easy bedside confirmation of suspected lesion

## SELECTED REFERENCES
1. Dubois J et al: Orbit and eyelid hemangiomas: is there a relationship between location and ocular problems? J Am Acad Dermatol. 55(4):614-9, 2006
2. Kavanagh EC et al: Imaging of the natural history of an orbital capillary hemangioma. Orbit. 25(1):69-72, 2006
3. Riveros LG et al: Primary intraosseous hemangioma of the orbit: an unusual presentation of an uncommon tumor. Can J Ophthalmol. 41(5):630-2, 2006
4. Schwartz SR et al: Risk factors for amblyopia in children with capillary hemangiomas of the eyelids and orbit. J AAPOS. 10(3):262-8, 2006
5. Verity DH et al: Natural history of periocular capillary haemangiomas: changes in internal blood velocity and lesion volume. Eye. 20(10):1228-37, 2006
6. Bilaniuk LT: Vascular lesions of the orbit in children. Neuroimaging Clin N Am. 15(1):107-20, 2005
7. Mierzwa ML et al: Radiation therapy for recurrent orbital hemangioma. Head Neck. 25(5):412-5, 2003
8. O'Keefe M et al: Capillary haemangioma of the eyelids and orbit: a clinical review of the safety and efficacy of intralesional steroid. Acta Ophthalmol Scand. 81(3):294-8, 2003
9. Rootman J et al: Vascular diseases. In: Diseases of the Orbit. Philadelphia, Lippincott, 2003
10. Waner M et al: The nonrandom distribution of facial hemangiomas. Arch Dermatol. 139(7):869-75, 2003
11. Sleep TJ et al: Doppler ultrasonography to aid diagnosis of orbital capillary haemangioma in neonates. Eye. 16(3):316-9, 2002
12. Bilaniuk LT: Orbital vascular lesions. Role of imaging. Radiol Clin North Am. 37(1):169-83, xi, 1999
13. Harris GJ: Orbital vascular malformations: a consensus statement on terminology and its clinical implications. Orbital Society. Am J Ophthalmol. 127(4):453-5, 1999
14. Walter JW et al: Genetic mapping of a novel familial form of infantile hemangioma. Am J Med Genet. 82(1):77-83, 1999
15. Yap EY et al: Periocular capillary hemangioma: a review for pediatricians and family physicians. Mayo Clin Proc. 73(8):753-9, 1998
16. Forbes G: Vascular lesions in the orbit. Neuroimaging Clin N Am. 6(1):113-22, 1996
17. Henderson GW: Vascular hamartomas, hyperplasias and neoplasms. In: Orbital Tumors. New York, Raven Press, 1994
18. Rootman J et al: Multidisciplinary approaches to complicated vascular lesions of the orbit. Ophthalmology. 99(9):1440-6, 1992

## IMAGE GALLERY

### Typical

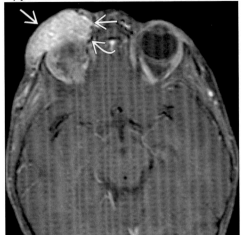 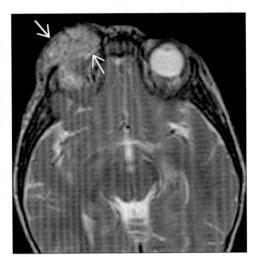

*(Left) Axial T1 C+ FS MR shows a homogeneously and intensely enhancing mass ➡ on the right forehead extending into the right orbit. Vascular flow voids ➡ are visible. (Right) Axial T2WI MR in same patient as previous image shows the mass ➡ to be somewhat heterogeneous and minimally hyperintense compared with brain. Hemangiomas often cross fascial planes.*

### Typical

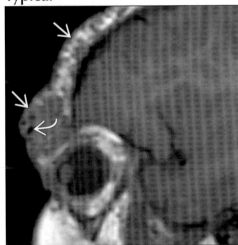 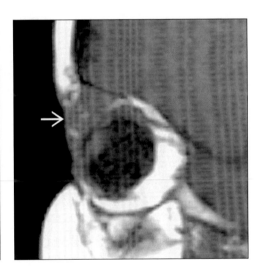

*(Left) Sagittal T1WI MR of same patient as previous two images shows a lobulated, irregular infiltrative mass ➡ in the scalp and forehead extending into the extraconal orbit. Note flow void ➡. (Right) Sagittal T1WI MR in a different patient shows an extraconal orbital hemangioma ➡ situated superior to the globe. Note distortion of the contour of the globe.*

### Typical

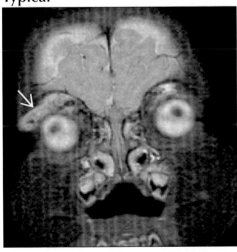 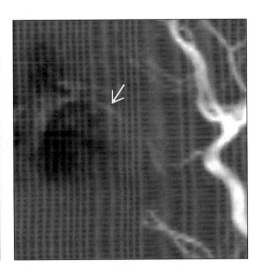

*(Left) Coronal STIR MR (same patient as previous image) shows the hemangioma ➡ to be heterogeneous and largely isointense to the unmyelinated brain. Note the hypointense vascular signal voids. (Right) Sagittal MRA (same patient as previous 2 images) shows probable arterial supply to the hemangioma via superior medial palpebral artery ➡, one of terminal branches of ophthalmic artery.*

# RETINOBLASTOMA

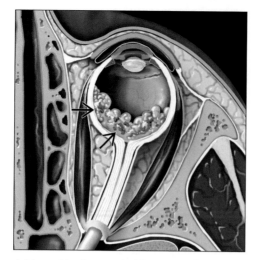

*Axial graphic shows retinoblastoma, with lobulated tumor extending through the limiting membrane into the vitreous. Punctate calcifications ➡ are characteristic.*

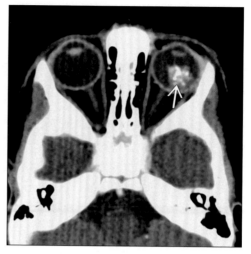

*Axial CECT shows a large, lobulated, partially calcified left intraocular mass ➡, typical of retinoblastoma.*

## TERMINOLOGY

### Abbreviations and Synonyms
- Retinoblastoma (RB)

### Definitions
- Malignant retinal neoplasm, arises from neuroectodermal cells
- Trilateral RB: Bilateral ocular tumors plus midline intracranial neuroblastic tumor, pineal > > suprasellar
- Retinocytoma: Rare benign variant, similar genetics

## IMAGING FINDINGS

### General Features
- Best diagnostic clue: Calcified intraocular mass
- Location
  - Unilateral in 70-75%
  - Bilateral in 25-40%
  - Trilateral disease rare
    - 5-15% of familial lesions
    - 80% pineal, 20% suprasellar
  - Optic nerve or intraorbital extension uncommon

- 10-15% of patients, poor prognostic factor
  - Leptomeningeal metastasis rare
    - 15-20% of patients with recurrent disease
  - Hematogenous metastasis rare
- Growth patterns
  - Endophytic form: Inward growth into vitreous
    - Associated with vitreous seeding
  - Exophytic form: Outward growth into subretinal space
    - Associated with retinal detachment
  - Diffuse infiltrating form: Plaque-like growth along retina
    - Rare (1-2%); often no Ca++; older children
    - Simulates inflammatory or other conditions

### CT Findings
- NECT: Calcified (90-95%) intraocular mass
- CECT: Variable enhancement of noncalcified portion

### MR Findings
- T1WI: Variable, mildly hyperintense relative to vitreous
- T2WI
  - Hypointense relative to vitreous
  - Helps distinguish from other congenital lesions

## DDx: Globe Calcification

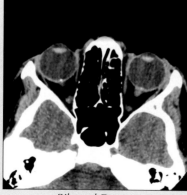

*Bilateral Drusen*

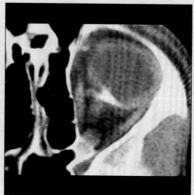

*Astrocytoma in TSC*

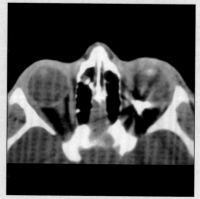

*Metallic FB - BB*

# RETINOBLASTOMA

## Key Facts

### Terminology
- Malignant retinal neoplasm, arises from neuroectodermal cells

### Imaging Findings
- Best diagnostic clue: Calcified intraocular mass
- Unilateral in 70-75%
- Hypointense relative to vitreous
- Moderate to marked heterogeneous enhancement
- CT best tool for identification of calcification
- MR best for assessing extraocular and intracranial disease

### Top Differential Diagnoses
- Retinal Astrocytoma
- Foreign Body (FB)
- Phthisis Bulbi

### Pathology
- RB1 gene codes for pRB tumor suppressor protein
- Sporadic nonfamilial form: 60%
- Familial hereditary form: 40%
- Most common malignant intraocular tumor of childhood; 3% of cancers in children under 15

### Clinical Issues
- Most common signs/symptoms: Leukocoria (white pupillary reflex): 60%
- 90-95% diagnosed by age 5 years
- 90% cure for noninvasive intraocular RB

### Diagnostic Checklist
- Check for intracranial trilateral or quadrilateral disease in pineal and suprasellar regions

II

2

55

---

- ○ Useful for demonstrating retinal detachment
- T1 C+
  - ○ Moderate to marked heterogeneous enhancement
  - ○ Best evaluates optic nerve and transscleral extension
  - ○ Anterior segment enhancement more aggressive tumor behavior
  - ○ Appearance after enucleation and hydroxyapatite orbital prosthesis
    - ▪ Expect contrast-enhancement of orbital prosthesis secondary to fibrovascular tissue infiltration

### Ultrasonographic Findings
- Echogenic, irregular mass with focal shadows
- Limited visualization of extra-ocular extension

### Imaging Recommendations
- Best imaging tool
  - ○ CT best tool for identification of calcification
  - ○ MR best for assessing extraocular and intracranial disease
- Protocol advice: Whole brain for trilateral disease, CSF seeding; FSE T2 and FS T1 Gd MR orbit

## DIFFERENTIAL DIAGNOSIS

### Optic Nerve Head Drusen
- Dystrophic calcification, most are idiopathic
- Most cases incidentally found on funduscopic exam: Pseudopapilledema

### Retinal Astrocytoma
- Rare; isolated or in association with tuberous sclerosis (TSC)
- With or without exudative retinal detachment, hemorrhage and calcification

### Foreign Body (FB)
- Metallic BB most common
- Intraocular associated with globe rupture

### Phthisis Bulbi
- End-stage shrinking and calcification of the globe secondary to destructive disease

- ○ Trauma, infection/inflammation, radiation

### Ocular Toxocariasis
- Sclerosing endophthalmitis due to Toxocara canis
- Uveoscleral enhancement; no Ca++ acutely

## PATHOLOGY

### General Features
- Genetics
  - ○ RB1 gene on chromosome 13 at q14 locus
    - ▪ RB1 gene codes for pRB tumor suppressor protein
    - ▪ Regulates cell growth, division, and apoptosis
    - ▪ Two hit theory: Lack of both RB1 alleles in embryonic retinoblast leads to absence of pRB, resulting in malignancy
    - ▪ Other cell line malignancies also related to RB1
  - ○ Somatic mosaicism in 10-20% of RB patients
- Etiology
  - ○ Sporadic nonfamilial form: 60%
    - ▪ Spontaneous somatic mutation or deletion of both copies of RB1 in a retinoblast
    - ▪ Majority (85%) of unilateral disease
  - ○ Familial hereditary form: 40%
    - ▪ Germline mutation or deletion of one copy of RB1, spontaneous mutation of other copy
    - ▪ Autosomal dominant
    - ▪ Positive family history in 5-10%
    - ▪ New germline mutations in 30-35%
    - ▪ Essentially all bilateral and multilateral disease
    - ▪ Minority (15%) of unilateral disease
- Epidemiology
  - ○ Most common malignant intraocular tumor of childhood; 3% of cancers in children under 15
  - ○ 1% of cancer deaths; 5% of childhood blindness
  - ○ Incidence of 1:15,000-30,000 live births
    - ▪ Has increased in past 60 years
- Associated abnormalities
  - ○ Risk of other nonocular malignances in patients with familial form
    - ▪ 20-30% in non-irradiated patients; 50-60% in irradiated patients

# RETINOBLASTOMA

- Within 30 years, average 10-13 years
  - Osteosarcoma, soft tissue sarcomas, melanoma
- 13q deletion syndrome: RB plus multiple organ system anomalies

## Gross Pathologic & Surgical Features
- Yellowish-white to pink irregular retinal mass

## Microscopic Features
- Small round cells, scant cytoplasm and large nuclei
- Flexner-Wintersteiner rosettes and fleurettes

## Staging, Grading or Classification Criteria
- Reese-Ellsworth classification
  - Groups I through V; based on size, location, and multifocality
  - More useful in radiation therapy management
- International classification (newer)
  - Groups A through E; based on size, retinal location, subretinal or vitreous seeding, and several specific prognostic features
  - More useful in chemotherapy management

## CLINICAL ISSUES

### Presentation
- Most common signs/symptoms: Leukocoria (white pupillary reflex): 60%
- Other signs/symptoms
  - Strabismus, severe vision loss, inflammatory signs (10%)
  - Less common: Anisocoria, heterochromia, glaucoma, cataract, nystagmus, proptosis

### Demographics
- Age
  - RB is congenital but usually not apparent at birth
  - Average age 13 months at diagnosis in US
    - Earlier if family history with routine screening
  - 90-95% diagnosed by age 5 years

### Natural History & Prognosis
- 90% cure for noninvasive intraocular RB
- Degree of nerve involvement correlates with survival
  - Superficial or no invasion: 90%; invasion to lamina cribrosa: 70%; invasion beyond lamina cribrosa: 60%; involvement at surgical margin: 20%
- Poor prognosis for extraocular disease
  - > 90% mortality
- Dismal prognosis for trilateral disease or CSF spread
  - < 24 month survival

### Treatment
- Chemotherapy (chemoreduction)
  - Recent advance; limits need for external radiation
  - Currently favored first line therapy for lower grade intraocular tumors
  - Used in conjunction with other local modalities to achieve cure
- External beam radiation therapy (EBRT)
  - Indicated for bulky tumors with seeding
  - Unfavorable complications, e.g., arrested bone growth and radiation-induced tumors
- Plaque radiotherapy

- Locally directed, I-215 or other isotope
- Selected solitary or small tumors
- Enucleation
  - Indicated when no chance of preserving useful vision due to tumor spread or retinal detachments
- Cryotherapy
  - Primary local treatment of small anterior tumors
- Photocoagulation
  - Primary local treatment of small posterior tumors

## DIAGNOSTIC CHECKLIST

### Consider
- Early diagnosis is crucial for good outcome
- Regular screening for children with family history
- Close surveillance until age 7 for development of metachronous multilateral tumors
- RB can mimic inflammatory disease, particularly diffuse form

### Image Interpretation Pearls
- Biopsy carries significant risk of seeding; therefore imaging diagnosis is crucial
- Check for intracranial trilateral or quadrilateral disease in pineal and suprasellar regions

## SELECTED REFERENCES

1. Provenzale JM et al: Trilateral retinoblastoma: clinical and radiologic progression. AJR Am J Roentgenol. 183(2):505-11, 2004
2. Galluzzi P et al: Retinoblastoma: Abnormal gadolinium enhancement of anterior segment of eyes at MR imaging with clinical and histopathologic correlation. Radiology. 228(3):683-90, 2003
3. Klapper SR et al: Hydroxyapatite orbital implant vascularization assessed by magnetic resonance imaging. Ophthal Plast Reconstr Surg. 19(1):46-52, 2003
4. Schueler AO et al: High resolution magnetic resonance imaging of retinoblastoma. Br J Ophthalmol. 87(3):330-5, 2003
5. Tateishi U et al: CT and MRI features of recurrent tumors and second primary neoplasms in pediatric patients with retinoblastoma. AJR Am J Roentgenol. 181(3):879-84, 2003
6. De Potter P: Current treatment of retinoblastoma. Curr Opin Ophthalmol. 13(5):331-6, 2002
7. Brisse HJ et al: Sonographic, CT, and MR imaging findings in diffuse infiltrative retinoblastoma: report of two cases with histologic comparison. AJNR Am J Neuroradiol. 22(3):499-504, 2001
8. Shields CL et al: Recent developments in the management of retinoblastoma. J Pediatr Ophthalmol Strabismus. 36(1):8-18; quiz 35-6, 1999
9. Kaufman LM et al: Retinoblastoma and simulating lesions. Role of CT, MR imaging and use of Gd-DTPA contrast enhancement. Radiol Clin North Am. 36(6):1101-17, 1998
10. Skulski M et al: Trilateral retinoblastoma with suprasellar involvement. Neuroradiology. 39(1):41-3, 1997
11. Wong FL et al: Cancer incidence after retinoblastoma. Radiation dose and sarcoma risk. JAMA. 278(15):1262-7, 1997
12. Provenzale JM et al: Radiologic-pathologic correlation. Bilateral retinoblastoma with coexistent pinealoblastoma (trilateral retinoblastoma). AJNR Am J Neuroradiol. 16(1):157-65, 1995

# RETINOBLASTOMA

## IMAGE GALLERY

### Typical

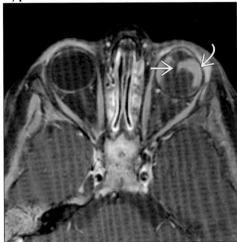

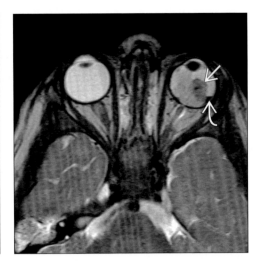

*(Left) Axial T1WI FS MR shows a hypointense, nonenhancing left intraocular mass with associated retinal detachment ➡ and hyperintense subretinal hemorrhage ➡. (Right) Axial T2WI MR shows hypointense T2 signal intensity within intraocular mass ➡, characteristic of retinoblastoma. Notice associated fluid-fluid level ➡ in the subretinal hemorrhage.*

### Typical

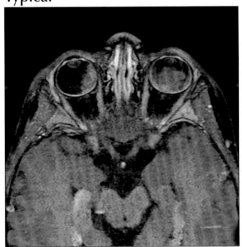

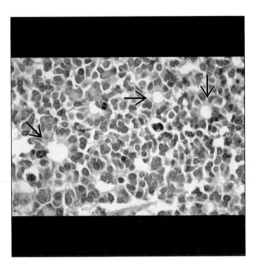

*(Left) Axial T1 C+ FS MR shows bilateral, enhancing intraocular masses without extension beyond the sclera or into the optic nerves in a child with bilateral retinoblastoma. (Right) Micropathology shows several Flexner-Wintersteiner rosettes ➡ in a sea of bluish-red cells with scant cytoplasm. (Courtesy B. Ey, MD).*

### Typical

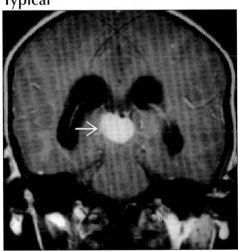

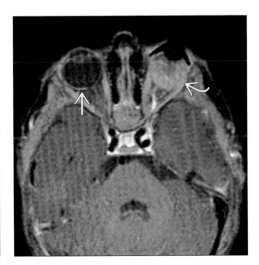

*(Left) Coronal T1 C+ MR shows a diffusely enhancing ➡ mass in the pineal region, in a child treated for bilateral retinoblastoma, consistent with trilateral retinoblastoma. (Courtesy B. Ey, MD). (Right) Axial T1WI FS MR shows contrast-enhancement of the left hydroxyapatite orbital implant ➡ in a patient with bilateral RB, residual disease in the right globe ➡.*

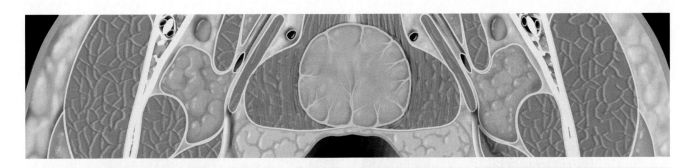

# SECTION 3: Suprahyoid & Infrahyoid Neck

# CONGENITAL LESIONS OF THE NECK

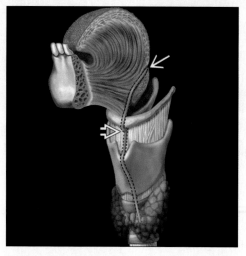

Sagittal oblique graphic shows path of thyroglossal duct as it descends from the foramen cecum at tongue base ➡, curves around hyoid bone ➡, then descends off midline to thyroid gland.

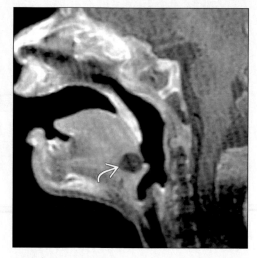

Sagittal T1 C+ FS MR shows an incidental hypointense cyst ➡ located in the posterior tongue at the foramen cecum. The patient was studied for a facial hemangioma.

## TERMINOLOGY

### Abbreviations
- First branchial cleft cyst (1st BCC)
- Second branchial cleft cyst (2nd BCC)
- Third branchial cleft cyst (3rd BCC)
- Fourth branchial anomaly (4th BA): From 4th branchial pouch, not cleft
- Thyroglossal duct cyst (TGDC)
- Cervical thymic cyst (CTC): From 3rd branchial pouch
- Lymphatic malformation (LM) = lymphangioma, cystic hygroma
- Venous vascular malformation (VVM) = cavernous hemangioma = misnomer
- Capillary malformation = port-wine stains, capillary hemangioma, nevus flammeus
- Infantile hemangioma = strawberry hemangioma, cutaneous hemangioma-vascular complex syndrome

### Definitions
- Branchial cleft cyst
  - Fluid-containing cyst with well-defined wall formed from failure of obliteration of a portion of branchial apparatus (cleft or pouch)
    - 1st BCC: Failure of obliteration of portion 1st branchial apparatus
    - 2nd BCC: Failure of obliteration of portion 2nd branchial apparatus
    - 3rd BCC: Failure of obliteration of portion 3rd branchial apparatus
- Branchial sinus
  - Congenital tract with one opening to skin surface or external auditory canal (1st BC sinus), pharynx (2nd BC sinus) or superolateral hypopharynx (3rd BC sinus)
  - 4th BA: Most commonly sinus tract from inferior tip of LEFT pyriform sinus to anterior thyroid bed
- Branchial fistula
  - Congenital residual tract with two openings, one to skin surface and one to external auditory canal (1st BC fistula) or pharynx (2-3rd BC fistula)

- By definition a branchial fistula arises as an epithelial-lined tract left behind when there is persistence of both a branchial cleft and its corresponding pharyngeal pouch
- Branchial fistula is a congenital malformation that connects the skin to the lumen of the foregut
- Thyroglossal duct cyst
  - Congenital cyst arising from failure of a segment of the thyroglossal duct to involute
- Cervical thymic cyst (3rd branchial anomaly)
  - Congenital cervical neck cyst resulting from incomplete obliteration of thymopharyngeal duct, a remnant of 3rd branchial pouch
- Vascular malformations
  - Lymphatic malformation: Unilocular or multilocular congenital cystic mass composed of endothelium-lined lymphatic channels that are separated by connective tissue stroma
  - Capillary malformation: Low-flow lesion that may be associated with distribution of trigeminal nerve in case of Sturge-Weber syndrome
  - Venous vascular malformation: Congenital low-flow soft tissue lesion supplied by small arteries
  - Arteriovenous malformation: High-flow congenital malformation resulting from abnormal blood vessel morphogenesis and arteriovenous malformations
- Infantile hemangioma: Congenital high-flow neoplasia that presents in early infancy, rapidly enlarges, then involutes by 8-10 years of age

## EMBRYOLOGY

### Embryologic Events
- Branchial apparatus
  - Branchial apparatus is 1st identified in 4th week of embryogenesis & is complete by 7th week
  - 1st branchial apparatus ectodermal portion forms external auditory canal & external layer of tympanic membrane
  - 2nd branchial arch overgrows the 3rd & 4th arches at about 6th week of fetal development

# CONGENITAL LESIONS OF THE NECK

## Differential Diagnosis

### Important Concepts
- Differentiate cyst versus sinus versus fistula
- Locations of branchial clefts and arches
- Location of thymopharyngeal, thyroglossal ducts
- Lymphatic system formation in head and neck

### Disorders of Branchial Apparatus
- 1st branchial cleft cyst, type 1
- 1st branchial cleft cyst, type 2
- 2nd branchial cleft cyst
- 3rd branchial cleft cyst
- 4th branchial apparatus anomaly (sinus tract with or without cyst)

### Disorders of Thymopharyngeal Duct
- Ectopic thymus
- Cervical thymic remnant

- Cervical thymic cyst (third pouch remnant)

### Disorders of Thyroglossal Duct
- Ectopic thyroid gland
- Thyroid tissue remnant
- Thyroglossal duct cyst

### Vascular/Lymphatic Malformations
- Lymphatic malformation
- Capillary malformation
- Venous vascular malformation
- Arteriovenous malformation

### Benign Masses
- Infantile hemangioma
  - Benign tumor; spontaneously regresses
- Dermoid

- - Cavity created by this embryologic event is referred to as cervical sinus of His
  - Cervical sinus of His covers 2nd, 3rd & 4th arches & clefts
- Thyroid gland migration, foramen cecum to low cervical neck
  - Median thyroid anlage buds from foramen cecum in midline at junction of anterior 2/3-posterior 1/3 of tongue
  - Thyroglossal duct diverticulum descends caudally in midline neck, migrates off midline as it reaches thyroid bed in lower cervical neck
  - Median thyroid anlage path passes along anterior surface of developing hyoid bone
  - When hyoid bone rotates to adult position, takes adherent tract under and deep to hyoid bone, placing this portion of tract into area just anterior to pre-epiglottic space of larynx
- Thymus descent into upper mediastinum
  - Develops from outpouching of ventral portions of 3rd pharyngeal pouches during 6th week of gestation
    - Outpouching elongates caudally
  - Thymic outpouchings are connected bilaterally to pharynx by thymopharyngeal ducts
  - Thymic primordia migrate caudally & medially
    - Obliterated thymopharyngeal ducts lie just below thyroid glands by middle of 7th week of embryogenesis
  - By end of 9th week gestation, thymic glands are in final anterior mediastinal location
- Lymphatic system formation in extracranial head & neck
  - Lymphatic system develops separately from veins initially within fetal mesenchyme
  - Lymphatic system forms communications with the venous system later

## Practical Implications
- 1st branchial apparatus anomalies
  - Failure of involution of 1st branchial apparatus components leads to 1st BC anomalies

- - Both type 1 & 2 1st BCC may communicate with bony-cartilaginous junction of external auditory canal
- 2nd, 3rd & 4th branchial apparatus anomalies
  - Vestigial remnant theory of formation of branchial cleft anomalies
  - Suggests that if any portion of the cervical sinus of His, branchial pouch or branchial cleft fails to involute during embryogenesis, this focus can become a cyst, sinus or fistula
    - When sinus of His fails to obliterate, branchial cleft cysts, fistulae or sinuses develop
  - 2nd, 3rd & 4th branchial anomalies result depending on area of sinus of His that does not involute completely
- Thyroglossal duct anomalies
  - Ectopic thyroid gland
    - Incomplete descent of thyroid into low neck
    - Can be seen anywhere along course from foramen cecum in tongue base to superior mediastinum
    - Most common location in neck is just deep to = "lingual thyroid" foramen cecum in tongue base
  - Thyroid tissue remnants
    - Sequestration of thyroid tissue along thyroglossal duct
    - Can be seen anywhere along course of thyroglossal duct from foramen cecum to thyroid bed of low cervical neck
    - Pyramidal lobe of thyroid is midline normal variant remnant of this process
    - Lingual thyroid gland from lack of migration of tissue
    - Thyroglossal duct cysts often have thyroid tissue in wall
  - Thyroglossal duct cyst
    - Results from failure of involution of portion of thyroglossal duct
    - Can occur anywhere along course of thyroglossal duct from foramen cecum at tongue base to just anterior to thyroid lobes
    - Most occur in midline in vicinity of hyoid bone

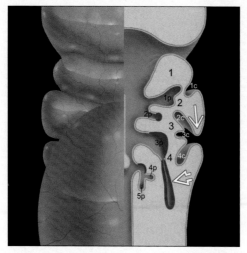
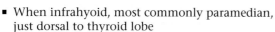

Anteroposterior graphic of a 6 week old fetus shows 2nd branchial arch ➡ growing inferiorly over 3rd and 4th arches, resulting in cavity (cervical sinus of His). Note developing thymopharyngeal duct ➡.

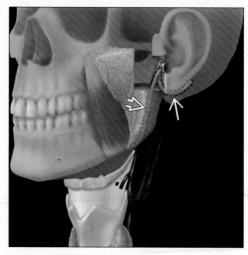

Graphic shows tract of type 1 1st BC anomaly ➡ from medial bony EAC toward retroauricular area. Tract of type 2 1st BC anomaly ➡ connects EAC to angle of mandible.

- When infrahyoid, most commonly paramedian, just dorsal to thyroid lobe
- Thymic anomalies
  - Ectopic thymus
    - Incomplete descent of thymus into chest
    - Rare congenital lesion
    - Found in cervicothoracic junction when present
  - Thymic tissue remnants
    - Sequestration of thymic tissue along thymopharyngeal duct course
    - Thymic gland remnants can be found anywhere along thymopharyngeal duct in lateral neck
    - Connected to mediastinal thymus or isolated
    - Solid thymic tissue rests can mimic tumor clinically & on imaging
  - Cervical thymic cyst
    - Failure of involution of thymopharyngeal duct in cervical neck or upper mediastinum
    - Cyst may be found anywhere along LEFT TGD
    - At level of thyroid gland, CTC may exactly mimic thyroid or parathyroid cyst
    - If large, present as dumbbell cyst in cervicothoracic junction
    - Mediastinal thymic cyst also found without cervical neck component
- Lymphatic system anomalies
  - Lymphatic malformation results from enlargement of isolated lymphatic channels that do not communicate with regional veins
  - 3 hypotheses for this malformation
    - Failure of primordial lymphatic sacs to drain into adjacent veins
    - Abnormal sequestration of lymphatic tissue
    - Abnormal budding of lymphatics from lymphatic primordia

## CUSTOM DIFFERENTIAL DIAGNOSIS

### Pediatric Cystic Neck Mass
- Congenital
  - 1st BCC

- 2nd BCC
- 3rd BCC
- TGDC
- Lymphatic malformation
- Thymic cyst
- Inflammatory
  - Retention cyst (vallecula, tonsil)
  - Ranula
- Infectious
  - Suppurative node
  - Abscess
- Vascular
  - Carotid artery pseudoaneurysm
  - Venous malformation
- Degenerative
  - Laryngocele
  - Thyroid cyst
- Benign tumor
  - Lymphoepithelial tumor
  - Cystic schwannoma
  - Neurofibroma
  - Dermoid
- Malignant tumor, primary
  - Mucoepidermoid
  - Angiosarcoma
- Malignant tumor, metastatic nodes
  - Papillary carcinoma of thyroid

## RELATED REFERENCES

1. Koch BL: Cystic malformations of the neck in children. Pediatr Radiol. 35(5):463-77, 2005
2. D'Souza AR et al: Updating concepts of first branchial cleft defects: a literature review. Int J Pediatr Otorhinolaryngol. 62(2):103-9, 2002
3. Mandell DL: Head and neck anomalies related to the branchial apparatus. Otolaryngol Clin North Am. 33(6):1309-32, 2000
4. Koeller KK et al: Congenital cystic masses of the neck: radiologic-pathologic correlation. Radiographics. 19(1):121-46; quiz 152-3, 1999
5. Mulliken JB et al: Classification of pediatric vascular lesions. Plast Reconstr Surg. 70(1):120-1, 1982

# CONGENITAL LESIONS OF THE NECK

## IMAGE GALLERY

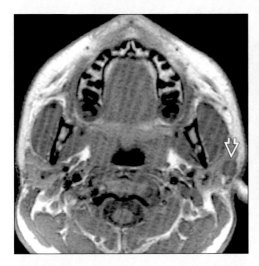
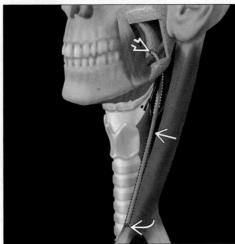

*(Left)* Axial T1WI MR shows large lesion ➡ arising in the lateral aspect of the left parotid gland. This is a focal enlargement of a tract starting at the EAC and terminating in anterolateral neck. *(Right)* Graphic of tract of 2nd branchial cleft fistula ➡ shows proximal opening ➡ in faucial tonsil and distal opening in anterior supraclavicular neck ➡.

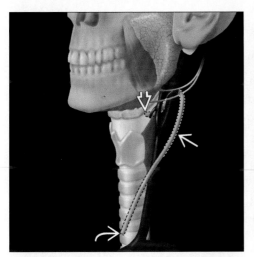
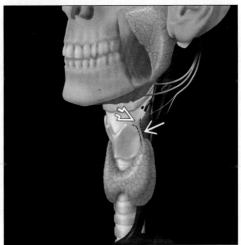

*(Left)* Sagittal oblique graphic of the neck shows tract of 3rd branchial cleft anomaly ➡ extending from cephalad aspect of lateral hypopharynx ➡ to skin of supraclavicular anterior neck ➡. *(Right)* Sagittal oblique graphic of neck shows tract of 4th branchial cleft anomaly ➡ extending from hypopharynx ➡ to location of left thyroid lobe. This lesion often presents with thyroiditis.

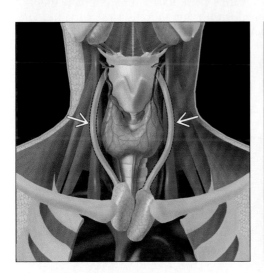
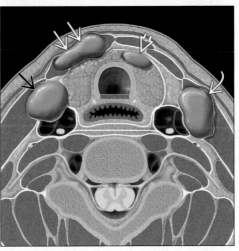

*(Left)* Anteroposterior graphic shows thymopharyngeal duct tracts ➡ extending from the lateral hypopharyngeal region to the location of the normal lobes of the thymus in the superior mediastinum. *(Right)* Axial graphic shows locations of 4 major congenital cystic lesions of neck. Infrahyoid 2nd & 3rd BCC ➡, infrahyoid TGDC ➡, 4th BCC ➡, and cervical thymic cyst ➡.

# LINGUAL THYROID

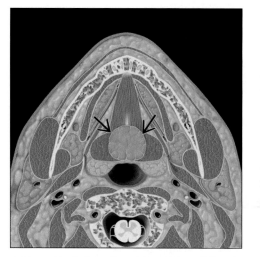

*Axial graphic depicts a lingual thyroid focus ➡ in the posterior midline of the tongue, just deep to location of foramen cecum.*

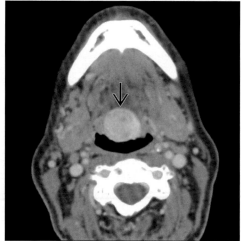

*Axial CECT shows a round to ovoid, well delineated enhancing mass in the posterior tongue ➡.*

## TERMINOLOGY

### Abbreviations and Synonyms
- Ectopic thyroid tissue, thyroid dysgenesis

### Definitions
- Lingual thyroid: Thyroid tissue in abnormal location in tongue base or floor of mouth

## IMAGING FINDINGS

### General Features
- Best diagnostic clue: Well-circumscribed midline or paramedian tongue mass, with density/intensity similar to normal thyroid tissue
- Location
  - Usually in midline dorsum of the tongue
  - Less commonly found in sublingual space or tongue root along course of thyroglossal duct
- Size: 1-3 cm
- Morphology: Well-circumscribed, round/ovoid

### CT Findings
- NECT
  - High density sharply marginated midline foramen cecum area lesion
    - High density secondary to iodine accumulation
- CECT: Avid homogeneous enhancement

### MR Findings
- T1WI: Increased signal intensity compared to tongue musculature
- T2WI: High signal midline mass
- T1 C+: Avid homogeneous enhancement

### Nuclear Medicine Findings
- Technetium 99m pertechnetate scan preferred over iodine 123 in children to confirm ectopic thyroid tissue
  - Uptake confirms gland-like nature of tongue mess
  - Not trapped within thyroid cells (unlike iodine) so less radiation to gland

---

## DDx: Solid Tongue Masses

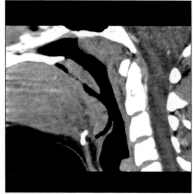

*Enlarged Lingual Tonsil*

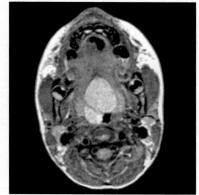

*Rhabdomyosarcoma*

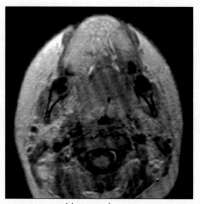

*Hemangioma*

# LINGUAL THYROID

## Key Facts

### Terminology
- Lingual thyroid: Thyroid tissue in abnormal location in tongue base or floor of mouth

### Imaging Findings
- Best diagnostic clue: Well-circumscribed midline or paramedian tongue mass, with density/intensity similar to normal thyroid tissue

### Top Differential Diagnoses
- Thyroglossal Duct Cyst (TGDC), Suprahyoid
- Dermoid or Epidermoid, Oral Cavity
- Enlarged Lingual Tonsil

### Diagnostic Checklist
- Lingual thyroid is only functioning thyroid tissue in 75% of cases

## DIFFERENTIAL DIAGNOSIS

### Thyroglossal Duct Cyst (TGDC), Suprahyoid
- Cystic midline mass along course of thyroglossal duct

### Dermoid or Epidermoid, Oral Cavity
- Cystic, well-demarcated mass ± fatty components

### Rhabdomyosarcoma
- Aggressive mass

### Hemangioma
- Hypervascular mass, infiltrative; more homogeneity and T2 bright signal than rhabdomyosarcoma

### Enlarged Lingual Tonsil
- Mucosal lesion; appearance similar to other (hypertrophied) lymphoid structures

## PATHOLOGY

### General Features
- Etiology
  - Arrest of thyroid anlage migration within tongue base between 3rd & 7th week of gestation
    - Complete arrest: No cervical thyroid (75%)
    - Partial arrest: Cervical thyroid components present (25%)
- Epidemiology
  - Most common location of ectopic thyroid tissue (90%)
  - Reported incidence: 1:3,000 to 1:10,000

## CLINICAL ISSUES

### Presentation
- Most common signs/symptoms
  - Dysphonia, throat fullness, dysphagia
  - Rare hyperthyroidism, or stridor in infants

### Natural History & Prognosis
- Lingual thyroid may expand rapidly during puberty

## DIAGNOSTIC CHECKLIST

### Image Interpretation Pearls
- If lingual thyroid identified on CECT, remember to comment on status of cervical thyroid tissues
  - Lingual thyroid is only functioning thyroid tissue in 75% of cases

## SELECTED REFERENCES

1. Aktolun C et al: Diagnosis of complete ectopic lingual thyroid with Tc-99m pertechnetate scintigraphy. Clin Nucl Med. 26(11):933-5, 2001
2. Massine RE et al: Lingual thyroid carcinoma: a case report and review of the literature. Thyroid. 11(12):1191-6, 2001
3. Takashima S et al: MR imaging of the lingual thyroid. Comparison to other submucosal lesions. Acta Radiol. 42(4):376-82, 2001

## IMAGE GALLERY

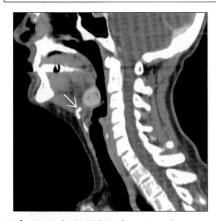
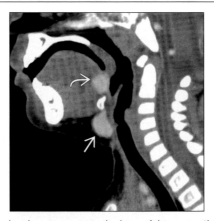
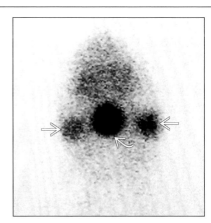

*(Left)* Sagittal 2D CECT reformation shows a round, enhancing mass in the base of the tongue/foramen cecum location, with absent thyroid in inferior neck. The hyoid bone ➡ is deformed. *(Center)* Sagittal CECT shows relatively homogeneous posterior ➡ and inferior ➡ midline masses in the midline. This was multifocal, ectopic thyroid tissue. *(Right)* Axial image from a Tc-99m pertechnetate nuclear scan demonstrates activity within a mass at the base of the tongue ➡. Radionuclide uptake also evident in the parotid glands ➡.

# DERMOID, AND EPIDERMOID ORAL CAVITY

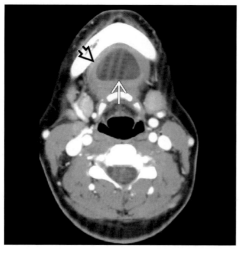

*Axial CECT shows a midline nonenhancing cystic mass in the floor of the mouth ➡, not associated with the hyoid bone. It is bordered by the mylohyoid muscle ⊳.*

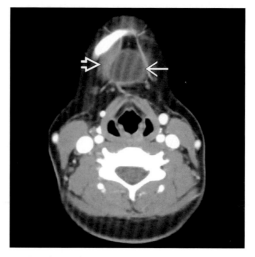

*Axial CECT in the same patient as previous image shows the inferior most extension of the dermoid ➡. Anterior belly of the digastric muscle ➡ is slightly bowed.*

## TERMINOLOGY

### Abbreviations and Synonyms
- Developmental oral cavity (OC) cyst, ectodermal inclusion cyst, dermoid cyst

### Definitions
- Cystic, OC lesion resulting from congenital epithelial inclusion or rest
  - Dermoid: Epithelial elements plus dermal substructure including dermal appendages
  - Epidermoid: Epithelial elements only

## IMAGING FINDINGS

### General Features
- Best diagnostic clue
  - Dermoid: Cystic, well-demarcated OC mass with fatty, fluid or mixed contents
  - Epidermoid: Cystic, well-demarcated OC mass with fluid contents only
- Location

  - Dermoid and epidermoid OC lesions most commonly involve floor of the mouth
    - Submandibular space (SMS), sublingual space (SLS) or root of tongue (ROT)
    - ROT: Potential space in inferior, midline tongue between genioglossus-geniohyoid muscles
- Size: Typically < 4 cm as clinically evident early
- Morphology
  - Ovoid or tubular
    - Most show thin definable wall (75%)
    - No nodular soft tissue in wall or outside cyst (80%)

### CT Findings
- NECT
  - Low density, unilocular, well-circumscribed mass
    - Dermoid: Fatty internal material, mixed density fluid, calcification (< 50%) all possible
    - Epidermoid: Fluid density material inside lesion without complex features
  - If dermoid contains no fatty elements, will be indistinguishable from epidermoid
- CECT
  - Lesion wall may be imperceptible

## DDx: Other Cystic Oral Masses

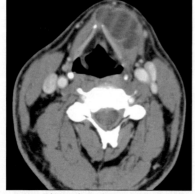

*Thyroglossal Duct Cyst*

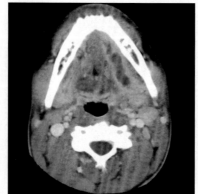

*Sialodochitis*

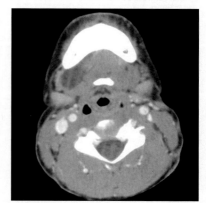

*Simple Ranula*

# DERMOID, AND EPIDERMOID ORAL CAVITY

## Key Facts

### Terminology
- Developmental oral cavity (OC) cyst, ectodermal inclusion cyst, dermoid cyst
- Cystic, OC lesion resulting from congenital epithelial inclusion or rest
- Dermoid: Epithelial elements plus dermal substructure including dermal appendages
- Epidermoid: Epithelial elements only

### Imaging Findings
- Dermoid: Cystic, well-demarcated OC mass with fatty, fluid or mixed contents
- Epidermoid: Cystic, well-demarcated OC mass with fluid contents only
- Dermoid and epidermoid OC lesions most commonly involve floor of the mouth

- Submandibular space (SMS), sublingual space (SLS) or root of tongue (ROT)
- If dermoid contains no fatty elements, will be indistinguishable from epidermoid
- If complex signal present, most likely dermoid, not epidermoid
- CECT = MR unless extensive dental amalgam

### Top Differential Diagnoses
- Thyroglossal Duct Cyst (TGDC), Suprahyoid
- Oral Cavity Lymphangioma
- Simple Ranula
- Diving Ranula
- Oral Cavity Abscess

---

- ○ Subtle rim-enhancement of wall sometimes seen

## MR Findings
- T1WI
  - ○ Dermoid: Well-circumscribed, SLS, SMS or ROT lesion with complex fluid
    - ▪ If fatty elements, focal or diffuse high signal present
  - ○ Epidermoid: Well-circumscribed SLS, SMS or ROT lesion with homogeneous fluid signal
    - ▪ If complex signal present, most likely dermoid, not epidermoid
    - ▪ Diffuse high signal may be from high protein fluid
- T2WI
  - ○ Dermoid: Heterogeneous high signal
    - ▪ Intermediate signal if fat
    - ▪ Focal areas of low signal if calcifications
  - ○ Epidermoid: Homogeneous high signal
- T1 C+
  - ○ Thin rim-enhancement or none
  - ○ If fat-saturation is used, areas of fat will be low signal in dermoid

## Ultrasonographic Findings
- Useful for evaluation of superficial lesions
- Dermoid: Mixed internal echoes from fat with echogenic foci with dense shadowing if calcifications
- Epidermoid: "Pseudosolid" appearance with uniform internal echoes
  - ○ Cellular material within cyst creates "pseudosolid" appearance
  - ○ Posterior wall echo enhancement is clue to cystic nature of lesion

## Imaging Recommendations
- Best imaging tool
  - ○ CECT = MR unless extensive dental amalgam
  - ○ MR used if dental amalgam obscures CECT
- Protocol advice
  - ○ Routine CECT of cervical soft tissues
  - ○ If use MR, get T1 pre-contrast & use fat-saturation techniques to diagnose dermoid

## DIFFERENTIAL DIAGNOSIS

### Thyroglossal Duct Cyst (TGDC), Suprahyoid
- Midline unilocular cystic mass between hyoid bone & foramen cecum
- In upper neck, paramedian anterior mass associated with hyoid bone
- No complex elements (no fat or calcifications)
- When in posterior tongue root, may mimic epidermoid

### Oral Cavity Lymphangioma
- Multilocular trans-spatial cystic mass
- Generally does not involve SLS

### Simple Ranula
- Unilateral low density/signal mass in SLS with thin, nonenhancing wall
- May exactly mimic epidermoid of SLS

### Diving Ranula
- Simple ranula that ruptures from SLS into SMS
- Comet-shaped unilocular mass with tail in collapsed SLS ("tail sign") & "head" in posterior SMS

### Oral Cavity Abscess
- Clinical setting of septic patient with painful OC mass is distinctive
- Rim-enhancing cystic mass often with extensive tongue & soft tissue cellulitis-edema

## PATHOLOGY

### General Features
- Etiology
  - ○ Congenital inclusion of dermal elements at site of embryonic 1st & 2nd second branchial arches
    - ▪ Sequestration of trapped surface ectoderm
- Epidemiology
  - ○ Present from birth; spontaneous occurrence
  - ○ Dermoid/epidermoid are least common of all congenital neck lesions

○ OC dermoids account for < 25% of all dermoids of H&N (orbit most common)

## Gross Pathologic & Surgical Features
- Oily or cheesy material, tan, yellow or white
  ○ May contain blood or chronic blood products
- Cyst wall ⇒ fibrous capsule; 2-6 mm in thickness

## Microscopic Features
- Epidermoid
  ○ Simple squamous cell epithelium with a fibrous wall
- Dermoid
  ○ Contains dermal structures including sebaceous glands, hair follicles, blood vessels, fat ± collagen
    ▪ Sweat glands in minority (20%)
    ▪ Lined by keratinizing squamous epithelium
- Teratoid cysts (rare lesion)
  ○ Contain elements from all 3 germ cell layers

## Staging, Grading or Classification Criteria
- Meyer Classification of Dysontogenetic Cysts of Floor of Mouth
  ○ Epidermoid: Lined with simple squamous epithelium & surrounding connective tissue
  ○ Dermoid: Epithelium-lined cyst that contains skin appendages
  ○ Teratoid: Epithelium-lined cyst that contains mesodermal or endodermal elements such as muscle, bones, teeth & mucous membranes

# CLINICAL ISSUES

## Presentation
- Most common signs/symptoms
  ○ Painless subcutaneous or submucosal mass (85-90%)
  ○ Other signs/symptoms
    ▪ Dysphagia; globus oral sensation
    ▪ Airway encroachment when large

## Demographics
- Age: All pediatric age groups, unusual before age 5 years

## Natural History & Prognosis
- Benign lesion, usually cosmetic considerations
- Very slow growth, dormant for years
  ○ Present during childhood but small & dormant
  ○ Becomes symptomatic during rapid growth phase in young adult
- Sudden growth or change following rupture
  ○ Significant inflammation & increased size (rare complication)

## Treatment
- Surgical resection is curative
  ○ Entire cyst must be removed to prevent recurrence
- Extracapsular excision can be performed by intraoral or external approach
  ○ Surgical approach may be decided by lesion position relative to mylohyoid muscle
    ▪ SLS: (Superomedial to mylohyoid muscle) intraoral approach; good cosmetic & functional results
    ▪ SMS: (Inferolateral to mylohyoid) submandibular approach
- Steroids or non-steroidal drugs to calm inflammation in ruptured lesions
- Post-operative complications are rare

# DIAGNOSTIC CHECKLIST

## Image Interpretation Pearls
- Cyst found in oral cavity
  ○ Sublingual space ± submandibular space
    ▪ SLS ranula, dermoid, epidermoid or lymphangioma
    ▪ Simple ranula may exactly mimic epidermoid (fluid only)
    ▪ Dermoid (complex elements) vs. lymphangioma (fluid only, multilocular, trans-spatial)
  ○ Root of tongue cyst
    ▪ Dermoid, epidermoid or suprahyoid TGDC
    ▪ Dermoid (complex elements) vs. epidermoid (fluid only)
    ▪ Suprahyoid TGDC: Along tract from hyoid bone to foramen cecum

# SELECTED REFERENCES

1. Din SU: Dermoid cyst of the floor of mouth. J Coll Physicians Surg Pak. 13(7):416-7, 2003
2. Ho MW et al: Simultaneous occurrence of sublingual dermoid cyst and oral alimentary tract cyst in an infant: a case report and review of the literature. Int J Paediatr Dent. 13(6):441-6, 2003
3. Longo F et al: Midline (dermoid) cysts of the floor of the mouth: report of 16 cases and review of surgical techniques. Plast Reconstr Surg. 112(6):1560-5, 2003
4. Fuchshuber S et al: Dermoid cyst of the floor of the mouth--a case report. Eur Arch Otorhinolaryngol. 259(2):60-2, 2002
5. Eaton D et al: Congenital foregut duplication cysts of the anterior tongue. Arch Otolaryngol Head Neck Surg. 127(12):1484-7, 2001
6. Mathews J et al: True lateral dermoid cyst of the floor of the mouth. J Laryngol Otol. 115(4):333-5, 2001
7. Myssiorek D et al: Intralingual dermoid cysts: a report of two new cases. Ear Nose Throat J. 79(5):380-3, 2000
8. Godden DR et al: Sliding dermoid cyst. A case report. Int J Oral Maxillofac Surg. 28(6):459-60, 1999
9. Yousem DM et al: Oral cavity and pharynx. Radiol Clin North Am. 36(5):967-81, vii, 1998
10. Miles LP et al: Congenital dermoid cyst of the tongue. J Laryngol Otol. 111(12):1179-82, 1997
11. Oygur T et al: Oral congenital dermoid cyst in the floor of the mouth of a newborn. The significance of gastrointestinal-type epithelium. Oral Surg Oral Med Oral Pathol. 74(5):627-30, 1992
12. Tuffin JR et al: True lateral dermoid cyst of the neck. Int J Oral Maxillofac Surg. 20(5):275-6, 1991
13. al-Khayat M et al: Midline sublingual dermoid cyst. J Laryngol Otol. 104(7):578-80, 1990
14. Arcand P et al: Congenital dermoid cyst of the oral cavity with gastric choristoma. J Otolaryngol. 17(5):219-22, 1988
15. Howell CJ: The sublingual dermoid cyst. Report of five cases and review of the literature. Oral Surg Oral Med Oral Pathol. 59(6):578-80, 1985
16. Gibson WS Jr et al: Congenital sublingual dermoid cyst. Arch Otolaryngol. 108(11):745-8, 1982

# DERMOID, AND EPIDERMOID ORAL CAVITY

## IMAGE GALLERY

### Typical

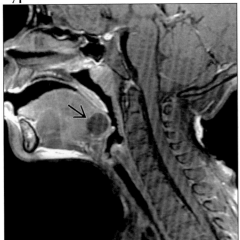
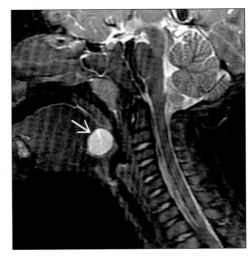

*(Left)* Sagittal T1WI FS MR shows a rounded, well-defined homogeneous mass ➡ at the base of the tongue just above the vallecula. Mass does not enhance. *(Right)* Sagittal T2WI FS MR (same patient as previous image) shows the ovoid dermoid ➡ at the tongue base to be homogeneously hyperintense.

### Typical

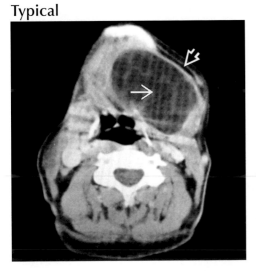
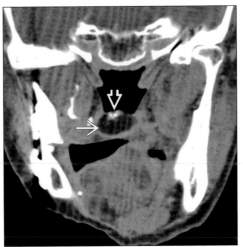

*(Left)* Axial CECT shows a compound dermoid of the floor of the mouth and left submandibular space ➡. Multiple rounded foci of low attenuation represent fat globules, "sack-of-marbles", appearance ➡. *(Right)* Coronal CECT demonstrates a superficial calcification ➡ within a hypodense posterior tongue dermoid ➡. The mass is primarily fatty with attenuation similar to subcutaneous fat.

### Variant

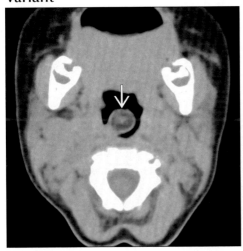
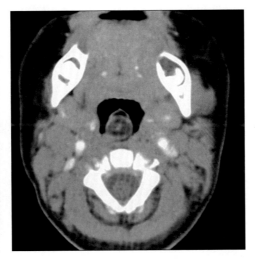

*(Left)* Axial NECT shows mixed hypo and isoattenuation pedunculated mass ➡ lying within the central oropharynx. *(Right)* Axial CECT (same mass as previous image), no enhancement evident. Characteristics are those of a dermoid. Pathology demonstrated skin covered mass with branchial cleft remnants.

# REACTIVE NODES/CERVICAL LYMPHADENITIS

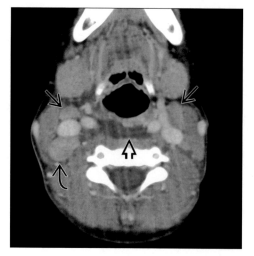

*Axial CECT shows enlarged, reactive bilateral internal jugular ➡ and right spinal accessory ➔ lymph nodes and retropharyngeal edema ▷.*

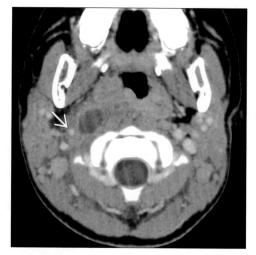

*Axial CECT shows large low attenuation right lateral retropharyngeal lymph node (phlegmon or early abscess) and decrease in right internal carotid artery caliber ➡ in the same patient as previous image.*

## TERMINOLOGY

### Abbreviations and Synonyms
- Reactive adenopathy, lymphadenitis

### Definitions
- Non-neoplastic enlargement of lymph nodes
  - Acute or chronic
  - Localized or generalized
  - Suppurative or nonsuppurative

## IMAGING FINDINGS

### General Features
- Best diagnostic clue
  - Well-defined multiple oval-shaped nodes, increased in number and/or size
  - Low attenuation center phlegmon vs. early suppuration (pus within lymph node)
- Location
  - Any nodal group in the head and neck
  - Lateral retropharyngeal nodes common in asymptomatic children

- Size
  - Large size range
  - May be multiple centimeters in child & still be reactive node
- Morphology: Well-defined oval shaped nodes rather than round

### CT Findings
- CECT
  - Variable enhancement, usually mild
  - Enhancing linear markings within hilum of node
  - +/- Associated enlargement of Waldeyer ring (nasopharyngeal adenoids, palatine tonsils, lingual tonsils)
    - Common in EBV/mononucleosis
  - +/- Stranding of adjacent fat = cellulitis
  - +/- Enlargement of adjacent muscles = myositis
  - +/- Thick enhancing nodal wall with central low attenuation = phlegmon vs. early abscess/suppuration
  - +/- Soft tissue abscess secondary to rupture of suppurative node into adjacent soft tissues

### MR Findings
- T1WI: Homogeneous low to intermediate signal

## DDx: Cervical Lymphadenopathy

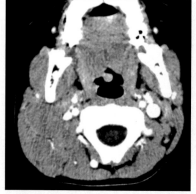

*Lymphoma*

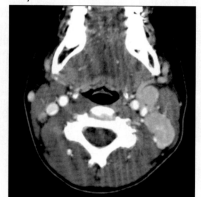

*Metastatic Thyroid Cancer*

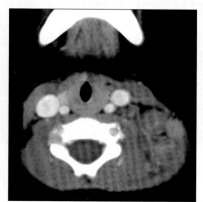

*Neuroblastoma*

# REACTIVE NODES/CERVICAL LYMPHADENITIS

## Key Facts

### Terminology
- Non-neoplastic enlargement of lymph nodes

### Imaging Findings
- Well-defined multiple oval-shaped nodes, increased in number and/or size
- Low attenuation center phlegmon vs. early suppuration (pus within lymph node)
- Variable enhancement, usually mild
- Enhancing linear markings within hilum of node

### Top Differential Diagnoses
- Lymphoma Nodes (HD or NHL)
- Metastatic Disease
- Posttransplant Lymphoproliferative Disorder (PTLD)

### Pathology
- Viral disease: EBV (most common), CMV, HSV, measles, HIV (rare in children)
- Bacterial disease: Streptococcus, Staphylococcus, Bartonella henselae (most common causative agent in cat scratch disease)
- Mycobacterium tuberculosis, atypical mycobacterium (nontuberculous mycobacterium) = M. avium-intracellulare (MAI), M. scrofulaceum, M. kansasii

### Diagnostic Checklist
- Lymph nodes with low attenuation centers and lack of surrounding cellulitis: Think atypical mycobacterium
- Cervical adenopathy plus Waldeyer ring hypertrophy: Think EBV or lymphoma

- T2WI
  - Homogeneous intermediate to high signal intensity
  - Central hyperintensity in suppurative node
- T1 C+
  - Variable enhancement, usually mild
  - Enhancing linear markings within node may be seen
  - Central nonenhancement in suppurative node
  - +/- Diffuse strandy soft tissue enhancement

## Ultrasonographic Findings
- Oval shaped nodes with echogenic vascular hilus
- Central hypoechogenicity in suppurative node or soft tissue abscess
- Most specific imaging modality: Phlegmon vs. abscess with drainable pus

## Nuclear Medicine Findings
- PET
  - Mild uptake of FDG may be seen
  - Marked uptake more likely with active granulomatous disease or tumor

## Imaging Recommendations
- Best imaging tool
  - CECT is first line tool for evaluation of adenopathy in the head and neck
    - Differentiates cellulitis vs. phlegmon vs. early abscess (low attenuation center suggests abscess, however may still be phlegmon without drainable pus)
    - Best evaluation of total extent of disease: Assess mediastinal, intraspinal, intracranial extension
    - Assess caliber of carotid artery and patency of jugular vein
- Protocol advice: Contrast-enhancement important to detect suppurative intranodal change and vessels

## DIFFERENTIAL DIAGNOSIS

### Lymphoma Nodes (HD or NHL)
- Multiple nodes enlarged ± enlargement of Waldeyer ring

- Homogeneous mild contrast-enhancement
- Systemic involvement common
- Unilateral or bilateral

### Metastatic Disease
- Neuroblastoma in young children
  - Metastatic cervical neuroblastoma much more common than primary cervical neuroblastoma
- Thyroid carcinoma in adolescents
- Nasopharyngeal carcinoma in adolescents
- Supraclavicular node suggests chest or body primary

### Posttransplant Lymphoproliferative Disorder (PTLD)
- Cervical lymphadenopathy
- Adenotonsillar hypertrophy, may lead to upper airway obstruction
- Associated findings: Sinusitis, otitis media

## PATHOLOGY

### General Features
- General path comments
  - Reactive nonsuppurative nodes are initial response to infection
    - May transform to phlegmon and then suppurative node with central intranodal abscess
- Etiology
  - Reactive adenopathy: Response to infectious agent, chemical, drug or foreign antigen
  - Frequently secondary to pharyngitis or tonsillitis
  - Occasionally secondary to dental disease in children
  - Most common infections in children
    - Viral disease: EBV (most common), CMV, HSV, measles, HIV (rare in children)
    - Bacterial disease: Streptococcus, Staphylococcus, Bartonella henselae (most common causative agent in cat scratch disease)
    - Mycobacterium tuberculosis, atypical mycobacterium (nontuberculous mycobacterium) = M. avium-intracellulare (MAI), M. scrofulaceum, M. kansasii

# REACTIVE NODES/CERVICAL LYMPHADENITIS

- Epidemiology: Common clinical problem in pediatric age group
- Associated abnormalities
  - Retropharyngeal edema common
  - Stranding of adjacent subcutaneous fat common with bacterial infection, rare with atypical mycobacteria
  - Lemierre syndrome = jugular vein septic thrombophlebitis secondary to pharyngotonsillitis with resultant septic emboli to lungs and large joints: Fusobacterium necrophorum most common agent
  - In patients with retropharyngeal infection, frequently see ipsilateral internal carotid artery narrowing

## Microscopic Features
- Nonspecific reaction patterns
  - Follicular hyperplasia, paracortical hyperplasia, sinus histiocytosis
  - Polymorphic population of lymphoid cells in different stages of transformation
- Granulomatous pattern with epithelioid cell granulomas ± necrotic material
  - Mycobacteria: Acid-fast bacilli with Ziehl-Neelsen stain in 25-56%
  - Cat scratch: Bartonella henselae or Bartonella quintana

## CLINICAL ISSUES

### Presentation
- Most common signs/symptoms
  - Firm sometimes fluctuant, freely mobile subcutaneous nodal masses
  - Other signs/symptoms
    - Bacterial adenitis usually painful
    - Nontuberculous mycobacteria (NTM) usually non-tender
    - Cat scratch disease: Scratch or bite 1-4 weeks prior to development of adenopathy
    - Acute infectious mononucleosis: Pharyngitis, abdominal pain, nonspecific prodrome
- Other signs/symptoms: Rarely central nervous system (CNS) complications: Bacterial abscess, viral encephalitis and cat scratch disease

### Demographics
- Age
  - Any age but most common in pediatric age group
  - Organisms have predilection for specific ages
    - Infants < 1 year: Staph. aureus, group B streptococcus, Kawasaki disease
    - Children 1-5 years: Staph. aureus, group A β-hemolytic streptococcus, atypical mycobacteria
    - 5-15 years: Anaerobic bacteria, mononucleosis, cat scratch disease, tuberculosis (TB)
- Ethnicity: In developing countries high incidence of M. tuberculosis

### Natural History & Prognosis
- Bacterial infection, NTM and cat scratch frequently progress to necrotic nodes

- Suppurative nodal rupture results in soft tissue abscess

## Treatment
- Antibiotics if bacterial cause suspected
- Many reactive nodes resolve spontaneously, including cat scratch disease
- Incision and drainage of large suppurative nodes and abscesses
- Atypical mycobacteria nodes may require excision to prevent recurrence or fistula/sinus tract
- Needle aspiration or nodal biopsy sometimes needed
  - Failed response to antibiotics, rapid increase in nodal size, hard matted nodes, associated mediastinal or abdominal adenopathy, generalized symptoms fever and weight loss
- Persistence of adenopathy requires repeat needle aspiration to rule out lymphoma, metastasis or TB

## DIAGNOSTIC CHECKLIST

### Image Interpretation Pearls
- Oval-shaped nodes are more likely benign and reactive
- Lymph nodes with low attenuation centers and lack of surrounding cellulitis: Think atypical mycobacterium
- Cervical adenopathy plus Waldeyer ring hypertrophy: Think EBV or lymphoma
- Low attenuation center suggests abscess, may still be phlegmon

## SELECTED REFERENCES

1. Herrmann BW et al: Otolaryngological manifestations of posttransplant lymphoproliferative disorder in pediatric thoracic transplant patients. Int J Pediatr Otorhinolaryngol. 70(2):303-10, 2006
2. Leung AK et al: Childhood cervical lymphadenopathy. J Pediatr Health Care. 18(1):3-7, 2004
3. Ramirez S et al: Increased diagnosis of Lemierre syndrome and other Fusobacterium necrophorum infections at a Children's Hospital. Pediatrics. 112(5):e380, 2003
4. Ahuja A et al: An overview of neck node sonography. Invest Radiol. 37(6):333-42, 2002
5. Ishikawa M et al: MR imaging of lymph nodes in the head and neck. Magn Reson Imaging Clin N Am. 10(3):527-42, 2002
6. Hudgins PA: Nodal and nonnodal inflammatory processes of the pediatric neck. Neuroimaging Clin N Am. 10(1):181-92, ix, 2000
7. Robson CD et al: Nontuberculous mycobacterial infection of the head and neck in immunocompetent children: CT and MR findings. AJNR Am J Neuroradiol. 20(10):1829-35, 1999
8. Shreve PD et al: Pitfalls in oncologic diagnosis with FDG PET imaging: physiologic and benign variants. Radiographics. 19(1):61-77; quiz 150-1, 1999
9. Stone ME et al: Correlation between computed tomography and surgical findings in retropharyngeal inflammatory processes in children. Int J Pediatr Otorhinolaryngol. 49(2):121-5, 1999
10. Hudgins PA et al: Internal carotid artery narrowing in children with retropharyngeal lymphadenitis and abscess. AJNR Am J Neuroradiol. 19(10):1841-3, 1998

# REACTIVE NODES/CERVICAL LYMPHADENITIS

## IMAGE GALLERY

### Typical

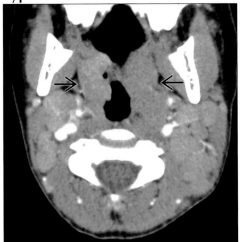 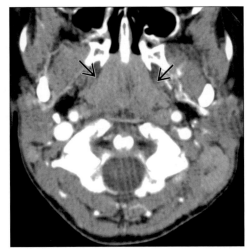

*(Left)* Axial CECT shows bilaterally enlarged reactive internal jugular and spinal accessory lymph nodes and bilateral enlargement of the palatine tonsils ➡ in a child with mononucleosis. *(Right)* Axial CECT shows symmetric enlargement of the nasopharyngeal adenoids ➡ in the same patient as previous image with mononucleosis.

### Typical

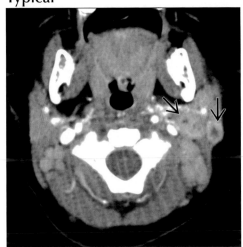 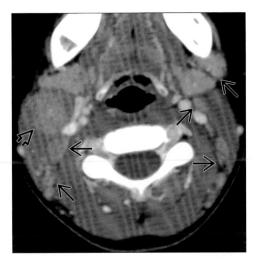

*(Left)* Axial CECT shows enlarged left lymph nodes with small areas of central necrosis ➡, without significant surrounding inflammation in a child with mycobacterium avium intracellulare. *(Right)* Axial CECT shows bilateral reactive lymphadenopathy ➡, with the largest node in the right jugulodigastric ➡, in a child with recent history of cat bite to the tongue.

### Typical

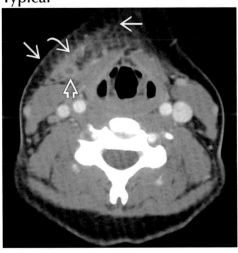 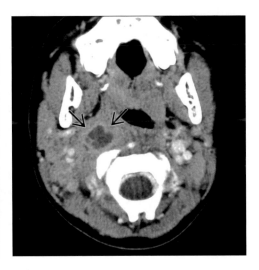

*(Left)* Axial CECT shows right neck cellulitis ➡, right platysma myositis ➡ and thrombus in the right anterior jugular vein ➡ in a patient with Lemierre syndrome. *(Right)* Axial CECT shows irregular, rim-enhancing low attenuation right lateral retropharyngeal suppurative collection ➡, found to be drainable abscess at surgery.

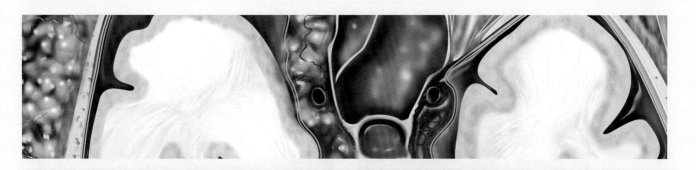

# SECTION 4: Multiple Regions, Head & Neck

# FIRST BRANCHIAL APPARATUS ANOMALIES

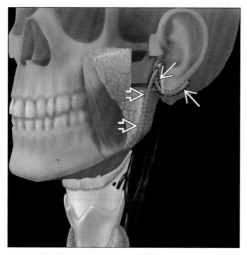

Sagittal oblique graphic shows potential locations of work type I ➡ and type II ➡ 1st branchial apparatus anomalies.

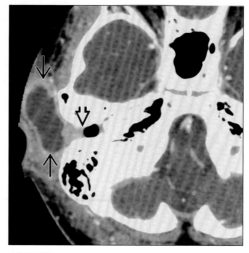

Axial CECT shows a rim enhancing fluid collection ➡ occluding the right external auditory canal ➡ in a patient with infected first branchial apparatus cyst.

## TERMINOLOGY

### Abbreviations and Synonyms
- First branchial apparatus cyst (BAC), branchial apparatus anomaly (BAA), branchial cleft cyst (BCC)
- Synonym: Cervicoaural cyst

### Definitions
- Most common 1st BAAs are cysts or sinuses
- 1st BAC: Benign, congenital cyst in or adjacent to parotid gland, EAC or pinna
  - Remnant of 1st branchial apparatus: Two most commonly used classifications
    - Work type I: Duplication of membranous EAC; ectodermal (cleft) origin
    - Work type II: Duplication of membranous EAC and cartilaginous pinna; skin (ectodermal cleft) and cartilage (mesodermal arch) origin; may also have contribution from the second arch
    - Arnot type I: Derived from buried rests of 1st branchial cleft (BC); intraparotid cyst or sinus
    - Arnot type II: Secondary to incomplete closure of the 1st BC; cyst or sinus in anterior triangle of neck ± communication with EAC

- 1st branchial apparatus sinus tract opens in region of parotid gland, EAC, parapharyngeal space or anterior triangle of the neck

## IMAGING FINDINGS

### General Features
- Best diagnostic clue: Cystic mass around pinna and EAC (type I) or extending from EAC to angle of mandible (type II)
- Location
  - Type I: Periauricular cyst or sinus tract
    - Anterior, inferior or posterior to pinna and concha
  - Type II: Periparotid
    - More intimately associated with parotid gland, medial or lateral to the facial nerve
    - Superficial, parotid & parapharyngeal spaces
- Size: Variable, but usually less than 3 cm
- Morphology: Well-circumscribed cyst

### CT Findings
- NECT
  - Low density cyst
  - If previously infected, can be isodense

## DDx: Cystic Parotid Masses

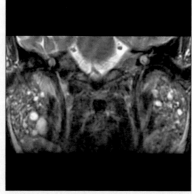

Cysts in HIV

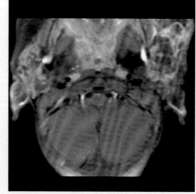

Bilateral VLM

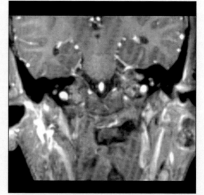

Pleomorphic Adenoma

# FIRST BRANCHIAL APPARATUS ANOMALIES

## Key Facts

### Terminology
- First branchial apparatus cyst (BAC), branchial apparatus anomaly (BAA), branchial cleft cyst (BCC)

### Imaging Findings
- Best diagnostic clue: Cystic mass around pinna and EAC (type I) or extending from EAC to angle of mandible (type II)
- Well-circumscribed, nonenhancing or rim-enhancing, low-density mass
- If infected, may have thick enhancing rim

### Top Differential Diagnoses
- Benign Lymphoepithelial Cysts
- Venolymphatic Malformation (VLM)
- Suppurative Adenopathy/Abscess
- Nontuberculous Mycobacterial Adenitis

### Pathology
- Remnant of 1st branchial apparatus
- Accounts for 8% of all branchial apparatus remnants
- Most common location for 1st BAC to terminate is in EAC between cartilaginous & bony portions

### Clinical Issues
- Soft, painless, compressible periauricular or periparotid suprahyoid neck mass

### Diagnostic Checklist
- Think of 1st BAC in patient with chronic unexplained otorrhea or recurrent parotid gland abscess
- Look for cyst in or adjacent to parotid gland, EAC or pinna, or rarely parapharyngeal

- CECT
  - Well-circumscribed, nonenhancing or rim-enhancing, low-density mass
  - If infected, may have thick enhancing rim
    - Surrounding induration suggests infection
  - 1st BAC, type I
    - Cyst anterior, inferior or posterior to EAC
    - Lesion may "beak" toward bony-cartilaginous junction of EAC
    - Often runs parallel to EAC
  - 1st BAC, type II
    - Cyst in superficial, parotid or parapharyngeal space
    - May be as low as posterior submandibular space
    - Deep projection may "beak" to bony-cartilaginous junction of EAC

## MR Findings
- T1WI: Low signal intensity unilocular cyst in characteristic locations
- T2WI
  - High signal intensity unilocular cyst in characteristic locations
  - May see sinus tract to skin, EAC or rarely parapharyngeal space
  - Absence of edema in surrounding soft tissues unless superinfection
- T1 C+
  - No wall enhancement is typical
  - Previous or concurrent infection may result in thick enhancing rim

## Ultrasonographic Findings
- Anechoic mass in periauricular or periparotid area

## Imaging Recommendations
- CECT usually adequate for evaluation of cyst
- Direct coronal or reformatted images (multidetector CT) helpful for evaluating relationship to EAC
- MR (particularly T2WI) better to evaluate small lesions and associated sinus tract

## DIFFERENTIAL DIAGNOSIS

### Benign Lymphoepithelial Cysts
- Single or multiple
- When multiple and bilateral, suspect HIV
  - Rare in children
  - Usually associated with cervical adenopathy and Waldeyer ring hypertrophy

### Venolymphatic Malformation (VLM)
- Usually multilocular, trans-spatial
- Contrast-enhancement of venous component
- No contrast-enhancement of lymphatic component

### Primary Parotid Neoplasms
- Uncommon in children; pleomorphic adenoma most common
- Solid much more common than cystic

### Suppurative Adenopathy/Abscess
- Clinical: Presents with marked tenderness and fever
- Imaging: Thick-walled, ovoid, cystic mass within parotid

### Nontuberculous Mycobacterial Adenitis
- Mycobacterium avium intracellulare (MAI)
- Rim enhancing with low attenuation nonenhancing center
- May lack surrounding inflammatory change
- May lack signs and symptoms of acute infection

## PATHOLOGY

### General Features
- General path comments
  - Embryology-anatomy
    - Remnant of 1st branchial apparatus
    - Cleft (ectoderm) of 1st apparatus gives rise to external auditory canal
    - Arch (mesoderm) gives rise to mandible, muscles of mastication, CN5, incus body, head of malleus

# FIRST BRANCHIAL APPARATUS ANOMALIES

- Pouch (endoderm) gives rise to eustachian tube, middle ear cavity, & mastoid air cells
  - Branchial remnant occurs if there is incomplete obliteration of 1st branchial apparatus
  - Isolated BCC has no internal (pharyngeal) or external (cutaneous) communication
  - BC fistula has both internal & external connections, from EAC lumen to skin
  - BC sinus opens externally or (rarely) internally, closed portion ends as blind pouch
  - 2/3 of 1st BC remnants are isolated cysts
- Epidemiology
  - Accounts for 8% of all branchial apparatus remnants
  - Type II > > type I 1st BAC
- Associated abnormalities: May be seen in association with other first branchial apparatus anomalies

## Gross Pathologic & Surgical Features
- Cystic neck mass
  - Easily dissected at surgery unless there has been repeated infection
- Contents of cyst usually thick mucus
- Cystic remnant may split facial nerve (CN7) trunk
- CN7 may be medial or lateral to 1st BAC
- Close proximity to CN7 makes surgery more difficult
- Most common location for 1st BAC to terminate is in EAC between cartilaginous & bony portions

## Microscopic Features
- Thin outer layer; fibrous pseudocapsule
- Inner layer; flat squamoid epithelium
- ± Germinal centers & lymphocytes in cyst wall

## CLINICAL ISSUES

## Presentation
- Most common signs/symptoms
  - Soft, painless, compressible periauricular or periparotid suprahyoid neck mass
  - Other signs/symptoms
    - Recurrent preauricular or periparotid swelling
    - Tender neck mass
    - Fever if infected
    - EAC or skin sinus tract rare
    - Chronic purulent ear drainage if ear sinus tract

## Demographics
- Age
  - Majority present < 10 years old
  - Presents earlier with sinus
  - When cyst only, may present later, even as adult
- Gender: No gender predilection

## Natural History & Prognosis
- May enlarge with upper respiratory tract infection
  - Lymph follicles in wall react, wall secretes
- Often incised & drained as an "abscess" only to recur
- Prognosis is excellent if completely resected
- May recur if residual cyst wall remains

## Treatment
- Complete surgical resection

- Proximity to facial nerve puts nerve at risk during surgery
  - Type I: Proximal facial nerve
  - Type II: More distal facial nerve branches

## DIAGNOSTIC CHECKLIST

### Consider
- Think of 1st BAC in patient with chronic unexplained otorrhea or recurrent parotid gland abscess
- Look for cyst in or adjacent to parotid gland, EAC or pinna, or rarely parapharyngeal

## SELECTED REFERENCES

1.  Koch BL: Cystic malformations of the neck in children. Pediatr Radiol. 35(5):463-77, 2005
2.  Daniel SJ et al: Surgical management of nonmalignant parotid masses in the pediatric population: the Montreal Children's Hospital's experience. J Otolaryngol. 32(1):51-4, 2003
3.  Gritzmann N et al: Sonography of soft tissue masses of the neck. J Clin Ultrasound. 30(6):356-73, 2002
4.  Nusbaum AO et al: Recurrence of a deep neck infection: a clinical indication of an underlying congenital lesion. Arch Otolaryngol Head Neck Surg. 125(12):1379-82, 1999
5.  Robson CD et al: Nontuberculous mycobacterial infection of the head and neck in immunocompetent children: CT and MR findings. AJNR Am J Neuroradiol. 20(10):1829-35, 1999
6.  Sichel JY et al: Clinical update on type II first branchial cleft cysts. Laryngoscope. 108(10):1524-7, 1998
7.  Triglia JM et al: First branchial cleft anomalies: a study of 39 cases and a review of the literature. Arch Otolaryngol Head Neck Surg. 124(3):291-5, 1998
8.  Nofsinger YC et al: Periauricular cysts and sinuses. Laryngoscope. 107(7):883-7, 1997
9.  Van der Goten A et al: First branchial complex anomalies: report of 3 cases. Eur Radiol. 7(1):102-5, 1997
10. Arndal H et al: First branchial cleft anomaly. Clin Otolaryngol. 21(3):203-7, 1996
11. Choi SS et al: Branchial anomalies: a review of 52 cases. Laryngoscope. 105(9 Pt 1):909-13, 1995
12. Mukherji SK et al: Evaluation of first branchial anomalies by CT and MR. J Comput Assist Tomogr. 17(4):576-81, 1993
13. Benson MT et al: Congenital anomalies of the branchial apparatus: embryology and pathologic anatomy. Radiographics. 12(5):943-60, 1992
14. Doi O et al: Branchial remnants: a review of 58 cases. J Pediatr Surg. 23(9):789-92, 1988
15. Finn DG et al: First branchial cleft cysts: clinical update. Laryngoscope. 97(2):136-40, 1987
16. Graham MD et al: First branchial cleft cyst presenting as a mass within the external auditory canal. Am J Otol. 6(6):500-2, 1985
17. Sherman NH et al: Ultrasound evaluation of neck masses in children. J Ultrasound Med. 4(3):127-34, 1985
18. Harnsberger HR et al: Branchial cleft anomalies and their mimics: computed tomographic evaluation. Radiology. 152(3):739-48, 1984
19. Olsen KD et al: First branchial cleft anomalies. Laryngoscope. 90(3):423-36, 1980
20. Wilson DB: Embryonic development of the head and neck: part 2, the branchial region. Head Neck Surg. 2(1):59-66, 1979

# FIRST BRANCHIAL APPARATUS ANOMALIES

## IMAGE GALLERY

### Typical

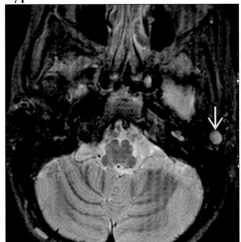 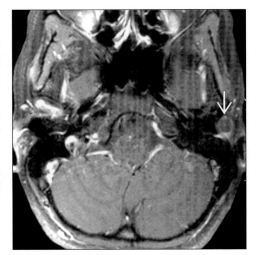

*(Left)* Axial T2WI MR shows a small well-defined preauricular cyst ➡, a Work type II first branchial apparatus cyst. *(Right)* Axial T1WI FS MR in the same patient as previous image shows the well-defined, nonenhancing left first branchial apparatus cyst ➡.

### Typical

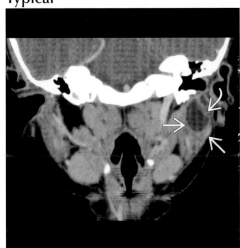 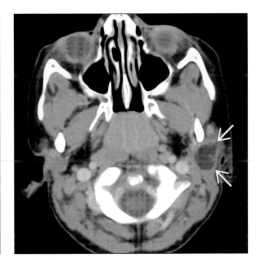

*(Left)* Coronal CECT shows a cyst ➡ inferior to the left EAC with a small tract ➡ extending toward the floor of the EAC. *(Right)* Axial CECT shows an irregularly shaped intraparotid first branchial apparatus cyst ➡. Note characteristic absence of enhancement.

### Typical

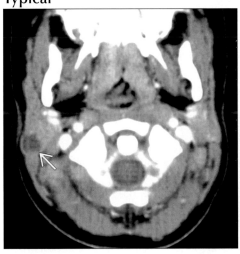 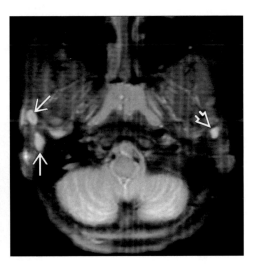

*(Left)* Axial CECT shows a well-defined first branchial apparatus cyst ➡ in the posterior aspect of the right parotid gland. *(Right)* Axial T2WI FS MR shows a well-defined bilobed right sided first branchial apparatus cyst ➡ and a smaller left sided first branchial apparatus cyst ➡.

# SECOND BRANCHIAL APPARATUS ANOMALIES

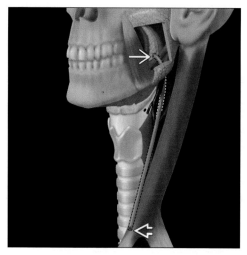

Sagittal oblique graphic shows 2nd BAC anterior to sternomastoid muscle and anterolateral to carotid space. Fistula tract may extend from faucial tonsil ➡ to low neck ➡.

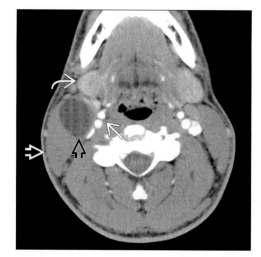

Axial CECT shows well-defined right BAC ➡ anterolateral to the carotid sheath ➡, anteromedial to SCM ➡ and posterolateral to the submandibular gland ➡.

## TERMINOLOGY

### Abbreviations and Synonyms
- Second branchial apparatus anomaly (BAA)
- Second branchial cleft cyst (BCC)
- Branchial apparatus cyst (BAC)
- Second branchial cleft remnant
- Second branchial cleft anomaly

### Definitions
- 2nd BAC: Most common branchial apparatus anomaly
  - Cystic remnant of cervical sinus of His: Derivative of 2nd, 3rd and 4th branchial clefts; and second branchial arch
- Sinus: Usually communicate externally along anterior margin of sternocleidomastoid muscle (SCM)
- Fistula: Communicate externally and internally
  - Secondary to persistence of both branchial cleft and pharyngeal pouch remnant
- Combinations
  - Cyst and sinus or fistula

## IMAGING FINDINGS

### General Features
- Best diagnostic clue: Cystic neck mass posterolateral to submandibular gland, lateral to carotid space, anterior (or anteromedial) to SCM
- Location
  - Bailey classification of second BACs
    - Type I: Deep to platysma muscle and anterior to SCM
    - Type II: Anterior to SCM, posterior to submandibular gland, lateral to carotid sheath
    - Type III: Protrudes between the internal and external carotid arteries, may extend to the lateral wall of pharynx or superiorly to skull base
    - Type IV: Adjacent to pharyngeal wall, probably remnant of second pharyngeal pouch
  - 2nd branchial apparatus fistula extends from anterior to the SCM, through carotid artery bifurcation & terminates in tonsillar fossa
- Size: Variable, may range from several cm to > 5 cm
- Morphology
  - Ovoid or rounded well-circumscribed cyst
  - Focal rim of cyst extending to carotid bifurcation

## DDx: Cystic Neck Masses

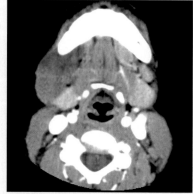

Lymphatic Malformation

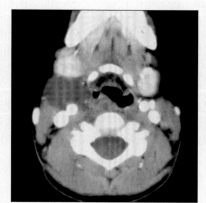

Thymic Cyst

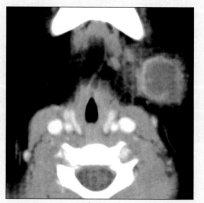

Abscess

# SECOND BRANCHIAL APPARATUS ANOMALIES

## Key Facts

### Terminology
- Second branchial apparatus anomaly (BAA)
- 2nd BAC: Most common branchial apparatus anomaly
- Cystic remnant of cervical sinus of His: Derivative of 2nd, 3rd and 4th branchial clefts; and second branchial arch

### Imaging Findings
- Best diagnostic clue: Cystic neck mass posterolateral to submandibular gland, lateral to carotid space, anterior (or anteromedial) to SCM
- NECT: Low density unilocular cyst
- If infected, wall is thicker & enhances with surrounding soft tissue cellulitis

### Top Differential Diagnoses
- Lymphatic Malformation (LM)
- Cervical Thymic Cyst
- Lymphadenopathy/Abscess
- Cystic Malignant Adenopathy

### Pathology
- 2nd BAC, sinus or fistulae
- Epidemiology: 2nd branchial apparatus anomalies account for up to 95% of all branchial apparatus anomalies

### Diagnostic Checklist
- Beware an adult with first presentation of "2nd BCC": Mass may be metastatic node from head & neck SCCa primary tumor or papillary thyroid carcinoma

- "Notch sign" pathognomonic for 2nd BCC

## CT Findings
- NECT: Low density unilocular cyst
- CECT
  - Low density cyst with nonenhancing wall
  - If infected, wall is thicker & enhances with surrounding soft tissue cellulitis

## MR Findings
- T1WI
  - Cyst is usually isointense to CSF
  - Infection; increase signal intensity/protein content
- T2WI: Hyperintense cyst, no discernible wall
- FLAIR: Cyst is iso- or slightly hyperintense to CSF
- T1 C+
  - No intrinsic contrast-enhancement
  - Peripheral wall enhancement if infected

## Ultrasonographic Findings
- Anechoic or hypoechoic thin-walled cyst
  - May give "pseudo-solid" US appearance
    - Real time will demonstrate mobile internal echoes to differentiate from solid lesion
- Thickened cyst wall if infected

## Imaging Recommendations
- CT, US or MR clearly demonstrate location of Bailey type I, II and III cysts
- May be difficult to visualize Bailey type IV cysts with US
- CT or MR best demonstrate associated findings of infection and rare type IV cysts

# DIFFERENTIAL DIAGNOSIS

## Lymphatic Malformation (LM)
- Unilocular or multilocular
- Frequently trans-spatial
- Fluid-fluid levels if intralesional hemorrhage
- Isolated to same location as 2nd branchial apparatus anomalies is uncommon

## Cervical Thymic Cyst
- Remnant of thymopharyngeal duct, derivative of 3rd pharyngeal pouch
- Left side more common than right
- Up to 50% extend into superior mediastinum

## Lymphadenopathy/Abscess
- Present with signs and symptoms of infection
- Irregular thick enhancing wall with nonenhancing central cavity
- Surrounding soft tissue induration except with mycobacterium
- Associated ipsilateral nonsuppurative adenopathy

## Cystic Malignant Adenopathy
- Necrotic mass with thick, enhancing wall
- Rare in children, occasional in teenagers
- Squamous cell carcinoma (SCCa) metastasis
- Papillary thyroid carcinoma (PTC) metastasis
- Others: Neuroblastoma, hepatoblastoma, testicular neoplasms

# PATHOLOGY

## General Features
- General path comments
  - Embryology
    - 2nd branchial arch overgrows 2nd, 3rd & 4th branchial clefts, forming the ectodermally lined cervical sinus of His
    - Remnant of second, third and fourth branchial clefts open into cervical sinus of His via cervical vesicles
    - Normal development cervical sinus of His and vesicles involute
    - Remnants of second branchial apparatus may form cyst, sinus or fistula
- Etiology
  - Remnants of cervical sinus of His or second branchial apparatus
    - 2nd BAC, sinus or fistulae

# SECOND BRANCHIAL APPARATUS ANOMALIES

- Epidemiology: 2nd branchial apparatus anomalies account for up to 95% of all branchial apparatus anomalies
- Associated abnormalities
  - Usually isolated lesion
  - May be part of branchio-otorenal (BOR) syndrome
    - Autosomal dominant inheritance
    - Bilateral branchial fistulas or cysts
    - Profound mixed hearing loss: Cochlear and semicircular canal malformations, stapes fixation
    - Renal anomalies: Dysplasia, aplasia, polycystic
    - Patulous eustachian tubes

## Gross Pathologic & Surgical Features

- Well-defined cyst in the locations described by Bailey
- Filled with cheesy material or serous, mucoid or purulent fluid

## Microscopic Features

- Squamous epithelial-lined cyst
- Lymphoid infiltrate in wall, often in form of germinal centers
  - Lymphoid tissue suggests epithelial rests may be entrapped within cervical lymph nodes during embryogenesis

## II 4 8

# CLINICAL ISSUES

## Presentation

- Most common signs/symptoms
  - Painless, compressible lateral neck mass in child or young adult
  - May enlarge during upper respiratory tract infection
    - Probably due to response of lymphoid tissue
  - Fever, tenderness and erythema if infected

## Demographics

- Age: Majority less than 5 years of age, second peak 2nd or 3rd decade

## Natural History & Prognosis

- Untreated, may become repeatedly infected & inflamed
- Recurrent inflammation = surgical resection more difficult
- Excellent prognosis if lesion is completely resected

## Treatment

- Complete surgical resection is treatment of choice
- Surgeon must dissect around cyst bed to exclude the possibility of an associated fistula or sinus
  - If a tract goes superomedially, it passes through carotid bifurcation into crypts of faucial palatine tonsil
  - If a tract goes inferiorly, it passes along anterior carotid space, reaching skin in supraclavicular area
    - If fistula present, usually identified at birth
    - Mucoid secretions are emitted from skin opening

# DIAGNOSTIC CHECKLIST

## Consider

- Infection if cyst wall enhances or surrounding cellulitis
- Does cyst appear adherent to internal jugular vein or carotid sheath?

## Image Interpretation Pearls

- Beware an adult with first presentation of "2nd BCC": Mass may be metastatic node from head & neck SCCa primary tumor or papillary thyroid carcinoma

# SELECTED REFERENCES

1. Koch BL: Cystic malformations of the neck in children. Pediatr Radiol. 35(5):463-77, 2005
2. Kemperman MH et al: Evidence of progression and fluctuation of hearing impairment in branchio-oto-renal syndrome. Int J Audiol. 43(9):523-32, 2004
3. Ceruti S et al: Temporal bone anomalies in the branchio-oto-renal syndrome: detailed computed tomographic and magnetic resonance imaging findings. Otol Neurotol. 23(2):200-7, 2002
4. Choo MJ et al: A case of second branchial cleft cyst with oropharyngeal presentation. J Korean Med Sci. 17(4):564-5, 2002
5. Kemperman MH et al: Inner ear anomalies are frequent but nonobligatory features of the branchio-oto-renal syndrome. Arch Otolaryngol Head Neck Surg. 128(9):1033-8, 2002
6. Shin JH et al: Parapharyngeal second branchial cyst manifesting as cranial nerve palsies: MR findings. AJNR Am J Neuroradiol. 22(3):510-2, 2001
7. Lev S et al: Imaging of cystic lesions. Radiol Clin North Am. 38(5):1013-27, 2000
8. Nusbaum AO et al: Recurrence of a deep neck infection: a clinical indication of an underlying congenital lesion. Arch Otolaryngol Head Neck Surg. 125(12):1379-82, 1999
9. Ahuja A et al: Solitary cystic nodal metastasis from occult papillary carcinoma of the thyroid mimicking a branchial cyst: a potential pitfall. Clin Radiol. 53(1):61-3, 1998
10. McDermott ID et al: Metastatic papillary thyroid carcinoma presenting as a typical branchial cyst. J Laryngol Otol. 110(5):490-2, 1996
11. Choi SS et al: Branchial anomalies: a review of 52 cases. Laryngoscope. 105(9 Pt 1):909-13, 1995
12. Benson MT et al: Congenital anomalies of the branchial apparatus: embryology and pathologic anatomy. Radiographics. 12(5):943-60, 1992
13. Doi O et al: Branchial remnants: a review of 58 cases. J Pediatr Surg. 23(9):789-92, 1988
14. Salazar JE et al: Second branchial cleft cyst: unusual location and a new CT diagnostic sign. AJR Am J Roentgenol. 145(5):965-6, 1985
15. Harnsberger HR et al: Branchial cleft anomalies and their mimics: computed tomographic evaluation. Radiology. 152(3):739-48, 1984
16. Gold BM: Second branchial cleft cyst and fistula. AJR Am J Roentgenol. 134(5):1067-9, 1980
17. Poswillo D: The pathogenesis of the first and second branchial arch syndrome. Oral Surg Oral Med Oral Pathol. 35(3):302-28, 1973
18. Bailey: Branchial cysts and other essays on surgical subjects in the faciocervical region: The clinical aspect of branchial cysts. London, Lewis. 1-18, 1929

# SECOND BRANCHIAL APPARATUS ANOMALIES

### Typical

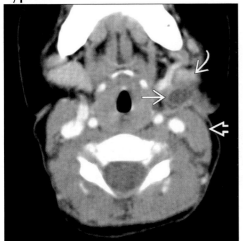 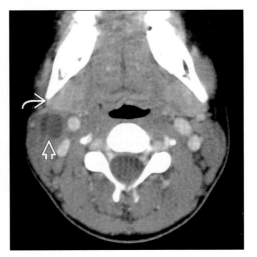

*(Left)* Axial CECT shows a small well-defined low attenuation, non-enhancing BAC ➡ anterior to the left SCM ➡ and posterior to the submandibular gland ➡. *(Right)* Axial CECT shows nonenhancing right BAC ➡ anterolateral to the carotid sheath, anteromedial to SCM and posterolateral to the submandibular gland ➡.

### Typical

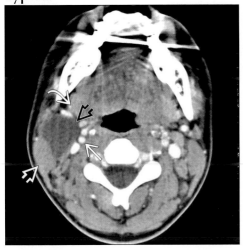 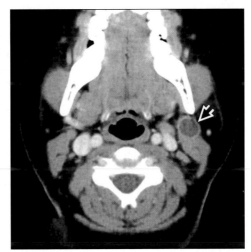

*(Left)* Axial CECT shows low attenuation non-enhancing right BAC ➡ anterolateral to the carotid sheath ➡, anteromedial to SCM ➡ and posterolateral to the submandibular gland ➡. *(Right)* Axial CECT shows left BAC with minimal rim enhancement ➡ in the classic location anterolateral to the carotid sheath and anteromedial to SCM.

### Typical

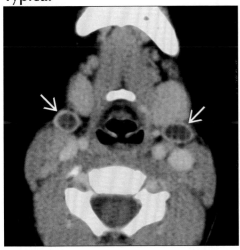 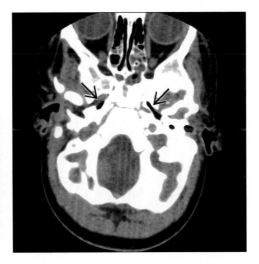

*(Left)* Axial CECT shows small bilateral branchial apparatus cysts ➡ in a child with branchio-otorenal (BOR) syndrome. *(Right)* Axial NECT shows typical prominence of the eustachian tubes ➡, in the same patient with BOR syndrome.

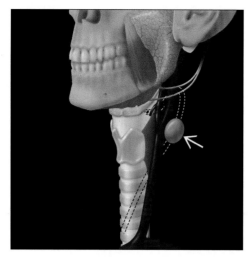

*Sagittal oblique graphic shows potential location of 3rd branchial cleft cysts, which occur most commonly in the upper posterior triangle ➡.*

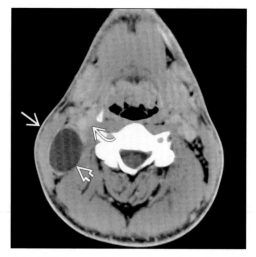

*Axial CECT shows well-defined, thin walled 3rd BCC ➡ in the right posterior cervical space, deep to the sternocleidomastoid muscle ➡ and posterolateral to the carotid sheath ➡.*

## TERMINOLOGY

### Abbreviations and Synonyms
- Cervical thymic cyst (CTC)
  - Thymopharyngeal duct cyst
- 3rd branchial cleft cyst (BCC)
  - Also called 3rd branchial apparatus cyst (BAC)

### Definitions
- Cervical thymic cyst: Cystic remnant of thymopharyngeal duct, derivative of 3rd pharyngeal pouch
- 3rd BAC: Cystic remnant of 3rd branchial cleft

## IMAGING FINDINGS

### General Features
- Best diagnostic clue
  - Cervical thymic cyst: Cystic lateral neck mass closely associated with carotid sheath
  - 3rd branchial cleft cyst: Unilocular cyst in upper posterior cervical space or lower anterior neck
- Location

  - Cervical thymic cyst
    - Anywhere along the tract of the thymopharyngeal duct from the pyriform sinus to the anterior mediastinum
    - Left more common than right
    - Up to 50% continuous with mediastinal thymus: Direct extension of cyst or via fibrous cord
    - Intimate association with carotid sheath, frequently splay the carotid artery and jugular vein
  - 3rd branchial cleft cyst
    - Upper neck posterior cervical space, lower neck anterior border sternocleidomastoid muscle
    - Rarely can be in submandibular space, just lateral to cephalad hypopharynx
- Size: Variable, usually 2-3 cm at presentation
- Morphology: Typically ovoid or round cyst

### CT Findings
- CECT
  - Rounded or ovoid sharply marginated lesions with central fluid attenuation
  - Cyst wall thin, no calcifications

---

## DDx: Cystic Neck Masses in Children

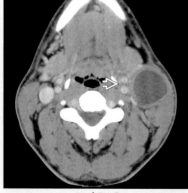

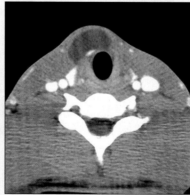

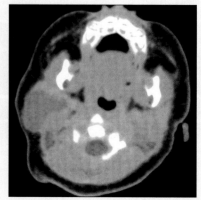

| 2nd BAC | TGDC | Lymphatic Malformation |

# THIRD BRANCHIAL APPARATUS ANOMALIES

## Key Facts

### Terminology
- Cervical thymic cyst: Cystic remnant of thymopharyngeal duct, derivative of 3rd pharyngeal pouch
- 3rd BAC: Cystic remnant of 3rd branchial cleft

### Imaging Findings
- Cervical thymic cyst: Cystic lateral neck mass closely associated with carotid sheath
- 3rd branchial cleft cyst: Unilocular cyst in upper posterior cervical space or lower anterior neck
- Size: Variable, usually 2-3 cm at presentation

### Top Differential Diagnoses
- 2nd Branchial Apparatus Cyst (BAC)
- Thyroglossal Duct Cyst (TGDC)
- Lymphatic Malformation (LM)

- Abscess

### Pathology
- Lymphoid tissue in walls of cyst with reactive lymphoid follicles

### Clinical Issues
- CTC and 3rd BAC: Good prognosis if completely resected

### Diagnostic Checklist
- If the cyst is intimately associated with the anterior carotid sheath, think CTC
- If the cyst extends from the anterior neck to the upper mediastinum, consider CTC
- If the cyst is in the posterior triangle of the upper neck, think 3rd BAC

- o If infected, cyst wall thickens, enhances and adjacent soft tissues show evidence of cellulitis
  - o CTC
    - ■ Closely associated with carotid sheath
    - ■ With or without continuation of cyst to the mediastinal thymus
    - ■ Solid components rare = aberrant thymic tissue, lymphoid aggregates or parathyroid tissue
  - o 3rd BAC
    - ■ Sternocleidomastoid muscle displaced laterally when cyst in high posterior neck
    - ■ Sternocleidomastoid muscle displaced posterolaterally when cyst in low anterior neck

### MR Findings
- T1WI
  - o Homogeneous T1 hypointense fluid contents
  - o Cyst wall thin or imperceptible
- T2WI
  - o Homogeneous T2 hyperintense fluid contents
  - o May see edema in surrounding tissues if infected
- T1 C+
  - o Thin, uniform minimally enhancing cyst wall
  - o If infected
    - ■ Cyst wall thickened & enhancing
    - ■ Fluid contents hyperintense relative to CSF
    - ■ Strandy enhancement in surrounding soft tissues

### Ultrasonographic Findings
- Thin walled hypoechoic mass

### Imaging Recommendations
- Best imaging tool: CECT or MR
- Protocol advice: Include upper mediastinum to demonstrate mediastinal extension in CTC

## DIFFERENTIAL DIAGNOSIS

### 2nd Branchial Apparatus Cyst (BAC)
- Most common branchial apparatus anomaly

- Usually lateral to carotid space, posterior to submandibular gland & anteromedial to sternomastoid muscle

### Thyroglossal Duct Cyst (TGDC)
- Midline or paramidline anterior neck cyst in child or young adult
- Anywhere along TGD from base of tongue (foramen cecum) to lower anterior neck in region of thyroid bed
- Embedded in strap muscles when infrahyoid

### Lymphatic Malformation (LM)
- Majority diagnosed under 2 years of age
- Unilocular or multilocular; focal or infiltrative
- Fluid-fluid levels if intralesional hemorrhage

### Abscess
- Present with signs and symptoms of infection
- Irregular thick enhancing wall, low attenuation center
- Surrounding soft tissue induration
- If associated with thyroid gland, think 4th brachial pouch anomaly

## PATHOLOGY

### General Features
- Etiology
  - o CTC
    - ■ Failure of obliteration of thymopharyngeal duct, remnant of 3rd pharyngeal pouch
  - o 3rd BCC
    - ■ Failure of obliteration of third branchial cleft or portion of cervical sinus of His
- Epidemiology
  - o CTC
    - ■ Rare
  - o 3rd BCC
    - ■ Rare lesion
    - ■ 3rd branchial cleft anomalies account for only 3% of all branchial anomalies
- Associated abnormalities
  - o 3rd branchial cleft sinus: Single opening

# THIRD BRANCHIAL APPARATUS ANOMALIES

- Some endopharyngeal in high lateral hypopharynx
- Others cutaneous in supraclavicular area anterior to carotid artery
- ○ 3rd branchial apparatus fistula: Two openings
  - One opening is endopharyngeal in high lateral hypopharynx
  - Second opening is cutaneous in supraclavicular area anterior to carotid artery

## Gross Pathologic & Surgical Features
- Smooth thin-walled cysts
  - ○ CTC may have cystic extension or fibrous cord to mediastinal thymus

## Microscopic Features
- CTC
  - ○ Hassall corpuscles in cyst wall diagnostic
    - Not always present if prior infection or hemorrhage
  - ○ Cholesterol crystals and granulomas in cyst wall common
    - Possibly related to prior hemorrhage
- 3rd BCC
  - ○ Lined by squamous epithelium (occasionally by columnar epithelium)
  - ○ Lymphoid tissue in walls of cyst with reactive lymphoid follicles

## CLINICAL ISSUES

### Presentation
- Most common signs/symptoms
  - ○ CTC
    - Enlarging, compressible mid to lower cervical mass
    - Other signs/symptoms: If large, may cause dysphagia or respiratory distress
  - ○ 3rd BAC
    - Fluctuant mass in posterolateral neck
    - May enlarge rapidly following an upper respiratory tract infection
    - Other signs/symptoms: Recurrent lateral neck or retropharyngeal abscesses, draining sinus along anterior margin of sternocleidomastoid muscle

### Demographics
- Age
  - ○ CTC
    - Most diagnosed between 2 and 15 years of age
  - ○ 3rd BAC
    - Frequently present in adulthood
    - Presentation of cysts in neonates & infants unusual
    - When sinus or fistula present, early presentation more common

### Natural History & Prognosis
- CTC and 3rd BAC: Good prognosis if completely resected

### Treatment
- CTC and 3rd BAC

- ○ Surgical resection

## DIAGNOSTIC CHECKLIST

### Consider
- If the cyst is intimately associated with the anterior carotid sheath, think CTC
- If the cyst extends from the anterior neck to the upper mediastinum, consider CTC
- If the cyst is in the posterior triangle of the upper neck, think 3rd BAC

## SELECTED REFERENCES

1. Koch BL: Cystic malformations of the neck in children. Pediatr Radiol. 35(5):463-77, 2005
2. Khariwala SS et al: Cervical presentations of thymic anomalies in children. Int J Pediatr Otorhinolaryngol. 68(7):909-14, 2004
3. Pereira KD et al: Management of anomalies of the third and fourth branchial pouches. Int J Pediatr Otorhinolaryngol. 68(1):43-50, 2004
4. Tsai CC et al: Branchial-cleft sinus presenting with a retropharyngeal abscess for a newborn: a case report. Am J Perinatol. 20(5):227-31, 2003
5. De Caluwe D et al: Cervical thymic cysts. Pediatr Surg Int. 18(5-6):477-9, 2002
6. Liberman M et al: Ten years of experience with third and fourth branchial remnants. J Pediatr Surg. 37(5):685-90, 2002
7. Huang RY et al: Third branchial cleft anomaly presenting as a retropharyngeal abscess. Int J Pediatr Otorhinolaryngol. 54(2-3):167-72, 2000
8. Mandell DL: Head and neck anomalies related to the branchial apparatus. Otolaryngol Clin North Am. 33(6):1309-32, 2000
9. Mukherji SK et al: Imaging of congenital anomalies of the branchial apparatus. Neuroimaging Clin N Am. 10(1):75-93, viii, 2000
10. Nicollas R et al: Congenital cysts and fistulas of the neck. Int J Pediatr Otorhinolaryngol. 55(2):117-24, 2000
11. Koeller KK et al: Congenital cystic masses of the neck: radiologic-pathologic correlation. Radiographics. 19(1):121-46; quiz 152-3, 1999
12. Millman B et al: Cervical thymic anomalies. Int J Pediatr Otorhinolaryngol. 47(1):29-39, 1999
13. Mouri N et al: Reappraisal of lateral cervical cysts in neonates: pyriform sinus cysts as an anatomy-based nomenclature. J Pediatr Surg. 33(7):1141-4, 1998
14. Edmonds JL et al: Third branchial anomalies. Avoiding recurrences. Arch Otolaryngol Head Neck Surg. 123(4):438-41, 1997
15. Kelley DJ et al: Cervicomediastinal thymic cysts. Int J Pediatr Otorhinolaryngol. 39(2):139-46, 1997
16. Nguyen Q et al: Cervical thymic cyst: case reports and review of the literature. Laryngoscope. 106(3 Pt 1):247-52, 1996
17. Benson MT et al: Congenital anomalies of the branchial apparatus: embryology and pathologic anatomy. Radiographics. 12(5):943-60, 1992
18. Cressman WR et al: Pathologic quiz case 1. Cervical thymic cyst. Arch Otolaryngol Head Neck Surg. 118(7):772-4, 1992
19. Zarbo RJ et al: Thymopharyngeal duct cyst: a form of cervical thymus. Ann Otol Rhinol Laryngol. 92(3 Pt 1):284-9, 1983
20. Guba AM Jr et al: Cervical presentation of thymic cysts. Am J Surg. 136(4):430-6, 1978

II

4

12

# THIRD BRANCHIAL APPARATUS ANOMALIES

## IMAGE GALLERY

### Typical

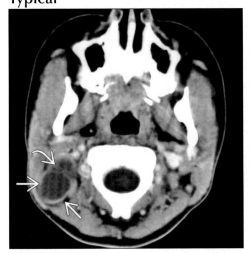

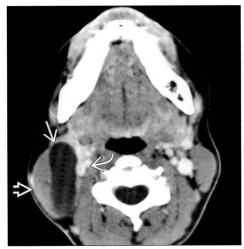

*(Left) Axial CECT shows a well-defined, low attenuation 3rd BCC with minimal peripheral contrast-enhancement ➡ and a few septations ➡ at the superior margin, suggesting prior infection. (Right) Axial CECT shows a well-defined, low attenuation 3rd BCC ➡ without significant contrast-enhancement, deep to the SCM ➡ and adjacent to the carotid space ➡.*

### Typical

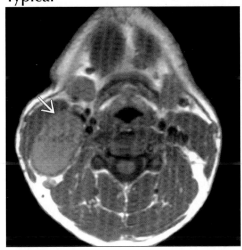

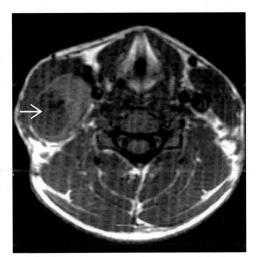

*(Left) Axial T1WI MR shows a 3rd BCC ➡ with hyperintense signal intensity indicating higher protein content likely related to prior infection or hemorrhage. (Right) Axial T1WI MR in the same patient as previous image, shows the inferior portion of the same 3rd BCC. On this image, the cyst is seen to be multiloculated with a central, more hypointense portion ➡.*

### Typical

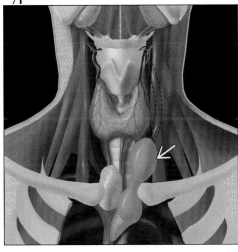

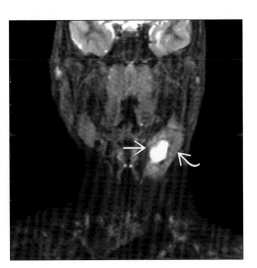

*(Left) Coronal graphic shows course of thymopharyngeal duct (a 3rd branchial pouch remnant) and typical appearance of a cervicothoracic dumbbell shaped thymic cyst ➡. (Right) Coronal STIR MR shows a periphery of solid thymic tissue ➡ and a medial cyst ➡ in this anomaly of the thymopharyngeal duct, a 3rd branchial pouch remnant.*

# FOURTH BRANCHIAL APPARATUS ANOMALIES

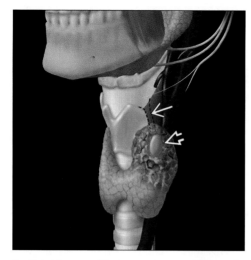

*Sagittal oblique graphic shows a sinus tract ➡ from the pyriform sinus to the left thyroid with associated cyst ⧐ and thyroiditis secondary to a 4th pharyngeal pouch remnant.*

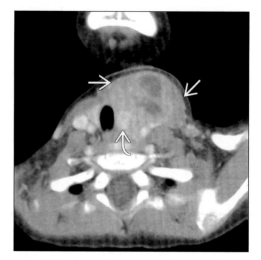

*Axial CECT shows a left anterior neck abscess ➡ with surrounding inflammation and a focal area of left lobe thyroiditis ➡, in a child with prior history of prior neck abscess.*

## TERMINOLOGY

### Abbreviations and Synonyms

- Sinus tract of pyriform sinus
- 4th branchial apparatus anomaly (BAA)
- 4th branchial apparatus cyst (BAC)
- 4th branchial cleft cyst (BCC): Misnomer because sinus tract is remnant of 4th pharyngeal pouch, not branchial cleft

### Definitions

- 4th BAC epithelial-lined cystic remnant of the fourth branchial pouch
  - Course from apex of pyriform sinus to upper aspect of the left thyroid lobe
- Branchial sinus tract: One opening-to-skin surface, external auditory canal, pharynx or hypopharynx
- Branchial fistula: Two openings - skin and lumen of the foregut
  - Arises as an epithelial-lined tract left behind when there is persistence of both a branchial cleft and its corresponding pharyngeal pouch

## IMAGING FINDINGS

### General Features

- Best diagnostic clue
  - Sinus tract extending from the apex of the pyriform sinus to the lower anterior neck after barium swallow
  - Abscess in or adjacent to anterior left thyroid lobe
- Location
  - May occur anywhere from left pyriform sinus apex to thyroid lobe
    - Commonly against or within superior aspect of the left lobe of thyroid gland or attached to thyroid cartilage
    - Upper end may communicate with or be adherent to pyriform sinus
- Size: Variable
- Morphology: Thin walled if not infected, thick enhancing wall if infected

### CT Findings

- CECT
  - Thin-walled cyst without significant enhancement

---

## DDx: Peri-Thyroidal Cysts

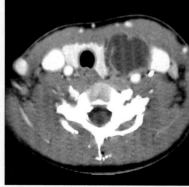

*Thymic Cyst*

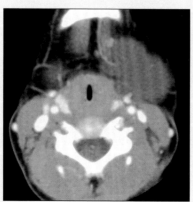

*Lymphatic Malformation*

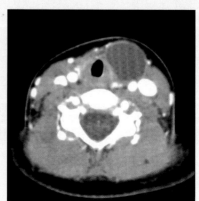

*Thyroglossal Duct Cyst*

# FOURTH BRANCHIAL APPARATUS ANOMALIES

## Key Facts

### Terminology

- 4th BAC epithelial-lined cystic remnant of the fourth branchial pouch
- Course from apex of pyriform sinus to upper aspect of the left thyroid lobe

### Imaging Findings

- Sinus tract extending from the apex of the pyriform sinus to the lower anterior neck after barium swallow
- Abscess in or adjacent to anterior left thyroid lobe
- Morphology: Thin walled if not infected, thick enhancing wall if infected
- CECT best demonstrates cyst or abscess
- Fluoroscopically guided barium swallow followed by noncontrast CT best demonstrates sinus tract

### Top Differential Diagnoses

- Cervical Thymic Cyst
- Lymphatic Malformation
- Thyroglossal Duct (TGD) Cyst
- Thyroid Colloid Cyst

### Clinical Issues

- Recurrent neck abscesses
- Recurrent suppurative thyroiditis
- If infected, initial treatment is antibiotics ± incision and drainage of abscess
- Complete resection of cyst & any associated sinus or fistula

### Diagnostic Checklist

- Left thyroid lobe abscess in pediatric patient should strongly suggest diagnosis of 4th BAA

- ○ Thick enhancing wall with surrounding cellulitis if infected
- NECT after barium swallow
  - ○ Barium filled tract extending from the apex of the pyriform sinus to the lower anterior neck

### MR Findings

- Thin-walled fluid signal intensity cyst if not infected
- Thick wall with increased signal intensity of fluid and surrounding cellulitis if infected

### Ultrasonographic Findings

- Thin walled echolucent cyst if not infected
- Internal echoes seen when infection or hemorrhage
- Thick walled abscess with hyperemic wall anterior to thyroid if infected

### Nuclear Medicine Findings

- Cold nodule on thyroid scan

### Fluoroscopic Findings

- Barium swallow
  - ○ Barium filled sinus tract extending from the apex of the pyriform sinus to the anterior lower neck
  - ○ If performed during acute infection, may not fill portions of sinus tract

### Imaging Recommendations

- Best imaging tool
  - ○ CECT best demonstrates cyst or abscess
  - ○ Fluoroscopically guided barium swallow followed by noncontrast CT best demonstrates sinus tract
  - ○ Direct injection of fistula best demonstrate course of fistula
- Protocol advice: Thin section post-contrast helical CT with multiplanar reconstructions very helpful

## DIFFERENTIAL DIAGNOSIS

### Cervical Thymic Cyst

- Congenital cyst: Remnant of thymopharyngeal duct, derivative of 3rd pharyngeal pouch
- Left side more common than right

- When confined to visceral space, may closely mimic 4th BAA
- Up to 50% of cervical thymic cysts extend into superior mediastinum

### Lymphatic Malformation

- Unilocular or multilocular
- Focal or infiltrative
- Fluid-fluid levels if intralesional hemorrhage

### Thyroglossal Duct (TGD) Cyst

- Anywhere along TGD from base of tongue (foramen cecum) to lower anterior neck in region of thyroid bed
- Infrahyoid TGD cyst
  - ○ Off-midline, anterior to thyroid lobe itself
  - ○ Closely related to thyroid cartilage or strap muscles

### Thyroid Colloid Cyst

- Uncommon in young children, most occur in older children and adults
- True thyroid cysts are rare
- Most "thyroid cysts" are degenerating adenomas
- May appear bright on T1 MR due to hemorrhage, colloid or high protein content

## PATHOLOGY

### General Features

- Etiology
  - ○ Controversial
    - ▪ Failure of obliteration of 4th branchial pouch
    - ▪ Failure of obliteration of distal cervical sinus of His
- Epidemiology
  - ○ Rarest of all forms of branchial apparatus anomalies (1-2% of all branchial anomalies)
  - ○ Most cases arise on LEFT
- Associated abnormalities
  - ○ 4th branchial sinus
    - ▪ When sinus connection with apex of pyriform sinus is maintained, infection is likely

■ Thyroiditis ± thyroid abscess possible in such circumstances
○ 4th branchial fistula
■ Term fistula denotes 2 openings, one in low anterior neck, 2nd into pyriform sinus apex

## Gross Pathologic & Surgical Features

• Anterolateral neck cyst or abscess; mostly found within anterior thyroid lobe
• Direct probing of the pyriform apex frequently demonstrates the fistula or sinus tract

## Microscopic Features

• Typically lined by non-keratinizing squamous epithelium
○ Occasionally lined by columnar epithelium
• Lymphoid tissue in cyst walls with reactive lymphoid follicles
• Thyroid follicles may be found in walls of cyst

## CLINICAL ISSUES

### Presentation

• Most common signs/symptoms
○ Recurrent neck abscesses
○ Recurrent suppurative thyroiditis
○ Fluctuant mass in lower third of neck anteromedial to sternocleidomastoid muscle; tender if infected
○ Throat pain
○ Dysphagia
○ Stridor

### Demographics

• Age
○ Most branchial sinuses & fistulae (all types) present in childhood
○ Most 4th branchial apparatus anomalies are diagnosed in infants and young children
• Gender: More common in females

### Natural History & Prognosis

• If sinus connection to pyriform sinus unrecognized & untreated, recurrent suppurative thyroiditis
• Recurrence likely if tract not resected & contains secretory epithelium

### Treatment

• If infected, initial treatment is antibiotics ± incision and drainage of abscess
• Complete resection of cyst & any associated sinus or fistula
• Pyriform sinus opening must be obliterated to prevent recurrence
• Thyroid lobectomy is required for lesions in thyroid lobe to prevent recurrence

## DIAGNOSTIC CHECKLIST

### Consider

• In any child with phlegmon or abscess in or anterior to left thyroid lobe or recurrent suppurative thyroiditis

## Image Interpretation Pearls

• Left thyroid lobe abscess in pediatric patient should strongly suggest diagnosis of 4th BAA

## SELECTED REFERENCES

1. Garrel R et al: Fourth branchial pouch sinus: from diagnosis to treatment. Otolaryngol Head Neck Surg. 134(1):157-63, 2006
2. Koch BL: Cystic malformations of the neck in children. Pediatr Radiol. 35(5):463-77, 2005
3. Jeyakumar A et al: Various presentations of fourth branchial pouch anomalies. Ear Nose Throat J. 83(9):640-2, 644, 2004
4. Pereira KD et al: Management of anomalies of the third and fourth branchial pouches. Int J Pediatr Otorhinolaryngol. 68(1): 43-50, 2004
5. Chaudhary N et al: Fistula of the fourth branchial pouch. Am J Otolaryngol. 24(4): 250-2, 2003
6. Wang HK et al: Imaging studies of pyriform sinus fistula. Pediatr Radiol. 33(5):328-33, 2003
7. Liberman M et al: Ten years of experience with third and fourth branchial remnants. J Pediatr Surg. 37(5): 685-90, 2002
8. Link TD et al: Fourth branchial pouch sinus: a diagnostic challenge. Plast Reconstr Surg. 108(3): 695-701, 2001
9. Minhas SS et al: Fourth branchial arch fistula and suppurative thyroiditis: a life-threatening infection. J Laryngol Otol. 115(12): 1029-31, 2001
10. Cases JA et al: Recurrent acute suppurative thyroiditis in an adult due to a fourth branchial pouch fistula. J Clin Endocrinol Metab. 85(3): 953-6, 2000
11. Mandell DL: Head and neck anomalies related to the branchial apparatus. Otolaryngol Clin North Am. 33(6): 1309-32, 2000
12. Nicollas R et al: Congenital cysts and fistulas of the neck. Int J Pediatr Otorhinolaryngol. 55(2): 117-24, 2000
13. Park SW et al: Neck infection associated with pyriform sinus fistula: imaging findings. AJNR Am J Neuroradiol. 21(5):817-22, 2000
14. Stone ME et al: A new role for computed tomography in the diagnosis and treatment of pyriform sinus fistula. Am J Otolaryngol. 21(5):323-5, 2000
15. Yang C et al: Fourth branchial arch sinus: clinical presentation, diagnostic workup, and surgical treatment. Laryngoscope. 109(3): 442-6, 1999
16. Nicollas R et al: Fourth branchial pouch anomalies: a study of six cases and review of the literature. Int J Pediatr Otorhinolaryngol. 44(1): 5-10, 1998
17. Cote DN et al: Fourth branchial cleft cysts. Otolaryngol Head Neck Surg. 114(1): 95-7, 1996
18. Choi SS et al: Branchial anomalies: a review of 52 cases. Laryngoscope. 105(9 Pt 1): 909-13, 1995
19. Benson MT et al: Congenital anomalies of the branchial apparatus: embryology and pathologic anatomy. Radiographics. 12(5):943-60, 1992
20. Rosenfeld RM et al: Fourth branchial pouch sinus: diagnosis and treatment. Otolaryngol Head Neck Surg. 105(1): 44-50, 1991
21. Godin MS et al: Fourth branchial pouch sinus: principles of diagnosis and management. Laryngoscope. 100(2 Pt 1): 174-8, 1990
22. Lucaya J et al: Congenital pyriform sinus fistula: a cause of acute left-sided suppurative thyroiditis and neck abscess in children. Pediatr Radiol. 21(1):27-9, 1990
23. Taylor WE Jr et al: Acute suppurative thyroiditis in children. Laryngoscope. 92(11):1269-73, 1982

# FOURTH BRANCHIAL APPARATUS ANOMALIES

## IMAGE GALLERY

### Typical

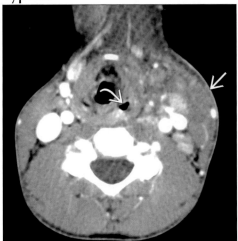 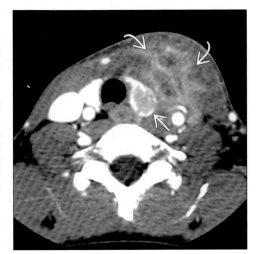

*(Left) Axial CECT shows ill-defined inflammation surrounding the apex of the left pyriform sinus ➡ and extending to involve the left SCM ➡ (myositis) and facial planes in the anterior neck. (Right) Axial CECT in the same patient as previous image shows left anterior neck phlegmon ➡, cellulitis and myositis with focal area of thyroiditis ➡ in the left thyroid lobe.*

### Typical

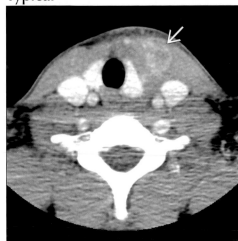 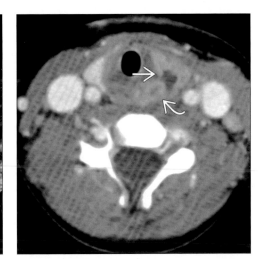

*(Left) Axial CECT shows focal phlegmon ➡, cellulitis and myositis anterior to the left lobe of the thyroid in a patient with sinus tract extending from the pyriform sinus apex. (Right) Axial CECT shows focal left lobe thyroiditis/abscess ➡ within low attenuation left lobe, and extrathyroid phlegmon ➡ secondary to a 4th branchial apparatus remnant sinus tract.*

### Typical

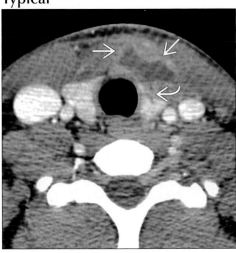 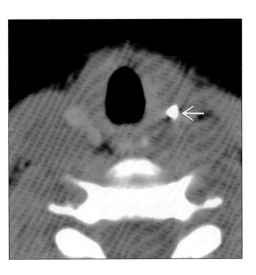

*(Left) Axial CECT shows focal ill-defined abscess ➡ with surrounding cellulitis in the anterior left neck. Notice small low attenuation tract ➡ extending into the upper left thyroid lobe. (Right) Axial NECT obtained after barium swallow shows contrast within the 4th branchial pouch remnant ➡ in a patient treated for left anterior neck abscess one month prior.*

# THYROGLOSSAL DUCT CYST

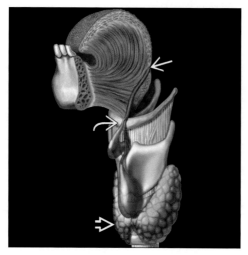

Sagittal oblique graphic shows course of TGDC, from foramen cecum ➡ to thyroid bed ➡. Note close relationship to mid-portion of hyoid bone ➡. Cyst can occur anywhere along tract.

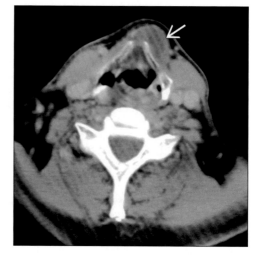

Axial CECT shows a fluid-intensity lesion ➡ in the strap muscles anterior and on the left side of the thyroid cartilage.

## TERMINOLOGY

### Abbreviations and Synonyms
- Thyroglossal duct cyst (TGDC)
- Thyroglossal duct remnant

### Definitions
- TGDC: Remnant of thyroglossal duct found between foramen cecum of tongue base & thyroid bed in infrahyoid neck

## IMAGING FINDINGS

### General Features
- Best diagnostic clue: Midline cystic neck mass embedded in infrahyoid strap muscles ("claw sign")
- Location
  - 20-25% in suprahyoid neck
  - Almost 50% at hyoid bone
  - About 25% in infrahyoid neck
  - Most in suprahyoid neck are midline
  - May be paramedian in infrahyoid neck
- Size: Usually between 2-4 cm, but may be smaller

- Morphology: Round or ovoid cyst

### CT Findings
- NECT: Low density (cystic) midline neck mass
- CECT
  - Benign-appearing, cystic neck mass
  - Low density mass, occasionally septated
  - Cystic midline neck mass with thin rim of peripheral enhancement
    - Wall may enhance if infected
  - Suprahyoid TGDC: Occurs at base of tongue or within posterior floor of mouth
  - At level of hyoid bone, found in midline abutting hyoid
    - May project into pre-epiglottic space
    - Usually anterior or ventral to hyoid bone
  - Infrahyoid TGDC: Embedded in strap muscles
    - More inferior the TGDC, the more paramedian
  - If associated thyroid carcinoma, solid eccentric mass, often with calcification within cyst

### MR Findings
- T1WI
  - Cyst usually with decreased signal intensity

---

## DDx: Thyroglossal Look Alikes

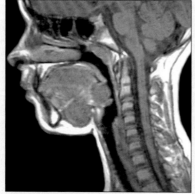

Lingual Thyroid

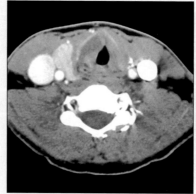

Laryngocele

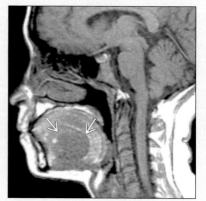

Dermoid of Tongue

# THYROGLOSSAL DUCT CYST

## Key Facts

### Terminology
- TGDC: Remnant of thyroglossal duct found between foramen cecum of tongue base & thyroid bed in infrahyoid neck

### Imaging Findings
- Best diagnostic clue: Midline cystic neck mass embedded in infrahyoid strap muscles ("claw sign")
- 20-25% in suprahyoid neck
- Almost 50% at hyoid bone
- About 25% in infrahyoid neck
- Wall may enhance if infected

### Top Differential Diagnoses
- Lingual or Sublingual Thyroid
- Dermoid or Epidermoid of Tongue
- Submandibular or Sublingual Space Abscess

- Delphian Chain Necrotic Node

### Pathology
- Failure of involution of TGD & persistent secretion of epithelial cells lining duct result in TGDC
- TGDC can occur anywhere along route of descent of TGD
- Most common congenital neck lesion

### Clinical Issues
- Entire cyst & midline portion of hyoid bone is resected

### Diagnostic Checklist
- Any associated nodularity or chunky calcification suggests associated thyroid carcinoma

- ○ May be hyperintense if filled with proteinaceous secretions
- T2WI: Homogeneously hyperintense
- T1 C+
  - ○ Nonenhancing cyst is norm
  - ○ Rim-enhancement if infected

## Ultrasonographic Findings
- Anechoic midline neck mass in close association with hyoid bone

## Imaging Recommendations
- TGDC in children have a classic clinical presentation
- CT or MR recommended if cyst is suprahyoid, or infected
- Sonography to confirm normal thyroid gland
- Nuclear scintigraphy only if unable to identify normal thyroid gland

# DIFFERENTIAL DIAGNOSIS

## Lingual or Sublingual Thyroid
- Ectopic thyroidal tissue enhances
- Appears solid on CT or MR imaging

## Dermoid or Epidermoid of Tongue
- Dermoid will be fat density on CT, hyperintense on T1 MR
- Epidermoid follows water density (CT) & signal (MR)
- Neither directly involves hyoid bone

## Submandibular or Sublingual Space Abscess
- Odontogenic, submandibular or sublingual gland initial infection
- Not embedded in strap muscles
- Thick enhancing wall around multiple fluid-pus collections

## Mixed Laryngocele
- Laryngocele can be traced back to laryngeal origin
- Laryngocele will not be embedded within strap muscles

## Delphian Chain Necrotic Node
- May be difficult to differentiate necrotic node from infected TGDC

# PATHOLOGY

## General Features
- General path comments
  - ○ Embryology-anatomy
    - ■ Thyroglossal duct (TGD) originates near foramen cecum, at posterior third of tongue
    - ■ Thyroid anlage arises at base of tongue, then descends to final location (thyroid bed) along TGD
    - ■ Descends through base of tongue, floor of mouth, around or through hyoid bone, anterior to strap muscles, to final position in thyroid bed anterior to thyroid or cricoid cartilage
    - ■ At 5-6 gestational weeks, TGD involutes, with foramen cecum & pyramidal thyroid lobe normal remnants
    - ■ Failure of involution, with persistent secretory activity, results in TGDC
- Genetics
  - ○ Familial cases occur (rare); usually autosomal dominant
  - ○ Thyroid developmental anomalies often occur in same family
- Etiology
  - ○ Failure of involution of TGD & persistent secretion of epithelial cells lining duct result in TGDC
  - ○ TGDC can occur anywhere along route of descent of TGD
  - ○ Ectopic thyroid tissue can also occur anywhere along this course
- Epidemiology
  - ○ Most common congenital neck lesion
    - ■ 90% of non-odontogenic congenital cysts
    - ■ 3 times as common as branchial cleft cysts
  - ○ At autopsy > 7% of population will have TGD remnant somewhere along course of tract

# THYROGLOSSAL DUCT CYST

○ < 1% TGDC have associated thyroid carcinoma
• Associated abnormalities
  ○ Thyroid agenesis, ectopia, pyramidal lobe
  ○ Occasionally associated with carcinoma
    ▪ Most commonly papillary carcinoma of the TGD

## Gross Pathologic & Surgical Features
• Smooth, benign-appearing cyst, with tract to hyoid bone ± foramen cecum

## Microscopic Features
• Cyst lined by respiratory or squamous epithelium
• Small deposits of thyroid tissue with colloid commonly associated
• Papillary carcinoma is most common associated malignancy

# CLINICAL ISSUES

## Presentation
• Most common signs/symptoms
  ○ Midline or paramedian doughy, compressible painless neck mass in child or young adult
  ○ Other signs/symptoms
    ▪ Recurrent appearance of midline neck mass with upper respiratory tract infections or trauma
    ▪ Often has a history of multiple prior incision & drainage procedures for "neck abscess"
  ○ Physical examination
    ▪ If TGDC around hyoid bone, cyst elevates when tongue is protruded

## Demographics
• Age
  ○ Age of presentation
    ▪ < 10 years (90%)
    ▪ 10% are 20-35 year olds
• Gender: M < F if hereditary form

## Natural History & Prognosis
• Recurrent, intermittent swelling of mass, usually following a minor upper respiratory infection
• Rapid enlarging mass suggests either infection or associated differentiated thyroid carcinoma
  ○ Carcinoma is associated with TGDC (< 1%)
  ○ Differentiated thyroid Ca (85% papillary carcinoma)

## Treatment
• Complete surgical resection, termed a "Sistrunk procedure"
  ○ Entire cyst & midline portion of hyoid bone is resected
  ○ Tract to foramen cecum dissected free, to prevent recurrence
  ○ Sistrunk procedure is treatment of choice
    ▪ Even if imaging shows no obvious connection to hyoid bone
    ▪ Exception is low infrahyoid neck TGDC
• Sistrunk procedure decreases recurrence rate from 50% to < 4%
• Prognosis is excellent with complete surgical resection
• Recurrences (incomplete resection) often complicated, lateral

# DIAGNOSTIC CHECKLIST

## Consider
• Relationship to hyoid bone important to note: Suprahyoid, hyoid or infrahyoid in location
• Any associated nodularity or chunky calcification suggests associated thyroid carcinoma
• Thyroid bed should be imaged, to be sure there is a thyroid gland present

# SELECTED REFERENCES

1. Falvo L et al: Papillary thyroid carcinoma in thyroglossal duct cyst: case reports and literature review. Int Surg. 91(3):141-6, 2006
2. Prasad KC et al: Thyroglossal duct cyst: an unusual presentation. Ear Nose Throat J. 85(7):454-6, 2006
3. Diaz MC et al: A thyroglossal duct cyst causing apnea and cyanosis in a neonate. Pediatr Emerg Care. 21(1):35-7, 2005
4. Koch BL: Cystic malformations of the neck in children. Pediatr Radiol. 35(5):463-77, 2005
5. Marianowski R et al: Risk factors for thyroglossal duct remnants after Sistrunk procedure in a pediatric population. Int J Pediatr Otorhinolaryngol. 67(1):19-23, 2003
6. Dedivitis RA et al: Thyroglossal duct: a review of 55 cases. J Am Coll Surg. 194(3):274-7, 2002
7. Dedivitis RA et al: Papillary thyroid carcinoma in thyroglossal duct cyst. Int Surg. 85(3):198-201, 2000
8. Glastonbury CM et al: The CT and MR imaging features of carcinoma arising in thyroglossal duct remnants. AJNR Am J Neuroradiol. 21(4):770-4, 2000
9. Sprinzl GM et al: Morphology of the human thyroglossal tract: a histologic and macroscopic study in infants and children. Ann Otol Rhinol Laryngol. 109(12 Pt 1):1135-9, 2000
10. Waddell A et al: Thyroglossal duct remnants. J Laryngol Otol. 114(2):128-9, 2000
11. Weber AL et al: The thyroid and parathyroid glands. CT and MR imaging and correlation with pathology and clinical findings. Radiol Clin North Am. 38(5):1105-29, 2000
12. Ewing CA et al: Presentations of thyroglossal duct cysts in adults. Eur Arch Otorhinolaryngol. 256(3):136-8, 1999
13. O'Hanlon DM et al: Aberrant thyroglossal cyst. J Laryngol Otol. 108(12):1105-7, 1994
14. Van Vuuren PA et al: Carcinoma arising in thyroglossal remnants. Clin Otolaryngol. 19(6):509-15, 1994
15. Chait P et al: Thyroglossal duct remnants. Arch Otolaryngol Head Neck Surg. 119(7):798, 1993
16. Maziak D et al: Management of papillary carcinoma arising in thyroglossal-duct anlage. Can J Surg. 35(5):522-5, 1992
17. Radkowski D et al: Thyroglossal duct remnants. Preoperative evaluation and management. Arch Otolaryngol Head Neck Surg. 117(12):1378-81, 1991
18. Pelausa ME et al: Sistrunk revisited: a 10-year review of revision thyroglossal duct surgery at Toronto's Hospital for Sick Children. J Otolaryngol. 18(7):325-33, 1989
19. Hoffman MA et al: Thyroglossal duct remnants in infants and children: reevaluation of histopathology and methods for resection. Ann Otol Rhinol Laryngol. 97(5 Pt 1):483-6, 1988
20. LaRouere MJ et al: Evaluation and management of a carcinoma arising in a thyroglossal duct cyst. Am J Otolaryngol. 8(6):351-5, 1987
21. Reede DL et al: CT of thyroglossal duct cysts. Radiology. 157(1):121-5, 1985
22. Guimaraes SB et al: Thyroglossal duct remnants in infants and children. Mayo Clin Proc. 47(2):117-20, 1972

# THYROGLOSSAL DUCT CYST

## IMAGE GALLERY

### Typical

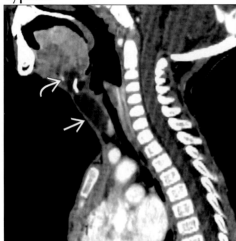

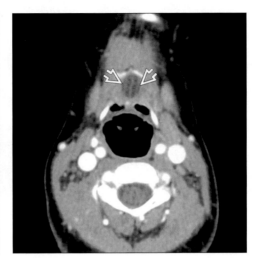

*(Left) Sagittal CECT reformation shows a cystic lesion in the midline with one component ➡ in the tongue base above the hyoid bone and a lower one ➡ in the strap muscles below the hyoid. (Right) Axial CECT (same patient as previous image) at the level of the vallecula shows a cystic structure ➡ in the midline, near the hyoid bone, where the thyroglossal duct attaches.*

### Typical

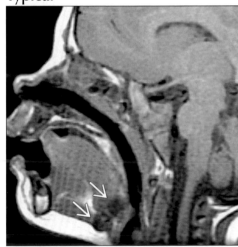

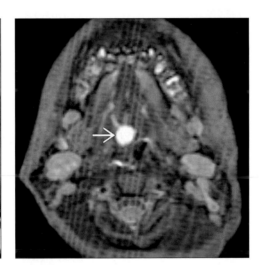

*(Left) Sagittal T1WI MR shows a hypointense, bilobed mass ➡ at the base of the tongue, just above the hyoid bone, a typical location for a thyroglossal duct cyst. (Right) Axial T2WI MR (same patient as previous image) shows the mass ➡ to be sharply defined and hyperintense. This appearance and location are strongly suggestive of thyroglossal duct cyst.*

### Typical

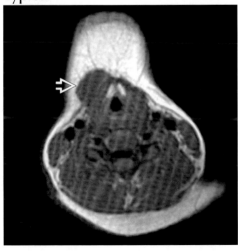

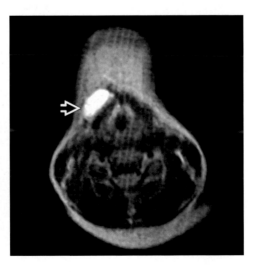

*(Left) Axial T1WI MR shows a well-defined, hypointense right anterior paramedian neck mass ➡ at the level of the hyoid bone. This is a typical appearance of paramedian thyroglossal duct cyst. (Right) Axial T2WI MR (same patient as previous image) shows the cyst ➡ becomes markedly hyperintense on this sequence. Note that it remains quite sharply demarcated from surrounding structures.*

# THYMIC CYST

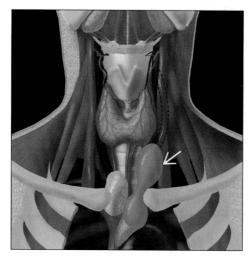

*Coronal graphic shows typical cervical thymic cyst ➡️ extending from the anterior mediastinum into the lower neck along the course of the thymopharyngeal duct.*

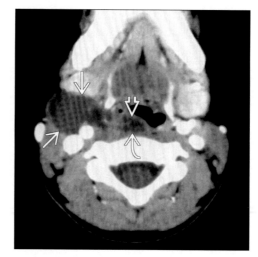

*Axial CECT shows the cyst ➡️ to be trans-spatial; it lies anterior to the right carotid sheath, extending into the retropharyngeal space ➡️ and compressing the airway ➡️.*

## TERMINOLOGY

### Abbreviations and Synonyms
- Cervical thymic cyst (CTC)
- Thymopharyngeal duct cyst
- Congenital thymic cyst

### Definitions
- Cystic remnant of thymopharyngeal duct, derivative of 3rd pharyngeal pouch
- Hassall corpuscles in cyst wall confirm diagnosis of CTC

## IMAGING FINDINGS

### General Features
- Best diagnostic clue
  - Cystic mass in lateral infrahyoid neck, in lateral visceral space or adjacent to carotid space
    - Closely associated with carotid sheath
- Location
  - Anywhere along thymopharyngeal duct from pyriform sinus to anterior mediastinum
  - Lateral left infrahyoid neck, at level of thyroid gland is most common location
  - May parallel sternocleidomastoid muscle, close to carotid sheath
  - Mediastinal thymic cyst may be found without cervical neck component
- Size: Variable, from several cm to very long, along course of thymopharyngeal duct
- Morphology
  - Usually large dominant cyst
  - May be multi-loculated
  - May splay carotid artery and jugular vein
  - Larger CTC may present as a dumbbell cervicothoracic mass, projecting from lower lateral cervical neck into superior mediastinum

### CT Findings
- CECT
  - Nonenhancing low attenuation left lateral neck cyst
    - Closely associated with carotid sheath common
    - Solid components rare = aberrant thymic tissue, lymphoid aggregates or parathyroid tissue
    - May be connected to mediastinal thymus directly, or by fibrous cord

## DDx: Lateral Cystic Neck Masses in Children

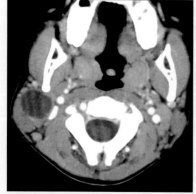

*2nd BAC*

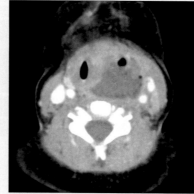

*Abscess 2° to 4th BAA*

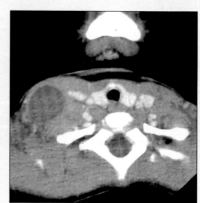

*Lymphatic Malformation*

II

4

22

# THYMIC CYST

## Key Facts

### Terminology
- Cystic remnant of thymopharyngeal duct, derivative of 3rd pharyngeal pouch
- Hassall corpuscles in cyst wall confirm diagnosis of CTC

### Imaging Findings
- Cystic mass in lateral infrahyoid neck, in lateral visceral space or adjacent to carotid space
- Lateral left infrahyoid neck, at level of thyroid gland is most common location
- Nonenhancing low attenuation left lateral neck cyst
- Closely associated with carotid sheath common
- May be connected to mediastinal thymus directly, or by fibrous cord

### Top Differential Diagnoses
- 2nd Branchial Apparatus Cyst (BAC)
- 4th Branchial Apparatus Anomaly
- Lymphatic Malformation (LM)
- Thyroid Cyst

### Pathology
- Remnants of thymopharyngeal duct result in CTC
- Rare lesion as compared with other congenital neck masses
- Smooth, thin-walled cervical cyst, often with caudal fibrous strand extending to mediastinal thymus
- Cyst wall may be nodular
- Hassall corpuscles in cyst wall confirm diagnosis

### Clinical Issues
- Often asymptomatic

## MR Findings
- T1WI
  - Homogeneous hypointense cyst most common
  - May be iso- to hyperintense if filled with blood products, proteinaceous fluid or cholesterol
  - Thin wall
  - Solid nodules usually isointense to muscle
- T2WI: Homogeneously hyperintense fluid contents
- T1 C+
  - Cystic component non-enhancing
  - Cyst wall or solid nodules may enhance slightly
  - If infected, cyst wall may be thickened and enhancing, surrounding soft tissue may be inflamed

## Ultrasonographic Findings
- Thin-walled anechoic or hypoechoic lateral neck mass
- Rarely have solid nodules in wall

## Imaging Recommendations
- Best imaging tool: CECT or MR preferable to ultrasound
- Protocol advice: Include upper mediastinum to demonstrate mediastinal extension

## DIFFERENTIAL DIAGNOSIS

### 2nd Branchial Apparatus Cyst (BAC)
- Most common branchial apparatus cyst
- Most common location = lateral to carotid sheath, anteromedial to SCM and posterior to submandibular gland
- When infrahyoid, anterior to carotid space
- May mimic CTC when found in lower neck on left

### 4th Branchial Apparatus Anomaly
- Primary location: Cyst or abscess anterior to the left thyroid lobe
- Often presents with suppurative thyroiditis
- Inflammation frequently extends to surround apex of pyriform sinus

## Lymphatic Malformation (LM)
- May affect any space in H&N
- When in PCS, abuts carotid space posteriorly
- Unilocular or multilocular
- Focal or infiltrative and transpatial
- Fluid-fluid levels common, secondary to intralesional hemorrhage

## Lateral Neck Abscess Unrelated to Branchial Apparatus Anomaly
- Present with signs and symptoms of infection
- Irregular, thick enhancing wall with low attenuation center
- If associated with thyroid gland, think 4th branchial pouch anomaly

## Thyroid Cyst
- Primary location: Intrathyroidal, left or right
- Large or hemorrhagic colloid cyst
- Usually more medial than CTC

## PATHOLOGY

### General Features
- General path comments
  - Embryology
    - Failure of obliteration of thymopharyngeal duct, a remnant of 3rd pharyngeal pouch
    - Thymopharyngeal duct arises from pyriform sinus, descends into mediastinum
    - Persistent sequestered remnants may occur from mandible to thoracic inlet
    - Thymus & parathyroid glands arise from 3rd & 4th pharyngeal pouches, respectively
    - Embryologic migration follows a caudal course along thymopharyngeal duct during 1st trimester
  - No malignant association
- Etiology
  - Remnants of thymopharyngeal duct result in CTC
  - Ectopic thymus may also occur along thymopharyngeal duct

# THYMIC CYST

- Epidemiology
  - Rare lesion as compared with other congenital neck masses
  - Almost always found in left side of neck

## Gross Pathologic & Surgical Features
- Smooth, thin-walled cervical cyst, often with caudal fibrous strand extending to mediastinal thymus
- Filled with brownish fluid
- Cyst wall may be nodular
- Associated with lymphoid tissue, parathyroid or thymic remnants
- Rarely may extend through thyrohyoid membrane into pyriform sinus

## Microscopic Features
- Hassall corpuscles in cyst wall confirm diagnosis
  - May not always be identifiable if prior hemorrhage or infection
- Cyst wall may contain
  - Lymphoid tissue
  - Parathyroid tissue
  - Thyroid tissue or thymic
  - Thymic tissue
  - Cholesterol crystals & granulomas, probably from prior hemorrhage

# CLINICAL ISSUES

## Presentation
- Most common signs/symptoms
  - Often asymptomatic
  - Gradually enlarging soft compressible mid- to lower cervical neck mass
  - When large, may cause dysphagia, respiratory distress or vocal cord paralysis
- Other presentations
  - Large, infantile, cervicothoracic thymic cyst may present with respiratory compromise
  - Rarely may be associated with disordered calcium metabolism, if parathyroid component is functioning

## Demographics
- Age
  - Most present between 2-15 years of age
  - Only 33% present after first decade
  - Rare reports of primary presentation in adulthood
- Gender: Slightly more common in males, for unknown reasons

## Natural History & Prognosis
- Excellent prognosis if completely resected
- Recurrence common if incompletely resected

## Treatment
- Complete surgical resection
- Large cervicothoracic thymic cyst may require H&N and thoracic surgery

# DIAGNOSTIC CHECKLIST

## Consider
- If cystic mass is intimately associated with anterior carotid sheath, think CTC
- If cystic mass extends from the anterior neck to the upper mediastinum, think CTC

## Image Interpretation Pearls
- Dumbbell-shaped left cervicothoracic cystic mass highly suggestive of either thymic cyst or lymphatic malformation
- If unilocular lesion with discrete margins, may be thymic cyst or unilocular lymphatic malformation

# SELECTED REFERENCES

1. Koch BL: Cystic malformations of the neck in children. Pediatr Radiol. 35(5):463-77, 2005
2. Khariwala SS et al: Cervical presentations of thymic anomalies in children. Int J Pediatr Otorhinolaryngol. 68(7):909-14, 2004
3. Pereira KD et al: Management of anomalies of the third and fourth branchial pouches. Int J Pediatr Otorhinolaryngol. 68(1):43-50, 2004
4. Liberman M et al: Ten years of experience with third and fourth branchial remnants. J Pediatr Surg. 37(5):685-90, 2002
5. Ozturk H et al: Multilocular cervical thymic cyst: an unusual neck mass in children. Int J Pediatr Otorhinolaryngol. 61(3): 249-52, 2001
6. Billings KR et al: Infected neonatal cervical thymic cyst. Otolaryngol Head Neck Surg. 123(5): 651-4, 2000
7. Koeller KK et al: Congenital cystic masses of the neck: radiologic-pathologic correlation. Radiographics. 19(1): 121-46; quiz 152-3, 1999
8. Millman B et al: Cervical thymic anomalies. Int J Pediatr Otorhinolaryngol. 47(1): 29-39, 1999
9. Hendrickson M et al: Congenital thymic cysts in children--mostly misdiagnosed. J Pediatr Surg. 33(6): 821-5, 1998
10. Hadi U et al: Valsalva-induced cervical thymic cyst. Otolaryngol Head Neck Surg. 117(6): S70-2, 1997
11. Kelley DJ et al: Cervicomediastinal thymic cysts. Int J Pediatr Otorhinolaryngol. 39(2):139-46, 1997
12. Nguyen Q et al: Cervical thymic cyst: case reports and review of the literature. Laryngoscope. 106(3 Pt 1):247-52, 1996
13. Burton EM et al: Cervical thymic cysts: CT appearance of two cases including a persistent thymopharyngeal duct cyst. Pediatr Radiol. 25(5): 363-5, 1995
14. Marra S et al: Cervical thymic cyst. Otolaryngol Head Neck Surg. 112(2): 338-40, 1995
15. Miller MB et al: Cervical thymic cyst. Otolaryngol Head Neck Surg. 112(4): 586-8, 1995
16. Benson MT et al: Congenital anomalies of the branchial apparatus: embryology and pathologic anatomy. Radiographics. 12(5):943-60, 1992
17. Zarbo RJ et al: Thymopharyngeal duct cyst: a form of cervical thymus. Ann Otol Rhinol Laryngol. 92(3 Pt 1):284-9, 1983
18. Guba AM Jr et al: Cervical presentation of thymic cysts. Am J Surg. 136(4):430-6, 1978
19. Tovi F et al: The aberrant cervical thymus. Embryology, Pathology, and clinical implications. Am J Surg. 136(5):631-7, 1978

# THYMIC CYST

## IMAGE GALLERY

### Typical

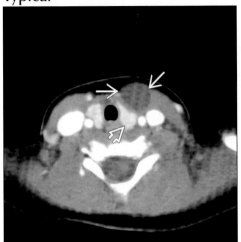

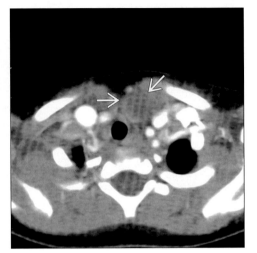

*(Left)* Axial CECT shows a well defined cystic mass ➔ closely applied to the anterior aspect of the carotid sheath and anterolateral to the left thyroid lobe ➔. *(Right)* Axial CECT of same patient as previous image shows the lowermost extension ➔. A tract extended from a lower neck cutaneous pit to the cyst, and from the upper cyst to the pharyngeal mucosa.

### Typical

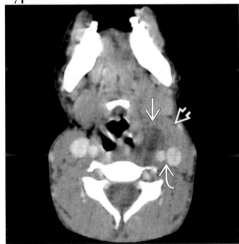

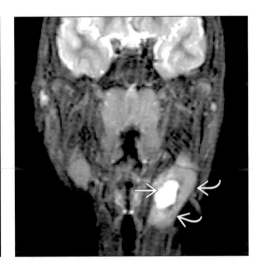

*(Left)* Axial CECT shows show a fluid collection ➔ in the left neck, anteromedial to the left carotid sheath ➔, with a crescent of ectopic thymus ➔ at the periphery. *(Right)* Coronal T2WI MR in the same patient as previous image better shows the full extent of the mass: The central cyst ➔ with a periphery of thymic tissue ➔.

### Typical

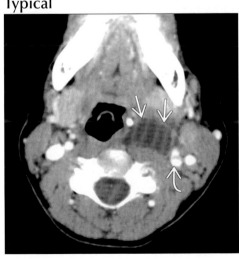

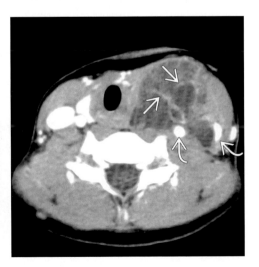

*(Left)* Axial CECT shows the superior extent of a thymic cyst ➔, situated anteromedial to the left carotid sheath ➔ and displacing the airway to the right. *(Right)* Axial CECT in the same patient as previous image shows the inferior extent of the cyst splaying the carotid sheath vessels ➔. The multiple septations ➔ are atypical and likely related to prior infection.

# VENOLYMPHATIC MALFORMATIONS

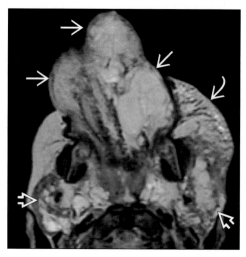

Axial T2WI MR shows multiloculated mass involving the tongue ➡, bilateral parapharyngeal and parotid spaces ➡ and left buccal space ➡.

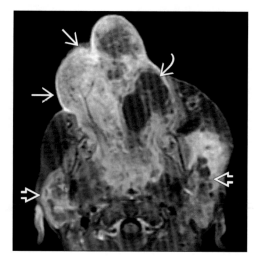

Axial T1 C+ FS MR shows enhancement of the venous component in the right tongue ➡, nonenhancing lymphatic components in the left tongue ➡, and mixed VLM in the parotid spaces ➡.

## TERMINOLOGY

### Abbreviations and Synonyms

- Synonyms
  - Lymphatic malformation (preferred term); cystic hygroma, lymphangioma
  - Venous malformation (preferred term); cavernous malformation, cavernous hemangioma (latter term should be avoided)
  - Venolymphatic malformation (preferred term); lymphaticovenous malformation
- Abbreviations
  - Lymphatic malformation (LM)
  - Venous malformation (VM)
  - Venolymphatic malformation (VLM)

### Definitions

- Vascular malformations: Congenital malformation; not a neoplasm; grow commensurate with the child
  - Lymphatic malformation
    - Abnormal collection of lymphatic vessels, microcystic or macrocystic; unifocal, multifocal or diffuse
  - Venous malformation

- Abnormal venous structures; unifocal, multifocal or diffuse
  - Arteriovenous malformation (AVM)
    - Direct connection of abnormal feeding arteries and draining veins without intervening capillary bed
  - Capillary malformation; port wine stain
    - Collection of tiny vessels within the dermis or within deep vascular malformations of all channel types
  - Mixed malformations: Most common venous and lymphatic = VLM

## IMAGING FINDINGS

### General Features

- Best diagnostic clue
  - Lymphatic malformation: Trans-spatial multicystic mass with fluid-fluid levels
    - Unilocular or multilocular nonenhancing cystic mass with imperceptible wall
    - Microcystic or macrocystic
    - Trans-spatial = cross multiple contiguous spaces

## DDx: Partially Cystic-Appearing Head & Neck Masses

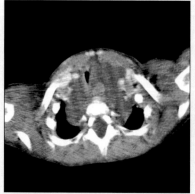
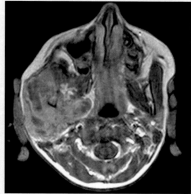
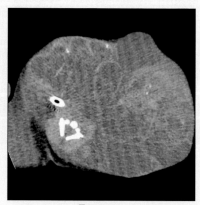

| Plexiform Neurofibroma | Sarcoma | Teratoma |

# VENOLYMPHATIC MALFORMATIONS

## Key Facts

### Terminology

- Vascular malformations: Congenital malformation; not a neoplasm; grow commensurate with the child
- Lymphatic malformation
- Venous malformation
- Arteriovenous malformation (AVM)
- Capillary malformation; port wine stain
- Mixed malformations: Most common venous and lymphatic = VLM

### Imaging Findings

- Lymphatic malformation: Trans-spatial multicystic mass with fluid-fluid levels
- Venous malformation: Lobulated soft tissue "mass" of venous channels
- Mixed venolymphatic malformation: Mixed cystic and enhancing venous trans-spatial mass

### Pathology

- 45% of children with periorbital LM have associated intracranial developmental venous anomalies
- 28% of children with venolymphatic malformations of the orbit have associated intracranial developmental venous anomalies

### Clinical Issues

- Lymphatic malformation
- Nontender, compressible soft tissue mass
- May rapidly increase in size in association with viral respiratory infection or intralesional hemorrhage
- Venous malformation
- Pain, soft tissue mass
- 90% of LM diagnosed before age 2 years

- Fluid-fluid levels typical if intralesional hemorrhage
- Septations may enhance
- If infected, wall and surrounding tissues may enhance
- Venous malformation: Lobulated soft tissue "mass" of venous channels
    - Phleboliths
    - May appear cystic on pre-contrast images
    - Variable contrast-enhancement
    - Osseous remodeling adjacent bone
    - Fat hypertrophy in adjacent soft tissues
    - May have enlarged draining veins
- Mixed venolymphatic malformation: Mixed cystic and enhancing venous trans-spatial mass
- Location
    - Any location in head and neck
        - Submandibular space, parotid space, masticator space, posterior cervical space, orbit, sublingual space, tongue, buccal space
        - Frequently trans-spatial
- Morphology
    - Solitary or multiple
    - Well-circumscribed or infiltrative

## Imaging Recommendations

- Best imaging tool
    - Lymphatic malformation
        - MR T2 best demonstrates extent of lesion and presence of fluid-fluid levels
        - Post-contrast T1WI with fat-saturation best demonstrates enhancing septations and enhancing venous component in mixed venolymphatic malformations
    - Venous vascular malformation
        - CT best demonstrates phleboliths
        - MR best demonstrates extent of lesion and best characterizes mixed venolymphatic malformations

## DIFFERENTIAL DIAGNOSIS

### Plexiform Neurofibroma (PF)

- Variable contrast-enhancement
    - May be hypointense on T2WI MR and low attenuation on CT
    - Suspect neurofibromatosis type 1 (NF1) if multiple or plexiform
- "Target sign" highly suggestive

### Sarcoma

- Heterogeneously enhancing soft tissue mass
    - Usually less intense enhancement than infantile hemangioma
    - Usually less homogeneous enhancement than infantile hemangioma
- ± Osseous destruction
- Usually lacks high flow vessels
    - Exception = alveolar soft part sarcoma

### Teratoma

- Frequently contain calcification
- Often large and infiltrative
- May cause significant airway and feeding issues when occur in head and neck

## PATHOLOGY

### General Features

- Genetics
    - LMs associated with Noonan syndrome, Turner syndrome and fetal alcohol syndrome
    - VMs associated with blue rubber bleb nevus syndrome, Turner syndrome, trisomy 13, 18 and 21
- Etiology
    - Lymphatic malformation
        - Failure of primordial lymphatic sacs to drain into the adjacent veins, abnormal sequestration of lymphatic tissue or abnormal budding of lymphatics
    - Venous vascular malformation
        - Anomalous congenital venous vascular rests

- Associated abnormalities
  - 45% of children with periorbital LM have associated intracranial developmental venous anomalies
  - 28% of children with venolymphatic malformations of the orbit have associated intracranial developmental venous anomalies
  - Klippel-Trenaunay syndrome
    - Combined low-flow vascular malformation and gigantism
    - Capillary-lymphaticovenous malformation
  - Parkes-Weber syndrome
    - Combined high-flow vascular malformation and gigantism
    - Capillary-lymphatic-arteriovenous malformation

## Microscopic Features
- Lymphatic malformation
  - Composed of primitive embryonic lymph sacs of varying sizes separated by connective tissue stroma
  - Increasing size of endothelial lined channels
    - Lymphangioma simplex
    - Cavernous lymphangioma
    - Cystic hygroma
- Venous malformation
  - Composed of venous channels of varying sizes and wall thickness, absent internal elastic lamina
  - Luminal thrombi = phleboliths

## CLINICAL ISSUES

## Presentation
- Most common signs/symptoms
  - Lymphatic malformation
    - Nontender, compressible soft tissue mass
    - May rapidly increase in size in association with viral respiratory infection or intralesional hemorrhage
  - Venous malformation
    - Pain, soft tissue mass

## Demographics
- Age
  - Most LM and VM identified at birth
  - 90% of LM diagnosed before age 2 years

## Treatment
- Lymphatic malformation
  - Surgical resection and/or percutaneous sclerotherapy
  - Recent literature describes success with radiofrequency ablation of microcystic LM of the oral cavity
- Venous malformation
  - Aimed at reduction of symptoms rather than total elimination of lesion
    - Aspirin to prevent thrombosis, elastic compression garments, percutaneous sclerotherapy, surgical resection

## DIAGNOSTIC CHECKLIST

## Image Interpretation Pearls
- Trans-spatial nonenhancing cystic mass in the head and neck, primary consideration lymphatic malformation
- Enhancing "mass" in the neck associated with calcifications, primary consideration venous malformation
- Mixed cystic and enhancing trans-spatial lesion in the head and neck, primary consideration mixed venous/lymphatic vascular malformation
- High flow vascular mass without significant soft tissue component consider arteriovenous malformation

## SELECTED REFERENCES

1. Grimmer JF et al: Radiofrequency ablation of microcystic lymphatic malformation in the oral cavity. Arch Otolaryngol Head Neck Surg. 132(11):1251-6, 2006
2. Greene AK et al: Periorbital lymphatic malformation: clinical course and management in 42 patients. Plast Reconstr Surg. 115(1):22-30, 2005
3. Koch BL: Cystic malformations of the neck in children. Pediatr Radiol. 35(5):463-77, 2005
4. Marler JJ et al: Current management of hemangiomas and vascular malformations. Clin Plast Surg. 32(1):99-116, ix, 2005
5. Lee BB et al: Advanced management of venous malformation with ethanol sclerotherapy: mid-term results. J Vasc Surg. 37(3):533-8, 2003
6. Donnelly LF et al: Vascular malformations and hemangiomas: a practical approach in a multidisciplinary clinic. AJR Am J Roentgenol. 174(3):597-608, 2000
7. Donnelly LF et al: Combined sonographic and fluoroscopic guidance: a modified technique for percutaneous sclerosis of low-flow vascular malformations. AJR Am J Roentgenol. 173(3):655-7, 1999
8. Burrows PE et al: Diagnostic imaging in the evaluation of vascular birthmarks. Dermatol Clin. 16(3):455-88, 1998
9. Fishman SJ et al: Vascular anomalies. A primer for pediatricians. Pediatr Clin North Am. 45(6):1455-77, 1998
10. Kohout MP et al: Arteriovenous malformations of the head and neck: natural history and management. Plast Reconstr Surg. 102(3):643-54, 1998
11. Barnes PD et al: Hemangiomas and vascular malformations of the head and neck: MR characterization. AJNR Am J Neuroradiol. 15(1):193-5, 1994
12. Fishman SJ et al: Hemangiomas and vascular malformations of infancy and childhood. Pediatr Clin North Am. 40(6):1177-200, 1993
13. Zadvinskis DP et al: Congenital malformations of the cervicothoracic lymphatic system: embryology and pathogenesis. Radiographics. 12(6):1175-89, 1992
14. Meyer JS et al: Biological classification of soft-tissue vascular anomalies: MR correlation. AJR Am J Roentgenol. 157(3):559-64, 1991
15. Mulliken JB et al: Hemangiomas and vascular malformations in infants and children: a classification based on endothelial characteristics. Plast Reconstr Surg. 69(3):412-22, 1982
16. Katz SE et al: Combined venous lymphatic malformations of the orbit (so-called lymphangiomas). Association with noncontiguous intracranial vascular anomalies.

# VENOLYMPHATIC MALFORMATIONS

## IMAGE GALLERY

### Typical

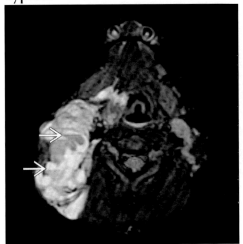
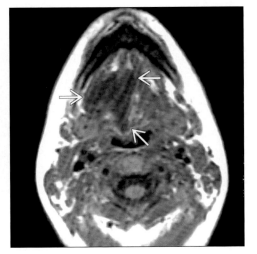

*(Left)* Axial STIR MR shows typical MR appearance of trans-spatial lymphatic malformation with fluid-fluid levels ➡ secondary to intralesional hemorrhage. *(Right)* Axial T1 C+ MR shows irregularly shaped nonenhancing unilocular, macrocystic lymphatic malformation ➡ in the floor of the mouth.

### Typical

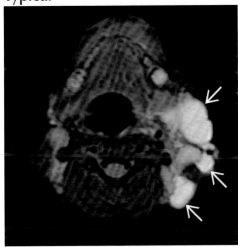
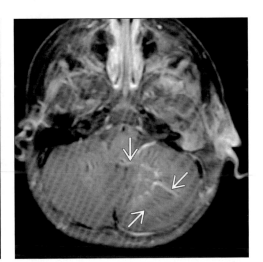

*(Left)* Axial STIR MR shows multiloculated transpatial VLM with multiple cysts ➡ that did not enhance after contrast. *(Right)* Axial T1 C+ FS MR in the same patient as previous image shows a large developmental venous anomaly ➡ in the left cerebellar hemisphere.

### Typical

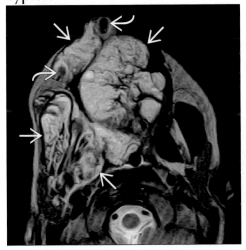
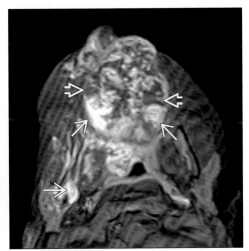

*(Left)* Axial T2WI MR shows a diffuse multiloculated VLM ➡ involving the right tongue and parapharyngeal, masticator and buccal spaces. Focal hypointensities ➡ likely represent phleboliths. *(Right)* Axial T1 C+ FS MR in the same patient as previous image shows contrast-enhancement of the venous component ➡ and no enhancement in the lymphatic component ➡.

# INFANTILE HEMANGIOMA

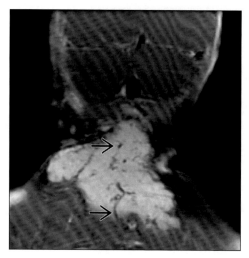

Coronal T1 C+ FS MR shows lobulated intensely enhancing infantile hemangioma of the neck, with high flow intralesional vessels ➡, in the posterior cervical space.

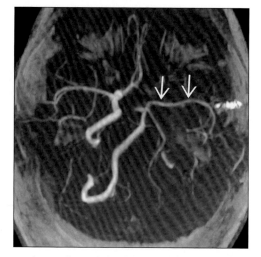

Axial MRA shows absent left internal carotid artery in a child with bilateral facial hemangiomas and PHACES syndrome. Right MCA ➡ fills from posterior circulation via posterior communicator.

## TERMINOLOGY

### Abbreviations and Synonyms

- Hemangioma of infancy (HI), capillary hemangioma, infantile hemangioma

### Definitions

- Benign neoplasm of proliferating endothelial cells
- Not a vascular malformation

## IMAGING FINDINGS

### General Features

- Best diagnostic clue
  - Well-defined mass with diffuse enhancement
  - High flow vessels in and adjacent to mass during proliferative phase (PP)
  - Decrease size with fatty replacement during involutional phase (IP)
- Location
  - 60% occur in head and neck (any space including parotid glands, orbit, nasal cavity, subglottic airway)
  - Other locations: Extremities, trunk, rarely cerebellopontine angle
- Size
  - Variable; small to very large
  - Depends on clinical phase: PP or IP
- Morphology
  - Majority are single lesions in subcutaneous tissues
  - Occasionally multiple, trans-spatial or deep
  - Associated abnormalities in PHACES syndrome
    - Posterior fossa and supratentorial brain malformations (Dandy Walker malformation, heterotopia)
    - Hemangiomas of the head and neck
    - Arterial stenosis, occlusion, aneurysm
    - Cardiovascular defects (aortic coarctation, cardiac anomalies)
    - Eye abnormalities (strabismus, amblyopia, proptosis)
    - Supra-umbilical raphe and sternal clefts
- CT findings
  - NECT
    - Intermediate attenuation without calcification
    - Rarely remodeling of adjacent osseous structures, no osseous erosion

## DDx: Enhancing Head and Neck Masses

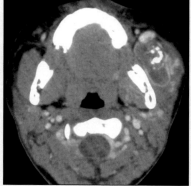

Venous Malformation

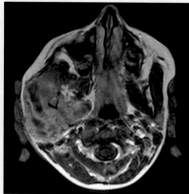

Ewing Sarcoma

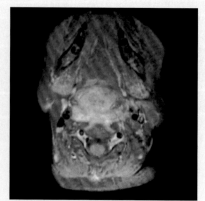

Plexiform Neurofibroma

# INFANTILE HEMANGIOMA

## Key Facts

### Terminology
- Hemangioma of infancy (HI), capillary hemangioma, infantile hemangioma
- Benign neoplasm of proliferating endothelial cells
- Not a vascular malformation

### Imaging Findings
- Well-defined mass with diffuse enhancement
- High flow vessels in and adjacent to mass during proliferative phase (PP)
- Decrease size with fatty replacement during involutional phase (IP)

### Top Differential Diagnoses
- Venous Malformation (VM)
- Sarcoma
- Plexiform Neurofibroma (NF)

- Arteriovenous Malformation (AVM)

### Pathology
- Incidence is 1-2% of neonates, 12% by age 1 year

### Clinical Issues
- Majority don't require treatment; expectant waiting

### Diagnostic Checklist
- Visible shortly after birth
- Parotid lesions: Evaluate facial nerve
- Phleboliths suggest venous malformation
- Older child or osseous destruction consider sarcoma
- Trans-spatial mass with cafe au lait skin lesions suggest plexiform neurofibroma
- Large vessels with little or ill-defined parenchymal mass suggest AVM

- Fatty infiltration during IP
  - ○ CECT
    - ■ Diffuse and prominent contrast-enhancement
    - ■ Prominent vessels in and adjacent to mass; PP
- MR findings
  - ○ T1WI: PP, isointense to muscle; IP, fatty replacement
  - ○ T2WI: Mildly hyperintense relative to muscle
  - ○ T1WI C+
    - ■ Intense contrast-enhancement
    - ■ Best appreciated on fat-saturation T1WI
    - ■ Serpiginous flow voids in and adjacent to mass
  - ○ MR GRE: High flow vessels in and adjacent to mass
  - ○ MRA: Stenosis, occlusion, agenesis, aneurysm (PHACES syndrome)
- Sonographic findings
  - ○ Soft tissue mass with prominent vessels
  - ○ Arterial and venous waveforms
  - ○ Mean venous peak velocities **not** elevated as might be identified in true arteriovenous malformation (AVM)
- Angiographic findings
  - ○ Not a primary imaging tool for diagnosis
  - ○ Hypervascular mass with prolonged capillary blush, without arteriovenous shunting

## Imaging Recommendations
- Best imaging tool
  - ○ MR or CT with contrast to identify diffuse contrast-enhancement
  - ○ Gradient-recalled echo sequences to identify intralesional and perilesional high flow vessels
  - ○ MRA to identify associated vascular abnormalities
  - ○ Imaging indications (most not imaged, diagnosed by history and physical examination)
    - ■ Suspect deep extension to identify total extent of lesion (particularly orbit and airway)
    - ■ Pretreatment if considering medical or surgical/laser treatment
    - ■ Assess response to treatment
    - ■ Atypical history, older patient or suspect neoplasm
- Protocol advice
  - ○ MR

- ■ Pre-contrast T1, FSE, STIR and SPGR images
- ■ Post-contrast T1 images with fat-suppression
- ■ MRA to identify associated vascular anomalies: Stenosis, occlusions, moyamoya, aneurysms
- ■ Parotid hemangiomas: Evaluate location of facial nerve
- ○ CT
  - ■ Post-contrast, pre-contrast if considering venous malformation in DDx to identify phleboliths
  - ■ CTA to identify associated vascular anomalies in suspected PHACES syndrome

## DIFFERENTIAL DIAGNOSIS

### Venous Malformation (VM)
- Congenital vascular malformation composed of large venous lakes
- Hyperintense T2, hypointense T1, diffuse post-contrast-enhancement
- Phleboliths
- Present often at birth and grow commensurate with child

### Sarcoma
- Older child
  - ○ Suspect if age, appearance, growth history, or imaging does not fit for infantile hemangioma
  - ○ Rhabdomyosarcoma, extra-osseous Ewing sarcoma, undifferentiated sarcoma
  - ○ Marked enhancement with prominent vessels suspect alveolar soft part sarcoma (ASPS)
  - ○ Mild to moderate enhancement frequently with osseous erosion suspect rhabdomyosarcoma

### Plexiform Neurofibroma (NF)
- Infiltrative, swirls, ill-defined margins frequently with trans-spatial involvement
- Associated with additional stigmata of neurofibromatosis type 1

# INFANTILE HEMANGIOMA

## Arteriovenous Malformation (AVM)

- Congenital vascular malformation composed of high flow feeding arteries, arteriovenous shunting and large draining veins

## PATHOLOGY

### General Features

- Genetics
  - Majority sporadic
  - Rare association with chromosome 5q31-q33
- Etiology: Proposed theory = clonal expansion of angioblasts with high expression of basic fibroblast growth factors and other angiogenesis markers
- Epidemiology
  - Most common head and neck tumor in infants
  - Incidence is 1-2% of neonates, 12% by age 1 year
  - More common in preterm infants, as high as 29% in infants weighing less than 1 kg

### Microscopic Features

- Prominent endothelial cells, pericytes, mast cells with mitotic figures and multi-laminated endothelial basement membrane

## CLINICAL ISSUES

### Presentation

- Most common signs/symptoms
  - During the proliferative phase (usually lasts up to 12 months), there is increase in size of soft tissue mass, typically with warm, reddish or "strawberry-like" cutaneous discoloration
  - Occasionally deep, present with overlying bluish coloration of the skin secondary to prominent draining veins
  - Spontaneous involution over the next several years
- Other signs/symptoms
  - Ulceration if associated breakdown of overlying subcutaneous fat
  - Airway obstruction with airway involvement
  - Proptosis if large orbital lesion
  - Associated abnormalities in PHACES syndrome

### Demographics

- Age: Typically inapparent at birth, usually presents with rapid growth within first few months of life
- Gender: More common in females than males (2.5:1)
- Ethnicity
  - Most frequent in Caucasians

### Natural History & Prognosis

- Proliferative phase during first year of life
- Involutional phase may last up to 12 years
- Large and segmental facial hemangiomas higher incidence of complications and need for treatment

### Treatment

- Majority don't require treatment; expectant waiting
- Treatment indications
  - Compromise vital structures such as optic nerve compression or airway obstruction
  - Significant skin ulceration
- Medical therapy
  - Steroids (systemic or intralesional), alpha interferon
- Procedural therapy
  - Laser, rarely surgical excision and embolization

## DIAGNOSTIC CHECKLIST

### Consider

- Visible shortly after birth
- Parotid lesions: Evaluate facial nerve
- Phleboliths suggest venous malformation
- Older child or osseous destruction consider sarcoma
- Trans-spatial mass with cafe au lait skin lesions suggest plexiform neurofibroma
- Large vessels with little or ill-defined parenchymal mass suggest AVM

## SELECTED REFERENCES

1. Judd CD et al: Intracranial infantile hemangiomas associated with PHACE syndrome: a report of four cases. AJNR in press, 2007
2. Drolet BA et al: Early stroke and cerebral vasculopathy in children with facial hemangiomas and PHACE association. Pediatrics. 117(3):959-64, 2006
3. Haggstrom AN et al: Patterns of infantile hemangiomas: new clues to hemangioma pathogenesis and embryonic facial development. Pediatrics. 117(3):698-703, 2006
4. Metry DW et al: A prospective study of PHACE syndrome in infantile hemangiomas: demographic features, clinical findings, and complications. Am J Med Genet A. 140(9):975-86, 2006
5. Rossi A et al: Agenesis of bilateral internal carotid arteries in the PHACE syndrome. AJNR Am J Neuroradiol. 27(8):1602, 2006
6. Kronenberg A et al: Ocular and systemic manifestations of PHACES (Posterior fossa malformations, Hemangiomas, Arterial anomalies, Cardiac defects and coarctation of the Aorta, Eye abnormalities, and Sternal abnormalities or ventral developmental defects) syndrome. J AAPOS. 9(2):169-73, 2005
7. Mulliken JB et al: Vascular anomalies. Curr Probl Surg. 37(8):517-84, 2000
8. Dubois J et al: Imaging and therapeutic approach of hemangiomas and vascular malformations in the pediatric age group. Pediatr Radiol. 29(12):879-93, 1999
9. Robertson RL et al: Head and neck vascular anomalies of childhood. Neuroimaging Clin N Am. 9(1):115-32, 1999
10. Burrows PE et al: Diagnostic imaging in the evaluation of vascular birthmarks. Dermatol Clin. 16(3):455-88, 1998
11. Yang WT et al: Sonographic features of head and neck hemangiomas and vascular malformations: review of 23 patients. J Ultrasound Med. 16(1):39-44, 1997
12. Mulliken JB: Cutaneous vascular anomalies. Semin Vasc Surg. 6(4):204-18, 1993
13. Meyer JS et al: Biological classification of soft-tissue vascular anomalies: MR correlation. AJR Am J Roentgenol. 157(3):559-64, 1991
14. Burrows PE et al: Childhood hemangiomas and vascular malformations: angiographic differentiation. AJR Am J Roentgenol. 141(3):483-8, 1983
15. Mulliken JB et al: Hemangiomas and vascular malformations in infants and children: a classification based on endothelial characteristics. Plast Reconstr Surg. 69(3):412-22, 1982

# INFANTILE HEMANGIOMA

## IMAGE GALLERY

### Typical

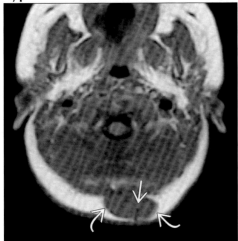
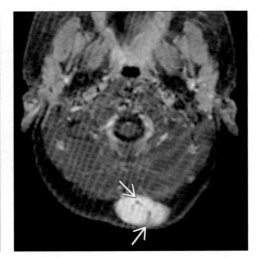

*(Left)* Axial T1WI MR shows a well-defined hypointense subcutaneous mass ➡ in the posterior neck. Note the linear signal voids ➡ representing large vessels. *(Right)* Axial T1 C+ MR in the same patient as previous image shows diffuse contrast-enhancement and again shows the small intralesional high flow vessels ➡.

### Typical

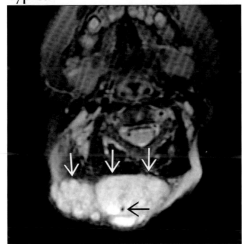
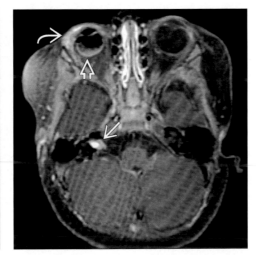

*(Left)* Axial T2WI FS MR shows a lobulated hyperintense infantile hemangioma ➡ in the posterior cervical space with an intralesional high flow vessel ➡, manifested as a flow void. *(Right)* Axial T1 C+ FS MR shows enhancing masses in the right IAC ➡ and preseptal orbit ➡, and small right globe with retinal detachment ➡, in a patient with PHACES syndrome.

### Typical

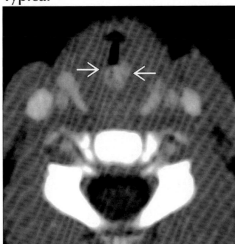
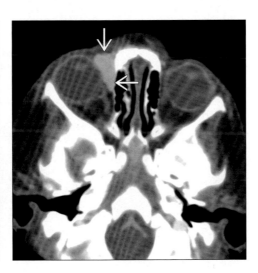

*(Left)* Axial CECT shows a small enhancing mass ➡ posterior to the larynx, causing some mass effect upon the larynx. This was a subglottic hemangioma ➡. *(Right)* Axial CECT shows a well-defined, enhancing mass ➡ in the medial extra-conal space of the right orbit. There is lateral deviation of the right globe and the right medial rectus muscle.

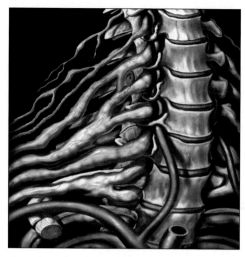

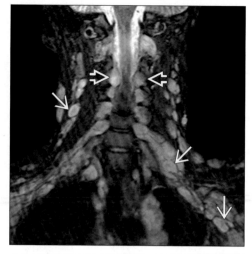

*Coronal graphic shows multilevel, lobulated, tortuous expansion of cervical nerve roots and trunks of the right brachial plexus.*

*Coronal T2WI FS MR shows multilevel, bilateral neurofibromas of the brachial plexus nerves (and others), some with a classic target appearance ➡, and some with intraspinal extension ➡.*

## TERMINOLOGY

### Abbreviations and Synonyms
- Neurofibromatosis 1 (NF1)
- von Recklinghausen disease, autosomal dominant neurofibromatosis

### Definitions
- Autosomal dominant neurocutaneous disorder (phakomatosis)
- Diagnostic NF1 criteria: Establish diagnosis if ≥ 2 present
  - > 6 café-au-lait spots measuring ≥ 5 mm in prepubertal and ≥ 15 mm in postpubertal patients
  - 2 or more neurofibromas (NF) or 1 plexiform NF
  - Axillary/inguinal freckling
  - Visual pathway glioma
  - 2 or more Lisch nodules (optic hamartomas)
  - Distinctive bony lesion
    - Sphenoid wing dysplasia
    - Thinning of long bones ± pseudoarthrosis
  - First degree relative with NF1

## IMAGING FINDINGS

### General Features
- Best diagnostic clue
  - Plexiform neurofibroma (PNF)
  - Multiple localized NFs
- Location
  - NFs and PNFs; any space in H&N
  - Other extracranial H&N manifestations of NF1
    - Orbit: Optic pathway glioma (OPG), sphenoid wing dysplasia, Lisch nodules, buphthalmos, large foramina with PNFs
    - Skull and skull base: Lambdoid suture defect; smooth, corticated enlargement skull base bony foramina with PNF infiltration of cranial nerves
    - Vascular dysplasia: ICA stenosis/occlusion and moyamoya; aneurysms and AV fistula rare
- Size
  - Localized NF: Millimeters to multiple centimeters
  - PNF: May reach large size
- Morphology
  - Localized NF: Ovoid to fusiform
  - PNF: Lobulated

## DDx: Other Manifestations of NF1

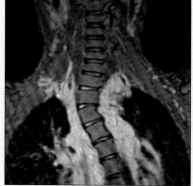

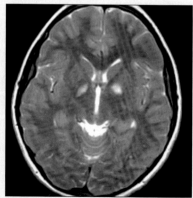

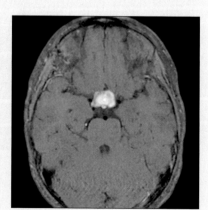

*Scoliosis*

*Typical GP Lesions*

*Optic Pathway Glioma*

# NEUROFIBROMATOSIS TYPE 1, H&N

## Key Facts

### Terminology
- von Recklinghausen disease, autosomal dominant neurofibromatosis

### Imaging Findings
- Plexiform neurofibroma (PNF)
- NFs and PNFs; any space in H&N
- Orbit: Optic pathway glioma (OPG), sphenoid wing dysplasia, Lisch nodules, buphthalmos, large foramina with PNFs
- Skull and skull base: Lambdoid suture defect; smooth, corticated enlargement skull base bony foramina with PNF infiltration of cranial nerves
- Vascular dysplasia: ICA stenosis/occlusion and moyamoya; aneurysms and AV fistula rare
- "Target" sign: Hypointense center, hyperintense periphery

- "Fascicular" sign: Multiple, small irregular hypointense foci (≈ fascicular bundles)

### Pathology
- Localized, plexiform or diffuse associated with NF1
- Most common autosomal dominant disorder occurring in 1:3,000-5,000

### Clinical Issues
- Majority of NF & PNF asymptomatic
- Cutaneous stigmata of NF1
- Sudden, painful ↑ size of stable NF suggests malignant transformation

### Diagnostic Checklist
- If patient has plexiform or multiple localized NFs, consider NF1

---

- ○ Malignant peripheral nerve sheath tumor (PNST): Invasive margins
- PNST = schwannoma, NF and PNF
  - ○ Localized NF
    - Multiple, well-circumscribed, smooth, fusiform, variably enhancing masses along course of nerves
    - Paraspinal NF may be dumbbell shaped ± smooth, corticated enlargement bony neural foramina
    - Schwannoma may be indistinguishable from NF
  - ○ Diffuse NF
    - Plaque-like thickening of skin with poorly defined, reticulated lesion in subcutaneous fat
  - ○ PNF
    - Multilevel, lobulated, tortuous, rope-like expansion within a major nerve distribution
    - Resembles "tangle of worms"
  - ○ Malignant PNST
    - Differentiation of benign from malignant PNST difficult on imaging alone
    - If large size (> 5 cm), heterogeneous with central necrosis, infiltrative margins and rapid growth, consider malignant PNST

## CT Findings
- CECT
  - ○ Localized NF & PNF
    - Frequently have low attenuation (5-25 HU)
    - "Target sign" where central tumor enhances relative to periphery
    - Paraspinal NF may be dumbbell shaped ± enlarged neural foramina

## MR Findings
- T2WI
  - ○ Localized NF & PNF
    - Hyperintense (diffuse neurofibromas often hypointense, likely from high collagen content)
    - "Target" sign: Hypointense center, hyperintense periphery
    - "Fascicular" sign: Multiple, small irregular hypointense foci (≈ fascicular bundles)
- T1 C+
  - ○ Localized NF & PNF

- Localized NF: Homogeneous or mildly heterogeneous enhancement, well circumscribed fusiform mass
- PNF: Heterogeneously enhancing, lobulated mass along course of peripheral nerve

## Imaging Recommendations
- Best imaging tool
  - ○ MR for tumor extent, especially when close to spine
  - ○ Bone CT delineates associated bone changes

---

# PATHOLOGY

## General Features
- General path comments
  - ○ Localized, plexiform or diffuse associated with NF1
  - ○ Localized neurofibroma
    - 90% are solitary & not associated with NF1
    - 10% associated with NF1 ⇒ more frequently are large, multiple & involve large deep nerves (brachial plexus)
    - Discrete NF; any age, most after puberty
    - New lesions may develop throughout life
  - ○ Plexiform neurofibroma
    - Characteristic & diagnostic feature of NF1
    - Any nerve (most common in H&N) ophthalmic division of CN5, brachial plexus, oral cavity (tongue, floor of mouth), scalp, cheek, retropharyngeal space
    - 5% risk of malignant transformation
  - ○ Diffuse neurofibroma
    - Majority (90%) isolated & not associated with NF1
    - Usually involves subcutaneous tissues of H&N
  - ○ Malignant peripheral nerve sheath tumor
    - 50% of malignant PNST associated with NF1
    - 5% patients with NF1 develop malignant PNST
    - Arise from malignant transformation of localized NF or PNF, rarely de novo
    - Most commonly involves major nerve trunks including brachial plexus
    - Usually develop in adults, rare in children
- Genetics

- ○ Autosomal dominant; 50% new mutations
- ○ Gene locus = chromosome 17q11.2
  - ■ "Nonsense mutation" of this gene leads to NF1
- • Etiology
  - ○ NF gene (a tumor suppressor gene) normally encodes production of "neurofibromin" that influences cell growth regulation
  - ○ NF gene "turned off" in NF1
    - ■ Results in cell proliferation & tumor development
- • Epidemiology
  - ○ Most common autosomal dominant disorder occurring in 1:3,000-5,000
  - ○ Most common neurocutaneous syndrome
  - ○ Most common inherited tumor syndrome
- • Other manifestations of NFI
  - ○ CNS
    - ■ Optic pathway gliomas, cerebral gliomas, hydrocephalus, cranial nerve schwannomas, vascular dysplasia
    - ■ Dynamic reactive/dysplastic lesions; white matter, dentate nucleus, globus pallidus (GP), brainstem, thalamus, hippocampus
  - ○ Spine
    - ■ Kyphoscoliosis, lateral thoracic meningocele, enlargement of spinal foramina
  - ○ Skeletal
    - ■ Pseudarthrosis, thinning of long bone cortex, bowing of long bones
  - ○ Vascular
    - ■ Vascular dysplasia; stenosis ± occlusion
    - ■ Renal artery stenosis, coarctation of aorta
  - ○ Neural crest tumors
    - ■ Pheochromocytoma 10 times ↑ in NF1 patients
    - ■ Parathyroid adenomas ↑ incidence
  - ○ Skin
    - ■ Cutaneous & subcutaneous neurofibromas, café-au-lait spots, axillary & inguinal freckling

## Gross Pathologic & Surgical Features

- • Localized neurofibroma
  - ○ Fusiform, firm, gray-white mass intermixed with nerve of origin
- • Plexiform neurofibroma
  - ○ Diffuse, tortuous, rope-like expansion of nerves resembling "tangle of worms"
  - ○ Involves adjacent skin, fascia & deeper tissues
- • Malignant PNST
  - ○ Fusiform, fleshy, tan-white mass with areas of necrosis & hemorrhage
  - ○ Nerve proximally & distally thickened due to spread of tumor along epineurium & perineurium

## Microscopic Features

- • Localized neurofibroma
  - ○ Schwann cells, fibroblasts, mast cells in matrix of collagen fibers & mucoid substance
  - ○ Axons usually embedded within tumor
- • Plexiform neurofibroma
  - ○ Schwann cells, perineural fibroblasts, grow along nerve fascicles
- • Malignant PNST
  - ○ Fibrosarcoma-like growth of spindle cells
  - ○ Considered high grade sarcomas

## Staging, Grading or Classification Criteria

- • Neurofibromas are WHO grade 1
- • Malignant PNST are WHO grade 3/4

# CLINICAL ISSUES

## Presentation

- • Most common signs/symptoms
  - ○ Majority of NF & PNF asymptomatic
  - ○ Cutaneous stigmata of NF1
  - ○ Sudden, painful ↑ size of stable NF suggests malignant transformation

## Demographics

- • Age: Any age, most common late childhood to early adult presentation

## Natural History & Prognosis

- • Slow growing unless malignant transformation

## Treatment

- • Resection NF that press on vital structures
- • Solitary NF resectable; PNF generally unresectable
- • Radiofrequency treatment in PNF may offer new hope

# DIAGNOSTIC CHECKLIST

## Consider

- • If patient has plexiform or multiple localized NFs, consider NF1

# SELECTED REFERENCES

1. Baujat B et al: Radiofrequency in the treatment of craniofacial plexiform neurofibromatosis: a pilot study. Plast Reconstr Surg. 117(4):1261-8, 2006
2. Ferner RE et al: Guidelines for the diagnosis and management of individuals with Neurofibromatosis 1 (NF1). J Med Genet. 2006
3. Mautner VF et al: MRI growth patterns of plexiform neurofibromas in patients with neurofibromatosis type 1. Neuroradiology. 48(3):160-5, 2006
4. Pacelli J et al: Brachial plexopathy due to malignant peripheral nerve sheath tumor in neurofibromatosis type 1: case report and subject review. Muscle Nerve. 33(5):697-700, 2006
5. Kim DH et al: A series of 397 peripheral neural sheath tumors: 30-year experience at Louisiana State University Health Sciences Center. J Neurosurg. 102(2):246-55, 2005
6. Jacquemin C et al: Orbit deformities in craniofacial neurofibromatosis type 1. AJNR Am J Neuroradiol. 24(8):1678-82, 2003
7. Fortman BJ et al: Neurofibromatosis type 1: a diagnostic mimicker at CT. Radiographics. 21(3):601-12, 2001
8. Lin J et al: Cross-sectional imaging of peripheral nerve sheath tumors: characteristic signs on CT, MR imaging, and sonography. AJR Am J Roentgenol. 176(1):75-82, 2001
9. Rapado F et al: Neurofibromatosis type 1 of the head and neck: dilemmas in management. J Laryngol Otol. 115(2):151-4, 2001
10. Gutmann DH et al: The diagnostic evaluation and multidisciplinary management of neurofibromatosis 1 and neurofibromatosis 2. JAMA. 278(1):51-7, 1997

# NEUROFIBROMATOSIS TYPE 1, H&N

## IMAGE GALLERY

### Typical

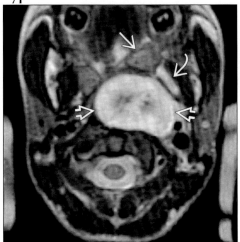

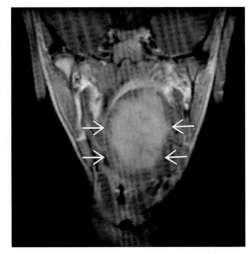

*(Left)* Axial T2WI MR shows a large, well-defined hyperintense solitary neurofibroma ➡ deviating the left palatine tonsil ➡ forward, and the adjacent parapharyngeal fat ➡ anterolaterally. *(Right)* Coronal T1 C+ FS MR in the same patient as previous image shows moderate, mildly heterogeneous contrast-enhancement, without intracranial extension of this solitary neurofibroma ➡.

### Typical

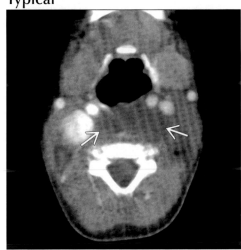

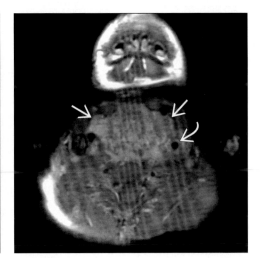

*(Left)* Axial CECT shows a lobulated, low attenuation prevertebral mass ➡ deviating the left carotid sheath vessels anteriorly. *(Right)* Axial T1 C+ FS MR shows a large plexiform neurofibroma ➡ in the anterior neck, involving multiple fascial spaces. Note how the cervical blood vessels ➡ are engulfed.

### Typical

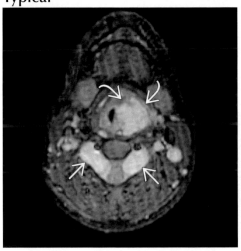

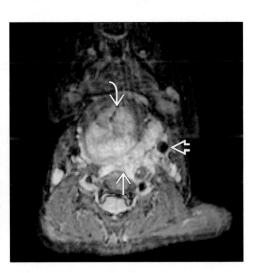

*(Left)* Axial T2WI FS MR shows bilateral localized neural foramen NFs ➡ and a plexiform NF in the infrahyoid visceral space ➡ deviating the airway to the right. *(Right)* Axial T1 C+ FS MR shows an infiltrative plexiform neurofibroma compressing the airway ➡, extending into the prevertebral space ➡ and nearly surrounding the left carotid artery ➡.

# BRACHIAL PLEXUS SCHWANNOMA

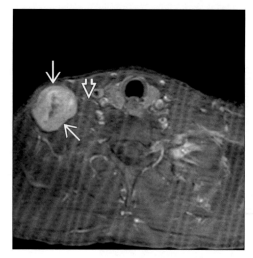

*Axial T1 C+ MR in a child with a neck mass shows a well-defined, enhancing mass ➡, with central necrosis in the lower right neck, adjacent to the anterior scalene muscle ⬌.*

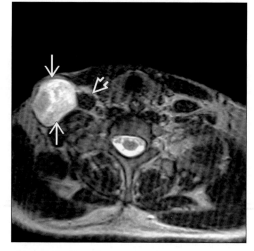

*Axial T2WI MR in the same patient as previous image shows the typical hyperintense signal of the well-defined brachial plexus schwannoma ➡ adjacent to the anterior scalene muscle ⬌.*

## TERMINOLOGY

### Abbreviations and Synonyms
- Neurilemoma ≈ schwannoma ≈ neurinoma

### Definitions
- Benign neoplasm of Schwann cell origin
- Benign peripheral nerve sheath tumors (PNST) = schwannoma, neurofibroma (NF) and plexiform NF

## IMAGING FINDINGS

### General Features
- Best diagnostic clue: Well-circumscribed, fusiform, T2 hyperintense, enhancing mass between anterior & middle scalene muscles
- Location
  - Anywhere along course of brachial plexus (BP, C5-T1) including intra- & extradural spaces, neural foramen, perivertebral space (PVS), posterior cervical space
  - Lesions within PVS are situated between anterior & middle scalene muscles

- Morphology
  - Fusiform mass oriented along nerve of origin
  - ± Dumbbell shape into enlarged neural foramen
  - Well-circumscribed, solid, enhancing mass
  - Cystic degeneration & hemorrhage common

### CT Findings
- NECT
  - Isodense to muscle, calcification uncommon
  - ± Smooth, corticated widening bony neural foramen
- CECT: Moderate to strong enhancement

### MR Findings
- T1WI: Isointense to muscle
- T2WI
  - Hyperintense
  - "Target" sign: Hypointense center, hyperintense periphery
  - "Fascicular" sign: Multiple, irregular, central hypointense foci
- T1 C+: Moderate to intense enhancement

### Imaging Recommendations
- Best imaging tool: High-resolution MR

---

## DDx: Brachial Plexus Masses

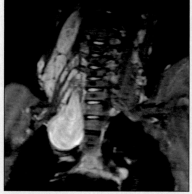

*Multiple Neurofibromas*

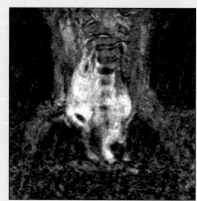

*Plexiform Neurofibroma*

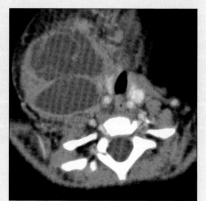

*Venolymphatic Malformation*

# BRACHIAL PLEXUS SCHWANNOMA

## Key Facts

### Terminology
- Benign neoplasm of Schwann cell origin

### Imaging Findings
- Best diagnostic clue: Well-circumscribed, fusiform, T2 hyperintense, enhancing mass between anterior & middle scalene muscles
- ± Dumbbell shape into enlarged neural foramen
- Cystic degeneration & hemorrhage common

- "Target" sign: Hypointense center, hyperintense periphery
- "Fascicular" sign: Multiple, irregular, central hypointense foci

### Top Differential Diagnoses
- Neurofibroma (NF)
- Plexiform Neurofibroma
- Malignant Peripheral Nerve Sheath Tumor
- Venolymphatic Malformation (VLM)

## DIFFERENTIAL DIAGNOSIS

### Neurofibroma (NF)
- May be indistinguishable from schwannoma
- "Target" appearance more common
- Cystic degeneration, hemorrhage uncommon

### Plexiform Neurofibroma
- Lobulated, bulky, multilevel expansion of affected nerves in patient with stigmata of NF1

### Malignant Peripheral Nerve Sheath Tumor
- Progressively enlarging, irregular, heterogeneous mass

### Venolymphatic Malformation (VLM)
- Microcystic or macrocystic nonenhancing lymphatic component mixed with enhancing venous component, ± phleboliths

## PATHOLOGY

### General Features
- Genetics: Solitary, usually sporadic, multiple occur in neurofibromatosis 2 and schwannomatosis
- Epidemiology: 5% of all benign soft tissue neoplasms

### Microscopic Features
- Alternating regions of high cellularity (Antoni A) & loose, myxoid, component (Antoni B)

## CLINICAL ISSUES

### Presentation
- Most common signs/symptoms: Painless, slow growing mass in lateral neck ± radiculopathy

### Demographics
- Age: Young adults 20–30 years of age

### Natural History & Prognosis
- Slow growing; malignant degeneration rare

## DIAGNOSTIC CHECKLIST

### Consider
- Fusiform T2 hyperintense mass between anterior and middle scalene muscle, consider schwannoma

## SELECTED REFERENCES

1. Baser ME et al: Increasing the specificity of diagnostic criteria for schwannomatosis. Neurology. 66(5):730-2, 2006
2. Beaman FD et al: Schwannoma: radiologic-pathologic correlation. Radiographics. 24(5):1477-81, 2004
3. Wittenberg KH et al: MR imaging of nontraumatic brachial plexopathies: frequency and spectrum of findings. Radiographics. 20(4):1023-32, 2000

## IMAGE GALLERY

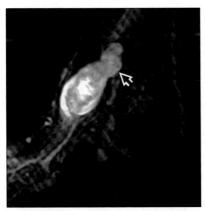 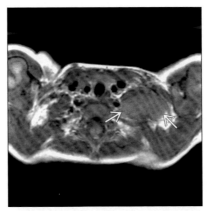 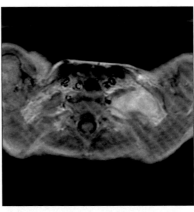

*(Left) Coronal T2WI FS MR shows a fusiform, slightly heterogeneous, dumbbell shaped right brachial plexus mass with a component extending into the spinal canal ➡ via an enlarged neural foramen. (Center) Axial T1WI MR in a child presenting with a left sided neck mass shows a large, homogeneous, oblong mass ➡ in the anterolateral left neck. (Right) Axial T1 C+ FS MR in the same patient as previous image shows that the mass enhances heterogeneously and displaces the anterior scalene muscle anteriorly. Child was eventually diagnosed with NF2.*

# FIBROMATOSIS COLLI

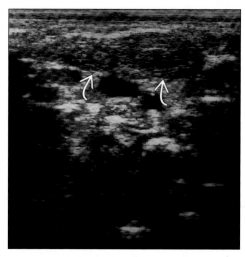

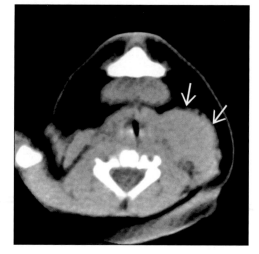

*Ultrasound through the middle portion of the neck shows smooth enlargement of the sternocleidomastoid muscle ➥. The surrounding tissues and underlying vessels appear normal.*

*Axial NECT (same patient as previous image) shows fusiform enlargement of the left sternocleidomastoid muscle ➥, similar in attenuation to the other neck muscles. No calcification is identified.*

## TERMINOLOGY

### Abbreviations and Synonyms
- Abbreviation: Fibromatosis colli (FColli)
- Synonyms: Sternocleidomastoid (SCM) or sternomastoid pseudotumor of infancy

### Definitions
- FColli: Non-neoplastic SCM muscle enlargement in early infancy
  - Likely related to injury during childbirth

## IMAGING FINDINGS

### General Features
- Best diagnostic clue: Non-tender sternocleidomastoid muscle enlargement without discrete mass in an infant
- Location
  - Mid to lower third of sternocleidomastoid muscle
  - Right > left; rarely bilateral
- Size
  - Variable

- Usually spans much of cervical portion of sternocleidomastoid muscle
- Morphology: Fusiform sternocleidomastoid muscle enlargement

### CT Findings
- NECT
  - Fusiform enlargement of affected SCM without discrete mass
  - Enlarged SCM is sharply defined
    - No inflammatory "stranding" in adjacent fat
  - No adenopathy
  - No calcifications
- CECT: Affected muscle enhances diffusely

### MR Findings
- T1WI
  - Fusiform enlargement of affected SCM
  - Mass is sharply marginated with normal surrounding tissue
  - Variable signal intensity
    - Usually isointense-hypointense to normal muscle
- T2WI
  - Variable signal intensity
    - Zones of hypointensity at maximal enlargement

## DDx: Anterior Neck Mass

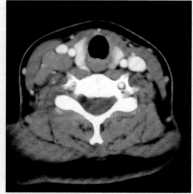

*Nodal Disease*

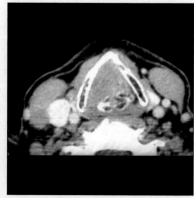

*Rhabdomyosarcoma*

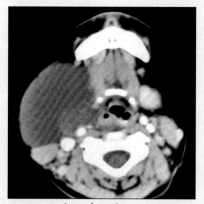

*Lymphangioma*

# FIBROMATOSIS COLLI

## Key Facts

### Terminology
- FColli: Non-neoplastic SCM muscle enlargement in early infancy

### Imaging Findings
- Best diagnostic clue: Non-tender sternocleidomastoid muscle enlargement without discrete mass in an infant
- Mid to lower third of sternocleidomastoid muscle
- Right > left; rarely bilateral
- Oval or fusiform unilateral sternocleidomastoid muscle enlargement
- No discrete mass or adenopathy
- Best imaging tool: Ultrasound confirms clinical suspicion

### Top Differential Diagnoses
- Lymphangioma
- Muscular Torticollis
- Myositis Related to Neck Infection
- Rhabdomyosarcoma
- Spinal Accessory Nodal Malignancy

### Pathology
- Fibrocollagenous infiltration of SCM
- When necessary, diagnosis can be confirmed by thin needle aspiration cytology
- Possibly precipitated by in utero head position and SCM compartment syndrome

### Clinical Issues
- Age: Most (70%) present by 2 months of age
- Mass appears within 2 weeks of delivery

- - Hypointense zones probably due to evolving fibrosis
  - Other regions are hyperintense to isointense compared with other muscles
  - ○ Adjacent soft tissues normal
    - Be aware that incidental "reactive" nodal enlargement in infants is common
    - Presence of adjacent nodes should not raise suspicion that this pseudotumor is a neoplasm
- T1 C+
  - ○ Affected muscle enhances diffusely
  - ○ Enhancement seen best if fat-suppression is used

### Radiographic Findings
- Radiography
  - ○ Lytic changes in clavicular head at muscle attachment reported
    - Rare plain film finding

### Ultrasonographic Findings
- Grayscale Ultrasound
  - ○ Oval or fusiform unilateral sternocleidomastoid muscle enlargement
  - ○ Variable echogenicity
    - Hyperechoic or mixed echogenicity common
  - ○ No discrete mass or adenopathy
  - ○ Affected sternomastoid muscle moves with respiration in same fashion as contralateral muscle

### Imaging Recommendations
- Best imaging tool: Ultrasound confirms clinical suspicion
- Protocol advice: Real time ultrasound mixed with a solid dose of clinical knowledge arrives at correct diagnosis

## DIFFERENTIAL DIAGNOSIS

### Pseudomass Due to Contralateral SCM Denervation
- CN11 injury causes SCM & trapezius to atrophy
- Normal SCM may appear large

### Lymphangioma
- Low density, separate from SCM
- Multiple fascial spaces

### Muscular Torticollis
- SCM "tightening" without palpable mass
- Most (> 70%) present after one year of age
- Some cases evolve from fibromatosis colli

### Myositis Related to Neck Infection
- Tenderness, cellulitis evident clinically
- Inflammatory changes in adjacent soft tissues at imaging
- Adenopathy conspicuous

### Rhabdomyosarcoma
- Rare in newborns
- More discrete mass with "aggressive" margins
- Trans-spatial mass common

### Spinal Accessory Nodal Malignancy
- Nodes enlarge deep to SCM muscle
- NHL, leukemia, metastatic neuroblastoma

### Teratoma
- Congenital tumor
- Associated with fat, calcification

## PATHOLOGY

### General Features
- General path comments
  - ○ Fibrocollagenous infiltration of SCM
  - ○ When necessary, diagnosis can be confirmed by thin needle aspiration cytology
    - Cytopathologists must be careful in interpreting cells as benign
    - Radiologist can help by suggesting diagnosis
- Genetics: At least one case of fibromatosis colli has been reported in siblings
- Etiology

# FIBROMATOSIS COLLI

○ Post-traumatic etiology with intramuscular hemorrhage & subsequent fibrosis
○ Possibly precipitated by in utero head position and SCM compartment syndrome
○ Associations
  ▪ Breech presentation
  ▪ Forceps delivery
• Epidemiology
  ○ Rare lesion
  ○ Affects 0.4% of infants

## Gross Pathologic & Surgical Features
• Enlargement, fibrosis of affected sternocleidomastoid muscle

## Microscopic Features
• Proliferation of spindle-cell fibroblasts
• Multinucleated giant cells (degenerating skeletal muscle)
• Collagen deposition
• Inflammatory changes rare

## CLINICAL ISSUES

### Presentation
• Most common signs/symptoms
  ○ Unilateral longitudinal cervical neck mass
  ○ Torticollis in up to 20%
• Clinical Profile: Infant with non-tender neck mass, following breach or forceps delivery

### Demographics
• Age: Most (70%) present by 2 months of age
• Gender: Slightly more common in males than females
• Ethnicity: No known ethnic predisposition

### Natural History & Prognosis
• Mass appears within 2 weeks of delivery
• Mass may increase in size for days to weeks after presentation
  ○ Usually regresses by 8 months of age
• Up to 20% progress to muscular torticollis despite conservative therapy
• Patients with unsuccessfully treated torticollis may develop distorted skull shape

### Treatment
• Watchful waiting for normal spontaneous resolution of problem
• Physical therapy
• Tenotomy for cases with torticollis that fail conservative therapy

## DIAGNOSTIC CHECKLIST

### Consider
• Is there a history of traumatic birth?
• Does imaging show mass confined to the sternocleidomastoid muscle?
  ○ If answer to both is yes, diagnosis is fibromatosis colli
• Is the mass tender?

• Are there other clinical or imaging signs of inflammation?
  ○ If the answer to both is yes, neck infection likely
• Does imaging show mass extending beyond the margins of sternocleidomastoid muscle?
  ○ Consider rhabdomyosarcoma or other tumor

## Image Interpretation Pearls
• Fusiform mass conforming to shape of sternocleidomastoid muscle = fibromatosis colli

## SELECTED REFERENCES

1. Kumar V et al: Bilateral sternocleidomastoid tumor of infancy. Int J Pediatr Otorhinolaryngol. 67(6):673-5, 2003
2. Sharma S et al: Fibromatosis colli in infants. A cytologic study of eight cases. Acta Cytol. 47(3):359-62, 2003
3. Kurtycz DF et al: Diagnosis of fibromatosis colli by fine-needle aspiration. Diagn Cytopathol. 23(5):338-42, 2000
4. Cheng JC et al: Sternocleidomastoid pseudotumor and congenital muscular torticollis in infants: a prospective study of 510 cases. J Pediatr. 134(6):712-6, 1999
5. Demirbilek S et al: Congenital muscular torticollis and sternomastoid tumor: results of nonoperative treatment. J Pediatr Surg. 34(4):549-51, 1999
6. Jaber MR et al: Sternocleidomastoid tumor of infancy: two cases of an interesting entity. Int J Pediatr Otorhinolaryngol. 47(3):269-74, 1999
7. Tufano RP et al: Bilateral sternocleidomastoid tumors of infancy. Int J Pediatr Otorhinolaryngol. 51(1):41-5, 1999
8. Ablin DS et al: Ultrasound and MR imaging of fibromatosis colli (sternomastoid tumor of infancy). Pediatr Radiol. 28(4):230-3, 1998
9. Bedi DG et al: Fibromatosis colli of infancy: variability of sonographic appearance. J Clin Ultrasound. 26(7):345-8, 1998
10. Eich GF et al: Fibrous tumours in children: imaging features of a heterogeneous group of disorders. Pediatr Radiol. 28(7):500-9, 1998
11. Snitzer EL et al: Magnetic resonance imaging appearance of fibromatosis colli. Magn Reson Imaging. 15(7):869-71, 1997
12. Vazquez E et al: US, CT, and MR imaging of neck lesions in children. Radiographics. 15(1):105-22, 1995
13. Youkilis RA et al: Ultrasonographic imaging of sternocleidomastoid tumor of infancy. Ann Otol Rhinol Laryngol. 104(4 Pt 1):323-5, 1995
14. Campbell RE et al: Image interpretation session: 1993. Fibromatosis colli. Radiographics. 14(1):208-9, 1994
15. Guarisco JL: Congenital head and neck masses in infants and children. Part II. Ear Nose Throat J. 70(2):75-82, 1991
16. Norton KI et al: Sternocleidomastoid tumor of infancy: CT manifestations. J Comput Assist Tomogr. 15(1):158-9, 1991
17. Crawford SC et al: Fibromatosis colli of infancy: CT and sonographic findings. AJR Am J Roentgenol. 151(6):1183-4, 1988
18. Glasier CM et al: High resolution ultrasound characterization of soft tissue masses in children. Pediatr Radiol. 17(3):233-7, 1987
19. Tom LW et al: The sternocleidomastoid tumor of infancy. Int J Pediatr Otorhinolaryngol. 13(3):245-55, 1987
20. Kraus R et al: Sonography of neck masses in children. AJR Am J Roentgenol. 146(3):609-13, 1986

# FIBROMATOSIS COLLI

## IMAGE GALLERY

### Typical

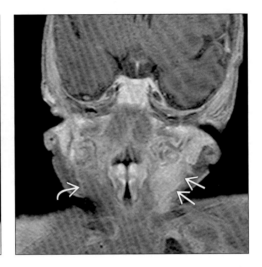

(Left) Sagittal T1WI MR shows diffuse enlargement of the left sternocleidomastoid muscle ➡, which is isointense to the other, non-involved muscles ➘.
(Right) Coronal T1 C+ FS MR (same patient as previous image) shows diffuse enlargement and enhancement of the left sternocleidomastoid muscle ➡, compared to the contralateral, non-involved muscle ➘.

### Typical

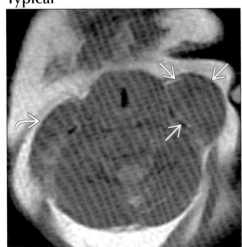
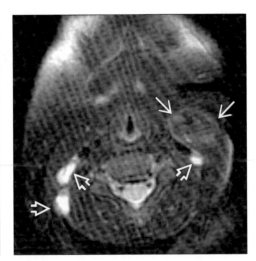

(Left) Axial T1WI MR shows typical MR appearance of fibromatosis colli with enlarged sternocleidomastoid muscle ➡ that is isointense to the contralateral muscle ➘.
(Right) Axial T2WI FS MR (same patient as previous image) shows that the muscle ➡ demonstrates heterogeneous mild hyperintensity. Note small cervical lymph nodes ➡ which are common in children of this age.

### Variant

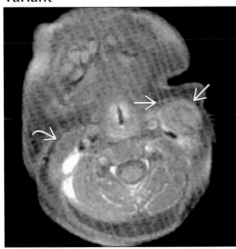
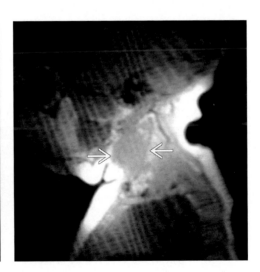

(Left) Axial T1 C+ FS MR (in same patient as previous image) shows heterogeneous signal intensity and contrast-enhancement ➡ in the affected sternocleidomastoid muscle as compared to the contralateral muscle ➘.
(Right) Sagittal T1WI MR shows variant MR appearance of fibromatosis colli with heterogeneous signal intensity ➡.

# RHABDOMYOSARCOMA

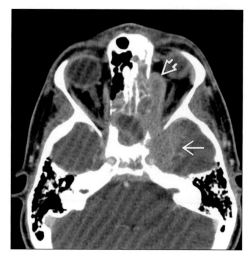

Axial CECT shows a heterogeneously enhancing parameningeal rhabdomyosarcoma, with osseous erosion and extension into the left middle cranial fossa ➥ and left orbit ➥.

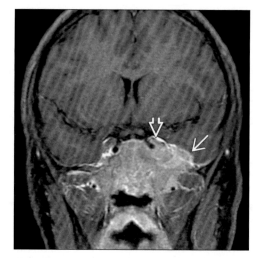

Coronal T1WI FS MR in the same patient as previous image, shows extensive tumor with left middle cranial fossa extension (displacing temporal lobe ➥) and invasion of the left cavernous sinus ➥.

## TERMINOLOGY

### Abbreviations and Synonyms
- Rhabdomyosarcoma (RMS)

### Definitions
- Malignant neoplasm of striated muscle, most common childhood soft tissue sarcoma

## IMAGING FINDINGS

### General Features
- Best diagnostic clue: Soft tissue mass with variable contrast enhancement ± bone destruction
- Location
  - Up to 40% occur in head/neck
    - Orbit
    - Parameningeal: Middle ear, paranasal sinus, nasopharynx (NP)
    - All other head and neck sites including cervical neck, nasal cavity
  - Up to 55% of parameningeal rhabdomyosarcomas have intracranial extension

- Size: Variable, may present earlier in orbit secondary to small space and early proptosis

### CT Findings
- Soft tissue mass with variable contrast-enhancement
- Osseous erosion common but does not occur in all cases

### MR Findings
- Relative to muscle; isointense T1WI, hyperintense T2WI
- Variable contrast-enhancement, ± intracranial extension in parameningeal RMS

### Imaging Recommendations
- Best imaging tool
  - CT best to evaluate osseous erosion
  - MR best to evaluate intracranial and perineural spread of RMS
- Protocol advice
  - Coronal postcontrast fat-saturation T1 imaging for intracranial disease assessment
  - Axial and coronal thin section bone algorithm for osseous erosion

## DDx: Non-Inflammatory Head/Neck Masses with Bone Destruction

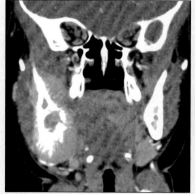

Metastatic NBL

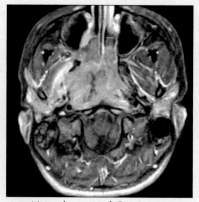

Nasopharyngeal Carcinoma

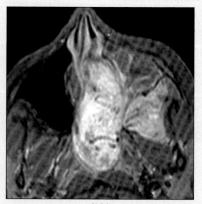

JNA

# RHABDOMYOSARCOMA

## Key Facts

### Terminology
- Rhabdomyosarcoma (RMS)
- Malignant neoplasm of striated muscle, most common childhood soft tissue sarcoma

### Imaging Findings
- Best diagnostic clue: Soft tissue mass with variable contrast enhancement ± bone destruction
- Up to 40% occur in head/neck
- Soft tissue mass with variable contrast-enhancement
- Osseous erosion common but does not occur in all cases
- Relative to muscle; isointense T1WI, hyperintense T2WI
- CT best to evaluate osseous erosion
- MR best to evaluate intracranial and perineural spread of RMS

### Top Differential Diagnoses
- Metastatic Neuroblastoma (NBL)
- Nasopharyngeal (NP) Carcinoma
- Juvenile Nasopharyngeal Angiofibroma (JNA)
- Leukemia
- Lymphoma
- Langerhans Cell Histiocytosis (LCH)

### Clinical Issues
- Symptoms variable, depend on location
- Orbit: Orbital mass, proptosis, decreased vision
- Sinonasal: Nasal obstruction, epistaxis, may present late with soft tissue facial mass
- Temporal bone: Postauricular mass, otitis media, external auditory canal mass
- Neck: Neck mass, pain, rarely airway compromise

○ Include neck to rule out cervical metastatic adenopathy

## DIFFERENTIAL DIAGNOSIS

### Metastatic Neuroblastoma (NBL)
- Most common malignant tumor in children less than one year of age
- Cervical primary lesions rare, most cervical disease is metastatic
- Metastatic disease to skull base frequently bilateral with enhancing masses, intracranial and/or extracranial extension, aggressive osseous erosion with spiculated periosteal reaction

### Nasopharyngeal (NP) Carcinoma
- NP mass with variable contrast-enhancement
- Central skull base erosion, widening of the petroclival fissure, extension to pterygopalatine fossa, masticator space, parapharyngeal space, unilateral or bilateral cervical adenopathy, lateral retropharyngeal adenopathy
- In children, most are 10-19 years of age
- In the United States, more common in African Americans than in Caucasians

### Juvenile Nasopharyngeal Angiofibroma (JNA)
- Presents with epistaxis or nasal obstruction in adolescent males
- Intensely enhancing mass with bone destruction and intralesional high flow vessels
  ○ Originates at sphenopalatine foramen on lateral nasopharyngeal wall, potential spread
    - Pterygopalatine and pterygomaxillary fissures into infratemporal fossa
    - Orbit via inferior orbital fissure
    - Intracranial
    - Sphenoid or ethmoid sinus

### Leukemia
- Granulocytic sarcoma = chloroma
- Soft tissue mass ± aggressive bone destruction

- Rare complication acute myeloid leukemia (AML) or chronic myeloid leukemia (CML)
- Most in adults, most in patients with AML
- In CML, ominous sign, usually heralds blast crisis
- In AML, does not affect overall prognosis
- Locations: Skull, face, orbit, paranasal sinuses, nasal cavity, nasopharynx, tonsil, mouth, lacrimal gland, salivary glands

### Lymphoma
- Accounts for approximately 50% of all head and neck malignancies in children
  ○ 50% Hodgkin disease (HD), 50% non-Hodgkin lymphoma (NHL)
  ○ Imaging characteristics similar, can not differentiate between HD and NHL
- Sinonasal, orbital or NP may cause osseous erosion
- Unilateral or bilateral cervical adenopathy, usually without osseous erosion

### Langerhans Cell Histiocytosis (LCH)
- Enhancing soft tissue mass with smooth osseous erosion
- In head and neck: Orbit, maxilla, mandible, temporal bone, cervical spine, calvaria

## PATHOLOGY

### General Features
- Genetics
  ○ Increased incidence in children with p53 tumor suppressor gene mutation
  ○ Most embryonal RMS have loss of heterozygosity (LOH) at 11p15 locus
  ○ PAX3-FKHR and variant PAX7-FKHR gene fusions in some with alveolar RMS
    - PAX3-FKHR gene fusion better prognosis
- Etiology: Originates from primitive mesenchymal cells committed to skeletal muscle differentiation (rhabdomyoblasts)
- Associated abnormalities

# RHABDOMYOSARCOMA

- ○ Rarely associated with neurofibromatosis type I, Li-Fraumeni and Beckwith-Wiedemann syndrome
- ○ Rarely associated with hereditary retinoblastoma
- ○ May occur as radiation induced second primary neoplasm

## Microscopic Features
- Rhabdomyoblasts in varying stages of differentiation
- Immunohistochemistry: Positive for desmin, vimentin and antibody to muscle-specific actin
- Histologic subtypes
  - ○ Embryonal RMS: Most common
    - ▪ Primitive cellular structure
    - ▪ Round or elongated cells with hyperchromic, irregular nuclei and frequent mitoses
    - ▪ Account for more that 50% of all RMS, 70-90% of which occur in head/neck or genitourinary tract
    - ▪ Botryoid RMS gross appearance similar to cluster of grapes, 75% arise in vagina, prostate or bladder, 25% in head/neck or bile ducts, most patients 2-5 years of age
  - ○ Alveolar RMS: Second most common
    - ▪ Most common in extremities and trunk
    - ▪ Usually occurs in patients 15-25 years of age
  - ○ Pleomorphic RMS: Least common
    - ▪ Usually in adults 40-60 years of age, rarely less than 15 years of age
    - ▪ Most arise in extremities, rarely in head/neck

## Staging, Grading or Classification Criteria
- Intergroup Rhabdomyosarcoma Study Group (IRSG)
  - ○ Group I: Localized tumor completely resected
  - ○ Group II: Gross total resection with microscopic residual disease
  - ○ Group III: Incomplete resection with gross residual disease
  - ○ Group IV: Distant metastases
- WHO Classification: 6 histologic subtypes
- TNM: Tumor site, size (5 cm), local invasion, lymph nodes, distant metastases

## CLINICAL ISSUES

### Presentation
- Most common signs/symptoms
  - ○ Symptoms variable, depend on location
    - ▪ Orbit: Orbital mass, proptosis, decreased vision
    - ▪ Sinonasal: Nasal obstruction, epistaxis, may present late with soft tissue facial mass
    - ▪ Temporal bone: Postauricular mass, otitis media, external auditory canal mass
    - ▪ Neck: Neck mass, pain, rarely airway compromise

### Demographics
- Age: 70% under 12 years, 43% under 5 years of age
- Ethnicity: More common in Caucasians

### Natural History & Prognosis
- Variable, depends on location and cell type
  - ○ Orbit: Best prognosis (80-90% disease-free survival)
  - ○ Parameningeal: Worst prognosis (40-50% disease free survival)

- ○ Alveolar worse prognosis than embryonal and pleomorphic

## Treatment
- Surgical debulking, chemotherapy, and/or radiation therapy

## DIAGNOSTIC CHECKLIST

### Consider
- Not always associated with bone destruction
  - ○ Beware of enhancing soft tissue mass without bone destruction, may simulate infantile hemangioma
    - ▪ Infantile hemangioma usually more intensely and homogeneously enhancing, with intralesional high flow vessels
    - ▪ Flow voids usually absent in sarcomas with the exception of alveolar soft part sarcomas

## SELECTED REFERENCES

1. Stambuk HE et al: Nasopharyngeal carcinoma: recognizing the radiographic features in children. AJNR Am J Neuroradiol. 26(6):1575-9, 2005
2. Breneman JC et al: Prognostic factors and clinical outcomes in children and adolescents with metastatic rhabdomyosarcoma--a report from the Intergroup Rhabdomyosarcoma Study IV. J Clin Oncol. 21(1):78-84, 2003
3. Tateishi U et al: CT and MRI features of recurrent tumors and second primary neoplasms in pediatric patients with retinoblastoma. AJR Am J Roentgenol. 181(3):879-84, 2003
4. Simon JH et al: Prognostic factors in head and neck rhabdomyosarcoma. Head Neck. 24(5):468-73, 2002
5. Sorensen PH et al: PAX3-FKHR and PAX7-FKHR gene fusions are prognostic indicators in alveolar rhabdomyosarcoma: a report from the children's oncology group. J Clin Oncol. 20(11):2672-9, 2002
6. McCarville MB et al: Rhabdomyosarcoma in pediatric patients: the good, the bad, and the unusual. AJR Am J Roentgenol. 176(6):1563-9, 2001
7. Koch BL: Langerhans histiocytosis of temporal bone: role of magnetic resonance imaging. Top Magn Reson Imaging. 11(1):66-74, 2000
8. Kraus DH et al: Pediatric rhabdomyosarcoma of the head and neck. Am J Surg. 174(5):556-60, 1997
9. Pappo AS et al: Biology and therapy of pediatric rhabdomyosarcoma. J Clin Oncol. 13(8):2123-39, 1995
10. Quraishi MS et al: Langerhans' cell histiocytosis: head and neck manifestations in children. Head Neck. 17(3):226-31, 1995
11. Castillo M et al: Rhabdomyosarcoma of the middle ear: imaging features in two children. AJNR Am J Neuroradiol. 14(3):730-3, 1993
12. Yousem DM et al: Rhabdomyosarcomas in the head and neck: MR imaging evaluation. Radiology. 177(3):683-6, 1990
13. Wiatrak BJ et al: Rhabdomyosarcoma of the ear and temporal bone. Laryngoscope. 99(11):1188-92, 1989
14. Latack JT et al: Imaging of rhabdomyosarcomas of the head and neck. AJNR Am J Neuroradiol. 8(2):353-9, 1987
15. Schwartz RH et al: Rhabdomyosarcoma of the middle ear: a wolf in sheep's clothing. Pediatrics. 65(6):1131-3, 1980
16. Abramson DH et al: Second tumors in nonirradiated bilateral retinoblastoma. Am J Ophthalmol. 87(5):624-7, 1979

# RHABDOMYOSARCOMA

## IMAGE GALLERY

### Typical

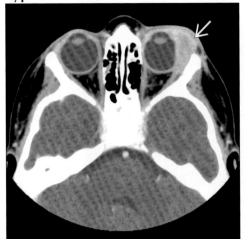

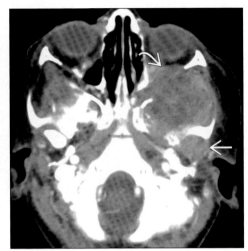

*(Left)* Axial CECT shows a moderately enhancing left orbital RMS ➡, deviating and compressing the left globe, without significant bone erosion or intracranial extension. *(Right)* Axial CECT shows heterogeneously enhancing left infratemporal fossa RMS eroding the floor of the middle cranial fossa and extending into the orbit ⇒ and temporomandibular joint ➡.

### Typical

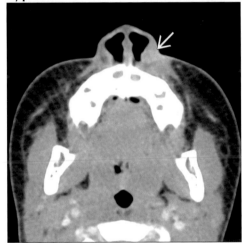

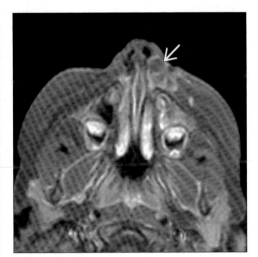

*(Left)* Axial CECT shows a heterogeneously enhancing, ill-defined RMS ➡ involving the left nasal ala and adjacent soft tissues without significant bone erosion. *(Right)* Axial T1 C+ FS MR in the same patient as previous image, shows heterogeneous contrast-enhancement of the well-defined left nasal ala RMS ➡.

### Typical

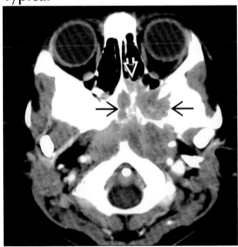

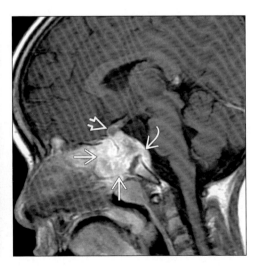

*(Left)* Axial CECT shows a heterogeneously enhancing rhabdomyosarcoma with significant erosion ➡ of the central skull base, extension into the left nasal cavity ⇒. *(Right)* Sagittal T1 C+ MR in the same patient as previous image, shows enhancing RMS displacing pituitary ⇒, destroying the sphenoid base ➡, with intracranial extension along the dorsal aspect of the clivus ➡.

# MELANOTIC NEUROECTODERMAL TUMORS

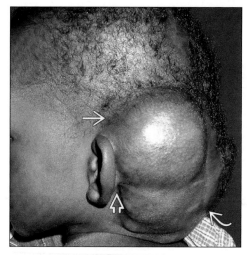

Lateral clinical photograph shows huge mass extending toward parietal squama superiorly ➡ and in upper neck inferiorly ➡ behind displaced left ear ➡. Overlying skin looks normal.

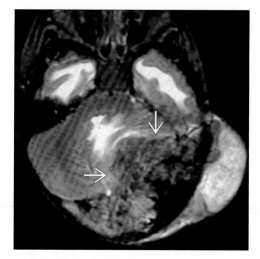

Axial T2WI FS MR shows huge occipital bone tumor with extensive intra- and extracranial components, compressing & likely infiltrating cerebellum: Loss of low signal dural lining ➡, edema.

## TERMINOLOGY

### Abbreviations and Synonyms
- Melanotic neuroectodermal tumor of infancy (MNTI)
- Previously, 23 different names including adamantinoma, retinal anlage tumor, melanotic progonoma

### Definitions
- Rare tumor of neural crest origin in infants; involves maxilla & jaw mostly, brain & calvarium less commonly

## IMAGING FINDINGS

### General Features
- Best diagnostic clue
  - MR is not specific
    - Iso-/high T1, low T2 (melanin) growing mass in infant, strongly enhanced
  - CT: Osteolysis with sclerotic margin, faint Ca++
- Location
  - Maxilla (65-70%), mandible (6-10%), calvarium-dura (10%), brain (5%); rare elsewhere
  - In calvarium: Anterior fontanel, parietooccipital
- Size: Depends on time of diagnosis
- Morphology
  - In skull, well demarcated benign osteolytic lesion
  - In brain usually malignant and infiltrative

### Imaging Recommendations
- Best imaging tool
  - MR: Signal changes of melanin
  - CT: Osteolysis with sclerotic margin
- Protocol advice: Look for meningeal, sinovenous involvement

## DIFFERENTIAL DIAGNOSIS

### Calvarium
- Other bone tumors: Ewing, neuroblastoma etc.

### Intracranial
- Pinealoblastoma, melanotic schwannoma
- Melanotic medulloblastoma of cerebellum (different immunoreactivity)

### DDx: Other Epidural Neoplasms

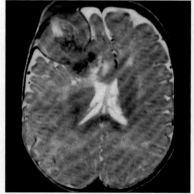

Ewing Sarcoma

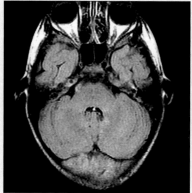

Metastatic Neuroblastoma

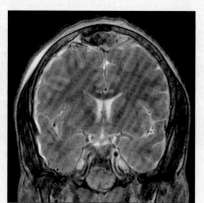

Extramedullary Hematopoiesis

# MELANOTIC NEUROECTODERMAL TUMORS

## Key Facts

### Terminology
- Rare tumor of neural crest origin in infants; involves maxilla & jaw mostly, brain & calvarium less commonly

### Imaging Findings
- Iso-/high T1, low T2 (melanin) growing mass in infant, strongly enhanced
- In skull, well demarcated benign osteolytic lesion
- In brain usually malignant and infiltrative

### Top Differential Diagnoses
- Other bone tumors: Ewing, neuroblastoma etc.
- Pinealoblastoma, melanotic schwannoma
- Neurocutaneous melanosis (diffuse meningeal involvement, cutaneous lesions)

### Clinical Issues
- Typically benign in face and calvarium
- Midline intra-arachnoidal often malignant

---

- Neurocutaneous melanosis (diffuse meningeal involvement, cutaneous lesions)

## PATHOLOGY

### General Features
- Etiology
  - Neural crest cells tumor
  - ↑ Vanillylmandelic acid (VMA) common
- Epidemiology: Only 355 cases reported since 1918

### Gross Pathologic & Surgical Features
- Rock-hard tumor of the calvarium or face
- Poorly circumscribed midline brain tumor

### Microscopic Features
- Tubular alveolar formations of large melanin-containing epithelial cells and cells resembling neuroblasts
- Cytologic diagnosis possible by needle aspiration

## CLINICAL ISSUES

### Presentation
- Most common signs/symptoms: Local mass effect
- Other signs/symptoms: Intracranial hypertension for midline brain tumors

### Demographics
- Age

  - Mostly infants
  - Less common in older children, unusual in adults
- Gender: No gender predilection

### Natural History & Prognosis
- Typically benign in face and calvarium
- Midline intra-arachnoidal often malignant

### Treatment
- Removal of circumscribed lesion
- Chemotherapy helpful in malignant forms

## SELECTED REFERENCES

1. Kruse-Losler B et al: Melanotic neuroectodermal tumor of infancy: systematic review of the literature and presentation of a case. Oral Surg Oral Med Oral Pathol Oral Radiol Endod. 102(2):204-16, 2006
2. Antunes AC et al: Melanotic neuroectodermal tumor of infancy: case report. Arq Neuropsiquiatr. 63(3A):670-2, 2005
3. George JC et al: Melanotic neuroectodermal tumor of infancy. AJNR Am J Neuroradiol. 16(6):1273-5, 1995
4. Kapadia SB et al: Melanotic neuroectodermal tumor of infancy. Clinicopathological, immunohistochemical, and flow cytometric study. Am J Surg Pathol. 17(6):566-73, 1993
5. Atkinson GO Jr et al: Melanotic neuroectodermal tumor of infancy. MR findings and a review of the literature. Pediatr Radiol. 20(1-2):20-2, 1989
6. Parizek J et al: Melanotic neuroectodermal neurocranial tumor of infancy of extra-intra-and subdural right temporal location: CT examination, surgical treatment, literature review. Neuropediatrics. 17(3):115-23, 1986

## IMAGE GALLERY

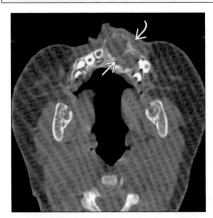 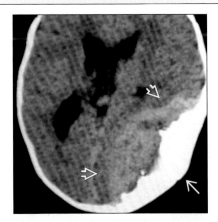 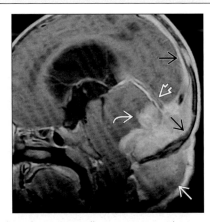

*(Left)* Axial bone CT shows most common appearance, location and age for melanotic neuroectodermal tumor: Maxillary expansion with osteolysis ➡, adjacent soft tissue changes ➡ in an infant. *(Center)* Axial NECT shows extensive bone expansion ➡ with ill-defined, slightly hyperdense (diffuse Ca++) intracranial component ➡ compressing dilated ventricles. *(Right)* Sagittal T1 C+ MR shows involvement of calvarium ➡. Extensive soft tissue masses displace occluded dural sinuses ➡, infiltrate cerebellum ➡ & invade cervical soft tissues ➡.

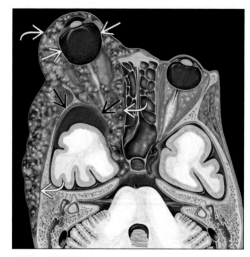

Axial graphic shows a transpatial plexiform neurofibroma ➡ and sphenoid wing dysplasia ➡ (which typically occur together), marked proptosis, and buphthalmos ➡.

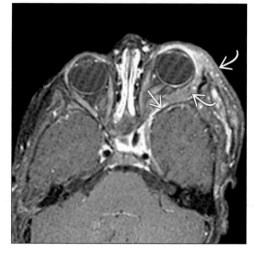

Axial T1 C+ FS MR shows left proptosis along with 2 commonly associated orbital findings in NF1: Large transpatial plexiform neurofibroma ➡ and sphenoid wing dysplasia ➡.

## TERMINOLOGY

### Abbreviations and Synonyms
- Neurofibromatosis, type 1 (NF1)
- von Recklinghausen disease

### Definitions
- Neurocutaneous disorder (inherited tumor syndrome)
- Inherited disease with distinct orbital manifestations

## IMAGING FINDINGS

### General Features
- Best diagnostic clue: NF1 orbital findings comprise constellation of features that are pathognomonic
- Location: Orbitofacial NF1 typically unilateral
- Plexiform neurofibroma (PNF)
  - PNF anywhere is pathognomonic for NF1
  - Serpentine, irregular infiltrative masses
  - Surround and engulf normal orbital structures
  - Associated with sphenoid dysplasia
  - Frequently trans-spatial, in face, orbit and temporal fossa

- Sphenoid dysplasia (SD)
  - Bony defects, decalcification, or remodeling of greater sphenoid wing
  - Enlargement of middle fossa with herniation of intracranial contents into orbit
- Buphthalmos (BUPH)
  - "Ox's eye", results from congenital glaucoma
  - Increased size of globe in front to back diameter
  - Thickening of uveal/scleral layer
  - Associated with anterior rim enlargement and anterior orbit PNF
- Optic pathway glioma (OPG)
  - Enlargement of intraorbital nerve ± any segment of optic pathway posteriorly

### CT Findings
- NECT
  - PNF: Hypodense infiltrative soft tissue masses
  - SD: Bony changes; proptosis may be marked
  - BUPH: Globe enlargement and scleral thickening

### MR Findings
- T1WI
  - PNF: Hypointense infiltrative soft tissue masses

## DDx: Orbital Masses

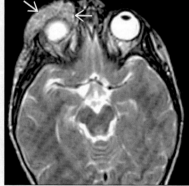

*Hemangioma*

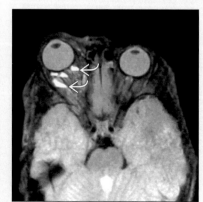

*Lymphangioma*

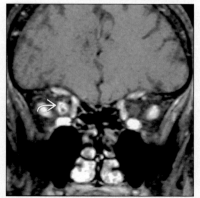

*Meningioma*

# NEUROFIBROMATOSIS TYPE 1, ORBIT

## Key Facts

### Imaging Findings
- Best diagnostic clue: NF1 orbital findings comprise constellation of features that are pathognomonic
- Plexiform neurofibroma (PNF)
- Sphenoid dysplasia (SD)
- Buphthalmos (BUPH)
- Optic pathway glioma (OPG)

### Pathology
- Disorder of histogenesis, classified as a neurocutaneous, or inherited tumor, syndrome
- Orbital features of NF1 have interrelated underlying pathology
- Autosomal dominant; variable expression
- 50% new mutations; gene locus = 17q11.2
- Most common inherited tumor syndrome
- Orbital involvement in approximately 33%

- May involve lid, conjunctiva, iris, choroid, ciliary body, periorbita, scalp, temporal fossa, and skull base
- Bony defect of posterior orbit; frequently associated with middle fossa arachnoid cyst

### Clinical Issues
- Eyelid, periorbital and facial soft tissue masses
- Proptosis and ptosis
- PNF, SD, BUPH, and OPG may not be evident at birth
- Decreased life expectancy
- Malignancy most common cause of death

### Diagnostic Checklist
- Although NF1 is inherited disorder, orbital manifestations are progressive and develop over time
- Rapid change in appearance of PNF worrisome for malignant degeneration

- ○ OPG: Enlarged isointense optic nerve ± low signal cysts
- T2WI
  - ○ PNF: Infiltrative irregular heterogeneously hyperintense mass
  - ○ OPG: Hyperintense enlarged optic nerve ± higher signal cystic regions
- T1 C+
  - ○ PNF: Variable
  - ○ OPG: Variable

## Radiographic Findings
- Radiography
  - ○ Defects of greater sphenoid wing
  - ○ Enlarged egg-shaped anterior orbital rim
  - ○ "Harlequin eye" appearance
  - ○ Optic canal and/or orbital fissure enlargement

## Ultrasonographic Findings
- PNF: Irregular, compressible, high reflectivity
- SD: Defect of posterior bony orbital wall
- BUPH: Increased axial globe length
- OPG: Smooth and regular, low reflectivity

## Imaging Recommendations
- Best imaging tool: MR preferred for assessing extent of PNF, OPG, other intracranial features of NF1
- Protocol advice: Dedicated orbital sequences if extensive abnormalities

# DIFFERENTIAL DIAGNOSIS

## General Comments
- Constellation of orbital NF1 findings is pathognomonic
- Orbital findings not isolated due to underlying complex and interactive pathogenesis
  - ○ In particular, SD and PNF intimately associated
- Only if findings isolated is there a differential

## Infiltrative Orbital Mass (DDx PNF)
- Capillary hemangioma
- Lymphangioma

- Rhabdomyosarcoma
- Hematologic malignancy
- Orbital cellulitis

## Sphenoid Bony Defect (DDx SD)
- Sphenoid cephalocele

## Globe Enlargement (DDx BUPH)
- Infantile glaucoma
- Other congenital and inherited syndromes

## Optic Nerve Enlargement (DDx OPG)
- Optic nerve sheath meningioma

# PATHOLOGY

## General Features
- General path comments
  - ○ Disorder of histogenesis, classified as a neurocutaneous, or inherited tumor, syndrome
  - ○ Orbital features of NF1 have interrelated underlying pathology
- Genetics
  - ○ Autosomal dominant; variable expression
  - ○ 50% new mutations; gene locus = 17q11.2
- Etiology: Loss of NF1 tumor suppressor gene function
- Epidemiology
  - ○ Most common inherited tumor syndrome
  - ○ Prevalence 1:2,000-5,000
  - ○ Orbital involvement in approximately 33%
- Associated abnormalities
  - ○ CNS tumors (often low grade), bright T2 foci on brain imaging or "NF spots" that resolve with age
  - ○ Diffuse neurofibromas; skeletal deformities

## Gross Pathologic & Surgical Features
- Plexiform neurofibroma
  - ○ Worm-like infiltrating subcutaneous mass
  - ○ May involve lid, conjunctiva, iris, choroid, ciliary body, periorbita, scalp, temporal fossa, and skull base
- Sphenoid dysplasia

# NEUROFIBROMATOSIS TYPE 1, ORBIT

○ Bony defect of posterior orbit; frequently associated with middle fossa arachnoid cyst
○ Enlargement of anterior orbital rim
• Buphthalmos
○ Associated with PNF in anterior orbit
• Optic pathway glioma
○ Diffuse fusiform nerve enlargement

## Microscopic Features
• Plexiform neurofibroma
○ Tortuous mass of enlarged peripheral nerve branches
○ Myxoid endoneural accumulation early
○ Schwann cell proliferation and collagen accumulation later
• Optic pathway glioma
○ Vast majority pilocytic astrocytomas
○ Spindle-shaped astrocytes with hyperplasia of fibroblasts and meningothelial cells
○ Circumferential perineural infiltration with arachnoid gliomatosis

## Staging, Grading or Classification Criteria
• Diagnostic criteria established by NIH consensus statement on neurofibromatosis

# CLINICAL ISSUES

## Presentation
• Most common signs/symptoms
○ Eyelid, periorbital and facial soft tissue masses
○ Proptosis and ptosis
• Other signs/symptoms: Lisch nodules, choroidal hamartomas, pulsatile exophthalmos
• Clinical Profile
○ PNF: Bulky soft tissue masses; "bag of worms" texture on palpation
○ SD: Pulsatile exophthalmos
○ BUPH: Enlarged eye; impaired vision
○ OPG: Asymptomatic, decreased vision or endocrine dysfunction

## Demographics
• Age
○ Cutaneous signs present at birth or 1st year
○ Tumors begin to appear in childhood
• Ethnicity: OPG risk lower in African descent

## Natural History & Prognosis
• PNF and SD are progressive developmental lesions rather than simply congenital defects
• 50% of OPG associated with NF1 may not progress
• PNF, SD, BUPH, and OPG may not be evident at birth
• Progressive lesions threaten vision
• 2-12% of PNF undergo sarcomatous degeneration (malignant peripheral nerve sheath tumor)
• Decreased life expectancy
○ Malignancy most common cause of death

## Treatment
• Plexiform neurofibroma
○ Not surgically curable due to infiltrative nature
○ Debulking may be required for vision or cosmesis
○ Anterior orbit and eyelid procedures most common

○ Radiation therapy not effective
• Sphenoid dysplasia
○ Transcranial reconstruction with grafts of severe posterior defects
○ Debulking of associated PNF
• Buphthalmos
○ Medical ± surgical therapy for glaucoma
• Optic pathway glioma
○ Observation unless vision threatened
○ Radiation or proton beam therapy and surgery for bulky tumors

# DIAGNOSTIC CHECKLIST

## Consider
• Although NF1 is inherited disorder, orbital manifestations are progressive and develop over time

## Image Interpretation Pearls
• Rapid change in appearance of PNF worrisome for malignant degeneration

# SELECTED REFERENCES

1. Lee V et al: Orbitotemporal neurofibromatosis. Clinical features and surgical management. Ophthalmology. 111(2):382-8, 2004
2. Jacquemin C et al: Orbit deformities in craniofacial neurofibromatosis type 1. AJNR Am J Neuroradiol. 24(8):1678-82, 2003
3. Rootman J: Neoplasia. In: Diseases of the Orbit. Philadelphia, Lippincott, 2003
4. Ferner RE et al: International consensus statement on malignant peripheral nerve sheath tumors in neurofibromatosis. Cancer Res. 62(5):1573-7, 2002
5. Jacquemin C et al: Reassessment of sphenoid dysplasia associated with neurofibromatosis type 1. AJNR Am J Neuroradiol. 23(4):644-8, 2002
6. Rasmussen SA et al: NF1 gene and neurofibromatosis 1. Am J Epidemiol. 151(1):33-40, 2000
7. Heinz GW et al: The effect of buphthalmos on orbital growth in early childhood: increased orbital soft tissue volume strongly correlates with increased orbital volume. J AAPOS. 2(1):39-42, 1998
8. Snyder BJ et al: Transcranial correction of orbital neurofibromatosis. Plast Reconstr Surg. 102(3):633-42, 1998
9. Krastinova-Lolov D et al: The surgical management of cranio-orbital neurofibromatosis. Ann Plast Surg. 36(3):263-9, 1996
10. Macfarlane R et al: Absence of the greater sphenoid wing in neurofibromatosis type I: congenital or acquired: case report. Neurosurgery. 37(1):129-33, 1995
11. Macfarlane R et al: Absence of the greater sphenoid wing in neurofibromatosis type I: congenital or acquired: case report. Neurosurgery. 37(1):129-33, 1995
12. Smith M et al: Imaging and differential diagnosis of the large eye. Radiographics. 14(4):721-8, 1994
13. Smith JL et al: Ocular pulsation in neurofibromatosis. A clinical/neuroradiologic correlation. J Clin Neuroophthalmol. 13(3):163-70, 1993
14. Consensus Development Conference: Neurofibromatosis. National Institutes of Health. 1(3):172-8, 1988
15. Reed D et al: Plexiform neurofibromatosis of the orbit: CT evaluation. AJNR Am J Neuroradiol. 7(2):259-63, 1986

## IMAGE GALLERY

### Typical

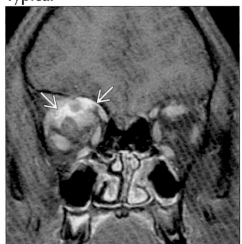

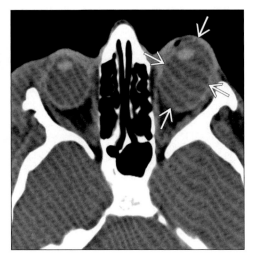

*(Left) Coronal T1 C+ FS MR shows an irregular, ill-defined enhancing plexiform neurofibroma ⇥ involving both the intra- and extraconal spaces of the right superior orbit. (Right) Axial NECT shows large, elongated left globe ⇥, diagnostic of buphthalmos. Mild left sphenoid wing dysplasia and associated left plexiform neurofibroma was seen on other images.*

### Typical

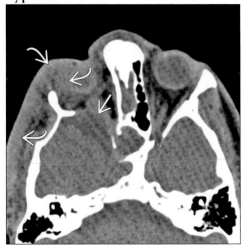

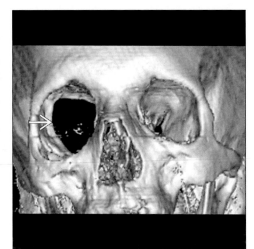

*(Left) Axial NECT shows a transpatial plexiform neurofibroma ⇥ in and around the right orbit. The sphenoid wing/lateral orbital wall are dysplastic. Temporal lobe herniates ⇥ into the orbit. (Right) Anteroposterior bone CT 3D surface reconstruction of same patient as previous image shows classic enlargement of the right orbit. Absence of the greater sphenoid wing creates defect ⇥ in back of orbit.*

### Typical

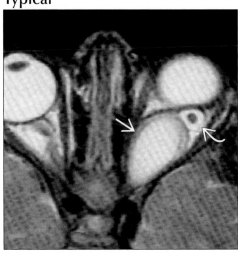

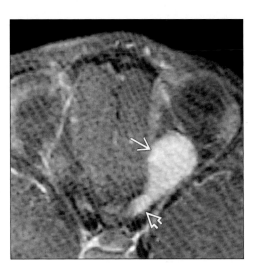

*(Left) Axial T2WI MR shows a hyperintense, enlarged left optic nerve ⇥, consistent with optic glioma. The optic sheath ⇥ distal to the tumor is markedly dilated. (Right) Axial T1 C+ FS MR of same patient as previous image shows an intensely enhancing large left optic nerve glioma ⇥ with the enlargement and enhancement extending through the optic foramen ⇥.*

# PART III
**Spine**

III
1

III
2

III
3

III
4

III
5

III
6

# SPINE & SPINAL CORD DEVELOPMENT

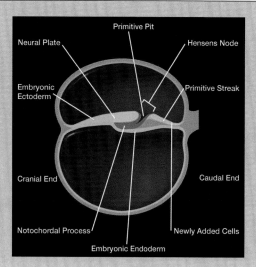

Graphic of early embryo shows notochordal process forming from cells migrating through primitive pit at the Hensens node. Ectoderm overlying notochordal process becomes neural plate.

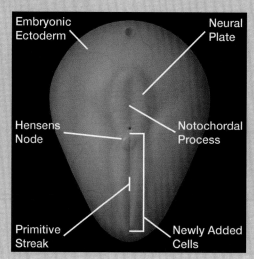

Graphic of the bilaminar embryo shows early CNS development. Ectoderm lying above the notochordal process (which will become notochord) becomes neuroectoderm and forms the neural plate.

## ANATOMY-BASED IMAGING ISSUES

### Key Concepts or Questions
- Classified according to embryologic event at which normal development goes awry
- Four main processes in spinal cord development
  - Notochord formation
    - Notochordal process forms due to migration of epiblastic cells from primitive streak through primitive node to intercalate between embryonic ectoderm and embryonic endoderm
    - Notochordal plate forms at rostral end of notochordal process; folds to become notochord
    - Notochord permits overlying ectoderm to become neuroectoderm (neural plate)
  - Neurulation
    - Edges of neural plate lift dorsally to form neural fold
    - Neural crest forms at junction between neuroectoderm and cutaneous ectoderm
    - Edges of neural fold approach each other in order to meet in midline
  - Disjunction of cutaneous ectoderm and neuroectoderm
    - As edges of neural folds meet, neuroectoderm, neural crest, and cutaneous ectoderm separate (disjunction)
    - Neuroectoderm becomes neural tube; neural crest forms spinal ganglia, leptomeninges, posterior elements of vertebrae, paraspinous muscles
  - Canalization and retrogressive differentiation
    - Caudalmost spinal cord (below S2) forms by different process
    - Communication with cord induces portion of pluripotential caudal cell mass to become neuroectoderm
    - Neuroectoderm in caudal cell mass fuses to caudalmost spinal cord
    - Cysts form in this part of cord, then coalesce to form rudimentary central canal
    - Caudalmost central canal may remain dilated as ventriculus terminalis

- Note that caudal cell mass also contributes to lower portions of genitourinary (GU) and gastrointestinal (GI) systems; essential to look for anomalies of these systems when malformations due to abnormal canalization/retrogressive differentiation are identified, and vice versa
- Spinal column development
  - Membranous development
    - Notochord separates from primitive gut and neural tube to create two zones: Ventral subchordal and dorsal epichordal
    - Zones are filled with mesenchyme, which migrates from initial location lateral to neural tube
    - Mesenchyme organizes into somites, separated by intersegmental fissures
    - Each somite dives into medial sclerotome (→ ipsilateral hemivertebra, directed by SHH) and lateral dermatomyotome (→ paraspinous muscles)
    - Other mesenchyme migrates dorsally to form precursors of neural arches after induction by BMP4
  - Chondrification
    - Sclerotomes separate transversely along intersegmental fissures
    - Inferior half of one sclerotome fuses with superior half of subjacent sclerotome → vertebral body
    - Process occurs bilaterally, symmetrically: Fusion of sclerotomes on one side form half of vertebral body on that side
    - Notochordal remnants persist between new vertebra → intervertebral discs
  - Ossification
    - Chondral skeleton ossifies
    - Starts in 3 centers: Middle of vertebral body and two vertebral arches
    - Ossification of the synchondroses between these ossification centers occur at variable ages, usually ages 4-7 yrs

### Imaging Approaches
- For evaluating spinal cord, filum
  - MR: Thin section (3 mm or less) sagittal T1 and T2 images

# SPINE & SPINAL CORD DEVELOPMENT

## Key Facts

### Concepts
- Spine malformations are classified according to embryologic event that goes wrong
- Five main processes in spine development
  - Notochord formation
  - Neurulation
  - Disjunction
  - Canalization and retrogressive differentiation
  - Spinal column development
- Imaging findings are best understood in light of these processes

### Imaging Spinal Malformations
- MR best shows malformations of cord, filum
  - Ultrasound is useful during first year after birth
- CT best shows malformations of spinal column

- CT myelography may be useful in severe scoliosis
- CSF flow more rapid in cervical, upper thoracic than lumbar regions
  - Beware CSF flow artifacts on T2 images

### Associated Anomalies
- Caudal cell mass also contributes to lower portions of spine, GU, GI systems
  - Look for anomalies of lower GI, GU systems when malformations due to abnormal canalization/retrogressive differentiation are identified, and vice versa
- Scoliosis: Look for underlying malformations
  - If atypical curve
  - If rapid progression
  - If neurologic signs/symptoms

- T1 best shows lipomas, subcutaneous segments of dermal sinuses
- T2 best shows bony/fibrous spurs (diastematomyelia), dermal sinuses within thecal sac
- MR: Axial T1 and T2 weighted images
  - T1 best shows fibrolipoma of filum, relationship of lipoma to placode
  - T2 best shows bony, fibrous spurs (diastematomyelia); size of filum; location of dermal sinus within sac
- Ultrasound: Excellent for evaluation on conus, filum in infants in first 6 months after birth
  - More difficult to detect multiple lesions
  - Useful until posterior elements begin to ossify
- For evaluating spinal column
  - Sagittal 3 mm T1 and STIR images
  - Coronal T1 images
    - Best shows hemivertebrae, butterfly vertebrae
    - Shows associated renal anomalies
    - Useful in programming planes for sagittal, axial images when scoliosis present
  - Bone CT is valuable adjunct for detail of bony anomalies
    - Better than MR or ultrasound; should always be obtained if surgery is needed
    - Multidetector helical scanners with sagittal and coronal reformations
    - But cord is not evaluated without intrathecal contrast
  - CT myelography occasionally useful for evaluation of neural structures in setting of severe scoliosis
    - Use multidetector helical scanner with reformations in multiple planes to optimally visualize vertebral column and contents
    - Also useful for foci of tethering (meningocele manque) in diastematomyelia

### Imaging Pitfalls
- Watch for CSF flow artifacts (signal voids) on T2 MR images
  - Signal void may resemble solid structure, mimic mass or second spinal cord (split cord malformation)

- Signal void most common in ventrolateral C-spine, dorsal T-spine
- Signal void least common in lower thoracic and lumbar regions
- Note: Signal voids may be in unusual locations in children with scoliosis

## PATHOLOGIC ISSUES

### General Pathologic Considerations
- Malformations result from disturbances of normal developmental processes described above

### Classification
- Malformations secondary to abnormal notochord development
  - Split cord malformations (diastematomyelia)
  - Split notochord syndromes
    - Neurenteric cyst
    - Dorsal enteric sinus, fistula
    - GI duplications, pulmonary sequestrations
- Malformations secondary to premature disjunction of neuroectoderm from cutaneous ectoderm
  - Lipomyelocele, lipomyelomeningocele
  - Subpial lipoma
- Malformations secondary to lack of disjunction of neuroectoderm from cutaneous ectoderm
  - Myelocele, myelomeningocele
  - Dorsal dermal sinus
  - Cervical myelocystocele
- Malformations secondary to abnormalities of caudal cell mass/canalization/retrogressive differentiation
  - Ventriculus terminalis
  - Filar cysts
  - Fibrolipoma of filum terminale
  - Tethered cord with terminal lipoma
  - Caudal regression syndrome/lumbosacral hypogenesis
  - Terminal myelocystocele
  - Sacrococcygeal teratoma

# SPINE & SPINAL CORD DEVELOPMENT

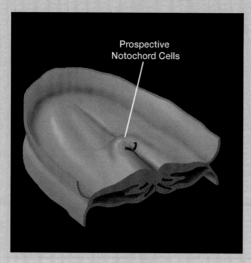

*Graphic with the yolk sac and amniotic cavity cut away shows how prospective notochordal cells migrate between ectoderm and entoderm to form notochordal process which will induce neuroectoderm.*

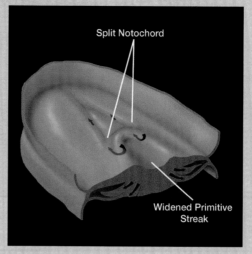

*Graphic shows how diastematomyelia is purported to develop. Adhesion between ectoderm and entoderm causes the notochord to focally split, resulting in two hemicords in a portion of the spine (diastematomyelia).*

## EMBRYOLOGY

### Embryologic Events
- Notochord development
  - Duplication or splitting of notochord results in formation of two spinal cords
- Neurulation
  - Causes of neurulation defects felt to be multifactorial
  - Genetic defects currently felt to be less important
  - Frequency of neurulation defects related to season, location, ethnicity, economic status, maternal age
  - Folic acid supplementation of maternal diet reduces incidence of neurulation defects
  - Other potential factors include methionine deficit, mutations
- Canalization and retrogressive differentiation
  - Defects in this process often result in Currarino triad
    - Caudal regression - often lumbosacral hypogenesis
    - Anorectal malformation - often anal atresia
    - Presacral mass - often sacrococcygeal teratoma
- Spinal column development
  - Defects most commonly result in congenital scoliosis

## CLINICAL IMPLICATIONS

### Clinical Importance
- Most spine malformations result in dysfunction of distal portions of spinal cord
- Clinical presentations include
  - Tethered cord syndrome: Lower extremity weakness, spasticity; low back pain; urinary or fecal incontinence
    - Tight filum terminale
    - Tethering with terminal lipoma
    - Lipomyelocele, lipomyelomeningocele
  - Orthopedic deformities of lower extremities: Club foot, congenital hip dislocation
    - Lumbosacral hypogenesis
    - Tethered cord from any cause (see above)

- Recurrent infections from seeding through dermal sinuses
  - Focal infection (cellulitis, abscess)
  - Widespread infection (meningitis)
- Large, fatty lumbosacral mass
  - Associated with lipomyelocele, lipomyelomeningocele
  - Sacral teratoma
- Cauda equina syndrome (hyporeflexia, lower extremity weakness)
  - Lumbar or sacral lipoma, (epi)dermoid
- Myelopathy (hyperreflexia, lower extremity weakness)
  - Cervical or thoracic lipoma, (epi)dermoid, tight filum terminale
- Scoliosis with rapid progression, abnormal curve, neurological signs/symptoms
  - Any cause of tethering
  - Malformations associated with vertebral anomalies: Hemivertebrae, butterfly vertebrae
- Cutaneous stigmata: Hypertrichosis, skin tag, hemangioma
  - Classically seen with diastematomyelia
  - Also seen with tight filum terminale, dermal sinus, lipomyeloceles, lipomyelomeningoceles

## RELATED REFERENCES

1. Schenk JP et al: Imaging of congenital anomalies and variations of the caudal spine and back in neonates and small infants. Eur J Radiol. 58(1):3-14, 2006
2. Barkovich AJ. Pediatric Neuroimaging, 4th Ed. Lippincott Williams & Wilkins, Philadelphia, 2005
3. Copp AJ: Neurulation in the cranial region--normal and abnormal. J Anat. 207(5):623-35, 2005
4. Kaplan KM et al: Embryology of the spine and associated congenital abnormalities. Spine J. 5(5):564-76, 2005
5. Martucciello G et al: Currarino syndrome: proposal of a diagnostic and therapeutic protocol. J Pediatr Surg. 39(9):1305-11, 2004
6. Giampietro PF et al: Congenital and idiopathic scoliosis: clinical and genetic aspects. Clin Med Res. 1(2):125-36, 2003

## IMAGE GALLERY

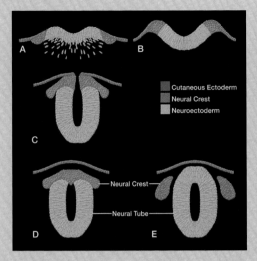

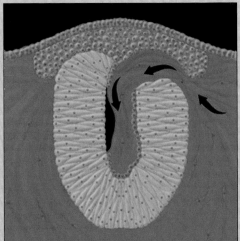

*(Left)* Graphic of neurulation. Neural plate (A) folds into neural fold (C) and then neural tube (E). When edges of fold meet, cutaneous ectoderm/neural crest separate (disjunction) from neuroectoderm to form skin/meninges. *(Right)* Graphic shows mesenchyme migrating (arrows) into central canal of developing neural tube after premature disjunction of neuroectoderm from skin. Ectopic mesenchyme become fat in spinal lipomas.

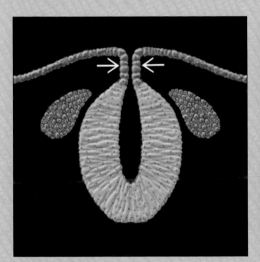

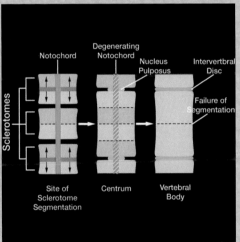

*(Left)* Graphic shows focal nondisjunction of neuroectoderm from cutaneous ectoderm. This results in an epithelium-lined tract ➡ connecting neural structures with skin: Dermal sinus tract. *(Right)* Graphic shows vertebral segmentation. After segmentation into sclerotomes, superior half of one sclerotome combines with inferior half of adjacent one to form vertebral body. Failure ⇒ nonsegmented ("fused") vertebrae without intervening disc.

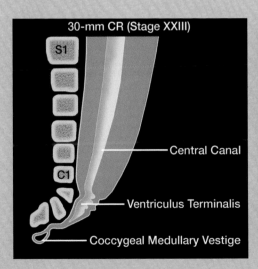

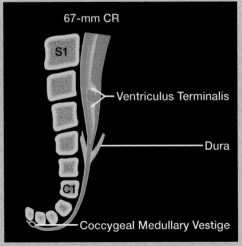

*(Left)* Graphic shows irregular caudalmost spinal cord, which is derived from the caudal cell mass in the lower sacral/coccygeal segments. Cord extends to sacrum without filum terminale. *(Right)* Graphic shows development of filum from apoptosis/elongation of cells in caudalmost spinal cord. Cord terminus moves rostrally with respect to vertebrae. Ventriculus terminalis may remain dilated.

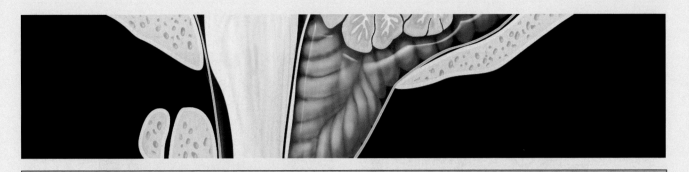

# SECTION 1: Craniocervical Junction

# CHIARI I MALFORMATION

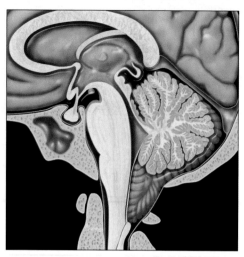

Sagittal graphic shows ectopic cerebellar tonsils displaced into the upper cervical canal. The 4th ventricle is in normal position.

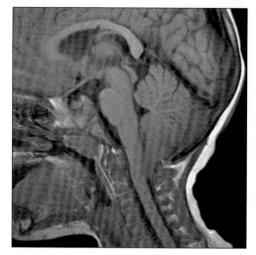

Sagittal T1WI MR shows ectopic cerebellar tonsillar displacement into cervical canal with ventral spinal cord displacement. Note retroflexed dens, foreshortened clivus, and normal 4th ventricle.

## TERMINOLOGY

### Abbreviations and Synonyms
- Chiari I malformation (CM I)

### Definitions
- Elongated, "peg-shaped" cerebellar tonsils extend below foramen magnum into cervical spinal canal

## IMAGING FINDINGS

### General Features
- Best diagnostic clue: Pointed cerebellar tonsils ≥ 5 mm below foramen magnum +/- syringohydromyelia (14-75%)
- Location: Craniovertebral junction (CVJ)
- Size: Tonsils > 5 mm below foramen magnum
- Morphology: Low-lying, pointed "peg-like" tonsils with oblique vertical sulci, elongated but normally located 4th ventricle

### CT Findings
- NECT: Small posterior fossa (PF) ⇒ low torcular, "crowded" foramen magnum, tonsillar ectopia, flattened spinal cord
- Bone CT
  - Often normal; abnormal cases ⇒ short clivus, CVJ segmentation/fusion anomalies, small posterior fossa

### MR Findings
- T1WI
  - Pointed (not rounded) tonsils ≥ 5 mm below foramen magnum
  - "Tight foramen magnum" with small/absent cisterns
  - +/- Elongation of 4th ventricle, hindbrain anomalies
- T2WI
  - Oblique tonsillar folia (like "sergeant's stripes")
  - +/- Short clivus ⇒ "apparent" descent of 4th ventricle, medulla
  - +/- Syringohydromyelia (14-75%)

## DDx: Chiari I Malformation

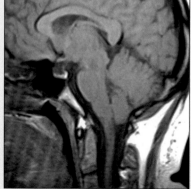

Normal Low Tonsils

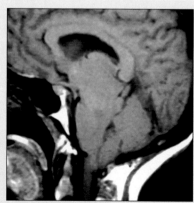

CSF Hypotension

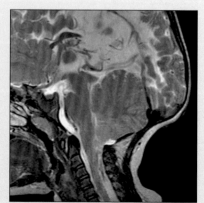

Chiari II Malformation

# CHIARI I MALFORMATION

## Key Facts

### Terminology
- Chiari I malformation (CM I)

### Imaging Findings
- Best diagnostic clue: Pointed cerebellar tonsils ≥ 5 mm below foramen magnum +/- syringohydromyelia (14-75%)
- "Tight foramen magnum" with small/absent cisterns
- +/- Elongation of 4th ventricle, hindbrain anomalies
- Oblique tonsillar folia (like "sergeant's stripes")

### Top Differential Diagnoses
- Normal Tonsillar Displacement Below Foramen Magnum
- Acquired Tonsillar Herniation ("Acquired Chiari I")
- Chiari II Malformation

### Pathology
- Diagnostic criteria: Herniation of at least one cerebellar tonsil > 5 mm or herniation of both tonsils 3 mm to 5 mm below a line connecting the basion with opisthion

### Clinical Issues
- Clinical Profile: Clinical CM I syndrome: Headache, pseudotumor-like episodes, Meniere disease-like syndrome, lower cranial nerve and spinal cord signs
- Increasing ectopia + time ⇒ ↑ likelihood symptoms

### Diagnostic Checklist
- Unless tonsils > 5 mm and/or pointed, probably not clinically significant Chiari I malformation
- Tonsillar herniation > 12 mm nearly always symptomatic

## Radiographic Findings
- Radiography: Normal or short clivus; +/- retroflexed dens, CVJ segmentation/fusion anomalies, small posterior fossa

## Non-Vascular Interventions
- Myelography: Low-lying tonsils efface cerebrospinal fluid (CSF) at foramen magnum

## Other Modality Findings
- Cine phase contrast (PC) MR: Disorganized CSF pulsation, ↑ brainstem/cerebellar tonsil motion ⇒ ↑ peak systolic velocity, ↓ flow through foramen magnum

## Imaging Recommendations
- Best imaging tool: MR imaging
- Protocol advice: Multiplanar T1WI, T2WI of spinal axis and posterior fossa, PC MR CSF flow study

## DIFFERENTIAL DIAGNOSIS

### Normal Tonsillar Displacement Below Foramen Magnum
- Tonsils may normally lie below foramen magnum
- Unless tonsils > 5 mm and/or pointed, probably not clinically significant Chiari I malformation

### Acquired Tonsillar Herniation ("Acquired Chiari I")
- Acquired basilar invagination (osteogenesis imperfecta, Paget disease, craniosynostosis, rickets, achondroplasia, acromegaly) ⇒ small posterior fossa
- "Pull from below" (LP shunt, CSF leak) 2° to intracranial hypotension
  - "Sagging" brainstem, tonsillar herniation, smooth dural enhancement, dilated epidural plexus, retrospinal C1/2 fluid collection, spinal hygroma
- "Push from above"
  - Chronic VP shunt; thick skull, premature sutural fusion, arachnoidal adhesions

- ↑ ICP, intracranial mass

### Chiari II Malformation
- Associated with myelomeningocele
- Beaked tectum, vermian ectopia, abnormal effaced 4th ventricle, medullary kink

## PATHOLOGY

### General Features
- General path comments
  - Underdeveloped occipital enchondrium ⇒ small posterior fossa vault, downward hindbrain herniation
  - Foramen magnum obstruction ⇒ decreased communication between cranial, spinal CSF compartments
- Genetics
  - Autosomal dominant inheritance with reduced penetrance, or autosomal recessive inheritance
  - Syndromic/familial associations (velocardiofacial/microdeletion chromosome 22, Williams syndrome, craniosynostosis, achondroplasia, Hajdu-Cheney syndrome, and Klippel-Feil syndrome)
- Etiology
  - Hydrodynamic theory
    - Systolic piston-like descent of impacted tonsils/medulla ⇒ plugs CSF pathway at foramen magnum
    - During diastole, rapid recoil of brain stem/tonsils disimpacts foramen magnum, permits normal CSF diastolic pulsation
  - Posterior fossa underdevelopment theory
    - Underdevelopment of occipital somites of para-axial mesoderm produce diminutive posterior fossa ⇒ 2° tonsillar herniation
- Epidemiology: Incidence 0.01-0.6% all age groups, 0.9% pediatric patient groups
- Associated abnormalities

# CHIARI I MALFORMATION

○ 4th occipital sclerotome syndromes (50%): Short clivus, craniovertebral segmentation/fusion anomalies
○ Osseous skull base/skeletal anomalies (25-50%)
  ■ Scoliosis +/- kyphosis (42%); left thoracic curve
  ■ Retroflexed odontoid process (26%)
  ■ Platybasia, basilar invagination (25-50%)
  ■ Klippel-Feil syndrome (5-10%)
  ■ Incomplete C1 ring ossification (5%)
  ■ Atlantooccipital assimilation (1-5%)
○ Syringomyelia (30-60%) ⇒ 60-90% in symptomatic CM I patients
  ■ Most common C4-6; holocord hydrosyringomyelia, cervical/upper-thoracic syrinx, syringobulbia uncommon
○ Hydrocephalus (11%)

## Gross Pathologic & Surgical Features
• Herniated, sclerotic tonsils grooved by opisthion
• Arachnoidal veils or scarring and adhesions at foramen magnum

## Microscopic Features
• Tonsillar softening or sclerosis with Purkinje/granular cell loss

## Staging, Grading or Classification Criteria
• Diagnostic criteria: Herniation of at least one cerebellar tonsil > 5 mm or herniation of both tonsils 3 mm to 5 mm below a line connecting the basion with opisthion
○ Herniation of both tonsils 3-5 mm below foramen magnum + syrinx, cervicomedullary kinking, 4th ventricular elongation, or pointed tonsils ⇒ congenital CM I
○ Tonsil herniation ≤ 5 mm does not exclude CM I

# CLINICAL ISSUES

## Presentation
• Most common signs/symptoms
○ Up to 50% asymptomatic (especially if ≤ 5 mm inferior displacement)
○ Symptomatic patients present with constellation of findings
  ■ Sudden death (rare)
  ■ Suboccipital headache, cranial nerve palsy, ocular disturbances, otoneurologic dysfunction, cord motor or sensory abnormalities, gait disturbance, neuropathic joint
  ■ Tonsillar herniation > 12 mm nearly always symptomatic; ~ 30% with tonsils 5-10 mm below foramen magnum asymptomatic
  ■ CM I patients with syrinx nearly always present with symptoms referable to syrinx; if the syrinx extends into medulla, bulbar symptoms predominate
○ Trauma is a common precipitating event for symptom onset (24%)
• Clinical Profile: Clinical CM I syndrome: Headache, pseudotumor-like episodes, Meniere disease-like syndrome, lower cranial nerve and spinal cord signs

## Demographics
• Age: 10 months → elderly; syrinx, congenital CVJ anomalies hasten presentation
• Gender: M < F (2:3)

## Natural History & Prognosis
• Natural history not clearly understood
○ Many patients asymptomatic for prolonged periods
○ Increasing ectopia + time ⇒ ↑ likelihood symptoms
• Children respond better to treatment than adults
• Degree of tonsillar herniation correlates with clinical severity

## Treatment
• Treating asymptomatic patients is controversial
○ "Radiographic" CM I (no syrinx), no corresponding clinical signs/symptoms → conservative management
○ Asymptomatic Chiari I + syrinx → consider decompression
• Symptomatic patients: PF decompression/resection of posterior arch C1, +/- duraplasty, cerebellar tonsil resection
○ > 90% ↓ brainstem signs
○ > 80% ↓ hydrosyringomyelia
○ +/- Scoliosis arrest
• Direct shunting of symptomatic syrinx obsolete; goal to restore normal CSF flow at foramen magnum

# DIAGNOSTIC CHECKLIST

## Consider
• Unless tonsils > 5 mm and/or pointed, probably not clinically significant Chiari I malformation

## Image Interpretation Pearls
• Tonsillar herniation > 12 mm nearly always symptomatic

# SELECTED REFERENCES

1. McGirt MJ et al: Correlation of cerebrospinal fluid flow dynamics and headache in Chiari I malformation. Neurosurgery. 56(4):716-21; discussion 716-21, 2005
2. Flynn JM et al: Predictors of progression of scoliosis after decompression of an Arnold Chiari I malformation. Spine. 29(3):286-92, 2004
3. Iskandar BJ et al: Foramen magnum cerebrospinal fluid flow characteristics in children with Chiari I malformation before and after craniocervical decompression. J Neurosurg. 101(2 Suppl):169-78, 2004
4. Tubbs RS et al: Arachnoid veils and the Chiari I malformation. J Neurosurg. 100(5 Suppl Pediatrics):465-7, 2004
5. Tubbs RS et al: Persistent syringomyelia following pediatric Chiari I decompression: radiological and surgical findings. J Neurosurg. 100(5 Suppl Pediatrics):460-4, 2004
6. Spiegel DA et al: Scoliotic curve patterns in patients with Chiari I malformation and/or syringomyelia. Spine. 28(18):2139-46, 2003
7. Tubbs RS et al: Surgical experience in 130 pediatric patients with Chiari I malformations. J Neurosurg. 99(2):291-6, 2003

## IMAGE GALLERY

### Typical

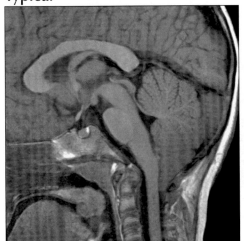
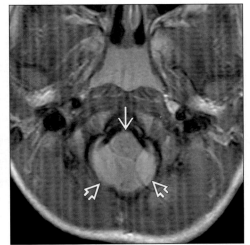

*(Left) Sagittal T1WI MR demonstrates tonsillar ectopia into the upper cervical canal. Note retroflexed dens and foreshortened clivus. Normal 4th ventricle and tectal plate distinguish from CM III. (Right) Axial T2WI MR depicts crowding of the medulla ➡ at the foramen magnum by the ectopic cerebellar tonsils ⇛.*

### Typical

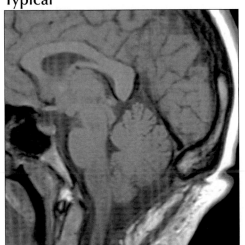
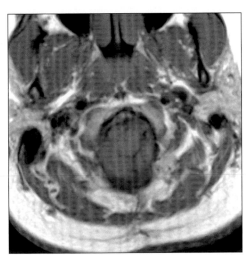

*(Left) Sagittal T1WI MR following surgical decompression of Chiari I malformation demonstrates expected post-operative changes from suboccipital craniectomy and resection of the posterior C1 ring. (Right) Axial T1WI MR reveals expected post-operative appearance after Chiari I decompression and resection of the posterior C1 ring.*

### Variant

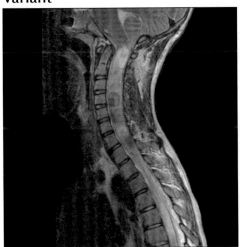
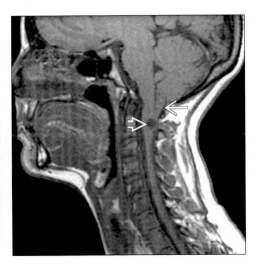

*(Left) Sagittal T2WI MR shows tonsillar ectopia and large cervical spinal cord syringohydromyelia. Note also associated foreshortened clivus and retroflexed odontoid process. (Right) Sagittal T1WI MR shows elongated ectopic cerebellar tonsils ➡, compression of craniovertebral CSF spaces, and focal cystic cord hydromyelia ⇛. The 4th ventricle is in normal position.*

# CHIARI II MALFORMATION

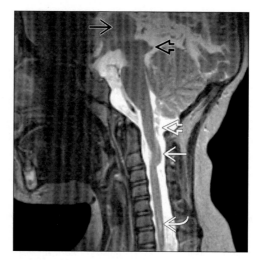

*Sagittal graphic shows herniation of the cerebellar vermis into the upper cervical canal. The medullary kink and beaked tectum with low-lying torcular herophili are characteristic of CM II.*

*Sagittal T2WI MR demonstrates cervicomedullary kink ➡, vermian displacement ⮞ through foramen magnum, large massa intermedia ➡, tectal beak ⮞, and small syringohydromyelia ➡.*

## TERMINOLOGY

### Abbreviations and Synonyms
- Synonyms: CM II, Arnold-Chiari malformation, Chiari type II

### Definitions
- Complex hindbrain malformation
  - Virtually 100% associated with neural tube closure defect (NTD), usually lumbar myelomeningocele (MMC)
    - Rare reports in closed spinal dysraphism; most probably misinterpreted Chiari I

## IMAGING FINDINGS

### General Features
- Best diagnostic clue: Cerebellar herniation with concurrent myelomeningocele
- Location: Posterior fossa (PF), upper cervical spine; syrinx may involve entire cord
- Size: Posterior fossa smaller than normal

- Morphology: Cerebellum "wraps" around medulla and "towers" through incisura, with beaked tectum and heart-shaped midbrain

### CT Findings
- NECT: Crowded posterior fossa, widened tentorial incisura, tectal beaking, and inferior vermian displacement
- Bone CT
  - Small posterior fossa
    - Low lying tentorium/torcular inserts near foramen magnum
    - Large, funnel-shaped foramen magnum with "notched" opisthion
    - Scalloped posterior petrous pyramids, clivus
  - Posterior C1 arch anomalies (66%), enlarged cervical canal
  - Irregular inner table 2° to Luckenshädel

### MR Findings
- T1WI
  - "Cascade" or "waterfall" of cerebellum/brainstem downwards
    - Uvula/nodulus/pyramid of vermis ⇒ sclerotic "peg"

## DDx: Chiari II Malformation

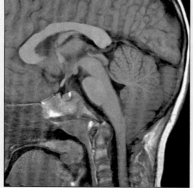

*Chiari I Malformation*

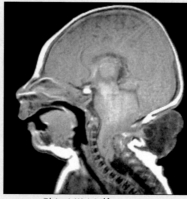

*Chiari III Malformation*

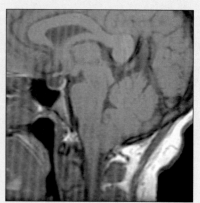

*CSF Hypotension*

# CHIARI II MALFORMATION

## Key Facts

### Terminology
- Synonyms: CM II, Arnold-Chiari malformation, Chiari type II
- Virtually 100% associated with neural tube closure defect (NTD), usually lumbar myelomeningocele (MMC)

### Imaging Findings
- Small posterior fossa
- "Cascade" or "waterfall" of cerebellum/brainstem downwards
- Medulla "heaps up" over cord tethered by dentate ligaments ⇒ cervicomedullary "kink" (70% )

### Top Differential Diagnoses
- Chiari I Malformation
- Chiari III Malformation

- Intracranial CSF Hypotension
- Multisutural Craniosynostosis Syndromes

### Pathology
- Secondary to sequelae of CSF leakage through open spinal dysraphism during gestation (4th fetal week)

### Clinical Issues
- Usually presents within context of known MMC
- Chiari II malformation most common cause of death in MMC

### Diagnostic Checklist
- Low torcular herophili indicates small posterior fossa
- CT or MR showing towering cerebellum, downward vermian displacement, +/- brainstem compression diagnostic of Chiari II

---

- Medulla "heaps up" over cord tethered by dentate ligaments ⇒ cervicomedullary "kink" (70% )
- "Towering" cerebellum ⇒ compresses midbrain, causes "beaked" tectum
- 4th ventricle elongated with no posterior point (fastigium)
  - Open dysraphism, MMC ~ 100% (lumbar > > cervical)
  - Hydrosyringomyelia (20-90%)
- T2WI
  - Similar to T1WI + hyperintense gliotic brain tissue
  - +/- 4th ventricular lesions (rare)
    - Roof of IV ventricle adjacent/within choroid plexus
    - Glial or arachnoidal cysts, glial or choroidal nodules, subependymoma
- Other MR findings
  - Phase contrast cine MR ⇒ restricted CSF flow through foramen magnum, decreased conus movement

### Radiographic Findings
- Radiography: Lateral skull ⇒ low torcular herophili, Luckenshädel (irregular linear skull markings, universal at birth, largely resolve by 6 months of age)

### Ultrasonographic Findings
- Grayscale Ultrasound
  - Fetal obstetrical ultrasound (US) provides early diagnosis
    - MMC may be identified as early as 10 weeks gestation
    - Characteristic brain findings ("lemon" and "banana" signs) seen as early as 12 weeks

### Imaging Recommendations
- Initial screening using MR imaging (brain and spine)
- Follow-up CT or MR to assess hydrocephalus status; MR for progressive brainstem or spinal symptoms

## DIFFERENTIAL DIAGNOSIS

### Chiari I Malformation
- No association with myelomeningocele
- 4th ventricle in normal position
- Tonsillar herniation (not vermis)

### Chiari III Malformation
- Chiari II malformation + cervical dysraphism, occipital cephalocele

### Intracranial CSF Hypotension
- Symptomatic expression of low CSF pressure; distinguishable by clinical onset and symptoms
- Slumping posterior fossa with pons compressed against clivus, dural thickening/enhancement

### Multisutural Craniosynostosis Syndromes
- Produce small posterior fossa, cerebellar herniation, ventriculomegaly

## PATHOLOGY

### General Features
- General path comments: Hydrocephalus and severity of brain malformation relate to size of PF, degree of caudal hindbrain descent
- Genetics
  - Methylene-Tetra-Hydrofolate-Reductase (MTHFR) mutations associated with abnormal folate metabolism
    - MTHFR mutations PLUS folate deficiency ⇒ ↑ risk NTD ⇒ Chiari II
    - 4-8% recurrence risk if one affected child
- Etiology
  - Secondary to sequelae of CSF leakage through open spinal dysraphism during gestation (4th fetal week)
    - Abnormal neurulation ⇒ CSF escapes through NTD ⇒ failure to maintain 4th ventricular distention ⇒ hypoplastic PF chondrocranium ⇒ displaced/distorted PF contents

# CHIARI II MALFORMATION

- Exceedingly rare cases of closed spinal dysraphism with Chiari II malformation may contradict this theory
  - Alternative theory proposes association between Chiari II malformation and myelomeningocele is due to rostral and caudal neural tube dysgenesis
- Epidemiology: Incidence: 0.44 per 1,000 births, ↓ with folate replacement therapy
- Associated abnormalities
  - Spine
    - Open dysraphism (MMC) ~ 100% (lumbar > > cervical)
    - Posterior arch C1 anomalies (66%)
    - Hydrosyringomyelia (20-90%)
    - Diastematomyelia (5%)
    - Klippel-Feil syndrome
    - Cervical myelocystocele
  - Brain/skull
    - Corpus callosum (CC) dysgenesis (90%), aqueductal stenosis, rhombencephalosynapsis, gray matter malformations, absent septum pellucidum, fused forniceal columns
    - Lacunar skull (Lückenschädel)

## Gross Pathologic & Surgical Features
- Small PF ⇒ contents shift down into cervical spinal canal
  - Cerebellar hemispheres/tonsils "wrap" around medulla
  - Pons/cranial nerve roots often elongated
  - Compressed/elongated/low IV ventricle ⇒ pouch in cervical canal
  - +/- Hydrosyringomyelia

## Microscopic Features
- Purkinje cell loss, sclerosis within herniated tissues

# CLINICAL ISSUES

## Presentation
- Most common signs/symptoms
  - Neonate: MMC, enlarging head circumference +/- hydrocephalus symptoms
  - Older child/adult: Clinical hydrocephalus, symptoms referable to tethered cord (MMC repair)
  - All age groups: Varying degrees of lower extremity paralysis/sphincter dysfunction/bulbar signs
- Clinical Profile
  - Usually presents within context of known MMC
    - Infants: Enlarging head circumference
    - Child/adult: Known Chiari II malformation, signs of hydrocephalus/shunt failure +/- bulbar symptoms
- Laboratory
  - Fetal screening: ↑ α-fetoprotein

## Demographics
- Age: Usually presents at birth with MMC +/- hydrocephalus
- Gender: M = F

## Natural History & Prognosis
- Chiari II malformation most common cause of death in MMC
  - Brainstem compression/hydrocephalus, intrinsic brainstem "wiring" defects
- Progression of spinal neurological deficits is rare; suspect hydrocephalus, associated undiagnosed spinal deformity (diastematomyelia), tethered cord

## Treatment
- Folate supplement for pregnant mothers (pre-conception ⇒ 6 weeks post conception) significantly decreases MMC risk
- Surgical management
  - Chiari decompression with resection of posterior foramen magnum, C1 ring
  - CSF diversion/shunting
  - Fetal MMC repair in selected patients may ameliorate Chiari II severity

# DIAGNOSTIC CHECKLIST

## Consider
- Brain/spinal axis MR to detect presence of Chiari II, assess severity, look for complications

## Image Interpretation Pearls
- Low torcular herophili indicates small posterior fossa
- CT or MR showing towering cerebellum, downward vermian displacement, +/- brainstem compression diagnostic of Chiari II

# SELECTED REFERENCES

1. Tubbs RS et al: Degree of tectal beaking correlates to the presence of nystagmus in children with Chiari II malformation. Childs Nerv Syst. 20(7):459-61, 2004
2. McLone DG et al: The Chiari II malformation: cause and impact. Childs Nerv Syst. 19(7-8):540-50, 2003
3. Sener RN et al: Rhombencephalosynapsis and a Chiari II malformation. J Comput Assist Tomogr. 27(2):257-9, 2003
4. Tubbs RS et al: Chiari II malformation and occult spinal dysraphism. Case reports and a review of the literature. Pediatr Neurosurg. 39(2):104-7, 2003
5. McDonnell GV et al: Prevalence of the Chiari/hydrosyringomyelia complex in adults with spina bifida: preliminary results. Eur J Pediatr Surg. 10 Suppl 1:18-9, 2000
6. McLone DG: Hydromyelia in a child with chiari II. Pediatr Neurosurg. 32(6):328, 2000
7. Northrup H et al: Spina bifida and other neural tube defects. Curr Probl Pediatr. 30(10):313-32, 2000
8. Piatt JH Jr et al: The Chiari II malformation: lesions discovered within the fourth ventricle. Pediatr Neurosurg. 30(2):79-85, 1999
9. Nishino A et al: Cervical myelocystocele with Chiari II malformation: magnetic resonance imaging and surgical treatment. Surg Neurol. 49(3):269-73, 1998
10. La Marca F et al: Presentation and management of hydromyelia in children with Chiari type-II malformation. Pediatr Neurosurg. 26(2):57-67, 1997
11. Shuman RM: The Chiari malformations: a constellation of anomalies. Semin Pediatr Neurol. 2(3):220-6, 1995
12. Ruge JR et al: Anatomical progression of the Chiari II malformation. Childs Nerv Syst. 8(2):86-91, 1992

## IMAGE GALLERY

### Typical

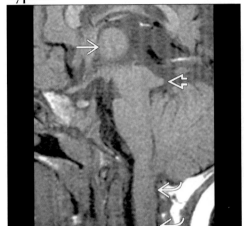
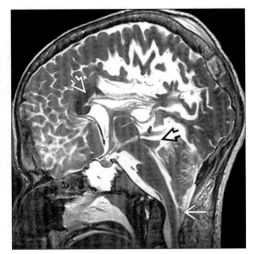

*(Left)* Sagittal T1WI MR through the craniovertebral junction shows characteristic beaked tectum ➡ and large massa intermedia ➡. Posterior fossa is crowded. Inferior vermis ➡ displaced. *(Right)* Sagittal T2WI MR reveals corpus callosum dysgenesis ➡, small posterior fossa, "beaked" tectum ➡, and downward shift of pons, 4th ventricle, and cerebellar vermis ➡.

### Typical

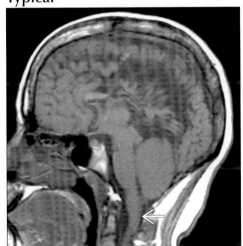
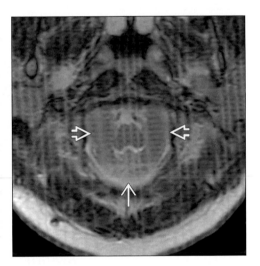

*(Left)* Sagittal T1WI MR shows mild CM II findings, including small posterior fossa, callosal dysgenesis, beaked tectum, large massa intermedia, small posterior fossa, and vermian ectopia to C2/3 ➡. *(Right)* Axial T2WI MR centered at the foramen magnum confirms brainstem crowding by the ectopic cerebellar vermis ➡ and tonsils ➡.

### Variant

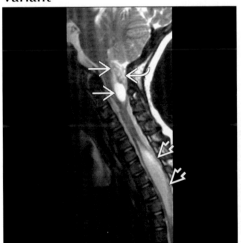
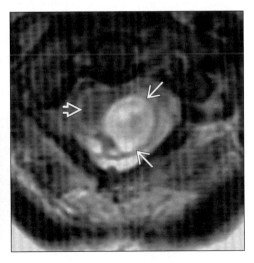

*(Left)* Sagittal T2WI MR shows small posterior fossa and vermian ectopia ➡. There is a large cervicothoracic cord syrinx ➡ with cervicomedullary extension (Note syringobulbia ➡). *(Right)* Axial T2WI MR in the same patient as previous image depicts eccentric intramedullary syringobulbia ➡ extending into the medulla ➡.

# CHIARI III MALFORMATION

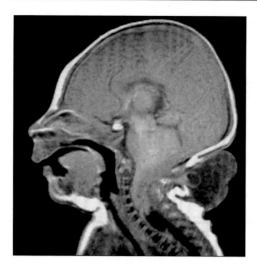 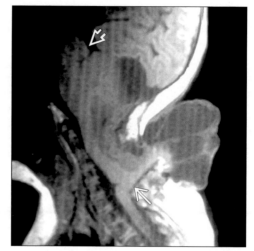

*Sagittal T1WI MR shows herniation of cerebellum through upper cervical spina bifida into meningeal sac. Note Chiari II features including vermian herniation, medullary kink, syrinx.*

*Sagittal T1WI MR reveals herniation of cerebellum, medulla, and meninges through a high cervical dysraphism. Note kinked medulla ➡ and tectal beaking ⇥.*

## TERMINOLOGY

### Abbreviations and Synonyms
- Synonyms: CM 3, Chiari III

### Definitions
- Chiari II malformation + high to mid-cervical cephalocele containing cerebellum

## IMAGING FINDINGS

### General Features
- Best diagnostic clue: Craniocervical junction (CCJ) or high cervical cephalocele containing cerebellum herniating into sac

### CT Findings
- Bone CT
  ○ Occipital +/- high cervical osseous dysraphism
  ○ Osseous Chiari II findings: Small posterior fossa, low torcular, scalloped clivus, Luckenshadel skull

### MR Findings
- T1WI
  ○ CCJ or high cervical cephalocele
    ▪ Meninges, cerebellum ± brainstem
    ▪ Cisterns, 4th ventricle, dural sinuses (50%)
  ○ ± Hydrocephalus
  ○ ± Intracranial Chiari II malformation
- T2WI: Neural tissue in sac ± high signal (gliosis)
- MRV: ± Veins within cephalocele

### Imaging Recommendations
- Best imaging tool: Multiplanar MR + MRV

## DIFFERENTIAL DIAGNOSIS

### Isolated Occipital Encephalocele
- Frequently tonsillar herniation
- Lacks intracranial Chiari II findings

### Syndromic Occipital Encephaloceles
- Iniencephaly: Occipital defect, ectatic foramen magnum +/- encephalocele, dorsal medullary cleft, cervical dysraphism/Klippel-Feil, severe cervicothoracic lordosis, fixed retroflexion of head
- Meckel-Gruber: Occipital encephalocele, multicystic kidney, polydactyly

### DDx: Chiari III Malformation

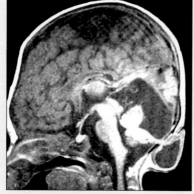 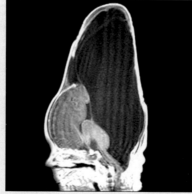 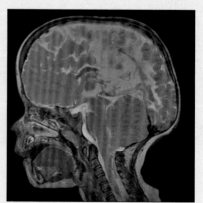

*Occipital Cephalocele*     *DWM + Occipital Cephalocele*     *Chiari II Malformation*

# CHIARI III MALFORMATION

## Key Facts

### Terminology
- Synonyms: CM 3, Chiari III
- Chiari II malformation + high to mid-cervical cephalocele containing cerebellum

### Imaging Findings
- CCJ or high cervical cephalocele
- ± Hydrocephalus
- ± Intracranial Chiari II malformation

### Top Differential Diagnoses
- Isolated Occipital Encephalocele
- Syndromic Occipital Encephaloceles

### Clinical Issues
- Dismal prognosis → early death, severe disability

### Diagnostic Checklist
- Occipital cephalocele containing cerebellum + intracranial Chiari II = Chiari III malformation

---

- Dandy-Walker malformation (DWM), Goldenhar-Gorlin, MURCS (Müllerian, renal, cervical-spine), Walker-Warburg, amniotic band

## PATHOLOGY

### General Features
- General path comments: Dysplastic cerebellar tissue ± brain stem herniating through dorsal cervical spina bifida
- Genetics: 677C ⇒ T mutation on methylene tetrahydrofolate reductase (MTHFR) gene (≤ 50%)
- Etiology
  ○ Maternal dietary folate deficiency, folate antagonists (antiepileptics)
  ○ Maternal hyperthermia
  ○ Toxins: Tripterygium wilfordii (Chinese herbs), arsenic
- Epidemiology: Rare; 1-1.5/150 Chiari cases
- Associated abnormalities: ↑ Amniotic homocysteine

### Gross Pathologic & Surgical Features
- Meninges, disorganized cerebellum +/- occipital/parietal brain tissue

### Microscopic Features
- Disorganized neuronal tissue
- Sac lining ± gray matter heterotopia

## CLINICAL ISSUES

### Presentation
- Most common signs/symptoms: Occipital encephalocele, microcephaly
- Other signs/symptoms: Respiratory deterioration, lower CN dysfunction
- Clinical Profile: Developmental delay, spasticity, hypotonia, seizures

### Demographics
- Age: Newborn
- Gender: M < F

### Natural History & Prognosis
- Dismal prognosis → early death, severe disability

### Treatment
- Surgical resection, repair of encephalocele
- CSF diversion for hydrocephalus

## DIAGNOSTIC CHECKLIST

### Image Interpretation Pearls
- Occipital cephalocele containing cerebellum + intracranial Chiari II = Chiari III malformation

## SELECTED REFERENCES

1. Cakirer S: Chiari III malformation: varieties of MRI appearances in two patients. Clin Imaging. 27(1):1-4, 2003

## IMAGE GALLERY

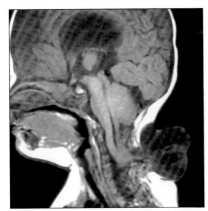 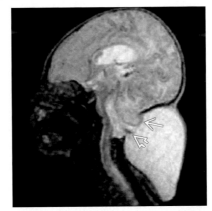 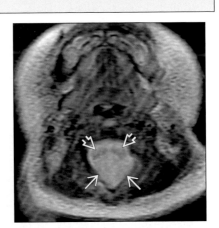

*(Left)* Sagittal T1WI MR demonstrates herniation of cerebellar tonsils/vermis and meninges through a mid-cervical dysraphic defect. CM2 findings are mild. *(Center)* Sagittal T2WI MR reveals herniation of cerebellar structures ➡ and occipital lobes ➡ through an upper cervical spina bifida to form a cephalocele. Brain stem is not herniated in this case. *(Right)* Axial T2WI MR (CM3 patient, cephalocele not shown) depicts cerebellar tissue herniation ➡ into upper cervical spinal canal and cervical spinal cord diaschisis ➡.

# CRANIOVERTEBRAL JUNCTION VARIANTS

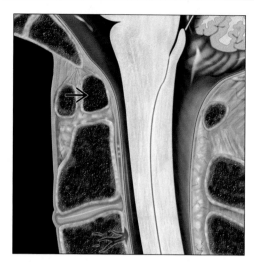

*Sagittal graphic shows an os odontoideum ➡ and enlarged anterior C1 ring suggesting a congenital origin. No static instability or CVJ stenosis in this case.*

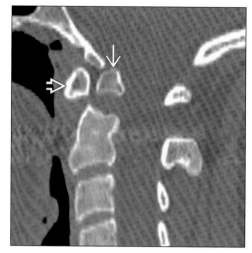

*Sagittal bone CT shows an os odontoideum ➡ with truncation of dens process. The clivus maintains normal relationship to the os. Enlarged anterior C1 ring ➡ supports congenital origin.*

## TERMINOLOGY

### Abbreviations and Synonyms
- Craniovertebral junction (CVJ) anomalies, craniocervical junction (CCJ) variants or anomalies

### Definitions
- Anatomical variations of skull base-cervical spine articulation

## IMAGING FINDINGS

### General Features
- Best diagnostic clue: Flattening or malformation of clivus, anterior C1 ring, or odontoid process
- Location: Craniovertebral junction
- Size: Variable with specific anatomical variation
- Morphology: Variable: Platybasia, segmentation and fusion anomalies, C1 or C2/dens anomalies

### CT Findings
- CECT
  - +/- Enhancing granulation tissue mass ("pannus")
    - Patients with reducible abnormalities have largest pannus
- Bone CT
  - Similar findings to plain radiographs; sagittal and coronal reformations minimize effect of overlapping structures

### MR Findings
- T1WI: Osseous anomalies +/- soft tissue granulation tissue, cord compression, hindbrain anomalies
- T2WI: Similar to T1WI; best shows spinal cord status
- T1 C+: +/- Enhancing "pannus"

### Radiographic Findings
- Radiography: Platybasia, basilar invagination, C1 ring assimilation, asymmetrical C1/2 articulation, backward tilt, hypoplasia/aplasia, or os odontoideum of odontoid process, C2/3 fusion (Klippel-Feil)

### Fluoroscopic Findings
- Variable instability of C0/1, C1/2 articulations with dynamic flexion and extension

## DDx: Congenital CVJ Variants

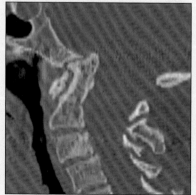

*Juvenile Chronic Arthritis*

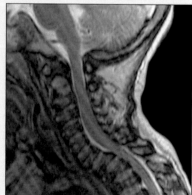

*Mucopolysaccharidosis*

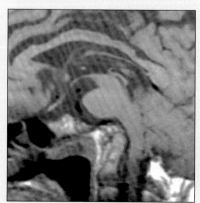

*Osteogenesis Imperfecta*

# CRANIOVERTEBRAL JUNCTION VARIANTS

## Key Facts

### Terminology
- Craniovertebral junction (CVJ) anomalies, craniocervical junction (CCJ) variants or anomalies

### Imaging Findings
- Best diagnostic clue: Flattening or malformation of clivus, anterior C1 ring, or odontoid process
- +/- Enhancing granulation tissue mass ("pannus")
- Best imaging tool: Bone CT with multiplanar reformations

### Top Differential Diagnoses
- Developmental CVJ Anomalies
- Inflammatory and Degenerative Arthritides
- Acquired Basilar Impression
- Trauma

### Pathology
- Severity ranges from benign, asymptomatic to potentially fatal instability ⇒ cord/brainstem compression

### Clinical Issues
- Gradual onset with localizing signs; some patients asymptomatic throughout life
- Occasionally neurological presentation is fulminant ⇒ quadriplegia, sudden death
- Undetected anomalies ⇒ risk for injury during minor trauma, anesthesia

### Diagnostic Checklist
- Dynamic flex-extend imaging determines stability, reducibility of abnormality

---

## Imaging Recommendations
- Best imaging tool: Bone CT with multiplanar reformations
- Protocol advice
  - Dynamic flexion/extension plain films demonstrate biomechanics, uncover instability
  - Multiplanar T1WI, T2WI to evaluate cord, soft tissues; flexion/extension MR delineates effect of position on neural compression
  - CT with multiplanar reformats to evaluate osseous structures for surgical planning

## DIFFERENTIAL DIAGNOSIS

### Developmental CVJ Anomalies
- CVJ stenosis or atlanto-axial instability 2° to achondroplasia, mucopolysaccharidosis, Down syndrome, or inborn errors of metabolism

### Inflammatory and Degenerative Arthritides
- Rheumatoid, reactive, or psoriatic arthritides, ankylosing spondylitis, degenerative arthritis (osteoarthritis)
- +/- CVJ fusion, anterior displacement of C1 ring from dens, basilar invagination → possible cord compression 2° to canal stenosis
- Clinical manifestations include myelopathy, pain, extremity deformity

### Acquired Basilar Impression
- Upward displacement of occipital condyles above plane of foramen magnum, radiological protrusion of dens tip above Chamberlain line
- 2° to bone softening; Paget disease, osteogenesis imperfecta, rickets, rheumatoid arthritis, hyperparathyroidism

### Trauma
- Fracture and/or ligamentous injury; CVJ injuries relatively uncommon but high morbidity/mortality
- Sharp, non-corticated margins argue against congenital anomaly

- Elicit appropriate history, clinical findings

## PATHOLOGY

### General Features
- General path comments
  - Congenital CVJ abnormalities uncommon
    - Severity ranges from benign, asymptomatic to potentially fatal instability ⇒ cord/brainstem compression
  - Type and severity of anomaly determined by anatomy relative to one or more standard "lines of reference"
    - Chamberlain line: Line drawn from opisthion to dorsal margin of hard palate
    - McGregor line: Line drawn from upper posterior hard palate to most caudad point of occiput
- Etiology: Maldevelopment/injury in developing CVJ neural and osseous tissue during 4th → 7th intrauterine weeks ⇒ hypoplasia, segmentation/fusion anomalies, CVJ ankylosis
- Epidemiology: Relatively uncommon: 0.14-0.25% pediatric population
- Associated abnormalities: Dwarfism, jaw anomalies, cleft palate, congenital ear deformities, short neck, Sprengel deformity, funnel chest, pes cavus, and syndactyly

### Gross Pathologic & Surgical Features
- Solid ankylosis or fibrous union in many irreducible anomalies
- Granulation tissue proliferation around motion areas in unstable or reducible anomalies

### Microscopic Features
- Variable components of histologically normal bone, fibrous tissue, and granulation tissue

### Staging, Grading or Classification Criteria
- Occipital sclerotome malformations

# CRANIOVERTEBRAL JUNCTION VARIANTS

○ Most occiput anomalies associated with ↓ skull base height +/- basilar invagination (odontoid tip > 4.5 mm above McGregor line)
  ▪ Condylus tertius, condylar hypoplasia, basiocciput hypoplasia, atlanto-occipital assimilation, bifid clivus
  ▪ Platybasia = congenital flattening of craniocervical angle > 135°
  ▪ Associated with hindbrain herniation, syringomyelia (≤ 30%)
- C1 ring anomalies
  ○ C1 assimilation ("occipitalized C1"): Segmentation failure → fibrous or osseous union between 1st spinal sclerotome and 4th occipital sclerotome
    ▪ +/- Occipitocervical synostosis; most C1 ring assimilations asymptomatic, more likely to be symptomatic if retro-odontoid AP canal diameter < 19 mm
  ○ C1 malformation: Aplasia, hypoplasia, cleft C1 arch, "split atlas" (anterior and posterior arch rachischisis)
  ○ Association with Klippel-Feil, basilar invagination, Chiari I malformation
- C2 anomalies: C1/2 segmentation failure, dens dysplasia
  ○ Majority confined to odontoid process; partial (hypoplasia) → complete absence (aplasia), ossiculum terminale persistens, os odontoideum
    ▪ Ossiculum terminale persistens: Ossification failure of terminal ossicle → incidental "notch" in dens tip
    ▪ Os odontoideum: Well-defined ossicle at dens tip + anterior C1 arch enlargement
  ○ Odontoid anomalies in association with ligamentous laxity → atlantoaxial instability; most common in Down syndrome, Morquio syndrome, Klippel-Feil syndrome, and skeletal dysplasias
    ▪ Incompetence of cruciate ligament → C1/2 instability, possible neurologic deficit or death

## CLINICAL ISSUES

### Presentation
- Most common signs/symptoms
  ○ Posterior occipital headache exacerbated by flexion/extension
  ○ Sub-occipital neck pain (85%); may clinically mimic "basilar migraine"
  ○ Myelopathy, brainstem/cranial nerve deficits, weakness, lower extremity ataxia
  ○ Vascular symptoms (15-20%); TIA, vertigo, visual symptoms with rotation or head manipulation
- Clinical Profile
  ○ Usually normal clinical appearance; obvious clinical dysmorphism implies syndromal association
  ○ Symptomatic presentation following mild trauma

### Demographics
- Age: Infancy → late adulthood depending on severity
- Gender: M = F

### Natural History & Prognosis
- Gradual onset with localizing signs; some patients asymptomatic throughout life

- Occasionally neurological presentation is fulminant ⇒ quadriplegia, sudden death
- Undetected anomalies ⇒ risk for injury during minor trauma, anesthesia
- Early diagnosis permits treatment before symptoms or permanent neurological sequelae

### Treatment
- Conservative approach initially unless unstable or neural deficits
  ○ Traction, cervical orthosis, activity restriction
- Symptomatic, refractory to conservative management
  ○ Skeletal traction to distinguish reducible from irreducible abnormalities, relieve symptoms pre-operatively
  ○ Correction of underlying biomechanical abnormality with decompression +/- fusion

## DIAGNOSTIC CHECKLIST

### Consider
- Look for combinations of anomalies based on known association patterns
- Impact of diagnosis must be customized to individual patient to develop best treatment approach

### Image Interpretation Pearls
- Dynamic flex-extend imaging determines stability, reducibility of abnormality
- CT with reformats indispensable to evaluate osseous abnormalities

## SELECTED REFERENCES

1. Naderi S et al: Anatomical and computed tomographic analysis of C1 vertebra. Clin Neurol Neurosurg. 105(4):245-8, 2003
2. Perez-Vallina JR et al: Congenital anomaly of craniovertebral junction: atlas-dens fusion with C1 anterior arch cleft. J Spinal Disord Tech. 15(1):84-7, 2002
3. Kim FM: Developmental anomalies of the craniocervical junction and cervical spine. Magn Reson Imaging Clin N Am. 8(3):651-74, 2000
4. Smoker WR: MR imaging of the craniovertebral junction. Magn Reson Imaging Clin N Am. 8(3):635-50, 2000
5. Taitz C: Bony observations of some morphological variations and anomalies of the craniovertebral region. Clin Anat. 13(5):354-60, 2000
6. Iwata A et al: Foramen magnum syndrome caused by atlanto-occipital assimilation. J Neurol Sci. 154(2):229-31, 1998
7. Menezes AH: Craniovertebral junction anomalies: diagnosis and management. Semin Pediatr Neurol. 4(3):209-23, 1997
8. Menezes AH: Primary craniovertebral anomalies and the hindbrain herniation syndrome (Chiari I): data base analysis. Pediatr Neurosurg. 23(5):260-9, 1995
9. Erbengi A et al: Congenital malformations of the craniovertebral junction: classification and surgical treatment. Acta Neurochir (Wien). 127(3-4):180-5, 1994
10. Smoker WR: Craniovertebral junction: normal anatomy, craniometry, and congenital anomalies. Radiographics. 14(2):255-77, 1994

## IMAGE GALLERY

### Variant

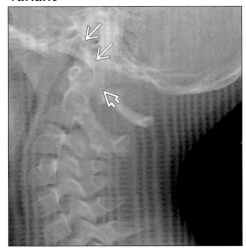
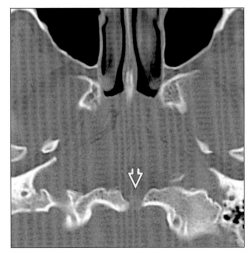

*(Left)* Lateral radiograph demonstrates anomalous flattening of the clivus ➡ relative to cervical spine and retroflexion of the odontoid process ⮞ compatible with platybasia. *(Right)* Axial bone CT demonstrates aberrant flattened, coronally oriented clivus with abnormal midline cleft ⮞.

### Variant

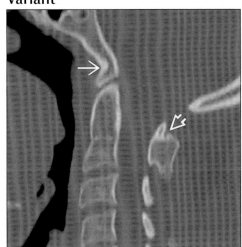
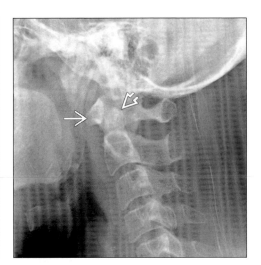

*(Left)* Sagittal bone CT reformation demonstrates assimilation of the anterior C1 ring with the clivus ⮞ as well as fusion of the posterior C1 ring with the C2 spinous process ⮞. *(Right)* Lateral radiograph depicts a congenitally hypoplastic dens process ⮞ with normal C1/2 alignment. The anterior C1 ring ➡ shows mild compensatory enlargement.

### Variant

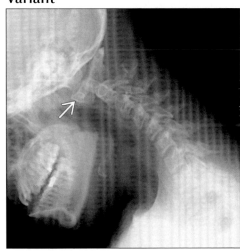
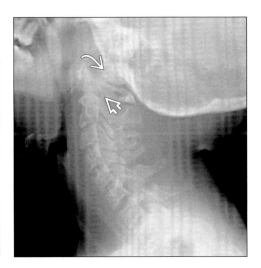

*(Left)* Lateral radiograph in cervical flexion (patient has Down syndrome) shows anterior subluxation of C1 anterior ring ➡ relative to dens (C2). *(Right)* Lateral radiograph of same patient as previous image in cervical extension shows reduction of C1/2 subluxation, but posterior displacement of occipital condyles ⮞ relative to C1 lateral masses ⮞.

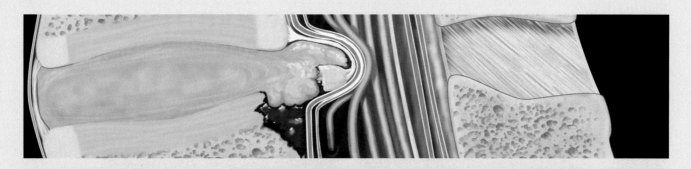

# SECTION 2: Vertebra

# POSTERIOR ELEMENT INCOMPLETE FUSION

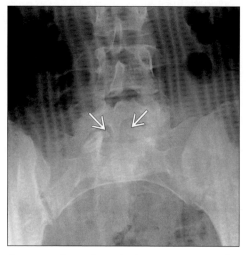

*Anteroposterior radiograph demonstrates incomplete posterior fusion of the S1 lamina ➡, which do not meet in the midline.*

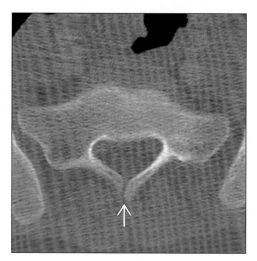

*Axial bone CT (10 year old male) depicts typical configuration of incomplete S1 posterior fusion ➡.*

## TERMINOLOGY

### Abbreviations and Synonyms
- Spina bifida occulta

### Definitions
- Spinous process/lamina fusion failure without underlying neural or dural abnormality

## IMAGING FINDINGS

### General Features
- Best diagnostic clue: Incomplete lumbosacral posterior element fusion
- Location: Lumbosacral junction (L5 > S1) > > cervical (C1 > C7 > T1), thoracic
- Morphology: Posterior elements do not fuse in midline; margins are rounded, well-corticated, and may overlap

### CT Findings
- Bone CT: Unfused spinous process/lamina approximate at midline

### MR Findings
- T1WI
  - Normal conus position, filum thickness
  - No abnormal neural, dural, or lipomatous tissue within posterior osseous defect
- T2WI: Same as T1WI

### Radiographic Findings
- Radiography
  - Unfused spinous process
  - Lamina approximate at midline

### Imaging Recommendations
- Best imaging tool: MR best for definitive exclusion of significant underlying abnormality

## DIFFERENTIAL DIAGNOSIS

### Normal Progression of Ossification
- Normal L5 laminae may remain unfused until 5-6 years of age

## DDx: Posterior Element Incomplete Fusion

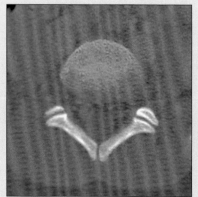

*Normal Ossification (5 years)*

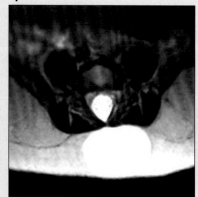

*Dorsal Meningocele*

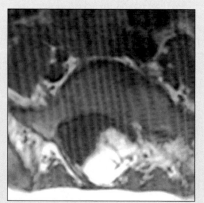

*Lipomyelomeningocele*

# POSTERIOR ELEMENT INCOMPLETE FUSION

## Key Facts

### Terminology
- Spina bifida occulta
- Spinous process/lamina fusion failure without underlying neural or dural abnormality

### Imaging Findings
- Location: Lumbosacral junction (L5 > S1) > > cervical (C1 > C7 > T1), thoracic
- Normal conus position, filum thickness

- No abnormal neural, dural, or lipomatous tissue within posterior osseous defect

### Top Differential Diagnoses
- Normal Progression of Ossification
- Closed Spinal Dysraphism (CSD)
- Surgical Laminectomy Defect

### Clinical Issues
- Usually asymptomatic if no cutaneous stigmata

## Closed Spinal Dysraphism (CSD)
- Lipoma, tethered cord, lipomyelomeningocele, dorsal meningocele, dorsal dermal sinus
- Search for clinical tethering, cutaneous stigmata

## Surgical Laminectomy Defect
- Surgical history present; look for incision scar, denervation of paraspinal muscles, laminectomy defect

## PATHOLOGY

### General Features
- Etiology: Unknown; probably not linked to neurulation process aberrations
- Epidemiology: Up to 30% US population

### Gross Pathologic & Surgical Features
- Non-fused spinous processes, lamina overlie normal dural sac

## CLINICAL ISSUES

### Presentation
- Most common signs/symptoms
  - Usually asymptomatic if no cutaneous stigmata
  - Skin dimples above gluteal cleft have higher incidence of associated abnormalities; merit further evaluation with MR

### Demographics
- Age: All; more common < 40 years of age
- Gender: M < F

### Natural History & Prognosis
- Usually incidental finding of no clinical significance

### Treatment
- Conservative

## DIAGNOSTIC CHECKLIST

### Consider
- Incomplete posterior fusion is an incidental finding, very rarely of neurological significance
  - MR best for definitive exclusion of significant underlying abnormality, but yield is low in absence of cutaneous stigmata or neurological deficits

## SELECTED REFERENCES

1. Frymoyer et al: The Adult Spine. Vol 2. 2nd ed. Philadelphia, Lippincott-Raven. 1923-6, 1997
2. Avrahami E et al: Spina bifida occulta of S1 is not an innocent finding. Spine. 19(1):12-5, 1994
3. Boone D et al: Spina bifida occulta: lesion or anomaly? Clin Radiol. 36(2):159-61, 1985

## IMAGE GALLERY

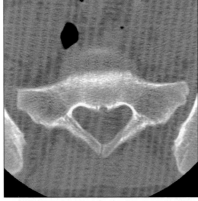 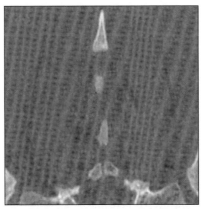 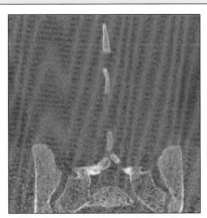

*(Left)* Axial bone CT (12 years) demonstrates characteristic appearance of unfused S1 posterior elements. *(Center)* Coronal bone CT (12 years) shows failure of the S1 posterior elements to unite in the midline at S1. The lamina do not show rotation or overlap. *(Right)* Coronal bone CT reveals failure of S1 posterior fusion. The laminae are rotated relative to each other, which may predispose to rotational forces and premature degenerative changes.

# FAILURE OF VERTEBRAL FORMATION

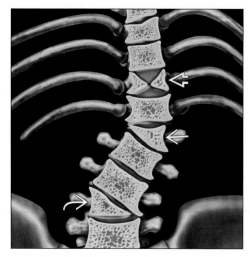

Coronal graphic demonstrates the most common forms of vertebral formation failure. There are segmented "balanced" L1 ➡ and L4 ➡ hemivertebra and a T11 ➡ butterfly vertebra.

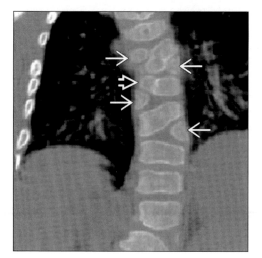

Coronal bone CT demonstrates extensive vertebral segmentation anomalies with multiple hemivertebrae ➡ and a butterfly vertebra ➡. This jumble of vertebrae produces a scoliotic curvature.

## TERMINOLOGY

### Abbreviations and Synonyms
- Segmentation and fusion anomaly (SFA), vertebral dysplasia, "disorganized spine"

### Definitions
- Partial or complete failure of vertebral formation
  - Partial formation failure ⇒ wedge vertebra
  - Complete formation failure ⇒ vertebral aplasia, hemivertebra, butterfly vertebra

## IMAGING FINDINGS

### General Features
- Best diagnostic clue: Sharply angulated, single curve, or focal scoliosis with deformed vertebral bodies
- Location: Thoracolumbar most common
- Size: Hemivertebra, butterfly vertebra generally smaller than normal vertebra
- Morphology: Incompletely formed vertebra; may be missing front, back, side, or middle of vertebral body

### CT Findings
- Bone CT
  - Sagittal or coronal vertebral clefts, hemivertebra, butterfly vertebra
    - Abnormal vertebra difficult to evaluate in axial plane; sagittal, coronal reformats most helpful
  - +/- Posterior element dysraphism, fusion anomalies
    - Most readily evaluated in axial plane

### MR Findings
- T1WI
  - Vertebral formation failure anomalies as with CT
  - Normal marrow, disc signal intensity
  - +/- Lipoma, tethered cord, diastematomyelia, spinal cord compression
- T2WI: Similar findings to T1WI

### Radiographic Findings
- Radiography
  - Vertebral formation failure anomalies
  - +/- Scoliosis
    - Paired bilateral hemivertebra ⇒ "balanced", scoliotic curves cancel out

## DDx: Failure of Vertebral Formation

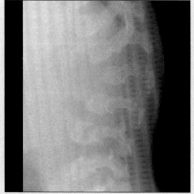

Hurler (MPS 1-H)

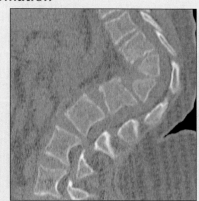

Achondroplasia

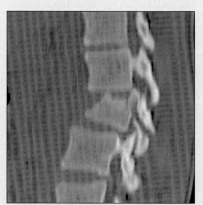

Burst Fracture

# FAILURE OF VERTEBRAL FORMATION

## Key Facts

### Terminology
- Segmentation and fusion anomaly (SFA), vertebral dysplasia, "disorganized spine"
- Partial or complete failure of vertebral formation

### Imaging Findings
- +/- Scoliosis
- Sagittal or coronal vertebral clefts, hemivertebra, butterfly vertebra
- +/- Lipoma, tethered cord, diastematomyelia, spinal cord compression

### Top Differential Diagnoses
- Inherited Spinal Dysplasias
- Vertebral Fracture

### Pathology
- Abnormal vertebrae may be supranumerary or replace normal vertebral body
- More severe SFA ⇒ higher likelihood of associated visceral anomalies

### Clinical Issues
- Abnormal spine curvature +/- neural deficits, limb or visceral abnormalities

### Diagnostic Checklist
- Look for concurrent segmentation failure, other neural and visceral anomalies
- Type of deformity determines propensity for scoliosis progression

- One or more unilateral hemivertebra ⇒ "unbalanced", uncompensated scoliotic curve
- Best modality for "counting" vertebral levels, determining presence and severity of scoliosis

### Imaging Recommendations
- Best imaging tool: MR imaging
- Protocol advice
  - Long-cassette weightbearing radiographs ⇒ quantitate scoliosis, "counting" to definitively localize abnormal vertebral levels
  - Multiplanar T1WI, T2WI MR ⇒ identify vertebral anomalies, evaluate spinal cord and soft tissues
    - Most vertebral and spinal cord anomalies seen best in coronal, sagittal planes
  - 3D Bone CT useful to characterize scoliosis and vertebral anomalies for pre-operative planning

## DIFFERENTIAL DIAGNOSIS

### Inherited Spinal Dysplasias
- Mucopolysaccharidosis, achondroplasia
- Distinguish by characteristic imaging, clinical, and laboratory findings

### Vertebral Fracture
- Pathologic or traumatic; history critical
- Two pedicles per level
- Noncorticated irregular fracture margins +/- soft tissue edema, cord injury

## PATHOLOGY

### General Features
- General path comments
  - Normal vertebral formation occurs over three sequential periods
    - Membrane development: Segmental formation of medial sclerotome (vertebral bodies) and lateral myotome (paraspinal muscles)

- Chondrification: Sclerotomes separate transversely, join with adjacent sclerotomal halves ⇒ paired chondrification sites develop in vertebral bodies and neural arches
- Ossification: Chondral skeleton ossifies from ossification center
  - Segmentation and fusion anomalies result from aberrant vertebral column formation
    - Abnormal vertebrae may be supranumerary or replace normal vertebral body
    - More severe SFA ⇒ higher likelihood of associated visceral anomalies
  - Imaging appearance of vertebral formation failure determined by deficient vertebral body portion
    - Lateral formation failure (common) ⇒ classic hemivertebrae of congenital scoliosis
    - Anterior formation failure (common) ⇒ sharply angulated kyphosis
    - Posterior formation failure (rare) ⇒ hyperlordotic curve
  - Hemivertebra variants subclassified as incarcerated, nonincarcerated, segmented, nonsegmented, or semisegmented
    - Incarcerated: Vertebral bodies above and below shaped to accommodate hemivertebrae ⇒ do not generally produce scoliosis
    - Nonincarcerated: Found at scoliosis apex, curve magnitude depends on size of wedged segment
    - Segmented ("free"): Discs above and below hemivertebra ⇒ progressive scoliosis 2° to unbalanced growth
    - Nonsegmented: Lack disc spaces between wedged, normal adjacent vertebral bodies
    - Semisegmented: Normal disc space on one side, nonsegmented on other side
  - Segmental spinal dysgenesis (SSD) = rare congenital abnormality in which one segment of vertebral column/spinal cord fails to develop properly
    - Spinal cord thinned or indiscernible at abnormality level; bulky, low-lying cord segment caudad to focal abnormality in most cases

- Severity of morphologic derangement correlates with residual spinal cord function, severity of clinical deficit
- Genetics
  - Deranged Pax-1 gene expression in developing vertebral column
  - Many syndromes manifest vertebral dysplasia
- Etiology
  - Total aplasia: Both chondral centers fail to develop early in development
  - Lateral hemivertebra: One chondral center does not develop; ossification center subsequently fails to develop on that side
  - Sagittal cleft ("butterfly") vertebra: Separate ossification centers form (but fail to unite) in each paired paramedian chondrification center
  - Coronal cleft vertebra: Formation and persistence of separate ventral and dorsal ossification centers
  - Posterior hemivertebra: Later failure during ossification stage
- Epidemiology
  - Isolated or syndromal, singular or multiple
  - Incidence increased with parental consanguinity, concurrent multisystem anomalies
- Associated abnormalities
  - Dysraphism, split notochord syndromes
    - Diastematomyelia, syrinx, tethered cord/fatty filum, congenital tumor, visceral organ anomalies
  - Other developmental vertebral abnormalities
    - Partial duplication (supernumerary hemivertebra)
    - Segmentation failure (block vertebra, posterior element dysraphism, pediculate bar, neural arch fusion)
  - Visceral abnormalities; 61% of congenital scoliosis patients

## Gross Pathologic & Surgical Features
- Normal bone density unless concurrent metabolic abnormality
- Surgical observations of vertebral configuration matches imaging findings

## Microscopic Features
- Normal bone histology unless concurrent metabolic abnormality

# CLINICAL ISSUES

## Presentation
- Most common signs/symptoms
  - Asymptomatic
  - Abnormal spine curvature +/- neural deficits, limb or visceral abnormalities
  - Other signs/symptoms
    - Respiratory failure (impeded chest movement 2° to fused ribs, kyphoscoliosis) ⇒ rare
- Clinical Profile
  - Most either asymptomatic or detected during scoliosis evaluation
  - Syndromal patients usually detected in infancy

## Demographics
- Age

- Usually diagnosed in infancy → early childhood
- Mild cases may present in adulthood
- Gender: M ≈ F

## Natural History & Prognosis
- Scoliosis is frequently progressive
  - Expectant watching, early intervention if warranted to prevent development of severe deformities

## Treatment
- Conservative in mild cases (orthotics, observation)
- Surgical resection and/or fusion to arrest/reverse kyphoscoliosis in moderate to severe cases

# DIAGNOSTIC CHECKLIST

## Consider
- Syndromal origin or association → important to look for and characterize visceral anomalies

## Image Interpretation Pearls
- Look for concurrent segmentation failure, other neural and visceral anomalies
- Type of deformity determines propensity for scoliosis progression

# SELECTED REFERENCES

1. Tsirikos AI et al: Congenital anomalies of the ribs and chest wall associated with congenital deformities of the spine. J Bone Joint Surg Am. 87(11):2523-36, 2005
2. Arlet V et al: Congenital scoliosis. Eur Spine J. 12(5):456-63, 2003
3. Isono M et al: Limited dorsal myeloschisis associated with multiple vertebral segmentation disorder. Pediatr Neurosurg. 36(1):44-7, 2002
4. Kim YJ et al: Surgical treatment of congenital kyphosis. Spine. 26(20):2251-7, 2001
5. Suh SW et al: Evaluating Congenital spine deformities for intraspinal anomalies with magnetic resonance imaging. J Pediatr Orthop. 21(4):525-31, 2001
6. Jaskwhich D et al: Congenital scoliosis. Curr Opin Pediatr. 12(1):61-6, 2000
7. McMaster MJ et al: Natural history of congenital kyphosis and kyphoscoliosis. A study of one hundred and twelve patients. J Bone Joint Surg Am. 81(10):1367-83, 1999
8. Hayman LA et al: Bony spine and costal elements, Part II. Int J Neurorad. 4(1):61-68, 1998
9. McMaster MJ: Congenital scoliosis caused by a unilateral failure of vertebral segmentation with contralateral hemivertebrae. Spine. 23(9):998-1005, 1998
10. Aslan Y et al: Multiple vertebral segmentation defects. Brief report of three patients and nosological considerations. Genet Couns. 8(3):241-8, 1997
11. Lopez BC et al: Inadequate PAX-1 gene expression as a cause of agenesis of the thoracolumbar spine with failure of segmentation. Case report. J Neurosurg. 86(6):1018-21, 1997
12. Martinez-Frias ML: Multiple vertebral segmentation defects and rib anomalies. Am J Med Genet. 66(1):91, 1996
13. Mortier GR et al: Multiple vertebral segmentation defects: analysis of 26 new patients and review of the literature. Am J Med Genet. 61(4):310-9, 1996
14. Mayfield JK et al: Congenital kyphosis due to defects of anterior segmentation. J Bone Joint Surg Am. 62(8):1291-301, 1980

# FAILURE OF VERTEBRAL FORMATION

## IMAGE GALLERY

### Typical

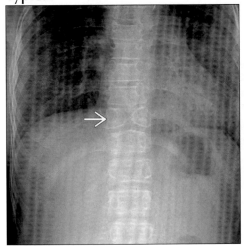
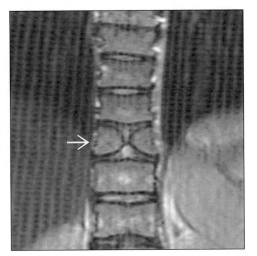

*(Left) Anteroposterior radiograph depicts a T10 butterfly vertebra ➡, with ossification of the right and left ossification centers but failure to join in the midline. (Right) Coronal T2WI MR confirms butterfly vertebral configuration ➡ as well as normal marrow signal within vertebral body. The adjacent disc spaces are dysmorphic but open.*

### Typical

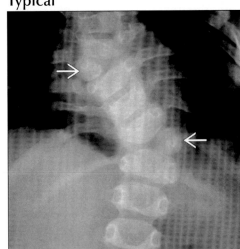
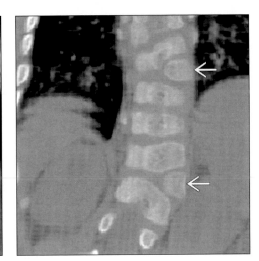

*(Left) Anteroposterior radiograph shows bilateral "balanced" hemivertebra ➡ in a patient with Klippel-Feil syndrome. These hemivertebra are on opposite sides and "cancel out" to limit spinal curve. (Right) Coronal bone CT reveals extensive vertebral segmentation anomalies with multiple hemivertebrae ➡ on the left side producing an "unbalanced" scoliotic curvature.*

### Typical

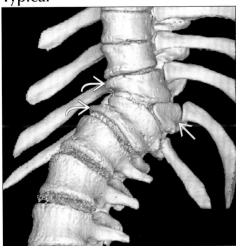
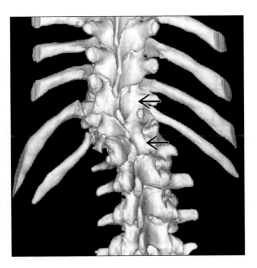

*(Left) 3D bone CT reformats nicely demonstrate relationship of left hemivertebra ➡ to adjacent vertebrae ➡, but underemphasize degree of fusion across the disc space. (Right) 3D bone CT reformats in posterior projection reveal right laminar osseous fusion bar ➡ contralateral to left hemivertebra and scoliotic curvature convex to the left.*

# PARTIAL VERTEBRAL DUPLICATION

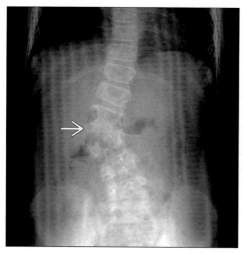

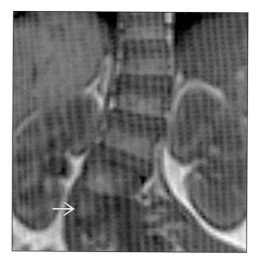

*Anteroposterior radiograph demonstrates a supernumerary L3 hemivertebra ➡ and five other typical (2 pedicle) lumbar vertebrae. The extra hemivertebra produces focal scoliotic curvature.*

*Coronal T1WI MR demonstrates normal marrow signal of the right L3 hemivertebra ➡ and confirms presence of a disc space above and below the supranumerary L3 vertebra.*

## TERMINOLOGY

### Abbreviations and Synonyms
- Supranumerary vertebra

### Definitions
- Partial duplication of vertebral column produces one or more supranumerary ("extra") vertebra

## IMAGING FINDINGS

### General Features
- Best diagnostic clue: Atypical scoliosis (sharply angulated, single curve, or focal) with one or more "extra" hemivertebra
- Location: Thoracolumbar > cervical

### CT Findings
- Bone CT: Supranumerary lateral hemivertebra

### MR Findings
- T1WI: Supranumerary lateral hemivertebra +/- dysraphism, spinal cord anomalies
- T2WI: Same as T1WI

### Radiographic Findings
- Radiography: Supranumerary hemivertebra with scoliosis

### Imaging Recommendations
- Plain films for counting, quantifying scoliosis
- Multiplanar MR imaging to assess for associated abnormalities

## DIFFERENTIAL DIAGNOSIS

### Hemivertebra
- Single pedicle
- Unilateral ossification center fails to form

### Butterfly Vertebra
- Two pedicles; looks like "bilateral hemivertebra"
- Separate bilateral ossification centers fail to unite

### Vertebral Fracture
- Noncorticated irregular margins +/- soft tissue edema, spinal cord injury
- Two pedicles at level, unlike hemivertebra

## DDx: Partial Vertebral Duplication

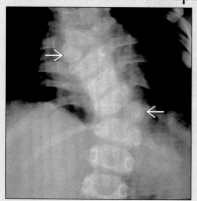

*Hemivertebrae*

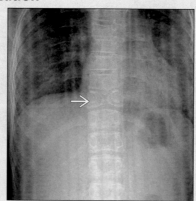

*Butterfly Vertebra*

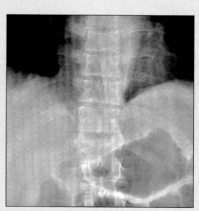

*Burst Fracture*

# PARTIAL VERTEBRAL DUPLICATION

## Key Facts

### Terminology
• Supranumerary vertebra
• Partial duplication of vertebral column produces one or more supranumerary ("extra") vertebra

### Imaging Findings
• Radiography: Supranumerary hemivertebra with scoliosis
• Bone CT: Supranumerary lateral hemivertebra

• T1WI: Supranumerary lateral hemivertebra +/- dysraphism, spinal cord anomalies

### Top Differential Diagnoses
• Hemivertebra
• Vertebral Fracture

### Diagnostic Checklist
• Supranumerary hemivertebra "missing" a pedicle on hypoplastic side; distinguishes from fracture

## PATHOLOGY

### General Features
• Etiology: Cervicothoracic or thoracolumbar junction segmentation variation ⇒ "extra" hemivertebra
• Associated abnormalities: Dysraphism, split notochord syndromes, caudal regression, other vertebral SFA, congenital tumors, visceral organ anomalies

### Gross Pathologic & Surgical Features
• Hemivertebra may be incorporated into adjacent vertebra ⇒ unbalanced block vertebra

## CLINICAL ISSUES

### Presentation
• Most common signs/symptoms
  ○ Asymptomatic
  ○ Neuromuscular scoliosis; usually progressive

### Demographics
• Age
  ○ More severe cases detected in infancy or childhood
  ○ Milder cases detected in adolescence during school scoliosis checks, by pediatrician, or incidentally during imaging
• Gender: M = F

### Natural History & Prognosis
• Variable; scoliosis may progress with growth, require treatment

### Treatment
• Conservative in mild cases
• Surgical fusion to arrest/reverse scoliosis in more severe cases

## DIAGNOSTIC CHECKLIST

### Consider
• Scoliosis pattern, exclude associated abnormalities

### Image Interpretation Pearls
• Supranumerary hemivertebra "missing" a pedicle on hypoplastic side; distinguishes from fracture

## SELECTED REFERENCES

1. Belmont PJ Jr et al: Intraspinal anomalies associated with isolated congenital hemivertebra: the role of routine magnetic resonance imaging. J Bone Joint Surg Am. 86-A(8):1704-10, 2004
2. Luboga S: Supernumerary lumbar vertebrae in human skeletons at the Galloway Osteological Collection of Makerere University, Kampala. East Afr Med J. 77(1):16-9, 2000
3. McMaster MJ: Congenital scoliosis caused by a unilateral failure of vertebral segmentation with contralateral hemivertebrae. Spine. 23(9):998-1005, 1998

## IMAGE GALLERY

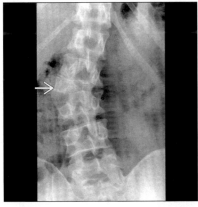 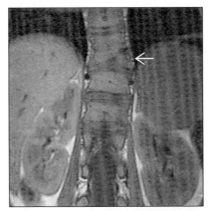 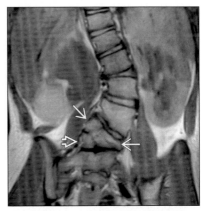

*(Left)* Anteroposterior radiograph reveals a supernumerary right L3 hemivertebra ➡ producing convex right focal scoliosis. *(Center)* Coronal T1WI MR shows a supernumerary left T10 hemivertebra ➡, confirmed by counting from plain films (not shown). Thoracic supranumerary vertebra are less common than lumbar. *(Right)* Coronal T1WI MR in a caudal regression patient reveals a tripediculate L5/L6 vertebra, consisting of a supranumerary right L6 hemivertebra ➡ that failed to segment from L5 ➡.

# VERTEBRAL SEGMENTATION FAILURE

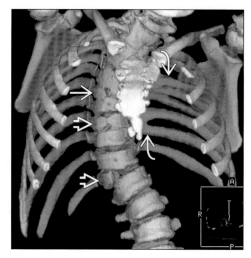
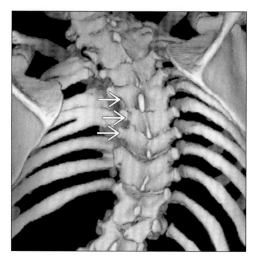

*Coronal bone CT shows coexisting segmentation failure ➡, failure of vertebral formation ⇨ with multiple abnormal fused ribs ↗ inhibiting axial skeletal growth ⇒ progressive scoliosis.*

*Coronal 3D bone CT reformats demonstrate multiple abnormal fused left posterior ribs and left laminar fusion bar ➡ at the concave apex of scoliotic curve.*

## TERMINOLOGY

### Abbreviations and Synonyms
- Segmentation anomaly, segmentation and fusion anomaly (SFA), "block vertebra", "disorganized spine"

### Definitions
- Vertebral column malformations (block vertebra, pediculate bar, neural arch fusion) resulting from deranged embryological development ⇒ failure of normal segmentation

## IMAGING FINDINGS

### General Features
- Best diagnostic clue: Sharply angulated, single curve, or focal scoliosis with abnormal fused vertebra
- Location: Lumbar > cervical > thoracic
- Size
  - Range from focal ⇒ extensive involvement
  - Block vertebra usually larger than a single normal vertebral body

- Morphology: Incomplete vertebral body segmentation, fused posterior elements, and large misshapen vertebral bodies incorporating one or more levels

### CT Findings
- Bone CT
  - Incomplete vertebral body segmentation
    - Large, misshapen vertebral bodies incorporating one or more levels
    - +/- Fused pedicles, ribs, posterior elements

### MR Findings
- T1WI
  - Deformed, fused vertebral bodies and posterior elements
  - Normal marrow signal intensity
  - +/- Scoliosis
- T2WI
  - Findings similar to T1WI
  - +/- Scoliosis, cord compression

### Radiographic Findings
- Radiography
  - Deformed, fused vertebra +/- scoliosis

## DDx: Vertebral Segmentation Failure

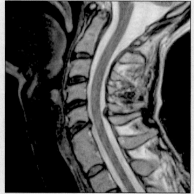
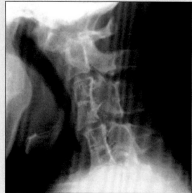
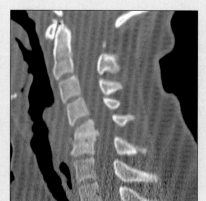

| *Surgical Fusion* | *Juvenile Chronic Arthritis* | *Chronic Discitis-Osteomyelitis* |

# VERTEBRAL SEGMENTATION FAILURE

## Key Facts

### Terminology
- Vertebral column malformations (block vertebra, pediculate bar, neural arch fusion) resulting from deranged embryological development ⇒ failure of normal segmentation

### Imaging Findings
- Best diagnostic clue: Sharply angulated, single curve, or focal scoliosis with abnormal fused vertebra
- Location: Lumbar > cervical > thoracic
- +/- Fused pedicles, ribs, posterior elements
- +/- Scoliosis, cord compression

### Top Differential Diagnoses
- Surgical Fusion
- Juvenile Chronic Arthritis
- Chronic Sequelae of Discitis

- Ankylosing Spondylitis

### Pathology
- Mildest (and most common) form is indeterminate (transitional) vertebrae at thoracolumbar, lumbosacral transition

### Clinical Issues
- Clinical Profile: Asymptomatic incidental detection or presents for evaluation of abnormal spine curvature

### Diagnostic Checklist
- Coronal MR, AP radiography best for detecting and characterizing SFAs, "counting" to determine abnormal vertebral levels

---

- Upright images with lateral and AP bending assess weightbearing effect on scoliosis

## Imaging Recommendations
- Weightbearing plain films to evaluate scoliosis, "count" to determine abnormal vertebral levels
- MR imaging
  - Multiplanar T1WI to evaluate vertebral anatomy
    - Vertebral anomalies seen best in coronal, sagittal planes
  - T2WI to evaluate spinal cord pathology, compression
- CT to characterize vertebral configuration
  - 3D CT useful for pre-operative planning

## DIFFERENTIAL DIAGNOSIS

### Surgical Fusion
- No "waist" at disc space level, facets infrequently ankylosed
- Surgical history key to making diagnosis

### Juvenile Chronic Arthritis
- Difficult to distinguish from cervical block vertebra
- Search for other affected joints, appropriate history

### Chronic Sequelae of Discitis
- Cortical endplate margins irregular, "waist" absent
- Search for history of prior spinal infection

### Ankylosing Spondylitis
- Delicate contiguous syndesmophytes ("bamboo spine") + symmetric SI joint disease
- HLA - B27 positive (95%)

## PATHOLOGY

### General Features
- General path comments
  - Normal embryology: Vertebral formation occurs over three sequential periods

- Membrane development: Segmental formation of medial sclerotome (vertebral bodies) and lateral myotome (paraspinal muscles)
- Chondrification: Sclerotomes separate transversely and join with adjacent sclerotomal halves ⇒ paired chondrification sites develop in vertebral bodies and neural arches
- Ossification: Chondral skeleton ossifies from ossification center
  - Segmentation and fusion anomalies result from aberrant vertebral column formation
  - Mildest (and most common) form is indeterminate (transitional) vertebrae at thoracolumbar, lumbosacral transition
- Genetics
  - Deranged Pax-1 gene expression ⇒ abnormal notochord signaling in developing vertebral column
  - Many syndromes associated with SFA
    - Klippel-Feil (cervical SFA): Common, gene locus 8q22.2
    - Spondylothoracic dysplasia (Jarcho-Levin): Uncommon, thoracic spine fusions in "crab-like" array with multiple rib fusions
- Etiology
  - Block vertebra: Segmentation failure of two or more vertebral somites
  - Posterior neural arch anomalies: Failure to unite in the midline ⇒ dysraphism +/- unilateral pedicle aplasia/hypoplasia
- Epidemiology
  - Isolated or syndromal, singular or multiple
  - SFAs account for 18% of scoliosis; incidence higher with multisystem abnormalities, parental consanguinity
- Associated abnormalities
  - Other neuraxis anomalies (40%)
    - Partial or complete failure of formation (vertebral aplasia, hemivertebra, butterfly vertebra)
    - Partial duplication (supernumerary hemivertebra)
    - Dysraphism, split notochord syndrome
  - Scoliosis

- ○ Renal, gastrointestinal (20%), congenital cardiac defects (10%)

## Gross Pathologic & Surgical Features
- Normal bone density unless concurrent metabolic abnormality
- Surgical observations of vertebral configuration match imaging findings

## Microscopic Features
- Normal bone histology unless concurrent metabolic abnormality

## Staging, Grading or Classification Criteria
- Block vertebra: Failure of ≥ 2 vertebral somites to segment
  - ○ Combined vertebrae may be normal height, short, or tall
  - ○ Disc space frequently rudimentary or absent
  - ○ Frequent association with hemivertebra/absent vertebra above or below block level, posterior element fusion
- Posterior neural arch anomalies
  - ○ Failure to unite in the midline ⇒ dysraphism (+/- unilateral pedicle aplasia/hypoplasia)
  - ○ Unfused spinous processes; L5, S1 > C1 > C7 > T1 > lower thoracic spine
  - ○ Multiple level posterior fusion ⇒ congenital vertebral bar

## CLINICAL ISSUES

### Presentation
- Most common signs/symptoms
  - ○ Asymptomatic
  - ○ Kyphoscoliosis
  - ○ Other signs/symptoms
    - ■ Neural deficits (usually myelopathic), limb or visceral anomalies
    - ■ Respiratory failure (rare, 2° impeded chest movement due to severe scoliosis, rib cage fusion)
- Clinical Profile: Asymptomatic incidental detection or presents for evaluation of abnormal spine curvature

### Demographics
- Age: Severe cases detected during infancy/childhood; mild cases may present as adults
- Gender: M ≈ F; dependent on syndromal association

### Natural History & Prognosis
- Scoliosis frequently progressive
  - ○ Unilateral unsegmented bar with contralateral hemivertebra ⇒ rapidly progressive, severely deforming congenital scoliosis
  - ○ Isolated block vertebra rarely produce scoliosis
- Abnormal segments may continue to fuse

### Treatment
- Conservative in mild cases (orthotics, observation)
- Surgical fusion to arrest/reverse kyphoscoliosis in moderate to severe cases

## DIAGNOSTIC CHECKLIST

### Consider
- Clinical manifestations variable, determined by type of SFA and syndromal association

### Image Interpretation Pearls
- Coronal MR, AP radiography best for detecting and characterizing SFAs, "counting" to determine abnormal vertebral levels

## SELECTED REFERENCES

1. Tsirikos AI et al: Congenital anomalies of the ribs and chest wall associated with congenital deformities of the spine. J Bone Joint Surg Am. 87(11):2523-36, 2005
2. Arlet V et al: Congenital scoliosis. Eur Spine J. 12(5):456-63, 2003
3. Cornier AS et al: Controversies surrounding Jarcho-Levin syndrome. Curr Opin Pediatr. 15(6):614-20, 2003
4. Isono M et al: Limited dorsal myeloschisis associated with multiple vertebral segmentation disorder. Pediatr Neurosurg. 36(1):44-7, 2002
5. Kim YJ et al: Surgical treatment of congenital kyphosis. Spine. 26(20):2251-7, 2001
6. Nagashima H et al: No neurological involvement for more than 40 years in Klippel-Feil syndrome with severe hypermobility of the upper cervical spine. Arch Orthop Trauma Surg. 121(1-2):99-101, 2001
7. Suh SW et al: Evaluating Congenital spine deformities for intraspinal anomalies with magnetic resonance imaging. J Pediatr Orthop. 21(4):525-31, 2001
8. Jaskwhich D et al: Congenital scoliosis. Curr Opin Pediatr. 12(1):61-6, 2000
9. Yildiran A et al: Semantic and nosological confusions on multiple vertebral segmentation defects. Pediatr Neurosurg. 33(3):168, 2000
10. McMaster MJ et al: Natural history of congenital kyphosis and kyphoscoliosis. A study of one hundred and twelve patients. J Bone Joint Surg Am. 81(10):1367-83, 1999
11. McMaster MJ: Congenital scoliosis caused by a unilateral failure of vertebral segmentation with contralateral hemivertebrae. Spine. 23(9):998-1005, 1998
12. Anderson PJ et al: The cervical spine in Crouzon syndrome. Spine. 22(4):402-5, 1997
13. Aslan Y et al: Multiple vertebral segmentation defects. Brief report of three patients and nosological considerations. Genet Couns. 8(3):241-8, 1997
14. Lopez BC et al: Inadequate PAX-1 gene expression as a cause of agenesis of the thoracolumbar spine with failure of segmentation. Case report. J Neurosurg. 86(6):1018-21, 1997
15. Mortier GR et al: Multiple vertebral segmentation defects: analysis of 26 new patients and review of the literature. Am J Med Genet. 61(4):310-9, 1996
16. Jansen BR et al: Discitis in childhood. 12-35-year follow-up of 35 patients. Acta Orthop Scand. 64(1):33-6, 1993
17. Lee CK et al: Isolated congenital cervical block vertebrae below the axis with neurological symptoms. Spine. 6(2):118-24, 1981
18. Mayfield JK et al: Congenital kyphosis due to defects of anterior segmentation. J Bone Joint Surg Am. 62(8):1291-301, 1980

# VERTEBRAL SEGMENTATION FAILURE

## IMAGE GALLERY

### Typical

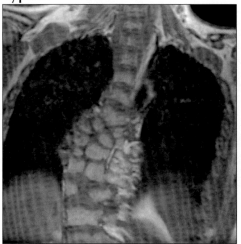
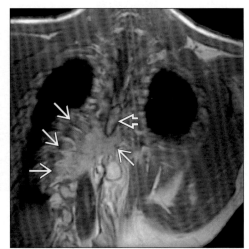

*(Left)* Coronal T1WI MR in a patient with diastematomyelia reveals multiple thoracic vertebral segmentation and fusion anomalies at apex of scoliotic curve. *(Right)* Coronal T1WI MR confirms multiple posterior element and rib fusions ➡ in conjunction with large osseous spur ⇨ (type 1 diastematomyelia patient).

### Typical

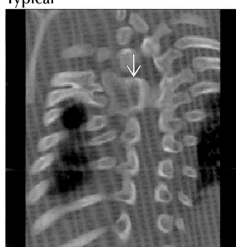
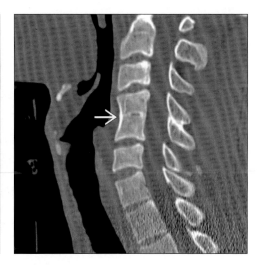

*(Left)* Coronal bone CT demonstrates a right pedicular bar ⇨ associated with multiple right posterior rib fusions. Pedicular bars predispose patient to progressive scoliotic curves. *(Right)* Sagittal bone CT in a patient with Klippel-Feil syndrome reveals mild single level congenital segmentation failure at C4-5. "Waist" ⇨ at rudimentary disc space and fused spinous processes are typical.

### Typical

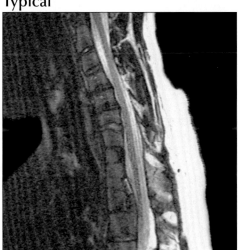
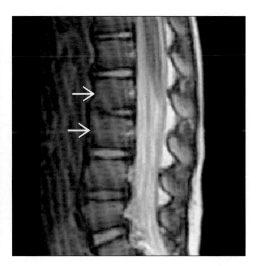

*(Left)* Sagittal T2WI MR in a patient with Klippel-Feil syndrome demonstrates extensive cervical and thoracic vertebral segmentation failure in conjunction with abnormal multilevel posterior element fusion. *(Right)* Sagittal T2WI MR shows very mild lumbar segmentation failure of the anterior L2 and L3 vertebra ➡, with a rudimentary anterior intervertebral disc and mild focal kyphosis.

# KLIPPEL-FEIL SPECTRUM

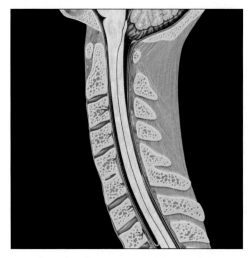

*Sagittal graphic shows congenital fusion of the C5-6 vertebrae and spinous processes, with characteristic rudimentary disc space and distinctive "waist" typical of congenital fusion.*

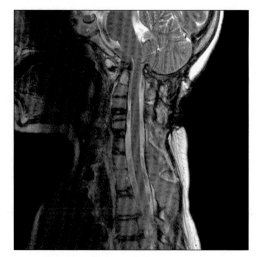

*Sagittal T2WI MR demonstrates severe KFS type 1 with multilevel cervical and thoracic segmentation failure. Anomalous CVJ anatomy narrows the upper cervical canal.*

## TERMINOLOGY

### Abbreviations and Synonyms
- Klippel-Feil syndrome, Klippel-Feil spectrum (KFS)

### Definitions
- Congenital spinal malformation characterized by segmentation failure of two or more cervical vertebra

## IMAGING FINDINGS

### General Features
- Best diagnostic clue: Single or multiple level congenital cervical segmentation and fusion anomalies
- Location: C2-3 (50%) > C5-6 (33%) > CVJ, upper thoracic spine
- Size
  - Vertebral bodies < normal size with tapered contour at affected disc space
  - Affected disc space reduced in height and diameter

- Morphology: Vertebral body narrowing ("wasp waist") at involved disc space +/- "fusion" of posterior elements

### CT Findings
- Bone CT
  - Typical osseous findings +/- degenerative changes
  - Sagittal, transverse spinal canal diameter usually normal
    - Canal enlargement ⇒ consider syringomyelia

### MR Findings
- T1WI
  - Cervical fusion(s): Vertebral bodies +/- facets, posterior elements
  - +/- Degenerative changes: Spondylosis, disc herniations common (especially lower cervical spine)
  - +/- CVJ osseous anomalies, Chiari I malformation
- T2WI
  - Osseous findings same as T1WI; normal marrow signal
  - +/- Cord or nerve root compression, syringomyelia, brainstem abnormalities, myeloschisis

## DDx: Klippel-Feil Spectrum

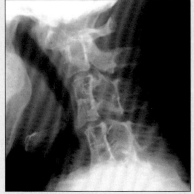

*Juvenile Chronic Arthritis*

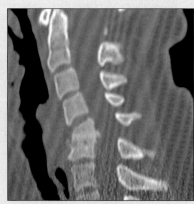

*Chronic Discitis*

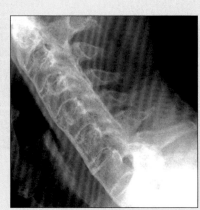

*Ankylosing Spondylitis*

# KLIPPEL-FEIL SPECTRUM

## Key Facts

### Terminology
- Klippel-Feil syndrome, Klippel-Feil spectrum (KFS)

### Imaging Findings
- Location: C2-3 (50%) > C5-6 (33%) > CVJ, upper thoracic spine
- Morphology: Vertebral body narrowing ("wasp waist") at involved disc space +/- "fusion" of posterior elements
- +/- Omovertebral bone

### Top Differential Diagnoses
- Juvenile Chronic Arthritis
- Chronic Sequelae of Discitis
- Surgical Fusion
- Ankylosing Spondylitis

### Pathology
- Caused by failure of normal segmentation of cervical somites (3rd → 8th weeks)
- Sporadic; familial genetic component with variable expression identified in many patients

### Clinical Issues
- Classic triad (33-50%): Short neck, low posterior hairline, and limited cervical motion
- Many patients have normal clinical appearance despite severity of involvement

### Diagnostic Checklist
- Much KFS morbidity and nearly all mortality related to visceral system dysfunction
- Look for instability, progressive degenerative changes, cord/brainstem compression

## Radiographic Findings
- Radiography
  - One or more fused vertebral levels with rudimentary, narrow disc space(s)
    - Disc space always abnormal; frequently fused facets, spinous processes as well
    - Adjacent mobile levels +/- accelerated degenerative changes
  - +/- Omovertebral bone
  - Flexion/extension films → lack of motion between fused levels, increased mobility at normal levels

## Imaging Recommendations
- Best imaging tool
  - Radiography to evaluate and follow instability, degenerative changes
  - MR to exclude cord compression, cord anomaly, detect degenerative changes
- Protocol advice
  - Serial neutral and flex/extend plain radiographs to detect progressive instability, degenerative disease
  - Multiplanar MR to evaluate canal compromise, cord compression, soft tissue degenerative changes
  - Ultrasound or CECT to detect and characterize associated visceral organ abnormalities

## DIFFERENTIAL DIAGNOSIS

### Juvenile Chronic Arthritis
- Difficult to distinguish from cervical block vertebra
- Search for other affected joints, appropriate history

### Chronic Sequelae of Discitis
- Irregular endplate margins, no "waist", +/- kyphosis
- Confirm history of prior spinal infection

### Surgical Fusion
- No disc space "waist", facets infrequently ankylosed
- Surgical history key to making diagnosis

### Ankylosing Spondylitis
- Delicate contiguous syndesmophytes ("bamboo spine") + symmetric SI joint disease
- HLA - B27 positive (95%)

## PATHOLOGY

### General Features
- General path comments
  - "Klippel-Feil syndrome" colloquially used for all patients with cervical congenital vertebral segmentation ("fusion") anomalies regardless of extent
  - Caused by failure of normal segmentation of cervical somites (3rd → 8th weeks)
- Genetics
  - Sporadic; familial genetic component with variable expression identified in many patients
    - C2/3 fusion (type 2) ⇒ autosomal dominant with variable penetrance
    - C5/6 fusion (type 2) ⇒ autosomal recessive
  - SGMI (chromosome 8) ⇒ 1st Klippel-Feil gene identified; gene expression overlaps all 3 KFS types
- Etiology
  - No universally accepted etiology; embryonic insult postulated between 4th → 8th weeks
    - Putative environmental causative factors include teratogens, maternal alcoholism
    - Association with other syndromes (fetal alcohol, Goldenhar, Wildervanck - cervical/oculo/acoustic)
- Epidemiology: 1/42,000 births
- Associated abnormalities
  - Hemivertebrae, butterfly vertebrae, spina bifida
  - Scoliosis (usually congenital) +/- kyphosis (60%)
  - Odontoid dysplasia, basilar impression, C1 assimilation, occipito-cervical instability
  - Syringomyelia, diastematomyelia (20%), Chiari I malformation (8%), neurenteric cyst or dermoid (rare)
  - Cervicomedullary neuroschisis +/- synkinesis (20%)

- ○ Sprengel deformity +/- omovertebral bone (15-30%); unilateral or bilateral
- ○ Sensorineural hearing loss (30%), GU tract abnormalities (35%), congenital heart disease (14%), upper extremity deformity, facial anomalies

## Gross Pathologic & Surgical Features
- Surgical observations correlate to imaging findings

## Microscopic Features
- Histologically normal bone, disc

## Staging, Grading or Classification Criteria
- Type 1 (9%): Massive fusion of cervical, upper thoracic spine → severe neurological impairment, frequent associated abnormalities
- Type 2 (84%): Fusion of two or more cervical vertebrae
- Type 3 (7%): Fusions involve cervical and lower thoracic/lumbar vertebrae

## CLINICAL ISSUES

### Presentation
- Most common signs/symptoms
  - ○ Cosmesis complaints, neck or radicular pain, slowly progressive or acute myelopathy
    - Multilevel involvement often noted in infancy/early childhood 2° to cosmetic deformity
  - ○ Neurologic problems in infancy, childhood usually 2° to CVJ abnormalities
  - ○ Lower cervical involvement becomes symptomatic due to degenerative changes/instability of adjacent segments in 4th/5th decade
  - ○ Other signs/symptoms
    - Vocal impairment (usually > 1 level fusion)
    - Synkinesia (mirror movements): 20%, upper > lower extremity, diminish with time
- Clinical Profile
  - ○ Classic triad (33-50%): Short neck, low posterior hairline, and limited cervical motion
  - ○ Wide variation in clinical and anatomical expression
    - Many patients have normal clinical appearance despite severity of involvement
    - Cervical motion limitation is most consistent clinical finding

### Demographics
- Age: Any age; most commonly 2nd → 3rd decade
- Gender: M ≤ F

### Natural History & Prognosis
- Accelerated spondylosis adjacent to fused segments
- Three patterns at greatest risk for future instability
  - ○ C0 → C3 fusion with occipitocervical synostosis
  - ○ Long cervical fusion + abnormal C0/1 junction
  - ○ Single open interspace between 2 fused segments
- ↑ Risk of neurological injury following minor trauma 2° hypermobility of cervical segments
  - ○ High risk patients: Two sets of block vertebra, occipitalization of atlas + basilar invagination, and cervical fusion + spinal stenosis

### Treatment
- Avoidance of contact sports, occupations and recreational activities at risk for head or neck trauma
- Activity modification, bracing, and traction may reduce symptoms
- Neurological lesion, significant pain despite conservative therapy, or progressive instability ⇒ decompression +/- spinal fusion

## DIAGNOSTIC CHECKLIST

### Consider
- Much KFS morbidity and nearly all mortality related to visceral system dysfunction

### Image Interpretation Pearls
- Look for instability, progressive degenerative changes, cord/brainstem compression

## SELECTED REFERENCES

1. Royal SA et al: Investigations into the association between cervicomedullary neuroschisis and mirror movements in patients with Klippel-Feil syndrome. AJNR Am J Neuroradiol. 23(4):724-9, 2002
2. Andronikou S et al: Klippel-Feil syndrome with cervical diastematomyelia in an 8-year-old boy. Pediatr Radiol. 31(9):636, 2001
3. Nagashima H et al: No neurological involvement for more than 40 years in Klippel-Feil syndrome with severe hypermobility of the upper cervical spine. Arch Orthop Trauma Surg. 121(1-2):99-101, 2001
4. Clark et al: The Cervical Spine. 3rd ed. Philadelphia, Lippincott-Raven. 339-348, 1998
5. Clarke RA et al: Heterogeneity in Klippel-Feil syndrome: a new classification. Pediatr Radiol. 28(12):967-74, 1998
6. Karasick D et al: The traumatized cervical spine in Klippel-Feil syndrome: imaging features. AJR Am J Roentgenol. 170(1):85-8, 1998
7. Rouvreau P et al: Assessment and neurologic involvement of patients with cervical spine congenital synostosis as in Klippel-Feil syndrome: study of 19 cases. J Pediatr Orthop B. 7(3):179-85, 1998
8. Theiss SM et al: The long-term follow-up of patients with Klippel-Feil syndrome and congenital scoliosis. Spine. 22(11):1219-22, 1997
9. Thomsen MN et al: Scoliosis and congenital anomalies associated with Klippel-Feil syndrome types I-III. Spine. 22(4):396-401, 1997
10. David KM et al: Split cervical spinal cord with Klippel-Feil syndrome: seven cases. Brain. 119 ( Pt 6):1859-72, 1996
11. Baba H et al: The cervical spine in the Klippel-Feil syndrome. A report of 57 cases. Int Orthop. 19(4):204-8, 1995
12. Guggenbuhl P et al: Adult-onset Klippel-Feil syndrome with inaugural neurologic symptoms: two case reports. Rev Rhum Engl Ed. 62(11):802-4, 1995
13. Guille JT et al: The natural history of Klippel-Feil syndrome: clinical, roentgenographic, and magnetic resonance imaging findings at adulthood. J Pediatr Orthop. 15(5):617-26, 1995
14. Pizzutillo PD et al: Risk factors in Klippel-Feil syndrome. Spine. 19(18):2110-6, 1994

## IMAGE GALLERY

### Typical

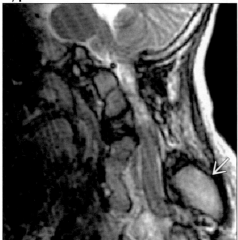

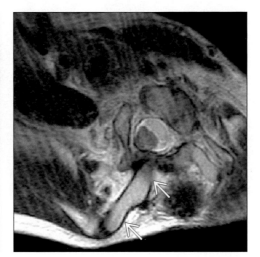

*(Left)* Sagittal T2WI MR reveals severe cervicothoracic scoliosis and multiple segmentation anomalies with characteristic bizarre vertebral appearance of severe KFS. Note the large omovertebral bone ➡️. *(Right)* Axial T2WI MR in a scoliotic severe KFS type 1 patient depicts an omovertebral bone ➡️ extending from the posterior vertebral elements to the scapula.

### Typical

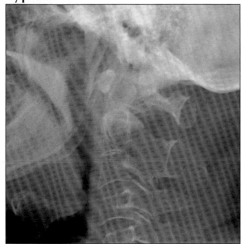

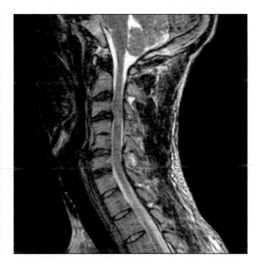

*(Left)* Lateral radiograph depicts an incidental congenital fusion of C2/3 in this KFS type 2 patient. Mild, single level fusion is the most commonly observed KFS variant. *(Right)* Sagittal T2WI MR shows congenital fusion of C4/5 (KFS type 2), with narrow waist and rudimentary disc. Disc herniation above the congenital fusion produces abnormal cord contour and signal.

### Typical

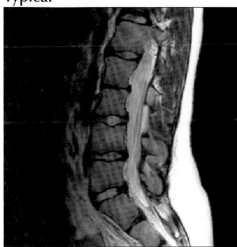

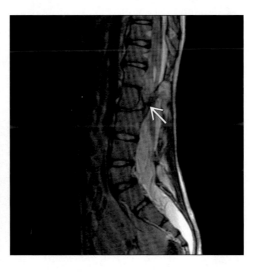

*(Left)* Sagittal T2WI MR shows most severe KFS subtype, type 3, with multiple lumbar segmentation anomalies. Segmentation failure extended to cervical and thoracic spine as well (not shown). *(Right)* Sagittal T2WI MR depicts severe KFS type 3, with cervical, thoracic, (not shown) and lumbar segmentation anomalies in conjunction with diastematomyelia ➡️.

# CONGENITAL SPINAL STENOSIS

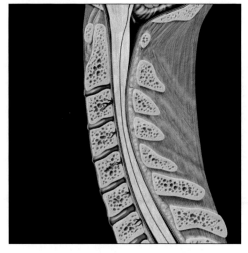

Sagittal graphic shows marked congenital AP narrowing of the central spinal canal. The shortening of the AP canal diameter is secondary to short pedicles.

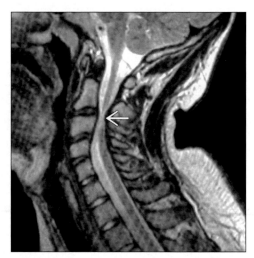

Sagittal T2WI MR shows severe congenital central canal stenosis at C2 and C3 producing spinal cord compression. High signal within flattened cord ➡ correlates with clinical myelopathy.

## TERMINOLOGY

### Abbreviations and Synonyms
- "Short pedicle" syndrome, congenital short pedicles, developmental spinal stenosis

### Definitions
- Reduced anteroposterior (AP) canal diameter 2° to short, squat pedicles and laterally directed laminae

## IMAGING FINDINGS

### General Features
- Best diagnostic clue: Short, thick pedicles producing narrowed AP spinal canal diameter
- Location: Lumbar > cervical > thoracic spine
- Size
  - Central canal diameter is smaller than normal
    - Cervical spine: Absolute AP diameter < 14 mm
    - Lumbar spine: Absolute AP diameter < 15 mm
- Morphology
  - Short thick pedicles
  - "Trefoil-shaped" lateral recesses
  - Laterally directed laminae

### CT Findings
- Bone CT
  - Short thick pedicles, "trefoil-shaped" lateral recesses, and laterally directed laminae
    - +/- Acquired disc, facet degenerative changes
  - Sagittal plane useful to survey extent of congenital narrowing
  - Axial plane best demonstrates reduced AP canal diameter, short thick pedicles

### MR Findings
- T1WI
  - Short AP diameter +/- superimposed acquired facet, disc degenerative changes
  - +/- Hypointense facet, vertebral body marrow changes indicative of superimposed degenerative changes
- T2WI
  - Similar osseous findings to T1WI MR
  - +/- Cord compression
- T2* GRE
  - Best depicts osseous structures

## DDx: Congenital Spinal Stenosis

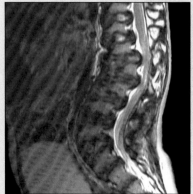

Mucopolysaccharidosis

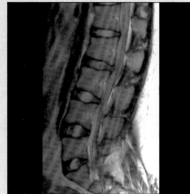

Achondroplasia

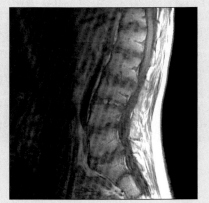

Homocystinuria

# CONGENITAL SPINAL STENOSIS

## Key Facts

### Terminology
- "Short pedicle" syndrome, congenital short pedicles, developmental spinal stenosis

### Imaging Findings
- Location: Lumbar > cervical > thoracic spine
- Short thick pedicles, "trefoil-shaped" lateral recesses, and laterally directed laminae

### Top Differential Diagnoses
- Inherited Spinal Stenosis
- Acquired Spinal Stenosis

### Clinical Issues
- Low back pain, radiating leg pain (unilateral or bilateral), +/- bladder and bowel dysfunction

- Neurogenic claudication: Radiating leg pain with walking, relieved by rest, bending forward
- Cauda equina syndrome (rare): Bilateral leg weakness, urinary retention due to atonic bladder
- Progressive myelopathy (spinal cord dysfunction) or reversible acute neurologic deficits ("stingers")

### Diagnostic Checklist
- Patients present at a younger age than typical for degenerative spine disease
- Congenital spinal stenosis may not produce symptoms until superimposed acquired degenerative changes accumulate
- Recognition of short thick pedicles, AP canal diameter reduction key to diagnosis

---

  ○ Caveat: Overestimates true degree of canal narrowing 2° to motion, susceptibility "blooming" artifact

## Radiographic Findings
- Radiography
  ○ Shortened AP distance between posterior vertebral body and spinolaminar line
    ▪ +/- Superimposed degenerative disc, facet disease
  ○ Lateral X-ray normally shows articular pillar ending before spinolaminar line
    ▪ Imaging pearl: If articular pillar takes up entire AP canal dimension on lateral X-ray, central canal stenosis is present

## Non-Vascular Interventions
- Myelography: Confirms shortened AP dimension, clarifies severity of neural compression

## Imaging Recommendations
- CT with sagittal and coronal reformats to evaluate osseous structures
  ○ Narrowed angle of laminae best appreciated in coronal plane
- MR imaging to assess degree/presence of spinal cord, dural sac compression
  ○ Also demonstrates osseous anatomy well; permits complete imaging assessment with a single imaging study
  ○ Sagittal MR best demonstrates AP canal narrowing, assesses for cord/cauda equina compression
  ○ Axial MR images confirm pedicle configuration, assess severity of canal narrowing

## DIFFERENTIAL DIAGNOSIS

### Inherited Spinal Stenosis
- Genetic predisposition
- Achondroplasia, mucopolysaccharidoses most common

- Frequently associated with characteristic brain, visceral, and/or extremity abnormalities enabling specific diagnosis

### Acquired Spinal Stenosis
- Normal pedicle length
- +/- Subluxation, spondylolysis, disc/facet degenerative changes

## PATHOLOGY

### General Features
- General path comments: Short, thickened pedicles
- Etiology: Idiopathic
- Epidemiology
  ○ Prevalence in general population difficult to establish; up to 30% of surgically proven lumbar stenosis in one study
    ▪ Not uncommonly seen in clinical practice during routine cervical or lumbar spine evaluation
    ▪ Congenital cervical stenosis reported in 7.6% of 262 high school and college football players
  ○ Symptomatic at earlier age than expected
- Associated abnormalities: Superimposed acquired (degenerative) stenosis

### Gross Pathologic & Surgical Features
- Sagittal canal narrowed 2° to short pedicles, thick laminae, and protrusion of inferior facet articular processes
- Lateral recess often narrowed 2° to co-existent hypertrophic superior facet articular processes

### Microscopic Features
- Histologically normal bone

### Staging, Grading or Classification Criteria
- Cervical spine
  ○ Torg ratio (AP canal diameter/AP vertebral body diameter) < 0.8
  ○ Absolute diameter < 14 mm

# CONGENITAL SPINAL STENOSIS

- Must take body habitus into account; relative dimension more important than absolute measurement
- Lumbar spine
  - Absolute AP diameter < 15 mm
    - Body habitus influences significance of measurement

## CLINICAL ISSUES

### Presentation
- Most common signs/symptoms
  - Lumbar
    - Low back pain, radiating leg pain (unilateral or bilateral), +/- bladder and bowel dysfunction
    - Neurogenic claudication: Radiating leg pain with walking, relieved by rest, bending forward
    - Cauda equina syndrome (rare): Bilateral leg weakness, urinary retention due to atonic bladder
  - Cervical
    - Radiating arm pain or numbness
    - Progressive myelopathy (spinal cord dysfunction) or reversible acute neurologic deficits ("stingers")
- Clinical Profile
  - Symptomatic cervical or lumbar stenosis symptoms at younger age than typical of degenerative stenosis
    - These patients typically lack complicating medical problems (diabetes or vascular insufficiency)
  - Athlete presents with temporary neurological deficit following physical contact that subsequently resolves

### Demographics
- Age: Symptoms may arise in teens; more commonly in 4th-5th decade
- Gender: M ≥ F
- Ethnicity: No ethnic or racial predilection

### Natural History & Prognosis
- May be incidental finding in younger patients
  - Borderline cases usually asymptomatic until superimposed acquired spinal degenerative disease occurs
- Many patients eventually develop symptomatic spinal stenosis
  - Minor superimposed acquired abnormalities (bulge, herniation, osteophyte) cause severe neurologic symptoms
- Early surgical treatment important for best outcome
  - Surgical decompression usually relieves symptoms effectively
  - Long term pain relief following surgery is common

### Treatment
- Lumbar: Decompressive laminectomy, posterior foraminotomy at involved levels
  - Risk of complications increases with more levels of decompression, diabetes, and long term steroid use
- Cervical: Posterior cervical laminectomy or laminoplasty
  - Same risk factors for complication as lumbar decompression

## DIAGNOSTIC CHECKLIST

### Consider
- Patients present at a younger age than typical for degenerative spine disease
- Congenital spinal stenosis may not produce symptoms until superimposed acquired degenerative changes accumulate

### Image Interpretation Pearls
- Recognition of short thick pedicles, AP canal diameter reduction key to diagnosis
- Look for superimposed degenerative changes

## SELECTED REFERENCES

1. Brigham CD et al: Permanent partial cervical spinal cord injury in a professional football player who had only congenital stenosis. A case report. J Bone Joint Surg Am. 85-A(8):1553-6, 2003
2. Allen CR et al: Transient quadriparesis in the athlete. Clin Sports Med. 21(1):15-27, 2002
3. Oguz H et al: Measurement of spinal canal diameters in young subjects with lumbosacral transitional vertebra. Eur Spine J. 11(2):115-8, 2002
4. Boockvar JA et al: Cervical spinal stenosis and sports-related cervical cord neurapraxia in children. Spine. 26(24):2709-12; discussion 2713, 2001
5. Shaffrey CI et al: Modified open-door laminoplasty for treatment of neurological deficits in younger patients with congenital spinal stenosis: analysis of clinical and radiographic data. J Neurosurg. 90(4 Suppl):170-7, 1999
6. Bey T et al: Spinal cord injury with a narrow spinal canal: utilizing Torg's ratio method of analyzing cervical spine radiographs. J Emerg Med. 16(1):79-82, 1998
7. Yoshida M et al: Indication and clinical results of laminoplasty for cervical myelopathy caused by disc herniation with developmental canal stenosis. Spine. 23(22):2391-7, 1998
8. Torg JS et al: Suggested management guidelines for participation in collision activities with congenital, developmental, or postinjury lesions involving the cervical spine. Med Sci Sports Exerc. 29(7 Suppl):S256-72, 1997
9. Azhar MM et al: Congenital spine deformity, congenital stenosis, diastematomyelia, and tight filum terminale in a workmen's compensation patient: a case report. Spine. 21(6):770-4, 1996
10. Ducker TB: Post-traumatic progressive cervical myelopathy in patient with congenital spinal stenosis. J Spinal Disord. 9(1):76; discussion 77-81, 1996
11. Lemaire JJ et al: Lumbar canal stenosis. Retrospective study of 158 operated cases. Neurochirurgie. 41(2):89-97, 1995
12. Torg JS: Cervical spinal stenosis with cord neurapraxia and transient quadriplegia. Sports Med. 20(6):429-34, 1995
13. Major NM et al: Central and foraminal stenosis of the lumbar spine. Neuroimaging Clinics of North America. 3(3):559-61, 1993
14. Smith MG et al: The prevalence of congenital cervical spinal stenosis in 262 college and high school football players. J Ky Med Assoc. 91(7):273-5, 1993
15. Scher AT: Spinal cord concussion in rugby players. Am J Sports Med. 19(5):485-8, 1991
16. Torg JS: Cervical spinal stenosis with cord neurapraxia and transient quadriplegia. Clin Sports Med. 9(2):279-96, 1990
17. Dauser RC et al: Symptomatic congenital spinal stenosis in a child. Neurosurgery. 11(1 Pt 1):61-3, 1982

# CONGENITAL SPINAL STENOSIS

## IMAGE GALLERY

### Typical

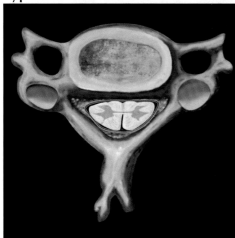
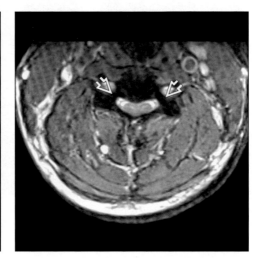

*(Left)* Axial graphic depicts congenital cervical AP spinal narrowing. The pedicles are thick and laterally directed, with resultant flattening of laminae and narrowing of AP canal diameter. *(Right)* Axial T2* GRE MR demonstrates that central canal stenosis is associated with short, laterally oriented pedicles ➡.

### Typical

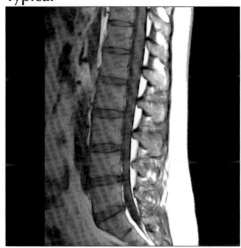
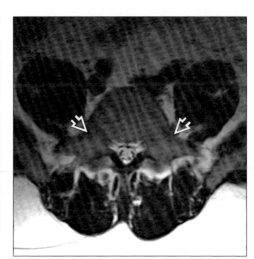

*(Left)* Sagittal T1WI MR depicts mild central canal narrowing in anteroposterior dimension. Unlike this case, the spinal canal should normally widen at the lumbosacral junction rather than taper. *(Right)* Axial T2WI MR at the lumbosacral junction confirms short, thickened, laterally directed pedicles ➡ with associated central anteroposterior spinal canal narrowing.

### Typical

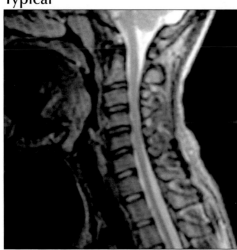
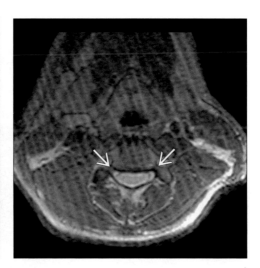

*(Left)* Sagittal T2WI MR demonstrates reduced AP diameter of the cervical central spinal canal. Relatively little encroachment into the canal by disc or fracture is needed to compress cord. *(Right)* Axial T2WI MR confirms reduced anteroposterior canal diameter is due to short pedicles ➡. No significant bony or soft tissue components of narrowing are present.

# SCOLIOSIS

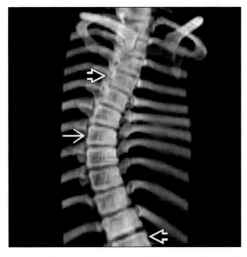

Coronal 3D reformatted bone CT image (idiopathic scoliosis) demonstrates rotation as well as scoliosis. ➡ placed on apical vertebra; ⇒ on terminal vertebrae.

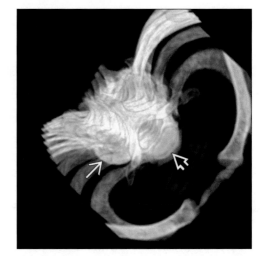

Axial 3D reformatted bone CT shows rotation of the apical vertebra ⇒ compared to the terminal vertebra ➡. 3D CT is valuable in surgical planning to determine amount of rotation.

## TERMINOLOGY

### Definitions
- General term for any lateral curvature of the spine
- Dextroscoliosis: Curve convex to the right
- Levoscoliosis: Curve convex to the left
- Kyphoscoliosis: Scoliosis with a component of kyphosis
- Rotoscoliosis: Scoliosis which includes rotation of the vertebrae
- S-curve scoliosis: Two adjacent curves, one to the right and one to the left
- C-curve scoliosis: Single curve
- Terminal vertebra: Most superior or inferior vertebra included in a curve
- Transitional vertebra: Vertebra between two curves
- Apical vertebra: Vertebra with greatest lateral displacement from the midline
- Primary curvature: Curvature with greatest angulation
- Secondary or compensatory curvature: Smaller curve which balances primary curvature

## IMAGING FINDINGS

### General Features
- Best diagnostic clue: Lateral curvature of the spine which returns to midline at ends of curve
- Location: Most commonly thoracic or thoracolumbar
- Size
  - Curve > 10°
  - May be > 90°
- Morphology
  - S-curve scoliosis
    - Idiopathic
    - Congenital
    - Syndromic
  - C-curve scoliosis
    - Neuromuscular
    - Neurofibromatosis
    - Scheuermann disease
    - Congenital
    - Syndromic
  - Short-curve scoliosis
    - Tumor
    - Trauma
    - Infection

## DDx: Scoliosis

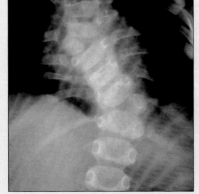

Congenital

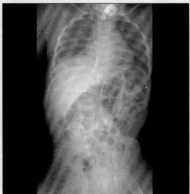

Neuromuscular

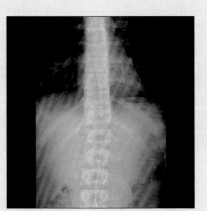

Scheuermann Disease

# SCOLIOSIS

## Key Facts

### Terminology
- General term for any lateral curvature of the spine

### Imaging Findings
- Location: Most commonly thoracic or thoracolumbar
- Standing PA radiograph of the full thoracic and lumbar spine on single cassette
- Method of Cobb is standard for measuring scoliosis
- Lateral radiograph to show sagittal plane abnormalities
- MR to screen for bone, cord abnormalities

### Top Differential Diagnoses
- Idiopathic Scoliosis
- Congenital Scoliosis
- Neuromuscular Scoliosis

- Scoliosis Due to Congenital Syndromes Without Vertebral Anomalies
- Scoliosis Due to Infection
- Scheuermann Disease
- Scoliosis Due to Tumor
- Scoliosis Due to Trauma
- Degenerative Scoliosis
- Compensatory Scoliosis

### Clinical Issues
- Idiopathic scoliosis asymptomatic
- Fusion for rapidly progressive curves, curves > 40°

### Diagnostic Checklist
- Short-curve scoliosis usually has underlying abnormalities

- Radiation
- Congenital
- Neuropathic

## CT Findings
- Bone CT
  - Shows congenital bone anomalies, tumor, infection, post-operative complications

## MR Findings
- Shows bone and spinal cord anomalies, syrinx, tumor, infection

## Radiographic Findings
- Radiography
  - Standing PA radiograph of the full thoracic and lumbar spine on single cassette
    - PA projection gives lower radiation dose to breasts than AP
    - Lifts used to equalize limb lengths if needed
  - Method of Cobb is standard for measuring scoliosis
    - Draw lines parallel to endplates of terminal vertebrae
    - If endplates difficult to see, use pedicles as landmarks
    - Cobb angle is angle between terminal endplates
    - Can also measure angle between two lines drawn perpendicular to endplates
    - Second method is easier with small curves
  - Choosing correct vertebrae to measure scoliosis critical to accuracy and monitoring
    - Terminal vertebra is one with greatest angle of endplate from horizontal
    - Rotoscoliosis: Terminal vertebra spinous process returns to midline
    - Interobserver variability 7-10°
  - Coned-down radiographs for better definition of vertebral abnormalities
  - Lateral radiograph to show sagittal plane abnormalities
    - Usually alters normal thoracic kyphosis, lumbar lordosis

  - Estimate rotational deformity by rib displacement on lateral radiograph

## Imaging Recommendations
- Best imaging tool: Radiography for initial diagnosis
- Protocol advice
  - MR to screen for bone, cord abnormalities
    - Coronal and sagittal T1WI and T2WI
    - Include craniocervical junction
    - Axial T2WI through areas of suspected abnormality
    - Axial T2WI through conus
  - CT for surgical planning
    - 1-3 mm multidetector CT with reformatted images
    - 3D helpful
  - CT for surgical complications
    - Thin, overlapping sections minimize artifact
    - Bone and soft tissue windows

# DIFFERENTIAL DIAGNOSIS

## Idiopathic Scoliosis
- Classic S-curve scoliosis
- Thoracic curve usually away from side of aortic arch

## Congenital Scoliosis
- 2° to abnormal vertebral segmentation
- Curve morphology highly variable

## Neuromuscular Scoliosis
- Neurologic disorders and muscular dystrophies
- Usually C-curve

## Scoliosis Due to Congenital Syndromes Without Vertebral Anomalies
- Neurofibromatosis, Marfan, osteogenesis imperfecta, diastrophic dwarfism, Ehlers-Danlos syndrome
- Frequently complex curvatures

## Scoliosis Due to Infection
- Painful; systemic signs may be absent
- Pyogenic bacteria, tuberculosis, fungi

- Usually short curve

## Scheuermann Disease
- 15% have scoliosis in addition to kyphosis
- Scoliosis generally mild

## Scoliosis Due to Tumor
- Painful
- Short curve
- Tumor may be occult on radiography
- Screen with MR

## Scoliosis Due to Trauma
- Usually see post-traumatic deformity
- Stress fracture may be occult cause

## Scoliosis Due to Radiation
- Usually avoided today by radiation port placement
- Radiation to entire vertebra rather than portion now preferred

## Degenerative Scoliosis
- Develops primarily in adults
- Degenerative disc disease, facet arthropathy
- May also have secondary degenerative disease from idiopathic scoliosis

## Neuropathic Spine
- Rapidly developing spine deformity
- Bony destruction seen on radiography

## Compensatory Scoliosis
- Due to limb length inequality
- Can be diagnosed on spine radiographs by relative positions of iliac crests

## Positional Scoliosis
- Poor positioning by radiology technologist
- Detected on supine radiographs, resolves on upright radiographs

## Iatrogenic Scoliosis
- Rib resection
- Level above lumbar fusion
- Hardware failure

## PATHOLOGY

### General Features
- Etiology: Causes listed above
- Epidemiology: Common

### Gross Pathologic & Surgical Features
- Deformity of trunk visible on physical examination

### Staging, Grading or Classification Criteria
- Etiology
- Direction of curve
- Severity of curve

## CLINICAL ISSUES

### Presentation
- Most common signs/symptoms

○ Visible deformity
○ Idiopathic scoliosis asymptomatic
○ Painful scoliosis indicates underlying abnormality

### Demographics
- Age: Usually presents in childhood or adolescence
- Gender: Idiopathic M:F = 1:7

### Natural History & Prognosis
- Most scoliosis is mild
- May progress rapidly, especially during growth spurts
- Degenerative disc disease common
  ○ Greatest along concave aspect of scoliosis
- Severe scoliosis
  ○ Respiratory compromise
  ○ Neurologic symptoms
  ○ Instability

### Treatment
- Bracing for curves > 25°
- Fusion for rapidly progressive curves, curves > 40°
- Vertical expansion prosthetic titanium rod (VEPTR) placement for respiratory insufficiency
- Observation for minor curves

## DIAGNOSTIC CHECKLIST

### Consider
- Short-curve scoliosis usually has underlying abnormalities

## SELECTED REFERENCES

1.  Wu J et al: Association of estrogen receptor gene polymorphisms with susceptibility to adolescent idiopathic scoliosis. Spine. 31(10):1131-6, 2006
2.  Arlet V et al: Congenital scoliosis. Eur Spine J. 12(5):456-63, 2003
3.  Ahn UM et al: The etiology of adolescent idiopathic scoliosis. Am J Orthop. 31(7):387-95, 2002
4.  Berven S et al: Neuromuscular scoliosis: causes of deformity and principles for evaluation and management. Semin Neurol. 22(2):167-78, 2002
5.  Cassar-Pullicino VN et al: Imaging in scoliosis: what, why and how? Clin Radiol. 57(7):543-62, 2002
6.  Do T: Orthopedic management of the muscular dystrophies. Curr Opin Pediatr. 14(1):50-3, 2002
7.  Lenke LG et al: Curve prevalence of a new classification of operative adolescent idiopathic scoliosis: does classification correlate with treatment? Spine. 27(6):604-11, 2002
8.  Redla S et al: Magnetic resonance imaging of scoliosis. Clin Radiol. 56(5):360-71, 2001
9.  Thomson JD et al: Scoliosis in cerebral palsy: an overview and recent results. J Pediatr Orthop B. 10(1):6-9, 2001
10. Lowe TG et al: Etiology of idiopathic scoliosis: current trends in research. J Bone Joint Surg Am. 82-A(8):1157-68, 2000
11. Mohaideen A et al: Not all rods are Harrington - an overview of spinal instrumentation in scoliosis treatment. Pediatr Radiol. 30(2):110-8, 2000
12. Roach JW: Adolescent idiopathic scoliosis. Orthop Clin North Am. 30(3):353-65, vii-viii, 1999
13. Kim HW et al: Spine update. The management of scoliosis in neurofibromatosis. Spine. 22(23):2770-6, 1997

# SCOLIOSIS

## IMAGE GALLERY

### Typical

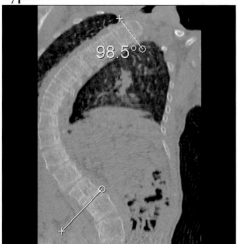

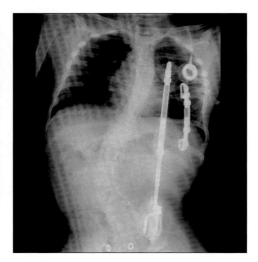

*(Left)* Coronal bone CT in a patient with C-shaped neuromuscular scoliosis 2° to cerebral palsy depicts method of Cobb. Angle between endplates of terminal vertebrae = 98.5°. *(Right)* Anteroposterior radiograph shows patient with neuromuscular scoliosis (spina bifida) and titanium expansion rods (VEPTR) placed for rib expansion to improve pulmonary function.

### Typical

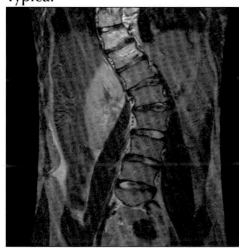

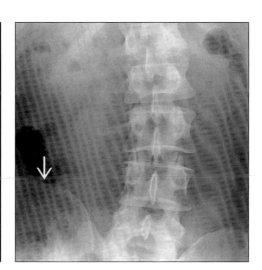

*(Left)* Coronal T2WI MR demonstrates S-shaped scoliosis and secondary degenerative changes of intervertebral discs and vertebral endplates in adolescent Marfan patient. *(Right)* Anteroposterior radiograph reveals apparent levoscoliosis. However, right iliac crest ➡ is higher than left, indicating scoliosis is actually compensatory for limb length inequality.

### Typical

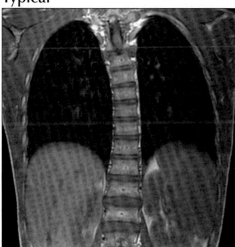

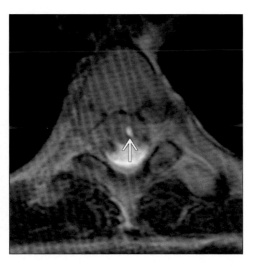

*(Left)* Coronal T1WI MR shows atypical convex left scoliosis in male patient with left sided aortic arch and neurological symptoms. Idiopathic thoracic curves are usually to opposite of side of arch. *(Right)* Axial T2WI MR in the same patient as previous image with atypical left scoliotic curvature demonstrates eccentric thoracic syrinx ➡. Underlying pathology should be suspected in atypical curves.

# CONGENITAL SCOLIOSIS AND KYPHOSIS

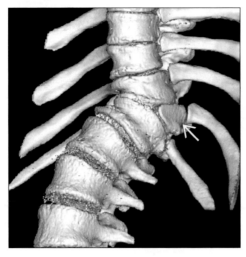

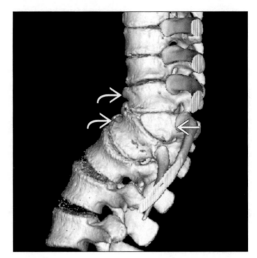

*3D bone CT reformat (congenital scoliosis) demonstrates focal short curve levoscoliosis secondary to an unbalanced left T11 hemivertebra →.*

*3D bone CT reformats (congenital kyphosis) shows an anterior thoracic hemivertebra → with incomplete segmentation of the adjacent vertebrae above and below → producing focal kyphosis.*

## TERMINOLOGY

### Definitions

- Spinal curvature 2° to congenital vertebral anomalies
- Failure of vertebral formation
  - Hemivertebra: Unilateral or anterior vertebral hypoplasia
  - Butterfly vertebra: Central vertebral cleft 2° to failure of central vertebral body development
- Vertebral segmentation failure
  - Block ("fused") vertebrae: Embryological vertebral segmentation failure rather than fusion
    - May affect vertebral body, posterior elements, or both
    - Affected vertebrae narrow in mediolateral, anteroposterior dimensions
    - ± Rudimentary intervertebral disc
  - Vertebral bar
    - Bony or cartilaginous connection between adjacent vertebrae
    - Often associated rib fusions

## IMAGING FINDINGS

### General Features

- Best diagnostic clue
  - Vertebral anomalies + scoliosis or kyphosis
  - Frequently short curve angulation, "bizarre" appearance
- Location: Thoracic > cervical, lumbar
- Morphology: Usually short curve scoliosis, but may have multiple curves if multiple anomalies present

### CT Findings

- Bone CT
  - Similar osseous findings to radiography
  - Coronal, sagittal reformatted images essential
  - 3D imaging helpful for surgical planning

### MR Findings

- T1WI
  - Similar morphological findings to CT
  - Evaluate bone morphology, exclude tumor, fatty filum, Chiari I malformation
- T2WI
  - Similar morphological findings to CT

## DDx: Congenital Kyphosis and Scoliosis

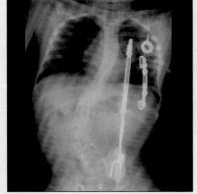

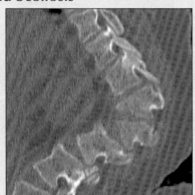

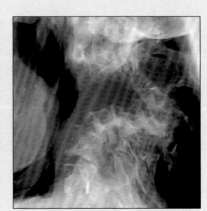

*Neuromuscular Scoliosis*

*Achondroplasia*

*Neurofibromatosis Type 1*

# CONGENITAL SCOLIOSIS AND KYPHOSIS

## Key Facts

### Terminology
- Spinal curvature 2° to congenital vertebral anomalies

### Imaging Findings
- Vertebral anomalies + scoliosis or kyphosis
- Frequently short curve angulation, "bizarre" appearance
- Location: Thoracic > cervical, lumbar
- Morphology: Usually short curve scoliosis, but may have multiple curves if multiple anomalies present

### Top Differential Diagnoses
- Idiopathic Scoliosis
- Neuromuscular Scoliosis
- Scoliosis Due to Syndromes
- Scoliosis Due to Trauma
- Idiopathic Kyphosis
- Scheuermann Kyphosis

### Pathology
- Failure of vertebral formation and segmentation may both be present
- Bar between vertebrae may be either cartilaginous or osseous

### Clinical Issues
- Clinical Profile: May be isolated anomaly or associated with multisystem anomalies (VACTERL)

### Diagnostic Checklist
- Angular curve on radiography without hemivertebra → probable bony bar
- Vertebral bars may be cartilaginous in young children
- Image entire spine to exclude additional bone or cord abnormalities, Chiari I malformation

---

- ○ Evaluate for tethered cord, syrinx, tumor

## Radiographic Findings
- Radiography
  - ○ Screen with full spine PA, lateral radiographs to "count" levels
  - ○ Vertebral anomalies often difficult to see; use coned-down radiographs, MR or CT to clarify

## Imaging Recommendations
- Best imaging tool
  - ○ Radiographs for surveying spinal axis, "counting" levels
  - ○ Multiplanar MR is best cross-sectional modality to evaluate full spine in children
    - Avoids CT radiation dose, excludes associated neural axis abnormalities
  - ○ CT with reformats is excellent for surgical planning because of superior spatial resolution, 3D rendering capabilities

## DIFFERENTIAL DIAGNOSIS

### Idiopathic Scoliosis
- S-shaped curve, no vertebral anomalies

### Neuromuscular Scoliosis
- Usually single, long thoracolumbar curve

### Scoliosis Due to Infection
- Short curve, painful
- Infection may be in disc or paraspinous tissues
- May result in vertebral body fusion

### Scoliosis Due to Syndromes
- E.g, neurofibromatosis, Marfan, osteogenesis imperfecta, diastrophic dwarfism, Ehlers-Danlos syndrome

### Scoliosis Due to Trauma
- Short curve scoliosis, vertebral body deformity, soft tissue traumatic changes

### Scoliosis Due to Radiation
- Short curve scoliosis, vertebral hypoplasia, history of radiation

### Limb Length Inequality
- Uneven height of iliac wings on standing film
- Use lifts under foot to equalize leg lengths, determine true scoliosis

### Idiopathic Kyphosis
- No vertebral anomalies

### Scheuermann Kyphosis
- Anterior vertebral wedging, endplate undulations
- 15% have scoliosis too

### Kyphosis Due to Tuberculosis
- May be severe ("gibbus") deformity
- Paraspinous cold abscess, endplate destruction → ± spinal fusion

### Juvenile Chronic Arthritis
- Fusion of vertebral bodies and facet joints
- Scoliosis or kyphosis may be present
- Onset later in childhood

### Ankylosing Spondylitis
- Kyphosis of upper thoracic spine
- Syndesmophytes at anterior vertebral margin mimics congenital bar

## PATHOLOGY

### General Features
- General path comments
  - ○ Curvature 2° to failure of development and/or failure of segmentation
  - ○ Failure of vertebral formation
    - Hypoplastic vertebra anteriorly or on one side (wedge vertebra)
    - Aplastic vertebra anteriorly or on one side (hemivertebra)

# CONGENITAL SCOLIOSIS AND KYPHOSIS

- Butterfly vertebra: Central cleft
- Supernumerary hemivertebrae
- Failure of vertebral segmentation
  - Vertebral body forms from half of two adjacent sclerotomes
  - Apparent congenital vertebral fusion is really failure of segmentation
  - Vertebral body, posterior elements, or both
- Failure of vertebral formation and segmentation may both be present
- Genetics
  - ± Chromosomal abnormalities
  - Usually not inherited
- Etiology: Fetal insult in 1st trimester → abnormal development and/or segmentation of vertebrae
- Epidemiology: Sporadic, uncommon
- Associated abnormalities
  - Klippel Feil (craniocervical, brainstem anomalies)
  - Syringohydromyelia
  - Diastematomyelia
  - Tethered spinal cord
  - Caudal regression
  - Hydrocephalus
  - Component of VACTERL association
    - Incidence of VACTERL 1.6/10,000 live births
    - Defective mesodermal development in early embryogenesis
    - Some cases inherited, others 2° to fetal insult
    - Patients have at least 3 of the following: Vertebral anomalies (37%), anal atresia (63%), cardiac anomalies (77%), tracheo-esophageal fistula (40%), renal and genitourinary anomalies (72%), radial ray hypoplasia (58%)

## Gross Pathologic & Surgical Features
- Bar between vertebrae may be either cartilaginous or osseous

## Microscopic Features
- Bone histologically normal

## Staging, Grading or Classification Criteria
- Classified by type and number of segmentation abnormalities present

# CLINICAL ISSUES

## Presentation
- Most common signs/symptoms: Visible spinal axis deformity
- Clinical Profile: May be isolated anomaly or associated with multisystem anomalies (VACTERL)

## Demographics
- Age: Present at birth; may not be clinically evident until later in childhood or adolescence
- Gender: M = F

## Natural History & Prognosis
- Kyphosis
  - Tendency to progress without treatment; fusion during childhood indicated
  - May lead to cord compression, paralysis

- Scoliosis
  - Difficult to predict which curves will progress
  - "Balanced" anomalies may grow fairly normally
    - E.g., contralateral hemivertebrae at adjacent levels
  - Hemivertebra not fused to adjacent levels causes rapidly progressive curve
  - Hemivertebra with contralateral failure of segmentation causes rapidly progressive curve

## Treatment
- Conservative management
  - Close clinical observation of scoliosis for progression
  - Brace of limited utility
- Surgical management
  - Kyphosis: Fusion to prevent paralysis
  - Scoliosis: Surgery for curves progressing > 10°/yr
    - Anterior or posterior fusion with instrumentation
    - Resection of vertebral bars, hemivertebrae
    - Hemiepiphysiodesis: Fuse growth plate on one side to prevent curve progression

# DIAGNOSTIC CHECKLIST

## Image Interpretation Pearls
- Angular curve on radiography without hemivertebra → probable bony bar
- Vertebral bars may be cartilaginous in young children
- Neural arch not fused in midline until ~ age 2 years; cleft on AP radiograph must not be confused with spinal anomaly
- Image entire spine to exclude additional bone or cord abnormalities, Chiari I malformation

# SELECTED REFERENCES

1. Arlet V et al: Congenital scoliosis. Eur Spine J. 12(5):456-63, 2003
2. Campbell RM Jr et al: Growth of the thoracic spine in congenital scoliosis after expansion thoracoplasty. J Bone Joint Surg Am. 85-A(3):409-20, 2003
3. Hedequist DJ et al: The correlation of preoperative three-dimensional computed tomography reconstructions with operative findings in congenital scoliosis. Spine. 28(22):2531-4; discussion 1, 2003
4. Kim YJ et al: Surgical treatment of congenital kyphosis. Spine. 26(20):2251-7, 2001
5. Redla S et al: Magnetic resonance imaging of scoliosis. Clin Radiol. 56(5):360-71, 2001
6. Jaskwhich D et al: Congenital scoliosis. Curr Opin Pediatr. 12(1):61-6, 2000
7. Oestreich AE et al: Scoliosis circa 2000: radiologic imaging perspective. I. Diagnosis and pretreatment evaluation. Skeletal Radiol. 27(11):591-605, 1998
8. Oestreich AE et al: Scoliosis circa 2000: radiologic imaging perspective. II. Treatment and follow-up. Skeletal Radiol. 27(12):651-6, 1998
9. Rittler M et al: VACTERL association, epidemiologic definition and delineation. Am J Med Genet. 63(4):529-36, 1996
10. Taybi H, Lachman RS: Radiology of syndromes, metabolic disorders, and skeletal dysplasias. 4th ed. St. Louis, Mosby. 510-12, 1996
11. Levine F et al: VACTERL association with high prenatal lead exposure: similarities to animal models of lead teratogenicity. Pediatrics. 87(3):390-2, 1991

# CONGENITAL SCOLIOSIS AND KYPHOSIS

## IMAGE GALLERY

### Typical

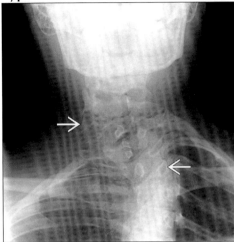 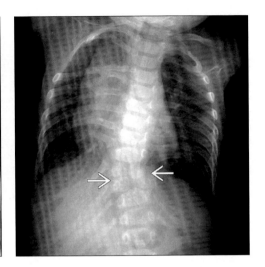

*(Left)* Anteroposterior radiograph shows bilateral cervical and thoracic hemivertebrae ➡ producing focal short curve cervical rightward curvature and leftward thoracic curvature. *(Right)* Anteroposterior radiograph demonstrates focal short curve thoracic scoliosis secondary to asymmetric congenital thoracic vertebral anomalies ➡.

### Typical

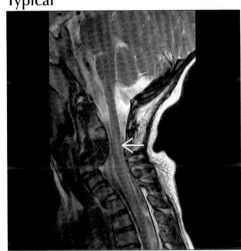 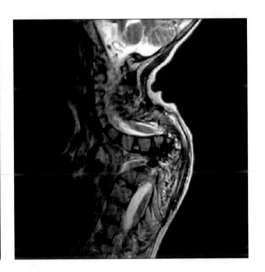

*(Left)* Sagittal T2WI MR (Larsen syndrome) depicts severe cervical kyphosis and exaggerated lordosis from congenital vertebral anomalies. Note focal cord thinning and abnormal signal intensity ➡. *(Right)* Sagittal T2WI MR (VACTERL) depicts severe acute-angle upper thoracic kyphoscoliosis (measured 49 degrees) resulting from associated anterior hemivertebra at the curve apex.

### Typical

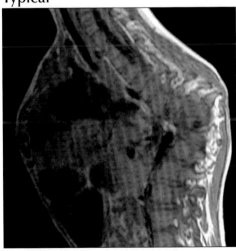 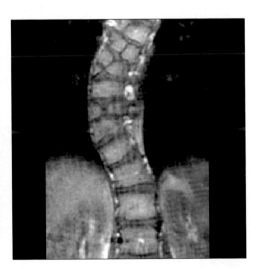

*(Left)* Sagittal T1WI MR (VACTERL) demonstrates severe acute-angle upper thoracic kyphoscoliosis resulting from an anterior hemivertebra located at the curve apex. *(Right)* Coronal T1WI MR demonstrates multiple congenital vertebral formation and segmentation anomalies producing convex rightward scoliotic curvature.

# SCHMORL NODE

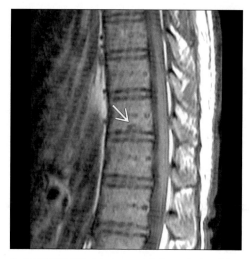

Sagittal T1WI MR shows a rounded vertebral endplate depression with semicircular hypointense line adjacent to endplate ➡, but no edematous marrow changes. Note contiguity with disc space.

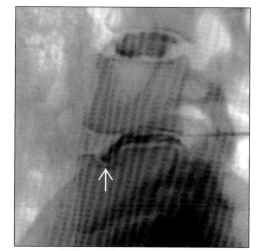

Lateral discogram reveals a superior endplate Schmorl node ➡. Contrast injected into the contiguous intervertebral disc fills herniated disc within the Schmorl node.

## TERMINOLOGY

### Abbreviations and Synonyms
- Intravertebral disc herniation

### Definitions
- Node within vertebral body from vertical disc extension through weakened vertebral endplate

## IMAGING FINDINGS

### General Features
- Best diagnostic clue: Focal invagination of endplate by disc material surrounded by either sclerotic (old) or abnormal bone (acute)
- Location: T8 → L1 most common
- Size: Variable; ranges from small (millimeters) to "giant"
- Morphology
  - Typically upwardly round or cone shaped endplate defect
  - Always contiguous with disc space

### CT Findings
- Bone CT
  - Axial: Island of low density surrounded by condensed bone
  - Sagittal, coronal reformats: End plate defect contiguous with disc space, capped by sclerotic bone
  - Schmorl node may calcify

### MR Findings
- T1WI
  - Focal vertebral endplate defect filled by disc
  - Marrow signal varies with injury stage
    - Low signal intensity edema within adjacent marrow (acute)
    - Normal marrow signal within adjacent marrow (chronic)
- T2WI
  - Focal vertebral endplate defect filled by disc
  - Marrow signal varies with injury stage
    - High signal intensity edema within adjacent marrow (acute)
    - Normal marrow signal within adjacent marrow (chronic)
- STIR: Similar findings to T2WI FS MR

## DDx: Schmorl Node

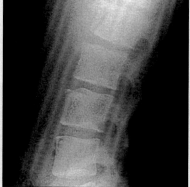

Limbus Vertebra

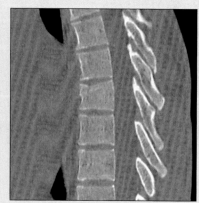

Acute Compression Fracture

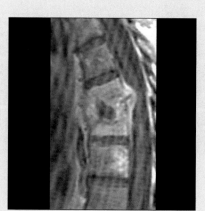

Discitis

# SCHMORL NODE

## Key Facts

### Terminology
- Intravertebral disc herniation

### Imaging Findings
- Location: T8 → L1 most common
- Well-corticated endplate contour defect extending from disc space → vertebral body spongiosa
- Focal vertebral endplate defect filled by disc
- Marrow signal varies with injury stage
- Enhancement varies with injury stage

### Top Differential Diagnoses
- Acute Compression Fracture
- Discitis
- Limbus Vertebrae
- Bone Island

### Pathology
- Secondary to repetitive stress of gravity on immature endplate
- Anulus biomechanically more resistant to mechanical failure than endplate in young individuals
- Focal weakness of endplate predisposes to Schmorl node formation
- Identified in up to 75% of normal spines

### Clinical Issues
- Sudden onset, localized, non-radiating pain, and tenderness in acute cases

### Diagnostic Checklist
- Schmorl node is always contiguous with parent disc
- Confirm contiguity with parent disc on all sequences to make diagnosis

- T1 C+
  - Enhancement varies with injury stage
    - Acute: Diffuse marrow enhancement
    - Subacute: Localized marginal contrast-enhancement
    - Chronic: No abnormal enhancement

## Radiographic Findings
- Radiography
  - Well-corticated endplate contour defect extending from disc space → vertebral body spongiosa
  - ± Sclerotic margins

## Nuclear Medicine Findings
- Bone Scan: ↑ Tc-99m MDP uptake in acute cases

## Imaging Recommendations
- Best imaging tool: MR best establishes presence or absence of edema, excludes Schmorl mimic
- Protocol advice: Multiplanar MR including fat suppressed fluid hyperintense sequence (T2WI FS MR or STIR) and T1 C+ FS MR if acute evaluation

# DIFFERENTIAL DIAGNOSIS

## Acute Compression Fracture
- Simulates diffuse edema of acute Schmorl node
- Lacks imploded disc nodule within abnormal marrow

## Discitis
- Both endplates show defect
- Disc signal diffusely abnormal

## Limbus Vertebrae
- Seen only at vertebral body corners
- Truncated anterior vertebral margin, with bone fragment anterior to defect

## Bone Island
- Sclerotic nodule without endplate defect

## Focal Fatty Marrow
- Hyperintense on T1WI

## Focal Metastasis
- Does not show contiguity with parent disc or disc signal intensity

## Type II Endplate Change
- Reactive change to disc degeneration; typically both adjacent vertebral bodies affected
- No focal end plate defect
- Granulation tissue, edema incited by degenerating disc
- Edema replaced by fat on follow-up MR studies

# PATHOLOGY

## General Features
- General path comments
  - Cartilaginous disc tissue with degenerative or inflammatory changes
    - Typical Schmorl node is a healed focal endplate fracture
    - Pathologic staging mirrors that of focal endplate fracture
- Genetics: Developmental, degenerative, traumatic, and disease influences
- Etiology
  - Secondary to repetitive stress of gravity on immature endplate
    - Anulus biomechanically more resistant to mechanical failure than endplate in young individuals
    - Focal weakness of endplate predisposes to Schmorl node formation
    - Acute axial traumatic load → Schmorl node formation with focal back pain
  - In some cases, endplate is weakened by osteopenia, neoplasm, or infection predisposing to Schmorl node formation
- Epidemiology
  - Identified in up to 75% of normal spines
  - May occur following single traumatic episode

## Gross Pathologic & Surgical Features
- Identical to end plate fracture

## Microscopic Features
- Fibrocartilaginous tissue surrounded by marrow with sclerotic cancellous bone or inflammatory changes

## Staging, Grading or Classification Criteria
- Vertebral body edema next to endplate following acute trauma, pain, no end plate defect on initial MR
- Subsequent formation of a chronic, asymptomatic Schmorl node on follow-up MR

## CLINICAL ISSUES

### Presentation
- Most common signs/symptoms
  - Sudden onset, localized, non-radiating pain, and tenderness in acute cases
  - Most cases found incidentally as chronic, "burned out" lesions
- Clinical Profile: Teenager involved in axial-loading sports

### Demographics
- Age
  - Adolescents and young adults
  - Most acute cases occur between 11-30 years
- Gender: M > F, up to 9:1 ratio

### Natural History & Prognosis
- Self-limited; good prognosis unless systemic osteopenia or pathologic lesion leads to recurrent compression fractures

### Treatment
- Observational, pain management in symptomatic cases
- Some preliminary reports describe vertebroplasty for selected refractory cases

## DIAGNOSTIC CHECKLIST

### Consider
- Follow-up MR in cases of unexplained vertebral body edema and localized pain

### Image Interpretation Pearls
- Schmorl node is always contiguous with parent disc
- Confirm contiguity with parent disc on all sequences to make diagnosis

## SELECTED REFERENCES

1. Masala S et al: Percutaneous vertebroplasty in painful schmorl nodes. Cardiovasc Intervent Radiol. 29(1):97-101, 2006
2. Peng B et al: The pathogenesis of Schmorl's nodes. J Bone Joint Surg Br. 85(6):879-82, 2003
3. Yamaguchi T et al: Schmorl's node developing in the lumbar vertebra affected with metastatic carcinoma: correlation magnetic resonance imaging with histological findings. Spine. 28(24):E503-5, 2003
4. Hauger O et al: Giant cystic Schmorl's nodes: imaging findings in six patients. AJR Am J Roentgenol. 176(4):969-72, 2001
5. Wagner AL et al: Relationship of Schmorl's nodes to vertebral body endplate fractures and acute endplate disk extrusions. AJNR Am J Neuroradiol. 21(2):276-81, 2000
6. Grive E et al: Radiologic findings in two cases of acute Schmorl's nodes. AJNR Am J Neuroradiol. 20(9):1717-21, 1999
7. Silberstein M et al: Spinal Schmorl's nodes: sagittal sectional imaging and pathological examination. Australas Radiol. 43(1):27-30, 1999
8. Fahey V et al: The pathogenesis of Schmorl's nodes in relation to acute trauma. An autopsy study. Spine. 23(21):2272-5, 1998
9. Seymour R et al: Magnetic resonance imaging of acute intraosseous disc herniation. Clin Radiol. 53(5):363-8, 1998
10. Swischuk LE et al: Disk degenerative disease in childhood: Scheuermann's disease, Schmorl's nodes, and the limbus vertebra: MRI findings in 12 patients. Pediatr Radiol. 28(5):334-8, 1998
11. Tribus CB: Scheuermann's kyphosis in adolescents and adults: diagnosis and management. J Am Acad Orthop Surg. 6(1):36-43, 1998
12. Stabler A et al: MR imaging of enhancing intraosseous disk herniation (Schmorl's nodes). AJR Am J Roentgenol. 168(4):933-8, 1997
13. Takahashi K et al: Schmorl's nodes and low-back pain. Analysis of magnetic resonance imaging findings in symptomatic and asymptomatic individuals. Eur Spine J. 4(1):56-9, 1995
14. Hamanishi C et al: Schmorl's nodes on magnetic resonance imaging. Their incidence and clinical relevance. Spine. 19(4):450-3, 1994
15. Jensen MC et al: Magnetic resonance imaging of the lumbar spine in people without back pain. N Engl J Med. 331(2):69-73, 1994
16. Takahashi K et al: A large painful Schmorl's node: a case report. J Spinal Disord. 7(1):77-81, 1994
17. Sward L: The thoracolumbar spine in young elite athletes. Current concepts on the effects of physical training. Sports Med. 13(5):357-64, 1992
18. Walters G et al: Magnetic resonance imaging of acute symptomatic Schmorl's node formation. Pediatr Emerg Care. 7(5):294-6, 1991
19. Sward L et al: Back pain and radiologic changes in the thoraco-lumbar spine of athletes. Spine. 15(2):124-9, 1990
20. Roberts S et al: Biochemical and structural properties of the cartilage end-plate and its relation to the intervertebral disc. Spine. 14(2):166-74, 1989
21. Kagen S et al: Focal uptake on bone imaging in an asymptomatic Schmorl's node. Clin Nucl Med. 13(8):615-6, 1988
22. Kornberg M: MRI diagnosis of traumatic Schmorl's node. A case report. Spine. 13(8):934-5, 1988
23. Yasuma T et al: Schmorl's nodes. Correlation of X-ray and histological findings in postmortem specimens. Acta Pathol Jpn. 38(6):723-33, 1988
24. Malmivaara A et al: Plain radiographic, discographic, and direct observations of Schmorl's nodes in the thoracolumbar junctional region of the cadaveric spine. Spine. 12(5):453-7, 1987
25. Lipson SJ et al: Symptomatic intravertebral disc herniation (Schmorl's node) in the cervical spine. Ann Rheum Dis. 44(12):857-9, 1985
26. Deeg HJ: Schmorl's nodule. N Engl J Med. 298(1):57, 1978

# SCHMORL NODE

## IMAGE GALLERY

### Typical

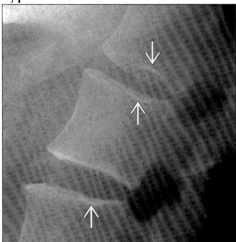
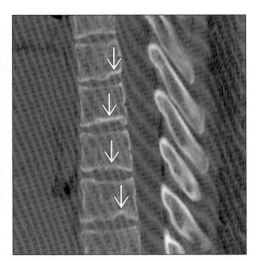

*(Left)* Lateral radiograph of the lumbar spine depicts multiple Schmorl nodes ➡, with characteristic sclerotic marginated saucer-shaped depressions within the vertebral endplates. *(Right)* Sagittal bone CT shows Schmorl nodes at multiple thoracic levels ➡ involving different vertebral endplate locations. Absence of wedge deformity and kyphosis excludes Scheuermann disease.

### Typical

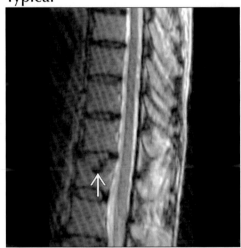
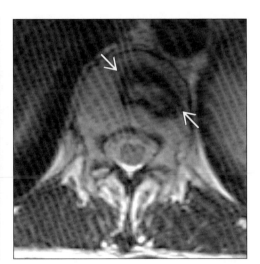

*(Left)* Sagittal T2WI MR shows a large chronic Schmorl node with "cup-shaped" vertebral endplate depression ➡. Note sclerotic margins, disc space contiguity, absence of adjacent marrow edema. *(Right)* Axial T2WI MR demonstrates a large chronic Schmorl node centered in the superior vertebral endplate ➡. Observe central marrow signal intensity with hypointense chronic sclerotic rim.

### Variant

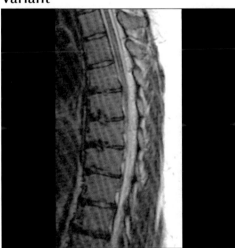
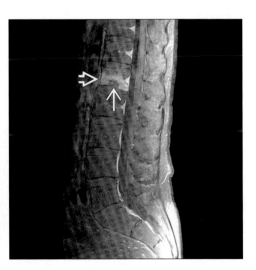

*(Left)* Sagittal T2WI MR (15 year old male) demonstrates multiple thoracic Schmorl nodes. Addition of anterior vertebral wedging and kyphosis is diagnostic of Scheuermann disease. *(Right)* Sagittal T1 C+ MR shows bone bruise adjacent to an acute Schmorl node ➡. Hyperintense edema around node with exuberant "band-like" abnormal marrow enhancement ➡ indicates acute injury.

# SCHEUERMANN DISEASE

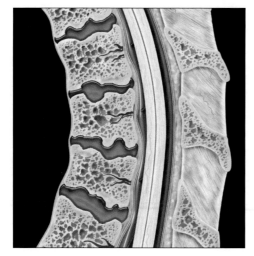

Sagittal graphic shows characteristic herniation of disc through vertebral endplates causing endplate irregularities and subcortical bone defects. Endplate undulations reflect bony reparative process.

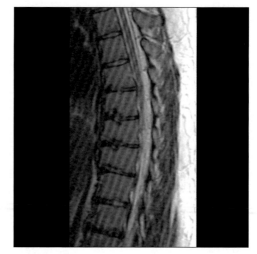

Sagittal T1WI MR in a 15 year old patient shows multilevel anterior thoracic vertebral wedging and endplate undulations with multiple Schmorl nodes producing mild abnormal kyphosis.

## TERMINOLOGY

### Abbreviations and Synonyms

- Juvenile kyphosis, Scheuermann juvenile kyphosis

### Definitions

- Anterior wedging of 3 or more adjacent thoracic vertebral bodies (≥ 5°), multiple Schmorl nodes, and endplate narrowing and undulation → secondary kyphosis
- Schmorl node: Invagination of disc material through vertebral body endplate

## IMAGING FINDINGS

### General Features

- Best diagnostic clue: Three or more adjacent wedged thoracic vertebral bodies (≥ 5° each), irregular, narrowed endplates pathognomonic
- Location: Thoracic (75%) > thoracolumbar (20-25%) > lumbar (< 5%) > > cervical (rare)
- Size
  - Normal thoracic kyphosis increases with age

  - Kyphosis > 40° considered abnormal

### CT Findings

- Bone CT
  - Endplate abnormalities more apparent than on radiography

### MR Findings

- T1WI
  - Schmorl nodes, disc herniations low signal intensity
  - +/- Discogenic sclerosis
- T2WI
  - Schmorl nodes may be low or high signal intensity
    - +/- Bone marrow edema adjacent to Schmorl nodes
  - Disc degeneration in 50% of involved discs
  - Disc herniations

### Radiographic Findings

- Radiography
  - 3 or more contiguous vertebrae, each ≥ 5° of kyphosis
  - Well-defined Schmorl nodes
  - +/- Limbus vertebrae

## DDx: Scheuermann Disease

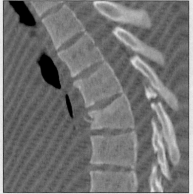

Compression Fracture

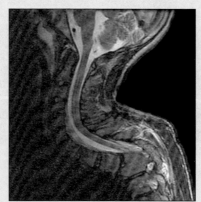

Post-Tuberculosis

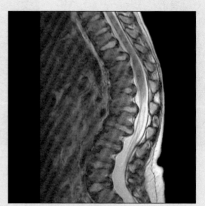

Spondyloepiphyseal Dysplasia

# SCHEUERMANN DISEASE

## Key Facts

### Imaging Findings
- Best diagnostic clue: Three or more adjacent wedged thoracic vertebral bodies (≥ 5° each), irregular, narrowed endplates pathognomonic
- Location: Thoracic (75%) > thoracolumbar (20-25%) > lumbar (< 5%) > > cervical (rare)
- Kyphosis > 40° considered abnormal
- 15% have scoliosis as well as kyphosis

### Top Differential Diagnoses
- Postural Kyphosis
- Wedge Compression Fractures
- Congenital Kyphosis
- Tuberculosis
- Osteogenesis Imperfecta Tarda
- Neuromuscular Disease
- Spondyloepiphyseal Dysplasia Tarda (SED)

### Pathology
- Disc extrusions through weakened regions of vertebral end plates
- Prevalence: 0.4-8% general population
- Peak incidence: 13-17 years

### Clinical Issues
- Thoracic spine pain and tenderness worsened by activity, abated by rest
- Increases in magnitude during adolescent growth spurt

### Diagnostic Checklist
- Radiography may show undulating endplates rather than discrete Schmorl nodes
- Schmorl nodes without anterior wedging not indicative of Scheuermann disease

---

- ○ Disc spaces narrowed, with greatest narrowing anteriorly
- ○ Undulation of endplates secondary to extensive disc invagination
- ○ Thoracic spine: Measure kyphosis from T3 to T12
- ○ Thoracolumbar or lumbar spine
  - ▪ Measure sagittal plane deformity from one vertebra above affected vertebrae to one vertebra below
  - ▪ Better estimate of functional kyphosis
  - ▪ Loss of normal lumbar lordosis functionally significant
- ○ 15% have scoliosis as well as kyphosis
  - ▪ Hyperextension lateral radiograph to assess flexibility of kyphosis

### Nuclear Medicine Findings
- Bone Scan: Normal or ↑ radiotracer uptake

### Other Modality Findings
- Normal bone mineral density (DEXA, CT bone densitometry)

### Imaging Recommendations
- Best imaging tool
  - ○ Plain radiograph for diagnosis
  - ○ MR to exclude disc herniation, cord abnormalities

## DIFFERENTIAL DIAGNOSIS

### Postural Kyphosis
- Vertebral endplates normal
- Deformity usually corrects in hyperextension unless long-standing

### Wedge Compression Fractures
- May involve contiguous levels
- Anterior vertebral cortex often shows angular deformity
- MR shows fracture lines, bone marrow edema

### Congenital Kyphosis
- Vertebral segmentation and fusion anomalies present

### Tuberculosis
- Kyphosis often severe
- Endplate destruction +/- vertebral fusion

### Osteogenesis Imperfecta Tarda
- Platyspondyly
- Severe osteopenia

### Neuromuscular Disease
- Persistence of infantile thoracolumbar kyphosis in nonambulatory patients
- Kyphoscoliosis

### Ankylosing Spondylitis (AS)
- Fusion of vertebral bodies
- Abnormalities of sacroiliac joints

### Spondyloepiphyseal Dysplasia Tarda (SED)
- Platyspondyly throughout spine
- Epiphyses abnormal

## PATHOLOGY

### General Features
- Genetics: Familial tendency
- Etiology
  - ○ Chronic repetitive trauma in a skeletally immature person
    - ▪ Weight lifting, gymnastics, other spine loading sports
    - ▪ Hard physical labor
  - ○ Disc extrusions through weakened regions of vertebral end plates
    - ▪ Disc space loss
    - ▪ Limbus vertebrae
    - ▪ Schmorl nodes
  - ○ Delayed growth in anterior portion of vertebrae causes wedging
- Epidemiology
  - ○ Prevalence: 0.4-8% general population
  - ○ Peak incidence: 13-17 years

# SCHEUERMANN DISEASE

## Gross Pathologic & Surgical Features
- Schmorl nodes invaginate into vertebral bodies through fissures in weakened growth plates
- Limbus vertebrae occur when disc material protrudes through growth plate of ring apophysis
- Thickened anterior longitudinal ligament (ALL) with narrowed intervertebral disks
- Vertebral bodies are wedged, and traumatic disk herniations through endplates are consistent findings

## Microscopic Features
- Vertebral body growth plates
  - Abnormal chondrocytes
  - Loose cartilage matrix
  - Diminished number or thickness of collagen fibers
  - Increased proteoglycan content
- Osteonecrosis, osteochondrosis not seen

## CLINICAL ISSUES

### Presentation
- Most common signs/symptoms
  - Kyphosis
    - Any degree of kyphosis > 40° is abnormal
    - Any degree of kyphosis at thoracolumbar junction or lumbar spine is abnormal
  - Other signs/symptoms
    - Thoracic spine pain and tenderness worsened by activity, abated by rest
    - Neurologic symptoms from kyphosis or from disc herniations
    - Fatigue
  - Pain, progressive deformity, neurologic compromise, cardiopulmonary complaints (rare), cosmetic issues

### Demographics
- Age
  - Develops in adolescence, may present later in life
  - Adolescents typically develop a progressive cosmetic deformity, which first brings them in for medical attention
  - Adults with long-standing deformity typically develop pain as an indication for treatment
- Gender: Actively debated, probably slight male predominance

### Natural History & Prognosis
- Increases in magnitude during adolescent growth spurt
- Mild progression after growth is complete
- Severe deformity uncommon
- Kyphosis greater than 70° has poor functional result
- Premature disc herniations related to degeneration, mechanical stress from spine deformity

### Treatment
- Observation
  - Indications
    - Growth still remains
    - Kyphotic deformity less than 50°
  - Elimination of the specific strenuous activity
  - Analgesics
  - Spine exercises

  - Follow-up until growth-plate fuses ≈ age 25
- Brace treatment
  - Indications
    - At least one year of growth remains
    - < 70° kyphosis
    - At least partial correction of kyphosis on hyperextension
- Surgical treatment
  - Uncommonly necessary
  - Indications
    - > 75° kyphosis in skeletally immature person
    - > 60° kyphosis in mature person
    - Excessive pain
    - Neurologic deficit
  - Posterior instrumentation and fusion
  - Anterior and posterior fusion for more severe kyphosis

## DIAGNOSTIC CHECKLIST

### Image Interpretation Pearls
- Radiography may show undulating endplates rather than discrete Schmorl nodes
- Schmorl nodes without anterior wedging not indicative of Scheuermann disease

## SELECTED REFERENCES

1. Arlet V et al: Scheuermann's kyphosis: surgical management. Eur Spine J. 14(9):817-27, 2005
2. Riaz S et al: Neurologic compression by thoracic disc in a case of scheuermann kyphosis - an infrequent combination. J Coll Physicians Surg Pak. 15(9):573-5, 2005
3. Faingold R et al: Imaging of low back pain in children and adolescents. Semin Ultrasound CT MR. 25(6):490-505, 2004
4. Lim M et al: Scheuermann kyphosis: safe and effective surgical treatment using multisegmental instrumentation. Spine. 29(16):1789-94, 2004
5. Soo CL et al: Scheuermann kyphosis: long-term follow-up. Spine J. 2(1):49-56, 2002
6. Stotts AK et al: Measurement of spinal kyphosis: implications for the management of Scheuermann's kyphosis. Spine. 27(19):2143-6, 2002
7. Wenger DR et al: Scheuermann kyphosis. Spine. 24(24):2630-9, 1999
8. Swischuk LE et al: Disk degenerative disease in childhood: Scheuermann's disease, Schmorl's nodes, and the limbus vertebra: MRI findings in 12 patients. Pediatr Radiol. 28(5):334-8, 1998
9. Tribus CB: Scheuermann's kyphosis in adolescents and adults: diagnosis and management. J Am Acad Orthop Surg. 6(1):36-43, 1998
10. Murray PM et al: The natural history and long-term follow-up of Scheuermann kyphosis. J Bone Joint Surg Am. 75(2):236-48, 1993
11. McKenzie L et al: Familial Scheuermann disease: a genetic and linkage study. J Med Genet. 29(1):41-5, 1992
12. Gilsanz V et al: Vertebral bone density in Scheuermann disease. J Bone Joint Surg Am. 71(6):894-7, 1989
13. Fon GT et al: Thoracic kyphosis: range in normal subjects. AJR Am J Roentgenol. 134(5):979-83, 1980

# SCHEUERMANN DISEASE

## IMAGE GALLERY

### Typical

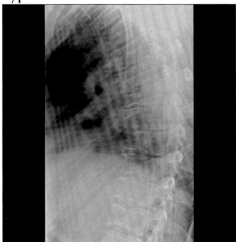 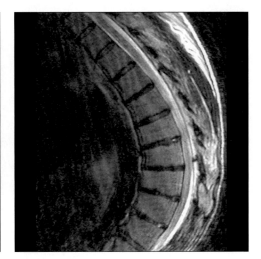

*(Left)* Lateral radiograph demonstrates thoracic kyphosis with anterior wedging and endplate irregularity characteristic of Scheuermann disease. *(Right)* Sagittal T2WI MR demonstrates marked thoracic kyphosis, with more than four consecutive thoracic vertebrae each wedged ≥ 5°. Endplates undulate, with several discrete Schmorl nodes.

### Typical

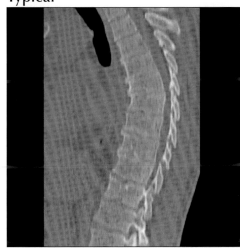 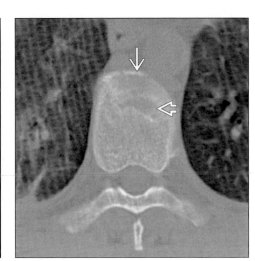

*(Left)* Sagittal bone CT depicts thoracic kyphosis with multilevel anterior vertebral body wedging and endplate irregularity. These findings are characteristic of Scheuermann disease. *(Right)* Axial bone CT confirms thoracic vertebral body ➡ anterior endplate irregularity and Schmorl node ➡.

### Variant

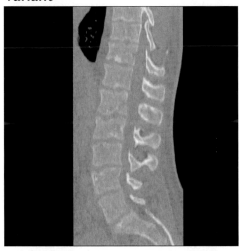 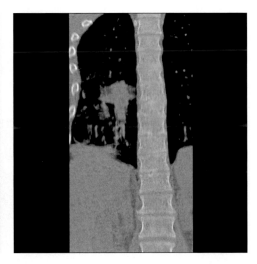

*(Left)* Sagittal bone CT demonstrates both thoracic and lumbar vertebral body wedging and endplate irregularity with multiple Schmorl nodes. *(Right)* Coronal bone CT confirms mild focal scoliosis with usual endplate irregularity. Scoliosis (15% of Scheuermann patients) is often mild and more focal compared to idiopathic scoliosis.

# ACHONDROPLASIA

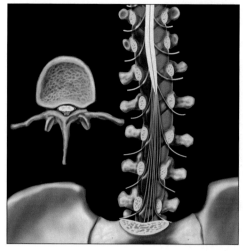

*Coronal graphic shows progressive caudad narrowing of interpediculate distance. Axial insert image shows spinal stenosis related to short pedicles & decreased interpediculate distance.*

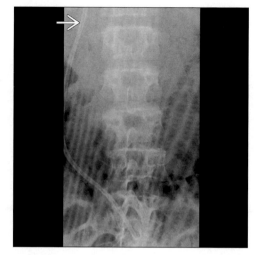

*Anteroposterior radiograph depicts classic progressive interpediculate distance narrowing caudally. Note VP shunt tubing ➡ to treat hydrocephalus resulting from foramen magnum stenosis.*

## TERMINOLOGY

### Abbreviations and Synonyms
- Synonym: Achondroplastic dwarfism

### Definitions
- Autosomal dominant dwarfism affecting spine, extremities
- Rhizomelic dwarfism; most severe growth disturbance occurs in proximal limbs

## IMAGING FINDINGS

### General Features
- Best diagnostic clue: Lumbar interpediculate distance progressively decreases in caudal direction (reversal of normal relationship)
- Location: Spine, skull, pelvis, extremities
- Morphology
  ○ Severe dwarfism involves trunk and extremities
  ○ Vertebral bodies mildly flattened with short pedicles
  ○ Lumbar hyperlordosis
  ○ Thoracolumbar kyphosis

### CT Findings
- NECT: Communicating hydrocephalus (uncommon)
- Bone CT
  ○ Small foramen magnum
  ○ Mildly flattened vertebral bodies
  ○ Bullet shaped vertebral bodies
  ○ Posterior vertebral body scalloping
  ○ Osseous spinal stenosis 2° to degenerative disease superimposed on congenital short pedicles
  ○ Deformity may lead to stress fractures

### MR Findings
- Morphologic changes as described for CT
- Compression of cervicomedullary junction, spinal cord, nerve roots ⇒ myelomalacia
- Disc herniations common

### Radiographic Findings
- Radiography
  ○ Lumbar interpedicular distance progressively decreases in caudad direction
  ○ Vertebral bodies slightly flattened with short pedicles
  ○ ± Bullet-shaped vertebral bodies

## DDx: Achondroplasia

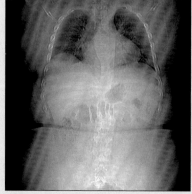

*Hypochondroplasia*

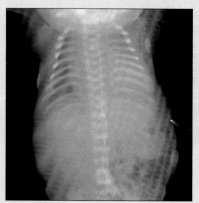

*Thanatophoric Dwarfism*

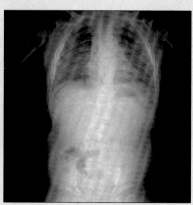

*SED Congenita*

# ACHONDROPLASIA

## Key Facts

### Terminology
- Autosomal dominant dwarfism affecting spine, extremities
- Rhizomelic dwarfism; most severe growth disturbance occurs in proximal limbs

### Imaging Findings
- Lumbar interpedicular distance progressively decreases in caudad direction
- Vertebral bodies slightly flattened with short pedicles
- ± Bullet-shaped vertebral bodies
- Thoracolumbar kyphosis
- Osseous spinal stenosis 2° to degenerative disease superimposed on congenital short pedicles
- Best imaging tool: Single AP "babygram" at birth shows skull, spine, pelvic abnormalities

### Top Differential Diagnoses
- Pseudoachondroplasia
- Hypochondroplasia
- Diastrophic Dysplasia
- Spondyloepiphyseal Dysplasia (SED) Congenita
- Thanatophoric Dysplasia
- Osteogenesis Imperfecta (OI)

### Pathology
- Autosomal dominant (usually spontaneous mutation)
- Epidemiology: Most common nonlethal skeletal dysplasia (1:26,000 live births)

### Diagnostic Checklist
- Most likely cause of short limbed dwarfism with normal ossification detected in 3rd trimester

---

- Usually seen in childhood, resolve by adulthood
  - Thoracolumbar kyphosis
    - Initially flexible deformity
    - May progress either to fixed gibbus deformity or resolve as child grows
  - Lumbar hyperlordosis
  - ± Mild scoliosis
  - ± Craniocervical stenosis; C1-2 instability rare
  - Extraspinal findings
    - "Champagne glass" pelvis: Pelvic inlet is flat and broad
    - Squared iliac wings
    - Shortened long bones, most prominent in proximal long bones ("rhizomelic")
    - Short ribs
    - "Trident hand": 2nd, 3rd and 4th digits equal in length
    - Enlarged skull
  - Bone mineral density normal

## Ultrasonographic Findings
- Growth disturbance evident in 3rd trimester obstetrical ultrasound
- Homozygous form may be diagnosed in 2nd trimester
- Ossification normal

## Non-Vascular Interventions
- Myelography
  - Spinal stenosis
  - Disc herniations common

## Imaging Recommendations
- Best imaging tool: Single AP "babygram" at birth shows skull, spine, pelvic abnormalities
- Protocol advice
  - 2-3 mm axial slices multidetector CT with sagittal and coronal reformats
  - Axial, sagittal MR through foramen magnum in all infants and children to assess for stenosis

# DIFFERENTIAL DIAGNOSIS

## Pseudoachondroplasia
- Facial features and skull normal
- Usually detected in early childhood rather than at birth
- Vertebral body flattening variably seen

## Hypochondroplasia
- Midface hypoplasia
- Similar to (but milder than) achondroplasia

## Diastrophic Dysplasia
- Facial features marked by micrognathia
- Flattened vertebral bodies; narrowed interpediculate distances
- Scoliosis and kyphosis
- C1-2 instability (uncommon in achondroplasia)
- Subluxations in extremities ("hitchhiker's thumb")
- Clubfoot

## Spondyloepiphyseal Dysplasia (SED) Congenita
- Facial features and skull normal
- Severe vertebral body flattening
- C1-2 instability, odontoid hypoplasia
- Flattening, delayed ossification of epiphyses
- Shortened long bones
- Absent pubic ossification (infants)

## Thanatophoric Dysplasia
- Lethal dwarfism
- Severe platyspondyly
- Long, narrow trunk
- Bell-shaped thorax
- ± "Cloverleaf" skull

## Osteogenesis Imperfecta (OI)
- Infantile form has short, thick bones, multiple fractures
- Milder forms present in childhood or adulthood with short stature, platyspondyly, osteopenia, fractures, bone deformities

# ACHONDROPLASIA

## PATHOLOGY

### General Features
- Genetics
  - Gene mapped to chromosome 4p16.3
  - Autosomal dominant (usually spontaneous mutation)
  - Same allele as hypochondroplasia, thanatophoric dwarfism
  - Homozygous form rare, much more severe than heterozygous
- Etiology: Fibroblast growth factor receptor abnormality
- Epidemiology: Most common nonlethal skeletal dysplasia (1:26,000 live births)

### Gross Pathologic & Surgical Features
- Spinal canal stenosis
  - Premature fusion of neural arch synchondroses
  - Short pedicles, thickened laminae
  - Disc bulges and herniations contribute to stenosis
  - Can occur at all spinal levels
  - Significant cause of morbidity in adults
- Foramen magnum stenosis
  - Found in almost all children with achondroplasia
  - Often resolves functionally as child grows
- Thoracolumbar kyphosis
  - Related to hypotonia in infants
  - Often resolves, but may develop fixed deformity
  - ~ 30% of adults

### Microscopic Features
- Disruption of growth plate enchondral ossification

## CLINICAL ISSUES

### Presentation
- Most common signs/symptoms: Dwarfism, characteristic facies evident at birth
- Other signs/symptoms
  - Sudden infant death
  - Infantile hypotonia
  - Sleep apnea in infants and children due to compression of cord at foramen magnum
  - Chest wall deformity may lead to respiratory difficulties
  - Spinal stenosis
  - Thoracolumbar kyphosis
  - Limb lengthening procedures can lead to neurologic symptoms
- Clinical Profile
  - Rhizomelic dwarfism apparent at birth
  - Frontal bossing and depressed nasal bridge characteristic
  - Intelligence normal
  - Obesity a common clinical problem
  - Probably overdiagnosed clinically

### Demographics
- Age: Congenital; diagnosis usually made in infancy
- Gender: M = F

### Natural History & Prognosis
- High morbidity from spinal stenosis

### Treatment
- Conservative
  - Growth hormone can promote growth of long bones
  - Kyphosis may be preventable by not allowing hypotonic infant to sit unassisted
  - Bracing, fusion for thoracolumbar kyphosis
- Surgical
  - Surgical decompression of foramen magnum in severe cases
  - VP shunt for symptomatic hydrocephalus
  - Surgical decompression for spinal stenosis
  - Ilizarov limb lengthening procedure controversial

## DIAGNOSTIC CHECKLIST

### Consider
- Most likely cause of short limbed dwarfism with normal ossification detected in 3rd trimester

### Image Interpretation Pearls
- Stress fracture or disc herniation may present acutely; best evaluated with CT or MR
- Spine imaging must include foramen magnum to evaluate for stenosis

## SELECTED REFERENCES

1. Moritani T et al: Magnetic resonance venography of achondroplasia: correlation of venous narrowing at the jugular foramen with hydrocephalus. Clin Imaging. 30(3):195-200, 2006
2. Misra SN et al: Thoracolumbar spinal deformity in achondroplasia. Neurosurg Focus. 14(1):e4, 2003
3. Park HW et al: Correction of lumbosacral hyperlordosis in achondroplasia. Clin Orthop. (414):242-9, 2003
4. Tanaka N et al: The comparison of the effects of short-term growth hormone treatment in patients with achondroplasia and with hypochondroplasia. Endocr J. 50(1):69-75, 2003
5. Thomeer RT et al: Surgical treatment of lumbar stenosis in achondroplasia. J Neurosurg. 96(3 Suppl):292-7, 2002
6. Gordon N: The neurological complications of achondroplasia. Brain Dev. 22(1):3-7, 2000
7. Keiper GL Jr et al: Achondroplasia and cervicomedullary compression: prospective evaluation and surgical treatment. Pediatr Neurosurg. 31(2):78-83, 1999
8. Lemyre E et al: Bone dysplasia series. Achondroplasia, hypochondroplasia and thanatophoric dysplasia: review and update. Can Assoc Radiol J. 50(3):185-97, 1999
9. Lachman RS: Neurologic abnormalities in the skeletal dysplasias: a clinical and radiological perspective. Am J Med Genet. 69(1):33-43, 1997
10. Taybi H et al: Radiology of syndromes, metabolic disorders, and skeletal dysplasias. 4th ed. St. Louis, Mosby. 748-55, 1996
11. Hall JG: Information update on Achondroplasia. Pediatrics. 95(4):620, 1995
12. Ryken TC et al: Cervicomedullary compression in achondroplasia. J Neurosurg. 81(1):43-8, 1994
13. Hecht JT et al: Neurologic morbidity associated with achondroplasia. J Child Neurol. 5(2):84-97, 1990

# ACHONDROPLASIA

## IMAGE GALLERY

### Typical

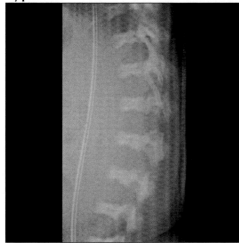
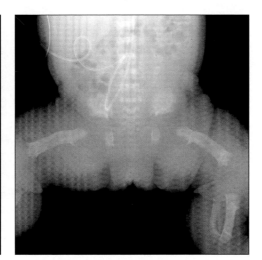

*(Left)* Lateral radiograph (neonate) demonstrates platyspondyly and distinctive notched endplates. These characteristic endplate changes resolve during childhood. *(Right)* Anteroposterior radiograph (neonate) shows characteristic achondroplasia findings at birth (flat vertebral bodies, narrow caudal interpediculate distance, pelvic/long bone deformities).

### Typical

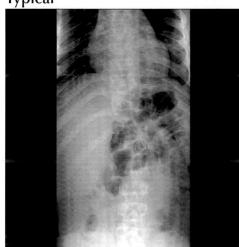
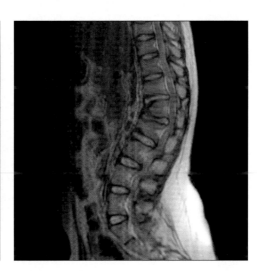

*(Left)* Anteroposterior radiograph demonstrates characteristic narrowing of the interpediculate distance in the distal lumbar spine, mild convex left scoliosis. *(Right)* Sagittal T2WI MR shows hypoplastic, bullet shaped L1 and L2 vertebra producing focal kyphosis. Spinal canal is narrowed due to short pedicles. Note posterior vertebral scalloping.

### Typical

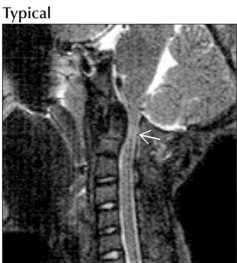
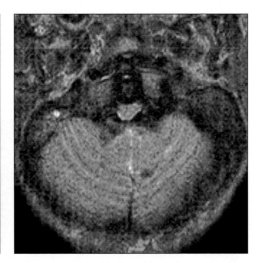

*(Left)* Sagittal T2WI MR depicts shortening of the AP diameter at the foramen magnum producing spinal stenosis, abnormal spinal cord T2 signal hyperintensity ➜. *(Right)* Axial T2WI MR in pediatric achondroplasia patient with myelopathy confirms moderately severe upper cervical spinal canal stenosis with narrowed AP diameter at the level of the dens.

# MUCOPOLYSACCHARIDOSES, SPINE

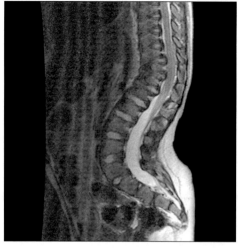

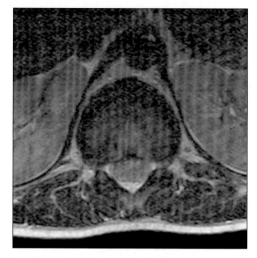

*Sagittal T2WI MR (MPS IV) demonstrates focal kyphosis at the thoracolumbar junction and prominent flattening of the vertebral bodies and accentuation of the intervertebral disc spaces.*

*Axial T2WI MR (MPS IV) confirms anteroposterior narrowing of the thoracolumbar central spinal canal, which is accentuated by short pedicles.*

## TERMINOLOGY

### Abbreviations and Synonyms
- Mucopolysaccharidoses (MPS), lysosomal storage disorder, "gargoylism"

### Definitions
- Inherited lysosomal storage disorders
  - Specific enzyme deficiency ⇒ inability to breakdown specific glycosaminoglycans (GAG)
  - Failure to break down GAG ⇒ intracellular accumulation and toxicity

## IMAGING FINDINGS

### General Features
- Best diagnostic clue: Dens hypoplasia, craniovertebral junction (CVJ) stenosis, and thickened dural ring at foramen magnum
- Location
  - Spine: CVJ, thoracolumbar spine, pelvis
  - Extraspinal: Brain, visceral organ deposition

- Size: Odontoid soft tissue mass varies from small to large; larger masses usually found in older patients
- Morphology
  - Craniocervical spine
    - Skull base thickening, occipital hypoplasia, short posterior C1 arch, odontoid hypoplasia +/- os odontoideum, ligamentous laxity, dural sac stenosis, and atlantoaxial instability
  - Thoracolumbar spine
    - Kyphosis, kyphoscoliosis
    - Platyspondyly, anterior beaking + thoracolumbar gibbus deformity (MPS I-H and IV)

### CT Findings
- CECT: CVJ central and foraminal narrowing, marked dural thickening without abnormal enhancement
- Bone CT
  - Abnormal dens ossification, marked laminar thickening, enlargement of medullary cavity

### MR Findings
- T1WI: Hypo- to isointense peri-odontoid soft tissue mass, hypointense thickened dura
- T2WI
  - Hypoplastic dens and peri-odontoid soft tissue mass

## DDx: Mucopolysaccharidosis

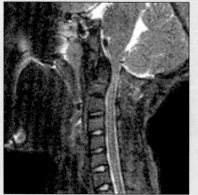

*Achondroplasia*

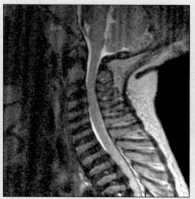

*Spondylometaphyseal Dysplasia*

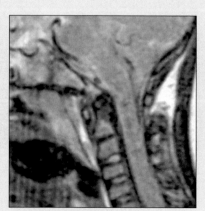

*Down Syndrome*

# MUCOPOLYSACCHARIDOSES, SPINE

## Key Facts

### Terminology
- Mucopolysaccharidoses (MPS), lysosomal storage disorder, "gargoylism"
- Inherited lysosomal storage disorders
- Specific enzyme deficiency ⇒ inability to breakdown specific glycosaminoglycans (GAG)

### Imaging Findings
- Best diagnostic clue: Dens hypoplasia, craniovertebral junction (CVJ) stenosis, and thickened dural ring at foramen magnum
- Platyspondyly, anterior beaking + thoracolumbar gibbus deformity (MPS I-H and IV)

### Top Differential Diagnoses
- GM1 Gangliosidosis
- Mucolipidosis III (Pseudo-Hurler Polydystrophy)

- Achondroplasia
- Down Syndrome
- Spondyloepiphyseal Dysplasia

### Pathology
- Odontoid hypoplasia, GAG deposition, +/- ligamentous laxity with reactive change produce soft tissue mass around dens

### Clinical Issues
- Premature death the rule; rate of deterioration depends on specific enzymatic deficiency

### Diagnostic Checklist
- Dens hypoplasia with mass and dural thickening suggests MPS syndrome

---

- Hypointense, thickened dura +/- cyst formation due to meningeal thickening (MPS 1-H, II)
- +/- Cord compression with hyperintense signal abnormality
- T1 C+: No abnormal enhancement, even if mass present
- MRS: Brain proton MRS may show diminished NAA/choline ratio, elevated glutamine/glutamate and inositol peak areas

### Radiographic Findings
- Radiography
  - Odontoid dysplasia +/- atlanto-axial subluxation
  - Dysplastic blunted spinous processes, wedged vertebral bodies, and spinal canal stenosis
  - Thoracolumbar inferior (MPS I-H) or central (MPS IV) vertebral beaking, gibbus deformity

### Fluoroscopic Findings
- +/- Dynamic CVJ instability on flexion-extension

### Imaging Recommendations
- Best imaging tool: MR imaging
- Protocol advice
  - Spine MR imaging to elucidate cause/site of cord compression
  - Plain radiographs to characterize osseous spine and limb abnormalities
  - Flexion-extension radiographs or fluoroscopy to detect craniovertebral instability

## DIFFERENTIAL DIAGNOSIS

### GM1 Gangliosidosis
- Shares features of vertebral beaking, upper lumbar gibbus, and dens hypoplasia
- Distinguish on clinical, genetic criteria

### Mucolipidosis III (Pseudo-Hurler Polydystrophy)
- Shares features of vertebral beaking, upper lumbar gibbus, and dens hypoplasia

- Distinguish on clinical, genetic criteria

### Achondroplasia
- Autosomal dominant disorder of enchondral bone formation
- Short broad pedicles and thickened laminae ⇒ spinal stenosis
- Distinguish on genetic, clinical criteria

### Down Syndrome
- +/- Dens hypoplasia without soft tissue dens mass or marrow deposition features
- Distinguish using genetic and clinical information

### Spondyloepiphyseal Dysplasia
- Autosomal dominant; presents at birth
- Flattening of vertebral bodies, dens hypoplasia, scoliosis
- Minimal hand and foot involvement

## PATHOLOGY

### General Features
- General path comments
  - GAG accumulates in most organs and ligaments
    - Coarse facies (hence the name "gargoylism")
    - Hepatosplenomegaly, umbilical hernia,
    - Skeletal dysotosis multiplex, joint contractures
    - Arterial wall (mid-aortic stenosis), cardiac valve thickening
    - Upper airway obstruction (38%); very difficult intubations
  - Odontoid hypoplasia, GAG deposition, +/- ligamentous laxity with reactive change produce soft tissue mass around dens
  - Biconvex ovoid, bullet shaped or rectangular vertebral bodies, vertebral beaking, posterior vertebral slip (MPS IV), large disc protrusions (MPS VI)
- Genetics: Autosomal recessive (except MPS II Hunters; X-linked recessive)
- Etiology: Inherited lysosomal enzyme deficiency

# MUCOPOLYSACCHARIDOSES, SPINE

- Epidemiology: MPS I-H (1:10,000 births), MPS IV (1:40,000 births) most common

## Gross Pathologic & Surgical Features
- CVJ stenosis ⇒ neurovascular compression, altered CSF dynamics ⇒ hydrocephalus, hydrosyringomyelia
- Dilated enlarged laminae medullary cavities
- Thickened dura may appear normal at surgery

## Microscopic Features
- Epidural/dural mucopolysaccharide deposition with elastic and collagenous proliferation

## Staging, Grading or Classification Criteria
- Hurler (MPS I-H), Hurler-Scheie (MPS 1-H/S): α-L-iduronidase (4p16.3)
- Hunter (MPS II): Iduronate 2-sulfatase (Xq28)
- Sanfillipo (MPS III): Heparin N-sulfatase (17q25.3)
- Morquio (MPS IV): Galactose 6-sulfatase (16q24.3)
- Scheie (MPS V)
- Maroteaux-Lamy (MPS VI): Arylsulfatase B (5q11-q13)
- Sly (MPS VII)

# CLINICAL ISSUES

## Presentation
- Most common signs/symptoms
  - Gradual subtle progressive myelopathy (often falsely attributed to lower extremity deformities)
    - Common with MPS I-H, II, III, and VII; uncommon with MPS IV, I H/S, VI unless associated with musculoskeletal deformities
    - Reduced exercise tolerance; may be earliest symptom
  - Clinical neurologic symptoms attributable to brain GAG deposition, myelination abnormalities, spinal deformities, and peripheral nerve entrapment
- Clinical Profile
  - Coarse facies with macroglossia, bushy eyebrows, flat nasal bridge (mild in MPS VI, VII)
  - Corneal clouding (except MPS II)
  - Significant mental retardation (except in MPS I H/S, IIb, IV)
  - Joint contractures, dysostosis multiplex (dominates in MPS IV, VI)
- Laboratory diagnosis: Measurement of specific urinary glycosaminoglycans
- Clinical diagnostic algorithm
  - Age, IQ, +/- corneal clouding, urinary GAG excretion, and specific clinical findings

## Demographics
- Age: Usually diagnosed in childhood; occasional mild cases diagnosed as adults
- Gender: M = F except MPS II (boys only ⇒ X-linked)

## Natural History & Prognosis
- Premature death the rule; rate of deterioration depends on specific enzymatic deficiency
- Slowly progressive cord compression ⇒ quadriparesis, sensory loss without treatment
  - Surgical results poor when performed late in disease course

- High spinal cord compression is major spinal cause of MPS complications and death
  - Apnea and sudden death may follow relatively minor trauma

## Treatment
- Options, risks, complications
  - Conservative (mild symptoms): External spinal bracing
  - Surgical (more severe symptoms)
    - Posterior occipitocervical decompression/stabilization
    - Transoral odontoid resection/posterior stabilization for symptomatic dens mass
  - Bone marrow transplant (BMT) or intravenous recombinant human enzyme
    - Decreases GAG accumulation in organs; ameliorates some but not all manifestations

# DIAGNOSTIC CHECKLIST

## Consider
- Successful diagnosis requires combination of clinical, imaging, and genetic/biochemical information

## Image Interpretation Pearls
- Dens hypoplasia with mass and dural thickening suggests MPS syndrome
- Vertebral beaking pattern may permit specific diagnosis

# SELECTED REFERENCES

1. Dickerman RD et al: Craniovertebral instability with spinal cord compression in a 17-month-old boy with Sly syndrome (mucopolysaccharidosis type VII): a surgical dilemma. Spine. 29(5):E92-4, 2004
2. Weisstein JS et al: Musculoskeletal manifestations of Hurler syndrome: long-term follow-up after bone marrow transplantation. J Pediatr Orthop. 24(1):97-101, 2004
3. Vougioukas VI et al: Neurosurgical interventions in children with Maroteaux-Lamy syndrome. Case report and review of the literature. Pediatr Neurosurg. 35(1):35-8, 2001
4. Chirossel JP et al: Management of craniocervical junction dislocation. Childs Nerv Syst. 16(10-11):697-701, 2000
5. Kim FM et al: Neuroimaging of scoliosis in childhood. Neuroimaging Clinics of North America. 9(1):213-14, 1999
6. Levin TL et al: Lumbar gibbus in storage diseases and bone dysplasias. Pediatr Radiol. 27(4): 289-94, 1997
7. Piccirilli CB et al: Cervical kyphotic myelopathy in a child with Morquio syndrome. Childs Nerv Syst. 12(2):114-6, 1996
8. Crockard HA et al: Craniovertebral junction anomalies in inherited disorders: part of the syndrome or caused by the disorder? Eur J Pediatr. 154(7):504-12, 1995
9. Vinchon M et al: Cervical myelopathy secondary to Hunter syndrome in an adult. AJNR Am J Neuroradiol. 16(7):1402-3, 1995
10. Blaser S et al: Neuroradiology of lysosomal disorders. Neuroimaging Clin NA. 4:283-98, 1994
11. Stevens JM et al: The odontoid process in Morquio-Brailsford's disease. The effects of occipitocervical fusion. J Bone Joint Surg Br. 73(5):851-8, 1991
12. Banna M et al: Compressive meningeal hypertrophy in mucopolysaccharidosis. AJNR Am J Neuroradiol. 8(2):385-6, 1987

# MUCOPOLYSACCHARIDOSES, SPINE

## IMAGE GALLERY

### Typical

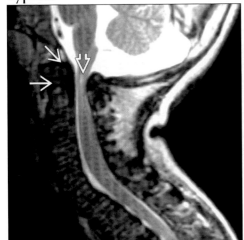 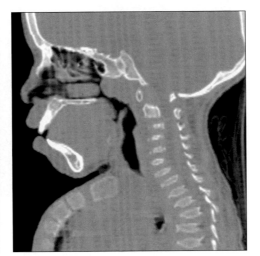

*(Left) Sagittal T2WI MR (MPS IV) demonstrates odontoid hypoplasia and markedly hypointense pannus ⇒ producing cord compression and abnormal cord T2 hyperintensity ⇛ at the CVJ. (Right) Sagittal bone CT (MPS IV) shows severe vertebral hypoplasia and malformation of the cervical vertebral bodies, with flattening and anterior beaking, characteristic of Morquio syndrome.*

### Variant

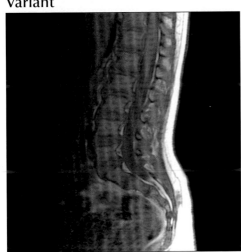 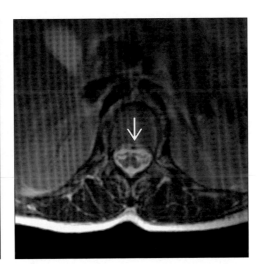

*(Left) Sagittal T1WI MR (MPS I-H) demonstrates posterior vertebral scalloping without dural dysplasia. The vertebral changes associated with Hurler syndrome are relatively subtle. (Right) Axial T2WI MR (MPS I-H) in a mildly affected patient confirms posterior vertebral scalloping ⇛ but no central spinal canal narrowing.*

### Variant

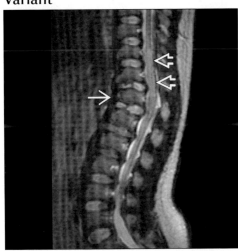 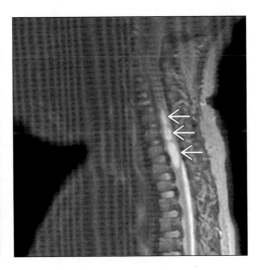

*(Left) Sagittal T2WI MR (MPS VI) shows anteriorly beaked vertebral bodies, canal stenosis, and focal lumbar kyphosis ⇒. Abnormal cord T2 signal intensity ⇛ represents secondary cord injury. (Right) Sagittal T2WI MR (MPS VI) reveals characteristic mucopolysaccharidosis vertebral changes. Hydrosyringomyelia (spanning from C5 to T1 ⇒) is an uncommon finding.*

# SICKLE CELL DISEASE, SPINE

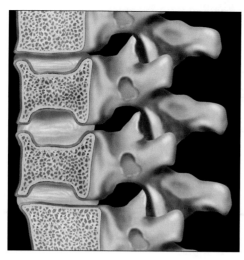

Sagittal graphic depicts multiple endplate compression fractures. SCD infarcts tend to affect central portion of vertebral body → focal central collapse, preservation of height peripherally.

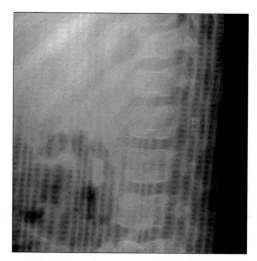

Lateral radiograph demonstrates multiple endplate middle compressions producing the classic "H-shaped" vertebra characteristic of SCD.

## TERMINOLOGY

### Abbreviations and Synonyms
- Synonyms: Sickle cell anemia (SCA), hemoglobin HbSS disease, HbSC disease

## IMAGING FINDINGS

### General Features
- Best diagnostic clue: "H-shaped" vertebral bodies
- Location: Spine: (43-70%)

### CT Findings
- Bone CT
  ○ Mottled sclerotic bone density

### MR Findings
- T1WI: Hypointense marrow (hyperplastic hematopoietic marrow, infarction, iron deposition, infection)
- T2WI: Variable hypointense (iron deposition) → hyperintense (infarct, osteomyelitis)

- T1 C+: Thin, linear serpentine (infarct) or diffuse/rim enhancement (osteomyelitis)

### Radiographic Findings
- Radiography: Osteopenia, "H-shaped" vertebrae, sclerosis, "bone-within-bone"

## DIFFERENTIAL DIAGNOSIS

### Thalassemia
- Avascular necrosis less common than in SCA

### Other Diagnoses May Mimic Radiographically, But Not Clinically
- Renal osteodystrophy
  ○ Thickened, dense vertebral endplates
- Osteopetrosis
  ○ Diffuse bone sclerosis
- Spondyloepiphyseal dysplasia (SED)
  ○ Cup shaped vertebral endplates
- Diffuse marrow replacement
  ○ Diffuse low signal marrow on T1WI MR

## DDx: Sickle Cell Disease

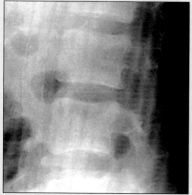

*Renal Osteodystrophy*

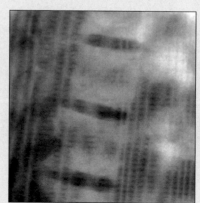

*Osteopetrosis*

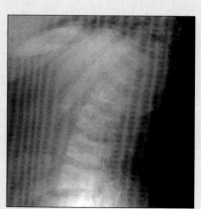

*Spondyloepiphyseal Dysplasia*

# SICKLE CELL DISEASE, SPINE

## Key Facts

### Terminology
- Synonyms: Sickle cell anemia (SCA), hemoglobin HbSS disease, HbSC disease

### Imaging Findings
- Best diagnostic clue: "H-shaped" vertebral bodies

### Top Differential Diagnoses
- Thalassemia
- Renal osteodystrophy

- Osteopetrosis
- Spondyloepiphyseal dysplasia (SED)
- Diffuse marrow replacement

### Pathology
- Sickled cells occlude small blood vessels → multisystem infarcts

### Diagnostic Checklist
- MR distinguishes acute infarction, osteomyelitis

## PATHOLOGY

### General Features
- Genetics
  - Autosomal recessive
    - Homozygous SCD: HbSS (sickle cell anemia)
    - Heterozygous SCD: HbSA (sickle cell trait, asymptomatic), HbSC (less severe form)
- Etiology
  - HbS structural defect: Valine substituted for glutamic acid (position 6)
    - Altered shape, plasticity of red blood cells
    - Sickled cells occlude small blood vessels → multisystem infarcts
- Epidemiology
  - 1% African-Americans HbSS, 8-13% HbSA
  - 3% African-Americans HbC carrier

## CLINICAL ISSUES

### Presentation
- Most common signs/symptoms
  - Sickle cell crisis
    - Acute, severe bone, abdomen, chest pain
- Clinical Profile
  - Recurrent crises, jaundice, growth retardation, stroke
  - Pneumococcal septicemia, meningitis, spinal osteomyelitis (rare, usually children)

### Demographics
- Age: Children protected during first 6 months by ↑ levels of fetal Hb (HbF)
- Ethnicity: African, Middle Eastern, and Eastern Mediterranean ethnicity

### Natural History & Prognosis
- Death < 50 years (HbSS)

### Treatment
- Sickle cell crisis: Oxygen, hydration, pain management

## DIAGNOSTIC CHECKLIST

### Image Interpretation Pearls
- MR distinguishes acute infarction, osteomyelitis

## SELECTED REFERENCES

1. Lonergan GJ et al: Sickle cell anemia. Radiographics. 21(4):971-94, 2001
2. States LJ: Imaging of metabolic bone disease and marrow disorders in children. Radiol Clin North Am. 39(4):749-72, 2001
3. Umans H et al: The diagnostic role of gadolinium enhanced MRI in distinguishing between acute medullary bone infarct and osteomyelitis. Magn Reson Imaging. 18(3):255-62, 2000
4. Levin TL et al: MR marrow signs of iron overload in transfusion-dependent patients with sickle cell disease. Pediatr Radiol. 25(8):614-9, 1995

## IMAGE GALLERY

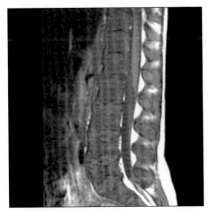 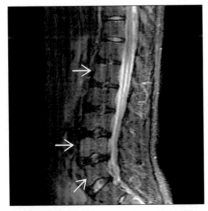 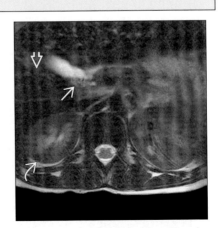

*(Left)* Sagittal T1WI MR shows characteristic "H"-shaped vertebrae at all lumbar levels. Note diffuse low marrow signal intensity deposition due to multiple transfusions & erythroid hyperplasia. *(Center)* Sagittal STIR MR shows multiple hyperintense bone infarcts ➡ superimposed on hypointense marrow from chronic iron deposition. Note characteristic "H-type" compression fxs. *(Right)* Axial T2WI MR shows dark marrow reflecting iron deposition. T2 shortening in liver ➡ & renal cortex ➡ reflect iron deposition in these organs. Gallstones ➡ common in SCD.

# OSTEOGENESIS IMPERFECTA

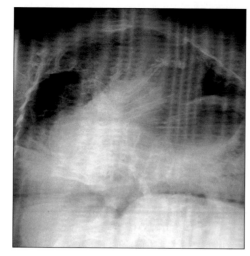

Anteroposterior radiograph (type I, adolescent) demonstrates severe osteopenia and kyphoscoliosis. Note multiple rib and clavicle fractures.

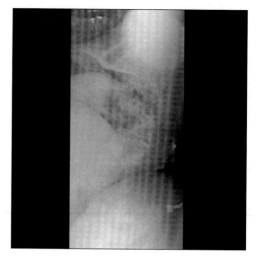

Sagittal radiograph (type I, adolescent) shows severe osteopenia & related kyphoscoliosis. It is difficult to identify individual endplates and posterior elements 2° to poor bone density.

## TERMINOLOGY

### Abbreviations and Synonyms
- Osteogenesis imperfecta (OI)
- "Brittle bone disease"

### Definitions
- Genetic disorder of type 1 collagen → bone fragility
- Codfish vertebra: Cupping of superior and inferior vertebral body endplates
- Terms "congenita" and "tarda" no longer used

## IMAGING FINDINGS

### General Features
- Best diagnostic clue: Severe osteopenia and multiple fractures
- Location: Entire skeleton
- Morphology: Multiple skeletal fractures

### CT Findings
- Bone CT
  - Thin bony cortices
  - Medullary cavity almost entirely filled with fat
    - Primary trabeculae sparse, but normally oriented
    - Secondary trabeculae almost absent
  - Basilar invagination
  - Kyphoscoliosis
  - Otosclerosis

### MR Findings
- Kyphoscoliosis
- Hydromyelia
- Abnormal marrow signal intensity due to fractures
- May be used to augment ultrasound for antenatal diagnosis

### Radiographic Findings
- Radiography
  - Vertebral fractures, vertebra plana, "codfish vertebrae"
  - Kyphoscoliosis
  - Osteoporosis
    - Cortical thinning, resorption of secondary trabeculae with prominent primary trabeculae
  - Multiple fractures of long bones and ribs
    - Bowing deformity due to microfractures as well as radiographically evident fractures

## DDx: Diffuse Vertebral Height Loss

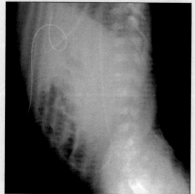

Thanatophoric Dwarfism

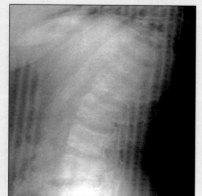

SED Congenita

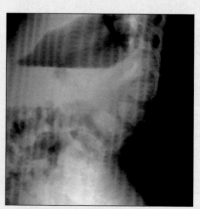

Achondroplasia

# OSTEOGENESIS IMPERFECTA

## Key Facts

### Terminology
- Osteogenesis imperfecta (OI)
- "Brittle bone disease"
- Genetic disorder of type 1 collagen → bone fragility
- Terms "congenita" and "tarda" no longer used

### Imaging Findings
- Best diagnostic clue: Severe osteopenia and multiple fractures
- Vertebral fractures, vertebra plana, "codfish vertebrae"
- Classified into 4 types based on clinical, genetic and radiographic criteria

### Top Differential Diagnoses
- Nonaccidental Trauma (NAT)
- Dwarfisms
- Osteoporosis

### Pathology
- Nearly all cases autosomal dominant
- Inherited or spontaneous mutation
- Epidemiology: 4/100,000 births

### Clinical Issues
- Multiple fractures
- Scoliosis
- ± Deafness, blue sclerae
- Severe forms previously lethal now may survive to adulthood
- Fractures often less common after puberty
- Growth retardation varies with severity of disease

### Diagnostic Checklist
- Nonaccidental trauma is main differential diagnosis

---

- ○ Enlarged epiphyses
- ○ "Popcorn" calcifications in metaphyses
  - Calcified cartilage nodules; due to fragmentation of growth plate from trauma
- ○ Growth retardation
- ○ Pelvis: Protrusio acetabulae, coxa vara
- ○ Increased anteroposterior chest diameter
- ○ Classified into 4 types based on clinical, genetic and radiographic criteria
  - Severe forms: Bones may be short, thickened due to multiple fractures in utero and early childhood
  - Milder forms: Bones thin and gracile

## Ultrasonographic Findings
- Grayscale Ultrasound
  - ○ Antenatal diagnosis in 2nd trimester
  - ○ Poorly ossified skull
  - ○ Short ribs
  - ○ Short, deformed limbs

## Nuclear Medicine Findings
- Bone Scan: Positive at fracture sites

## Other Modality Findings
- Bone densitometry with dual energy X-ray absorptiometry (DEXA) or CT
  - ○ Used to aid diagnosis in mild forms, follow response to treatment

## Imaging Recommendations
- Best imaging tool: Radiography
- Protocol advice: Low kVp technique to compensate for osteoporosis

## DIFFERENTIAL DIAGNOSIS

### Nonaccidental Trauma (NAT)
- Normal bone mineral density
- Fractures may otherwise appear identical
- Careful history, family evaluation needed
- Genetic testing may be useful

### Dwarfisms
- Loss of vertebral body height
- Short stature
- Scoliosis
- Bone density variable
- Common causes
  - ○ Thanatophoric dwarfism
  - ○ Achondroplasia
  - ○ Spondyloepiphyseal dysplasia (SED)

### Osteoporosis
- Thinned bone cortices, accentuation of primary trabeculae, resorption of secondary trabeculae
- Radiography insensitive for diagnosis; better evaluated by bone densitometry
- Codfish vertebrae, compression fractures
- Causes
  - ○ Senile
  - ○ Cushing disease
  - ○ Hyperparathyroidism
  - ○ Cerebral palsy
  - ○ Paralysis
  - ○ Disuse
  - ○ Malabsorption syndromes

## PATHOLOGY

### General Features
- General path comments
  - ○ Abnormal type I collagen
  - ○ Type I collagen found in bone, skin, sclerae
- Genetics
  - ○ Nearly all cases autosomal dominant
  - ○ Inherited or spontaneous mutation
- Etiology: Numerous type I collagen mutations ⇒ "brittle" bone
- Epidemiology: 4/100,000 births
- Associated abnormalities
  - ○ Blue sclerae
  - ○ Early hearing loss
  - ○ Brittle teeth

# OSTEOGENESIS IMPERFECTA

○ Thin, fragile skin
○ Joint laxity
○ Respiratory, cardiac problems

## Gross Pathologic & Surgical Features
• Thin, eggshell-like bone cortices
• Decreased medullary trabeculae
• Recent or healed fractures
• Bowing, angulation of bones
• Overgrowth of epiphyses

## Microscopic Features
• Lack of organized trabeculae
• Prominent osteoid seams
• Morphologically normal osteoblasts, increased in number
• Growth-plate fragmentation
  ○ Due to trauma
  ○ Results in "popcorn" calcifications in metaphyses seen on radiographs
  ○ Contributes to growth disturbance

## Staging, Grading or Classification Criteria
• Type I: Most common type
  ○ Thin, gracile long bones
  ○ High fracture risk in childhood, decreases after puberty
  ○ Kyphoscoliosis, wormian bones
  ○ Blue sclerae
• Type II: Often lethal early in life
  ○ Short, broad, deformed bones at birth due to multiple fractures
• Type III: Autosomal recessive; rare
  ○ Fractures at birth, kyphoscoliosis
• Type IV: Similar to type I
  ○ Kyphoscoliosis, wormian bones
  ○ Sclerae usually normal in adulthood, may be blue in childhood
• Recently types V-VII have been proposed, not distinguishable radiographically
  ○ These types do not localize to genes for type I collagen; etiology unknown

## CLINICAL ISSUES

### Presentation
• Most common signs/symptoms
  ○ Multiple fractures
  ○ Scoliosis
  ○ ± Deafness, blue sclerae
  ○ Short stature secondary to fractures, kyphoscoliosis, growth plate abnormalities
• Clinical Profile
  ○ Diagnosis suggested by radiographs, confirmed by
    ▪ Skin biopsy
    ▪ Genetic testing
    ▪ Caveat: Both tests may be falsely negative

### Demographics
• Age
  ○ Often evident at birth
  ○ Mild cases may first present in adulthood
• Gender: M = F

## Natural History & Prognosis
• Severe forms previously lethal now may survive to adulthood
• Fractures often less common after puberty
• Growth retardation varies with severity of disease

## Treatment
• Conservative management
  ○ Bisphosphonates used for medical therapy with some success
  ○ Prolonged immobilization avoided because of resultant worsening of osteoporosis
• Surgical management
  ○ Intramedullary rod placement for long bone fractures
    ▪ Least invasive internal fixation for rapid mobilization
    ▪ Helps prevent progression of deformity, further fractures
  ○ Spinal fusion for scoliosis
  ○ High risk of hardware mechanical failure

## DIAGNOSTIC CHECKLIST

### Consider
• Nonaccidental trauma is main differential diagnosis

## SELECTED REFERENCES

1. Daivajna S et al: Surgical management of severe cervical kyphosis with myelopathy in osteogenesis imperfecta: a case report. Spine. 30(7):E191-4, 2005
2. Grissom LE et al: Bone densitometry in pediatric patients treated with pamidronate. Pediatr Radiol. 35(5):511-7, 2005
3. Janus GJ et al: Osteogenesis imperfecta in childhood: MR imaging of basilar impression. Eur J Radiol. 47(1):19-24, 2003
4. Teng SW et al: Initial experience using magnetic resonance imaging in prenatal diagnosis of osteogenesis imperfecta type II: a case report. Clin Imaging. 27(1):55-8, 2003
5. Zeitlin L et al: Modern approach to children with osteogenesis imperfecta. J Pediatr Orthop B. 12(2):77-87, 2003
6. Glorieux FH et al: Osteogenesis imperfecta type VI: a form of brittle bone disease with a mineralization defect. J Bone Miner Res. 17(1):30-8, 2002
7. Marlowe A et al: Testing for osteogenesis imperfecta in cases of suspected non-accidental injury. J Med Genet. 39(6):382-6, 2002
8. Ward LM et al: Osteogenesis imperfecta type VII: an autosomal recessive form of brittle bone disease. Bone. 31(1):12-8, 2002
9. Glorieux FH et al: Type V osteogenesis imperfecta: a new form of brittle bone disease. J Bone Miner Res. 15(9):1650-8, 2000
10. Widmann RF et al: Spinal deformity, pulmonary compromise, and quality of life in osteogenesis imperfecta. Spine. 24(16):1673-8, 1999
11. Moore MS et al: The role of dual energy x-ray absorptiometry in aiding the diagnosis of pediatric osteogenesis imperfecta. Am J Orthop. 27(12):797-801, 1998

# OSTEOGENESIS IMPERFECTA

## IMAGE GALLERY

### Typical

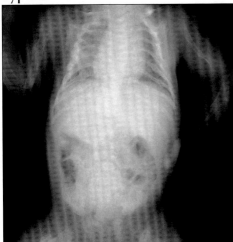
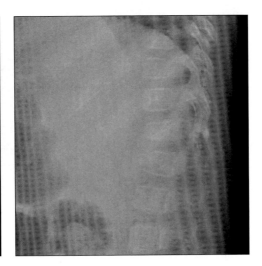

*(Left)* Anteroposterior radiograph (type II, 1 year old) shows scoliosis, not present at birth, has developed. Left humerus is gracile, right is broad; both show fractures. *(Right)* Lateral radiograph (type I, infant) admitted for NAT workup shows osteopenia & T12 compression fracture. Multiple rib fractures, femoral coxa vara, & wormian bones (not shown) confirm OI.

### Typical

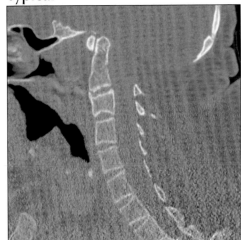
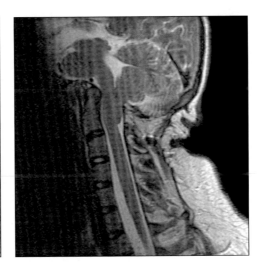

*(Left)* Sagittal bone CT (type I, young adult) shows severe osteopenia and cranial settling with platybasia and basilar invagination. Brainstem compression would be expected. *(Right)* Sagittal T2WI MR (type I, young adult) shows cranial settling with platybasia and basilar invagination producing brainstem compression and tonsillar displacement into upper cervical canal.

### Typical

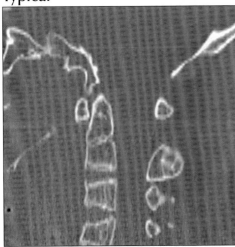
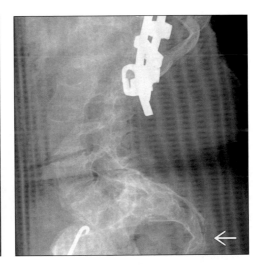

*(Left)* Sagittal bone CT (type 1) of the cervical spine depicts cortical thinning, vertebral body wedging at multiple levels. Secondary trabeculae are not seen, and primary trabeculae are sparse. *(Right)* Lateral radiograph (type 1, young adult) reveals severe osteopenia & cupping of vertebral endplates throughout lumbar spine. Sacral insufficiency fracture is also evident ➡.

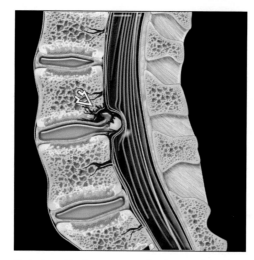

*Sagittal graphic shows an acute lumbar apophyseal ring fracture involving the posterior inferior corner ➡ with displacement and associated hemorrhage; the thecal sac is compressed.*

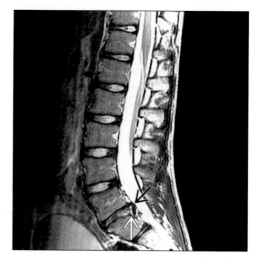

*Sagittal T2WI MR shows a L5 PAR fracture. A small disc protrusion ⇗ is evident. The posterior superior endplate of S1 ➡ is distorted. A bone fragment was seen on CT.*

## TERMINOLOGY

### Abbreviations and Synonyms
- Vertebral apophyseal fracture (fx), limbus vertebra (LV)
- Endplate avulsion fx, corner fx, slipped vertebral apophysis, lumbar posterior marginal node

### Definitions
- Fx or avulsion of vertebral ring apophysis (RA) due to injury in immature skeleton
  - Fx of anterior ring termed limbus vertebra (LV)
  - Fx of posterior ring termed posterior apophyseal ring fx (PAR-fx)

## IMAGING FINDINGS

### General Features
- Best diagnostic clue: Concentric bone fragment displaced from endplate margin
- Location
  - Lumbosacral spine most common; rare thoracic > cervical
  - L3-S1; PAR-fx commonly L4, S1
  - Inferior or superior endplate may be involved; LV usually superior
  - Fractured apophyseal fragment usually midline
- Size: Fragment size can vary
- Morphology: Rim-like morphology typical, but fragment(s) may be amorphous

### CT Findings
- NECT
  - Acute
    - PAR-fx: Arc-shaped or rectangular bone fragment posterior to dorsal endplate margin
    - Vertebral donor site occasionally not identified
    - LV: Same as PAR-fx except located anteriorly, ± mild kyphosis
  - Subacute - chronic
    - Sclerosis of fragment and donor site margins
    - Donor defect often enlarges, particularly LV

### MR Findings
- T1WI
  - Corner defect in marrow of parent vertebral body (VB) with disc extending into defect
  - Hypointense bone fragment

## DDx: Disc/End Plate Pathology

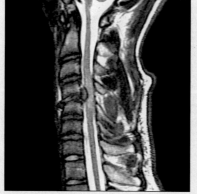

*Disc Herniation*

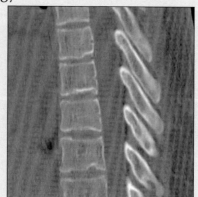

*Schmorl Nodes*

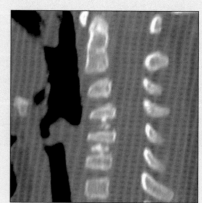

*Disc Calcification*

# APOPHYSEAL RING FRACTURE

## Key Facts

### Terminology

- Vertebral apophyseal fracture (fx), limbus vertebra (LV)
- Endplate avulsion fx, corner fx, slipped vertebral apophysis, lumbar posterior marginal node
- Fx or avulsion of vertebral ring apophysis (RA) due to injury in immature skeleton

### Imaging Findings

- Inferior or superior endplate may be involved; LV usually superior
- Corner defect in marrow of parent vertebral body (VB) with disc extending into defect
- Hypointense bone fragment
- Defect in endplate; hyperintense disc between fragment and VB
- T1 C+: Enhancement of donor site marrow if acute fx

- Best imaging tool: CT with bone as well as soft tissue windows
- Protocol advice: Thin-sections, sagittal reformations

### Top Differential Diagnoses

- Compression/Flexion Fracture of Anterior End Plate Corner
- Schmorl Node
- Disc Calcification or Ossification
- Calcified Disc Fragment; Posterior Osteophyte

### Diagnostic Checklist

- MR more sensitive in young children (RA not ossified)
- FS T2/STIR essential to assess for associated ligamentous injury

- T2WI
  - Defect in endplate; hyperintense disc between fragment and VB
  - High signal in subjacent marrow on T2WI in acute cases
- STIR: Same as T2WI, edema accentuated
- T2* GRE: Accentuation of sclerotic bone margins in chronic lesions
- T1 C+: Enhancement of donor site marrow if acute fx
- ↓ T1/T2 merges with adjacent ligaments
- PAR-fx: Commonly associated variable-sized posterior disc protrusion
  - Disc between fragment and vertebral body uncommon finding
  - Fx fragment plus Sharpey fibers = "Y or 7" shape on sagittal MR
- Disc height loss common, ± disc desiccation (↓ T2): Both ↑ over time

### Radiographic Findings

- Radiography: Bone fragments displaced from corner defect of endplate; bone fragment not identified > 50%

### Nuclear Medicine Findings

- Bone Scan: Increased radionuclide uptake in acute lesions

### Non-Vascular Interventions

- Myelography: Epidural defect on contrast column in PAR-fx

### Other Modality Findings

- Discography (LV): Contrasts diffuses into space between fragment & vertebral body

### Imaging Recommendations

- Best imaging tool: CT with bone as well as soft tissue windows
- Protocol advice: Thin-sections, sagittal reformations

## DIFFERENTIAL DIAGNOSIS

### Compression/Flexion Fracture of Anterior End Plate Corner

- Seen in older children, adults, after apophysis fused

### Schmorl Node

- End plate defect is within the interspace, not at endplate corner
- Associated edema and contrast-enhancement when acute

### Disc Calcification or Ossification

- Painful childhood nucleus pulposus calcification of unknown etiology
  - Multilevel common, cervical > thoracic, occasionally asymptomatic
  - Spontaneous resolution of calcifications and symptoms

### Calcified Disc Fragment; Posterior Osteophyte

- Sequelae long-standing degenerative disc disease, usually adult
- Fragment at level of disc, not above or below
- May see marrow if ossified

### Disc Herniation

- Uncommon in adolescents, rare (traumatic) in first decade

## PATHOLOGY

### General Features

- General path comments
  - Embryology-anatomy
    - Superior & inferior surface of developing VB covered by thin, peripherally thickened, cartilage plate ⇒ cartilaginous marginal ridge
    - Endochondral ossification of marginal ridge begins at 7-9 yrs ⇒ RA

# APOPHYSEAL RING FRACTURE

- RA seen as small bony triangles at corners of vertebral body (XR, sag/cor recon CT)
- RA separated from vertebral body by thin cartilage layer until apophysis fuses to vertebral body at 18-20 yrs ⇒ relative weak point in disc/vertebral body complex until fusion occurs
- Outermost fibers of annulus fibrosus (Sharpey fibers) embedded in RA, attaching disc to spine
- Genetics: Often seen with Scheuermann disease
- Etiology
  ○ LV: Herniation of nucleus pulposus (NP) between RA and vertebral body
  ○ PAR-fx: Two possible mechanisms described
    - Same as LV or herniating NP spares Sharpey fibers & avulses RA
- Epidemiology: 20% prevalence PAR-fx teen lumbar disc surgeries (33% in 14-17 yrs)
- Associated abnormalities
  ○ Disc herniation
  ○ Kyphosis

## Gross Pathologic & Surgical Features
- Displaced bony/cartilaginous rim fragment with or without disc material
- Sharpey fibers and posterior longitudinal ligament usually intact

## Microscopic Features
- Cancellous bone, hyaline cartilage, & acellular hyaline tissue (disc)
- Basophilic degeneration & foci hemorrhage in hyaline cartilage common

## Staging, Grading or Classification Criteria
- I: Avulsion posterior cortical vertebral rim (most common)
- II: Central cortical and cancellous bone fx
- III: Lateralized chip fx
- IV: Spans entire posterior vertebral margin

## CLINICAL ISSUES

### Presentation
- Most common signs/symptoms: Back pain in acute (adolescent) cases
- Clinical Profile: Adolescent athlete with acute low back pain
- PAR-fx: Principal presentation
  ○ Acute > > prolonged history of central low back pain ± sciatica
    - 66% had minor trauma or lifting event (weight-lifting, gymnastics)
  ○ Physical exam (PE) findings: Similar to herniated nucleus pulposus
- LV: No inciting event; chronic hx back pain; occasionally incidental finding
  ○ PE: ↓ ROM, ± kyphosis & pain with palpation of spinous processes
- Majority patients with Par-fx/LV report engagement in sporting activities

### Demographics
- Age: Late childhood through adolescence

- Gender: M > F (up to 85% males in PAR-fx group)

## Natural History & Prognosis
- Reports document evolution LV into anteriorly located Schmorl node
- LV: Symptoms resolve months (usual) to years (rare)
- PAR-fx: Good-excellent with surgery; occasional mild, short term deficits

## Treatment
- LV: Conservative - analgesics & limitation physical activity in acute setting
- PAR-fx: Surgical therapy mainstay, conservative rarely successful
  ○ Uni- or bilateral laminotomy with removal bone fragment, ± disc

## DIAGNOSTIC CHECKLIST

### Consider
- Obtaining bone scan to ascertain chronicity

### Image Interpretation Pearls
- MR more sensitive in young children (RA not ossified)
- FS T2/STIR essential to assess for associated ligamentous injury

## SELECTED REFERENCES

1. Sairyo K et al: Three-dimensional finite element analysis of the pediatric lumbar spine. Part I: pathomechanism of apophyseal bony ring fracture. Eur Spine J. 15(6):923-9, 2006
2. Asazuma T et al: Lumbar disc herniation associated with separation of the posterior ring apophysis: analysis of five surgical cases and review of the literature. Acta Neurochir (Wien). 145(6):461-6; discussion 466, 2003
3. Mendez JS et al: Limbus lumbar and sacral vertebral fractures. Neurol Res. 24(2):139-44, 2002
4. Bonic EE et al: Posterior limbus fractures: five case reports and a review of selected published cases. J Manipulative Physiol Ther. 21(4):281-7, 1998
5. Martinez-Lage JF et al: Avulsed lumbar vertebral rim plate in an adolescent: trauma or malformation? Childs Nerv Syst. 14(3):131-4, 1998
6. Swischuk LE et al: Disk degenerative disease in childhood: Scheuermann's disease, Schmorl's nodes, and the limbus vertebra: MRI findings in 12 patients. Pediatr Radiol. 28(5):334-8, 1998
7. Swischuk LE et al: Disk degenerative disease in childhood: Scheuermann's disease, Schmorl's nodes, and the limbus vertebra: MRI findings in 12 patients. Pediatr Radiol. 28(5):334-8, 1998
8. Talha A et al: Fracture of the vertebral limbus. Eur Spine J. 6(5):347-50, 1997
9. Henales V et al: Intervertebral disc herniations (limbus vertebrae) in pediatric patients: report of 15 cases. Pediatr Radiol. 23(8):608-10, 1993
10. Wagner A et al: Diagnostic imaging in fracture of lumbar vertebral ring apophyses. Acta Radiol. 33(1):72-5, 1992
11. Jonsson K et al: Avulsion of the cervical spinal ring apophyses: acute and chronic appearance. Skeletal Radiol. 20(3):207-10, 1991
12. Banerian KG et al: Association of vertebral end plate fracture with pediatric lumbar intervertebral disk herniation: value of CT and MR imaging. Radiology. 177(3):763-5, 1990

# APOPHYSEAL RING FRACTURE

## IMAGE GALLERY

### Typical

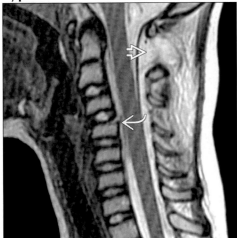

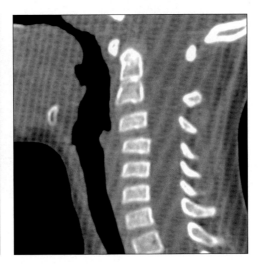

*(Left)* Sagittal T2WI MR in a 5 year old shows avulsion of the posterior superior marginal ridge of C4 ➘. Abnormal widening and disruption of the ligaments between C1 and C2 posteriorly ➔ is evident. *(Right)* Sagittal bone CT reconstruction in the same child as previous image shows posterior distraction at C1-C2. Anterolisthesis and abnormal angulation at C3-C4 are evident; the PAR fracture of C4 is not appreciated.

### Typical

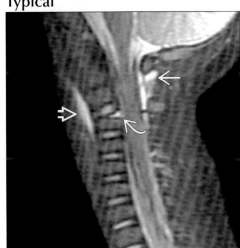

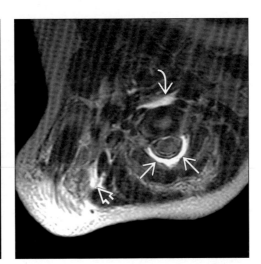

*(Left)* Sagittal STIR MR in an 8 month old shows avulsion of the posterior superior marginal ridge of C3 ➘. Note posterior ligamentous injury between C1 and C2 ➔, and prevertebral edema ➔. *(Right)* Axial T2WI MR shows edema in prevertebral soft tissues ➘ and lateral right neck ➔. At surgery, the dura mater was torn, with T2 bright CSF ➔ accumulating in the epidural space.

### Typical

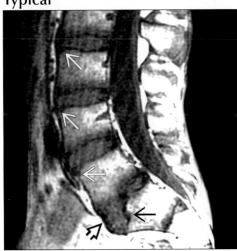

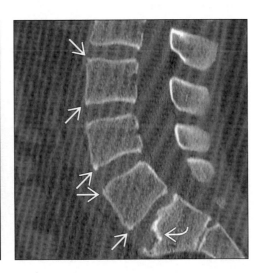

*(Left)* Sagittal T1WI MR in a 13 year old shows a limbus vertebra at S1 with anterior L5-S1 disc herniating inferiorly ➘ between ring apophysis and the S1 vertebral body. Note corner defect in the marrow of S1 ➘, and small ring apophyses ➔ at other levels. *(Right)* Sagittal bone CT in the same patient shows a cortical defect with sclerotic margins in the anterior corner of S1 ➘. Multiple ring apophyses are also seen ➔.

# SPONDYLOLISTHESIS

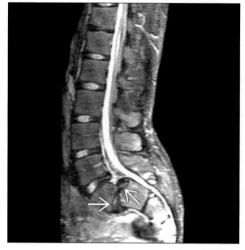

*Sagittal STIR MR shows almost 50% anterior slippage of L5 on S1. The L5-S1 disc ➡ has a bilobed shape and shows low T2 signal (degeneration). The spinal canal narrows at S1.*

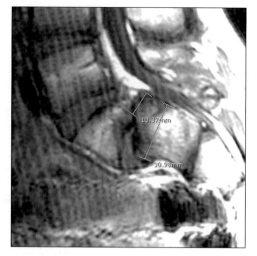

*Sagittal T1WI MR shows the measurement technique (extent of forward translation divided by the AP diameter of the caudal segment) used to grade spondylolisthesis, almost 50% in this case.*

## TERMINOLOGY

### Definitions
- Translation (forward slippage) of one vertebral segment relative to the next caudal segment
  - Low grade: Forward slippage less than 50% of the transverse width of the caudal segment
  - High grade: 50% or more forward slippage
- Spondyloptosis: Vertebral body displaced completely anteriorly, with inferior displacement to level of vertebral body below

## IMAGING FINDINGS

### General Features
- Best diagnostic clue: Displacement of posterior cortex of vertebral body on lateral radiograph
- Location: Most common in lower lumbar spine

### CT Findings
- Evaluate for pars intermedia defects, fractures; dysplasia of posterior elements
- Foraminal narrowing; spinal stenosis
- Disc space loss, disc bulge, degenerative changes

### MR Findings
- Sagittal, axial T1WI and T2WI to evaluate disc herniation, spinal stenosis and neural foraminal encroachment

### Radiographic Findings
- Radiography
  - Evaluate percentage or grade of listhesis on neutral, flexion and extension lateral
  - Lateral flexion and extension to evaluate for instability
  - "Napoleon's hat" sign
    - Severe spondylolisthesis results in focal kyphosis
    - Kyphotic, subluxed vertebra resembles an upside down curved hat on AP radiographs
  - Evaluate for fracture, spondylolysis
  - Degenerative: Degenerative disc disease and facet osteoarthritis present

### Imaging Recommendations
- Best imaging tool: CT scan; MR when neurologic signs and symptoms present

---

## DDx: Vertebral Malalignment

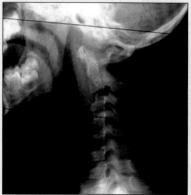
*C2-C3 Subluxation*

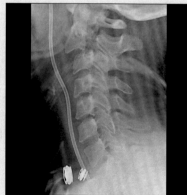
*Hangman's Fracture*

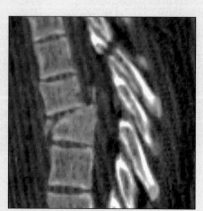
*Traumatic Listhesis*

# SPONDYLOLISTHESIS

## Key Facts

### Terminology
- Translation (forward slippage) of one vertebral segment relative to the next caudal segment

### Imaging Findings
- Best diagnostic clue: Displacement of posterior cortex of vertebral body on lateral radiograph
- Evaluate percentage or grade of listhesis on neutral, flexion and extension lateral

- Protocol advice: Obtain stack axial images as well as axials angled through intervertebral disc

### Pathology
- Grade I: < 25% displacement vertebral body
- Grade II: 25-50% displacement vertebral body
- Grade III: 50-75% displacement vertebral body
- Grade IV: 75-100% displacement vertebral body
- Grade V: Spondyloptosis

- Protocol advice: Obtain stack axial images as well as axials angled through intervertebral disc

- Grade II: 25-50% displacement vertebral body
- Grade III: 50-75% displacement vertebral body
- Grade IV: 75-100% displacement vertebral body
- Grade V: Spondyloptosis

## DIFFERENTIAL DIAGNOSIS

### Physiologic Motion
- Slight subluxations normal in children

### Vertebral Body Fracture/Dislocation
- Fracture often best seen on CT

## PATHOLOGY

### General Features
- Etiology
  - Dysplastic
    - Abnormal development of posterior elements, intact pars interarticularis
  - Developmental
    - No history of repetitive trauma; hereditary
  - Traumatic
    - Acute vs. chronic (repetitive) stress
  - Pathologic
    - Insufficiency of posterior elements from underlying bone pathology
  - Other: Post surgical, neuropathic, degenerative
- Associated abnormalities: Scoliosis may develop

### Staging, Grading or Classification Criteria
- Grade I: < 25% displacement vertebral body

## CLINICAL ISSUES

### Presentation
- Most common signs/symptoms: Back pain, radiculopathy, neurogenic claudication

### Natural History & Prognosis
- Progression common with high grade displacement and when secondary to congenital bone dysplasia

## DIAGNOSTIC CHECKLIST

### Consider
- Perform CT to differentiate pars defect from dysplasia as underlying etiology

## SELECTED REFERENCES

1. Cavalier R et al: Spondylolysis and spondylolisthesis in children and adolescents: I. Diagnosis, natural history, and nonsurgical management. J Am Acad Orthop Surg. 14(7):417-24, 2006
2. Herman MJ et al: Spondylolysis and spondylolisthesis in the child and adolescent: a new classification. Clin Orthop Relat Res. (434):46-54, 2005

## IMAGE GALLERY

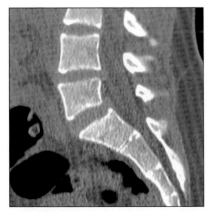 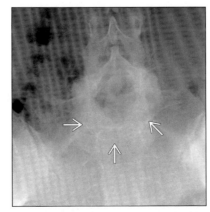 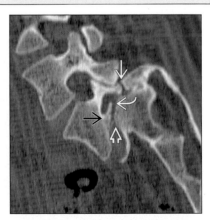

*(Left)* Sagittal NECT in a 15 year old shows a grade 1 spondylolisthesis. Low grade forward slippage of the L5 vertebra over S1 is evident. Bilateral spondylolytic defects were identified. *(Center)* Anteroposterior radiograph shows grade 4 spondylolisthesis causing "Napoleon's hat" appearance; rotated & anteriorly subluxed body of L5 ➡ is superimposed on S1. *(Right)* Sagittal bone CT shows high grade spondylolisthesis; posterior margin of L5 ➡ is almost aligned with anterior margin of S1 ➡. Spondylolytic defect ➡ & osteophyte ➡ are evident.

# SPONDYLOLYSIS

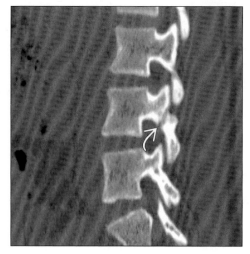

*Sagittal NECT shows a stress fracture of the pars interarticularis of L4. A defect is seen in the PI ➤ on these reconstructed images, without a well-defined bony gap or adjacent sclerosis.*

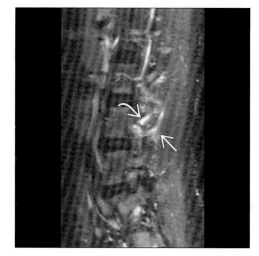

*Sagittal STIR MR (same patient as previous image) shows bright signal within the pars defect ➤. Edema is evident in the L4-L5 intervertebral foramen and in soft tissues inferior to the L4 lamina ➤.*

## TERMINOLOGY

### Abbreviations and Synonyms
- Isthmic spondylolysis; dysplastic spondylolysis

### Definitions
- Defect or abnormality in pars interarticularis (PI) and surrounding lamina and pedicle
  - Stress reaction: Intraosseous edema w/surrounding sclerosis without cortical or trabecular disruption
  - Stress fracture: Disruption of trabecular or cortical bone of the pars without a bony gap or lysis
  - Spondylolytic defect (nonunion): Complete disruption of the PI with a gap & surrounding sclerosis at the edges of the defect

## IMAGING FINDINGS

### General Features
- Best diagnostic clue: Defect in the PI, best seen on standing spot lateral and supine oblique views of the lumbosacral (LS) junction
- Location

- Most common at L5: 82%
- L4 second most common: 11%
- 10-15% unilateral defects
  - Unilateral healing or union of fractures that were initially bilateral

### CT Findings
- Bone CT
  - Stress reaction: Localized sclerosis without trabecular or cortical disruption
  - Stress fracture: Cortical or trabecular disruption of PI with minimal sclerosis or lysis of the fracture gap
  - Spondylolytic defect: Pars disruption with surrounding sclerosis
    - "Incomplete ring" sign on axial imaging
    - May simulate facet joints
    - Pars defects well seen on oblique reformation

### MR Findings
- T1WI
  - Spondylolytic defect: Focally decreased signal in PI on sagittal and axial imaging
  - Stress reaction not identified
- T2WI
  - Spondylolytic defect: Usually no edema

## DDx: Facet/Pedicle Pathology

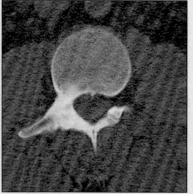

*Agenetic Pedicle*

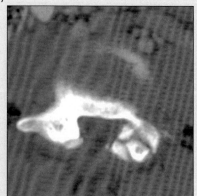

*Post Surgical Fragmentation*

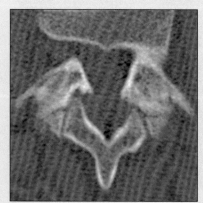

*Facet Fractures*

# SPONDYLOLYSIS

## Key Facts

### Terminology
- Defect or abnormality in pars interarticularis (PI) and surrounding lamina and pedicle
- Stress reaction: Intraosseous edema w/surrounding sclerosis without cortical or trabecular disruption
- Stress fracture: Disruption of trabecular or cortical bone of the pars without a bony gap or lysis
- Spondylolytic defect (nonunion): Complete disruption of the PI with a gap & surrounding sclerosis at the edges of the defect

### Imaging Findings
- Most common at L5: 82%
- 10-15% unilateral defects
- Spondylolytic defect: Focally decreased signal in PI on sagittal and axial imaging

- STIR: Stress reaction, fracture: Marrow edema, edema in tissues adjacent to pedicle, PI
- SPECT increases sensitivity

### Top Differential Diagnoses
- Other Causes of Sclerotic Pedicle

### Pathology
- Dysplastic spondylolysis/spondylolisthesis
- Developmental spondylolysis/spondylolisthesis
- Traumatic spondylolysis/spondylolisthesis
- Pathologic spondylolysis/spondylolisthesis

### Diagnostic Checklist
- Look for edema of pedicle and integrity of pars interarticularis on sagittal MR

○ Stress reaction, fracture: Hyperintensity of the pedicles (± lamina)
- STIR: Stress reaction, fracture: Marrow edema, edema in tissues adjacent to pedicle, PI

## Radiographic Findings
- Radiography
  ○ Ipsilateral pedicle hypertrophy and sclerosis
  ○ Radiolucent band in PI on oblique views of lumbar spine (stress fracture, spondylolytic defect)
    ▪ Discontinuity in the neck of "Scotty dog"
    ▪ Oblique lucency at base of laminae on lateral view
  ○ Contralateral pedicle and lamina hypertrophy and sclerosis (unilateral spondylolytic defect)
  ○ Increased incidence of spina bifida occulta, scoliosis

## Nuclear Medicine Findings
- Bone Scan
  ○ Indicated in evaluation when radiographs are inconclusive
  ○ Foci of increased radiotracer uptake in posterior elements (PI, lamina, pedicle)
    ▪ Suggests stress reaction, stress fracture or symptomatic spondylolytic defect
    ▪ SPECT increases sensitivity
    ▪ Spondylolytic defect + negative SPECT: Suggests spondylolysis is an incidental finding, not the source of pain/symptoms

## Imaging Recommendations
- Best imaging tool
  ○ Axial thin-section CT with bone algorithm
    ▪ Sagittal & oblique reformations best to show defect
- Protocol advice: Do SPECT (↑ uptake) or MR (hyperintense on STIR) for suspected stress reaction or stress fracture

## DIFFERENTIAL DIAGNOSIS

### Other Causes of Sclerotic Pedicle
- Infection

- Agenetic/hypoplastic pedicle/facet (contralateral sclerosis)
- Tumor (osteoid osteoma, osteoblastoma)
- Dysplasia (fibrous dysplasia, tuberous sclerosis)

### Mimickers of Spondylolysis on Sagittal MR
- Partial volume averaging of superior facet spur lateral to PI
- Partial facetectomy
- Sclerosing lesions (e.g., osteoid osteoma)

## PATHOLOGY

### General Features
- Genetics
  ○ Predisposing familial conditions to spondylolysis
    ▪ Marfan syndrome
    ▪ Osteogenesis imperfecta
    ▪ Osteopetrosis
    ▪ Other inherited traits
- Etiology
  ○ Dysplastic spondylolysis/spondylolisthesis
    ▪ Failure of normal development of posterior elements of the lumber spine with an intact PI
  ○ Developmental spondylolysis/spondylolisthesis
    ▪ Spondylolytic defect diagnosed incidentally
    ▪ Hereditary: 26% incidence of spondylolysis/spondylolisthesis in first-degree relatives
  ○ Traumatic spondylolysis/spondylolisthesis
    ▪ Acute: Acute fracture, results from high-energy trauma (e.g., MVA); uncommon in pediatrics
    ▪ Chronic: Repeated micro-fractures of PI lead to fatigue fracture; history of participation in sports/activity that involves repetitive loading of the lumbar spine
  ○ Pathologic spondylolysis/spondylolisthesis
    ▪ Insufficiency of pedicle/pars/lamina from underlying bone pathology
    ▪ See with osteogenesis imperfecta, osteopetrosis, neoplasm, osteoporosis
- Epidemiology
  ○ Prevalence of 4.4% at age 6

# SPONDYLOLYSIS

○ 5-7% in general population
   ■ 22-44% in competitive athletes in diving, weight lifting, wrestling
• Associated abnormalities
   ○ Scoliosis
   ○ 50% with spondylolisthesis
   ○ Spina bifida occulta
   ○ Scheuermann disease

## Microscopic Features
• New bone and cartilaginous matrix if healing present
• Fibrocartilaginous tissue within pars defects if not healed

## Staging, Grading or Classification Criteria
• Recent reclassification of spondylolysis/spondylolisthesis in 4 types based on etiology and specific morphologic changes
   ○ Type 1: Dysplastic
   ○ Type 2: Developmental
   ○ Type 3: Traumatic (acute vs. chronic)
   ○ Type 4: Pathologic

# CLINICAL ISSUES

## Presentation
• Most common signs/symptoms
   ○ Developmental spondylolysis/spondylolisthesis
      ■ Most without symptoms
   ○ Chronic traumatic spondylolysis/spondylolisthesis
      ■ Participation in gymnastics, weight lifting, wrestling, football, etc., starting at a young age
      ■ Training more than 15 hours per week
      ■ Repetitive exposure to rotation, flexion-extension, and hyperextension
      ■ Chronic or intermittent low back pain
      ■ Usually presents during adolescent growth spurt
      ■ Pain exacerbated by rigorous activities

## Demographics
• Age: 8-20 years

## Natural History & Prognosis
• Chronic traumatic stress reaction/fracture can progress to spondylolytic defect

## Treatment
• Conservative measures indicated for chronic traumatic spondylolysis & for symptomatic developmental spondylolysis
   ○ Activity restriction, spinal immobilization for up to 3 months
   ○ Anti-inflammatory medication, epidural steroid injection
   ○ Excellent outcome in > 80%
   ○ Low grade (< 50%) spondylolisthesis: Same treatment
• Surgical intervention indicated
   ○ For patient with persistent pain and impairment despite conservative treatment
   ○ For most acute traumatic spondylolysis/spondylolisthesis

• In cases of spondylolisthesis, surgical intervention indicated for
   ○ Low grade (< 50%) displacement with persistent pain and impairment despite conservative treatment
   ○ High-grade (> 50%) displacement
   ○ Worsening slippage
   ○ Presence of progressive neurologic deficits
   ○ Preserve neural function and prevent instability

# DIAGNOSTIC CHECKLIST

## Consider
• SPECT or MR in adolescent back pain with normal CT

## Image Interpretation Pearls
• Look for edema of pedicle and integrity of pars interarticularis on sagittal MR

# SELECTED REFERENCES

1. Sairyo K et al: MRI signal changes of the pedicle as an indicator for early diagnosis of spondylolysis in children and adolescents: a clinical and biomechanical study. Spine. 31(2):206-11, 2006
2. Takemitsu M et al: Low back pain in pediatric athletes with unilateral tracer uptake at the pars interarticularis on single photon emission computed tomography. Spine. 31(8):909-14, 2006
3. Ulibarri JA et al: Biomechanical and clinical evaluation of a novel technique for surgical repair of spondylolysis in adolescents. Spine. 31(18):2067-72, 2006
4. Herman MJ et al: Spondylolysis and spondylolisthesis in the child and adolescent: a new classification. Clin Orthop Relat Res. (434):46-54, 2005
5. McTimoney CA et al: Current evaluation and management of spondylolysis and spondylolisthesis. Curr Sports Med Rep. 2(1):41-6, 2003
6. Merbs CF: Asymmetrical spondylolysis. Am J Phys Anthropol. 119(2):156-74, 2002
7. Logroscino G et al: Spondylolysis and spondylolisthesis in the pediatric and adolescent population. Childs Nerv Syst. 17(11):644-55, 2001
8. Saifuddin A et al: The value of lumbar spine MRI in the assessment of the pars interarticularis. Clin Radiol. 52(9):666-71, 1997
9. Ulmer JL et al: MR imaging of lumbar spondylolysis: the importance of ancillary observations. AJR Am J Roentgenol. 169(1):233-9, 1997
10. Jinkins JR et al: Spondylolysis, spondylolisthesis, and associated nerve root entrapment in the lumbosacral spine: MR evaluation. AJR Am J Roentgenol. 159(4):799-803, 1992
11. Danielson BI et al: Radiologic progression of isthmic lumbar spondylolisthesis in young patients. Spine. 16(4):422-5, 1991
12. Frennered AK et al: Natural history of symptomatic isthmic low-grade spondylolisthesis in children and adolescents: a seven-year follow-up study. J Pediatr Orthop. 11(2):209-13, 1991
13. Rossi F et al: Lumbar spondylolysis: occurrence in competitive athletes. Updated achievements in a series of 390 cases. J Sports Med Phys Fitness. 30(4):450-2, 1990
14. Johnson DW et al: MR imaging of the pars interarticularis. AJR Am J Roentgenol. 152(2):327-32, 1989

# SPONDYLOLYSIS

## IMAGE GALLERY

### Typical

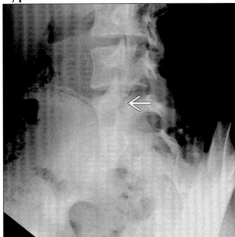

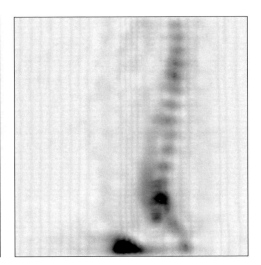

*(Left)* Sagittal oblique radiograph shows a defect in the pars interarticularis of L5 ➡️, featuring the typical discontinuity in the neck of the "Scotty dog" seen with a spondylolytic defect. *(Right)* Sagittal bone scan in the same patient as previous image shows increased uptake in the pars interarticularis of L5. Increased uptake establishes that there is active bone deposition within the defect.

### Typical

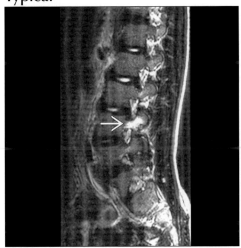

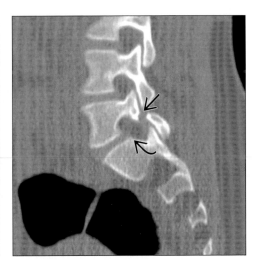

*(Left)* Sagittal T2WI MR shows abnormal signal in the pedicle and lamina of L4 ➡️. No cortical disruption was seen on CT. Findings are consistent with a stress reaction. *(Right)* Sagittal NECT shows well corticated defect of PI of L5 ➡️, typical of a spondylolytic defect. Bone scan was normal. L5-S1 neural foramen is elongated ➡️, indicative of a spondylolisthesis.

### Typical

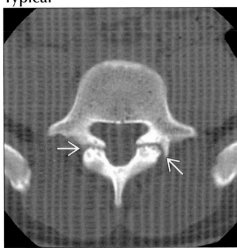

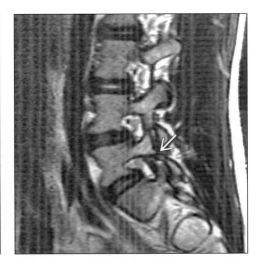

*(Left)* Axial bone CT shows bilateral L5 spondylolytic defects in an adolescent with back pain. A complete bony gap ➡️ is evident, with surrounding sclerosis. *(Right)* Sagittal T2WI MR in same patient as previous image shows difficulty of MR diagnosis of a spondylolytic defect. Defect ➡️ is poorly perceived as there is no abnormal signal, only irregular appearance of the PI.

# PYOGENIC OSTEOMYELITIS

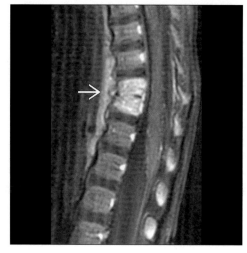

Sagittal T1WI FS MR in an 11 month old shows diffuse enhancement of T11 and 12 vertebral bodies. The disc space is narrowed and enhances. Note thickening of the prevertebral soft tissues ➡.

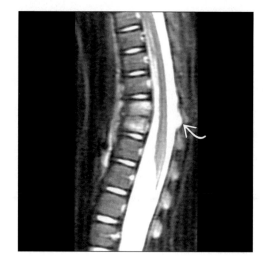

Sagittal STIR MR shows diffuse increased T2 in the involved vertebral bodies, with mild collapse, resulting in kyphotic angulation. Note inflammation in the epidural space posteriorly ➡.

## TERMINOLOGY

### Abbreviations and Synonyms
- Pyogenic spondylodiscitis

### Definitions
- Spondylodiscitis: Infection of vertebrae and intervertebral disc
- Discitis: Infection isolated to the intervertebral disc

## IMAGING FINDINGS

### General Features
- Best diagnostic clue: Ill-defined hypointense vertebral marrow on T1WI with loss of endplate definition on both sides of the disc
- Location
  ○ All spinal segments involved
    ▪ Lumbar (56%) > thoracic (35%) > cervical spine (10%)
- Size
  ○ 2 adjacent vertebrae with intervening disc
    ▪ 2/3 of pyogenic spondylodiscitis

- Morphology
  ○ Decreased disc height
  ○ Loss of vertebral endplate cortex
  ○ Ill-defined marrow signal alteration
  ○ Bone destruction, vertebral collapse
  ○ Paraspinal ± epidural infiltrative soft tissue ± loculated fluid collection
    ▪ In 75% of pyogenic vertebral osteomyelitis
  ○ Variable spinal canal narrowing

### CT Findings
- NECT
  ○ Iso- to hypodense paraspinal/epidural soft tissue edema, masses
    ▪ ± Soft tissue gas
- CECT: Enhancing disc, marrow, and paravertebral/epidural soft tissue
- Bone CT
  ○ Endplate osteolytic/osteosclerotic changes
  ○ Bony sequestra
  ○ Spinal deformity best seen on coronal and sagittal reformation

### MR Findings
- Disc space narrowing

## DDx: Mimics of Pyogenic Osteomyelitis

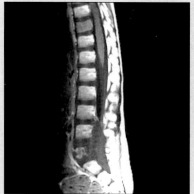

*Lymphoma*

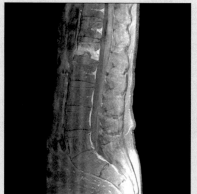

*Acute Schmorl Node*

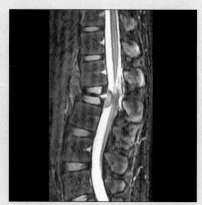

*Tuberculosis*

# PYOGENIC OSTEOMYELITIS

## Key Facts

### Terminology
- Pyogenic spondylodiscitis
- Spondylodiscitis: Infection of vertebrae and intervertebral disc

### Imaging Findings
- Lumbar (56%) > thoracic (35%) > cervical spine (10%)
- 2 adjacent vertebrae with intervening disc
- Decreased disc height
- Loss of vertebral endplate cortex
- Ill-defined marrow signal alteration
- Bone destruction, vertebral collapse
- Paraspinal ± epidural infiltrative soft tissue ± loculated fluid collection
- CECT: Enhancing disc, marrow, and paravertebral/epidural soft tissue

- Paraspinal and epidural granulation tissue vs. abscess ⇒ cord compression

### Top Differential Diagnoses
- Acute Schmorl Node
- Erosive Intervertebral Osteochondrosis
- Tuberculous Vertebral Osteomyelitis
- Vertebral Infarction with Sickle Cell Disease
- Spinal Neuropathic Arthropathy

### Pathology
- Intervertebral disc often first site of infection in children due to presence of vascularity

### Clinical Issues
- Acute or chronic pain (local or radicular)
- Focal spinal tenderness
- Fever (not always)

---

- ○ Hypointense on T1WI
- ○ Variable, typically hyperintense on T2WI
- ○ Post-gadolinium enhancement usually diffuse, can be patchy
- Vertebral marrow signal abnormality abutting disc
  - ○ Hypointense on T1WI
  - ○ Hyperintense on fat-saturated T2WI or STIR
  - ○ Avid enhancement with gadolinium
- Paraspinal and epidural granulation tissue vs. abscess ⇒ cord compression
  - ○ Isointense to muscle on T1WI
  - ○ Hyperintense on T2WI
  - ○ Diffuse vs. rim-enhancement

### Radiographic Findings
- Radiography
  - ○ Negative up to 2-8 weeks after onset of symptoms
  - ○ Initial endplate and vertebral osteolysis followed by increased bone density
  - ○ Paraspinal soft tissue density
  - ○ Fusion across disc space late in disease course

### Ultrasonographic Findings
- Grayscale Ultrasound: Anechoic or hypoechoic paraspinal abscess
- Color Doppler: Hyperemia and increased vascularity surrounding abscess

### Nuclear Medicine Findings
- Bone Scan: 3 phase technetium Tc-99m methylene diphosphonate (MDP) scan shows arterial hyperemia and progressive skeletal radionuclide uptake
- Gallium scan
  - ○ Increased uptake of gallium citrate (Ga-67)
    - ■ Increased sensitivity with SPECT
  - ○ May be used in combination with bone scan

### Imaging Recommendations
- Best imaging tool
  - ○ Sagittal and axial T2WI and T1WI MR
    - ■ Sensitivity 96%, specificity 92%, accuracy 94%
  - ○ Tc-99m MDP scan good alternative
    - ■ Sensitivity and specificity in low 90%

- Protocol advice
  - ○ STIR or FSE T2 with fat suppression most sensitive for marrow edema and epidural involvement
  - ○ Post-gadolinium T1WI with fat suppression also improves MR sensitivity

## DIFFERENTIAL DIAGNOSIS

### Acute Schmorl Node
- Enhancement of disc and adjacent vertebral body
- Edema within the vertebral body localized in distribution, does not reach the opposite end plate

### Erosive Intervertebral Osteochondrosis
- Acute, inflammatory disc degeneration, without production of typical osteophytes
- Edema of the vertebral bone marrow adjacent to the end plates, enhancement of disc
- Most common at L4-L5, L5-S1

### Tuberculous Vertebral Osteomyelitis
- Mid-thoracic or thoracolumbar > lumbar, cervical
- Vertebral collapse and gibbus deformity
- ± Endplate destructive changes
- Subligamentous spread of infection
- Large dissecting paraspinal abscesses out of proportion to vertebral involvement

### Vertebral Infarction with Sickle Cell Disease
- Low intensity T1 signal of marrow (hyperplasia)
- Focal areas of further decreased T1 with infarction (recent or remote)
- Focal increased T2 signal (edema) and enhancement with acute infarction

### Spinal Metastases
- Non-contiguous vertebral involvement
- Posterior elements commonly affected
- Disc space preserved

### Degenerative End Plate Changes
- Occasionally seen in older children
- Disc desiccation

- ○ Hypointense on T1WI and T2WI
- ○ Mild post-gadolinium enhancement, often linear
- Vertebral endplates preserved
- Degenerative marrow pattern

## Spinal Neuropathic Arthropathy
- Sequela of spinal cord injury
- Disc space loss/T2 hyperintensity, endplate erosion/sclerosis, osteophytosis, soft tissue mass
- Greater debris, disorganization, vacuum disc, facet involvement and spondylolisthesis than seen in spondylodiscitis

## Chronic Hemodialysis Spondyloarthropathy
- Cervical spine most common
- Disc space loss, endplate erosion, vertebral destruction
- Prevalence increased with patient age and duration of dialysis

## PATHOLOGY

### General Features
- General path comments
  - ○ Along a spectrum of suppurative infection involving disc, vertebrae, and adjacent soft tissue
  - ○ Intervertebral discs of neonates and infants well vascularized
    - ■ Enhancement of discs normally seen at MR up to age 2 years
    - ■ Vascularization regresses by age 13 years
- Etiology
  - ○ Staphylococcus aureus is the most common pathogen
    - ■ Escherichia coli most common within gram-negative bacilli
    - ■ Salmonella more common in patients with sickle cell disease
  - ○ Bacteremia from an extraspinal primary source
    - ■ Most common route of infection
    - ■ GU or GI tract, lungs, cardiac, mucous/cutaneous sources
    - ■ Vascularized subchondral bone adjacent to endplate seeded primarily
    - ■ Secondary infection of intervertebral disc and adjacent vertebra
    - ■ Intervertebral disc often first site of infection in children due to presence of vascularity
  - ○ Direct inoculation from penetrating trauma, surgical intervention, or diagnostic procedures
    - ■ Epidural injection/catheter
  - ○ Extension from adjacent infection in paraspinal soft tissues
- Associated abnormalities
  - ○ Spinal meningitis, abscess
  - ○ Myelitis

### Gross Pathologic & Surgical Features
- Necrotic bone
- Suppurative soft tissue

### Microscopic Features
- Bone/disc fragments
- Leukocytes, micro-organisms, cellular debris

- Vascular proliferation

## CLINICAL ISSUES

### Presentation
- Most common signs/symptoms
  - ○ Acute or chronic pain (local or radicular)
  - ○ Focal spinal tenderness
  - ○ Fever (not always)
  - ○ Other signs/symptoms
    - ■ Myelopathy if cord compromised
    - ■ Elevated erythrocyte sedimentation rate, C-reactive protein, and white cell count
- Clinical Profile: Average duration of symptoms for 7 weeks before diagnosis

### Natural History & Prognosis
- Vertebral collapse
- Irreversible neurological deficits
- Favorable outcome with resolution of symptoms if prompt diagnosis and treatment
- Recurrence due to incomplete treatment: 2-8%

### Treatment
- Early empiric antibiotics with broad spectrum coverage until causative pathogen isolated
  - ○ Coverage should be effective against staphylococci, gram negatives, and anaerobes
- Organism specific parenteral antibiotics for 6-8 weeks
- Spinal immobilization with bracing for 6-12 weeks
- Surgical treatment
  - ○ Laminectomy, debridement, ± stabilization
  - ○ Especially if epidural abscess, instability present

## DIAGNOSTIC CHECKLIST

### Image Interpretation Pearls
- Earliest MR findings: Marrow edema, enhancement of disc/adjacent vertebra
- Differentiate epidural abscess from solid granulation tissue with enhanced fat-sat T1 images
- Enhancing disc with endplate erosion, adjacent vertebral marrow edema and soft tissue swelling/inflammation highly suggestive of vertebral osteomyelitis

## SELECTED REFERENCES

1. James SL et al: Imaging of infectious spinal disorders in children and adults. Eur J Radiol. 58(1):27-40, 2006
2. Ledermann HP et al: MR imaging findings in spinal infections: rules or myths? Radiology. 228(2):506-14, 2003
3. Stabler A et al: Imaging of spinal infection. Radiol Clin North Am. 39(1):115-35, 2001
4. Carragee EJ: The clinical use of magnetic resonance imaging in pyogenic vertebral osteomyelitis. Spine. 22(7):780-5, 1997
5. Dagirmanjian A et al: MR imaging of vertebral osteomyelitis revisited. AJR Am J Roentgenol. 167(6):1539-43, 1996
6. Thrush A et al: MR imaging of infectious spondylitis. AJNR Am J Neuroradiol. 11(6):1171-80, 1990

# PYOGENIC OSTEOMYELITIS

## IMAGE GALLERY

### Typical

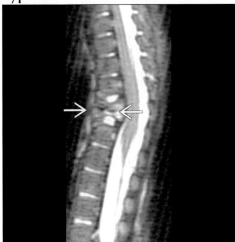 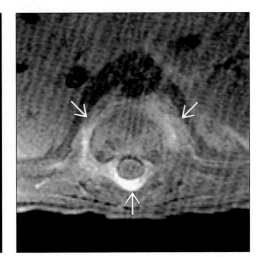

*(Left)* Sagittal STIR MR in an 11 week old with staph aureus septicemia shows marked collapse of the T11 and T12 vertebrae. The intervertebral disc ➡ is slit like, destroyed. *(Right)* Axial T1WI FS MR at T11-T12 (same patient as previous image) shows epidural and paravertebral cellulitis. Solid enhancing granulation tissue ➡ surrounds infected bone/disc. No ring-enhancing abscess is seen.

### Typical

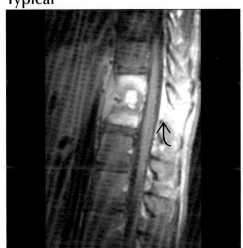 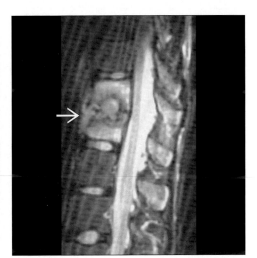

*(Left)* Sagittal T1WI FS MR shows diffuse enhancement of T11 and T12, more focally intense in middle of the disc space. Note inflammation in posterior epidural space/interspinous soft tissues ➡. *(Right)* Sagittal T2WI FS MR (same patient as previous image) shows total destruction of the disc space, end plate erosions, a prevertebral inflammatory mass ➡ and diffuse marrow edema.

### Variant

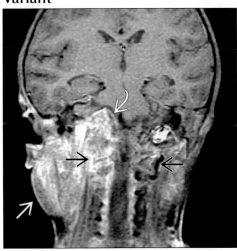 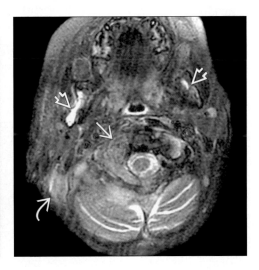

*(Left)* Coronal T1WI FS MR in 4 year old shows extensive osteomyelitis of base of skull ➡, C1, C2 ➡ vertebrae, and articular pillars of C3, C4. Note large, inflammatory soft tissue mass ➡. *(Right)* Axial T2WI FS MR (same patient as previous image) shows increased T2 of the C1 vertebra ➡, with surrounding cellulitis/myositis ➡. Lesions are also evident in the mandibles bilaterally ➡.

# OSTEOID OSTEOMA

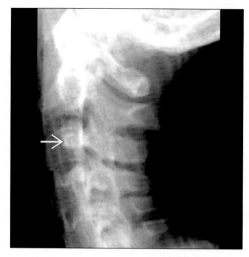

*Lateral radiograph in a 13 year old boy with neck pain shows sclerosis ➡ with some central lucency in the posterior body of C3.*

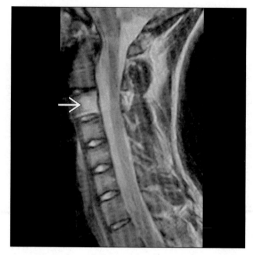

*Sagittal T2WI MR (same patient as previous) shows hyperintensity in the same region of the C3 vertebral body ➡. Edematous reaction to prostaglandin release is a major MR finding in osteoid osteoma.*

## TERMINOLOGY

### Abbreviations and Synonyms
- Osteoid osteoma (OO)

### Definitions
- Benign osteoid-producing tumor < 1.5 cm in size
- Tumor is often called a "nidus" to distinguish it from the surrounding sclerotic, reactive bone

## IMAGING FINDINGS

### General Features
- Best diagnostic clue: Small radiolucent tumor nidus with surrounding sclerosis
- Location
  - 10% of OO occur in spine
  - Almost all involve neural arch
  - Involvement of vertebral body rare
  - 59% lumbar, 27% cervical, 12% thoracic, 2% sacrum
- Size: < 1.5 cm nidus; larger lesions called osteoblastoma
- Morphology: Nidus round or oval

### CT Findings
- CECT
  - Variable enhancement
    - Contrast administration may obscure bony matrix
- Bone CT
  - Central nidus
    - Variable amount of ossification in the nidus
    - Nidus usually predominantly lucent
    - Occasionally nidus is sclerotic
  - Wide peripheral zone of reactive sclerosis surrounds nidus
  - Periosteal reaction variably present, usually unilaminar
  - Soft tissue mass or pleural thickening/effusion often seen
  - Bones adjacent to OO may show sclerosis, periosteal reaction
    - Ribs, adjacent vertebrae affected
  - Ossification of ligamentum flavum has been reported

### MR Findings
- T1WI

## DDx: Lytic Vertebral Lesions

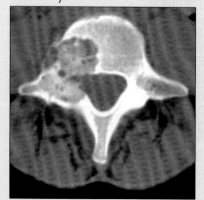

*Osteoblastoma*

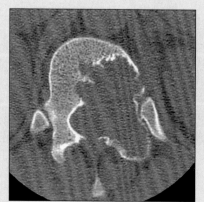

*Aneurysmal Bone Cyst*

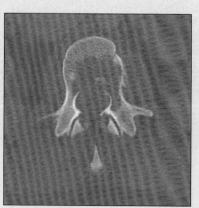

*Ewing Sarcoma*

# OSTEOID OSTEOMA

## Key Facts

### Terminology
- Benign osteoid-producing tumor < 1.5 cm in size
- Tumor is often called a "nidus" to distinguish it from the surrounding sclerotic, reactive bone

### Imaging Findings
- Best diagnostic clue: Small radiolucent tumor nidus with surrounding sclerosis
- 10% of OO occur in spine
- Central, lucent tumor nidus often obscured by reactive sclerosis
- Focal scoliosis concave on side of tumor

### Top Differential Diagnoses
- Osteoblastoma
- Stress Fracture of Pedicle or Lamina
- Unilateral Spondylolysis

- Unilateral Absent Pedicle or Pars Interarticularis
- Aneurysmal Bone Cyst (ABC)
- Osteomyelitis

### Pathology
- Epidemiology: 12% of all benign skeletal neoplasms

### Clinical Issues
- Most common signs/symptoms: Night pain relieved by aspirin, NSAIDs
- 70% have scoliosis related to muscle spasm, concave on side of tumor
- Gait disturbance, muscle atrophy, torticollis sometimes seen
- Majority occur in second decade of life

---

- Hypo- or isointense nidus and surrounding reactive zone
- Cortical thickening
- Thoracic OO: Pleural thickening and/or effusion
- T2WI
  - Nidus varies from hypointense to hyperintense
  - Surrounding hyperintensity is reactive host response related to prostaglandin release
    - Reactive zone involves much larger area than the tumor
    - Reactive zone may extend to adjacent vertebrae, ribs, and paraspinous soft tissues
    - Severe reactive response may lead to misdiagnosis of malignancy or infection
- T1 C+
  - Contrast-enhancement improves sensitivity of MR
  - Rapid enhancement pattern typical in nidus: Best seen on dynamic scans
  - Reactive zone enhances more slowly
  - These criteria reportedly result in equal conspicuity of lesion compared to CT
  - However, avid enhancement of reactive zone may obscure nidus relative to marrow fat signal
  - Note that this dedicated protocol centered at a specific level requires a pretest diagnosis of probable OO
- Literature reports high rate of missed MR diagnosis of OO
  - Lesion may not be seen due to small size of nidus
    - Thin shape, oblique orientation of posterior elements
    - Partial volume averaging with adjacent structures
    - Improve visualization with thin slices, 3-3.5 mm
    - Axial, coronal and sagittal planes
  - Lesion misidentified as reactive zone rather than nidus
    - Misdiagnosis of infection or malignancy common

### Radiographic Findings
- Radiography
  - Central, lucent tumor nidus often obscured by reactive sclerosis
  - Focal scoliosis concave on side of tumor

### Nuclear Medicine Findings
- Bone Scan: Positive on all 3 phases of Tc-99m MDP bone scan

### Imaging Recommendations
- Bone CT with 1 mm helical sections/reformations, IV contrast not needed

## DIFFERENTIAL DIAGNOSIS

### Osteoblastoma
- Larger (> 1.5 cm)
- Expansile lesion of neural arch/pedicle
- Also a benign tumor of the osteoblast

### Stress Fracture of Pedicle or Lamina
- Sclerosis around fracture mimics reactive sclerosis around osteoid osteoma
- CT with MPR or high-resolution MR will show fracture line
- May occur in patients with pre-existing scoliosis, due to altered stresses
- Pain related to activity, improves at night

### Unilateral Spondylolysis
- Linear defect pars interarticularis
- Contralateral side is sclerotic
- Painful
- Presents in young patients
- Scoliosis may develop
- May be diagnosed on oblique radiographs, CT

### Unilateral Absent Pedicle or Pars Interarticularis
- Contralateral side is sclerotic
- Congenital absence of pedicle or pars interarticularis confirmed on CT

### Aneurysmal Bone Cyst (ABC)
- Usually much larger
- Expansile lesion, thins and expands cortex
- Sharply defined, narrow zone of transition

# OSTEOID OSTEOMA

- No associated soft tissue mass
- Often secondary to other lesion

## Osteomyelitis

- Sequestrum or focal abscess can mimic nidus of osteoid osteoma
- Usually involves vertebral bodies
- MR, bone scan may appear very similar
- CT usually shows endplate destruction or destructive arthritis of facet joints
- Sequestrum tends to have irregular shape
- Often presents with night pain relieved by aspirin, NSAIDs

## Ewing Sarcoma

- Diffuse edema may involve adjacent vertebral bodies and ribs
- Pleural thickening, effusion
- Centered in vertebral body
- No nidus on CT scan

# PATHOLOGY

## General Features

- Etiology: Benign tumor of osteoblastic origin
- Epidemiology: 12% of all benign skeletal neoplasms

## Gross Pathologic & Surgical Features

- Sharply-demarcated, round, pink-red mass (nidus)
- Nidus can be shelled out from surrounding, sclerotic reactive bone which does not contain tumor

## Microscopic Features

- Web of osteoid trabeculae showing variable amounts of mineralization
- Vascular, fibrous connective tissue
- Similar histologically to osteoblastoma
- No malignant potential
- Reactive zone may contain lymphocytes and plasmocytes

# CLINICAL ISSUES

## Presentation

- Most common signs/symptoms: Night pain relieved by aspirin, NSAIDs
- Clinical Profile
  - 70% have scoliosis related to muscle spasm, concave on side of tumor
  - Gait disturbance, muscle atrophy, torticollis sometimes seen

## Demographics

- Age
  - Majority occur in second decade of life
  - Has been reported as late as seventh decade, but very rare
- Gender: M:F = 2-3:1

## Natural History & Prognosis

- Resection is curative in most cases
  - Entire nidus must be removed or recurrence is probable

- Radionuclide labeling can be used to localize intra-operatively
- Spontaneous healing has been reported

## Treatment

- Open excision
  - Proximity to vertebral artery should be noted in cervical OO
- CT-guided percutaneous excision
- Radiofrequency ablation
- Conservative observation (patients with well controlled symptoms)

# DIAGNOSTIC CHECKLIST

## Consider

- Important cause of painful scoliosis in a child or young adult

## Image Interpretation Pearls

- Thin-section CT most accurate in visualizing nidus
- Edema of adjacent bones on MR mimics extension of infection across discs and joints

# SELECTED REFERENCES

1. Cantwell CP et al: MRI features after radiofrequency ablation of osteoid osteoma with cooled probes and impedance-control energy delivery. AJR Am J Roentgenol. 186(5):1220-7, 2006
2. Liu PT et al: Imaging of osteoid osteoma with dynamic gadolinium-enhanced MR imaging. Radiology. 227(3):691-700, 2003
3. Davies M et al: The diagnostic accuracy of MR imaging in osteoid osteoma. Skeletal Radiol. 31(10):559-69, 2002
4. Scuotto A et al: Unusual manifestation of vertebral osteoid osteoma: case report. Eur Radiol. 12(1):109-12, 2002
5. Lefton DR et al: Vertebral osteoid osteoma masquerading as a malignant bone or soft-tissue tumor on MRI. Pediatr Radiol. 31(2):72-5, 2001
6. Cove JA et al: Osteoid osteoma of the spine treated with percutaneous computed tomography-guided thermocoagulation. Spine. 25(10):1283-6, 2000
7. Gangi A et al: Percutaneous laser photocoagulation of spinal osteoid osteomas under CT guidance. AJNR Am J Neuroradiol. 19(10):1955-8, 1998
8. Radcliffe SN et al: Osteoid osteoma: the difficult diagnosis. Eur J Radiol. 28(1):67-79, 1998
9. Assoun J et al: Osteoid osteoma: MR imaging versus CT. Radiology. 191(1):217-23, 1994
10. Zambelli PY et al: Osteoid osteoma or osteoblastoma of the cervical spine in relation to the vertebral artery. J Pediatr Orthop. 14(6):788-92, 1994
11. Greenspan A: Benign bone-forming lesions: osteoma, osteoid osteoma, and osteoblastoma. Clinical, imaging, pathologic, and differential considerations. Skeletal Radiol. 22(7):485-500, 1993
12. Woods ER et al: Reactive soft-tissue mass associated with osteoid osteoma: correlation of MR imaging features with pathologic findings. Radiology. 186(1):221-5, 1993
13. Raskas DS et al: Osteoid osteoma and osteoblastoma of the spine. J Spinal Disord. 5(2): 204-11, 1992
14. Afshani E et al: Common causes of low back pain in children. Radiographics. 11(2): 269-91, 1991
15. Crim JR et al: Widespread inflammatory response to osteoblastoma: the flare phenomenon. Radiology. 177(3):835-6, 1990

# OSTEOID OSTEOMA

## IMAGE GALLERY

### Typical

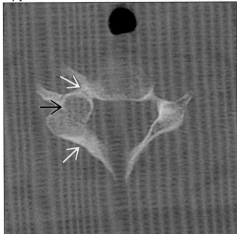

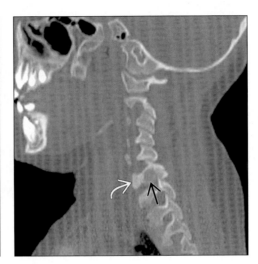

*(Left) Axial bone CT shows an expansile lesion of the right C6 pedicle ➡, with small calcific flecks characteristic of osteoid osteoma. Adjacent sclerosis ➡ is due to prostaglandin release. (Right) Sagittal bone CT reformatted image shows lucency ➡ of C6 vertebral body at the site of the tumor. Note the sclerosis ➡ of adjacent bone.*

### Typical

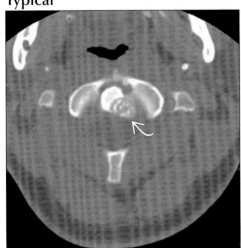

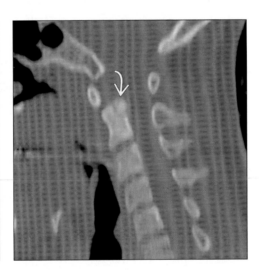

*(Left) Axial NECT shows a lytic lesion ➡ with multiple regions of central hyperdensity in C2 at the junction of the dens and the vertebral body. (Right) Sagittal NECT reformatted image (same patient as previous) shows that the lesion erodes the posterior cortex of the bone. Note central foci of hyperdensity in the largely hypodense lesion ➡.*

### Typical

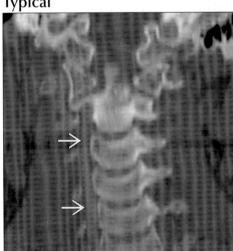

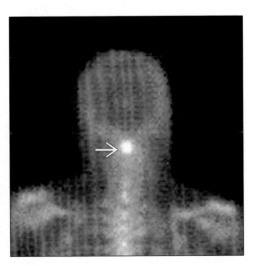

*(Left) Coronal CECT reformatted image (same patient as previous) shows the hypodense lesion with hyperdense foci. Note the enhancing vertebral artery ➡. Contrast was given for surgical planning. (Right) Coronal bone scan (same patient as previous) shows markedly increased uptake of radionuclide tracer ➡ at the site of the C2 osteoid osteoma.*

# OSTEOBLASTOMA

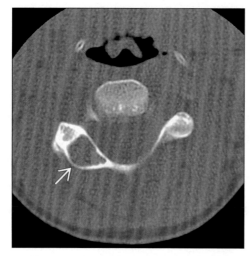

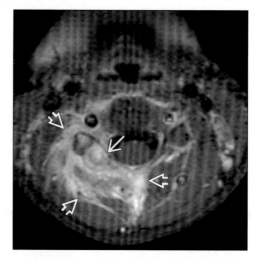

*Axial bone CT of a 6 year old shows a well defined, 12 mm long, expansile lytic lesion of the right lamina ➔ of C4. The surrounding bone demonstrates mild sclerosis.*

*Axial T1WI FS MR shows enhancement of the bone tumor ➔. An extensive enhancing inflammatory response ➔ is evident in the surrounding soft tissues.*

## TERMINOLOGY

### Abbreviations and Synonyms
- Osteoblastoma (OB); giant osteoid osteoma

### Definitions
- Benign tumor forming osteoid
- Differentiated grossly from osteoid osteoma by larger size (usually > 2 cm)

## IMAGING FINDINGS

### General Features
- Best diagnostic clue: Expansile lytic mass occurring in posterior elements
- Location
  - 40% of osteoblastomas occur in the spine
    - 40% cervical, 25% lumbar, 20% thoracic, 15-20% sacrum
  - Originate in neural arch
  - May be centered in pedicle, lamina, transverse or spinous process, articular pillar, or pars interarticularis
  - Often extend into vertebral body
- Size: > 2 cm, range 2-8 cm
- Morphology: Ovoid lytic lesion, often markedly expansile, with variable sclerotic margin

### CT Findings
- CECT: Heterogeneous enhancement obscures bone matrix
- Bone CT
  - Most common appearance
    - Well-circumscribed, expansile lesion of neural arch
    - Often extends into vertebral body
    - Narrow zone of transition, sclerotic rim
  - Aggressive osteoblastoma
    - Cortical breakthrough, wide zone of transition
  - Matrix mineralization
    - Variable amount of mineralization
    - May see small, irregular trabeculae
    - Can be difficult to distinguish from calcified cartilage of chondrosarcoma, enchondroma
  - Inflammatory response may spread far beyond lesion

## DDx: Lesions Involving the Posterior Vertebral Elements

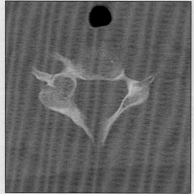

*Osteoid Osteoma*

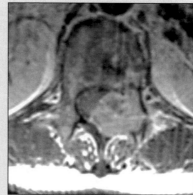

*Aneurysmal Bone Cyst*

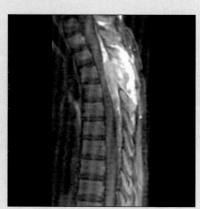

*Langerhans Cell Histiocytosis*

# OSTEOBLASTOMA

## Key Facts

### Terminology
- Osteoblastoma (OB); giant osteoid osteoma
- Benign tumor forming osteoid

### Imaging Findings
- 40% of osteoblastomas occur in the spine
- Originate in neural arch
- Matrix often not visible on spine radiographs, better seen on CT
- Scoliosis in 50-60% of cases
- May be occult on radiographs; obtain CT in every case of young patient with painful scoliosis
- Well-circumscribed, expansile lesion of neural arch
- Often extends into vertebral body
- Narrow zone of transition, sclerotic rim
- Variable amount of mineralization
- Inflammatory response may spread far beyond lesion

- May have aneurysmal bone cyst component
- Peritumoral edema may obscure lesion, mimic malignancy or infection on MR

### Top Differential Diagnoses
- Osteoid Osteoma (OO)
- Aneurysmal Bone Cyst (ABC)
- Giant Cell Tumor
- MR appearance of OB may mimic infection because of inflammatory change in adjacent bones
- Osteogenic Sarcoma (OGS)
- Langerhans Cell Histiocytosis (LCH)

### Clinical Issues
- Age: 90% in 2nd-3rd decades of life
- 10-15% recurrence for typical OB
- 50% recurrence for aggressive OB

---

- Widespread, ill-defined sclerotic bone around lesion
- Periosteal reaction adjacent ribs
- Pleural thickening/effusion
- Ossification of ligamentum flavum

## MR Findings
- T1WI: Low/intermediate signal
- T2WI
  - Intermediate/high signal intensity
  - Low signal areas of bone matrix
  - May have aneurysmal bone cyst component
    - Fluid-fluid levels
  - Extensive peritumoral edema common ("flare phenomenon")
  - Peritumoral edema may involve adjacent bones and soft tissues
  - Peritumoral edema may obscure lesion, mimic malignancy or infection on MR
  - Pleural effusions common with thoracic OB
- T1 C+
  - Variable enhancement
  - Peritumoral edema may enhance

## Radiographic Findings
- Radiography
  - Geographic lesion
  - Expansile
  - Matrix often not visible on spine radiographs, better seen on CT
  - Usually radiolucent, occasionally sclerotic
  - AP radiograph
    - Lucent or sclerotic pedicle
    - Expansion lateral process
    - Scoliosis in 50-60% of cases
    - Scoliosis concave on side of tumor
  - Lateral radiograph
    - Expanded pedicle, lamina, or spinous process
    - Sharply demarcated lucency posterior portion vertebral body
  - May be occult on radiographs; obtain CT in every case of young patient with painful scoliosis

## Nuclear Medicine Findings
- Bone Scan: Positive 3 phase bone scan

## Angiographic Findings
- Intense tumor blush

## Imaging Recommendations
- CT with sagittal, coronal reformations

## DIFFERENTIAL DIAGNOSIS

### Osteoid Osteoma (OO)
- Smaller (< 1.5 cm)
- Round nidus with surrounding sclerotic bone
- Same age group
- Pain usually more intense
- Scoliosis common

### Aneurysmal Bone Cyst (ABC)
- Expansile lesion of posterior elements
- ABC component present in 10-15% of OB
- ABC may also be isolated, or associated with other tumors
- Multiple blood-filled cavities with fluid-fluid levels
- Matrix absent in ABC without OB

### Giant Cell Tumor
- Common in 2nd, 3rd decades
- More common in sacrum than vertebrae
- Destructive, lytic mass ± poorly defined margins

### Infection
- MR appearance of OB may mimic infection because of inflammatory change in adjacent bones
- Distinction between OB & infection easily made on CT

### Osteogenic Sarcoma (OGS)
- Sarcoma containing bone matrix
- Rare in spine
- More aggressive appearance on radiographs, CT
- Wider zone of transition
- Cortical breakthrough rather than cortical expansion

# OSTEOBLASTOMA

- Involves neural arch and/or vertebral body

## Langerhans Cell Histiocytosis (LCH)
- Usually presents with vertebral body involvement, vertebra plana
- Primary localization in the posterior elements less common presentation

## Chordoma
- Involves vertebral body rather than posterior elements
- Common in sacrum, rare in vertebrae
- No matrix: Purely lytic tumor

## Fibrous Dysplasia
- Rare in spine
- Expansile lesion of posterior elements
- May be lytic, or contain "ground-glass" matrix or tiny trabeculae of bone

## Metastasis
- Rare in children compared to adults
- Usually destroys cortex rather than expanding
- Most common from Ewing sarcoma, neuroblastoma

## Chondrosarcoma
- Rare in spine
- Involves vertebral body and/or posterior elements
- May have fairly unaggressive features on imaging studies
- Cartilage calcification in arcs and rings

## PATHOLOGY

### General Features
- General path comments
  - Prostaglandins released by tumor cause extensive peritumoral edema
  - Pain usually less intense than with OO

### Gross Pathologic & Surgical Features
- Friable, highly vascular tumor
- Red color due to vascularity
- Well demarcated from surrounding host bone

### Microscopic Features
- Prominent osteoblasts
- Rims of osteoblasts along trabeculae
- Vascular fibrous stroma
- Woven bone matrix of variable quantity
- Cartilage absent
- ABC component found in 10-15%
- "Aggressive" OB
  - Same features as above, plus
  - More nuclear pleomorphism
  - Epithelioid osteoblasts

### Staging, Grading or Classification Criteria
- Classic osteoblastoma
- Aggressive osteoblastoma
  - Borderline lesion with osteosarcoma
  - Locally aggressive but does not metastasize
  - Sometimes called pseudomalignant OB

## CLINICAL ISSUES

### Presentation
- Most common signs/symptoms
  - Dull, localized pain
  - Scoliosis concave on side of tumor
  - Neurologic symptoms due to compression of cord, nerve roots
- Painful scoliosis; other causes include
  - Trauma
  - OO, other tumors
  - Infection
  - Spondylolysis
  - Renal or retroperitoneal abnormality

### Demographics
- Age: 90% in 2nd-3rd decades of life
- Gender: M:F = 2-2.5:1

### Natural History & Prognosis
- Grow slowly
- 10-15% recurrence for typical OB
- 50% recurrence for aggressive OB

### Treatment
- Curettage with bone graft or methylmethacrylate placement
- Pre-operative embolization may be useful

## DIAGNOSTIC CHECKLIST

### Image Interpretation Pearls
- Aggressive OB is difficult on imaging and histology to distinguish from osteogenic sarcoma
  - Wide zone of transition suspicious for osteogenic sarcoma
- OB is important cause of painful scoliosis

## SELECTED REFERENCES
1. Zileli M et al: Osteoid osteomas and osteoblastomas of the spine. Neurosurg Focus. 15(5):E5, 2003
2. Ozaki T et al: Osteoid osteoma and osteoblastoma of the spine: experiences with 22 patients. Clin Orthop Relat Res. (397):394-402, 2002
3. Biagini R et al: Osteoid osteoma and osteoblastoma of the sacrum. Orthopedics. 24(11):1061-4, 2001
4. Okuda S et al: Ossification of the ligamentum flavum associated with osteoblastoma: a report of three cases. Skeletal Radiol. 30(7):402-6, 2001
5. Shaikh MI et al: Spinal osteoblastoma: CT and MR imaging with pathological correlation. Skeletal Radiol. 28(1):33-40, 1999
6. Saifuddin A et al: Osteoid osteoma and osteoblastoma of the spine. Factors associated with the presence of scoliosis. Spine. 23(1):47-53, 1998
7. Cheung FM et al: Diagnostic criteria for pseudomalignant osteoblastoma. Histopathology. 31(2):196-200, 1997
8. Greenspan A: Benign bone-forming lesions: osteoma, osteoid osteoma, and osteoblastoma. Skeletal Radiol. 22(7):485-500, 1993
9. Crim JR et al: Widespread inflammatory response to osteoblastoma: the flare phenomenon. Radiology. 177(3):835-6, 1990

# OSTEOBLASTOMA

## IMAGE GALLERY

### Typical

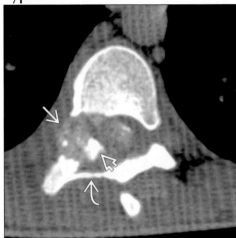

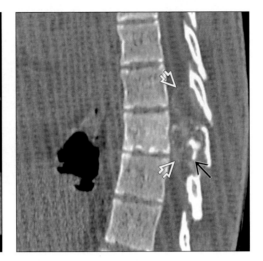

*(Left)* *Axial NECT shows replacement of a thoracic pedicle by an expansile, lytic mass* ➡. *Bone matrix material is seen in the adjacent epidural space* ➡. *The adjacent lamina* ➡ *is eroded.* *(Right)* *Sagittal bone CT (same patient as previous image) shows extensive tumor mass in the epidural space; both dense* ➡ *and faint* ➡ *mineralization are evident. The lamina is eroded.*

### Typical

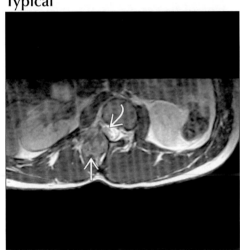

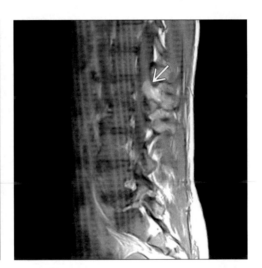

*(Left)* *Axial T2WI MR shows mass expanding the L2 lamina. The tumor* ➡ *is well circumscribed, displays mostly low T2 signal, and narrows spinal canal* ➡. *There is no edema in adjacent bone.* *(Right)* *Sagittal T1 C+ MR (same patient as previous image) shows moderate enhancement* ➡ *following gadolinium injection.*

### Variant

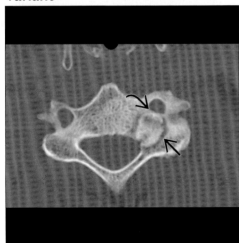

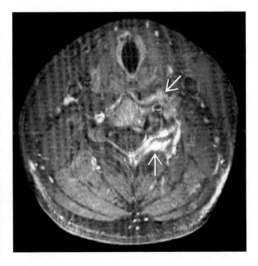

*(Left)* *Axial bone CT shows a mildly sclerotic cervical lesion with a surrounding lucent rim* ➡. *Mild expansion is evident, with mass effect on the foramen transversarium* ➡. *(Right)* *Axial T1WI FS MR shows low T1 signal (minimal to no enhancement) of the bone lesion. Enhancing peritumoral edema/inflammatory reaction* ➡ *are evident.*

# ANEURYSMAL BONE CYST

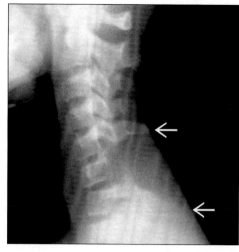

Lateral radiograph of a 13 year old shows complete lysis of posterior elements of C6. The expansile nature of the mass is inferred by displacement of the spinous processes of C5 and C7 ➡.

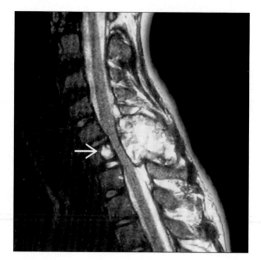

Sagittal T2WI MR shows the hyperintense mass replacing the spinous process of C6, with extension in the epidural space and cord compression. The lesion extends into the posterior body ➡.

## TERMINOLOGY

### Abbreviations and Synonyms
- Aneurysmal bone cyst (ABC)

### Definitions
- Expansile benign neoplasm containing thin-walled, blood-filled cavities

## IMAGING FINDINGS

### General Features
- Best diagnostic clue: Expansile multiloculated neural arch mass with fluid-fluid levels
- Location
  - 10-30% of ABC occur in spine/sacrum
  - Arise in neural arch
  - 75-90% extend into vertebral body

### CT Findings
- NECT
  - Balloon-like expansile remodeling of bone
  - Thinned, "eggshell" cortex
  - Focal cortical destruction common
  - Narrow, nonsclerotic zone of transition
  - Fluid-fluid levels caused by hemorrhage, blood product sedimentation
  - Tumor matrix absent
  - Thin bony septa may be present
  - Commonly extends into epidural space, may severely narrow spinal canal
- CECT
  - Periphery and septa enhance
  - Solid ABC variant enhances diffusely

### MR Findings
- T1WI
  - Lobulated neural arch mass ± extension into vertebral body
  - Cystic spaces of varying sizes within mass
    - Contain fluid-fluid levels due to blood products
    - Cysts separated by septae of varying thickness
  - Part or all of mass may be solid
    - Signal intensity can be high or medium
  - Hypointense rim around mass
    - Rim of periosteum visible on MR even when no cortex visible on CT

## DDx: Lytic, Expansile Spinal Masses

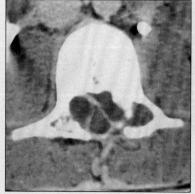

Hydatid Disease

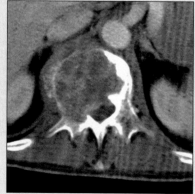

Giant Cell Tumor

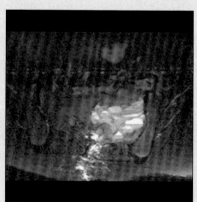

Telangiectatic Osteosarcoma

# ANEURYSMAL BONE CYST

## Key Facts

### Terminology
- Aneurysmal bone cyst (ABC)
- Expansile benign neoplasm containing thin-walled, blood-filled cavities

### Imaging Findings
- 10-30% of ABC occur in spine/sacrum
- Arise in neural arch
- 75-90% extend into vertebral body
- Balloon-like expansile remodeling of bone
- Centered in neural arch, extends into vertebral body
- Absent pedicle sign: Expansion of pedicle results in loss of pedicle contour on AP radiographs
- Cortical thinning
- Focal cortical destruction common
- Fluid-fluid levels caused by hemorrhage, blood product sedimentation

- Tumor matrix absent
- Commonly extends into epidural space, may severely narrow spinal canal

### Top Differential Diagnoses
- Osteoblastoma
- Giant Cell Tumor (GCT)
- Telangiectatic Osteogenic Sarcoma (OGS)
- Hydatid Disease
- Metastases
- Plasmacytoma

### Clinical Issues
- Back pain, most severe at night
- Scoliosis
- Neurologic signs and symptoms from root and/or cord compression

---

- o Epidural extension well seen
- T2WI
  - o Cystic spaces of varying sizes
  - o Fluid-fluid levels due to blood products
  - o Intensities vary with stage of blood degradation
  - o Hypointense rim around mass
  - o Epidural extension well seen
- STIR: Similar to T2WI
- T1 C+
  - o Enhancement at periphery, septa between cysts
  - o Diffuse enhancement in solid ABC variant

## Radiographic Findings
- Radiography
  - o Balloon-like expansile remodeling of bone
    - Centered in neural arch, extends into vertebral body
  - o Absent pedicle sign: Expansion of pedicle results in loss of pedicle contour on AP radiographs
  - o Cortical thinning
  - o Focal cortical destruction common
  - o Rare: Vertebral body collapse ("vertebra plana")
  - o Rare: Extends to more than 1 vertebral level
  - o Rare: Involves adjacent ribs

## Nuclear Medicine Findings
- Bone Scan
  - o Positive 3 phase bone scan
    - May have rim of activity around photopenic region ("donut sign")

## Angiographic Findings
- Conventional
  - o Hypervascular
  - o Vessels more prominent at periphery, drape around lesion

## Imaging Recommendations
- CT best for diagnosis based on specific imaging features
- CT best to differentiate from telangiectatic osteosarcoma
  - o Narrow zone of transition in ABC

- o Absence of infiltration into surrounding soft tissues
- MR shows epidural extent, spinal cord compromise

## DIFFERENTIAL DIAGNOSIS

### Osteoblastoma
- Same age range
- Expansile lesion of neural arch
- Bone matrix is visible on plain films or CT
- May be associated with ABC

### Giant Cell Tumor (GCT)
- Slightly older patients
- Involves vertebral body rather than neural arch
- Expansile, lytic lesion ± soft tissue mass
- May be associated with ABC

### Telangiectatic Osteogenic Sarcoma (OGS)
- Same age range or older
- Involves vertebral body and/or neural arch
- Also shows fluid-fluid levels
- Has more permeative bone destruction
- Wider zone of transition
- Infiltrates into surrounding soft tissues

### Hydatid Disease
- Spine affected in 50% of bone infection by echinococcosis
- Presents with cysts in the posterior elements, epidural, paravertebral tissues

### Metastases
- Uncommon in children
- Involves vertebral body ± neural arch
- Destructive lesion with associated soft tissue mass
- Rare: Vascular metastasis can have fluid levels
- Less expansile, more permeative

### Plasmacytoma
- Very rare in patients younger than 30 years
- Solitary plasmacytoma can have expansile appearance
- Involves vertebral body, usually spares neural arch

# ANEURYSMAL BONE CYST

## Tarlov Cyst
- Perineural cyst occurring in sacrum, arising in neural foramina
- Causes bone expansion, cortical breakthrough
- No enhancement
- Simple fluid on all pulse sequences

## PATHOLOGY

### General Features
- General path comments
  - Not a true tumor; an expansile vascular lesion of unknown cause
  - "Expansile" appearance reflects containment of lesion by appositional periosteal new bone
- Etiology
  - 3 theories
  - 1: Results from trauma + local circulatory disturbance
  - 2: Underlying tumor induces vascular process (venous obstruction or AV fistulae)
    - 5-35% of ABC associated with other tumor, most commonly GCT or OB
  - 3: Neoplasm with cytogenetic abnormalities
    - More than 1/2 cases show abnormality in chromosomes 17p or 16
- Epidemiology
  - 1-2% of primary bone tumors are ABC
  - 10-20% involve the spine or sacrum

### Gross Pathologic & Surgical Features
- Spongy, red mass
- Multiple blood-filled spaces

### Microscopic Features
- Typical
  - Cystic component predominates
    - Cavernous, communicating blood-filled cavities of variable sizes, filled with unclotted blood
    - Lined by fibroblasts, giant cells, histiocytes, hemosiderin
  - Solid components
    - Septations interposed between blood-filled spaces
    - Contain bland stroma with fibrous tissue, reactive bone, giant cells
- Solid ABC is rare variant
  - 5-8% of all ABCs
  - Solid component predominates
  - Propensity for spine

## CLINICAL ISSUES

### Presentation
- Most common signs/symptoms
  - Back pain, most severe at night
  - Other signs/symptoms
    - Scoliosis
    - Neurologic signs and symptoms from root and/or cord compression
    - Pathologic fracture

- Clinical Profile: Young patient with back pain of insidious onset

### Demographics
- Gender: Slightly more common in females
- Familial incidence has been reported

### Natural History & Prognosis
- Long term history of untreated ABC variable
  - Grows initially, then usually stabilizes
  - No malignant degeneration
- Recurrence rate 20-30% (increased if incomplete excision)

### Treatment
- Embolization
  - Curative as sole therapy in some cases
  - Can also be used pre-operatively
- Surgical excision
- May require instrumentation for stabilization of spine
- Radiation therapy may predispose to radiation-induced sarcoma

## DIAGNOSTIC CHECKLIST

### Consider
- "Absent pedicle" sign caused by: ABC, osteoblastoma, lytic OGS, metastasis, trauma, congenital absence of pedicle

### Image Interpretation Pearls
- Evaluation of pedicles on AP radiograph should be part of routine on every patient

## SELECTED REFERENCES

1. Mankin HJ et al: Aneurysmal bone cyst: a review of 150 patients. J Clin Oncol. 23(27):6756-62, 2005
2. Fares Y et al: Spinal hydatid disease and its neurological complications. Scand J Infect Dis. 35(6-7):394-6, 2003
3. Garneti N et al: Cervical spondyloptosis caused by an aneurysmal bone cyst: a case report. Spine. 28(4):E68-70, 2003
4. Lomasney LM et al: Fibrous dysplasia complicated by aneurysmal bone cyst formation affecting multiple cervical vertebrae. Skeletal Radiol. 32(9):533-6, 2003
5. Pogoda P et al: Aneurysmal bone cysts of the sacrum. Clinical report and review of the literature. Arch Orthop Trauma Surg. 123(5):247-51, 2003
6. Chan MS et al: Spinal aneurysmal bone cyst causing acute cord compression without vertebral collapse: CT and MRI findings. Pediatr Radiol. 32(8):601-4, 2002
7. Boriani S et al: Aneurysmal bone cyst of the mobile spine: report on 41 cases. Spine. 26(1):27-35, 2001
8. Papagelopoulos PJ et al: Treatment of aneurysmal bone cysts of the pelvis and sacrum. J Bone Joint Surg Am. 83-A(11):1674-81, 2001
9. DiCaprio MR et al: Aneurysmal bone cyst of the spine with familial incidence. Spine. 25(12):1589-92, 2000
10. Murphey MD et al: From the archives of the AFIP. Primary tumors of the spine: radiologic pathologic correlation. Radiographics. 16(5):1131-58, 1996
11. Kransdorf MJ et al: Aneurysmal bone cyst: concept, controversy, clinical presentation, and imaging. AJR Am J Roentgenol. 164(3):573-80, 1995

# ANEURYSMAL BONE CYST

## IMAGE GALLERY

### Typical

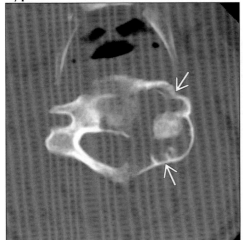
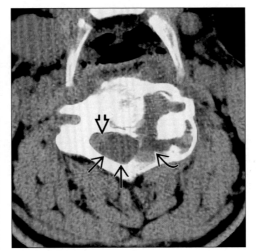

*(Left)* Axial bone CT of a 14 year old shows an expansile, lytic mass ➡ in an upper cervical vertebra. The lesion involves posterior elements on the left and the right side of the vertebral body. *(Right)* Axial NECT reveals fluid-fluid levels ➡ with hyperdense dependent material. Hypodense tumor ➡ occupies most of the spinal canal; spinal cord ⊡ is severely compressed/displaced.

### Typical

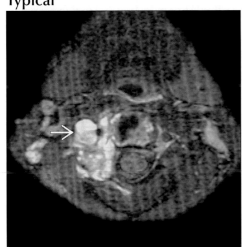
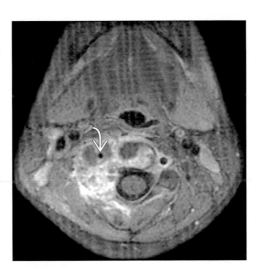

*(Left)* Axial STIR MR of a 9 year old shows a mass in the right posterior elements and the body of C3. Mixed bright and dark signal components are evident. Note fluid-fluid level ➡. *(Right)* Axial T1WI FS MR shows irregular enhancement of the solid aspects of the mass. The cystic portions do not enhance. The right vertebral artery ➡ is encased by tumor.

### Typical

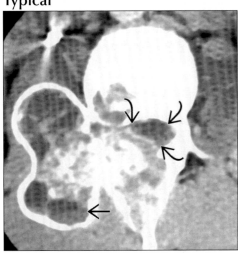
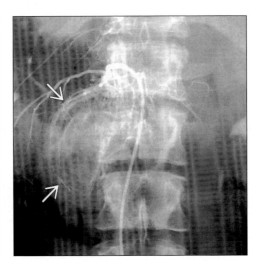

*(Left)* Axial CECT shows a large, expansile lesion of L2, with destruction of right pedicle, lamina, transverse and spinous process. Note fluid-fluid level ➡ and thecal sac ➡ compression. *(Right)* Anteroposterior angiography shows the moderate neovascularity of the mass. Vessels are draped around the periphery of the mass ➡. The right sided pedicle is absent.

# OSTEOCHONDROMA

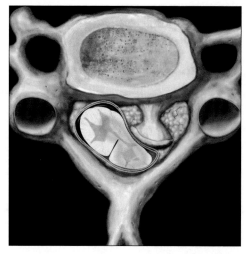

*Axial graphic shows a typical osteochondroma (exostosis) protruding into central canal, producing spinal cord compression. Note the thin cartilaginous "mushroom" cap.*

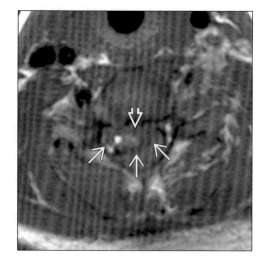

*Axial T1WI MR shows marrow space ⟹ and predominately hypointense cartilaginous cap ⟹. Markedly hypointense peripheral margin of cartilaginous cap is fibrocartilaginous perichondrium.*

## TERMINOLOGY

### Abbreviations and Synonyms
- Osteochondroma (OC), osteocartilaginous exostosis, exostosis
- Hereditary multiple exostoses (HME) = familial osteochondromatosis, diaphyseal aclasis

### Definitions
- Cartilage-covered osseous excrescence contiguous with parent bone

## IMAGING FINDINGS

### General Features
- Best diagnostic clue: Sessile or pedunculated osseous "cauliflower" lesion with marrow/cortical continuity with parent vertebra
- Location
  - Bones forming through endochondral ossification
    - Metaphysis of long tubular bones (85%) common, particularly knee
  - < 5% occur in spine
    - Cervical (50%, C2 predilection) > thoracic (T8 > T4 > other levels) > lumbar > > sacrum
    - Spinous/transverse processes > vertebral body
- Size: Vary dramatically; 1-10 cm

### CT Findings
- CECT: Sessile or pedunculated osseous projection +/- heterogeneous enhancement, cartilaginous cap Ca++
- Bone CT
  - Marrow/cortex continuity with parent bone
  - +/- Chondroid matrix ⇒ "arcs and rings", flocculent Ca++

### MR Findings
- T1WI
  - Central hyperintensity surrounded by hypointense cortex
  - Hypo/isointense hyaline cartilage cap
- T2WI
  - Central iso- to hyperintense signal surrounded by hypointense cortex
  - Hyperintense hyaline cartilage cap
- T1 C+: +/- Septal and peripheral cartilage cap enhancement

---

## DDx: Spinal Osteochondroma

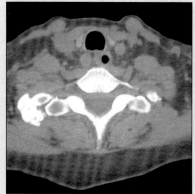

*Scleroderma*

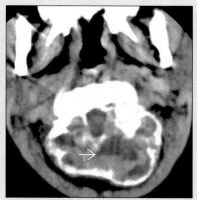

*Aneurysmal Bone Cyst*

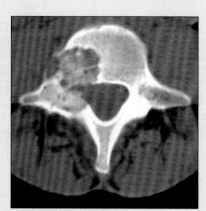

*Osteoblastoma*

# OSTEOCHONDROMA

## Key Facts

### Terminology
- Osteochondroma (OC), osteocartilaginous exostosis, exostosis
- Hereditary multiple exostoses (HME) = familial osteochondromatosis, diaphyseal aclasis

### Imaging Findings
- Best diagnostic clue: Sessile or pedunculated osseous "cauliflower" lesion with marrow/cortical continuity with parent vertebra
- Cervical (50%, C2 predilection) > thoracic (T8 > T4 > other levels) > lumbar > > sacrum
- Spinous/transverse processes > vertebral body

### Top Differential Diagnoses
- Metabolic and Connective Tissue Diseases
- Aneurysmal Bone Cyst (ABC)
- Osteoblastoma
- Chondrosarcoma

### Pathology
- Narrow stalk (pedunculated) or broad attachment base (sessile) contiguous with vertebral cortex, medullary space

### Clinical Issues
- Asymptomatic incidental diagnosis on radiography
- Palpable mass
- Myelopathy; onset often follows trauma

### Diagnostic Checklist
- Multiplicity → consider HME
- Interpret cartilage thickness in context of patient age
- Cartilage cap > 1.5 cm in adults raises concern for malignant transformation (chondrosarcoma)

## Radiographic Findings
- Radiography
  - Sessile/pedunculated osseous protuberance with flaring of parent bone cortex at OC attachment
  - Cartilage cap visible only if extensively mineralized

## Ultrasonographic Findings
- Grayscale Ultrasound
  - Hypoechoic nonmineralized cartilage cap easily distinguished from hyperechoic surrounding fat, muscle
  - Cartilage cap mineralization and osseous stalk → posterior acoustic shadowing

## Nuclear Medicine Findings
- Bone Scan
  - Variable; direct correlation with enchondral bone formation
    - ↑ Radionuclide uptake = metabolically active osteochondroma
    - No ↑ radionuclide uptake = quiescent osteochondroma

## Imaging Recommendations
- Best imaging tool: MR imaging
- Protocol advice
  - MR to measure cartilage cap, determine status of regional neural and musculoskeletal tissue
  - Bone CT to assess mineralization, confirm continuity with vertebral marrow space

## DIFFERENTIAL DIAGNOSIS

### Metabolic and Connective Tissue Diseases
- E.g., calcium metabolism disorders (hyperparathyroidism), dermatomyositis, scleroderma
- Sheet or tumoral calcification, abnormal lab studies

### Aneurysmal Bone Cyst (ABC)
- Expansile, multicystic; fluid-fluid levels

### Osteoblastoma
- Expansile lesion of neural arch/pedicle

### Chondrosarcoma
- Isolated or 2° malignant OC degeneration
- Lytic destructive lesion with sclerotic margins, soft tissue mass
- Chondroid matrix ("rings and arcs", 50%)

## PATHOLOGY

### General Features
- General path comments
  - Benign cartilaginous bone tumor
    - 9% of all bone tumors, most common benign bone tumor (30-45%)
    - Rapid growth, new pain, continued growth of cartilage cap > 1.5 cm thickness after skeletal maturity imply malignant transformation to chondrosarcoma
    - OC complications include deformity, fracture, vascular compromise, neurologic sequelae, overlying bursa formation, and malignant transformation
  - Vertebral OC rare; 1-5% of sporadic OC, 1–9% OC in HME
    - Narrow stalk (pedunculated) or broad attachment base (sessile) contiguous with vertebral cortex, medullary space
    - Hyaline cartilage cap thickness proportional to patient age
  - Many spinal OC are neurologically asymptomatic, produce mechanical impingement symptoms
    - Symptomatic OC arising from posterior vertebral body protrude into canal → cord compression, myelopathy
- Genetics
  - Hereditary multiple exostoses
    - Autosomal dominant, EXT gene locus chromosomes 8, 11, and 19 (tumor suppressor sites)

# OSTEOCHONDROMA

- Inactivation of one EXT gene → exostosis; subsequent inactivation of 2nd EXT gene → malignant transformation
- Etiology
  - Idiopathic, trauma, perichondrial ring deficiency, radiation induced (dose-dependent)
    - Peripheral portion of epiphyseal cartilage herniates out of growth plate
    - Metaplastic cartilage is stimulated; enchondral bone formation → bony stalk
  - Radiation-induced OC
    - Most common benign radiation-induced tumor; prevalence 6-24%
    - Radiation dose 1,500–5,500 cGy; occur at treatment field periphery, latent period 3-17 years, patients generally < 2 years old at time of XRT
    - Pathologically and radiographically identical to other exostoses
- Epidemiology
  - Prevalence of solitary OC unknown since many asymptomatic
  - Prevalence of HME 1:50,000 to 1:100,000 in Western populations; up to 1:1,000 in ethnic Chamorros

## Gross Pathologic & Surgical Features
- Osseous excrescence with cortex, medullary cavity contiguous with parent bone
- Cartilage cap ranges from thick bosselated glistening blue-gray surface (young patients) to several millimeters thick or entirely absent (adults)

## Microscopic Features
- Mature cartilaginous, cancellous, and cortical bone
- Cartilage cap histology reflects classic growth plate zones

# CLINICAL ISSUES

## Presentation
- Most common signs/symptoms
  - Asymptomatic incidental diagnosis on radiography
  - Palpable mass
  - Myelopathy; onset often follows trauma
  - Other signs/symptoms
    - Cranial nerve deficits (dysphagia, hoarseness), pharyngeal mass, scoliosis, radiculopathy
- Clinical Profile
  - Many solitary OC patients present with painless slowly growing mass, but may manifest identical symptoms to HME patients
  - HME patients more often symptomatic; many exostoses produce impingement, other symptoms referable to OC location
    - Mechanical pain → 2° to bursitis over exostosis, surrounding tendon/muscle/neural irritation, OC stalk fracture, or infarct/ischemic necrosis

## Demographics
- Age
  - Peak age = 10-30 years
  - Most HME patients diagnosed by age 5 years, virtually all by 12 years
- Gender: M:F = 3:1

## Natural History & Prognosis
- Post-surgical local recurrence rate < 2%
- Benign lesions; no propensity for metastasis
- Malignant transformation < 1% solitary lesions; 3-5% HME
  - Markers for possible malignant degeneration
    - Growth or new pain after skeletal maturity, ↑ cartilage cap thickness (> 1.5 cm in adults)

## Treatment
- Conservative management in asymptomatic patients
- Surgical excision, deformity correction in symptomatic patients

# DIAGNOSTIC CHECKLIST

## Consider
- Multiplicity → consider HME
- Interpret cartilage thickness in context of patient age

## Image Interpretation Pearls
- Cartilage cap > 1.5 cm in adults raises concern for malignant transformation (chondrosarcoma)
- Radiologic features pathognomonic, reflect pathologic appearance

# SELECTED REFERENCES

1. Bess RS et al: Spinal exostoses: analysis of twelve cases and review of the literature. Spine. 30(7):774-80, 2005
2. Faik A et al: Spinal cord compression due to vertebral osteochondroma: report of two cases. Joint Bone Spine. 72(2):177-9, 2005
3. Korinth MC et al: Cervical cord exostosis compressing the axis in a boy with hereditary multiple exostoses. Case illustration. J Neurosurg. 100(2 Suppl Pediatrics):223, 2004
4. Taitz J et al: Osteochondroma after total body irradiation: an age-related complication. Pediatr Blood Cancer. 42(3):225-9, 2004
5. Fiechtl JF et al: Spinal osteochondroma presenting as atypical spinal curvature: a case report. Spine. 28(13):E252-5, 2003
6. Jones KB et al: Of hedgehogs and hereditary bone tumors: re-examination of the pathogenesis of osteochondromas. Iowa Orthop J. 23:87-95, 2003
7. Pierz KA et al: Hereditary multiple exostoses: one center's experience and review of etiology. Clin Orthop. (401):49-59, 2002
8. Sharma MC et al: Osteochondroma of the spine: an enigmatic tumor of the spinal cord. A series of 10 cases. J Neurosurg Sci. 46(2):66-70; discussion 70, 2002
9. Jose Alcaraz Mexia M et al: Osteochondroma of the thoracic spine and scoliosis. Spine. 26(9):1082-5, 2001
10. Murphey MD et al: Imaging of osteochondroma: variants and complications with radiologic-pathologic correlation. Radiographics. 20(5):1407-34, 2000
11. Ratliff J et al: Osteochondroma of the C5 lamina with cord compression: case report and review of the literature. Spine. 25(10):1293-5, 2000
12. Silber JS et al: A solitary osteochondroma of the pediatric thoracic spine: a case report and review of the literature. Am J Orthop. 29(9):711-4, 2000
13. Wuyts W et al: Molecular basis of multiple exostoses: mutations in the EXT1 and EXT2 genes. Hum Mutat. 15(3):220-7, 2000

# OSTEOCHONDROMA

## IMAGE GALLERY

### Typical

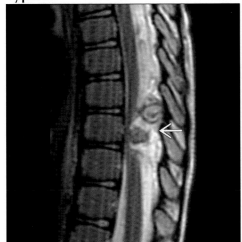
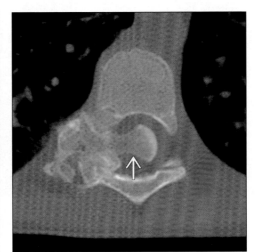

*(Left)* Sagittal T2WI MR depicts a heterogeneous extradural mass ⇒ compressing spinal cord against ventral spinal canal. No abnormalities of the vertebral bodies are detected. *(Right)* Axial bone CT confirms mature ossification contiguous with vertebral marrow space and characteristic "mushroom" configuration ⇒ of ossified osteochondroma (exostosis).

### Typical

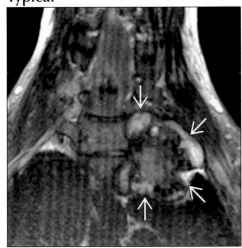
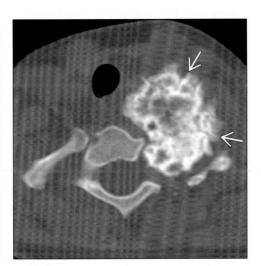

*(Left)* Coronal T2WI MR demonstrates a large peduncular rib osteochondroma a HME patient reveals characteristic T2 hyperintensity of the cartilaginous cap ⇒. *(Right)* Axial bone CT shows large left T1 exostosis with typical "cauliflower" ossification ⇒. Patient presented with brachial plexopathy secondary to regional neural compression.

### Variant

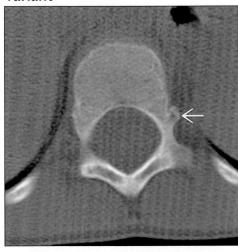
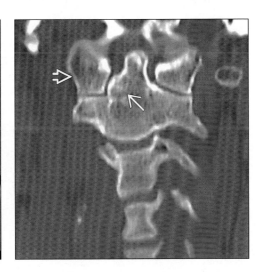

*(Left)* Axial bone CT demonstrates small exostosis of the left pedicle ⇒. Other CT slices (not shown) revealed numerous other exostoses, compatible with typical findings of HME. *(Right)* Coronal bone CT demonstrates a sessile osteochondroma at the C2 dens base ⇒ that remodels and laterally displaces the right C1 lateral mass ⇒.

# OSTEOSARCOMA

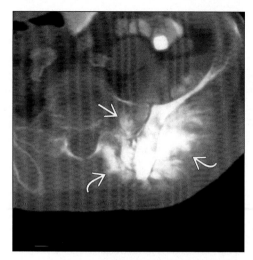

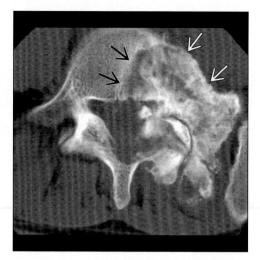

*Axial bone CT shows sclerotic sarcoma involving sacrum ➡ and iliac bone. Osteoid-containing tumor breaks through cortex into the surrounding soft tissues ➡.*

*Axial bone CT shows osteoid containing tumor in the left side of L5, expanding the vertebral body ➡. Note the moth eaten bone destruction and wide zone of transition ➡.*

## TERMINOLOGY

### Abbreviations and Synonyms
- Osteogenic sarcoma, osteosarcoma (OS)

### Definitions
- Sarcoma containing osteoid produced directly by the malignant cells

## IMAGING FINDINGS

### General Features
- Best diagnostic clue: Aggressive lesion forming immature bone
- Location
  - 4% of all primary OS occur in spine and sacrum
  - 79% arise in posterior elements
  - 17% involve 2 adjacent spinal levels
  - 84% invade spinal canal
- Size: Several centimeters at presentation

### CT Findings
- CECT: Contrast administration tends to obscure bone matrix and is not recommended
- Bone CT
  - Best visualization of bone matrix, wide zone of transition, soft tissue mass
  - Moth eaten bone destruction

### MR Findings
- T1WI
  - Low signal intensity: Mineralized tumor
  - Low-intermediate signal intensity: Solid, nonmineralized tumor
- T2WI
  - Low signal intensity: Mineralized tumor
  - High signal intensity: Nonmineralized tumor, soft tissue mass
  - Fluid/fluid levels seen in telangiectatic OS
- Appearance similar to other sarcomas; use CT for matrix visualization

### Radiographic Findings
- Radiography
  - Wide zone of transition

## DDx: Vertebral Tumors

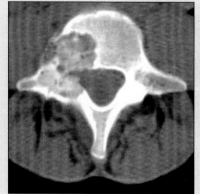

*Osteoblastoma*

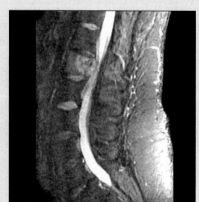

*Ewing Sarcoma*

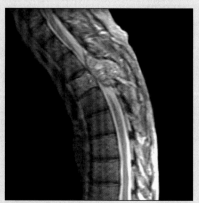

*Chondrosarcoma*

# OSTEOSARCOMA

## Key Facts

### Terminology
- Sarcoma containing osteoid produced directly by the malignant cells

### Imaging Findings
- 4% of all primary OS occur in spine and sacrum
- 79% arise in posterior elements
- 17% involve 2 adjacent spinal levels
- 84% invade spinal canal
- Wide zone of transition
- Permeative appearance
- Cortical breakthrough and soft tissue mass
- 80% have bone matrix seen on radiographs and/or CT scan
- 20% have lytic appearance without visible bone matrix
- Best imaging tool: CT scan

### Top Differential Diagnoses
- Sclerotic Metastasis
- Osteoblastoma (OB)
- Aneurysmal Bone Cyst (ABC)
- Osteomyelitis
- Ewing Sarcoma
- Chondrosarcoma
- Lymphoma

### Pathology
- Epidemiology: OS is second most common primary bone malignancy (after multiple myeloma)

### Clinical Issues
- Insidious onset of back pain
- Median survival 23 months in recent series
- Lower survival rate in sacral tumors

---

- ○ Permeative appearance
- ○ Cortical breakthrough and soft tissue mass
- ○ 80% have bone matrix seen on radiographs and/or CT scan
- ○ 20% have lytic appearance without visible bone matrix

### Nuclear Medicine Findings
- PET: Useful in evaluating tumor recurrence
- Bone Scan
  - ○ Increased uptake on all three phases
  - ○ For staging, detection of skip lesions, metastases

### Imaging Recommendations
- Best imaging tool: CT scan
- Protocol advice
  - ○ CT 1-3 mm with reformatted images
  - ○ MR useful to evaluate for cord, nerve root compression
  - ○ Staging should also include bone scan and chest CT

## DIFFERENTIAL DIAGNOSIS

### Sclerotic Metastasis
- Most commonly medulloblastoma
- Sclerosis reactive; doesn't extend beyond borders of bone
- Often multiple

### Osteoblastoma (OB)
- Expansile, bone-forming lesion in posterior elements
- Can extend into vertebral body
- Aggressive osteoblastoma mimics OS on imaging studies
- Difficult histologic differential diagnosis

### Aneurysmal Bone Cyst (ABC)
- Expansile lesion centered in posterior elements
- Fluid-fluid levels similar to telangiectatic OS
- Can break through cortex
- Zone of transition is narrow, unlike telangiectatic OS

### Osteomyelitis
- Occasionally sclerotic
- Usually involves 2 contiguous vertebrae and intervening disc space

### Ewing Sarcoma
- Can rarely be sclerotic
- Tends to permeate through cortex rather than cause a large visible area of destruction

### Chondrosarcoma
- Ring and arc calcifications

### Lymphoma
- Moth-eaten lytic bone destruction
- Can rarely be sclerotic

### Malignant Giant Cell Tumor
- Rare; most common in sacrum
- Lytic, aggressive mass without bone matrix formation
- Histologically similar to giant-cell rich OS

### Giant Bone Island
- Sclerotic focus in medullary bone
- Mature cortical bone
- Shows "brush border": Trabeculae merge with adjacent bone

## PATHOLOGY

### General Features
- General path comments
  - ○ Malignant tumor which produces osteoid directly from neoplastic cells
  - ○ Matrix (material produced by tumor cells) is immature, woven osteoid
  - ○ Other malignant tumors (e.g., chondrosarcoma) may contain bone but osteoid is not produced by the malignant cells
  - ○ Secondary osteosarcoma occurs in Paget disease, irradiated bone, bone infarct

# OSTEOSARCOMA

- Genetics: Alterations of Rb genes in OS that develops in association with retinoblastoma
- Etiology
  - Primary OS has unknown etiology: Most cases
  - Secondary OS has predisposing factors (Paget disease, bone infarct, radiation)
  - May be associated with retinoblastoma
- Epidemiology: OS is second most common primary bone malignancy (after multiple myeloma)

## Gross Pathologic & Surgical Features
- Heterogeneous mass with ossified and non-ossified components
- Ossified areas: Yellow-white, firm, may be as hard as cortical bone
- Less ossified areas: Soft, tan, with foci of hemorrhage and necrosis
- May break through cortex ⇒ large extraosseous tumor mass
- Necrosis common

## Microscopic Features
- Pluripotential neoplasm
- Malignant cells produce some osteoid in all subtypes, but it may be difficult to find
- Classic: High degree anaplasia, high mitotic rate
- Tumor cells may be spindle or round, size varies from small to giant
- Telangiectatic OS
  - Dilated vascular channels lined by multinucleated giant cells
  - Stroma forms osteoid, which may not be a prominent feature

## Staging, Grading or Classification Criteria
- Classified by predominant histologic cell type
  - Osteoblastic (conventional), chondroblastic, fibroblastic, telangiectatic, small cell, giant cell, epithelioid
  - Surface OS not reported in spine
- Surgical staging for malignant musculoskeletal tumors
  - Stage Ia: Low grade, intracompartmental
  - Stage Ib: Low grade, extracompartmental
  - Stage IIa: High grade, intracompartmental
  - Stage IIb: High grade, extracompartmental
  - Stage IIIa: Low or high grade, intracompartmental, metastases
  - Stage IIIb: Low or high grade, extracompartmental, metastases

# CLINICAL ISSUES

## Presentation
- Most common signs/symptoms
  - Insidious onset of back pain
  - Pain greatest at night
  - Radicular pain
  - Paraplegia
- Clinical Profile
  - Pathologic fracture
  - Pulmonary metastases common, can cause pneumothorax (calcifying)
  - Increased serum alkaline phosphatase

## Demographics
- Age
  - Spine OS has peak incidence in 4th decade
  - Later peak incidence than for appendicular OS
  - Wide age range: Children and adults
- Gender: M = F

## Natural History & Prognosis
- Median survival 23 months in recent series
- Lower survival rate in sacral tumors
- Survival rate lower than for peripheral OS due to difficulty of surgical resection
- Metastases: Bone, lung, liver
- 3% of 10 year survivors of all OS develop a second malignancy

## Treatment
- Surgical resection with wide margins
- Adjuvant and neoadjuvant chemotherapy
- Biopsies must be planned with future tumor excision in mind

# DIAGNOSTIC CHECKLIST

## Image Interpretation Pearls
- All telangiectatic OS are lytic on radiographs and CT, but not all lytic OS are telangiectatic

# SELECTED REFERENCES

1. Murakami H et al: Complete segmental resection of the spine, including the spinal cord, for telangiectatic osteosarcoma: a report of 2 cases. Spine. 31(4):E117-22, 2006
2. Ilaslan H et al: Primary vertebral osteosarcoma: imaging findings. Radiology. 230(3):697-702, 2004
3. Brenner W et al: PET imaging of osteosarcoma. J Nucl Med. 44(6):930-42, 2003
4. Aung L et al: Second malignant neoplasms in long-term survivors of osteosarcoma: Memorial Sloan-Kettering Cancer Center Experience. Cancer. 95(8):1728-34, 2002
5. Bredella MA et al: Value of FDG PET in conjunction with MR imaging for evaluating therapy response in patients with musculoskeletal sarcomas. AJR Am J Roentgenol. 179(5):1145-50, 2002
6. Ozaki T et al: Osteosarcoma of the spine: experience of the Cooperative Osteosarcoma Study Group. Cancer. 94(4):1069-77, 2002
7. Iwata A et al: Osteosarcoma as a second malignancy after treatment for neuroblastoma. Pediatr Hematol Oncol. 18(7):465-9, 2001
8. Yamamoto T et al: Sacral radiculopathy secondary to multicentric osteosarcoma. Spine. 26(15):1729-32, 2001
9. Bramwell VH: Osteosarcomas and other cancers of bone. Curr Opin Oncol. 12(4):330-6, 2000
10. Vuillemin-Bodaghi V et al: Multifocal osteogenic sarcoma in Paget's disease. Skeletal Radiol. 29(6):349-53, 2000
11. Unni KK: Osteosarcoma of bone. J Orthop Sci. 3(5):287-94, 1998
12. Rosenberg ZS et al: Osteosarcoma: Subtle, rare, and misleading plain film features. Am J Roentgenol. 165:1209-14, 1995
13. Barwick KW et al: Primary osteogenic sarcoma of the vertebral column: a clinicopathologic correlation of ten patients. Cancer. 46(3):595-604, 1980

# OSTEOSARCOMA

## IMAGE GALLERY

### Typical

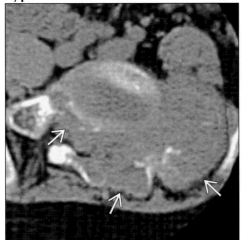

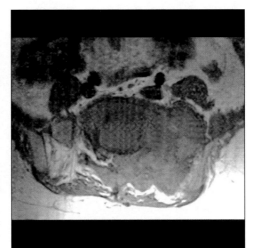

*(Left)* Axial NECT shows extensive extraosseous tumor ➡ after breaking through the cortex. Some types of OS, such as this one, contain only a small amount of osteoid. *(Right)* Axial PD/Intermediate MR shows extensive tumor involvement of the lateral aspect of S1. Mineralization is difficult to see on MR, which is more useful for assessing extent of canal invasion.

### Typical

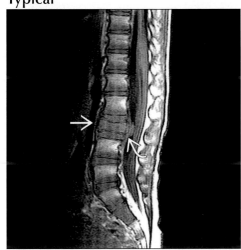

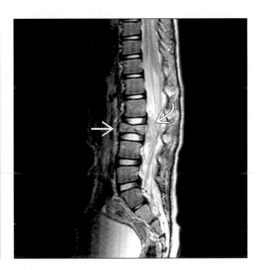

*(Left)* Sagittal T1WI MR shows compression deformity of L3 ➡, which is hypointense compared with other vertebrae. Tumor permeates through the cortex into the spinal canal ➡. *(Right)* Sagittal STIR MR shows bone marrow of L3 is replaced by diffuse tumor ➡ which permeates through the cortex into the spinal canal ➡, indicating an aggressive process.

### Typical

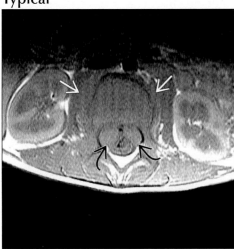

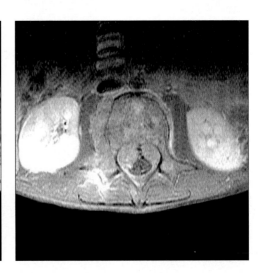

*(Left)* Axial T1WI MR (same patient as previous image) shows that the tumor has permeated the vertebral body and broken through cortex into the paraspinous regions ➡ and epidural space ➡. *(Right)* Axial T1 C+ FS MR in the same patient as the previous figure shows heterogeneous enhancement of the permeative tumor within and surrounding the vertebral body.

# CHORDOMA

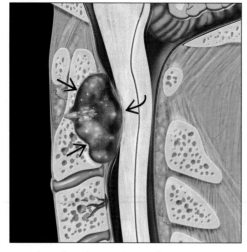

Sagittal graphic of cervical spine depicts an extradural soft tissue mass ➡ with center in posterior body of C2 producing bone destruction, epidural extension, and cord compression ➘.

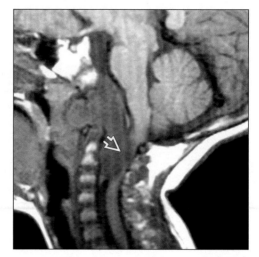

Sagittal T1WI MR shows a hypointense destructive mass engulfing the distal clivus and anterior C1 arch. Posterior extension ➡ compresses spinal cord.

## TERMINOLOGY

### Definitions
- Malignant clival or vertebral tumor arising from notochord remnants

## IMAGING FINDINGS

### General Features
- Best diagnostic clue: T2 hyperintense (to intervertebral discs) multilobular, septated mass centered in posterior vertebral body
- Location
  - Majority of pediatric chordomas arise in spheno-occipital region
  - In adults, sacrococcygeal > spheno-occipital >> vertebral body
- Size: Usually at least several centimeters at presentation
- Morphology
  - Midline multilobular soft tissue mass with osseous destruction
    - Extend into disc → involve 2 or more adjacent vertebrae
    - Extend into epidural/perivertebral space → cord compression
    - Extend along nerve roots → enlarge neural foramina

### CT Findings
- NECT
  - Destructive mass
    - Lysis of bone + hypodense soft tissue mass
  - ± Marginal sclerosis (40-60%)
  - Amorphous intratumoral Ca++
    - 2° to bone destruction, not matrix
  - Variable location
    - Sacrum > 70%
    - Vertebra (C > L > T) 30%
- CECT
  - Variable soft tissue enhancement
    - Many do not enhance at all
  - ± Heterogeneous areas of cystic necrosis

### MR Findings
- T1WI: Heterogeneous hypo- or isointense (relative to marrow) multilobulated mass

## DDx: Chordoma

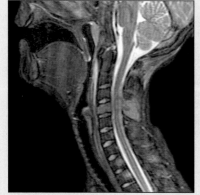

Ewing Sarcoma

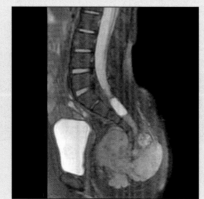

Rhabdomyosarcoma

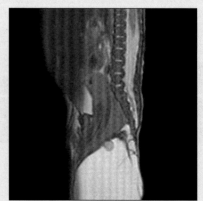

Sacrococcygeal Teratoma

# CHORDOMA

## Key Facts

### Terminology
- Malignant clival or vertebral tumor arising from notochord remnants

### Imaging Findings
- Best diagnostic clue: T2 hyperintense (to intervertebral discs) multilobular, septated mass centered in posterior vertebral body
- Majority of pediatric chordomas arise in spheno-occipital region
- Amorphous intratumoral Ca++

### Top Differential Diagnoses
- Chondrosarcoma
- Metastases/Ewing Sarcoma/Lymphoma
- Sacrococcygeal Teratoma
- Giant Cell Tumor

- Ecchordosis Physaliphora

### Pathology
- 2-4% of primary malignant bone neoplasms
- Incidence 0.08 per 100,000
- Histologic identification of physaliphorous cell confirms diagnosis

### Clinical Issues
- More common in adults than in children
- < 5% occur in children

### Diagnostic Checklist
- T2 hyperintense mass ("light bulb") with calcification, septations, minimal enhancement = chordoma/chondroid tumor

- T2WI
  - Heterogeneous multilobulated mass
  - Hyperintense to CSF, intervertebral discs
  - Hypointense fibrous septations
- T1 C+
  - Variable: Pediatric chordomas enhance less than adult chordomas
    - Many do not enhance at all

## Radiographic Findings
- Radiography
  - Heterogeneous, lytic destruction of sacrum or vertebral body
  - ± Marginal sclerosis

## Nuclear Medicine Findings
- Bone Scan: ↓ Radiotracer uptake

## Imaging Recommendations
- Best imaging tool: Multiplanar MR imaging
- Protocol advice
  - MR for soft tissue (STIR/fat-saturated T2WI, contrast-enhanced T1WI)
  - Bone CT for osseous margins

## DIFFERENTIAL DIAGNOSIS

### Chondrosarcoma
- Neural arch > vertebral body
- ± Chondroid matrix (rings and arcs)
- Similar MR characteristics (greater enhancement)

### Metastases/Ewing Sarcoma/Lymphoma
- Multifocal disease; heterogeneous T2 signal (usually lower signal intensity than chordoma)
- Less sharply defined margins

### Sacrococcygeal Teratoma
- Heterogeneous MR signal (fat = T1 hyperintense)

### Giant Cell Tumor
- Heterogeneous MR signal with blood products, hypointense T2 signal

### Ecchordosis Physaliphora
- Benign, nonneoplastic ectopic notochordal remnant(s)
- Rare (~ 2% of autopsies)
- Usually found at skull base/C2, but can occur anywhere (including intradural)

## PATHOLOGY

### General Features
- General path comments
  - Location
    - Sacrococcygeal (50%) > spheno-occipital (35%) > vertebral body (15%)
    - Vertebral body: Cervical (20-50%) > lumbar > thoracic
- Genetics
  - Losses on chromosomal arms 3p (50%) and 1p (44%)
  - Gains on 7q (69%), 20 (50%), 5q (38%), and 12q (38%)
- Etiology
  - Derived from notochord remnants
    - Notochord (column of cells ventral to neural tube) arises during 3rd gestational week, disappears by 7th week
    - Notochordal rests may persist in axial skeleton (dorsum sellae to coccyx)
- Epidemiology
  - 2-4% of primary malignant bone neoplasms
  - Incidence 0.08 per 100,000
  - < 5% of chordomas present in childhood

### Gross Pathologic & Surgical Features
- Lobulated grayish, soft, gelatinous mass

### Microscopic Features
- Histologic identification of physaliphorous cell confirms diagnosis
- 3 types described

# CHORDOMA

- Typical: Lobules, sheets, and cords of clear cells with intracytoplasmic vacuoles (physaliphorous cells); abundant mucin
- Chondroid: Hyaline cartilage (usually spheno-occipital)
- Dedifferentiated: Sarcomatous elements (rare, highly malignant)
- Immunohistochemistry: + Cytokeratin, + epithelial membrane antigen

## Staging, Grading or Classification Criteria
- Enneking system for staging musculoskeletal sarcomas
  - Grade of biologic aggressiveness
  - Anatomic setting
  - Presence of metastasis

# CLINICAL ISSUES

## Presentation
- Most common signs/symptoms
  - Cranial neuropathy
    - Many cervical chordomas extend into skull base
  - Pain, numbness, weakness, incontinence (location dependent)
  - Sacral or gluteal mass
- Other signs/symptoms: ± Autonomic dysfunction

## Demographics
- Age
  - More common in adults than in children
    - Peak incidence 5th-6th decades
  - < 5% occur in children
- Gender
  - M:F = 2:1 in vertebral body
  - No gender predilection in sacrum
- Ethnicity: Rare in African-Americans

## Natural History & Prognosis
- Slow-growing
  - Pediatric chordomas may behave more aggressively than in adults
- Distant metastases 5-40% (lung, liver, lymph nodes, bone)
- Poor prognostic factors
  - Large size
  - Subtotal resection, local recurrence
  - Microscopic necrosis
  - Ki-67 index > 5%
- Survival
  - 5 year up to 67-84%
  - 10 year ~ 40%

## Treatment
- Surgical resection with adjuvant radiation therapy (XRT)
  - En bloc resection yields best outcome
- Recurrence common
  - Local (90%)
  - Regional lymph nodes (5%)
  - Distant metastases (5%); lung, bone
  - 5 year survival after relapse (5-7%)

# DIAGNOSTIC CHECKLIST

## Consider
- T2 hyperintense mass ("light bulb") with calcification, septations, minimal enhancement = chordoma/chondroid tumor

## Image Interpretation Pearls
- Recurrence (seeding) along operative tract is not uncommon
  - Modify imaging field-of-view to include operative approach

# SELECTED REFERENCES

1. Hoch BL et al: Base of skull chordomas in children and adolescents: a clinicopathologic study of 73 cases. Am J Surg Pathol. 30(7):811-8, 2006
2. Pamir MN et al: Analysis of radiological features relative to histopathology in 42 skull-base chordomas and chondrosarcomas. Eur J Radiol. 58(3):461-70, 2006
3. Noel G et al: Chordomas of the base of the skull and upper cervical spine. One hundred patients irradiated by a 3D conformal technique combining photon and proton beams. Acta Oncol. 44(7):700-8, 2005
4. Mehnert F et al: Retroclival ecchordosis physaliphora: MR imaging and review of the literature. AJNR Am J Neuroradiol. 25(10):1851-5, 2004
5. Baratti D et al: Chordoma: natural history and results in 28 patients treated at a single institution. Ann Surg Oncol. 10(3):291-6, 2003
6. Smolders D et al: Value of MRI in the diagnosis of non-clival, non-sacral chordoma. Skeletal Radiol. 32(6):343-50, 2003
7. Bayar MA et al: Spinal chordoma of the terminal filum. Case report. J Neurosurg. 96(2 Suppl):236-8, 2002
8. Carpentier A et al: Suboccipital and cervical chordomas: the value of aggressive treatment at first presentation of the disease. J Neurosurg. 97(5):1070-7, 2002
9. Delank KS et al: Metastasizing chordoma of the lumbar spine. Eur Spine J. 11(2):167-71, 2002
10. Steenberghs J et al: Intradural chordoma without bone involvement. Case report and review of the literature. J Neurosurg. 97(1 Suppl):94-7, 2002
11. Arnautovic KI et al: Surgical seeding of chordomas. J Neurosurg. 95(5):798-803, 2001
12. Crapanzano JP et al: Chordoma: a cytologic study with histologic and radiologic correlation. Cancer. 93(1):40-51, 2001
13. McMaster ML et al: Chordoma: incidence and survival patterns in the United States, 1973-1995. Cancer Causes Control. 12(1):1-11, 2001
14. Scheil S et al: Genome-wide analysis of sixteen chordomas by comparative genomic hybridization and cytogenetics of the first human chordoma cell line, U-CH1. Genes Chromosomes Cancer. 32(3):203-11, 2001
15. Bergh P et al: Prognostic factors in chordoma of the sacrum and mobile spine: a study of 39 patients. Cancer. 88(9):2122-34, 2000
16. Wippold FJ 2nd et al: Clinical and imaging features of cervical chordoma. AJR Am J Roentgenol. 172(5):1423-6, 1999
17. Murphy JM et al: CT and MRI appearances of a thoracic chordoma. Eur Radiol. 8(9):1677-9, 1998
18. Ng SH et al: Cervical ecchordosis physaliphora: CT and MR features. Br J Radiol. 71(843):329-31, 1998

# CHORDOMA

## IMAGE GALLERY

### Typical

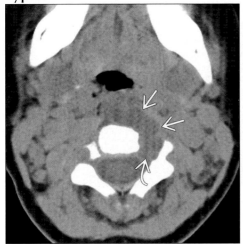
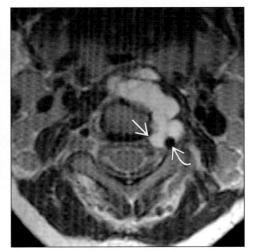

*(Left)* Axial NECT depicts a hypodense noncalcified pre- and paraspinal mass ➡ extending into the left C2 neural foramen ➡. *(Right)* Axial T2WI MR in same patient as previous image confirms T2 hyperintense C2 mass. Note extension into the left neural foramen ➡, partially engulfing vertebral artery ➡.

### Typical

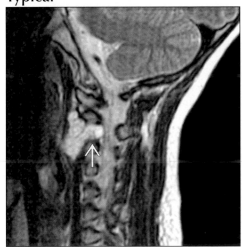
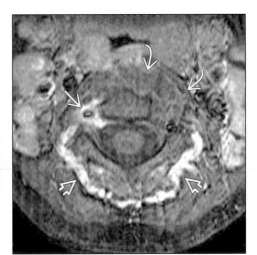

*(Left)* Sagittal T2WI MR in same patient as previous image demonstrates T2 hyperintense mass with hypointense internal septations extending into the C2 neural foramen ➡. *(Right)* Axial T1 C+ FS MR in same patient as previous image reveals mild heterogeneous enhancement of mass ➡. Note engorgement of enhancing venous plexus ➡ and paraspinal veins ➡.

### Typical

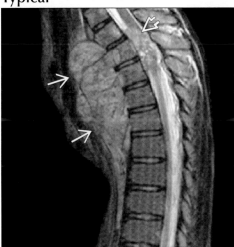
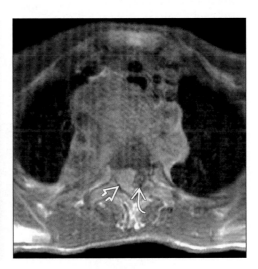

*(Left)* Sagittal T2WI MR in 14 year old male with myelopathy shows a large hyperintense destructive vertebral mass ➡ producing canal compromise and cord compression ➡. *(Courtesy J. Ross, MD)*. *(Right)* Axial T1 C+ MR confirms a large destructive enhancing vertebral mass with epidural extension ➡ producing spinal cord ➡ displacement and compression. *(Courtesy J. Ross, MD)*.

# EWING SARCOMA

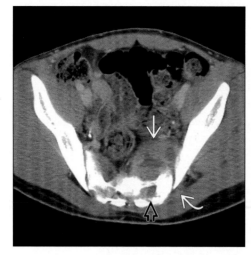

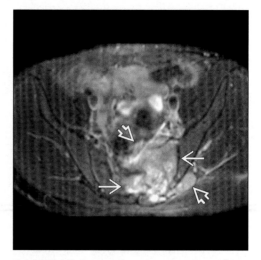

*Axial CECT shows a soft tissue mass arising from the left hemisacrum, with a dominant presacral ➜ component; intrasacral ⟱ and posterolateral parasacral infiltration ➜ is evident.*

*Axial STIR MR (same patient as previous image) better demonstrates the extensive infiltration of the sacral body and the left hemisacrum ➜, along with the parasacral soft tissue involvement ➜.*

## TERMINOLOGY

### Abbreviations and Synonyms
- Ewing sarcoma, Ewing tumor

### Definitions
- Round cell sarcoma of bone

## IMAGING FINDINGS

### General Features
- Best diagnostic clue: Permeative lytic lesion of vertebral body or sacrum
- Location
  - Spine: 5-10% of all Ewing tumor
  - Involve vertebral body before neural arch
  - Sacrum more common site than spine
  - May involve adjacent bones: Vertebrae, ribs, or ilium
  - Contiguous spread along peripheral nerves from spine or sacral primary
  - May originate in soft tissues

### CT Findings
- CECT
  - Heterogeneous enhancement
  - Areas of central necrosis common
- Bone CT
  - Permeative intramedullary mass ± soft tissue mass
  - Tiny perforations through cortex more common than widespread breakthrough
  - Rarely sclerotic; no ossification in soft tissue mass

### MR Findings
- T1WI
  - Intermediate to low signal intensity
  - Hypointense compared to surrounding bone marrow
  - Cortex often appears thinned but intact despite extraosseous tumor spread
- T2WI
  - Intermediate to high signal intensity
  - Cannot reliably distinguish between tumor/peritumoral edema
- STIR: Tumor more conspicuous than on T2WI
- T1 C+
  - Moderate enhancement
  - Areas of necrosis

## DDx: Sacral Masses in Children

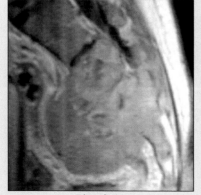

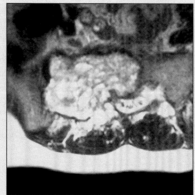

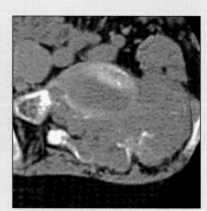

*Chordoma*

*Giant Cell Tumor*

*Lytic Osteosarcoma*

# EWING SARCOMA

## Key Facts

### Terminology
- Round cell sarcoma of bone

### Imaging Findings
- Centered in vertebral body or sacrum
- Permeative/moth eaten bone destruction
- Wide zone of transition
- Tiny perforations of cortex rather than extensive loss of cortical bone radiographically
- 50% have extraosseous, noncalcified, soft tissue mass
- MR best shows involvement of adjacent bones & soft tissues

### Top Differential Diagnoses
- Primitive Neuroectodermal Tumor (PNET)
- Langerhans Cell Histiocytosis
- Other Small Round Cell Tumors

- Osteomyelitis
- Osteogenic Sarcoma (OGS)
- Other Primary Sarcomas and Metastatic Disease

### Pathology
- Primitive neuroectodermal tumor (PNET) is closely related tumor
- 6th most common malignant bone tumor

### Clinical Issues
- Localized pain
- Fever, leukocytosis, elevated ESR (simulating osteomyelitis)
- Prognosis worse in spinal than peripheral Ewing sarcoma because of difficulty of surgical resection
- Significant risk of second malignancy

---

  ○ Cannot reliably distinguish between tumor/peritumoral edema

### Radiographic Findings
- Radiography
  ○ Centered in vertebral body or sacrum
  ○ Permeative/moth eaten bone destruction
  ○ Wide zone of transition
  ○ Tiny perforations of cortex rather than extensive loss of cortical bone radiographically
  ○ 50% have extraosseous, noncalcified, soft tissue mass
  ○ 5% sclerotic (represents host reaction, not tumor matrix)
  ○ May cause vertebra plana
  ○ May involve 2 or more adjacent bones
  ○ If adjacent vertebrae involved, do not see disc height loss and peridiscal erosions as in osteomyelitis

### Nuclear Medicine Findings
- PET: Increased FDG uptake of tumor, metastases
- Bone Scan: Positive 3-phase bone scan

### Imaging Recommendations
- Best imaging tool
  ○ MR best shows involvement of adjacent bones & soft tissues
    - CT can underestimate soft tissue involvement
  ○ MR may overestimate tumor size due to peritumoral edema
- Protocol advice
  ○ MR to determine extent of tumor
    - Sagittal T1WI
    - Axial and sagittal STIR, post-contrast T1WI
  ○ CT useful to confirm absence of tumor matrix, distinguish from osteosarcoma

## DIFFERENTIAL DIAGNOSIS

### Primitive Neuroectodermal Tumor (PNET)
- Clinically/radiologically identical to Ewing sarcoma
- Arises in extraskeletal soft tissues

- Greater neuroectodermal differentiation of tumor cells

### Langerhans Cell Histiocytosis
- May have identical radiographic appearance
- May form discrete geographic lytic lesion

### Other Small Round Cell Tumors
- Lymphoma, leukemia, metastatic neuroblastoma
- Have same radiographic appearance as Ewing sarcoma
- Ill-defined lytic lesion showing permeative pattern
- Involve vertebral body more than neural arch
- Often involve multiple vertebrae

### Osteomyelitis
- Ill-defined lytic lesion showing permeative pattern
- May be more geographic (intraosseous abscess with peripheral enhancement)
- Involves vertebral body more than neural arch
- Discocentric: Extends from one vertebral body to adjacent vertebra across disc
- Disc height loss, enhancement of disc on MR, endplate erosions
- Soft tissue mass common

### Osteogenic Sarcoma (OGS)
- Ill-defined lytic lesion showing permeative pattern
- 80% show bone matrix on radiographs or CT
- Involves vertebral body or neural arch
- May involve adjacent vertebral body

### Other Primary Sarcomas and Metastatic Disease
- Includes
  ○ Chondrosarcoma
  ○ Malignant fibrous histiocytoma
  ○ Malignant giant cell tumor (GCT)
- Ill-defined lytic lesion showing permeative pattern
- Tend to have more focal and complete cortical destruction
- Involve vertebral body, ± neural arch

# EWING SARCOMA

## PATHOLOGY

### General Features
- General path comments
  - Prototype of non-hematologic small round cell tumor
  - Primitive neuroectodermal tumor (PNET) is closely related tumor
- Genetics: Reciprocal translocation between EWS gene on chromosome 22 and EWS-like genes on chromosome 11
- Etiology: Undifferentiated mesenchymal cells with slight differentiation toward neuroectodermal cells
- Epidemiology
  - Annual incidence of Ewing sarcoma all locations: 3/1,000,000 Caucasian children < 15 years old
  - 6th most common malignant bone tumor

### Gross Pathologic & Surgical Features
- Grayish white tumor
- Poorly demarcated
- Areas of hemorrhage, cyst formation, necrosis

### Microscopic Features
- Small, round cells (2-3 times larger than lymphocytes), meager cytoplasm
- Cell outlines indistinct
- Round nuclei, frequent indentations, high mitotic rate
- Solid sheets of cells divided into irregular masses by fibrous strands
- Features which distinguish PNET from Ewing sarcoma
  - PNET forms rosettes of cells
  - PNET is positive for 2 or more neuroectodermal markers
  - Distinction most reliably made with fluorescence in situ hybridization (FISH)

## CLINICAL ISSUES

### Presentation
- Most common signs/symptoms
  - Localized pain
  - Fever, leukocytosis, elevated ESR (simulating osteomyelitis)
  - Vertebra plana
  - Neurologic symptoms ranging from radiculopathy to paralysis

### Demographics
- Age
  - 90% of all Ewing sarcoma patients present before 20 years
  - Spine and sacral lesions often in older patients than peripheral Ewing sarcoma
- Gender: M:F = 2:1

### Natural History & Prognosis
- Metastases to lung, regional lymph nodes, and other bones in 30% at presentation
- Prognosis worse in spinal than peripheral Ewing sarcoma because of difficulty of surgical resection
- Significant risk of second malignancy

- Current treatments yield long term survival > 50% of patients with localized disease at presentation
- Complications common > 5 years after treatment
  - Local recurrence
  - Metastases
  - Treatment complications
  - Second malignancies

### Treatment
- Surgery or radiotherapy; without chemotherapy universally fatal
- Neoadjuvant chemotherapy given prior to surgery
- Surgical resection with wide margins
- Radiation therapy for surgically inaccessible lesions, stage III disease, poor response to chemotherapy

## DIAGNOSTIC CHECKLIST

### Image Interpretation Pearls
- Always consider osteomyelitis and other small round cell tumors in imaging differential diagnosis

## SELECTED REFERENCES

1. Bacci G et al: Long-term outcome for patients with non-metastatic Ewing's sarcoma treated with adjuvant and neoadjuvant chemotherapies. 402 patients treated at Rizzoli between 1972 and 1992. Eur J Cancer. 40(1):73-83, 2004
2. Bacci G et al: Therapy and survival after recurrence of Ewing's tumors: the Rizzoli experience in 195 patients treated with adjuvant and neoadjuvant chemotherapy from 1979 to 1997. Ann Oncol. 14(11):1654-9, 2003
3. Burchill SA: Ewing's sarcoma: diagnostic, prognostic, and therapeutic implications of molecular abnormalities. J Clin Pathol. 56(2):96-102, 2003
4. Fuchs B et al: Complications in long-term survivors of Ewing sarcoma. Cancer. 98(12):2687-92, 2003
5. Fuchs B et al: Ewing's sarcoma and the development of secondary malignancies. Clin Orthop. (415):82-9, 2003
6. Harimaya K et al: Primitive neuroectodermal tumor and extraskeletal Ewing sarcoma arising primarily around the spinal column: report of four cases and a review of the literature. Spine. 28(19):E408-12, 2003
7. Goktepe AS et al: Paraplegia: an unusual presentation of Ewing's sarcoma. Spinal Cord. 40(7):367-9, 2002
8. Hawkins DS et al: Evaluation of chemotherapy response in pediatric bone sarcomas by [F-18]-fluorodeoxy-D-glucose positron emission tomography. Cancer. 94(12):3277-84, 2002
9. Hoffer FA: Primary skeletal neoplasms: osteosarcoma and ewing sarcoma. Top Magn Reson Imaging. 13(4):231-9, 2002
10. Paulussen M et al: Ewing tumour: incidence, prognosis and treatment options. Paediatr Drugs. 3(12):899-913, 2001
11. Venkateswaran L et al: Primary Ewing tumor of the vertebrae: clinical characteristics, prognostic factors, and outcome. Med Pediatr Oncol. 37(1):30-5, 2001
12. Downing JR et al: Detection of the (11;22)(q24;q12) translocation of Ewing's sarcoma and peripheral neuroectodermal tumor by reverse transcription polymerase chain reaction. Am J Pathol. 143(5):1294-300, 1993
13. Eggli KD et al: Ewing's sarcoma. Radiol Clin North Am. 31(2):325-37, 1993
14. Boyko OB et al: MR imaging of osteogenic and Ewing's sarcoma. AJR Am J Roentgenol. 148(2):317-22, 1987

# EWING SARCOMA

## IMAGE GALLERY

### Typical

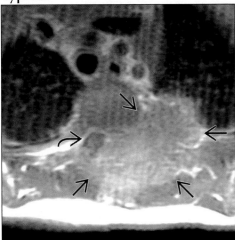
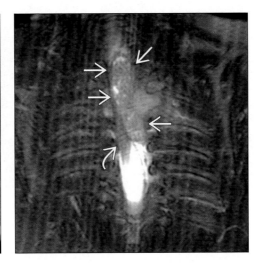

*(Left)* Axial T1 C+ MR in a 6 month old shows a large soft tissue mass ➡ in the upper thoracic spine. The mass infiltrates the epidural space and displaces the spinal cord ➡ to the right. *(Right)* Coronal STIR MR demonstrates low T2 signal typical of cellular tumors. The epidural component ➡ extends over several vertebral segments. Displaced spinal cord ➡ is evident inferiorly.

### Typical

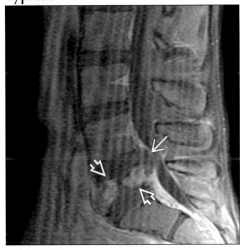
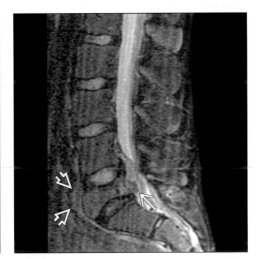

*(Left)* Sagittal T1 C+ FS MR shows abnormal enhancement and near complete collapse (vertebra plana) of the L5 body ➡. Non-enhancing epidural component ➡ is evident at the L4-L5 disc level. *(Right)* Sagittal T2WI FS MR (same patient as previous image) shows extensive epidural infiltration ➡. A prevertebral component ➡ is again appreciated. Adjacent intervertebral discs are not involved.

### Variant

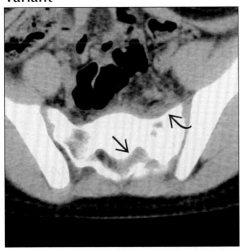
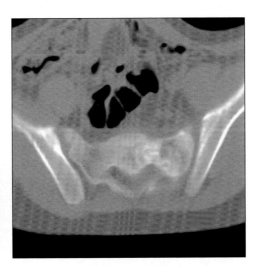

*(Left)* Axial NECT of a sacral Ewing sarcoma in a 7 year old shows infiltration of the intrasacral epidural fat planes ➡ and mild changes in the prevertebral soft tissues on the left ➡. *(Right)* Axial bone CT reveals unusual mixed lytic and sclerotic appearance. The permeative character of tumor spread is evident, with infiltration of soft tissue planes adjacent to fairly intact bone.

# KYPHOSIS

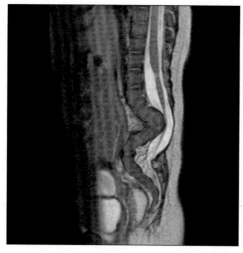 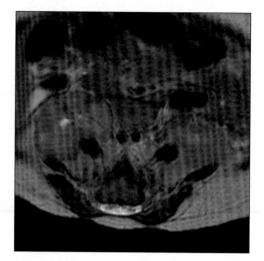

*Sagittal T2WI MR in post-operative myelomeningocele patient shows posterior dysraphism extending from L2 to L5, and severe focal kyphosis centered at L3. The distal cord is draped over L3.*

*Axial T2WI MR in post-operative myelomeningocele patient shows posterior dysraphism and severe spinal stenosis at L3 level, the apex of severe focal kyphosis.*

## TERMINOLOGY

### Definitions

- Increased apex dorsal curvature of spine (sagittal plane)
- Gibbus deformity: Extreme, angular focal kyphosis

## IMAGING FINDINGS

### General Features

- Best diagnostic clue: Increased Cobb angle on lateral radiograph
- Location
  - Normal thoracic spine kyphosis < 40°
  - Normal lumbar spine lordosis = 25-35°
  - Normal cervical spine = mild lordosis, large range of motion
- Morphology: Sagittal plane curvature changes gradually from cervical lordosis → thoracic kyphosis → lumbar lordosis

### CT Findings

- Bone CT
  - Kyphosis often underestimated because of supine position

### MR Findings

- Same as CT

### Radiographic Findings

- Radiography
  - Measure using method of Cobb
  - Determining ends of curve
    - Thoracic kyphosis measured from T3 → T12
    - Fracture: Measure from 1 level above fracture → 1 level below
    - Other deformity: Measure points of greatest inclination from horizontal
  - Determine flexibility of curve
    - Lateral radiograph in full extension
    - Decrease in kyphosis measured

### Imaging Recommendations

- Best imaging tool: CT with sagittal, coronal reformations

---

### DDx: Kyphosis Causes

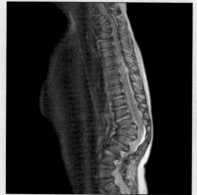 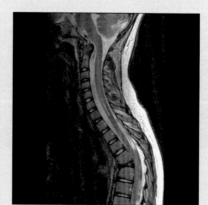 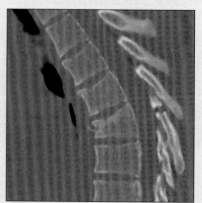

*Mucopolysaccharidosis*     *Congenital Hemivertebra*     *Compression Fractures*

# KYPHOSIS

## Key Facts

**Terminology**
- Increased apex dorsal curvature of spine (sagittal plane)

**Imaging Findings**
- Normal thoracic spine kyphosis < 40°
- Normal lumbar spine lordosis = 25-35°

**Top Differential Diagnoses**
- Positional Kyphosis

**Pathology**
- Traumatic
- Congenital
- Developmental
- Infectious
- Neoplastic
- Iatrogenic

**Diagnostic Checklist**
- Progressive kyphosis warrants CT scan

## DIFFERENTIAL DIAGNOSIS

### Positional Kyphosis
- Poor positioning of uncooperative patient

## PATHOLOGY

### General Features
- General path comments
  - Infant spine has C-shaped curve
  - Lumbar, cervical lordosis develop with erect posture
- Etiology
  - Traumatic
    - Compression, burst or chance fracture
    - Ligamentous injury
  - Congenital
    - Posterior hemivertebra
    - Syndromes: Achondroplasia, Marfan, Ehlers-Danlos, neurofibromatosis
    - Osteogenesis imperfecta
  - Developmental
    - Scheuermann disease, postural (idiopathic) kyphosis, neurogenic kyphosis
  - Infectious
    - Pyogenic, tubercular (gibbus deformity)
  - Neoplastic
    - Primary or metastatic tumors
  - Iatrogenic
    - Post-surgical, post-radiation

### Staging, Grading or Classification Criteria
- Flexible vs. rigid (lateral radiograph in full extension)

## CLINICAL ISSUES

### Demographics
- Age
  - Child: Consider neurogenic, congenital causes
  - Adolescent or young adult: Consider Scheuermann, postural, post-traumatic

### Natural History & Prognosis
- Premature degenerative disease, neurologic compromise

### Treatment
- Treatment of underlying etiology
- Brace vs. fusion

## DIAGNOSTIC CHECKLIST

### Consider
- Progressive kyphosis warrants CT scan

## SELECTED REFERENCES

1. Betz RR: Kyphosis of the thoracic and thoracolumbar spine in the pediatric patient: normal sagittal parameters and scope of the problem. Instr Course Lect. 53:479-84, 2004

## IMAGE GALLERY

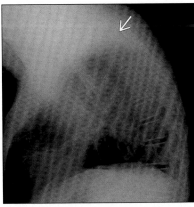 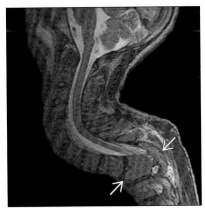 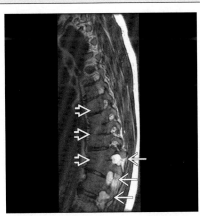

*(Left)* Anteroposterior radiograph shows severe focal post-tubercular kyphosis (apex ➡) of upper thoracic spine in a patient with acquired kyphosis and paralysis developing over several weeks. *(Center)* Sagittal T2WI MR (in a TB patient) shows severe focal kyphosis, abnormal vertebral fusion ➡ in recently paralyzed refugee who rapidly developed kyphosis over a few weeks. *(Right)* Sagittal T2WI MR shows kyphosis secondary to congenital vertebral segmentation failure ➡. Associated arachnoid cyst is seen to extend through several neural foramina ➡.

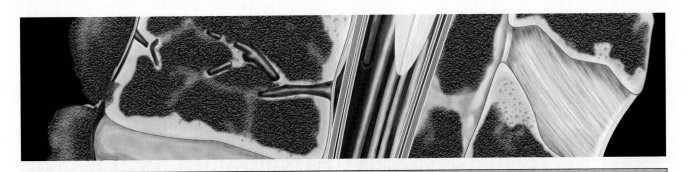

# SECTION 3: Extradural Space

# OCCULT INTRASACRAL MENINGOCELE

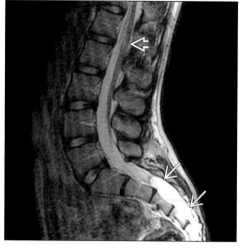

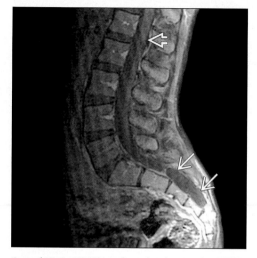

*Sagittal T2WI MR depicts a sacral cyst ➡ that remodels the distal sacral canal and is more hyperintense than CSF in the thecal sac. Spinal cord termination ⬌ is at L1/2.*

*Sagittal T1 C+ FS MR confirms that the sacral cyst ➡ is separate from the thecal sac, with mild enhancement of the cyst margins. Spinal cord termination ⬌ is at L1/2.*

## TERMINOLOGY

### Abbreviations and Synonyms
- Occult intrasacral meningocele (OIM), sacral meningeal cyst, type 1B meningeal cyst

### Definitions
- Spinal extradural arachnoid cyst localized to sacrum

## IMAGING FINDINGS

### General Features
- Best diagnostic clue: Smooth, cystic enlargement of central sacral canal
- Location: Sacrum
- Size: Expands but does not transgress margins of sacrum
- Morphology: Sacral extradural meningeal cyst; no internal neural elements

### CT Findings
- NECT
  - Cerebrospinal fluid (CSF) density cyst enlarges sacral canal
  - Nerve roots displaced by extradural cyst
- CECT: No cyst enhancement
- Bone CT
  - Smooth remodeling, enlargement of sacral canal
  - No expansion or remodeling of neural foramina

### MR Findings
- T1WI: CSF signal intensity extradural sacral cyst adjacent to distal thecal sac
- T2WI
  - Cyst follows CSF signal intensity
  - No neural elements within cyst
- DWI: Hypointense signal intensity excludes epidermoid tumor
- T1 C+: No cyst enhancement

### Radiographic Findings
- Radiography: Sacral canal enlargement and posterior vertebral scalloping

### Ultrasonographic Findings
- Grayscale Ultrasound: Hypoechoic intrasacral cyst without intrinsic neural elements

## DDx: Occult Intrasacral Meningocele

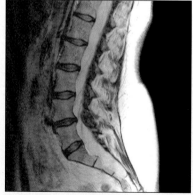

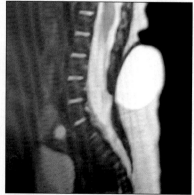

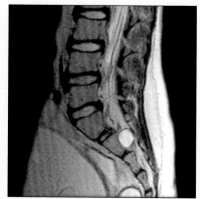

*Dural Dysplasia*

*Dorsal Meningocele*

*Tarlov Cyst*

# OCCULT INTRASACRAL MENINGOCELE

## Key Facts

### Terminology
- Occult intrasacral meningocele (OIM), sacral meningeal cyst, type 1B meningeal cyst

### Imaging Findings
- Best diagnostic clue: Smooth, cystic enlargement of central sacral canal
- Cyst follows CSF signal intensity
- No neural elements within cyst

### Top Differential Diagnoses
- Dural Dysplasia
- Dorsal Meningocele
- Tarlov Cyst

### Pathology
- Extradural arachnoid cyst

- No herniation of meninges, hence not a true meningocele
- Cyst is connected to thecal sac by a pedicle that permits contiguous CSF flow
- CSF pulsation +/- raised intraspinal pressure (across stenotic pedicle) pressure erodes and remodels sacral canal

### Clinical Issues
- Most patients are asymptomatic and need no specific treatment
- Symptomatic patients or very large cysts may require surgery

### Diagnostic Checklist
- MR best modality for diagnosis of sacral cyst, pre-operative planning

## Non-Vascular Interventions
- Myelography
  - Enlargement of distal sacral canal, extradural compression of distal contrast-filled thecal sac
    - +/- Contrast opacification of cyst (if isthmus large enough)

## Other Modality Findings
- CSF cine phase contrast flow sensitive imaging may help define cyst walls by depicting differential CSF pulsation

## Imaging Recommendations
- Best imaging tool
  - Magnetic resonance imaging best modality for initial diagnosis
  - CT myelography may help reveal connection between cyst and subarachnoid space
- Protocol advice: Sagittal and axial T1WI and T2WI to identify cyst, clarify relationship to adjacent structures

## DIFFERENTIAL DIAGNOSIS

### Dural Dysplasia
- Vertebral scalloping usually present in lumbar spine as well as sacrum, +/- lateral meningocele
- Search for characteristic imaging and clinical stigmata of etiological disorder

### Dorsal Meningocele
- True meningocele; protrudes through dorsal dysraphism into subcutaneous tissues

### Tarlov Cyst
- Etiologically similar to OIM; congenital dilatation of nerve root meningeal sleeves
- Large cysts may remodel sacrum, but will be eccentrically centered over neural foramen
- Frequently multiple

## PATHOLOGY

### General Features
- General path comments
  - Extradural arachnoid cyst
    - No herniation of meninges, hence not a true meningocele
    - No neuronal elements within cyst
  - Cyst is connected to thecal sac by a pedicle that permits contiguous CSF flow
  - CSF pulsation +/- raised intraspinal pressure (across stenotic pedicle) pressure erodes and remodels sacral canal
- Etiology: Diverticulum of sacral subarachnoid space ⇒ expands into sacral cyst 2° to valve-like mechanism ⇒ secondary remodeling of sacral canal
- Epidemiology
  - Spinal meningeal cysts are uncommon
    - Comprise 1-3% of all spinal tumors
  - Prevalence of occult sacral meningocele unknown, but < prevalence of Tarlov cyst
- Associated abnormalities
  - Tarlov cyst(s)
  - Posterior spinal dysraphism
  - Tethered cord syndrome

### Gross Pathologic & Surgical Features
- Sacral laminectomy ⇒ thinned sacral vertebral laminae
  - Cyst may be attached to distal thecal sac by a narrow pedicle that permits one-way (mostly) CSF flow into cyst
  - Symptomatic cysts less likely to communicate with subarachnoid space than asymptomatic cysts

### Microscopic Features
- Cyst is lined by fibrous connective tissue +/- single inner layer of arachnoid membrane

### Staging, Grading or Classification Criteria
- Nabors classification: Type IB meningeal cyst

# OCCULT INTRASACRAL MENINGOCELE

## CLINICAL ISSUES

### Presentation
- Most common signs/symptoms
  - Asymptomatic; incidental discovery on MR
  - Symptomatic: Chronic low back pain, sciatica, perineal paresthesias, and bladder dysfunction
  - Less common signs/symptoms
    - Intermittent, severe lower back pain
    - Atypical bowel symptoms, severe constipation, and stool incontinence
    - Tethered cord syndrome
- Clinical Profile
  - Specific symptoms are referable to sacral root compression
  - May be exacerbated by positional change or Valsalva maneuver

### Demographics
- Age
  - Teen → elderly
  - Rarely diagnosed in children
- Gender: Some series report M > F, others M < F

### Natural History & Prognosis
- Most patients are asymptomatic and need no specific treatment
  - Asymptomatic cysts are most commonly identified and referred to specialists following incidental discovery on MR
- Symptomatic patients or very large cysts may require surgery
  - Indications for operative intervention include increased cyst size on serial exams, or onset of symptoms referable to cyst
  - Good prognosis for recovery following surgery

### Treatment
- Conservative approach recommended for asymptomatic cysts, especially when small
- Symptomatic cysts may require treatment
  - Percutaneous cyst aspiration may relieve symptoms temporarily
    - May be used as diagnostic test prior to definitive therapy
    - Percutaneous cyst aspiration with fibrin glue therapy may produce definitive long-lasting symptom reduction
  - Operative therapy ⇒ sacral laminectomy to expose, resect cyst
    - May not be necessary to completely resect entire cyst
    - Primary goal is to close dural defect ⇒ eradicate one-way valve communication, prevent cyst recurrence
    - If adhesions prevent full excision, may partially resect posterior wall or marsupialize cyst to subarachnoid space

## DIAGNOSTIC CHECKLIST

### Consider
- MR best modality for diagnosis of sacral cyst, pre-operative planning
- Definitive cyst characterization based on operative inspection, histological examination

### Image Interpretation Pearls
- Classic appearance is an intrasacral cyst producing smooth sacral canal expansion with outward displacement of nerve roots
- OIM centered in midline; center over neural foramen implies Tarlov cyst

## SELECTED REFERENCES

1. Apel K et al: Extradural spinal arachnoid cysts associated with spina bifida occulta. Acta Neurochir (Wien). 148(2):221-226, 2006
2. Kilickesmez O et al: Expanding occult intrasacral meningocele associated with diastematomyelia and multiple vertebral anomalies. Case report. J Neurosurg. 101(1 Suppl):108-11, 2004
3. Nishio Y et al: A case of occult intrasacral meningocele presented with atypical bowel symptoms. Childs Nerv Syst. 20(1):65-7, 2004
4. Sato et al: Spinal Extradural Meningeal Cyst: Correct Radiological and Histopathological Diagnosis. Neurosurg Focus. 13(4), 2002
5. Diel J et al: The sacrum: pathologic spectrum, multimodality imaging, and subspecialty approach. Radiographics. 21(1):83-104, 2001
6. Patel MR et al: Percutaneous fibrin glue therapy of meningeal cysts of the sacral spine. AJR Am J Roentgenol. 168(2):367-70, 1997
7. Okada T et al: Occult intrasacral meningocele associated with spina bifida: a case report. Surg Neurol. 46(2):147-9, 1996
8. Doi H et al: Occult intrasacral meningocele with tethered cord--case report. Neurol Med Chir (Tokyo). 35(5):321-4, 1995
9. Tatagiba M et al: Management of occult intrasacral meningocele associated with lumbar disc prolapse. Neurosurg Rev. 17(4):313-5, 1994
10. Davis SW et al: Sacral meningeal cysts: evaluation with MR imaging. Radiology. 187(2):445-8, 1993
11. Bayar MA et al: Management problems in cases with a combination of asymptomatic occult intrasacral meningocele and disc prolapse. Acta Neurochir (Wien). 108(1-2):67-9, 1991
12. Doty JR et al: Occult intrasacral meningocele: clinical and radiographic diagnosis. Neurosurgery. 24(4):616-25, 1989
13. Nabors MW et al: Updated assessment and current classification of spinal meningeal cysts. J Neurosurg. 68(3):366-77, 1988
14. Goyal RN et al: Intraspinal cysts: a classification and literature review. Spine. 12:209-13, 1987
15. Genest AS: Occult intrasacral meningocele. Spine. 9(1):101-3, 1984
16. Grivegnee A et al: Comparative aspects of occult intrasacral meningocele with conventional X-ray, myelography and CT. Neuroradiology. 22(1):33-7, 1981
17. Fortuna A et al: Arachnoid diverticula: a unitary approach to spinal cysts communicating with the subarachnoid space. Acta Neurochir. 39:259-68, 1977
18. Lombardi G et al: Congenital cysts of the spinal membranes and roots. Br J Radiol. 36:197-205, 1963

# OCCULT INTRASACRAL MENINGOCELE

## IMAGE GALLERY

### Variant

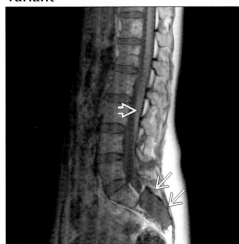
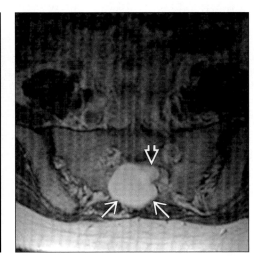

**3**

5

*(Left)* Sagittal T1WI MR demonstrates an intrasacral meningocele ➡ producing tethering of the low-lying spinal cord ➡, which correlated well with clinical findings. *(Right)* Axial T2WI MR confirms cyst localization within sacrum ➡. There is smooth enlargement of the sacral canal and displacement of the thecal sac ➡.

### Variant

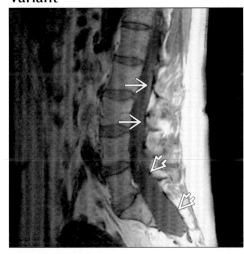
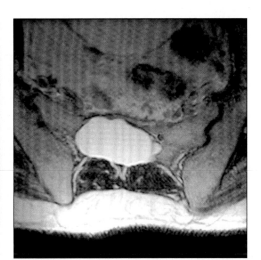

*(Left)* Sagittal T1WI MR reveals a large occult intrasacral meningocele ➡ that extensively remodels the sacrum. The spinal cord ➡ is low-lying and thinned. *(Right)* Axial T2WI MR shows a large sacral cyst, with characteristic extensive osseous remodeling and canal expansion. The posterior elements are thinned but remain intact.

### Variant

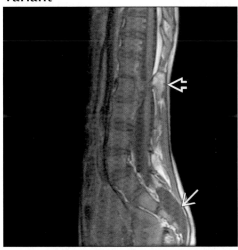
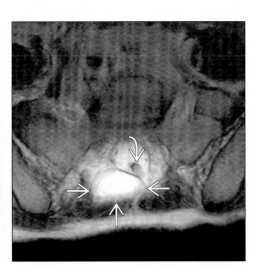

*(Left)* Sagittal T1WI MR (Klippel-Feil patient with diastematomyelia ➡) demonstrates a low-lying hydromyelic tethered spinal cord and fluid intensity cyst ➡ in the terminal sacral canal. *(Right)* Axial T2WI MR shows a low-lying spinal cord ➡ and cyst ➡ signal intensity slightly higher than CSF. There is remodeling and enlargement of the sacral central canal.

# SACROCOCCYGEAL TERATOMA

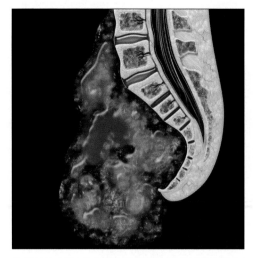

Sagittal graphic depicts a typical large, heterogeneous, partially cystic sacrococcygeal teratoma located anterior to the sacrum. Note characteristic lack of osseous sacral invasion.

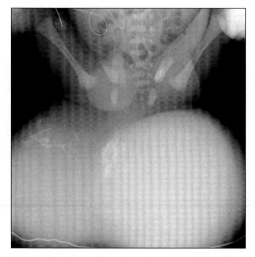

Anteroposterior radiograph demonstrates a large, calcified pelvic mass originating from the perineum without osseous sacral anomaly. Surgical resection confirmed sacrococcygeal teratoma.

## TERMINOLOGY

### Abbreviations and Synonyms
- Sacral germ-cell tumor (SGT), germ cell tumor of coccyx

### Definitions
- Congenital sacral tumor containing elements of all three germ layers

## IMAGING FINDINGS

### General Features
- Best diagnostic clue: Large, heterogeneous sacral mass in an infant
- Location: Sacrum/coccyx
- Size
  - Usually large at diagnosis
    - Mature teratomas mean ~ 7.5 cm
    - Immature teratomas mean ~ 11.6 cm
- Morphology: Heterogeneous mass containing calcifications, mixed solid and cystic components, fat-debris levels, bone, hair, teeth, and/or cartilage

### CT Findings
- CECT
  - Complex mixed attenuation cystic/solid pelvic mass with enhancement of solid portions
    - Calcifications (≤ 60%); small punctate foci → well formed teeth, bones
    - Calcium (hyperdense), fluid (hypodense), and fat (markedly hypodense)

### MR Findings
- T1WI: Heterogeneous mixed signal intensity; fat (hyperintense), soft tissue (isointense), cyst fluid (hypointense), and calcium (markedly hypointense)
- T2WI: Heterogeneous signal intensity; fat (hyperintense), soft tissue (isointense), cyst fluid (hyperintense), and calcium (markedly hypointense)
- T2* GRE: Shows calcifications, hemorrhage best
- T1 C+: Heterogeneous enhancement of solid portions

### Radiographic Findings
- Radiography: Soft tissue mass, calcifications (≤ 60%)

### Ultrasonographic Findings
- Grayscale Ultrasound

## DDx: Cystic Presacral and Pelvic Masses

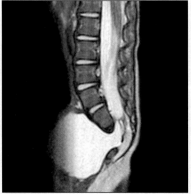

Anterior Sacral Meningocele

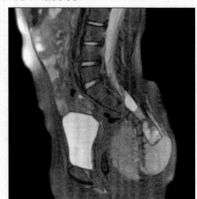

Rhabdomyosarcoma

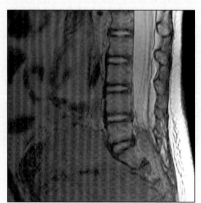

Neuroblastoma

# SACROCOCCYGEAL TERATOMA

## Key Facts

### Terminology
- Sacral germ-cell tumor (SGT), germ cell tumor of coccyx

### Imaging Findings
- Usually large at diagnosis
- Complex mixed attenuation cystic/solid pelvic mass with enhancement of solid portions
- Calcifications ($\le$ 60%); small punctate foci → well formed teeth, bones

### Top Differential Diagnoses
- Anterior Sacral Meningocele (ASM)
- Chordoma
- Neuroblastoma
- Exophytic Rhabdomyosarcoma

### Pathology
- Most common newborn tumor
- Malignant risk ↑ with age at diagnosis, higher surgical subtype, male gender, presence of necrosis or hemorrhage
- Epidemiology: 1:35,000 to 40,000 births

### Clinical Issues
- Most common: Neonate with large sacral mass noted prenatally or at time of delivery
- Less common: Newborn with buttock asymmetry or presacral tumor presenting in infancy

### Diagnostic Checklist
- AAP type influences prognosis, treatment approach
- Heterogeneous sacral tumor +/- calcification, cysts, hemorrhage suggests diagnosis

○ Complex mixed hypo-/hyperechoic sacral mass
  ■ Obstetrical: In-utero diagnosis ⇒ cesarian section, possible fetal surgery or radiofrequency ablation (RFA)
  ■ Post-natal: Visualization hampered by fat/calcium shadowing, posterior bone elements, large size

## Imaging Recommendations
- Best imaging tool
  ○ Prenatal: Obstetrical ultrasound +/- fetal MR
  ○ Post-natal: MR
- Protocol advice
  ○ MR +/- CT to determine full extent of mass, treatment planning
    ■ Sagittal and axial MR imaging for surgical planning
    ■ CT with oral/IV contrast to delineate extent of bone destruction, calcifications

## DIFFERENTIAL DIAGNOSIS

### Anterior Sacral Meningocele (ASM)
- Cystic mass; no solid component or enhancement
- Enlarges with Valsalva maneuver

### Chordoma
- Mixed solid/cystic destructive sacral mass
- Rare in children; peak incidence 5th → 6th decade
- T2WI → markedly hyperintense
- Bone CT → destructive margins

### Neuroblastoma
- Smaller, more homogeneous than SGT
- Cellular appearance on MR, variable enhancement

### Exophytic Rhabdomyosarcoma
- Aggressive appearing tumor without calcium, bone, or hair
- Cellular appearance on MR, variable enhancement

## PATHOLOGY

### General Features
- General path comments
  ○ Most common newborn tumor
    ■ 80% mature, 20% immature; immature teratomas have greater risk of malignancy
  ○ Malignancy risk 10% at term; ↑ to 65-90% if diagnosed > 2 months
    ■ Malignant risk ↑ with age at diagnosis, higher surgical subtype, male gender, presence of necrosis or hemorrhage
- Genetics
  ○ Most cases are sporadic; some syndromic associations (Currarino triad)
  ○ Scattered reports of autosomal dominant parent-child associations
    ■ Congenital sacral deformities, anorectal stenosis, vesicoureteral reflux, retrorectal abscess, and skin dimple
- Etiology
  ○ Originate from totipotential cell rests at caudal spine/notochord (Hensen node)
    ■ Degree of totipotential cell differentiation ⇒ tumor type
    ■ Less differentiated ⇒ more malignant
  ○ Alternative hypothesis: "Twinning" accident ⇒ incomplete separation during embryogenesis
- Epidemiology: 1:35,000 to 40,000 births
- Associated abnormalities: Currarino triad, anorectal or genitourinary abnormalities (10%)

### Gross Pathologic & Surgical Features
- Benign teratomas (83%)
  ○ Heterogeneous noninvasive, partially cystic, calcified soft tissue mass; rarely invade spinal canal
  ○ Multiple tissue types show varying stages of differentiation, maturation
- Malignant teratomas (17%)
  ○ More commonly intrasacral, locally aggressive

○ Malignancy postulated to arise from differentiated cell lines within teratoma ⇒ neuroblastoma, adenocarcinoma, or rhabdomyosarcoma, embryonal cell carcinoma, or anaplastic carcinoma

## Microscopic Features
- Elements derived from all three germ layers (endoderm, mesoderm, and ectoderm)

## Staging, Grading or Classification Criteria
- Four surgical subtypes (Altman/AAP classification)
  ○ Type I: Primarily external (47%) ⇒ best prognosis
  ○ Type II: Dumbbell shape, equal external/internal portions (34%)
  ○ Type III: Primarily internal within abdomen/pelvis (9%)
  ○ Type IV: Entirely internal; no visible external component (10%) ⇒ worst prognosis

## CLINICAL ISSUES

### Presentation
- Most common signs/symptoms
  ○ Back/pelvic mass in a newborn
    ■ Exophytic masses easily diagnosed, but internal (type III, IV) occult ⇒ delayed diagnosis
  ○ In-utero presentation
    ■ Polyhydramnios, high output cardiac failure with hydrops, hepatomegaly, placentomegaly, tumor hemorrhage → anemia or nonimmune hydrops fetalis
  ○ Urinary retention, constipation (larger tumors)
- Clinical Profile
  ○ Most common: Neonate with large sacral mass noted prenatally or at time of delivery
  ○ Less common: Newborn with buttock asymmetry or presacral tumor presenting in infancy
- Laboratory
  ○ Post-op tumor markers: Serum α-fetoprotein (AFP), β-human chorionic gonadotropin (HCG)

### Demographics
- Age: 50-70% diagnosed in-utero or during first days of life, 80% by 6 months, and fewer than 10% beyond 2 years
- Gender: M:F = 1:4

### Natural History & Prognosis
- Prognosis excellent in benign tumors
  ○ Mature or mostly cystic ⇒ good prognosis
  ○ Immature teratomas ⇒ greater risk of malignancy if not totally resected
- Malignant tumors have variable prognosis; later diagnosis (> 1st birthday), internal location ⇒ worse prognosis
- Fetal mortality rate 20-65% (2° to polyhydramnios, tumor hemorrhage, high-output cardiac failure)
  ○ Hydrops fetalis portends grim prognosis; > 30 weeks gestation ⇒ 25% mortality, < 30 weeks gestation ⇒ 93% mortality
- Postpartum morbidity attributable to associated congenital anomalies, recurrence, tumor mass effects, or intra-operative/post-operative complications

### Treatment
- Surgery alone curative if entire benign tumor and coccyx removed; recurs if coccyx not resected
- Cytoreduction surgery + radiation, chemotherapy may be palliative for malignant tumors; early diagnosis, resection best chance for cure
- Fetal surgery (RFA) offered at some specialized centers; good outcome requires careful patient selection

## DIAGNOSTIC CHECKLIST

### Consider
- Imaging goals: Imperative to confirm diagnosis, determine intra/extrapelvic extent and size, relationship to adjacent structures, and presence/absence of metastatic disease
- AAP type influences prognosis, treatment approach

### Image Interpretation Pearls
- Heterogeneous sacral tumor +/- calcification, cysts, hemorrhage suggests diagnosis

## SELECTED REFERENCES

1. Woodward PJ et al: From the archives of the AFIP: a comprehensive review of fetal tumors with pathologic correlation. Radiographics. 25(1):215-42, 2005
2. Sebire NJ et al: Sacrococcygeal tumors in infancy and childhood; a retrospective histopathological review of 85 cases. Fetal Pediatr Pathol. 23(5-6):295-303, 2004
3. Graf JL et al: Fetal sacrococcygeal teratoma. World J Surg. 27(1):84-6, 2003
4. Hirose S et al: Fetal surgery for sacrococcygeal teratoma. Clin Perinatol. 30(3):493-506, 2003
5. Avni FE et al: MR imaging of fetal sacrococcygeal teratoma: diagnosis and assessment. AJR Am J Roentgenol. 178(1):179-83, 2002
6. Axt-Fliedner R et al: Prenatal diagnosis of sacrococcygeal teratoma: a review of cases between 1993 and 2000. Clin Exp Obstet Gynecol. 29(1):15-8, 2002
7. Monteiro M et al: Case report: sacrococcygeal teratoma with malignant transformation in an adult female: CT and MRI findings. Br J Radiol. 75(895):620-3, 2002
8. Perrelli L et al: Sacrococcygeal teratoma. Outcome and management. An analysis of 17 cases. J Perinat Med. 30(2):179-84, 2002
9. Paek BW et al: Radiofrequency ablation of human fetal sacrococcygeal teratoma. Am J Obstet Gynecol. 184(3):503-7, 2001
10. Holterman AX et al: The natural history of sacrococcygeal teratomas diagnosed through routine obstetric sonogram: a single institution experience. J Pediatr Surg. 33(6):899-903, 1998
11. Schropp KP et al: Sacrococcygeal teratoma: the experience of four decades. J Pediatr Surg. 27(8):1075-8; discussion 1078-9, 1992
12. Wells RG et al: Imaging of sacrococcygeal germ cell tumors. Radiographics. 10(4):701-13, 1990
13. Altman RP et al: Sacrococcygeal teratoma: American Academy of Pediatrics Surgical Section Survey-1973. J Pediatr Surg. 9(3):389-98, 1974

# SACROCOCCYGEAL TERATOMA

## IMAGE GALLERY

### Other

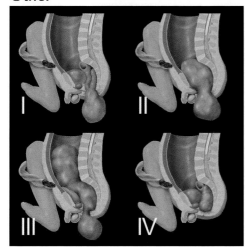

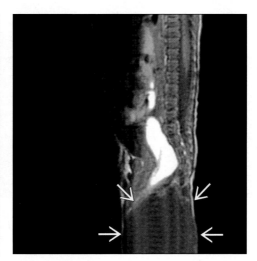

*(Left)* Sagittal graphic depicts the four AAP subtypes. Type I is nearly entirely internal, II is approximately half internal and half external, while III is mostly and IV entirely internal. *(Right)* Sagittal T1WI MR shows a predominately cystic external (type I) sacrococcygeal teratoma ➡ contiguous with the coccyx. Hyperintense signal intensity within rectum represents meconium.

### Typical

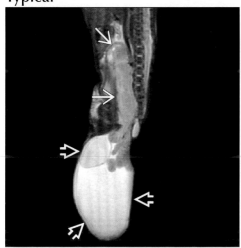

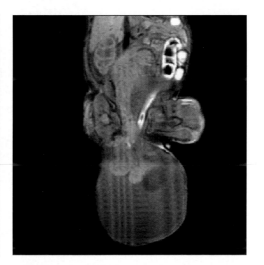

*(Left)* Sagittal T2WI MR shows a mixed cystic/solid pelvic mass that is ~ 50% internal (AAP type II). The internal portion ➡ is solid and the external portion ⮕ mostly cystic. *(Right)* Coronal T1 C+ FS MR confirms a mixed cystic and enhancing solid tissue mass. Note that the cystic portions demonstrate differing signal intensities reflecting varied proteinaceous content.

### Typical

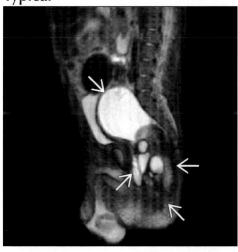

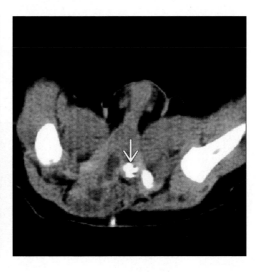

*(Left)* Sagittal T2WI FS MR reveals a predominately internal (type III) mixed cystic and solid presacral pelvic tumor ➡ that displaces the pelvic viscera anteriorly. *(Right)* Axial CECT demonstrates a predominately internal type III mixed cystic and enhancing solid pelvic tumor with a large chunky tumor calcification ➡.

# EPIDURAL LIPOMATOSIS

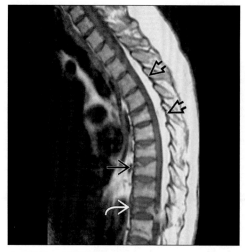

*Sagittal T1WI MR shows large mass ▷ of hyperintense fat in the dorsal epidural space. Endplate fractures ▣→ and compression fractures ▣ of vertebrae are seen in the lower thoracic spine.*

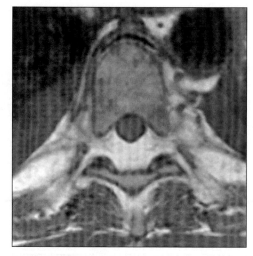

*Axial T1WI MR shows better the large mass of epidural fat dorsal to and compressing the thecal sac in this child who has received long-standing high dose steroids for Crohn Disease.*

## TERMINOLOGY

### Abbreviations and Synonyms
- Spinal epidural lipomatosis (SEL)

### Definitions
- Excessive accumulation of intraspinal fat causing cord compression and neurologic deficits

## IMAGING FINDINGS

### General Features
- Best diagnostic clue: Abundant epidural fat in mid-thoracic and distal lumbar spinal canal compressing thecal sac
- Location
  - Thoracic spine: 58-61%
    - T6-8
    - Dorsal to spinal cord
  - Lumbar spine: 39-42%
    - L4-5
    - Circumferential surrounding thecal sac
- Size

  - Epidural fat ≥ 7 mm thick in thoracic spine
  - Over multiple vertebral segments
- Morphology
  - "Y" sign
    - "Y" shaped configuration to lumbar thecal sac on axial imaging

### CT Findings
- NECT
  - Increased fat density in spinal canal
  - Cord compression
  - Tapered caudal thecal sac
- CECT: No enhancement
- Bone CT
  - No bony erosion

### MR Findings
- T1WI
  - Homogeneous, hyperintense tissue surrounding and compressing spinal cord
  - Hypointense with fat-suppression
- T2WI: Intermediate signal intensity
- STIR: Hypointense
- T1 C+: No enhancement
- Homogeneous

## DDx: Epidural Lipomatosis

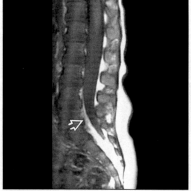

*Epidural Abscess*

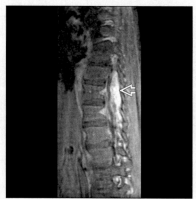

*Neuroblastoma*

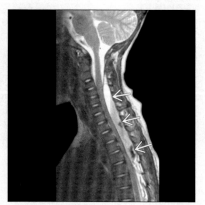

*Epidural Hematoma*

# EPIDURAL LIPOMATOSIS

## Key Facts

### Terminology
- Excessive accumulation of intraspinal fat causing cord compression and neurologic deficits

### Imaging Findings
- Best diagnostic clue: Abundant epidural fat in mid-thoracic and distal lumbar spinal canal compressing thecal sac
- Thoracic spine: 58-61%
- Lumbar spine: 39-42%
- Epidural fat ≥ 7 mm thick in thoracic spine
- Homogeneous, hyperintense tissue surrounding and compressing spinal cord
- Mass effect on thecal sac and nerve roots

### Top Differential Diagnoses
- Subacute Epidural Hematoma

- Spinal Angiolipoma
- Epidural Tumor: PNET, Neuroblastoma, Lymphoma
- Epidural Abscess

### Pathology
- Long term exogenous steroid administration
- Excessive endogenous steroid production

### Clinical Issues
- Lower extremity weakness: > 85%

### Diagnostic Checklist
- Excessive extradural fat in dorsal midthoracic spine and caudal lumbar spine diagnostic of SEL

---

- Mass effect on thecal sac and nerve roots
  - Compressed/obliterated CSF
  - Cord compression
  - Crowded cauda equina

## Radiographic Findings
- Radiography
  - Osteopenia from exogenous or endogenous steroids
  - Vertebral compression fractures

## Non-Vascular Interventions
- Myelography
  - Often normal
  - Effacement of cerebral spinal fluid (CSF)

## Imaging Recommendations
- Best imaging tool: Sagittal and axial T1WI and T2WI MR
- Protocol advice: Fat-suppression to confirm adipose tissue

## DIFFERENTIAL DIAGNOSIS

### Subacute Epidural Hematoma
- Hyperintense on T1WI
  - Hyperintense even with fat-suppression
- Heterogeneous with hypointense foci on T2WI
  - Fluid-fluid levels
- Acute onset of symptoms

### Spinal Angiolipoma
- Benign neoplasm with varying proportion of adipose and vascular elements
- Mid-thoracic region most common
- Infiltrative type invades surrounding bone
- Hyperintense on T1WI
  - Slightly or moderately hypointense to epidural fat
  - Heterogeneous due to vascular elements
- Iso- to slightly hypointense to epidural fat on T2WI
- Diffuse post-contrast-enhancement
  - Better visualized with fat-suppression

### Epidural Tumor: PNET, Neuroblastoma, Lymphoma
- Hypointense to epidural fat on T1WI and T2WI
  - Soft tissue signal intensity
- Vertebral and paraspinal involvement
  - Not limited to spinal canal
- Avid post-gadolinium enhancement

### Epidural Abscess
- Most common in ventral epidural space
  - Associated with discitis/osteomyelitis
    - Enhancing disk
  - Smudging of epidural fat by abscess/inflammation
- Posterolateral spinal canal from septic facet joint
- Hypointense on T1WI
- Hyperintense on T2WI

## PATHOLOGY

### General Features
- General path comments
  - Increased fat tissue in spinal canal
  - Typically in thoracic and lumbar regions
- Genetics: No genetic predisposition
- Etiology
  - Long term exogenous steroid administration
    - 75% of reported cases
    - Treatment of kidney disease, systemic lupus erythematosus, etc.
    - No definite correlation with dosage and duration of steroid use
  - Association with epidural steroid injection also reported
  - Excessive endogenous steroid production
    - Cushing disease
    - Hypothyroidism
    - Other endocrinopathies
  - General obesity
  - Idiopathic
- Epidemiology: Uncommon in pediatrics; more frequent in adults

# EPIDURAL LIPOMATOSIS

- Associated abnormalities
  - Vertebral compression fractures
    - Steroid related osteoporosis
  - Syrinx
- Anatomy
  - Meningovertebral ligaments in lumbar spine
    - Median, paramedian, lateral aspects of ventral and dorsal epidural space
    - Anchor dura to spinal canal
    - May form septum, partitioning epidural space

## Gross Pathologic & Surgical Features
- Abundant adipose tissue external to thecal sac
- No capsule

## Microscopic Features
- Hypertrophied fat cells

# CLINICAL ISSUES

## Presentation
- Most common signs/symptoms
  - Lower extremity weakness: > 85%
  - Back pain: 64%
- Other signs/symptoms
  - Decreased sensation, polyradiculopathy
    - Altered reflexes, Incontinence
- Clinical Profile: Gradual progression of symptoms

## Demographics
- Age
  - Mean age at presentation: 43 yo
    - Slightly younger for thoracic SEL
    - Older (50s) for lumbar SEL
    - Uncommon in children
- Gender: M > F
- Ethnicity: No racial predilection

## Natural History & Prognosis
- > 80% with post-surgical symptomatic relief
  - Pre-surgical low steroid dose and idiopathic SEL have better prognosis
- Post-surgical mortality: 22%
  - Immunocompromised state from chronic steroid use

## Treatment
- Correction of underlying endocrinopathies
- Discontinuing exogenous steroids
- Weight reduction in case of general obesity
- Surgical intervention
  - Indicated when cord compression and radiculopathy present
  - Multilevel laminectomy, Fat debulking
  - Posterolateral fusion to maintain stability

# DIAGNOSTIC CHECKLIST

## Consider
- Fat suppression to distinguish from epidural hematoma

## Image Interpretation Pearls
- Excessive extradural fat in dorsal midthoracic spine and caudal lumbar spine diagnostic of SEL

# SELECTED REFERENCES

1. Kano K et al: Spinal epidural lipomatosis in children with renal diseases receiving steroid therapy. Pediatr Nephrol. 20(2):184-9, 2005
2. Fassett DR et al: Spinal epidural lipomatosis: a review of its causes and recommendations for treatment. Neurosurg Focus. 16(4):Article 11, 2004
3. Geers C et al: Polygonal deformation of the dural sac in lumbar epidural lipomatosis: anatomic explanation by the presence of meningovertebral ligaments. AJNR Am J Neuroradiol. 24(7):1276-82, 2003
4. Payer M et al: Idiopathic symptomatic epidural lipomatosis of the lumbar spine. Acta Neurochir (Wien). 145(4):315-20; discussion 321, 2003
5. Dumont-Fischer D et al: Spinal epidural lipomatosis revealing endogenous Cushing's syndrome. Joint Bone Spine. 69(2):222-5, 2002
6. Munoz A et al: Symptomatic epidural lipomatosis of the spinal cord in a child: MR demonstration of spinal cord injury. Pediatr Radiol. 32(12):865-8, 2002
7. Lisai P et al: Cauda Equina Syndrome Secondary to Idiopathic Spinal Epidural Lipomatosis. Spine. 26:307-9, 2001
8. Citow JS et al: Thoracic epidural lipomatosis with associated syrinx: case report. Surg Neurol. 53(6):589-91, 2000
9. McCullen GM et al: Epidural lipomatosis complicating lumbar steroid injections. J Spinal Disord. 12(6):526-9, 1999
10. Robertson SC et al: Idiopathic spinal epidural lipomatosis. Neurosurgery. 41(1):68-74; discussion 74-5, 1997
11. Benamou PH et al: Epidural lipomatosis not induced by corticosteroid therapy. Three cases including one in a patient with primary Cushing's disease (review of the literature). Rev Rhum Engl Ed. 63(3):207-12, 1996
12. Hierholzer J et al: Epidural lipomatosis: case report and literature review. Neuroradiology. 38(4):343-8, 1996
13. Kumar K et al: Symptomatic Epidural lipomatosis Secondary to Obesity. J Neurosurg. 85:348-50, 1996
14. Provenzale JM et al: Spinal angiolipomas: MR features. AJNR Am J Neuroradiol. 17(4):713-9, 1996
15. Zentner J et al: Spinal epidural lipomatosis as a complication of prolonged corticosteroid therapy. J Neurosurg Sci. 39(1):81-5, 1995
16. Kuhn MJ et al: Lumbar epidural lipomatosis: the "Y" sign of thecal sac compression. Comput Med Imaging Graph. 18(5):367-72, 1994
17. Preul MC et al: Spinal angiolipomas. Report of three cases. J Neurosurg. 78(2):280-6, 1993
18. Roy-Camille R et al: Symptomatic spinal epidural lipomatosis induced by a long-term steroid treatment. Review of the literature and report of two additional cases. Spine. 16(12):1365-71, 1991
19. Healy ME et al: Demonstration by magnetic resonance of symptomatic spinal epidural lipomatosis. Neurosurgery. 21(3):414-5, 1987
20. Randall BC et al: Epidural lipomatosis with lumbar radiculopathy: CT appearance. J Comput Assist Tomogr. 10(6):1039-41, 1986

# EPIDURAL LIPOMATOSIS

## IMAGE GALLERY

### Typical

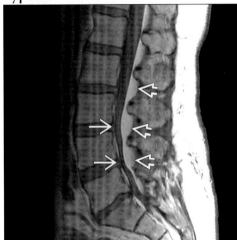

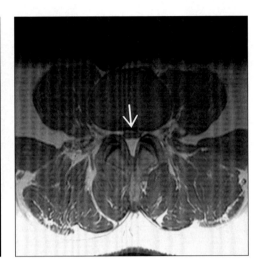

*(Left)* Sagittal T1WI MR shows dorsal epidural fat ➡ compressing the thecal sac at L3-4 and L4-5 levels ➡ in this adolescent with rheumatoid arthritis. *(Right)* Axial T1WI MR shows the severity of the spinal stenosis ➡ resulting from the dorsal epidural fat at L4-5.

### Typical

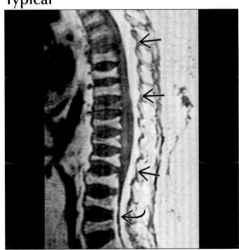

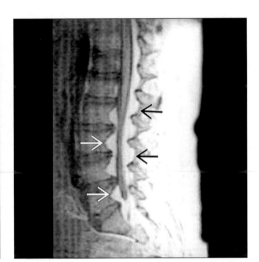

*(Left)* Sagittal T1WI MR shows many compression deformities from chronic steroid use for renal failure. Extensive dorsal epidural fat ➡ present; markedly thins thecal sac ➡ at lumbar levels. *(Right)* Sagittal T1WI MR shows extensive narrowing of the lumbar thecal sac due to excessive fat deposition in the ventral ➡ and dorsal ➡ epidural spaces.

### Typical

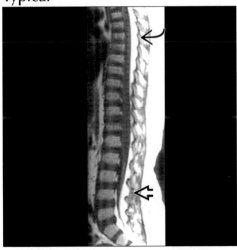

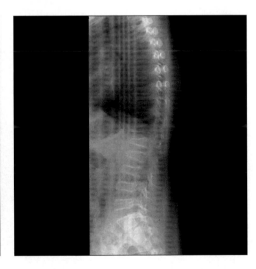

*(Left)* Sagittal T1WI MR shows two large areas of dorsal epidural fat, one at the thoracic level ➡ and one at the lumbar level ➡. These are the most common levels of involvement. *(Right)* Lateral radiograph shows severe osteopenia and multiple compression deformities in this adolescent with history of chronic steroid use for renal disease.

# LANGERHANS CELL HISTIOCYTOSIS, SPINE

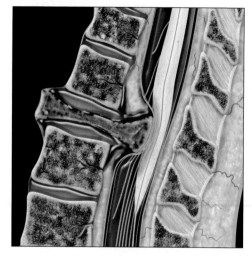

Sagittal graphic shows focal vertebral body marrow infiltration with pathologic fracture producing disc-sparing vertebra plana. Epidural extension produces ventral cord compression.

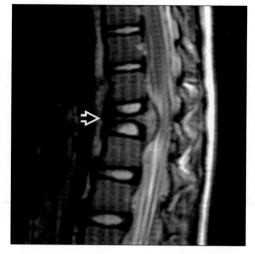

Sagittal T2WI MR shows the classic imaging appearance of LCH: Disc-sparing vertebra plana ➡ with small epidural component. Mild kyphosis is also present.

## TERMINOLOGY

### Abbreviations and Synonyms
- Langerhans cell histiocytosis (LCH)
- Synonym: Histiocytosis X
- Eosinophilic granuloma: Historical term used to describe LCH limited to bone

### Definitions
- Spinal LCH: Abnormal histiocyte proliferation producing granulomatous spinal lesions

## IMAGING FINDINGS

### General Features
- Best diagnostic clue: Disc-sparing vertebra plana in a child
- Location
  - Skull > long bones > spine > pelvis, ribs
  - Spine: Thoracic (54%) > lumbar (35%) > cervical
    - Vertebral body (posterior element more common in cervical spine)
- Morphology
  - Vertebra plana: Collapse of vertebral body to thin disc; adjacent discs normal
  - Other: Destructive lytic lesion
    - More common in cervical spine (commonly C1, C2)
  - Small paraspinal/epidural soft tissue component common

### CT Findings
- NECT: Bone CT: Vertebra plana or lytic vertebral lesion
- CECT: Enhancement of lesion +/- paraspinal, epidural soft tissue component

### MR Findings
- T1WI: Hypointense vertebral mass +/- pathologic fracture, paraspinal/epidural extension
- T2WI
  - Heterogeneously hyperintense vertebral mass
  - Disc spaces generally spared
- T1 C+
  - Homogeneous enhancement
  - Enhancement typically absent in chronic lesions

## DDx: Vertebra Plana

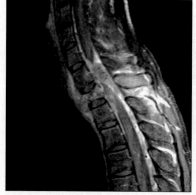

*Ewing Sarcoma*

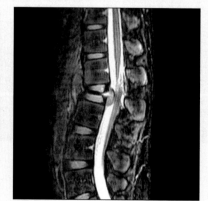

*Tuberculosis*

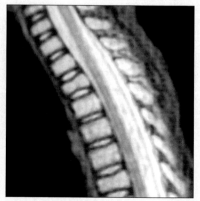

*Leukemia*

# LANGERHANS CELL HISTIOCYTOSIS, SPINE

## Key Facts

### Terminology
- Langerhans cell histiocytosis (LCH)
- Spinal LCH: Abnormal histiocyte proliferation producing granulomatous spinal lesions

### Imaging Findings
- Best diagnostic clue: Disc-sparing vertebra plana in a child
- Skull > long bones > spine > pelvis, ribs
- Spine: Thoracic (54%) > lumbar (35%) > cervical
- Vertebra plana: Collapse of vertebral body to thin disc; adjacent discs normal

### Top Differential Diagnoses
- Ewing Sarcoma
- Metastases, Neuroblastoma, Hemopoietic Malignancies

- Osteomyelitis
- Giant Cell Tumor

### Pathology
- Caused by monoclonal proliferation and accumulation of Langerhans cells in various tissues

### Clinical Issues
- Clinical Profile: Older child with back pain
- Spontaneous resolution of lesions common

### Diagnostic Checklist
- Unexplained vertebral compression fractures in children merit evaluation to exclude LCH or leukemia
- LCH most common cause vertebra plana in child

## Radiographic Findings
- Radiography
  - Vertebra plana or lytic destructive vertebral lesion
  - +/- Scoliosis, kyphosis

## Nuclear Medicine Findings
- Bone Scan
  - Variable: Lesions may be hot, cold, or mixed ("ring")
  - False negatives common (35%)

## Imaging Recommendations
- Best imaging tool: MR
- Protocol advice
  - Skeletal survey: Search for other lesions, confirm dx
  - MR C+: Evaluate soft tissues, epidural extension
  - Bone algorithm CT with multiplanar reformats to define osseous destruction, vertebral height loss

## DIFFERENTIAL DIAGNOSIS

### Ewing Sarcoma
- Permeative bone destruction not limited to vertebral body
- Associated moderate-large soft tissue mass

### Metastases, Neuroblastoma, Hemopoietic Malignancies
- Multifocal disease
- Widespread abnormal marrow signal, enhancement with extensive disease

### Osteomyelitis
- Endplate destruction with abnormal adjacent disc
- Disc may be spared in tuberculous spondylitis

### Giant Cell Tumor
- Expansile, lytic vertebral lesion + soft tissue mass
- Uncommon in pediatric population
- Sacrum most common spinal location

## PATHOLOGY

### General Features
- General path comments
  - Caused by monoclonal proliferation and accumulation of Langerhans cells in various tissues
  - Less than 1% of biopsy-proven primary bone lesions; vertebral involvement 6%
  - Embryology-anatomy
    - Langerhans cell (LC): Subset of non-phagocytic histiocyte (dendritic cell)
    - LC precursors originate in bone marrow; mature into LCs in lymph nodes, spleen, lung, skin; predominate in skin
    - LCs express variety of surface antigens; thought to play role in immune response
- Genetics: Sporadic, non-hereditary
- Etiology
  - PCR-based assay demonstrates all LCH forms are clonal ⇒ LCH probably clonal neoplasia rather than reactive disorder as previously believed
  - Clonal proliferation may result from exposure to infectious agents (e.g., viruses), immune system dysfunction, neoplastic mechanisms, genetic factors
- Epidemiology: 0.05-0.5/100,000 children/year
- Associated abnormalities
  - Pituitary-hypothalamic axis → diabetes insipidus
  - Temporal bone involvement → deafness
  - Orbital involvement → proptosis
  - Cutaneous LCH (≤ 50%)
  - Lung involvement (20-40%); male predominance, older age (20-40 years), smoking association
  - Gastrointestinal bleeding, liver/spleen abnormalities
  - Lymph node enlargement +/- suppuration, chronic drainage (30%)

### Gross Pathologic & Surgical Features
- Yellow, gray, or brown mass
- Variable hemorrhage, cyst formation

# LANGERHANS CELL HISTIOCYTOSIS, SPINE

## Microscopic Features

- Light microscopy: Pleocytic infiltrate of LCs, eosinophils, giant cells, foamy cells +/- bone necrosis
  - LC: Dendritic cell with grooved nucleus, pale cytoplasm; often found in sheets, clusters
- Immunohistochemistry: LC is S-100 and CD1a reactive
- Electron microscopy: Birbeck granules = racquet-shaped cytoplasmic inclusions unique to LC

## Staging, Grading or Classification Criteria

- Historically LCH divided into 3 named categories based on age, severity, extent of involvement
  - Eosinophilic granuloma (EG, 70%): Benign form confined to bone; older children
  - Hand-Schüller-Christian (HSC, 20%): Classic triad of exophthalmos, diabetes insipidus, bone destruction; younger children
  - Letterer-Siwe (LS, 10%): Disseminated form with involvement of visceral organs; infants
- Revised criteria according to disease extent
  - Single system disease
    - Limited to skin, bone, or lymph nodes
    - Can be uni- or multifocal within each system
  - Multisystem disease
    - Involving 2 or more systems (skin, lymph node, bone, visceral organs, lung, marrow)
    - Ranges from few systems to disseminated disease

## CLINICAL ISSUES

### Presentation

- Most common signs/symptoms
  - Back/neck pain
  - Additional lesions detected on skeletal survey may be asymptomatic
- Other signs/symptoms: Torticollis, radiculopathy
- Clinical Profile: Older child with back pain
- ~ 60% with spinal lesions have additional bone lesions on skeletal survey (polyostotic > monostotic)
- ~ 10% with spinal lesions have extraskeletal disease

### Demographics

- Age
  - Single system skeletal disease (EG): 5-15 years
  - Multisystem disease, no dissemination (HSC): 1-5 y
  - Acute, disseminated disease (LS): < 3 years
  - Adult disease uncommon; often limited to lungs
- Gender: M:F = 2:1

### Natural History & Prognosis

- Natural history: Variable
  - Disease confined to bone
    - Spontaneous resolution of lesions common
    - Regression usually begins after ~ 3 months, may take up to 2 years
    - 18-63% reconstitution of vertebral body height before skeletal maturity; 72-97% after
    - New lesions may develop, usually within 1-2 years
- Prognosis: Variable; depends on age, number of organs involved, extent of organ damage
  - Single system LCH in older child ⇒ excellent prognosis

- Infant with disseminated disease, organ dysfunction ⇒ poor prognosis; most die within 1-2 years

### Treatment

- Spinal LCH
  - Conservative: Observation +/- bracing
  - +/- Curettage, fusion, external beam radiotherapy, chemotherapy, steroids in patients with neurological deficits or conservative treatment

## DIAGNOSTIC CHECKLIST

### Consider

- Unexplained vertebral compression fractures in children merit evaluation to exclude LCH or leukemia
- LCH most common cause vertebra plana in child

### Image Interpretation Pearls

- Disc-sparing vertebra plana with relative absence of epidural mass classic for LCH

## SELECTED REFERENCES

1. Azouz EM et al: Langerhans' cell histiocytosis: pathology, imaging and treatment of skeletal involvement. Pediatr Radiol. 35(2):103-15, 2005
2. Tanaka N et al: Langerhans cell histiocytosis of the atlas. A report of three cases. J Bone Joint Surg Am. 87(10):2313-7, 2005
3. Garg S et al: Langerhans cell histiocytosis of the spine in children. Long-term follow-up. J Bone Joint Surg Am. 86-A(8):1740-50, 2004
4. Kuhn J et al: Caffey's Pediatric Diagnostic Imaging. 10th ed. Philadelphia, Mosby. 704, 2004
5. Simanski C et al: The Langerhans' cell histiocytosis (eosinophilic granuloma) of the cervical spine: a rare diagnosis of cervical pain. Magn Reson Imaging. 22(4):589-94, 2004
6. Tan G et al: Langerhans cell histiocytosis of the cervical spine: a single institution experience in four patients. J Pediatr Orthop B. 13(2):123-6, 2004
7. Fernando Ugarriza L et al: Solitary eosinophilic granuloma of the cervicothoracic junction causing neurological deficit. Br J Neurosurg. 17(2):178-81, 2003
8. Puertas EB et al: Surgical treatment of eosinophilic granuloma in the thoracic spine in patients with neurological lesions. J Pediatr Orthop B. 12(5):303-6, 2003
9. Bertram C et al: Eosinophilic granuloma of the cervical spine. Spine. 27(13):1408-13, 2002
10. Graham D et al: Greenfield's Neuropathology. 7th ed. London, Arnold. 1017-18, 2002
11. Kamimura M et al: Eosinophilic granuloma of the spine: early spontaneous disappearance of tumor detected on magnetic resonance imaging. Case report. J Neurosurg. 93(2 Suppl):312-6, 2000
12. Reddy PK et al: Eosinophilic granuloma of spine in adults: a case report and review of literature. Spinal Cord. 38(12):766-8, 2000
13. Yeom JS et al: Langerhans' cell histiocytosis of the spine. Analysis of twenty-three cases. Spine. 24(16):1740-9, 1999
14. Kandoi M et al: Rapidly progressive polyostotic eosinophilic granuloma involving spine: a case report. Indian J Med Sci. 52(1):22-4, 1998
15. Raab P et al: Vertebral remodeling in eosinophilic granuloma of the spine. A long-term follow-up. Spine. 23(12):1351-4, 1998

# LANGERHANS CELL HISTIOCYTOSIS, SPINE

## IMAGE GALLERY

### Typical

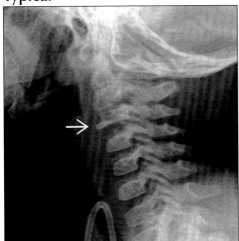
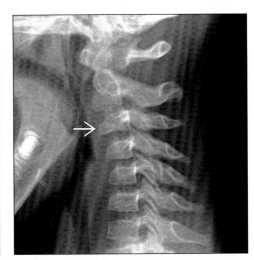

(**Left**) Lateral radiograph shows typical C3 vertebral plana ➡ in a child with multiple other skeletal lesions. (**Right**) Lateral radiograph in the same patient as previous image three years later shows considerable vertebral body reconstitution ➡.

### Typical

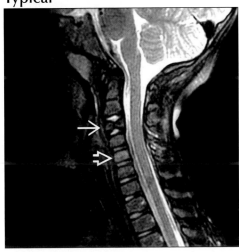
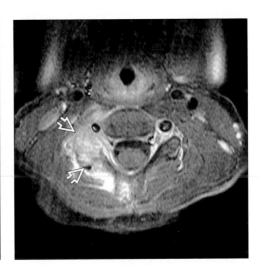

(**Left**) Sagittal T2WI FS MR shows natural history of LCH. A chronic lesion with mild residual vertebral deformity ➡ is present at C3. Abnormal signal ➡ can barely be detected at C5. (**Right**) Axial T1 C+ FS MR in same patient as previous image shows enhancing lesion ➡ of C5 facet and lamina. Posterior element involvement is more common in the cervical spine.

### Typical

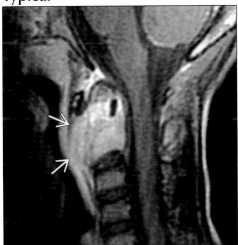
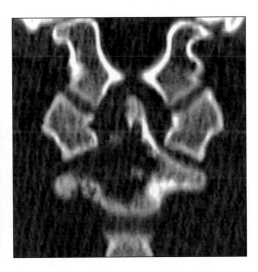

(**Left**) Sagittal T1 C+ MR shows enhancing C2 mass ➡ with prevertebral soft tissue extension. The adjacent disc is spared. The absence of vertebral body height loss is typical of LCH in the axis. (**Right**) Coronal bone CT in the same patient as previous image shows lytic destruction of the body of C2 and dens without vertebral body height loss.

# EXTRAMEDULLARY HEMATOPOIESIS, SPINE

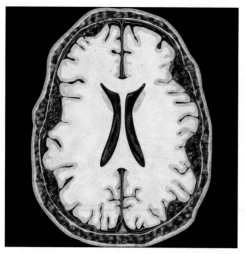

Axial graphic shows multiple dural masses and diploic space expansion due to extramedullary hematopoiesis.

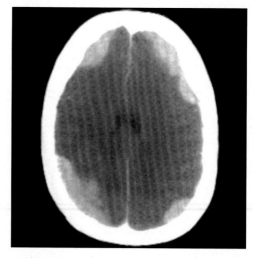

Axial NECT shows multiple hyperdense dural masses due to extramedullary hematopoiesis in a patient with myelofibrosis.

## TERMINOLOGY

### Abbreviations and Synonyms
- Extramedullary hematopoiesis (EMH)
- Extramedullary erythropoiesis

### Definitions
- Dural, epidural or paravertebral proliferation of hematopoietic tissue in response to profound chronic anemia

## IMAGING FINDINGS

### General Features
- Best diagnostic clue: Dural (intracranial), epidural (spine) or paraspinal (spine) masses with associated diffuse marrow hypointensity in patient with chronic anemia
- Location
  ○ Intracranial
    ■ Dura (including falx)
    ■ Parenchyma
    ■ Optic nerve sheath
    ■ Diploic space of skull
  ○ Spine
    ■ Mid thoracic > cervical, lumbar
    ■ Epidural or paravertebral
  ○ Other
    ■ Anterior ribs, liver, spleen, lymph nodes, kidney, adrenals, pleura, intestine, skin, thyroid, breast, maxillary antra
- Size
  ○ Intracranial: Variably sized multifocal dural masses
  ○ Spine: Variably sized multi-segmental masses
- Morphology
  ○ Well-circumscribed
  ○ Homogeneous
  ○ Lobular soft tissue mass

### CT Findings
- NECT
  ○ Soft tissue density (spine) to high attenuation (intracranial)
  ○ Intracranial: Dural mass ± compression or displacement of brain
  ○ Spine: Central canal narrowing, ± cord displacement and compression

## DDx: Cellular Masses

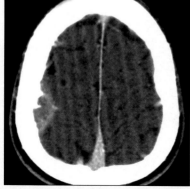

*Neuroblastoma*

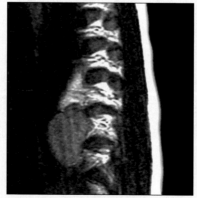

*Neuroblastoma*

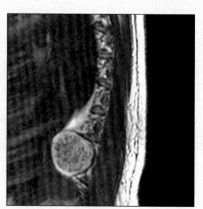

*Schwannoma*

# EXTRAMEDULLARY HEMATOPOIESIS, SPINE

## Key Facts

### Imaging Findings

- Best diagnostic clue: Dural (intracranial), epidural (spine) or paraspinal (spine) masses with associated diffuse marrow hypointensity in patient with chronic anemia
- Soft tissue density (spine) to high attenuation (intracranial)
- T1WI: Isointense to cortex or cord
- May be markedly hypointense due to increased iron content in hematopoietic tissue
- T1 C+: Minimal to marked enhancement
- Variable mass effect on brain and spinal cord
- Diffuse marrow hypointensity on all sequences
- Technetium sulfur colloid scan (Tc-99m-SC) diagnostic

### Pathology

- Ectopic hematopoietic rests stimulated in response to chronic anemic states
- Intracranial involvement rare
- Spinal involvement most common after hepatosplenic EMH

### Clinical Issues

- Clinical Profile: Suspect EMH in patient with chronic anemia with headache or back pain

### Diagnostic Checklist

- Consider if dural/epidural/paraspinal mass in patient with chronic anemia

- CECT: Mild to intense enhancement
- Bone CT
  - No bony erosion
  - No calcifications

## MR Findings

- T1WI: Isointense to cortex or cord
- T2WI
  - Iso- to mildly hyperintense to cortex or cord
  - May be markedly hypointense due to increased iron content in hematopoietic tissue
- STIR: Iso- to hyperintense
- T1 C+: Minimal to marked enhancement
- Variable mass effect on brain and spinal cord
  - Intracranial
    - Intracranial dural involvement most common in thalassemia (50%) and myelofibrosis (31%)
  - Spine
    - Cord compression most commonly reported with β-thalassemia
    - Intramedullary T2 hyperintensity may be present due to edema or myelomalacia
    - Nerve root compression may occur
- Diffuse marrow hypointensity on all sequences

## Radiographic Findings

- Radiography: Spine: Bilateral (a)symmetrically or unilateral widened paraspinal stripe on radiograph

## Nuclear Medicine Findings

- PET
  - Technetium sulfur colloid scan (Tc-99m-SC) diagnostic
    - Foci of intracranial dural or spinal epidural/paraspinal uptake correspond to EMH

## Non-Vascular Interventions

- Myelography: Spine: Nonspecific epidural mass effacing central canal

## Imaging Recommendations

- Best imaging tool: MR with gadolinium

## DIFFERENTIAL DIAGNOSIS

### Epidural Hematoma (Intracranial)

- Often hyperintense on T1WI, blooms on T2*, peripheral enhancement

### Tumors (Intracranial and Spine)

- Meningioma, PNET, lymphoma, myeloma, leukemia, extraosseous Ewing, neuroblastoma
- Imaging may be indistinguishable but no history of chronic anemia

### Phlegmon/Abscess (Intracranial and Spine)

- Associated with infectious spondylitis with destructive changes in vertebrae in spine
- Peripheral enhancement

### Neurogenic Tumor (Spine)

- Often at a single level
- Multiple neurofibromas in neurofibromatosis type 1
- Widened intervertebral foramina

### Lateral Meningocele (Spine)

- Fluid signal on MR

## PATHOLOGY

### General Features

- General path comments: Compensatory mechanism that attempts to maintain erythrogenesis necessary for circulatory demands in chronic anemia
- Etiology
  - Ectopic hematopoietic rests stimulated in response to chronic anemic states
    - Intermediate β-thalassemia: Most common
    - Sickle cell anemia
    - Polycythemia vera
    - Myelofibrosis with myeloid metaplasia
  - Source of extra-vertebral hematopoiesis controversial
    - Embryonic hematopoietic rests in epidural space
    - Direct extension of hematopoietic marrow from vertebrae into epidural space

# EXTRAMEDULLARY HEMATOPOIESIS, SPINE

- Fetal hematopoietic capacity of dura
- ○ Other possible theory: Stem cells differentiate into hematopoietic cells
  - Stimulated by unknown factors
- Epidemiology
  - ○ Intracranial involvement rare
  - ○ Spinal involvement most common after hepatosplenic EMH
    - Spinal EMH: 27% of non-hepatosplenic involvement
- Associated abnormalities: Hemothorax can occur with paraspinal EMH

## Gross Pathologic & Surgical Features
- Discrete flesh colored mass

## Microscopic Features
- Resembles bone marrow on biopsy: Trilineage hematopoiesis erythroid and granulocytic precursors, megakaryocytes

## CLINICAL ISSUES

### Presentation
- Most common signs/symptoms
  - ○ Intracranial: Headache, seizures, hemiplegia, altered consciousness, cranial nerve deficits, some asymptomatic
  - ○ Spine: Back ± radicular pain, paraparesis, sensory deficit, gait disturbance, bladder and/or bowel dysfunction, diminished deep tendon reflexes
- Other signs/symptoms: Anemia, pancytopenia
- Clinical Profile: Suspect EMH in patient with chronic anemia with headache or back pain

### Demographics
- Age: More common in adults
- Gender: No gender predilection
- Ethnicity
  - ○ Some hemoglobinopathies more common in certain ethnic groups
    - Sickle cell disease: African-Americans
    - Thalassemia: Races along Eastern Mediterranean Sea; Greek, Italian, Persian, etc.

### Natural History & Prognosis
- Excellent prognosis: Resolution of symptoms 3-7 days after radiotherapy
  - ○ Overall prognosis limited by underlying hemoglobinopathy or myeloproliferative disorder

### Treatment
- Low dose radiation treatment of choice since hematopoietic tissue highly radiosensitive
- Surgery considered if neurologic emergency
- Hypertransfusion or cytotoxic drugs may be used

## DIAGNOSTIC CHECKLIST

### Image Interpretation Pearls
- Consider if dural/epidural/paraspinal mass in patient with chronic anemia

## SELECTED REFERENCES

1. Collins WO et al: Extramedullary hematopoiesis of the paranasal sinuses in sickle cell disease. Otolaryngol Head Neck Surg. 132(6):954-6, 2005
2. Haidar S et al: Intracranial involvement in extramedullary hematopoiesis: case report and review of the literature. Pediatr Radiol. 35(6):630-4, 2005
3. Salehi SA et al: Spinal cord compression in beta-thalassemia: case report and review of the literature. Spinal Cord. 42(2):117-23, 2004
4. Chehal A et al: Hypertransfusion: a successful method of treatment in thalassemia intermedia patients with spinal cord compression secondary to extramedullary hematopoiesis. Spine. 28(13):E245-9, 2003
5. Koch CA et al: Nonhepatosplenic extramedullary hematopoiesis: associated diseases, pathology, clinical course, and treatment. Mayo Clin Proc. 78(10):1223-33, 2003
6. Cario H et al: Treatment with hydroxyurea in thalassemia intermedia with paravertebral pseudotumors of extramedullary hematopoiesis. Ann Hematol. 81(8):478-82, 2002
7. Chourmouzi D et al: MRI findings of extramedullary haemopoiesis. Eur Radiol. 11(9):1803-6, 2001
8. Elgin VE et al: Extramedullary hematopoiesis within a frontoethmoidal encephalocele in a newborn with holoprosencephaly. Pediatr Dev Pathol. 4(3):289-97, 2001
9. Kapelushnik J et al: Upper airway obstruction-related sleep apnea in a child with thalassemia intermedia. J Pediatr Hematol Oncol. 23(8):525-6, 2001
10. Alorainy IA et al: MRI features of epidural extramedullary hematopoiesis. Eur J Radiol. 35(1):8-11, 2000
11. Aydingoz U et al: Spinal cord compression due to epidural extramedullary haematopoiesis in thalassaemia: MRI. Neuroradiology. 39(12):870-2, 1997
12. Dibbern DA Jr et al: MR of thoracic cord compression caused by epidural extramedullary hematopoiesis in myelodysplastic syndrome. AJNR Am J Neuroradiol. 18(2):363-6, 1997
13. Guermazi A et al: Imaging of spinal cord compression due to thoracic extramedullary haematopoiesis in myelofibrosis. Neuroradiology. 39(10):733-6, 1997
14. Kalina P et al: Cord compression by extramedullary hematopoiesis in polycythemia vera. AJR Am J Roentgenol. 164(4):1027-8, 1995
15. Papavasiliou C: Clinical expressions of the expansion of the bone marrow in the chronic anemias: the role of radiotherapy. Int J Radiat Oncol Biol Phys. 28(3):605-12, 1994
16. Kalina P et al: MR of extramedullary hematopoiesis causing cord compression in beta-thalassemia. AJNR Am J Neuroradiol. 13(5):1407-9, 1992
17. Konstantopoulos K et al: A case of spinal cord compression by extramedullary haemopoiesis in a thalassaemic patient: a putative role for hydroxyurea? Haematologica. 77(4):352-4, 1992
18. Gouliamos A et al: Low back pain due to extramedullary hemopoiesis. Neuroradiology. 33(3):284-5, 1991
19. Kaufmann T et al: The role of radiation therapy in the management of hematopoietic neurologic complications in thalassemia. Acta Haematol. 85(3):156-9, 1991
20. Papavasiliou C et al: Masses of myeloadipose tissue: radiological and clinical considerations. Int J Radiat Oncol Biol Phys. 19(4):985-93, 1990

# EXTRAMEDULLARY HEMATOPOIESIS, SPINE

## IMAGE GALLERY

### Typical

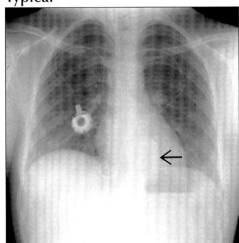

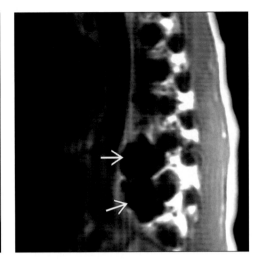

*(Left)* Anteroposterior radiograph in a teenage girl with beta thalassemia shows a left paraspinal mass ➡. *(Right)* Sagittal T1WI MR (same patient as previous image) shows low signal intensity masses ➡ in the left paraspinous soft tissues.

### Typical

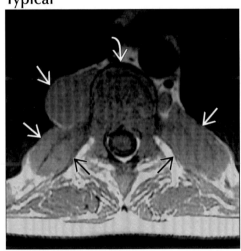

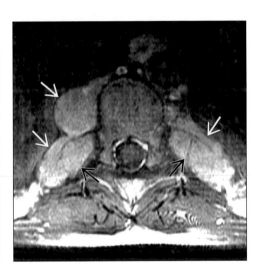

*(Left)* Axial T1WI MR shows multiple bilateral paraspinal masses ➡, bilateral expansion within the marrow of the ribs ➡, and ventral expansion ➡ of marrow in vertebral body. *(Right)* Axial T1 C+ MR (same patient as previous image) shows enhancement of the bilateral paraspinal masses ➡ and region of the expanded bilateral proximal ribs ➡.

### Typical

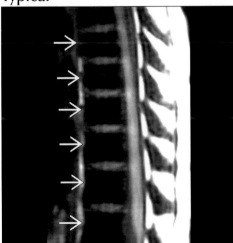

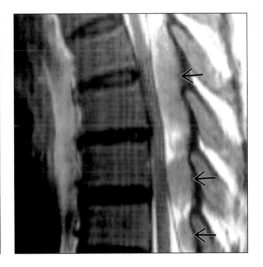

*(Left)* Sagittal T2WI MR shows markedly decreased signal intensity ➡ in all vertebral bodies due to replacement of yellow marrow with hematopoietic red marrow. *(Right)* Sagittal T2WI MR shows multiple hypointense epidural masses ➡ of low T2 signal signal intensity in the dorsal epidural space in this child with severe chronic anemia.

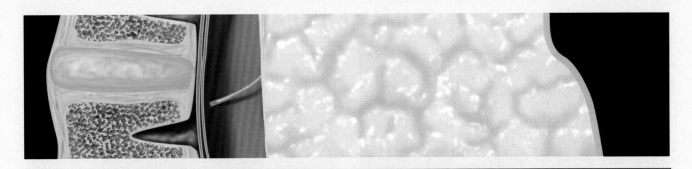

# SECTION 4: Intradural Extramedullary Space

# SPINAL LIPOMA

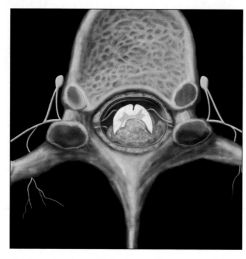

*Axial graphic demonstrates incomplete closure of dorsal spinal cord around a juxtamedullary conus lipoma. The dorsal nerve roots course through the lipoma.*

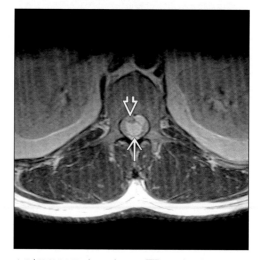

*Axial T2WI MR shows lipoma ⇨ is subpial, intradural location, dorsal to conus ⇨. Note chemical shift artifact, confirming presence of fat.*

## TERMINOLOGY

### Abbreviations and Synonyms
- Intradural (juxtamedullary, subpial) or terminal lipoma

### Definitions
- Spinal lipoma intimately associated with spinal cord (intradural) or distal cord/filum insertion (terminal)

## IMAGING FINDINGS

### General Features
- Best diagnostic clue: Hyperintense (T1WI) intradural mass
- Location
  - Intradural
    - Thoracic (30%) > cervicothoracic (24%) > cervical (12%) > lumbosacral spine
    - Dorsal (73%) > lateral/anterolateral (25%) > anterior (2%)
  - Terminal
    - Lumbosacral

- Size: Range: Tiny → huge
- Morphology: Lipoma invaginates into cord substance (intradural lipoma) or tether cord with extension through dorsal dysraphism into subcutaneous fat (terminal lipoma)

### CT Findings
- NECT
  - Intradural lipoma: Focal lobulated hypodense intradural mass +/- central canal, neural foraminal widening at lipoma level
  - Terminal lipoma: Elongated hypodense mass at filum termination; may extend into subcutaneous fat through dysraphic defect

### MR Findings
- T1WI
  - Intradural lipoma
    - Lobulated ovoid/rounded intradural hyperintense mass intimately associated with cord
    - +/- Canal widening, local dysraphism
    - ↓ Signal intensity on fat saturation sequences
  - Terminal lipoma

---

## DDx: Spinal Lipoma

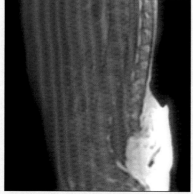

*Lipomyelomeningocele*

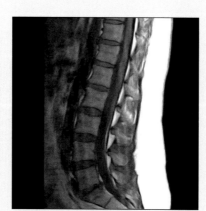

*Filum Fibrolipoma*

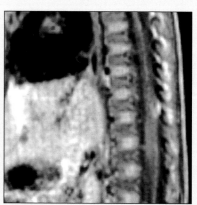

*Dermoid*

# SPINAL LIPOMA

## Key Facts

### Terminology
- Spinal lipoma intimately associated with spinal cord (intradural) or distal cord/filum insertion (terminal)

### Imaging Findings
- Best diagnostic clue: Hyperintense (T1WI) intradural mass
- Grayscale Ultrasound: Echogenic intraspinal mass +/- reduced conus motion

### Top Differential Diagnoses
- Lipomyelocele/Lipomyelomeningocele
- Filum Fibrolipoma
- Dermoid Cyst

### Pathology
- Composed of normal fat

- Arise from premature separation (dysjunction) of cutaneous ectoderm from neuroectoderm during neurulation

### Clinical Issues
- Intradural lipoma: Patient complains of weakness and sensory anomalies referable to lesion level
- Terminal lipoma: Patient presents with clinical appearance of "tethered cord syndrome" and (frequently) cutaneous stigmata

### Diagnostic Checklist
- Profound hypodensity on CT myelography and T1WI hyperintensity distinctively characteristic of lipoma
- Use chemical fat-saturation or inversion recovery MR technique to confirm fat content

- Hyperintense mass attached to distal cord/filum; extends through lumbosacral dysraphism ⇒ subcutaneous fat
- Thin, "stretched" cord usually tethered +/- syrinx
- T2WI
  - Similar signal intensity, imaging appearance to T1WI
  - +/- Spinal cord compression (intradural) ⇒ hyperintense cord signal
- STIR: ↓ Signal intensity confirms fat
- T1 C+: No lipoma enhancement

## Radiographic Findings
- Radiography
  - Intradural lipoma
    - Hypodense mass +/- dysraphism; posterior elements generally intact but show focal canal widening 2° to bony erosion
  - Terminal lipoma
    - Hypodense mass +/- posterior dysraphism

## Ultrasonographic Findings
- Grayscale Ultrasound: Echogenic intraspinal mass +/- reduced conus motion

## Non-Vascular Interventions
- Myelography
  - Intradural or terminal hypodense mass partially surrounded by hyperdense contrast
  - Large tumors may produce spinal block

## Other Modality Findings
- Sagittal PC MR: Decreased conus motion ⇒ tethered cord

## Imaging Recommendations
- Best imaging tool: MR imaging
- Protocol advice
  - Ultrasound in infants for screening; confirm with MR if positive
  - Sagittal, axial T1WI to define lipoma(s) extent and relationship to neural placode, adjacent tissues
    - Image through tip of thecal sac to avoid missing fibrolipoma or terminal lipoma

## DIFFERENTIAL DIAGNOSIS

### Lipomyelocele/Lipomyelomeningocele
- Skin covered (closed) neural placode-lipoma complex contiguous with subcutaneous fat through dysraphic defect
- Mass often palpable +/- cutaneous stigmata

### Filum Fibrolipoma
- Common; 4-6% population, mostly asymptomatic but symptomatic patients present at any age with "tethered cord"
- Hyperintense/hypodense mass in filum +/- tethering, low-lying conus

### Dermoid Cyst
- Mixed density/signal intensity mass; lack of homogeneous hyperintensity +/- dermal sinus help to distinguish

## PATHOLOGY

### General Features
- General path comments
  - Three main types of spinal lipomas: Intradural, lipomyelo(meningo)cele/terminal lipoma, and filum lipoma
  - Composed of normal fat
    - Fat cells ↑ in size considerably during infancy; tiny lipomas in neonates may grow substantially during infancy
    - Conversely, lipomas ↓ in size if patient loses weight
- Etiology
  - Arise from premature separation (dysjunction) of cutaneous ectoderm from neuroectoderm during neurulation
    - Surrounding mesenchyme enters ependyma-lined central spinal canal, impeding closure of neural folds ⇒ open placode
    - Mesenchyme differentiates into fat

- Similar mechanism ⇒ dermal sinus tract; explains their frequent association
- Epidemiology
  - Intradural lipoma (4%)
    - < 1% of primary intraspinal tumors
  - Lipomyelo(meningo)cele (includes terminal lipoma) (84%)
  - Filum lipoma (12%)
- Associated abnormalities
  - Intradural lipoma: +/- Localized dysraphism at lipoma level; segmentation anomalies rare
  - Terminal lipoma: Sacral hypogenesis, anorectal malformations, genitourinary (GU) malformations (5-10%), terminal diastematomyelia, epidermoid, dermal sinus, angioma, arachnoid cyst
    - Sacral anomalies much more likely if GU, anorectal malformations present (≥ 90%)

## Gross Pathologic & Surgical Features

- Intradural lipoma
  - Partially encapsulated sessile (55%) or exophytic (45%) juxtamedullary fatty mass entirely enclosed within dural sac
  - Midline spinal cord "open"; subpial lipoma nestled between open lips
- Terminal lipoma
  - Delicately encapsulated fatty mass attached to cord/filum; frequently contiguous with subcutaneous fat through dorsal lumbosacral dysraphism
    - Rotation uncommon (unlike LMMC)
  - Cord almost always tethered; stretched and thinned +/- hydrosyringomyelia (20%)

## Microscopic Features

- Homogeneous mass of mature fat separated into globules by strands of fibrous tissue
  - +/- Calcification, ossification, muscle fibers, nerves, glial tissue, arachnoid, ependyma

# CLINICAL ISSUES

## Presentation

- Most common signs/symptoms
  - Cervical, thoracic intradural lipoma: Slow ascending mono- or paraparesis, spasticity, cutaneous sensory loss, deep sensory loss
  - Lumbosacral intradural lipoma: Flaccid lower extremity paralysis, sphincter dysfunction
  - Terminal lipoma: Bowel/bladder dysfunction, lower extremity weakness/sensory abnormality, foot deformity, scoliosis
  - Symptoms may be exacerbated by pregnancy
- Clinical Profile
  - Intradural lipoma: Patient complains of weakness and sensory anomalies referable to lesion level
    - Overlying skin usually looks normal; no cutaneous stigmata
  - Terminal lipoma: Patient presents with clinical appearance of "tethered cord syndrome" and (frequently) cutaneous stigmata

## Demographics

- Age
  - 3 age peaks for presentation
    - < 5 years (24%)
    - 2nd → 3rd decades (55%)
    - 5th decade (16%)
- Gender
  - Intradural: M ≤ F
  - Terminal: M < F

## Natural History & Prognosis

- Small lipomas may grow dramatically during infancy
- Very rarely, lipomas may spontaneously regress
- Symptomatic patients unlikely to improve spontaneously without intervention
  - Caveat: Lipomas may shrink if patient loses weight

## Treatment

- Surgical resection, untethering of cord (if applicable)
- Weight loss may be conservative management method to avoid surgery in highly selected obese patients

# DIAGNOSTIC CHECKLIST

## Consider

- Follow-up even small lipomas in neonates; they may grow significantly!

## Image Interpretation Pearls

- Profound hypodensity on CT myelography and T1WI hyperintensity distinctively characteristic of lipoma
- Use chemical fat-saturation or inversion recovery MR technique to confirm fat content

# SELECTED REFERENCES

1. Hashiguchi K et al: Usefulness of constructive interference in steady-state magnetic resonance imaging in the presurgical examination for lumbosacral lipoma. J Neurosurg. 103(6 Suppl):537-43, 2005
2. Morimoto K et al: Spinal lipomas in children--surgical management and long-term follow-up. Pediatr Neurosurg. 41(2):84-7, 2005
3. Kulkarni AV et al: Conservative management of asymptomatic spinal lipomas of the conus. Neurosurgery. 54(4):868-73; discussion 873-5, 2004
4. Pierre-Kahn A et al: Lumbosacral lipomas: in utero diagnosis and prognosis. Childs Nerv Syst. 19(7-8):551-4, 2003
5. Arai H et al: Surgical experience of 120 patients with lumbosacral lipomas. Acta Neurochir (Wien). 143(9):857-64, 2001
6. Bulsara KR et al: Clinical outcome differences for lipomyelomeningoceles, intraspinal lipomas, and lipomas of the filum terminale. Neurosurg Rev. 24(4):192-4, 2001
7. Endoh M et al: Spontaneous shrinkage of lumbosacral lipoma in conjunction with a general decrease in body fat: case report. Neurosurgery. 43(1):150-1; discussion 151-2, 1998
8. Byrne RW et al: Operative resection of 100 spinal lipomas in infants less than 1 year of age. Pediatr Neurosurg. 23(4):182-6; discussion 186-7, 1995
9. Aoki N: Rapid growth of intraspinal lipoma demonstrated by magnetic resonance imaging. Surg Neurol. 34(2):107-10, 1990

# SPINAL LIPOMA

## IMAGE GALLERY

### Typical

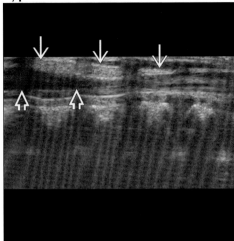
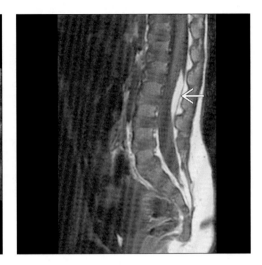

*(Left) Sagittal ultrasound demonstrates a hyperechoic dorsal juxtamedullary lipoma ➡ extending along dorsal surface of conus ➡. (Right) Sagittal T1WI MR show the typical hyperintense appearance of a dorsal conus juxtamedullary lipoma ➡. The conus is low-lying, at L2/3 level.*

### Variant

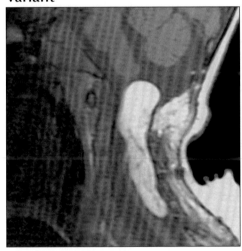
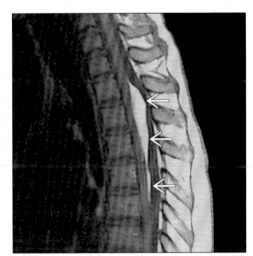

*(Left) Sagittal T1WI MR demonstrates a hyperintense intradural lipoma intimately associated with the cervical spinal cord. No posterior dysraphism was identified. (Right) Sagittal T1WI MR depict a dorsal hyperintense intradural subpial lipoma ➡ with mild spinal cord distortion but normal cord signal. Note remodeling of spinal canal, widened AP diameter.*

### Variant

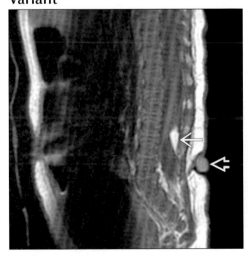
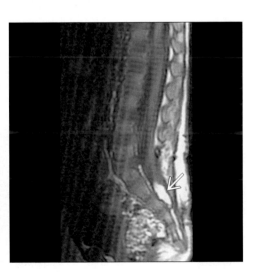

*(Left) Sagittal T1WI MR shows a low-lying spinal cord tethered by small subpial lipoma ➡ in conjunction with a dorsal dermal sinus tract. Skin opening of tract is marked by Vitamin E capsule ➡. (Right) Sagittal T1WI MR shows low spinal cord termination, tethered by a hyperintense terminal lipoma ➡. No sacral dysgenesis was identified.*

# FILUM TERMINALE FIBROLIPOMA

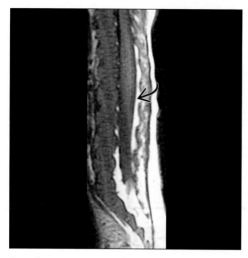

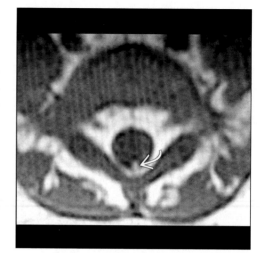

*Sagittal T1WI MR in an infant with anal atresia shows normal-appearing conus ⇗ at L2. The filum is often difficult to see well on sagittal images, particularly in infants.*

*Axial T1WI MR in the same patient as previous image shows an enlarged, fat-containing filum terminale ⇗, which often cannot be seen on sagittal images.*

## TERMINOLOGY

### Abbreviations and Synonyms
- Fibrolipoma of filum terminale, fatty filum terminale, "fat in the filum"

### Definitions
- Presence of fat within normal sized or slightly enlarged filum terminale
- Often asymptomatic; may be associated with signs, symptoms of tethered cord

## IMAGING FINDINGS

### General Features
- Best diagnostic clue: Linear hyperintensity within large filum terminale on T1WI
- Location: Filum terminale (conus level to caudal end of thecal sac)
- Size
  - 1-5 mm diameter
  - Variable length

- Morphology: Linear, rostro-caudal "stripe" of high signal on T1WI

### CT Findings
- NECT: Punctate fat attenuation in dorsal aspect of lumbar thecal sac
- CECT: No enhancement

### MR Findings
- T1WI
  - Linear high signal oriented in rostral to caudal direction
    - May occur anywhere from below conus to sacrum
    - May be difficult to see on sagittal images, as filum is often located very posteriorly
    - Always acquire axial images from conus to bottom of S1
  - Filum has low signal on fat suppressed sequence
  - Conus may be at normal level (above lower endplate of L2) or low
    - When associated with low conus, more likely symptomatic
  - Dural sac frequently widened
    - Dorsal dura tented posteriorly by filum
    - Tenting of dura seen best on axial images

## DDx: Hyperintense Lesions in Caudal Spine

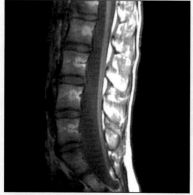

*Terminal Lipoma*

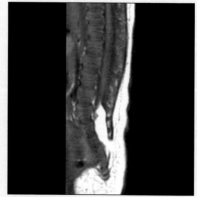

*Terminal Lipomyelocele*

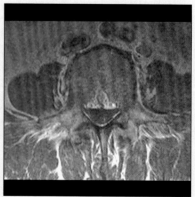

*Enhancing Vein*

# FILUM TERMINALE FIBROLIPOMA

## Key Facts

### Terminology
- Fibrolipoma of filum terminale, fatty filum terminale, "fat in the filum"
- Presence of fat within normal sized or slightly enlarged filum terminale

### Imaging Findings
- Best diagnostic clue: Linear hyperintensity within large filum terminale on T1WI
- MR imaging: T1WI shows typical fat appearance, slightly enlarged filum focally or diffusely
- Acquire sagittal and axial T1WI

### Top Differential Diagnoses
- Subpial Lipoma
- Tethered Cord with Terminal Lipoma
- Lipomyelocele

- Intrathecal Vein
- Sacrococcygeal Teratoma

### Pathology
- Disruption of cellular architecture throughout filum
- Often seen in association with diastematomyelia
- Cause is thought to be disruption of normal retrogressive differentiation of distal spinal cord
- Some fat in filum in 4-6% of autopsy subjects
- Fibrolipomas constitute 12% of intradural lipomas

### Diagnostic Checklist
- Suspect fibrolipoma if conus is elongated or filum looks too dorsal or too straight
- Always acquire axial T1 and T2 weighted images through L5-S1 to look for fatty or thick filum

---

- Dilated central canal seen in conus in 20%
  - May indicate tethering
- T2WI
  - Filum may appear too thick
  - Chemical shift artifact, especially on axial images, may cause fat to look displaced
  - Dural sac frequently widened
    - Dorsal dura may be tented posteriorly by filum
    - Tenting of dura seen best on axial images
- T1 C+: No enhancement
- MR Cine
  - Quantitative cardiac gated phase contrast imaging may be useful to predict associated tethering of cord
  - If cord is tethered, magnitude of pulsations is reduced

## Radiographic Findings
- Radiography
  - Often asymmetric spina bifida occulta
    - Seen in 20%

## Imaging Recommendations
- Best imaging tool
  - MR imaging: T1WI shows typical fat appearance, slightly enlarged filum focally or diffusely
    - Best to acquire sagittal and axial images
- Protocol advice
  - Acquire sagittal and axial T1WI
  - Axial T2WI from conus to bottom of S1
  - Add fat suppressed sequence if uncertain of T1WI signal etiology

## DIFFERENTIAL DIAGNOSIS

### Subpial Lipoma
- Larger lipomatous mass (> few mm)
- Involves spinal cord, not filum terminale
- Not associated with tethered cord

### Tethered Cord with Terminal Lipoma
- Cord extends to sacrum
- Thick lipoma at caudal termination

- Indistinct cord termination; conus with smooth transition to filum
  - Filum begins where nerve roots stop coming off

### Lipomyelocele
- Dysraphic spinal cord associated with lipomatous mass
- Cord forms neural placode
  - Lipoma is dorsal to placode
  - Subarachnoid space is ventral to placode
- Lipoma extends dorsally through spina bifida

### Intrathecal Vein
- Normal finding; not associated with neurologic signs or symptoms
- Runs parallel to nerve root; exits via neural foramen
- Does not suppress with fat-saturation

### Sacrococcygeal Teratoma
- Bulky mass
- Cystic and solid components, as well as fat

## PATHOLOGY

### General Features
- General path comments
  - Fatty infiltration of filum
  - Disruption of cellular architecture throughout filum
  - Often seen in association with diastematomyelia
- Etiology
  - Cause is thought to be disruption of normal retrogressive differentiation of distal spinal cord
  - Normally, cells in most distal cord arise from pluripotential cells in caudal cell mass
    - Cells in caudal aspects of spinal cord undergo apoptosis
    - Filum elongates due to apoptosis and elongation of cells
    - Cystic areas within developing filum coalesce into ependyma-lined central canal
    - Level of conus "ascends" relative to spinal column
    - Tip of conus above L2-L3 interspace in 99% after birth

- ○ Fibrolipomas may result from incomplete apoptosis
  - ▪ Fibers in filum do not elongate, causing tethering
- ○ As a result of disruption of normal development, various abnormalities may be found
  - ▪ Fatty filum: Fat may be localized in the filum or diffuse from conus to end of thecal sac
  - ▪ Filar cyst(s)
  - ▪ Low-lying conus
  - ▪ Dilated central canal in conus
- ○ When filum fails to elongate, tethering effect is transmitted to conus medullaris
  - ▪ Stretching of axons results in abnormal oxidative metabolism in conus
- Epidemiology
  - ○ Some fat in filum in 4-6% of autopsy subjects
  - ○ Fibrolipomas constitute 12% of intradural lipomas
- Associated abnormalities
  - ○ Spina bifida occulta seen in 20%
  - ○ Cutaneous stigmata uncommon
  - ○ Other spinal anomalies (see below)

## Gross Pathologic & Surgical Features

- Variable amount of fat within thickened filum terminale
- Conus may be at normal position or low-lying
- Fibrolipoma often present when other malformations present
  - ○ Diastematomyelia
  - ○ Dorsal dermal sinus

## Microscopic Features

- Filum: Fibrous tissue mixed with typical fat cells

## CLINICAL ISSUES

### Presentation

- Most common signs/symptoms
  - ○ May be discovered incidentally
  - ○ Back pain, motor dysfunction if cord is tethered
  - ○ Urinary or fecal incontinence in severe cases

### Demographics

- Age
  - ○ Any
  - ○ Percentage of asymptomatic patients decreases with increasing age
- Gender: M = F

### Natural History & Prognosis

- If cord is tethered, can become symptomatic at any age
- If symptoms develop, they progress unless tethering is released

### Treatment

- Options, risks, complications
  - ○ Treatment of asymptomatic fatty filum is controversial
    - ▪ Symptoms do not regress after treatment
    - ▪ Many remain asymptomatic
    - ▪ Urodynamic testing can help to identify presymptomatic patients with tethered cords
- Treatment (if necessary) is transection of filum

- Some patients with bladder, bowel dysfunction improve after untethering of cord

## DIAGNOSTIC CHECKLIST

### Consider

- Intraspinal lipoma if other congenital spine lesion and filum > 1 mm in thickness
- Look for fibrolipoma if scoliosis is atypical
  - ○ Consider direction of curvature, age, associated signs, symptoms

### Image Interpretation Pearls

- Suspect fibrolipoma if conus is elongated or filum looks too dorsal or too straight
- Always acquire axial T1 and T2 weighted images through L5-S1 to look for fatty or thick filum

## SELECTED REFERENCES

1. Metcalfe PD et al: Treatment of the occult tethered spinal cord for neuropathic bladder: results of sectioning the filum terminale. J Urol. 176(4 Pt 2):1826-9; discussion 1830, 2006
2. Steinbok P et al: Occult tethered cord syndrome: a survey of practice patterns. J Neurosurg. 104(5 Suppl):309-13, 2006
3. Rinaldi F et al: Tethered cord syndrome. J Neurosurg Sci. 49(4):131-5; discussion 135, 2005
4. Rosahl SK et al: High-resolution constructive interference in steady-state imaging in tethered cord syndrome: technical note. Surg Neurol. 63(4):372-4, 2005
5. Shaya MR et al: Diffuse back pain and urological symptoms: recognizing tethered cord syndrome early. J La State Med Soc. 157(1):39-41, 2005
6. Michelson DJ et al: Tethered cord syndrome in childhood: diagnostic features and relationship to congenital anomalies. Neurol Res. 26(7):745-53, 2004
7. Nogueira M et al: Tethered cord in children: a clinical classification with urodynamic correlation. J Urol. 172(4 Pt 2):1677-80; discussion 1680, 2004
8. Schaan M et al: Intraoperative urodynamics in spinal cord surgery: a study of feasibility. Eur Spine J. 13(1):39-43, 2004
9. Yamada S et al: Pathophysiology of tethered cord syndrome and other complex factors. Neurol Res. 26(7):722-6, 2004
10. Bulsara KR et al: Clinical outcome differences for lipomyelomeningoceles, intraspinal lipomas, and lipomas of the filum terminale. Neurosurg Rev. 24(4): 192-4, 2001
11. La Marca F et al: Spinal lipomas in children: outcome of 270 procedures. Pediatr Neurosurg. 26(1): 8-16, 1997
12. Johnson DL et al: Predicting outcome in the tethered cord syndrome: a study of cord motion. Pediatr Neurosurg. 22(3):115-9, 1995
13. Brown E et al: Prevalence of incidental intraspinal lipoma of the lumbosacral spine as determined by MRI. Spine. 19(7): 833-6, 1994
14. McCullough DC et al: Toward the prediction of neurological injury from tethered spinal cord: investigation of cord motion with magnetic resonance. Pediatr Neurosurg. 16(1):3-7; discussion 7, 1990-1991
15. Moufarrij NA et al: Correlation between magnetic resonance imaging and surgical findings in the tethered spinal cord. Neurosurgery. 25(3): 341-6, 1989

# FILUM TERMINALE FIBROLIPOMA

## IMAGE GALLERY

### Typical

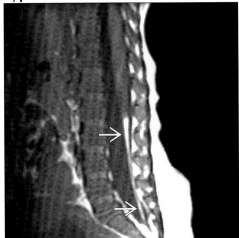 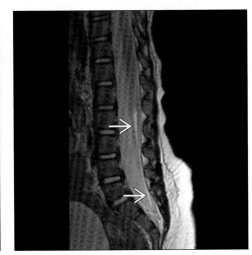

*(Left)* Sagittal T1WI MR shows the conus terminating at L2 and a fatty, thickened filum terminale ➡ extending from the conus tip to the end of the thecal sac. *(Right)* Sagittal T2WI MR in the same patient as previous image shows the hyperintense fat ➡ to be slightly mismapped compared with the T1WI due to chemical shift effects.

### Typical

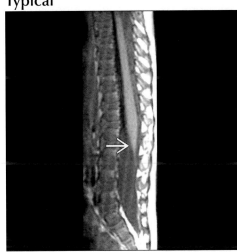 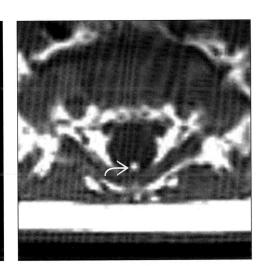

*(Left)* Sagittal T1WI MR shows a stretched, elongated conus medullaris ➡ that is commonly associated with tethering of the spinal cord. The conus tip is at the L3 level, which is too caudal. *(Right)* Axial T1WI MR shows the thick, fatty filum ➡ situated within the posterior aspect of the thecal sac at the level of the S1 vertebral body.

### Typical

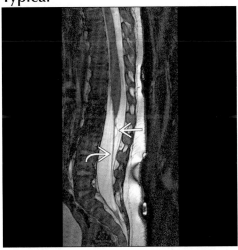 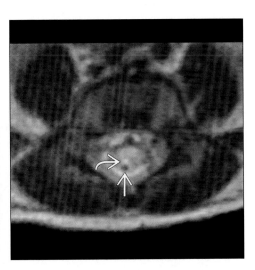

*(Left)* Sagittal T2WI MR using a steady state technique shows a straight, thickened filum ➡ and small filar cysts ➡. Filar cysts are poorly seen on routine T2WIs. *(Right)* Axial T2WI MR in same patient as previous image shows thickened filum terminale ➡ as focus of hypointensity larger than nerve roots. Note chemical shift artifact with fat signal ➡ mismapped ventrally.

# ANGIOLIPOMA

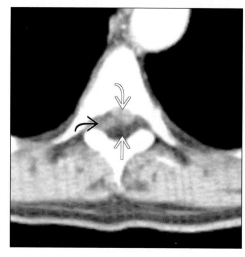

*Axial CECT shows the fat attenuation ➡ of a dorsal mass with a more soft tissue component ➡ along right dorsal epidural space. The mass displaces and compresses the spinal cord ➡.*

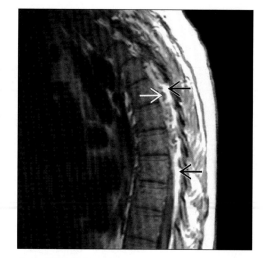

*Sagittal T1WI MR in the same patient as previous image shows a large heterogeneous dorsal epidural T1 hyperintense mass ➡ compressing the spinal cord. Curvilinear flow voids ➡ are evident.*

## TERMINOLOGY

### Abbreviations and Synonyms
- Angiolipoma (AL), vascular lipoma, hemangiolipoma, fibromyolipoma, angiomyolipoma

### Definitions
- Benign tumor of adipose and vascular elements

## IMAGING FINDINGS

### General Features
- Best diagnostic clue: Epidural heterogeneous fatty lesion on T1 showing enhancement on fat-suppressed T1WI
- Location
  - Uncommon tumors of extremities, trunk, neck
  - Spine involvement uncommon: Extradural > > intramedullary
  - C6 ⇒ L4 level
  - Report of mediastinal angiolipoma with spinal canal extension
- Size
  - Extend over 1-4 vertebral body segments
  - Average extent > 2 vertebral body length
- Morphology: Focal or infiltrating mass showing heterogeneous fat signal

### CT Findings
- NECT
  - CT shows extradural mass of fat attenuation (-20 to -60 HU)
  - Scattered soft tissue reticulation
  - Slight to intense enhancement
  - Rare calcification
  - Rare bony remodeling

### MR Findings
- T1WI
  - 40% hyperintense on T1WI, 70% with heterogeneous signal
  - Heterogeneity thought related to capillary and venous channels
  - Prominence of vascular component may result in isointense (cf. muscle) T1 signal
  - Cord compression common in symptomatic cases
- T2WI: Mild increase signal relative to CSF

## DDx: Hyperintense Epidural Lesions

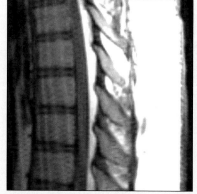

*Epidural Lipomatosis*

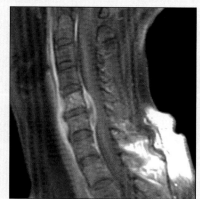

*Epidural Abscess*

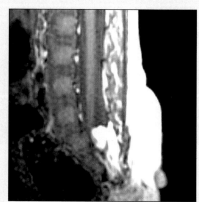

*Intrathecal Lipoma*

# ANGIOLIPOMA

## Key Facts

### Terminology
- Angiolipoma (AL), vascular lipoma, hemangiolipoma, fibromyolipoma, angiomyolipoma

### Imaging Findings
- Best diagnostic clue: Epidural heterogeneous fatty lesion on T1 showing enhancement on fat-suppressed T1WI
- Extend over 1-4 vertebral body segments
- CT shows extradural mass of fat attenuation (-20 to -60 HU)
- Scattered soft tissue reticulation
- 40% hyperintense on T1WI, 70% with heterogeneous signal
- Cord compression common in symptomatic cases
- T1 C+: Fat-suppressed T1WI most useful for lesion definition, showing heterogeneous enhancement

### Top Differential Diagnoses
- Epidural Lipomatosis
- Lipoma
- Liposarcoma
- Hematoma
- Abscess

### Pathology
- Noninfiltrating more common than infiltrating

### Clinical Issues
- Clinical Profile: Slowly progressive paraparesis with back pain

### Diagnostic Checklist
- Can be mistaken for a malignant tumor when vascular component dominates

- PD/Intermediate: Increased signal relative to CSF, but decreased signal relative to fat
- T1 C+: Fat-suppressed T1WI most useful for lesion definition, showing heterogeneous enhancement

## Imaging Recommendations
- Best imaging tool: MR ± contrast
- Protocol advice
  - Axial, sagittal T1 and T2 weighted images pre-contrast
  - Axial and sagittal post-contrast fat-suppressed T1WI

# DIFFERENTIAL DIAGNOSIS

## Epidural Lipomatosis
- Homogeneous fat signal, without enhancement
- Typical history of steroid use
- Typical dorsal thoracic epidural location

## Lipoma
- Little or no enhancement, minimal septations
- May be intradural, extradural or subcutaneous
  - Rarely exclusively epidural
- Distinguishable microscopically, with AL showing vessels branching pattern and fibrous scarring

## Liposarcoma
- May have irregular thickened septa, with areas of T2 hyperintensity
- Liposarcomas show cellular pleomorphism and mitotic activity
- May show considerable T1 isointense (to muscle) tissue

## Hematoma
- No suppression with fat-sat
- No enhancement, unless more chronic
- May show low signal on T2* images

## Abscess
- May show heterogeneous T1 signal within epidural fat, with focal areas of low signal
- Prominent peripheral enhancement

- May show heterogeneous signal and enhancement, like angiolipoma

# PATHOLOGY

## General Features
- General path comments
  - Benign tumor usually found in extremities, trunk or neck
  - Spine angiolipomas rare
    - ~ 100 case reports in literature, 7 in children
  - Noninfiltrating more common than infiltrating
    - Noninfiltrating more common in posterior thoracic epidural space, no bone destruction
    - Infiltrating more common in anterior epidural space, may destroy adjacent bone
  - Noninfiltrating form may occur at multiple sites in subcutaneous tissues
- Genetics
  - Subcutaneous angiolipomas show predominately normal karyotype
    - Contrasted with characteristic chromosomal aberrations in other lipomatous lesions such as lipoma, lipoblastoma, hibernomas
  - Rare familial occurrence of angiolipomas
- Etiology
  - Etiology unknown, with several theories
    - May originate from primitive pluripotential mesenchymal cells
    - Congenital malformation
    - Hamartomatous lesion, enlarging in response to normal growth/injury/inflammation
- Epidemiology
  - Rare, approximately 0.2-1% of all spinal tumors
  - 2-3% of extradural tumors
  - Noninfiltrating; more common in spine
  - Typically mid-thoracic, but can occur any where in spine
  - CNS involvement rare

# ANGIOLIPOMA

## Gross Pathologic & Surgical Features
- Gross features of fatty tissue, although may show port wine or dark brown coloration

## Microscopic Features
- Presence of mature adipocytes and vascular tissues
  - Vascular proliferation with microthrombi
  - Consistent marker of angiolipomas is presence of fibrin microthrombi in vascular channels
    - Associated with disrupted endothelial cells
- Vessels variously described as sinusoids, thin-walled, thick walled with smooth muscle proliferation
- Mitoses and pleomorphism not present
- Features vary
  - Predominately lipomatous with few small angiomatous regions
  - Predominately vascular with small lipomatous component

## CLINICAL ISSUES

### Presentation
- Most common signs/symptoms
  - Nonspecific back pain
  - Other signs/symptoms: Cord compression
    - Progressive paraparesis
    - Symptoms may progress with pregnancy
    - Acute onset of symptoms may occur due to degeneration, or hemorrhage into lesion
- Clinical Profile: Slowly progressive paraparesis with back pain

### Demographics
- Age
  - 5th decade, although may occur in children or adults
  - In children mean age 11.2 years (range 4-18 years)
- Gender: M:F ~ 1:1.6 overall but 2:1 in children

### Natural History & Prognosis
- Slowly progressive
- Bone infiltration associated with more aggressive behavior and worse prognosis

### Treatment
- Surgical excision
  - Noninfiltrating low rate of recurrence following excision
  - Infiltrative 50% recurrence rate
- Partial resection may give good symptomatic relief in infiltrative form but goal total resection
- Degree of hypointensity on T1WI predictive of degree of vascularity encountered at surgery

## DIAGNOSTIC CHECKLIST

### Consider
- Not to be confused with angiomyolipoma, which is seen in tuberous sclerosis, and occurs in kidney

## Image Interpretation Pearls
- Fatty epidural lesion with variable enhancement compressing cord
- Can be mistaken for a malignant tumor when vascular component dominates

## SELECTED REFERENCES
1. Dogan S et al: Lumbar spinal extradural angiolipomas. Two case reports. Neurol Med Chir (Tokyo). 46(3):157-60, 2006
2. Hattori H: Epidural angiolipoma is histologically distinct from its cutaneous counterpart in the calibre and density of its vascular component; a case report with review of the literature. J Clin Pathol. 58(8):882-3, 2005
3. Rabin D et al: Infiltrating spinal angiolipoma: a case report and review of the literature. J Spinal Disord Tech. 17(5):456-61, 2004
4. Rocchi G et al: Lumbar spinal angiolipomas: report of two cases and review of the literature. Spinal Cord. 42(5):313-6, 2004
5. Samdani AF et al: Spinal angiolipoma: case report and review of the literature. Acta Neurochir (Wien). 146(3):299-302; discussion 302, 2004
6. Turgut M: Spinal extradural angiolipoma, with a literature review. Childs Nerv Syst. 20(2):73-4, 2004
7. Leu NH et al: MR imaging of an infiltrating spinal epidural angiolipoma. AJNR Am J Neuroradiol. 24(5):1008-11, 2003
8. Gelabert-Gonzalez M et al: Spinal extradural angiolipoma, with a literature review. Childs Nerv Syst. 18(12):725-8, 2002
9. Amlashi SF et al: Spinal epidural angiolipoma. J Neuroradiol. 28(4): 253-6, 2001
10. Choi JY et al: Angiolipoma of the posterior mediastinum with extension into the spinal canal: a case report. Korean J Radiol. 1(4): 212-4, 2000
11. Klisch J et al: Radiological and histological findings in spinal intramedullary angiolipoma. Neuroradiology. 41(8): 584-7, 1999
12. Labram EK et al: Revisited: spinal angiolipoma--three additional cases. Br J Neurosurg. 13(1): 25-9, 1999
13. Oge HK et al: Spinal angiolipoma: case report and review of literature. J Spinal Disord. 12(4): 353-6, 1999
14. Sciot R et al: Cytogenetic analysis of subcutaneous angiolipoma: further evidence supporting its difference from ordinary pure lipomas: a report of the CHAMP Study Group. Am J Surg Pathol. 21(4):441-4, 1997
15. Fletcher CD et al: Correlation between clinicopathological features and karyotype in lipomatous tumors. A report of 178 cases from the Chromosomes and Morphology (CHAMP) Collaborative Study Group. Am J Pathol. 148(2):623-30, 1996
16. Provenzale JM et al: Spinal angiolipomas: MR features. AJNR Am J Neuroradiol. 17(4): 713-9, 1996
17. Weiss SW: Lipomatous tumors. Monogr Pathol. 38:207-39, 1996
18. Shibata Y et al: Thoracic epidural angiolipoma--case report. Neurol Med Chir (Tokyo). 33(5): 316-9, 1993
19. Pagni CA et al: Spinal epidural angiolipoma: rare or unreported? Neurosurgery. 31(4): 758-64; discussion 764, 1992
20. Stranjalis G et al: MRI in the diagnosis of spinal extradural angiolipoma. Br J Neurosurg. 6(5):481-3, 1992
21. Weill A et al: Spinal angiolipomas: CT and MR aspects. J Comput Assist Tomogr. 15(1): 83-5, 1991
22. Dixon AY et al: Angiolipomas: an ultrastructural and clinicopathological study. Hum Pathol. 12(8):739-47, 1981

# ANGIOLIPOMA

## IMAGE GALLERY

### Typical

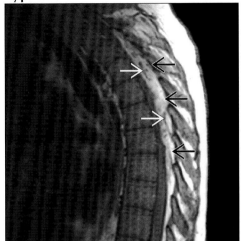

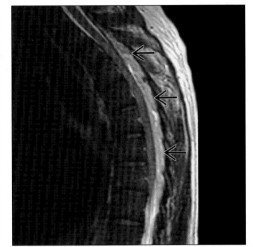

*(Left)* Sagittal T1WI MR in same patient as first page shows thoracic cord being compressed by a large heterogeneous dorsal epidural T1 hyperintense mass ➡. Note serpentine structures ➡ within the fat. *(Right)* Sagittal T2WI MR in same patient as previous image shows that the epidural mass ➡ remains isointense to fat with heterogeneous signal.

### Typical

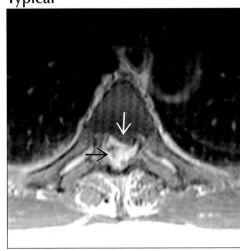

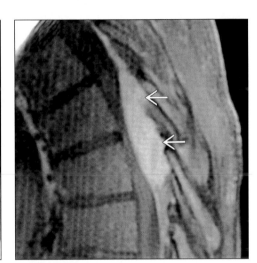

*(Left)* Axial T1 C+ MR in the same patient as previous image shows the hyperintense mass ➡ lying dorsally within the spinal canal and compressing the spinal cord ➡ while displacing it ventrally. *(Right)* Sagittal T1 C+ FS MR shows intense enhancement of a dorsal epidural mass ➡ (pre-contrast T1 showed the mass close in signal to muscle). This likely reflects the vascular character of this lesion.

### Typical

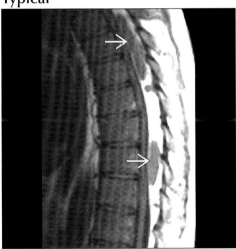

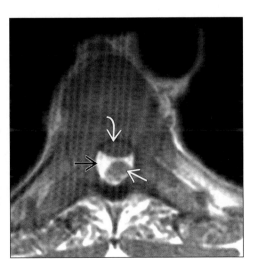

*(Left)* Sagittal T1WI MR shows islands ➡ of predominately T1 hyperintense mass intermixed with fat involving a long segment of the thoracic dorsal epidural space, with moderate cord compression. *(Right)* Axial T1WI MR in the same patient as previous image shows the islands of intermediate T1 signal ➡, that are likely more vascular components, intermixed with fat ➡ and compressing the cord ➡ ventrally.

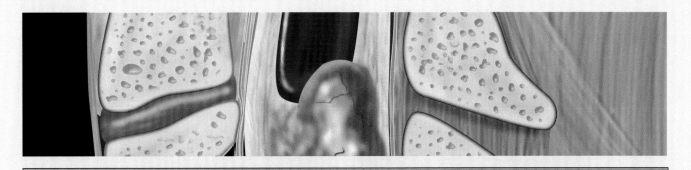

# SECTION 5: Intramedullary Space

# VENTRICULUS TERMINALIS

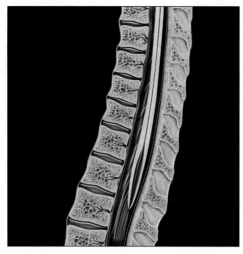

Sagittal graphic demonstrates uncomplicated fusiform dilatation of the distal central cord canal. Lack of haustration and confinement to the conus is typical of ventriculus terminalis.

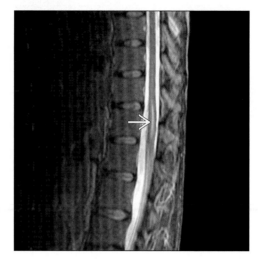

Sagittal T2WI MR shows mild fusiform dilatation of distal central canal ➔ at conus level. No cord signal abnormality, mass, or dilatation of proximal cord is seen to suggest it is a syrinx.

## TERMINOLOGY

### Abbreviations and Synonyms
- 5th ventricle, terminal ventricle

### Definitions
- Expanded central canal of spinal cord at conus/proximal filum level

## IMAGING FINDINGS

### General Features
- Best diagnostic clue: Mild cystic dilatation of distal central spinal cord canal without cord signal abnormality or enhancement
- Location: Distal spinal cord, at conus medullaris and origin of filum terminale
- Size: 2-4 mm (transverse); rarely exceeds 2 cms in length
- Morphology
  - Central intramedullary fluid with smooth, regular margins and no mass
  - Conus terminates at normal level (T12 → L2)

### CT Findings
- CECT
  - Fluid density in central canal of caudal most spinal cord
  - No mass lesion or enhancement

### MR Findings
- T1WI
  - Hypointense fluid in dilated central canal of distal spinal cord
    - Beware phase ghosting or truncation (Gibb) artifact mimicking central canal dilatation
  - Conus terminates at normal level
  - No filum terminale thickening or lipoma
- T2WI
  - Hyperintense (CSF intensity) fluid in dilated central canal of distal spinal cord
  - No septations within dilated central canal
- T1 C+: No nodular or ring enhancement

### Ultrasonographic Findings
- Grayscale Ultrasound
  - Mild anechoic non-septated central canal dilatation within normally situated conus

## DDx: Ventriculus Terminalis

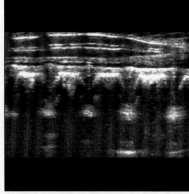

*Transient Neonatal Dilation*

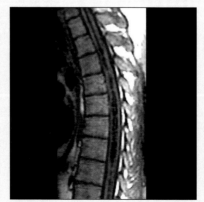

*Syringomyelia*

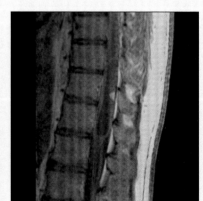

*Hemangioblastoma*

# VENTRICULUS TERMINALIS

## Key Facts

### Terminology
- 5th ventricle, terminal ventricle

### Imaging Findings
- Best diagnostic clue: Mild cystic dilatation of distal central spinal cord canal without cord signal abnormality or enhancement
- Size: 2-4 mm (transverse); rarely exceeds 2 cms in length
- Conus terminates at normal level (T12 → L2)

### Top Differential Diagnoses
- Transient Dilatation of the Central Canal
- Hydrosyringomyelia
- Cystic Spinal Cord Neoplasm
- Myelomalacia

### Pathology
- Simple CSF filled central canal of conus medullaris
- Normal cord microscopic histology

### Clinical Issues
- Incidental finding on imaging performed for unrelated indications
- Clinical Profile: Patient is asymptomatic or presents with nonspecific neurological symptoms

### Diagnostic Checklist
- Most important imaging goal is to distinguish from cystic cord neoplasm or syrinx
- Isolated mild dilatation of distal central canal in a normally located conus is nearly always an incidental normal finding

---

- ○ Normal nerve root and conus pulsation
- ○ Filum normal thickness without fat
- M-mode: May be used to confirm normal nerve root and conus pulsation

## Imaging Recommendations
- Best imaging tool: MR imaging in sagittal and axial planes
- Newborns
  - ○ Ultrasound to screen for congenital anomalies
    - Distinguish ventriculus terminalis from syrinx or cord neoplasm
    - Abnormal findings should be confirmed with MR imaging
- Infants (with positive ultrasound studies) and children
  - ○ Thin-section sagittal T1WI & T2WI MR imaging (3 mm slice thickness)
  - ○ Axial T1WI & T2WI (4 mm slice thickness) distal cord to sacrum
    - Best to exclude occult dysraphism, lipoma, or thick filum
  - ○ T1 C+ MR in sagittal, axial planes to exclude mass

## DIFFERENTIAL DIAGNOSIS

### Transient Dilatation of the Central Canal
- Normal variant
- Slight dilatation of central canal in a newborn
- Disappears in first weeks of life

### Hydrosyringomyelia
- Cystic expansion of distal one-third (or more) of spinal cord
- Isolated finding, or associated with congenital spine anomalies (up to 30% of patients)

### Cystic Spinal Cord Neoplasm
- Astrocytoma, ependymoma, hemangioblastoma
- Differentiated by cord signal abnormality and expansion, contrast-enhancement in solid portions

### Myelomalacia
- History of trauma, vascular accident, or other cord insult
- Cord atrophy, +/- T2 hyperintensity

## PATHOLOGY

### General Features
- General path comments
  - ○ CSF filled cavity at conus medullaris level
    - Enclosed by ependyma
    - Normally present as either virtual cavity or ependymal residue
  - ○ Size variable throughout life; smallest in middle-age and largest in early childhood, old age
- Etiology
  - ○ Forms during embryogenesis (9th week) via canalization and retrogressive differentiation of caudal spinal cord
    - Represents point of union between central canal portion formed by neurulation and portion formed by caudal cell mass canalization
    - Usually regresses in size during 1st weeks after birth; persistence leads to identification in children or adults
- Epidemiology
  - ○ Identified at all ages, but most commonly before 5 years of age
    - 2.6% of normal children (under 5 years) have a visible ventriculus terminalis on MR
    - Less commonly identified in adults; primarily an autopsy curiosity before widespread availability of MR imaging
- Associated abnormalities: Occasionally identified in conjunction with caudal regression or tethered cord

### Gross Pathologic & Surgical Features
- Simple CSF filled central canal of conus medullaris
- No gliosis or neoplasm

# VENTRICULUS TERMINALIS

## Microscopic Features
- Normal cord microscopic histology
  - Cystic cavity lined by ependymal cells
  - No gliosis or neoplasm

## CLINICAL ISSUES

### Presentation
- Most common signs/symptoms
  - Incidental finding on imaging performed for unrelated indications
    - Usually identified during sciatica work-up
  - Rarely becomes abnormally dilated and symptomatic, necessitating treatment
    - Bilateral sciatica
    - Lower extremity weakness
    - Urinary retention
- Clinical Profile: Patient is asymptomatic or presents with nonspecific neurological symptoms

### Demographics
- Age: Most commonly identified under age 5; may be found at any age
- Gender: M = F

### Natural History & Prognosis
- No effect on mortality or morbidity
  - Most commonly either stable in size or regresses; size progression not reported
- Rare symptomatic surgical cases show symptom improvement post-operatively

### Treatment
- No treatment indicated for asymptomatic incidental finding
  - MR follow-up if deemed necessary based on clinical findings
- Surgical decompression and management of associated abnormalities in rare symptomatic cases
  - Cyst fenestration +/- cyst shunting to the subarachnoid space, pleural cavity, or peritoneal cavity

## DIAGNOSTIC CHECKLIST

### Consider
- Most important imaging goal is to distinguish from cystic cord neoplasm or syrinx
- Asymptomatic patients require no further imaging evaluation
- Symptomatic patients should be monitored using clinical and MR follow-up unless degree of cyst expansion prompts surgical drainage

### Image Interpretation Pearls
- Isolated mild dilatation of distal central canal in a normally located conus is nearly always an incidental normal finding
  - Calcification, septations, nodules, enhancement, or eccentric location all argue against ventriculus terminalis and prompt further evaluation
  - Beware of truncation or phase ghosting artifact mimicking a dilated terminal ventricle or syrinx
- Exclude other unsuspected abnormalities that may predispose to syrinx or cord tethering before attributing finding to incidental dilatation of ventriculus terminalis

## SELECTED REFERENCES

1. Dullerud R et al: MR imaging of ventriculus terminalis of the conus medullaris. A report of two operated patients and a review of the literature. Acta Radiol. 44(4):444-6, 2003
2. Celli P et al: Cyst of the medullary conus: malformative persistence of terminal ventricle or compressive dilatation? Neurosurg Rev. 25(1-2):103-6, 2002
3. Kriss VM et al: Sonographic appearance of the ventriculus terminalis cyst in the neonatal spinal cord. J Ultrasound Med. 19(3):207-9, 2000
4. Tortori-Donati P et al: Spinal dysraphism: a review of neuroradiological features with embryological correlations and proposal for a new classification. Neuroradiology. 42(7):471-91, 2000
5. Unsinn KM et al: US of the spinal cord in newborns: spectrum of normal findings, variants, congenital anomalies, and acquired diseases. Radiographics. 20(4):923-38, 2000
6. Matsubayashi R et al: Cystic dilatation of ventriculus terminalis in adults: MRI. Neuroradiology. 40(1):45-7, 1998
7. Truong BC et al: Dilation of the ventriculus terminalis: sonographic findings. J Ultrasound Med. 17(11):713-5, 1998
8. Agrillo U et al: Symptomatic cystic dilatation of V ventricle: case report and review of the literature. Eur Spine J. 6(4):281-3, 1997
9. Tindall et al: The Practice of Neurosurgery. Baltimore, Williams and Wilkins. 2797, 1996
10. Unsinn KM et al: Sonography of the ventriculus terminalis in newborns. AJNR Am J Neuroradiol. 17(5):1003-4, 1996
11. Unsinn KM et al: Ventriculus terminalis of the spinal cord in the neonate: a normal variant on sonography. AJR Am J Roentgenol. 167(5):1341, 1996
12. Coleman LT et al: Ventriculus terminalis of the conus medullaris: MR findings in children. AJNR Am J Neuroradiol. 16(7):1421-6, 1995
13. Kriss VM et al: The ventriculus terminalis of the spinal cord in the neonate: a normal variant on sonography. AJR Am J Roentgenol. 165(6):1491-3, 1995
14. Rypens F et al: Atypical and equivocal sonographic features of the spinal cord in neonates. Pediatr Radiol. 25(6):429-32, 1995
15. Iskander BJ et al. Terminal hydrosyringomyelia and occult spinal dysraphism. J Neurosurg. 81:513-19, 1994
16. Choi BH et al: The ventriculus terminalis and filum terminale of the human spinal cord. Hum Pathol. 23(8):916-20, 1992
17. Sigal R et al: Ventriculus terminalis of the conus medullaris: MR imaging in four patients with congenital dilatation. AJNR Am J Neuroradiol. 12(4):733-7, 1991
18. Stewart DH Jr et al: Surgical drainage of cyst of the conus medullaris. Report of three cases. J Neurosurg. 33(1):106-10, 1970

# VENTRICULUS TERMINALIS

## IMAGE GALLERY

### Typical

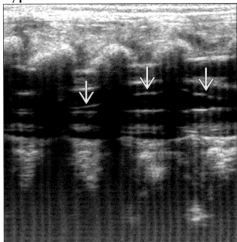
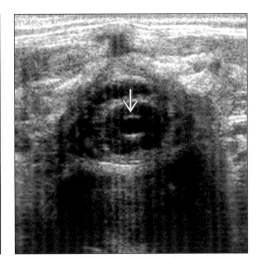

*(Left)* Sagittal ultrasound demonstrates incidental detection of fusiform dilatation ➔ of the distal central canal of the spinal cord confined to the conus in patient imaged for coccygeal dimple. *(Right)* Axial ultrasound in same patient confirms localization of central canal dilatation ➔ to the conus.

### Typical

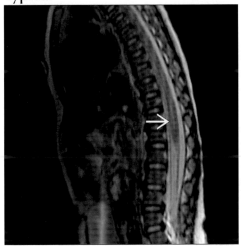
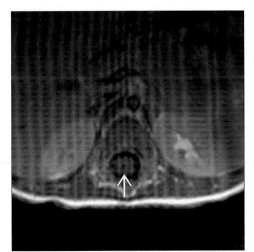

*(Left)* Sagittal T2WI MR in an infant with mild dilatation of the distal central spinal cord canal ➔ shows normal cord termination at L1-2 without radiologic tethering or abnormal lesion. *(Right)* Axial T1 C+ MR confirms central location of CSF dilatation ➔ and absence of abnormal nodular enhancement. There is mild dilatation of the left renal collecting system from hydronephrosis, which along with neurogenic bladder (not shown) led to the initial imaging consultation.

III

5

5

### Variant

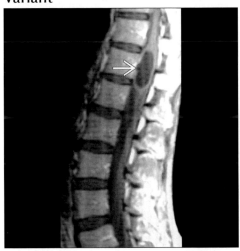
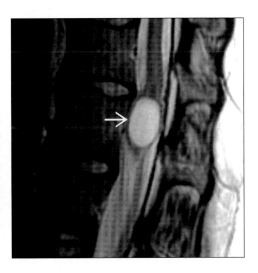

*(Left)* Sagittal T1 C+ MR shows cystic dilatation ➔ of the central canal confined to the conus. No nodule or abnormal enhancement of the cyst was identified. *(Right)* Sagittal T2WI MR shows cystic expansion of the ventriculus terminalis, or "5th ventricle" ➔. The dilatation is within the central canal, confined to the conus only.

# SYRINGOMYELIA

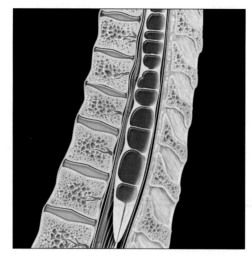

*Sagittal graphic demonstrates a large, sacculated, "beaded" syrinx extending to the conus level. Despite the loculated appearance, the syrinx fluid spaces are contiguous.*

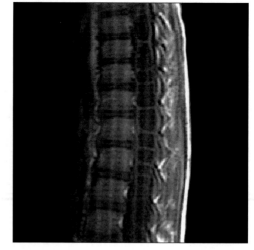

*Sagittal T1 C+ MR demonstrates a sacculated holocord syrinx extending to the conus tip. This represents hydromyelia secondary to Chiari I malformation (not shown).*

## TERMINOLOGY

### Abbreviations and Synonyms
- Hydromyelia, syringohydromyelia, syrinx

### Definitions
- Hydromyelia: Cystic central canal dilatation
- Syringomyelia: Cystic spinal cord cavity not contiguous with central cord canal
  - Syringobulbia: Brainstem syrinx extension
  - Syringocephaly: Brain/cerebral peduncle syrinx extension
- Syringohydromyelia: Features of both syringomyelia and hydromyelia

## IMAGING FINDINGS

### General Features
- Best diagnostic clue: Expanded spinal cord with dilated, beaded, or sacculated cystic cavity
- Location: Intramedullary spinal cord
- Size: Small → markedly dilated

- Morphology: Cystic intramedullary lesion; small syrinxes are tubular, large are "beaded" or "loculated with septations"

### CT Findings
- CECT: Cord expansion, nonenhancing cerebrospinal fluid (CSF) density spinal cord cavitation
- Bone CT
  - Normal or canal enlargement, vertebral scalloping (severe, long-standing syrinx)

### MR Findings
- T1WI
  - Hypointense spinal cord cleft
    - Sagittal images demonstrate longitudinal extent
    - Axial images confirm syrinx topology, clarify relationship to adjacent structures
- T2WI
  - Hyperintense intramedullary cavity +/- adjacent gliosis, myelomalacia
    - +/- Arachnoidal adhesions, cord tethering or edema
- T1 C+: Nonenhancing cavity; enhancement suggests inflammatory or neoplastic lesion

---

## DDx: Spinal Cord Cysts

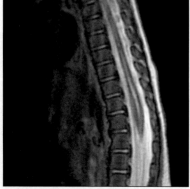

*Ventriculus Terminalis*

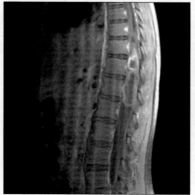

*Astrocytoma*

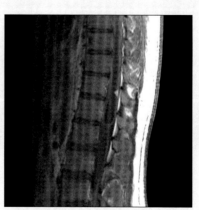

*Hemangioblastoma*

# SYRINGOMYELIA

## Key Facts

### Terminology
- Hydromyelia, syringohydromyelia, syrinx
- Hydromyelia: Cystic central canal dilatation
- Syringomyelia: Cystic spinal cord cavity not contiguous with central cord canal

### Imaging Findings
- Best diagnostic clue: Expanded spinal cord with dilated, beaded, or sacculated cystic cavity
- Sagittal images demonstrate longitudinal extent
- Axial images confirm syrinx topology, clarify relationship to adjacent structures

### Top Differential Diagnoses
- Ventriculus Terminalis
- Cystic Spinal Cord Tumor
- Myelomalacia

### Pathology
- Longitudinally oriented CSF-filled cavity +/- surrounding gliosis, myelomalacia

### Clinical Issues
- "Cloak-like" pain and temperature sensory loss with preservation of position sense, proprioception, light touch
- Distal upper extremity weakness, gait instability
- Mechanical spinal pain, radicular pain, spastic paraparesis, scoliosis

### Diagnostic Checklist
- Despite septated appearance, large syrinx cavities usually contiguous
- Contrast administration essential to exclude tumor in complicated cavitary lesions

## Radiographic Findings
- Radiography
  - Normal or wide osseous canal
  - +/- Atrophic neuroarthropathy (cervical syrinx)

## Ultrasonographic Findings
- Grayscale Ultrasound: Hypoechoic intramedullary cavitation or central canal dilatation

## Non-Vascular Interventions
- Myelography
  - Expanded spinal cord +/- spinal canal widening
  - Delayed syrinx contrast uptake

## Other Modality Findings
- 2D MR cine phase contrast (PC) CSF flow study
  - +/- Abnormal CSF dynamics across tonsils (Chiari I)
  - Normal conus motion argues against tethered cord
  - Larger syrinx commonly shows internal CSF flow

## Imaging Recommendations
- Best imaging tool: MR imaging
- Protocol advice
  - Sagittal and axial T1WI, T2WI, T1 C+ MR
  - Cine PC CSF flow MR

# DIFFERENTIAL DIAGNOSIS

## Ventriculus Terminalis
- Asymptomatic (normal) dilatation of terminal cord central canal only

## Cystic Spinal Cord Tumor
- Cord expansion, cystic cavity surrounded by abnormal T2 signal, nodular enhancement

## Myelomalacia
- Cord volume loss, gliosis
- No CSF signal cavitation on T1WI

# PATHOLOGY

## General Features
- General path comments
  - Longitudinally oriented CSF-filled cavity +/- surrounding gliosis, myelomalacia
  - Associated with scoliosis (↑ with left curve, high or low apex/end vertebra, male sex, Chiari I or II malformation)
  - Hydromyelia: Dilated ependymal-lined central canal
    - "Spinal cord hydrocephalus"
    - Central canal patency determines syrinx location, extent
    - Slit-like central canal remnant detected in small percentage of asymptomatic adults
  - Syringomyelia: Paracentral spinal cord cavitation lined by gliotic parenchyma independent of central canal
    - +/- Eccentric extension into anterior commissure, posterior horn
    - ↑ Intramedullary pressure → neurological dysfunction 2° to compression of long tracts, neurons, and microcirculation
- Etiology
  - Likely multifactorial; two most popular theories not mutually exclusive
    - Abnormal subarachnoid space (arachnoid adhesions, mass, Chiari malformation, spinal dysraphism, diastematomyelia) drives CSF into central canal through perivascular spaces → formation, enlargement of syrinx
    - Cord destruction 2° to primary disease process (trauma, infectious or inflammatory myelitis, spondylosis) → cord cavitation
- Epidemiology
  - Primary syrinx usually in young patients
    - ↑ Prevalence with basilar invagination, Chiari I or II malformation
  - Secondary syrinx at any age; timing of appearance determined by primary disease behavior
    - 25% spinal cord injury (SCI) patients → syrinx

# SYRINGOMYELIA

- Associated abnormalities: Hydrocephalus, Chiari I or II malformation, myelomeningocele or other spinal dysraphism, tethered cord, congenital scoliosis

## Gross Pathologic & Surgical Features
- Dilated cavity +/- contiguous with central canal
- +/- Arachnoid adhesions, mass lesion, tethered cord, Chiari malformation, blood products/trauma detritus

## Microscopic Features
- Central canal dilatation may communicate directly with 4th ventricle
  - Cavity lined by ependyma; length influenced by age-related central canal stenosis
- Noncommunicating (isolated) central canal dilation below syrinx-free cord segment
  - Variable distance below 4th ventricle; cavity margins defined by adjacent central canal stenosis
  - +/- Paracentral dissection into parenchyma, gliosis
- Extracanalicular (parenchymal) syrinx non-contiguous with central canal
  - Watershed spinal cord area +/- myelomalacia, paracentral dissection lined by glial or fibroglial tissue, rupture into spinal subarachnoid space, central chromatolysis, neuronophagia, Wallerian degeneration

## CLINICAL ISSUES

### Presentation
- Most common signs/symptoms
  - "Cloak-like" pain and temperature sensory loss with preservation of position sense, proprioception, light touch
  - Distal upper extremity weakness, gait instability
  - Other signs/symptoms
    - Mechanical spinal pain, radicular pain, spastic paraparesis, scoliosis
    - Cranial neuropathy (2° to syringobulbia)
- Clinical Profile
  - Symmetrically enlarged central cavity asymptomatic or presents with nonspecific neurological signs (spasticity, weakness, segmental pain)
  - Paracentral cavitation associated with combination of long tract and segmental signs referable to level, side, and quadrant of spinal cord cavitation

### Demographics
- Age: Usual presentation in late adolescence or early adulthood; uncommon in childhood
- Gender: M = F

### Natural History & Prognosis
- Variable; dependent on underlying etiology
  - Chronic, slow progression usual; occasional acute course
  - Spontaneous resolution rare
- +/- Reversibility after Chiari decompression, mass removal, adhesion lysis, or cord untethering
  - Long term improvement < 50%
  - Sensory disturbances, dysesthesias, pain more likely to improve than motor weakness or gait disturbance

- CSF diastolic flow determines cyst size, biological behavior
  - Diastolic flow velocity ↓ after successful surgery; persistent ↑ implies poor outcome

## Treatment
- Primarily address underlying causative etiology
  - Correct osseous deformities, decompress/untether spinal cord, lyse adhesions
  - Consider syrinx drainage with indwelling catheter only if not possible to restore normal cord CSF dynamics

## DIAGNOSTIC CHECKLIST

### Consider
- Syrinx etiology influences treatment approach
- Despite septated appearance, large syrinx cavities usually contiguous

### Image Interpretation Pearls
- Simple syringomyelia rarely enhances or produces diagnostic dilemma
- Contrast administration essential to exclude tumor in complicated cavitary lesions

## SELECTED REFERENCES

1. Aryan HE et al: Syringocephaly. J Clin Neurosci. 11(4):421-3, 2004
2. Piatt JH Jr: Syringomyelia complicating myelomeningocele: review of the evidence. J Neurosurg. 100(2 Suppl):101-9, 2004
3. Brodbelt AR et al: Post-traumatic syringomyelia: a review. J Clin Neurosci. 10(4):401-8, 2003
4. Kyoshima K et al: Spontaneous resolution of syringomyelia: report of two cases and review of the literature. Neurosurgery. 53(3):762-8; discussion 768-9, 2003
5. Ozerdemoglu RA et al: Scoliosis associated with syringomyelia: clinical and radiologic correlation. Spine. 28(13):1410-7, 2003
6. Holly LT et al: Slitlike syrinx cavities: a persistent central canal. J Neurosurg. 97(2 Suppl):161-5, 2002
7. Klekamp J et al: Syringomyelia associated with foramen magnum arachnoiditis. J Neurosurg. 97(3 Suppl):317-22, 2002
8. Klekamp J: The pathophysiology of syringomyelia - historical overview and current concept. Acta Neurochir (Wien). 144(7):649-64, 2002
9. Klekamp J et al: Spontaneous resolution of Chiari I malformation and syringomyelia: case report and review of the literature. Neurosurgery. 48(3):664-7, 2001
10. Vinas FC et al: Spontaneous resolution of a syrinx. J Clin Neurosci. 8(2):170-2, 2001
11. Brugieres P et al: CSF flow measurement in syringomyelia. AJNR. 21(10):1785-92, 2000
12. Fischbein NJ et al: The "presyrinx" state: a reversible myelopathic condition that may precede syringomyelia. AJNR Am J Neuroradiol. 20(1):7-20, 1999
13. Levy LM: MR imaging of cerebrospinal fluid flow and spinal cord motion in neurologic disorders of the spine. Magn Reson Imaging Clin N Am. 7(3):573-87, 1999
14. Milhorat TH et al: Pathological basis of spinal cord cavitation in syringomyelia: analysis of 105 autopsy cases. J Neurosurg. 82(5):802-12, 1995

# SYRINGOMYELIA

## IMAGE GALLERY

### Typical

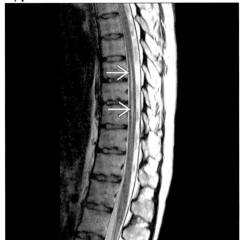

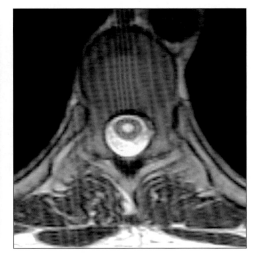

*(Left)* Sagittal T2WI MR demonstrates characteristic central fusiform high signal intensity ➡ dilatation of the central canal of the spinal cord. *(Right)* Axial T2WI MR confirms characteristic central fusiform high signal intensity dilatation of central canal of the spinal cord. No eccentricity of the "cyst" or cord volume loss is present.

### Variant

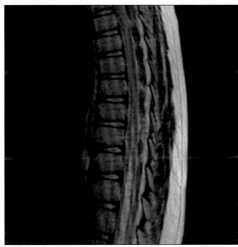

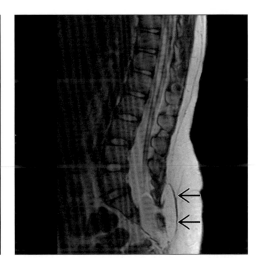

*(Left)* Sagittal T2WI MR demonstrates CSF signal intensity dilatation of central cord canal. It is difficult to determine whether this best represents hydro- or syringomyelia (syringohydromyelia). *(Right)* Sagittal T2WI MR depicts syrinx extension into the conus, which is low-lying and inserts into a distal lipomatous malformation ➡.

### Variant

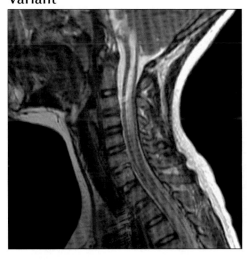

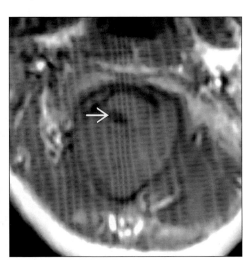

*(Left)* Sagittal T2WI MR demonstrates hyperintense CSF signal dilatation of the central brain stem and spinal cord, extending from the medulla (syringobulbia) into the thoracic spinal cord. *(Right)* Axial T1WI MR confirms eccentric cystic extension of cord cavitation ➡ into the medulla, characteristic of syringobulbia.

# GUILLAIN-BARRE SYNDROME

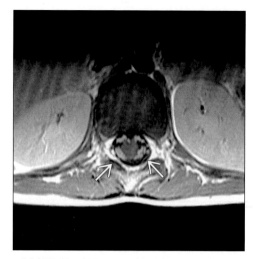

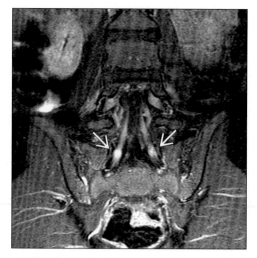

*Axial T1 C+ MR shows bilateral symmetrical enhancement of ventral and dorsal nerve roots ➡ in relation to lower cord, characteristic of GBS; also enhancement of anterior spinal artery.*

*Axial T1 C+ FS MR in same patient as previous image, shows that enhancement extends from roots to spinal ganglion and to proximal spinal nerve ➡.*

## TERMINOLOGY

### Abbreviations and Synonyms
- Guillain-Barré syndrome (GBS)
- Acute inflammatory demyelinating polyradiculoneuropathy (AIDP)
- Ascending paralysis

### Definitions
- Autoimmune post-infectious or post-vaccinial acute inflammatory demyelination of peripheral nerves, nerve roots, cranial nerves

## IMAGING FINDINGS

### General Features
- Best diagnostic clue: Smooth diffuse enhancement of the nerve roots (cranial and spinal)
- Location
  - Any level possible
  - Conspicuous at cauda equina but thoracic, cervical nerve roots, & posterior fossa "cranial nerves" (actually roots) involved as well

- Size: Nerve roots appear mildly enlarged
- Morphology: Symmetrical, smooth enhancement of roots (all, or only ventral or dorsal)

### CT Findings
- CECT: Of no value

### MR Findings
- T1WI
  - May show slight enlargement of roots, mostly on parasagittal cuts
  - May be used to evaluate enhancement
- T2WI
  - Should see normal conus
  - Excludes flaccid paralysis due to myelitis
- T1 C+
  - Avid enhancement of cauda equina
    - Roots may be slightly thickened, but not nodular
    - Compare with cord intensity
  - Axial images show symmetrical enhancement of cauda equina
    - May be global, or predominate either on anterior or posterior roots
  - Thoracic, cervical, posterior fossa roots commonly involved as well

## DDx: Other Radicular Enhancements

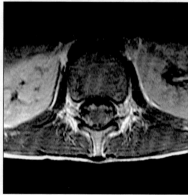

*CIDP*

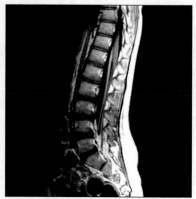

*Mitochondriopathy*

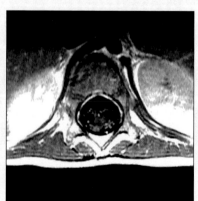

*Seeding From Ependymoma*

# GUILLAIN-BARRE SYNDROME

## Key Facts

### Terminology
- Autoimmune post-infectious or post-vaccinial acute inflammatory demyelination of peripheral nerves, nerve roots, cranial nerves

### Imaging Findings
- Best diagnostic clue: Smooth diffuse enhancement of the nerve roots (cranial and spinal)
- Avid enhancement of cauda equina
- Roots may be slightly thickened, but not nodular
- Axial images show symmetrical enhancement of cauda equina

### Top Differential Diagnoses
- Myelitis
- Chronic Polyneuropathies
- Metabolic Diseases

- Carcinomatous or Lymphomatous Meningitis
- Bacterial or Granulomatous Meningitis
- Chemical or Post-Surgical Arachnoiditis
- Vasculitic Neuropathy
- Physiological Nerve Root Enhancement

### Pathology
- Inflammatory (postulated autoimmune or viral) demyelination

### Clinical Issues
- Most patients somewhat better by 2-3 months
- Permanent deficits in 5-10%
- Mortality up to 8%

### Diagnostic Checklist
- Always check the cauda equina in case of acute paralysis

---

- Enhancement of pial surface of distal cord reported

### Non-Vascular Interventions
- Myelography
  - Useless; contrast agent in CSF may deteriorate nerve function
  - Lumbar puncture typically done in early stages to assess spinal fluid chemistry, protein levels, bacteriology

### Imaging Recommendations
- Best imaging tool: MR axial T1 with contrast
- Protocol advice: Fat-saturation for better imaging

## DIFFERENTIAL DIAGNOSIS

### Myelitis
- Symptomatology may be the same at the acute stage

### Chronic Polyneuropathies
- Subacute inflammatory demyelinating polyradiculoneuropathy (SIDP)
- Chronic inflammatory demyelinating polyradiculoneuropathy (CIDP)
  - Both show slow onset, more protracted course
- Hereditary polyneuropathies
  - Charcot-Marie-Tooth, Dejerine-Sottas

### Metabolic Diseases
- Radicular enhancement may be observed in mitochondriopathies, Krabbe disease etc.

### Carcinomatous or Lymphomatous Meningitis
- Enhancement is frequently more nodular than GBS, less symmetrical
- Conus deposits frequently cause T2 signal abnormality

### Bacterial or Granulomatous Meningitis
- Acute onset; fever, headache, + LP
- Meningeal, not radicular, enhancement, not necessarily symmetrical

### Chemical or Post-Surgical Arachnoiditis
- Hemorrhage-induced arachnoidal inflammation
- Chemotherapy; systemic (vincristine neuropathy), or intrathecal
- Post-operative up to 6 weeks

### Vasculitic Neuropathy
- Polyarteritis nodosa or Churg-Strauss most commonly
- Cranial nerves & respiratory nerves frequently spared

### Physiological Nerve Root Enhancement
- Much more subtle enhancement of normal roots
- Radiculo-medullary arteries have a consistent anatomical course
- Absent clinical syndrome

## PATHOLOGY

### General Features
- General path comments
  - Lesions are scattered throughout peripheral nerves, nerve roots, cranial nerves
  - Inflammatory changes and demyelination
- Genetics
  - May be first presentation of genetic or hereditary disorders
    - 17p12 mutation
    - Reported association between HLA typing and Guillain-Barré subtypes
- Etiology
  - Inflammatory (postulated autoimmune or viral) demyelination
    - Antecedent event or "trigger" in 70%; usually recent viral illness
    - Campylobacter jejuni: 1/3 have antibodies against nerve gangliosides which cross-react with C. jejuni liposaccharide constituent
    - Vaccination (influenza, others) found also
  - Both cell-mediated and humoral mechanisms involved in pathogenesis

# GUILLAIN-BARRE SYNDROME

- o More tenuous association with prior recent surgery or systemic illness
- Epidemiology
  - o Incidence: 0.5-1.5:100,000 in children < 18 years
  - o Affects all ages, races, socioeconomic status
  - o Most common cause of acute paralysis in Western countries

## Gross Pathologic & Surgical Features
- Thickened nerve roots

## Microscopic Features
- Focal segmental demyelination
- Perivascular and endoneural lymphocytic/monocytic (macrophages) infiltrates
- Axonal degeneration in conjunction with segmental demyelination in severe cases

## Staging, Grading or Classification Criteria
- Three forms of GBS
  - o True acute inflammatory demyelinating polyradiculoneuropathy (AIDP)
  - o Axonal forms
    - Pure acute motor axonal neuropathy (3%)
    - Associated motor-sensory axonal neuropathy
  - o Miller-Fisher syndrome: Ophthalmoplegia-ataxia-areflexia (involvement of posterior sensory columns)
- Spectrum of disease extends to subacute inflammatory demyelinating polyradiculoneuropathy (SIDP)
  - o Which itself bridges to chronic inflammatory demyelinating polyradiculopathy (CIDP)
  - o Both entities exhibit slower onset, protracted course, exacerbations, lesser cranial nerve involvement

## CLINICAL ISSUES

### Presentation
- Most common signs/symptoms
  - o Distal paraesthesias rapidly followed by "ascending paralysis"
    - Typically bilateral and symmetrical
  - o Ascent up to brainstem to involve cranial nerves
    - Respiratory paralysis requiring ventilator in severe cases
    - Facial nerves 50%, ophthalmoplegia 10-20%
  - o Sensory disturbances: Pain, sensory loss, numbness tingling
- Other signs/symptoms: Autonomic disturbances

### Demographics
- Age: Typically children & young adults
- Gender: No preference
- Ethnicity: All

### Natural History & Prognosis
- Clinical nadir at 4 weeks
- Most patients somewhat better by 2-3 months
  - o 30-50% have persistent symptoms at 1 year
  - o Permanent deficits in 5-10%
- 2-10% relapse
  - o 6% develop chronic course resembling CIDP

- o Earliest stages of SIDP, CIDP may be indistinguishable clinically from Guillain-Barré
- Mortality up to 8%

## Treatment
- Medical management with plasma exchange or intravenous gamma globulin
- No proven benefit from corticosteroid administration
- Intensive care management in severe cases

## DIAGNOSTIC CHECKLIST

### Consider
- Always check the cauda equina in case of acute paralysis

### Image Interpretation Pearls
- Symmetrical diffuse enhancement of roots of cauda equina

## SELECTED REFERENCES

1. Ryan MM: Guillain-Barre syndrome in childhood. J Paediatr Child Health. 41(5-6):237-41, 2005
2. Takahashi M et al: Epidemiology of Campylobacter jejuni isolated from patients with Guillain-Barre and Fisher syndromes in Japan. J Clin Microbiol. 43(1):335-9, 2005
3. Hung PL et al: A clinical and electrophysiologic survey of childhood Guillain-Barre syndrome. Pediatr Neurol. 30(2):86-91, 2004
4. Inoue N et al: MR imaging findings of spinal posterior column involvement in a case of Miller Fisher syndrome. AJNR Am J Neuroradiol. 25(4):645-8, 2004
5. Chang YW et al: Spinal MRI of vincristine neuropathy mimicking Guillain-Barre syndrome. Pediatr Radiol. 33(11):791-3, 2003
6. Coskun A et al: Childhood Guillain-Barre syndrome. MR imaging in diagnosis and follow-up. Acta Radiol. 44(2):230-5, 2003
7. Haber P et al: Influenza vaccination and Guillain Barre syndrome. Clin Immunol. 109(3):359; author reply 360-1, 2003
8. Molinero MR et al: Epidemiology of childhood Guillain-Barre syndrome as a cause of acute flaccid paralysis in Honduras: 1989-1999. J Child Neurol. 18(11):741-7, 2003
9. Oh SJ et al: Subacute inflammatory demyelinating polyneuropathy. Neurology. 61(11):1507-12, 2003
10. Wilmshurst JM et al: Lower limb and back pain in Guillain-Barre syndrome and associated contrast enhancement in MRI of the cauda equina. Acta Paediatr. 90(6):691-4, 2001
11. Berciano J et al: Perineurium contributes to axonal damage in acute inflammatory demyelinating polyneuropathy. Neurology. 55(4):552-9, 2000
12. Jones HR Jr: Guillain-Barre syndrome: perspectives with infants and children. Semin Pediatr Neurol. 7(2):91-102, 2000
13. Duarte J et al: Hypertrophy of multiple cranial nerves and spinal roots in chronic inflammatory demyelinating neuropathy. J Neurol Neurosurg Psychiatry. 67(5):685-7, 1999
14. Iwata F et al: MR imaging in Guillain-Barre syndrome. Pediatr Radiol. 27(1):36-8, 1997
15. Gorson KC et al: Prospective evaluation of MRI lumbosacral nerve root enhancement in acute Guillain-Barre syndrome. Neurology. 47(3):813-7, 1996

# GUILLAIN-BARRE SYNDROME

## IMAGE GALLERY

### Typical

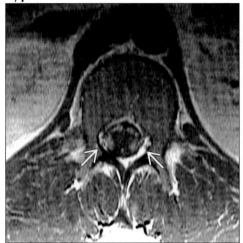 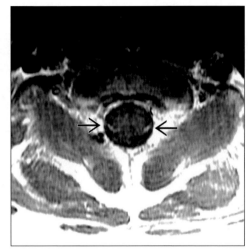

*(Left)* Axial T1 C+ MR shows global symmetrical enhancement of the roots of cauda equina at level of distal cord ➡. *(Right)* Axial T1 C+ MR in same patient as previous image, shows enhancement ➡ of the dorsal (sensory) roots at cervical level as well.

### Typical

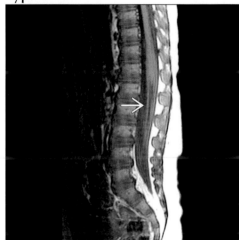 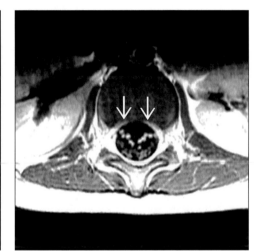

*(Left)* Sagittal T1WI MR shows ventral root of cauda equina ➡ somewhat prominent, thickened. *(Right)* Axial T1 C+ MR shows symmetrical enhancement of ventral (motor) roots only ➡.

### Typical

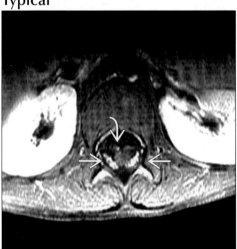 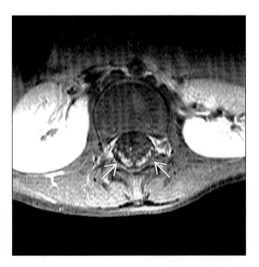

*(Left)* Axial T1 C+ FS MR shows enhancement of the dorsal (sensory) roots only ➡ at level of distal cord; note the anterior spinal artery ➡. *(Right)* Axial T1 C+ FS MR in same patient as previous image, shows same pattern ➡ at level of the upper filum.

# ADEM, SPINAL CORD

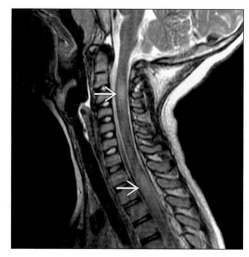
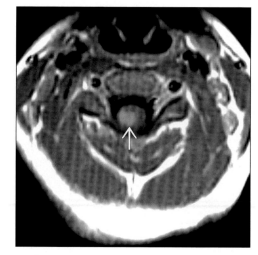

Sagittal T2WI MR shows focal spinal cord T2 hyperintensities ➡ at C3 and at T2 with mild mass effect. These lesions enhanced homogeneously and additional lesions were present in the brain.

Axial T1 C+ MR in same patient as previous image shows homogeneous lesion enhancement ➡ in the right lateral aspects of the cord resulting from acute inflammation and blood-cord barrier breakdown.

## TERMINOLOGY

### Abbreviations and Synonyms
- Acute disseminated encephalomyelitis (ADEM)

### Definitions
- Para/postinfectious immune-mediated inflammatory disorder of the white matter

## IMAGING FINDINGS

### General Features
- Best diagnostic clue
  - Multifocal lesions with relatively little mass effect
  - Brain almost always involved
- Location
  - ~ 20% of patients with cerebral ADEM present with cord involvement
  - Anywhere in the spinal cord but thoracic > cervical
  - Involvement of entire cord possible
  - Gray and/or white matter of cord involved
  - If segmental typically involves 2-3 vertebral bodies in length

- Size: Segmental > punctate, may involve entire cord
- Morphology: Plump lesions with feathery edges

### CT Findings
- CECT: May see (multi)focal intramedullary enhancement

### MR Findings
- T1WI: Focal low signal and slight cord swelling
- T2WI
  - Multifocal flame-shaped white matter lesions with slight cord swelling
  - Dorsal white matter more voluminous
  - May see gray matter involvement
- PD/Intermediate: Sometimes depict the lesions more sensitively
- T2* GRE: Same as T2WI, not as sensitive
- DWI: Variable from increased to decreased
- T1 C+
  - Variable enhancement, depending on stage of disease
  - Punctate, ring-shaped, or fluffy enhancement
  - May see nerve enhancement

## DDx: Cord Lesions

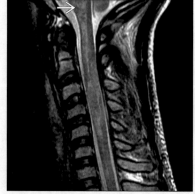
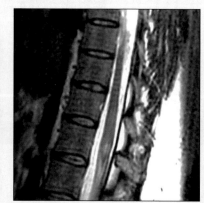
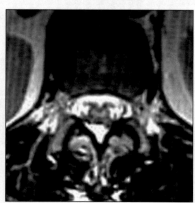

| Transverse Myelitis | Multiple Sclerosis | Cord Infarct |

# ADEM, SPINAL CORD

## Key Facts

### Terminology
- Acute disseminated encephalomyelitis (ADEM)
- Para/postinfectious immune-mediated inflammatory disorder of the white matter

### Imaging Findings
- Multifocal lesions with relatively little mass effect
- Brain almost always involved
- Anywhere in the spinal cord but thoracic > cervical
- Multifocal flame-shaped white matter lesions with slight cord swelling
- Variable enhancement, depending on stage of disease

### Top Differential Diagnoses
- Viral or Idiopathic Transverse Myelitis
- Multiple Sclerosis
- Immune-Mediated Vasculitis

### Pathology
- Autoimmune process producing inflammatory reaction

### Clinical Issues
- Paresis
- 75% have severe mental status changes
- Abnormal CSF
- Usually no oligoclonal bands
- Typically childhood or young adult
- Up to 90% have good or complete recovery

### Diagnostic Checklist
- Re-scanning if initially negative
- Caution: ADEM can mimic cord neoplasm!

---

### Non-Vascular Interventions
- Myelography: May see focal cord swelling

### Imaging Recommendations
- Best imaging tool: Pre- and post-contrast MR
- Protocol advice: Include brain MR whenever suspicious cord lesions found

## DIFFERENTIAL DIAGNOSIS

### Viral or Idiopathic Transverse Myelitis
- Usually single lesion
- Mono- to multisegmental

### Multiple Sclerosis
- Indistinguishable on single study
- Optic nerve involvement more common in MS but bilateral optic nerve involvement more common in ADEM
- Not encephalopathic (encephalopathy necessary for diagnosis of ADEM)
- < 2 vertebral segments in length
- < 1/2 cross-sectional area of cord
- 90% associated intracranial lesions
- Relapsing-remitting course suggests MS

### Immune-Mediated Vasculitis
- Systemic lupus erythematosus

### Devic Disease
- Optic neuritis but no brain lesions
- Cavitation more common

### Cord Infarct
- Stroke-like, acute presentation
- Focal, segmental lesion in gray matter
- Typically conus involvement

### Chronic Inflammatory Demyelinating Polyneuropathy
- Typically no demyelinating lesions
- Hypertrophic nerve roots

### Spinal Cord Neoplasm
- Cord expansion invariably present
- +/- Diffuse or nodular contrast enhancement
- Slower clinical progression

### Dural Arterial Venous Fistula (AVF)
- Dural AVF often show distal cord signal increase only, not multi-focal
  - Stuttering course of paresis
  - No cranial nerve findings
  - Signal abnormality spares cord periphery
  - Abnormal flow voids dorsal to conus

## PATHOLOGY

### General Features
- General path comments
  - Tumefactive swelling in some larger, acute lesions
    - Most lesions show no gross features
- Genetics: HLA-DR linkage in some
- Etiology
  - Autoimmune process producing inflammatory reaction
  - Infection during preceding month in 55%
  - 35% nonspecific URI, 26% no defined prodrome, 12% vaccine, 11% GI illness, 5% varicella, 2% HSV, 1% mumps, 1% rubella
  - Predisposing infection
    - Chickenpox, mycoplasma, influenza, Epstein-Barr virus, measles, mumps, rubella, coxsackie B, cytomegalovirus, herpes simplex virus, hepatitis A virus, adenovirus, Borrelia, nonspecific infections of the upper respiratory tract
  - Post-vaccinial association in some reported cases
    - Polio vaccine (40-50 days after), plasma-derived form of Hepatitis B vaccine (1-3 weeks after), tetanus (acutely after), rubella vaccine, rabies vaccine, smallpox vaccine, influenza vaccine, following intravenous immunoglobulin administration, sporadically after other vaccines
- Epidemiology: Unknown

- Increasingly recognized
  - More sensitive imaging tools

## Gross Pathologic & Surgical Features
- Slight swelling to tumefactive necrosis

## Microscopic Features
- Acute myelin loss
- Lymphocytic infiltrate
- Axonal preservation
- Astroglial reaction, proliferation
- +/- Necrosis
- Perivascular lymphocytic infiltration

## CLINICAL ISSUES

### Presentation
- Most common signs/symptoms
  - Paresis
  - Cranial nerve palsies
  - Symptoms are typically more obvious 1-2 days after diagnosis and can progress for up to 2 weeks
- Other signs/symptoms
  - Due to brain involvement
    - Decreased consciousness, behavior changes
    - Focal neurologic deficits
    - Seizures
  - 55% have brainstem dysfunction
  - 75% have severe mental status changes
- Clinical Profile
  - Usual prodromal phase 12-14 days prior to neurologic symptoms
    - Fever
    - Malaise
    - Myalgia
  - Abnormal CSF
    - Increased protein
    - Usually no oligoclonal bands
    - Leukocytosis

### Demographics
- Age
  - Typically childhood or young adult
  - Mean age 5.3 +/- 3.9 years
- Gender: Some reports suggest male predominance
- Ethnicity: All

### Natural History & Prognosis
- Typically monophasic (90%)
- Acute relapsing-remitting disseminated encephalomyelitis (ARDEM) occurs in small fraction
- Up to 90% have good or complete recovery
- 11% have residual deficits and neurological syndromes
- May see cord atrophy in chronic phase

### Treatment
- Corticosteroids (typically pulsed intravenous)
- Immunomodulation, supportive
- Plasmapheresis in fulminant cases

III

5

16

## DIAGNOSTIC CHECKLIST

### Consider
- Re-scanning if initially negative
  - Typically delay between clinical onset and appearance of imaging findings
- MR of the brain to look for associated cerebral involvement

### Image Interpretation Pearls
- Check thin-section intracranial slices on T1 C+ for cranial nerve enhancement
- Caution: ADEM can mimic cord neoplasm!

## SELECTED REFERENCES

1. Mikaeloff Y et al: First episode of acute CNS inflammatory demyelination in childhood: prognostic factors for multiple sclerosis and disability. J Pediatr. 144(2):246-52, 2004
2. Dale RC: Acute disseminated encephalomyelitis. Semin Pediatr Infect Dis. 14(2):90-5, 2003
3. Garg RK: Acute disseminated encephalomyelitis. Postgrad Med J. 79(927):11-7, 2003
4. Idrissova ZhR et al: Acute disseminated encephalomyelitis in children: clinical features and HLA-DR linkage. Eur J Neurol. 10(5):537-46, 2003
5. Miravalle A et al: Encephalitis complicating smallpox vaccination. Arch Neurol. 60(7):925-8, 2003
6. Au WY et al: Acute disseminated encephalomyelitis after para-influenza infection post bone marrow transplantation. Leuk Lymphoma. 43(2):455-7, 2002
7. Inglese M et al: Magnetization transfer and diffusion tensor MR imaging of acute disseminated encephalomyelitis. AJNR Am J Neuroradiol. 23(2):267-72, 2002
8. Khong PL et al: Childhood acute disseminated encephalomyelitis: the role of brain and spinal cord MRI. Pediatr Radiol. 32(1):59-66, 2002
9. Khong PL et al: Childhood acute disseminated encephalomyelitis: the role of brain and spinal cord MRI. Pediatr Radiol. 32(1):59-66, 2002
10. Murthy SN et al: Acute disseminated encephalomyelitis in children. Pediatrics. 110(2 Pt 1):e21, 2002
11. Tenembaum S et al: Acute disseminated encephalomyelitis: a long-term follow-up study of 84 pediatric patients. Neurology. 59(8):1224-31, 2002
12. Arya SC: Acute disseminated encephalomyelitis associated with poliomyelitis vaccine. Pediatr Neurol. 24(4):325, 2001
13. Bastianello S: Magnetic resonance imaging of MS-like disease. Neurol Sci. 22 Suppl 2:S103-7, 2001
14. Singh S et al: Acute disseminated encephalomyelitis and multiple sclerosis: magnetic resonance imaging differentiation. Australas Radiol. 44(4):404-11, 2000
15. Tsuru T et al: Acute disseminated encephalomyelitis after live rubella vaccination. Brain Dev. 22(4):259-61, 2000
16. Pradhan S et al: Intravenous immunoglobulin therapy in acute disseminated encephalomyelitis. J Neurol Sci. 165(1):56-61, 1999
17. Kumada S et al: Encephalomyelitis subsequent to mycoplasma infection with elevated serum anti-Gal C antibody. Pediatr Neurol. 16(3):241-4, 1997
18. Baum PA et al: Deep gray matter involvement in children with acute disseminated encephalomyelitis. AJNR Am J Neuroradiol. 15(7):1275-83, 1994

## IMAGE GALLERY

### Typical

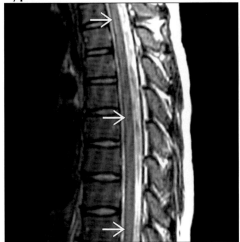

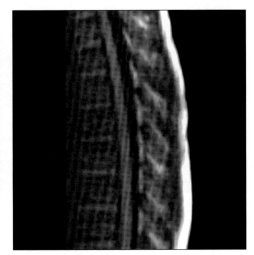

*(Left)* Sagittal T2WI MR shows diffuse hyperintensity ➡ within the cord without mass effect. There was no enhancement post-contrast. Lesions were also present in the brain. *(Right)* Sagittal DWI MR in the same patient as previous image shows no evidence of reduced diffusion in the affected areas of the spinal cord. Of note, this patient had full clinical recovery.

### Typical

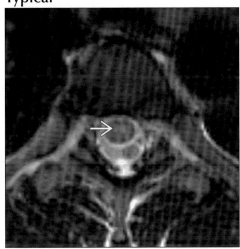

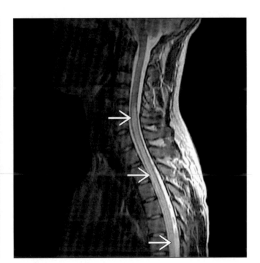

*(Left)* Axial T2WI MR in the same patient as previous image shows increased signal intensity ➡ in the central gray matter, mimicking a cord infarct. No white matter involvement was identified. *(Right)* Sagittal T2WI MR shows diffuse expansion and increased signal intensity in the central thoracic spinal cord ➡ after a rabies vaccination. Intracranial lesions were also present.

### Typical

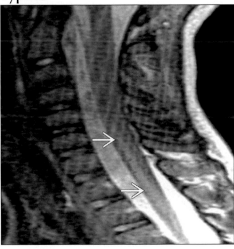

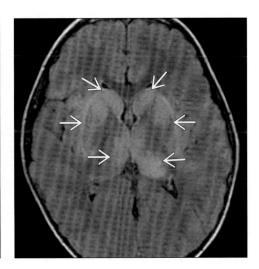

*(Left)* Sagittal T2WI MR shows diffusely increased signal in the lower cervical spinal cord ➡ without associated mass effect. There was no contrast-enhancement. *(Right)* Axial FLAIR MR in the same patient as previous image shows bilateral involvement of thalami, putamina, and caudate heads ➡. Deep gray nuclei are involved in up to 50% of children with ADEM.

# IDIOPATHIC ACUTE TRANSVERSE MYELITIS

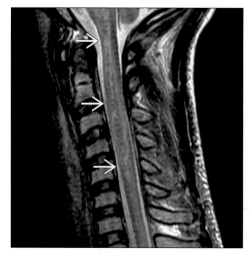

*Sagittal T2WI MR at presentation shows diffuse increased signal ⇒ within the cervical cord extending over 4 vertebral levels, involving the brainstem and causing mild cord expansion.*

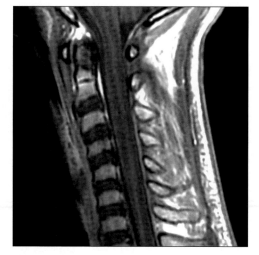

*Sagittal T1 C+ MR at presentation in same child as previous image shows no contrast-enhancement. Enhancement is not always present initially; repeat imaging at 2-7 days may be needed.*

## TERMINOLOGY

### Abbreviations and Synonyms
- Idiopathic acute transverse myelitis (IATM)
- Idiopathic transverse myelopathy (broader term)

### Definitions
- Inflammatory disorder resulting in bilateral motor, sensory, and autonomic dysfunction
- Diagnosis of exclusion

## IMAGING FINDINGS

### General Features
- Best diagnostic clue: Central cord lesion > 2 vertebral segments ± patchy enhancement
- Location
  ○ Thoracic more common (conus especially)
  ○ 10% in cervical cord
  ○ Central cord location
- Size
  ○ > 2/3 cross-sectional area
  ○ > 2 vertebral segments in length, often 3 to 4

- Morphology: Well-circumscribed

### MR Findings
- T1WI
  ○ Smooth cord expansion; less extensive T1 than T2 abnormality
  ○ Iso- to hypointense
- T2WI
  ○ High T2 signal intensity
  ○ ± Central dot sign (central gray surrounded by edema)
- STIR: Hyperintense
- T1 C+
  ○ Variable post-gadolinium enhancement
    ■ None, focal nodular, subtle diffuse, patchy, peripheral or meningeal enhancement
  ○ More frequent in subacute than acute and chronic stage
  ○ Resolves over time
  ○ Not predictive of clinical course
  ○ Enhancement more common when cord enlargement present
  ○ Enhancing area less extensive than T2 hyperintensity

### DDx: Intramedullary Lesions

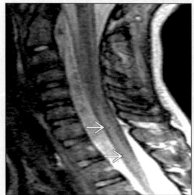

*ADEM*

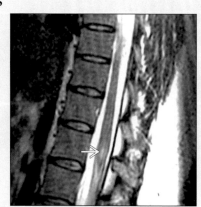

*Multiple Sclerosis*

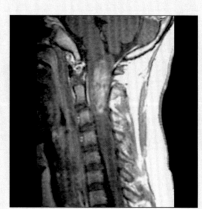

*Astrocytoma*

# IDIOPATHIC ACUTE TRANSVERSE MYELITIS

## Key Facts

### Terminology
- Inflammatory disorder resulting in bilateral motor, sensory, and autonomic dysfunction
- Diagnosis of exclusion

### Imaging Findings
- Best diagnostic clue: Central cord lesion > 2 vertebral segments ± patchy enhancement
- Thoracic more common (conus especially)
- Central cord location
- > 2/3 cross-sectional area
- > 2 vertebral segments in length, often 3 to 4
- Smooth cord expansion; less extensive T1 than T2 abnormality
- High T2 signal intensity
- Variable post-gadolinium enhancement
- Up to 40-50% of cases not demonstrated by MR

### Top Differential Diagnoses
- Acute Disseminated Encephalomyelitis (ADEM)
- Multiple Sclerosis
- Devic Disease (Neuromyelitis Optica)
- Spinal Cord Infarct
- Spinal Cord Neoplasm

### Diagnostic Checklist
- Brain MR to exclude intracranial lesions associated with MS or ADEM
- Peripheral enhancement in centrally located T2 hyperintensity more characteristic of IATM
- Central enhancement in peripherally located T2 hyperintensity more characteristic of multiple sclerosis
- Caution: IATM can mimic cord neoplasm!

---

- Solitary or multifocal lesions
- Up to 40-50% of cases not demonstrated by MR

### Imaging Recommendations
- Best imaging tool: MR
- Protocol advice: Sagittal and axial T2WI and T1WI with gadolinium

## DIFFERENTIAL DIAGNOSIS

### Acute Disseminated Encephalomyelitis (ADEM)
- Associated brain involvement on MR
- Mental status change, seizure

### Multiple Sclerosis
- Peripheral location in cord
- Less than two vertebral segments in length
- Less than half cross-sectional area of cord
- 90% with associated intracranial lesions
- Relapsing and remitting clinical course

### Devic Disease (Neuromyelitis Optica)
- Optic neuritis but no brain lesions

### Spinal Cord Infarct
- Ventral cord location
- Motor signs greater than sensory
- Nadir less than 4 hours

### Chronic Inflammatory Demyelinating Polyneuropathy (CIDP)
- Hypertrophic nerve roots
- Typically no demyelinating lesions

### Spinal Cord Neoplasm
- Cord expansion invariably present
- ± Diffuse or nodular contrast-enhancement
- Slower clinical progression

### Syringohydromyelia
- Well-defined central cystic lesion

## PATHOLOGY

### General Features
- General path comments
  - Perivascular inflammation
  - Demyelination
- Genetics: No familial predisposition
- Etiology
  - Possible association with previous viral infection or vaccination in some cases
  - Autoimmune phenomenon with formation of antigen-antibody complexes
  - Small vessel vasculopathy resulting in cord ischemia
  - Associated demyelinating process
- Epidemiology
  - 4.6 new cases of transverse myelitis per million people per year in US
    - 1,400 new cases per year
  - Majority of cases occurred in late winter through spring in one series
- Associated abnormalities
  - Depression
    - Life time risk > 50%
    - Correlates with severity of sensory symptoms

### Microscopic Features
- Necrosis of gray and white matter
- Destruction of neurons, axons, and myelin
- Astrocytic gliosis
- Perivascular lymphocytic infiltrate

## CLINICAL ISSUES

### Presentation
- Most common signs/symptoms
  - Sensory deficit
    - Loss of pain and temperature sensation
    - Clearly defined upper level
    - Ascending paresthesia in bilateral lower extremities
    - Band-like dysesthesia

# IDIOPATHIC ACUTE TRANSVERSE MYELITIS

- ○ Acute to subacute onset of symptoms
- Other signs/symptoms
  - ○ Paraplegia or quadriplegia
  - ○ Back ± radicular pain
  - ○ Bladder and bowl dysfunction
  - ○ Urgency, incontinence, retention
  - ○ Hypotonia and hyporeflexia initially
  - ○ Spasticity and hyperreflexia over time
- Clinical Profile
  - ○ Prodrome of generalized body aches
  - ○ Preceding viral-like illness
  - ○ Rapid progression to maximal neurologic deficits within days
  - ○ Inclusion criteria
    - Sensory, motor, or autonomic dysfunction attributable to spinal cord
    - Bilateral signs and symptoms
    - Well-defined sensory level
    - Compressive etiology excluded by neuroimaging
    - MR or myelography
    - Cord inflammation confirmed by cerebral spinal fluid (CSF) pleocytosis, elevated IgG index, or gadolinium enhancement
    - May repeat MR ± lumbar puncture between 2-7 days if signs of inflammation absent initially
    - Progression to nadir between 4 hours to 21 days from onset (usually 24 hours)
    - Symptoms must progress if they are present upon awakening
  - ○ Exclusion criteria
    - History of spinal radiation within past 10 years
    - Cord ischemia and infarction due to anterior spinal artery thrombosis
    - Cord arterial venous malformations
    - Connective tissue diseases
    - Sarcoidosis, SLE, Sjögren syndrome, etc.
    - CNS infections
    - Syphilis, Lyme disease, mycoplasma, HIV, HTLV-1, other viral infections: VZV, EBV, CMV, etc.
    - Brain MR suggestive of multiple sclerosis
    - Clinical optic neuritis

## Demographics

- Age
  - ○ All ages can be affected
  - ○ Two peaks: 10-19 and 30-39 years old
- Gender: No gender predilection
- Ethnicity: No racial predilection

## Natural History & Prognosis

- One third or more → good to complete recovery
  - ○ Symptomatic improvement starting 2-12 weeks after onset
  - ○ Children have better prognosis than adults
- One third → fair recovery
  - ○ Residual spasticity and urinary dysfunction
- One third → poor recovery
  - ○ Persistent complete deficits
- Factors portending poor prognosis
  - ○ Rapid clinical deterioration
  - ○ Back pain
  - ○ Spinal shock: Loss of motor, sensation, sphincter control, and areflexia

- ○ MR signal alteration > 10 spinal segments
- ○ Significant denervation on electromyogram
- ○ Abnormal somatosensory evoked potential
- Typically monophasic especially in children
  - ○ Multiple sclerosis: Progression to multiple sclerosis in 2-10% of cases of transverse myelitis

## Treatment

- High dose intravenous steroid pulse therapy
- Physical therapy

## DIAGNOSTIC CHECKLIST

### Consider

- Brain MR to exclude intracranial lesions associated with MS or ADEM

### Image Interpretation Pearls

- Peripheral enhancement in centrally located T2 hyperintensity more characteristic of IATM
- Central enhancement in peripherally located T2 hyperintensity more characteristic of multiple sclerosis
- Caution: IATM can mimic cord neoplasm!

## SELECTED REFERENCES

1. Bruna J et al: Idiopathic acute transverse myelitis: a clinical study and prognostic markers in 45 cases. Mult Scler. 12(2):169-73, 2006
2. Chan KH et al: Idiopathic inflammatory demyelinating disorders after acute transverse myelitis. Eur J Neurol. 13(8):862-8, 2006
3. de Seze J et al: Idiopathic acute transverse myelitis: application of the recent diagnostic criteria. Neurology. 65(12):1950-3, 2005
4. Harzheim M et al: Discriminatory features of acute transverse myelitis: a retrospective analysis of 45 patients. J Neurol Sci. 217(2):217-23, 2004
5. Andronikou S et al: MRI findings in acute idiopathic transverse myelopathy in children. Pediatr Radiol. 33(9):624-9, 2003
6. Banit DM et al: Recurrent transverse myelitis after lumbar spine surgery: a case report. Spine. 28(9):E165-8, 2003
7. Kim KK: Idiopathic recurrent transverse myelitis. Arch Neurol. 60(9):1290-4, 2003
8. Kerr DA et al: Immunopathogenesis of acute transverse myelitis. Curr Opin Neurol. 15(3):339-47, 2002
9. Transverse Myelitis Consortium Working Group: Proposed diagnostic criteria and nosology of acute transverse myelitis. Neurology. 59(4):499-505, 2002
10. Scotti G et al: Diagnosis and differential diagnosis of acute transverse myelopathy. The role of neuroradiological investigations and review of the literature. Neurol Sci. 22 Suppl 2:S69-73, 2001
11. Misra UK et al: Role of MRI in acute transverse myelitis. Neurol India. 47(4):253-4, 1999
12. Murthy JM et al: Acute transverse myelitis: MR characteristics. Neurol India. 47(4):290-3, 1999
13. Isoda H et al: MR imaging of acute transverse myelitis (myelopathy). Radiat Med. 16(3):179-86, 1998
14. Choi KH et al: Idiopathic transverse myelitis: MR characteristics. AJNR Am J Neuroradiol. 17:1151-60, 1996
15. Misra UK et al: A clinical, MRI and neurophysiological study of acute transverse myelitis. J Neurol Sci. 138(1-2):150-6, 1996
16. Tartaglino LM et al: Idiopathic acute transverse myelitis: MR imaging findings. Radiology. 201(3):661-9, 1996

# IDIOPATHIC ACUTE TRANSVERSE MYELITIS

## IMAGE GALLERY

### Typical

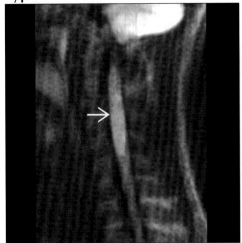
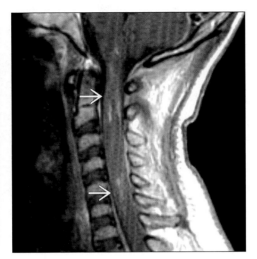

*(Left) Sagittal DWI MR in same child as previous images shows increased signal ➡ resulting from decreased diffusion. Areas of rapid demyelination may be associated with decreased diffusion. (Right) Sagittal T1 C+ MR 2 days after figure 2 now shows patchy enhancement ➡ which is evidence of blood brain barrier breakdown due to inflammation.*

### Variant

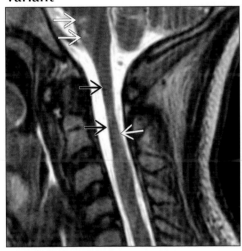
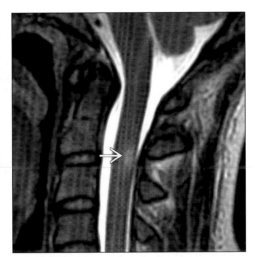

*(Left) Sagittal T2WI MR in same child as previous image 2 months after onset shows marked volume loss ➡ and gliosis ➡ in after resolution of the acute process. This child was left with a significant neurologic deficit. (Right) Sagittal T2WI MR shows focal dorsal T2 hyperintensity ➡ that enhanced after contrast (not shown). This is atypical in extent and location. This patient is at risk for MS.*

### Typical

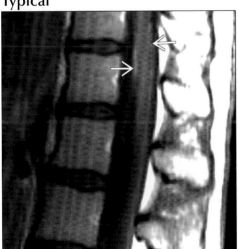
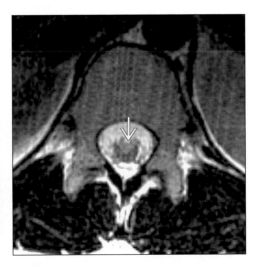

*(Left) Sagittal T1 C+ MR in a child with acute onset of lower extremity weakness shows dorsal and ventral meningeal enhancement ➡ at the level of the conus. (Right) Axial T2WI MR in the same child as previous image shows T2 hyperintensity ➡ in the conus. This case is slightly atypical in location as it involves primarily the anterior conus similar to Guillain-Barre.*

# ASTROCYTOMA, SPINAL CORD

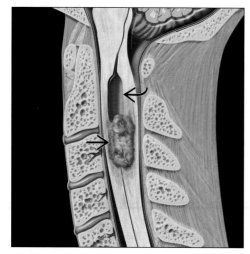

*Sagittal graphic of cervical spine shows solid mass ➡ with cystic component ⇨ within cervical cord.*

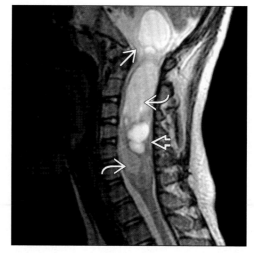

*Sagittal T2WI MR shows heterogeneous mass within cervical cord extending to medulla with a large dorsal cyst ➡. Core of tumor is variably hyperintense ➡ & contains two cysts ➡.*

## TERMINOLOGY

### Abbreviations and Synonyms
- Intramedullary glioma

### Definitions
- Primary neoplasm of astrocytic origin within spinal cord

## IMAGING FINDINGS

### General Features
- Best diagnostic clue: Enhancing infiltrating mass expanding cord
- Location
  - Intradural intramedullary
  - Cervical cord astrocytomas often extend to medulla oblongata
- Size
  - Usually 4 vertebral bodies or less
  - May be extensive, especially with pilocytic histology
- Morphology
  - Fusiform expansion of cord, with enhancing component of variable morphology
  - Occasionally asymmetric, even exophytic

### CT Findings
- NECT: ± Expansion, remodeling of bony canal

### MR Findings
- T1WI
  - Cord expansion
    - Usually < 4 vertebral bodies
    - Occasionally multisegmental, even holocord (more common with pilocytic astrocytoma)
  - Solid portion hypo/isointense, blood products uncommon
  - ± Cyst in/adjacent to tumor (especially medulla oblongata)
  - Edema, syrinx above and below the lesion
  - Sometimes hyperintense proteinaceous subarachnoid CSF below the mass
- T2WI
  - Hyperintense on PD, T2WI
  - Edema, tumor cysts (brighter than CSF), syrinx (CSF-like)
- T1 C+

---

## DDx: Other Spinal Cord Masses

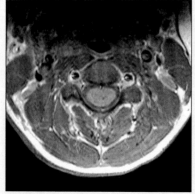

*Cervical Ependymoma*

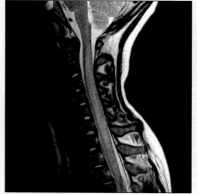

*Acute Transverse Myelitis*

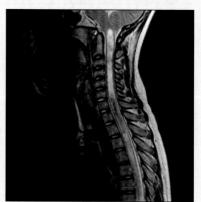

*Syrinx & Chiari I*

# ASTROCYTOMA, SPINAL CORD

## Key Facts

### Terminology
- Intramedullary glioma

### Imaging Findings
- Best diagnostic clue: Enhancing infiltrating mass expanding cord
- Occasionally asymmetric, even exophytic
- Almost always enhances densely
- Focus of enhancement is target for biopsy

### Top Differential Diagnoses
- Other Spinal Cord Tumors
- Syringohydromyelia
- Autoimmune or Inflammatory Myelitis
- Cord ischemia/infarction
- Vascular malformation

### Pathology
- Most common cord neoplasm in children
- 80-90% low grade
- Subarachnoid dissemination may occur, sometimes prominent, with malignant but also with low grade tumors

### Clinical Issues
- Slow onset of myelopathy: Pain, paresthesia, spasticity
- Most common intramedullary tumor in children

### Diagnostic Checklist
- MR at first suggestion of myelopathy
- Syrinx without clear explanation should lead to consider tumor

---

   ○ Almost always enhances densely
- Mild/moderate → intense enhancement
- Partial or total enhancement
- Heterogeneous/infiltrating or homogeneous/sharply-delineated
- Focus of enhancement is target for biopsy

### Radiographic Findings
- Radiography
  - Enlargement of spinal canal (late)
  - Scoliosis without bony cause

### Non-Vascular Interventions
- Myelography: Enlarged cord shadow, effacing contrast in surrounding thecal sac

### Imaging Recommendations
- Best imaging tool: Contrast-enhanced MR
- Protocol advice: Always look for upper and lower limits of tumor

## DIFFERENTIAL DIAGNOSIS

### Other Spinal Cord Tumors
- Ependymoma
  - Uncommon in children
  - Intense, sharply delineated enhancement
  - Central → eccentric growth pattern
  - Hemorrhage more common
- Other neoplasms
  - Ganglioglioma, mixed glioma
    - Typically indistinguishable
  - Hemangioblastoma
    - Older children
    - Often associated with von Hippel Lindau syndrome
    - Densely enhanced nodule
    - Large associated blood vessels
    - Huge cysts possible

### Syringohydromyelia
- CSF-like cyst; no enhancement
- Look for explanatory lesion: Chiari I, dysraphism

### Autoimmune or Inflammatory Myelitis
- Demyelinating disease
  - Acute transverse myelitis (ATM)
    - Acute onset, previous febrile episode or vaccination
    - Long cord segment (> 3 vertebral bodies), no cyst
    - ± Patchy, ill-defined enhancement if acute
    - May be part of ADEM
  - Infectious myelitis
    - Clinical context
    - Rapid onset
  - Multiple sclerosis
    - Typically multifocal, 90% brain involvement
    - Short cord segment (< 3 vertebral bodies)
    - Cord may show focal swelling, flame shaped

### Vascular Diseases
- Cord ischemia/infarction
  - Abrupt onset
  - Risk factors, uncommon in children
- Infectious vasculitis causes cord swelling and edema
- Vascular malformation
  - Prominent radiculo-medullary vessels, flow voids
  - Intramedullary hemorrhage

## PATHOLOGY

### General Features
- General path comments
  - Eccentric → central growth pattern (starts eccentric)
  - Bony spinal canal often enlarged, remodeled
  - Cervical > thoracic
- Etiology: No specific cause known
- Epidemiology
  - Most common cord neoplasm in children
    - 30-35% of intraspinal neoplasms
    - > 60% of intramedullary tumors
  - Intramedullary spinal cord tumors (IMSCTs) = 5-10% of all CNS tumors
  - Association with NF1, NF2

# ASTROCYTOMA, SPINAL CORD

## Gross Pathologic & Surgical Features
- Expanded cord

## Microscopic Features
- Juvenile pilocytic astrocytoma (JPA, grade I)
  - Rosenthal fibers
  - Glomeruloid/hyalinized vessels
  - Low prevalence of nuclear atypia/mitoses
  - Sometimes extensive (holocord)
- Fibrillary astrocytoma (grade II)
  - Increased cellularity
  - Variable atypia/mitoses
  - More parenchymal infiltration

## Staging, Grading or Classification Criteria
- 80-90% low grade
  - Pilocytic astrocytoma = grade I (most common)
  - Fibrillary astrocytoma = grade II
  - Ganglioglioma: Astrocytoma with ganglionic cells
    - Commonly JPA
    - Often slow growing, thus spinal canal enlargement, scoliosis common
  - Mixed gliomas also occur
- High grade: 10-15%
  - Anaplastic astrocytomas (grade III)
  - Glioblastoma (grade IV) do occur in cord
- Subarachnoid dissemination may occur, sometimes prominent, with malignant but also with low grade tumors

# CLINICAL ISSUES

## Presentation
- Most common signs/symptoms
  - Slow onset of myelopathy: Pain, paresthesia, spasticity
  - Torticollis
- Other signs/symptoms
  - Progressive scoliosis without bony explanation
  - Spinal cord tumors may generate hydrocephalus
- Clinical Profile: Insidious onset of myelopathy in adolescent or young adult

## Demographics
- Age
  - Most common intramedullary tumor in children
  - 60% of IMSCTs in children are astrocytomas, 30% ependymomas
- Gender: M > F = 1.3:1

## Natural History & Prognosis
- Most are slow-growing
- Malignant tumors may cause rapid neurologic deterioration
- Survival varies with tumor histology/grade, & gross total resection
  - 80% 5 year survival for low grade
  - 30% 5 year survival for high grade
  - Recurrences often develop late
- Post-operative neurologic function determined largely by degree of pre-operative deficit

## Treatment
- Obtain tissue diagnosis
- Microsurgical resection (low grade tumors)
  - Intraoperative US, evoked potentials helpful
- Adjuvant therapy
  - Radiotherapy, chemotherapy may help (controversial)

# DIAGNOSTIC CHECKLIST

## Consider
- MR at first suggestion of myelopathy

## Image Interpretation Pearls
- Syrinx without clear explanation should lead to consider tumor
- Scoliosis without spinal malformation + enlarged canal = tumor is likely

# SELECTED REFERENCES

1. Loh JK et al: Primary spinal tumors in children. J Clin Neurosci. 12(3):246-8, 2005
2. Saito R et al: Symptomatic spinal dissemination of malignant astrocytoma. J Neurooncol. 61(3):227-35, 2003
3. Santi M et al: Spinal cord malignant astrocytomas. Clinicopathologic features in 36 cases. Cancer. 98(3):554-61, 2003
4. Brotchi J: Intrinsic spinal cord tumor resection. Neurosurgery. 50(5):1059-63, 2002
5. Constantini S et al: Radical excision of intramedullary spinal cord tumors: surgical morbidity and long-term follow-up evaluation in 164 children and young adults. J Neurosurg. 93(2 Suppl):183-93, 2000
6. Houten JK et al: Pediatric intramedullary spinal cord tumors: special considerations. J Neurooncol. 47(3):225-30, 2000
7. Houten JK et al: Spinal cord astrocytomas: presentation, management & outcome. J Neurooncol. 47(3):219-24, 2000
8. Koeller KK et al: From the archives of the AFIP: neoplasms of the spinal cord & filum terminale: Radiologic-pathologic correlation. RadioGraphics. 20:1721-49, 2000
9. Lowe GM: Magnetic resonance imaging of intramedullary spinal cord tumors. J Neurooncol. 47(3):195-210, 2000
10. Miller DC: Surgical pathology of intramedullary spinal cord neoplasms. J Neurooncol. 47(3):189-94, 2000
11. Nishio S et al: Spinal cord gliomas: management and outcome with reference to adjuvant therapy. J Clin Neurosci. 7(1):20-3, 2000
12. Strik HM et al: A case of spinal glioblastoma multiforme: immunohistochemical study and review of the literature. J Neurooncol. 50(3):239-43, 2000
13. Baleriaux DL: Spinal cord tumors. Eur Radiol. 9(7):1252-8, 1999
14. Bourgouin PM et al: A pattern approach to the differential diagnosis of intramedullary spinal cord lesions on MR imaging. AJR Am J Roentgenol. 170(6):1645-9, 1998
15. Squires LA et al: Diffuse infiltrating astrocytoma of the cervicomedullary region: clinicopathologic entity. Pediatr Neurosurg. 27(3):153-9, 1997
16. Constantini S et al: Intramedullary spinal cord tumors in children under the age of 3 years. J Neurosurg. 85(6):1036-43, 1996
17. Minehan KJ et al: Spinal cord astrocytoma: pathological and treatment considerations. J Neurosurg. 83(4):590-5, 1995

## IMAGE GALLERY

### Typical

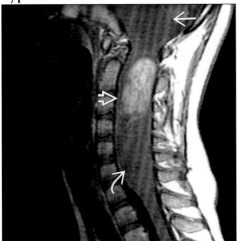

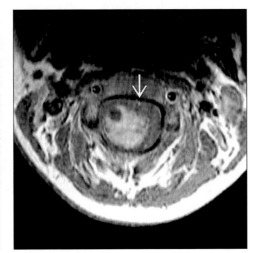

*(Left)* Sagittal T1 C+ MR in same patient as previous image shows enhancement of upper solid portion of tumor ➡. Lower portion ➡ & cystic medullary component ➡ do not enhance and likely have different histology. *(Right)* Axial T1 C+ MR shows that the tumor is excentric: Spinal artery ➡ shifted to the left. Eccentricity is not commonly seen in ependymomas. Note mild spinal canal enlargement.

### Typical

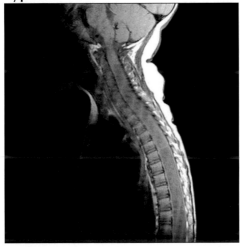

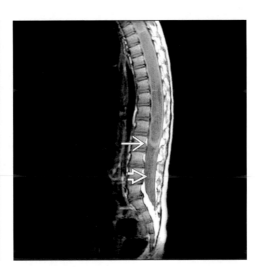

*(Left)* Sagittal T1WI MR shows holocord astrocytoma. This extensive tumor of cervical & thoracic segments of cord in toddler appears homogeneous. Note enlarged spinal canal. *(Right)* Sagittal T1WI MR in same patient as previous image shows caudal extension of tumor down to conus ➡. Lumbar subarachnoid CSF ➡ is isointense to cord, due to high protein content (CSF block).

### Typical

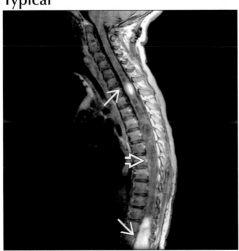

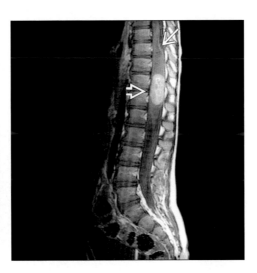

*(Left)* Sagittal T1 C+ MR shows cervicothoracic astrocytoma with enhancing upper and lower nodules ➡ separated by multicystic appearing, non-enhancing intermediate segment ➡. *(Right)* Sagittal T1 C+ MR shows astrocytoma restricted to lumbar enlargement, with clear upper limit ➡ and normal-looking thoracic cord. Note enhancing caudal component ➡.

# EPENDYMOMA, CELLULAR, SPINAL CORD

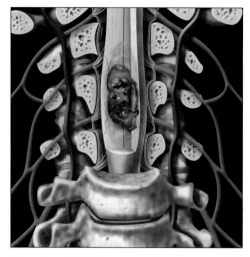

Coronal graphic depicts an ependymoma centered in the cervical spinal cord with mild cord expansion. Cranial and rostral cysts as well as hemorrhagic products are associated with this mass.

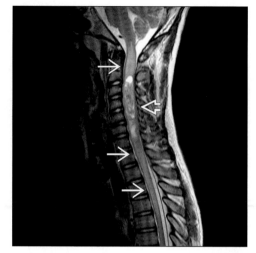

Sagittal T2WI MR shows heterogeneous C2-C7 mass ➡ effacing subarachnoid space but without significant spinal canal enlargement. Note adjacent superior and inferior cord edema ➡.

## TERMINOLOGY

### Abbreviations and Synonyms
- Cord ependymoma

### Definitions
- Ependymal tumor of spinal cord
  - Excludes myxopapillary ependymoma of filum terminale

## IMAGING FINDINGS

### General Features
- Best diagnostic clue: Circumscribed, enhancing cord mass with hemorrhage
- Location: Cervical > thoracic > conus
- Size
  - Multisegmental
    - Typically 3-4 segments
- Morphology
  - Well-circumscribed
  - Symmetric cord expansion
  - May have exophytic component
  - May be cystic, or associated with cysts

### CT Findings
- NECT
  - Spinal canal widening
    - Thinned pedicles
    - Widened interpediculate distance
    - Posterior vertebral scalloping
- CECT: May show symmetrically enlarged spinal cord with well-circumscribed enhancement

### MR Findings
- T1WI
  - Isointense or slightly hypointense to spinal cord
  - Hemorrhage hyperintense
  - Cord atrophy may be present
    - Correlates with surgical morbidity
  - Hypointense cysts
- T2WI
  - Hyperintense
  - Polar (rostral or caudal) or intratumoral cysts: 50-90%
  - Syrinx in adjacent cord
  - Focal hyper/hypointensity: Blood products

## DDx: Other Masses of Spinal Cord

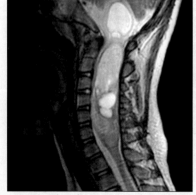

Juvenile Pilocytic Astrocytoma

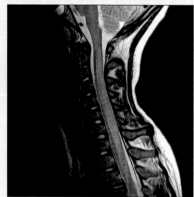

Acute Transverse Myelitis

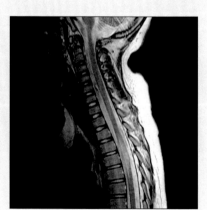

Toxocara Migrans

# EPENDYMOMA, CELLULAR, SPINAL CORD

## Key Facts

### Terminology
- Ependymal tumor of spinal cord
- Excludes myxopapillary ependymoma of filum terminale

### Imaging Findings
- Best diagnostic clue: Circumscribed, enhancing cord mass with hemorrhage
- Focal hyper/hypointensity: Blood products
- Intense, well-delineated compact homogeneous enhancement: 50%
- Fusiform cord enlargement

### Top Differential Diagnoses
- Other Spinal Cord Tumors
- Inflammatory/Demyelinating Cord Diseases
- Spinal Cord Ischemia and Infarct

### Pathology
- Four ependymoma subtypes: Cellular, papillary, clear-cell, tanycytic

### Clinical Issues
- Most common signs/symptoms: Neck or back pain, torticollis
- Progressive spasticity, paraparesis, paresthesia
- Progressive scoliosis
- Clinical Profile: Delay in diagnosis due to slow growth
- 5 year survival: 85%
- Treat by surgical resection

### Diagnostic Checklist
- Consider spinal cord tumor in any cord lesion
- Peripheral hemorrhage: Ependymoma likely

---

- ▪ "Cap sign": Hemosiderin at cranial or caudal margin
  - ▪ 20-64% of cord ependymomas
  - ○ Adjacent cord edema
- T1 C+
  - ○ Intense, well-delineated compact homogeneous enhancement: 50%
  - ○ Nodular, peripheral, heterogeneous enhancement possible
  - ○ Minimal or no enhancement rare

### Radiographic Findings
- Radiography
  - ○ Spinal canal widening: 20% (late), vertebral scalloping
  - ○ Scoliosis

### Non-Vascular Interventions
- Myelography
  - ○ Fusiform cord enlargement
  - ○ Partial or complete block of intrathecal contrast

### Imaging Recommendations
- Best imaging tool: MR in sagittal and axial planes with gadolinium
- Protocol advice: Fat suppression with T2WI and T1WI plus gadolinium

## DIFFERENTIAL DIAGNOSIS

### Other Spinal Cord Tumors
- Astrocytoma
  - ○ Most common primary cord neoplasm in children, typically grade I (juvenile pilocytic astrocytoma)
  - ○ May be indistinguishable
  - ○ Often more extensive, may be holocord
  - ○ More often eccentric, infiltrative with indistinct margins
  - ○ Hemorrhage uncommon
- Ganglioglioma
  - ○ Similar to astrocytoma
  - ○ Bony changes more common (slow growing tumor)

- High grade gliomas: Anaplastic astrocytoma (grade III), glioblastoma multiforme (grade IV)
- Hemangioblastomas
  - ○ Cyst with enhancing highly vascular nodule, flow voids may be present
    - ▪ More extensive surrounding edema
    - ▪ Thoracic > cervical
    - ▪ Older patients, associated with von Hippel-Lindau disease

### Inflammatory/Demyelinating Cord Diseases
- Diagnoses of exclusion
- Acute transverse myelitis
  - ○ Immuno-allergic: Acute onset, often previous infection, vaccination
  - ○ Cord expansion less pronounced, thoracic > cervical
  - ○ Bilateral, centrally located, 2/3 of cord section, 3-4 vertebral segments in length
  - ○ Variable enhancement
- ADEM
  - ○ Immuno-allergic: Acute onset, previous febrile episode or vaccination common
  - ○ Myelitis associated with multiple areas of brain demyelination
- Acute cord infection
- MS
  - ○ Often multifocal, 90% have brain lesions
  - ○ Ill-defined lesions more often peripheral, posterolateral
  - ○ Typically < 2 vertebral segments in length
  - ○ Faint nodular or patchy enhancement

### Spinal Cord Ischemia and Infarct
- Sudden onset of symptoms
- Posterior columns typically spared in anterior spinal infarct

## PATHOLOGY

### General Features
- General path comments

# EPENDYMOMA, CELLULAR, SPINAL CORD

○ Four ependymoma subtypes: Cellular, papillary, clear-cell, tanycytic
  ▪ Cellular usual cord tumor subtype
- Genetics
  ○ Myriad tumoral genetic abnormalities
  ○ Cord ependymomas genetically different from intracranial lesions
    ▪ Gain on chromosomes 2, 7, 12, etc.
    ▪ Structural abnormalities: Chromosomes 1, 6, 17, etc.
  ○ Ependymoma associated with NF2
    ▪ Deletions, translocations of chromosome 22
- Epidemiology: Extremely uncommon in children, except in NF2
- Associated abnormalities
  ○ NF2
    ▪ Schwannomas: Multiple, sensory nerve roots (cranial, spinal)
    ▪ Meningiomas: Multiple, often invasive (cranial, spinal)

## Gross Pathologic & Surgical Features
- Soft red or grayish-purple mass
  ○ Small blood vessels on tumor surface
- Well-circumscribed
  ○ May be encapsulated, relatively easy to remove
- Cystic change common
- Hemorrhage at tumor periphery

## Microscopic Features
- Perivascular pseudorosettes
  ○ True ependymal rosettes less common
- Moderate cellularity with low mitotic activity
- Occasional nuclear atypia
- Immunohistochemistry: Positive for GFAP, S-100, vimentin

## Staging, Grading or Classification Criteria
- Most are WHO grade II
- Rare: WHO grade III (anaplastic ependymoma)

# CLINICAL ISSUES

## Presentation
- Most common signs/symptoms: Neck or back pain, torticollis
- Other signs/symptoms
  ○ Progressive spasticity, paraparesis, paresthesia
  ○ Progressive scoliosis
- Clinical Profile: Delay in diagnosis due to slow growth

## Demographics
- Age: Teenagers
- Gender: Slight male predilection
- Ethnicity: No racial predilection

## Natural History & Prognosis
- Less pre-operative neurologic deficit at presentation, better post-operative outcome
- Thoracic tumors have worse surgical outcome
- Rarely metastasis
  ○ Lung, skin, kidney, lymph nodes
- 5 year survival: 85%

## Treatment
- Treat by surgical resection
  ○ Gross total resection in > 85% of cases
- Radiotherapy for subtotal resection or recurrent disease
- Unproven benefit: Chemotherapy for failed surgery and radiotherapy

# DIAGNOSTIC CHECKLIST

## Consider
- Consider spinal cord tumor in any cord lesion

## Image Interpretation Pearls
- Peripheral hemorrhage: Ependymoma likely

# SELECTED REFERENCES

1. Loh JK et al: Primary spinal tumors in children. J Clin Neurosci. 12(3):246-8, 2005
2. Chamberlain MC: Ependymomas. Curr Neurol Neurosci Rep. 3(3):193-9, 2003
3. Sun B et al: MRI features of intramedullary spinal cord ependymomas. J Neuroimaging. 13(4):346-51, 2003
4. Carter M et al: Genetic abnormalities detected in ependymomas by comparative genomic hybridisation. Br J Cancer. 86(6):929-39, 2002
5. Choi JY et al: Intracranial and spinal ependymomas: review of MR images in 61 patients. Korean J Radiol. 3(4):219-28, 2002
6. Hanbali F et al: Spinal cord ependymoma: radical surgical resection and outcome. Neurosurgery. 51(5):1162-72; discussion 1172-4, 2002
7. Jeuken JW et al: Correlation between localization, age, and chromosomal imbalances in ependymal tumours as detected by CGH. J Pathol. 197(2):238-44, 2002
8. Takeuchi H et al: Epithelial differentiation and proliferative potential in spinal ependymomas. J Neurooncol. 58(1):13-9, 2002
9. Hirose Y et al: Chromosomal abnormalities subdivide ependymal tumors into clinically relevant groups. Am J Pathol. 158(3):1137-43, 2001
10. Houten JK et al: Pediatric intramedullary spinal cord tumors: special considerations. J Neurooncol. 47(3):225-30, 2000
11. Koeller KK et al: Neoplasms of the spinal cord and filum terminale: radiologic-pathologic correlation. Radiographics. 20(6):1721-49, 2000
12. Miyazawa N et al: MRI at 1.5 T of intramedullary ependymoma and classification of pattern of contrast enhancement. Neuroradiology. 42(11):828-32, 2000
13. Bourgouin PM et al: A pattern approach to the differential diagnosis of intramedullary spinal cord lesions on MR imaging. AJR Am J Roentgenol. 170(6):1645-9, 1998
14. Constantini S et al: Intramedullary spinal cord tumors in children under the age of 3 years. J Neurosurg. 85(6):1036-43, 1996
15. Kahan H et al: MR characteristics of histopathologic subtypes of spinal ependymoma. AJNR Am J Neuroradiol. 17(1):143-50, 1996
16. Fine MJ et al: Spinal cord ependymomas: MR imaging features. Radiology. 197(3):655-8, 1995
17. Nemoto Y et al: Intramedullary spinal cord tumors: significance of associated hemorrhage at MR imaging. Radiology. 182(3):793-6, 1992

III

5

28

## IMAGE GALLERY

### Typical

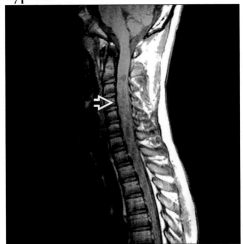
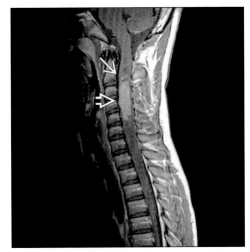

*(Left)* Sagittal T1WI MR in same patient as previous image shows corresponding signal heterogeneity, mostly isointense ➡, indicating tumor cellularity. The mildly enlarged cord effaces the subarachnoid spaces. *(Right)* Sagittal T1 C+ MR corresponding slice shows well demarcated, compact, enhancing component ➡ occupying most of cord. Some enhancement is seen around adjacent cystic-looking structure ➡.

### Typical

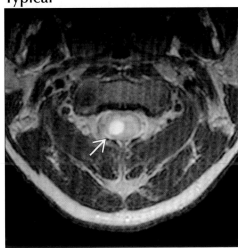
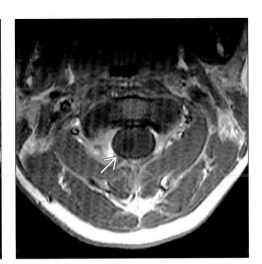

*(Left)* Axial T2WI MR at C2 level shows cyst with higher signal than CSF ➡, presumably degraded blood or proteinaceous fluid. Note edema in the enlarged surrounding cord. *(Right)* Axial T1 C+ MR at same level shows the cyst ➡ to be hypointense, which is not suggestive of hemorrhage. Thus, it is likely proteinaceous.

### Typical

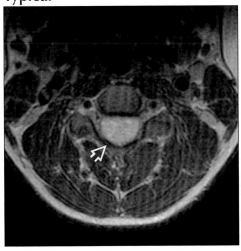
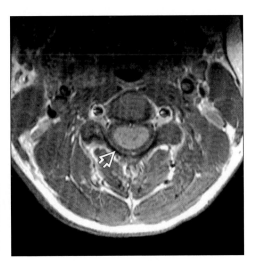

*(Left)* Axial T2WI MR at the mid-cervical level (through nodule) shows heterogeneous structure of the lesion with irregular high signal ➡ suggesting cellular tumor with edema. *(Right)* Axial T1 C+ MR at same level shows intense quite homogeneous enhancement ➡ occupying most of anteroposterior extent of the cord section.

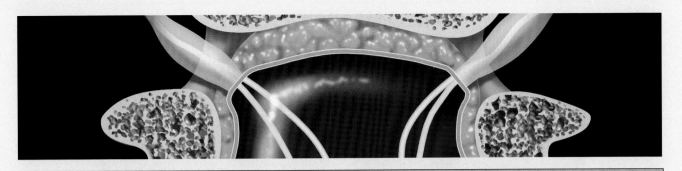

# SECTION 6: Multiple Regions, Spine

# MYELOMENINGOCELE

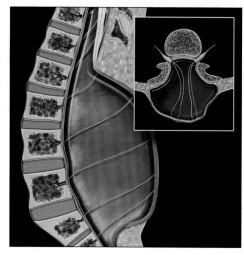

Sagittal graphic shows a patulous dural sac (without skin covering) protruding through a dysraphic defect. Inset shows open dysraphism, with nerve roots dangling from red ventral placode.

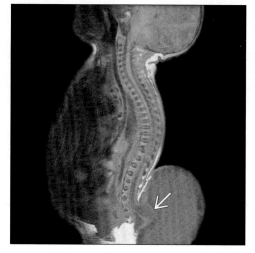

Sagittal T1WI MR shows typical Chiari II malformation findings as well as a large myelomeningocele with internal neural elements ➡ protruding through a posterior dysraphic defect.

## TERMINOLOGY

### Abbreviations and Synonyms
- Myelomeningocele (MMC), meningomyelocele, open spinal dysraphism (OSD), spina bifida aperta, spina bifida cystica

### Definitions
- Posterior spinal defect lacking skin covering ⇒ neural tissue, CSF, and meninges exposed to air

## IMAGING FINDINGS

### General Features
- Best diagnostic clue: Wide osseous dysraphism, low-lying cord/roots, post-operative skin closure changes
- Location: Lumbosacral (44%) > thoracolumbar (32%) > lumbar (22%) > thoracic (2%)
- Size: Small ⇒ large, depending on extent of neural tube defect
- Morphology: Exposed CSF sac + neural elements protrude through wide dorsal dysraphism

### CT Findings
- NECT
  - Wide posterior osseous dysraphism, skin covered CSF sac (post-operative)
  - Associated anomalies, post-operative complications
    - Spine CT: Diastematomyelia spur, dural constriction, or cord ischemia sequelae (abrupt cord termination)
    - Head CT: Hydrocephalus from VP shunt failure

### MR Findings
- T1WI
  - Wide spinal dysraphism, flared laminae, low-lying cord/roots; skin covered CSF sac (post-operative)
  - Loss of normal posterior epidural fat segmentation at anomaly level (sagittal imaging)
    - Epidural fat contiguous on two or more adjacent levels ⇒ suspicious for dysraphism
- T2WI: Nerve roots originate from ventral placode surface; ventral roots exit medial to dorsal roots

### Radiographic Findings
- Radiography
  - Posterior spina bifida with wide eversion of laminae

## DDx: Myelomeningocele

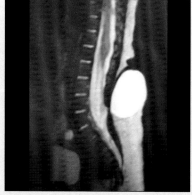

*Dorsal Meningocele*

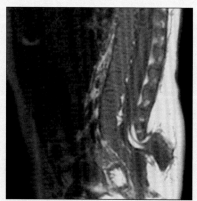

*Lipomyelomeningocele*

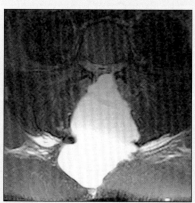

*Pseudomeningocele*

# MYELOMENINGOCELE

## Key Facts

### Terminology
- Myelomeningocele (MMC), meningomyelocele, open spinal dysraphism (OSD), spina bifida aperta, spina bifida cystica
- Posterior spinal defect lacking skin covering ⇒ neural tissue, CSF, and meninges exposed to air

### Imaging Findings
- Best diagnostic clue: Wide osseous dysraphism, low-lying cord/roots, post-operative skin closure changes

### Top Differential Diagnoses
- Dorsal Meningocele
- Closed (Occult) Spinal Dysraphism
- Post-Operative Pseudomeningocele

### Pathology
- Red, exposed neural placode leaking CSF protrudes through osseous midline defect

### Clinical Issues
- Lesion level determines severity of neurological deficits
- Stable post-operative deficit expected → best possible outcome

### Diagnostic Checklist
- Imaging untreated MMC seldom indicated
- MMC patients frequently have other CNS abnormalities; neurological deterioration requires assessment of entire craniospinal axis
- Low-lying cord on MR imaging does not always equate to clinical tethering

---

  - ○ Most rostral normal lamina = superior margin of myeloschisis defect

## Ultrasonographic Findings
- Grayscale Ultrasound
  - ○ Obstetrical ultrasound ⇒ antenatal diagnosis
    - ■ Open neural arch, flared laminae, protruding myelomeningocele sac, and Chiari II brain findings ("lemon" sign, "banana" sign, hydrocephalus)

## Non-Vascular Interventions
- Myelography: +/- CSF loculations, absence of CSF between placode and dura, low-lying cord

## Other Modality Findings
- Sagittal cine phase contrast MR ⇒ diminished conus pulsation may indicate tethering

## Imaging Recommendations
- Best imaging tool: MR imaging
- Protocol advice
  - ○ Obstetrical ultrasound: Initial MMC diagnosis, delivery planning (cesarean section), triaging for possible fetal surgery
  - ○ Head CT: Hydrocephalus evaluation
  - ○ MR: Sagittal and axial T1WI and T2WI; must include entire sacrum

## DIFFERENTIAL DIAGNOSIS

### Dorsal Meningocele
- Meninges protrude through dorsal dysraphism into subcutaneous fat
- Skin covered, usually does not contain neural elements

### Closed (Occult) Spinal Dysraphism
- Dorsal osseous dysraphism; cord may be low-lying
- Skin or other cutaneous derivative (e.g., lipoma) covers neural elements

### Post-Operative Pseudomeningocele
- History, clinical exam permit distinction
- Look for surgical laminectomy defect, absence of spina bifida osseous changes

## PATHOLOGY

### General Features
- General path comments
  - ○ Diajunction = normal neural tube separation from overlying ectoderm during neural tube closure
  - ○ Open neural tube defects (NTD) arise from disjunction failure ⇒ neural placode
    - ■ Anterior placode surface ⇒ external pia mater cord surface
    - ■ Posterior placode surface ⇒ internal neural tube ependyma
  - ○ Placode may be segmental or terminal
    - ■ Segmental (lumbar, thoracolumbar, thoracic) ⇒ spinal cord continues distally
    - ■ Terminal (lumbosacral, sacral) ⇒ placode at end of spinal cord
- Genetics
  - ○ Pax 3 paired box gene derangements
  - ○ Methylene-tetra-hydrofolate-reductase (MTHFR) mutations associated with abnormal folate metabolism
    - ■ MTHFR mutations + folate deficiency ⇒ increased risk of NTD
  - ○ Trisomy 13, 18 (14% of NTD fetuses)
- Etiology
  - ○ Lack of complex carbohydrate molecule expression on neuroectodermal cell surface ⇒ failed neural tube closure
  - ○ NTD deficits worsened by chronic mechanical injury, amniotic fluid chemical trauma
- Epidemiology
  - ○ Incidence 0.44-0.6:1,000 live births
  - ○ Maternal folate deficiency, obesity, anti-epileptic therapy (lowers folate bioavailability)
- Associated abnormalities

- Kyphoscoliosis: Neuromuscular imbalance +/- vertebral segmentation anomalies
  - Developmental (65%): Neuromuscular imbalance, anterior displacement of spinal extensor muscles
  - Congenital (30%): Congenital osseous anomalies (hemivertebrae, bony bar)
- Diastematomyelia, dermal sinus (31-46%)
  - Cord split above (31%), below (25%), or at (22%) MMC level
  - Hemimyelocele variant (10%) → asymmetric deficits
- Syrinx (30-75%)
- Chiari II malformation (≈ 100%), hydrocephalus requiring shunting (80%)
- Orthopedic abnormalities (80%); 2° to muscular imbalance

## Gross Pathologic & Surgical Features
- Red, exposed neural placode leaking CSF protrudes through osseous midline defect
- Spinal cord always physically tethered; +/- clinical neurologic deterioration

## Microscopic Features
- Purkinje cell loss, sclerosis of herniated posterior fossa tissues related to Chiari II malformation

# CLINICAL ISSUES

## Presentation
- Most common signs/symptoms
  - Stable neurological deficits expected following closure
    - Neurological deterioration ⇒ imaging evaluation for tethered cord, dural ring constriction, cord ischemia, or syringohydromyelia
- Clinical Profile
  - Newborn with midline raw, red, exposed neural placode
    - Lesion level determines severity of neurological deficits
    - Hydrocephalus 2° to Chiari II malformation
  - Post-operative: Fixed paraparesis and sensory deficits concomitant with defect level, large heads (hydrocephalus), neurologically induced orthopedic disorders, neurogenic bladder (90%), +/- kyphoscoliosis
- Laboratory findings: Elevated maternal serum alpha fetoprotein (AFP)

## Demographics
- Age: Always present at birth
- Gender: M < F (1:3)
- Ethnicity: ↑ Frequency in Irish/Welsh populations (4-8x), families with other affected children (7-15x)

## Natural History & Prognosis
- Stable post-operative deficit expected → best possible outcome
  - Hydrocephalus, tethered cord determine prognosis for deterioration
  - Neurological deterioration suggests complication

- Tethering by scar or second (unrecognized) malformation → most common
- Constricting post-operative dural ring
- Cord compression by epidermoid/dermoid tumor or arachnoid cyst
- Cord ischemia
- Syringohydromyelia (29-77%)
- Hydrocephalus related to Chiari II malformation is the most common cause of death in MMC patients

## Treatment
- Folate supplementation to pregnant/conceiving women
- MMC closure < 48 hours to stabilize neural deficits, prevent infection
  - Some tertiary centers perform in-utero surgical repair; may lessen Chiari II, neurological deficit severity
- Subsequent management revolves around treating post-operative complications
  - Cord untethering, hydrocephalus management, treatment of kyphoscoliosis

# DIAGNOSTIC CHECKLIST

## Consider
- Imaging untreated MMC seldom indicated
- MMC patients frequently have other CNS abnormalities; neurological deterioration requires assessment of entire craniospinal axis
- Cord re-tethering = most common spinal cause of delayed deterioration

## Image Interpretation Pearls
- Low-lying cord on MR imaging does not always equate to clinical tethering

# SELECTED REFERENCES

1. Dias MS: Neurosurgical causes of scoliosis in patients with myelomeningocele: an evidence-based literature review. J Neurosurg. 103(1 Suppl):24-35, 2005
2. Hudgins RJ et al: Tethered spinal cord following repair of myelomeningocele. Neurosurg Focus. 16(2):E7, 2004
3. Piatt JH Jr: Syringomyelia complicating myelomeningocele: review of the evidence. J Neurosurg. 100(2 Suppl Pediatrics):101-9, 2004
4. Tulipan N: Intrauterine closure of myelomeningocele: an update. Neurosurg Focus. 16(2):E2, 2004
5. Rintoul NE et al: A new look at myelomeningoceles: functional level, vertebral level, shunting, and the implications for fetal intervention. Pediatrics. 109(3):409-13, 2002
6. Trivedi J et al: Clinical and radiographic predictors of scoliosis in patients with myelomeningocele. J Bone Joint Surg Am. 84-A(8):1389-94, 2002
7. Bowman RM et al: Spina bifida outcome: a 25-year prospective. Pediatr Neurosurg. 34(3):114-20, 2001
8. Tortori-Donati P et al: Spinal dysraphism: a review of neuroradiological features with embryological correlations and proposal for a new classification. Neuroradiology. 42(7):471-91, 2000
9. Shaw GM et al: Risk of neural tube defect-affected pregnancies among obese women. JAMA. 275(14):1093-6, 1996

# MYELOMENINGOCELE

## IMAGE GALLERY

### Typical

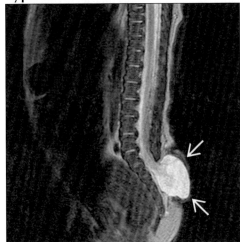 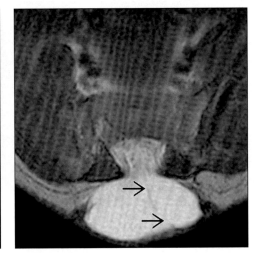

*(Left)* Sagittal T2WI MR of an unrepaired sacral myelomeningocele shows open spinal dysraphism and CSF-filled myelomeningocele sac containing nerve roots inserting onto dorsal neural placode ➡. *(Right)* Axial T2WI MR confirms characteristic wide spinal dysraphism and nerve roots ➡ dangling from the ventral placode.

### Typical

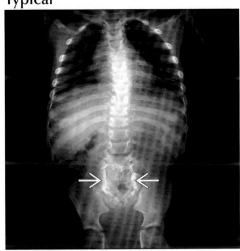 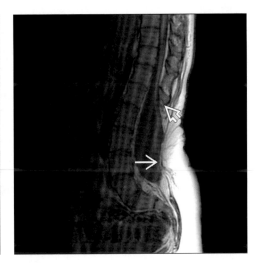

*(Left)* Anteroposterior radiograph demonstrates wide posterior spinal dysraphism ➡. The sacrum is also hypoplastic, indicating concurrent caudal regression syndrome. *(Right)* Sagittal T1WI MR illustrates capacious spinal canal and thinned spinal cord scarred into surgical closure. Note small syrinx in distal cord ➡. ➡ Marks last intact posterior element.

### Variant

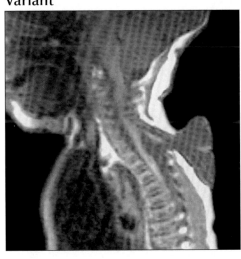 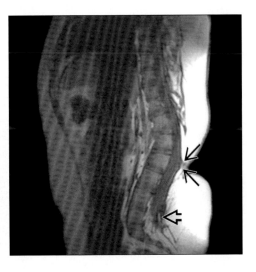

*(Left)* Sagittal T1WI MR demonstrates a cervicothoracic myelomeningocele. The neural elements are drawn into the CSF-filled sac, which is not skin covered. *(Right)* Sagittal T1WI MR shows an attenuated spinal cord with segmental adhesion to myelomeningocele closure ➡. Spinal cord continues past neural placode to terminate in small terminal lipoma ➡.

# LIPOMYELOMENINGOCELE

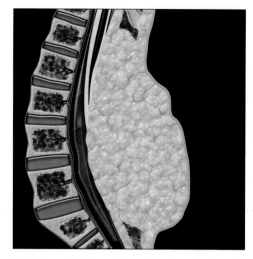

*Sagittal graphic demonstrates a low-lying, hydromyelic spinal cord terminating in a large dorsal lipomatous malformation, extending through a dysraphic defect to blend with subcutaneous fat.*

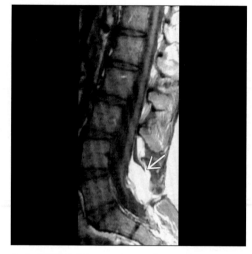

*Sagittal T1WI MR reveals an elongated spinal cord inserting into a transitional lipoma →. The last fused posterior elements are at L3, with lipoma extending through the dysraphic defect.*

## TERMINOLOGY

### Abbreviations and Synonyms
- Lipomyelomeningocele (LMMC), lipomyelocele (LMC), lipomyeloschisis

### Definitions
- Lipomyelocele: Neural placode-lipoma complex contiguous with subcutaneous fat through dysraphic defect, attaching to and tethering spinal cord
- Lipomyelomeningocele: Lipomyelocele + meningocele, enlargement of subarachnoid space, displacement of neural placode outside of spinal canal

## IMAGING FINDINGS

### General Features
- Best diagnostic clue: Subcutaneous fatty mass contiguous with neural placode through posterior dysraphism
- Location: Lumbosacral
- Size: Subcutaneous mass varies from nearly imperceptible ⇒ large

- Morphology: Tethered low lying spinal cord inserts into lipoma through dysraphic defect

### CT Findings
- NECT
  - Ventral neural placode/tethered cord +/- terminal hydromyelia, cord myeloschisis
  - Hypodense dorsal lipoma is contiguous with subcutaneous fat through posterior spina bifida
- Bone CT
  - Multilevel dysraphism, enlarged canal at placode level

### MR Findings
- T1WI
  - Hyperintense lipoma contiguous with subcutaneous fat, tethered cord/placode
    - Herniation of placode-lipoma complex immediately inferior to last intact lamina above dorsal defect
    - Lipoma usually dorsal; may be rotated (40%)
    - +/- Intramedullary, intradural, or extradural lipoma - actually occult extension from LMMC rather than discrete second lesion

## DDx: Lipomyelomeningocele

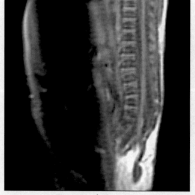

*Terminal Lipoma*

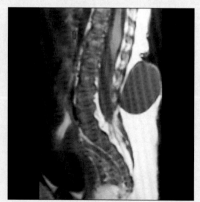

*Dorsal Meningocele*

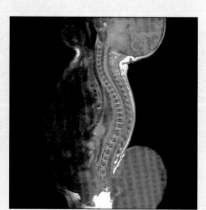

*Myelomeningocele*

# LIPOMYELOMENINGOCELE

## Key Facts

### Terminology
- Lipomyelomeningocele (LMMC), lipomyelocele (LMC), lipomyeloschisis

### Imaging Findings
- Best diagnostic clue: Subcutaneous fatty mass contiguous with neural placode through posterior dysraphism
- Ventral neural placode/tethered cord +/- terminal hydromyelia, cord myeloschisis

### Top Differential Diagnoses
- Intradural (Juxtamedullary) Lipoma
- Terminal Lipoma
- Dorsal Meningocele
- Myelocele/Myelomeningocele

### Pathology
- Cord always tethered
- Lipoma may be asymmetric (40%), rotating placode and elongating roots on one side, shortening on other

### Clinical Issues
- Soft midline or paramedian skin covered mass above buttocks
- Cutaneous stigmata (50%); hemangioma, dimple, dermal sinus, skin tag, hairy patch

### Diagnostic Checklist
- Determination of re-tethering following surgery primarily clinical diagnosis; use imaging to search for complications

---

- Cord tethering +/- myeloschisis, terminal hydromyelia
- T2WI: Hyperintense lipoma; neural elements isointense on background of hyperintense CSF
- STIR: Lipoma → hypointense, confirming fat composition

### Radiographic Findings
- Radiography: Multilevel dorsal spinal dysraphism +/- hypodense soft tissue mass

### Ultrasonographic Findings
- Grayscale Ultrasound: Echogenic intradural spinal mass contiguous with tethered cord through dorsal dysraphism

### Non-Vascular Interventions
- Myelography: Dorsal dysraphism + dilated thecal sac; low lying conus inserts into hypodense lipoma

### Imaging Recommendations
- Best imaging tool: MR imaging
- STIR or chemical fat-saturated techniques confirm fat composition

## DIFFERENTIAL DIAGNOSIS

### Intradural (Juxtamedullary) Lipoma
- Enclosed by intact dura; cutaneous manifestations unusual
- Cervical, thoracic spine most common

### Terminal Lipoma
- Lipoma tethers low lying conus, stretching cord
- No spinal canal enlargement
- Rotation of lipoma, vertebral segmentation and fusion anomalies (SFA) rare

### Dorsal Meningocele
- Skin covered, no fat elements
- More limited dysraphic defect

### Myelocele/Myelomeningocele
- Clinically open dysraphism; no skin or subcutaneous fat covering, no lipoma

## PATHOLOGY

### General Features
- General path comments
  - LMC and LMMC are analogous to myelocele and myelomeningocele respectively except that a lipoma is attached to dorsal placode surface and intact skin overlies lesion
  - Cord always tethered
- Etiology
  - Neural tube normally forms by infolding and closure of neural ectoderm as it separates from cutaneous ectoderm during 3rd and 4th week ⇒ neurulation and disjunction
    - In LMMC, premature disjunction of neural ectoderm from cutaneous ectoderm ⇒ mesenchymal tissue direct access to incompletely closed neural tube
    - Mesenchyme is incorporated between neural folds
    - Neural folds remain open, forming neural placode at site of premature disjunction
    - Ependymal lining of primitive neural tube induces mesenchyme to form fat ⇒ lipoma
- Epidemiology
  - 20-56% of occult spinal dysraphism; 20% of skin covered lumbosacral masses
  - Recurrence risk estimated from 2-5% in siblings
  - Incidence not impacted by folate supplementation to pregnant women (unlike MMC)
- Associated abnormalities
  - +/- Intramedullary, intradural, or extradural lipoma → occult extension of LMMC
  - Butterfly vertebrae, hemivertebrae, fused vertebrae (≤ 43%)
  - Sacral abnormalities (≤ 50%); confluent foramina and partial sacral dysgenesis

- ○ Anorectal and GU abnormalities (5-10%); if concurrent sacral anomalies → 90%
- ○ Terminal diastematomyelia (≤ 10%)
- ○ (Epi)dermoid tumor, dermal sinus, angioma, arachnoid cyst (rare)
- ○ Arteriovenous malformation (very rare)

## Gross Pathologic & Surgical Features
- Canal enlarged at placode, spina bifida level
- Lipoma may envelop both dorsal and ventral nerve roots, dorsal nerve roots only, or filum terminale/conus
- Dura deficient at spina bifida zone → does not close neural tube
  - ○ Attached to lateral margin of neural placode, posterior to dorsal nerve roots as they emerge from cord
- Lipoma may be asymmetric (40%), rotating placode and elongating roots on one side, shortening on other
  - ○ Predisposes to operative injury, incomplete tether release

## Microscopic Features
- Dorsal placode surface adjacent to lipoma has no ependymal lining; covered by connective tissue mixed with islands of glial cells, smooth muscle fibers

## Staging, Grading or Classification Criteria
- Dorsal lipoma: Attached to placode above conus medullaris
- Transitional lipoma: Attached to placode and to conus (involves cauda equina)
- Terminal lipoma: Attaches at termination of conus

**III**

**6**

**8**

# CLINICAL ISSUES

## Presentation
- Most common signs/symptoms: Back/leg pain, scoliosis, lower extremity paraparesis, sacral sensory loss, limb atrophy, orthopedic foot deformity, bladder/bowel dysfunction
- Clinical Profile
  - ○ Soft midline or paramedian skin covered mass above buttocks
    - ▪ Lumbosacral mass: Clinical attention within 6 months
    - ▪ No mass: Present with neurological deficits (5 years ⇒ adulthood)
  - ○ Cutaneous stigmata (50%); hemangioma, dimple, dermal sinus, skin tag, hairy patch

## Demographics
- Age: Infancy (most common) ⇒ adulthood
- Gender: M < F

## Natural History & Prognosis
- Potentially irreversible progressive neurological impairment (cord tethering, enlarging lipoma)
  - ○ Lipoma grows with infant
  - ○ Bladder dysfunction usually persists if cord not released early
- ≤ 45% of children neurologically normal at diagnosis

- ○ 16-88% develop neurological symptoms if left untreated
- ○ Most symptoms progress if untreated
- Neurologically intact patients at surgery usually remain intact on long term follow-up
- Post-operative exam should not deteriorate with longitudinal growth; neurological decline raises suspicion of re-tethering, warrants repeat imaging
- Symptomatic re-tethering common; weeks to years after initial surgery
  - ○ Median time between initial procedure and reoperation for re-tethering ⇒ 52 months

## Treatment
- Early prophylactic surgery (< 1 year of age) to untether cord, resect lipoma, and reconstruct dura

# DIAGNOSTIC CHECKLIST

## Consider
- Presence/absence of placode rotation important pre-operative information for surgeon

## Image Interpretation Pearls
- Determination of re-tethering following surgery primarily clinical diagnosis; use imaging to search for complications

# SELECTED REFERENCES

1. Forrester MB et al: Precurrence risk of neural tube defects in siblings of infants with lipomyelomeningocele. Genet Med. 7(6):457, 2005
2. Kannu P et al: Familial lipomyelomeningocele: a further report. Am J Med Genet A. 132(1):90-2, 2005
3. Rossi A et al: Spinal dysraphism: MR imaging rationale. J Neuroradiol. 31(1):3-24, 2004
4. Schoenmakers MA et al: Long-term outcome of neurosurgical untethering on neurosegmental motor and ambulation levels. Dev Med Child Neurol. 45(8):551-5, 2003
5. Bulsara KR et al: Clinical outcome differences for lipomyelomeningoceles, intraspinal lipomas, and lipomas of the filum terminale. Neurosurg Rev. 24(4):192-4, 2001
6. Tortori-Donati P et al: Magnetic resonance imaging of spinal dysraphism. Top Magn Reson Imaging. 12(6):375-409, 2001
7. Cochrane DD et al: The patterns of late deterioration in patients with transitional lipomyelomeningocele. Eur J Pediatr Surg. 10 Suppl 1:13-7, 2000
8. Colak A et al: Recurrent tethering: a common long-term problem after lipomyelomeningocele repair. Pediatr Neurosurg. 29(4):184-90, 1998
9. Wu HY et al: Long-term benefits of early neurosurgery for lipomyelomeningocele. J Urol. 160(2):511-4, 1998
10. Chreston J et al: Sonographic detection of lipomyelomeningocele: a retrospective documentation. J Clin Ultrasound. 25(1):50-1, 1997
11. Herman JM et al: Analysis of 153 patients with myelomeningocele or spinal lipoma reoperated upon for a tethered cord. Presentation, management and outcome. Pediatr Neurosurg. 19(5):243-9, 1993
12. Kanev PM et al: Management and long-term follow-up review of children with lipomyelomeningocele, 1952-1987. J Neurosurg. 73(1):48-52, 1990

# LIPOMYELOMENINGOCELE

## IMAGE GALLERY

### Typical

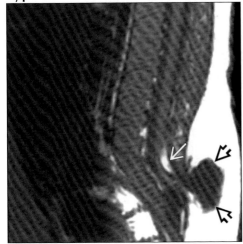
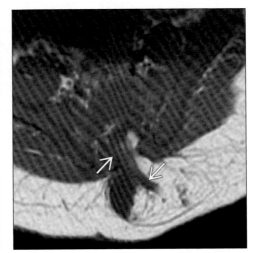

*(Left)* Sagittal T1WI MR demonstrates an elongated spinal cord with distal lipoma ➡️, that "balloons" through a posterior dysraphic defect into a CSF signal cyst ⮞, within the subcutaneous fat. *(Right)* Axial T1WI MR demonstrates insertion of the distal cord ➡️ into the rotated lipoma. The majority of the lipoma and cyst reside within the subcutaneous tissues.

### Typical

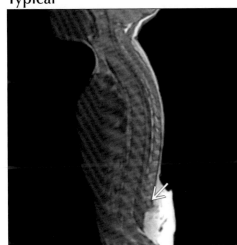
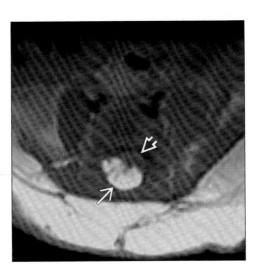

*(Left)* Sagittal T1WI MR shows an elongated spinal cord inserting into a large terminal lipomatous mass contiguous with subcutaneous fat. The last intact posterior elements are at L4 ➡️. *(Right)* Axial T1WI MR at the neural placode demonstrates fat invaginating into the neural placode, and rotation of the lipoma ➡️ and placode ⮞.

### Variant

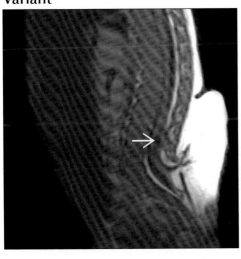
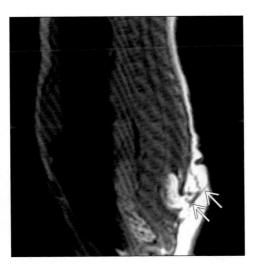

*(Left)* Sagittal T1WI MR reveals a low lying hydromyelic ➡️ spinal cord inserting into a lumbosacral lipomatous mass that extends into contiguous large subcutaneous lipoma. *(Right)* Sagittal T1WI MR reveals a low-lying spinal cord and dorsal lipoma extending through dysraphic defect into subcutaneous fat. Note hypointense dermal sinus tract ➡️ extends into the lipoma.

# DORSAL DERMAL SINUS

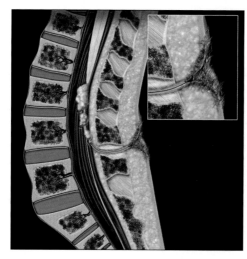

Sagittal graphic shows a dermal sinus with epidermoid extending from skin surface into spinal canal to terminate at conus. Skin dimple with hemangioma and hairy tuft mark sinus opening.

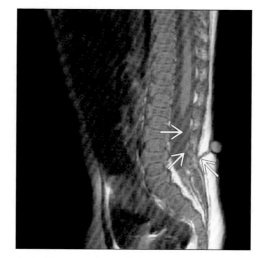

Sagittal T1WI MR shows a hypointense linear sinus tract → extending from skin surface dimple at L4-5, through L4-5 posterior elements into thecal sac, and terminating at conus.

## TERMINOLOGY

### Abbreviations and Synonyms
- Dermal sinus tract (DST)

### Definitions
- Midline/paramedian stratified squamous epithelial-lined sinus tract extending inward from skin surface for a variable distance

## IMAGING FINDINGS

### General Features
- Best diagnostic clue: Hypointense curvilinear tract superimposed on hyperintense subcutaneous fat
- Location: Lumbosacral (60%) > occipital (25%) > thoracic (10%) > cervical (1%)
- Size: Tract is thin (several mm); length variable
- Morphology
  ○ Subcutaneous tract +/- dysraphism
  ○ Length of tract varies; may end in subcutaneous tissue or extend to neural tissue

- Usually terminates conus medullaris (lumbosacral lesions) or central spinal canal (cervical, thoracic lesions)

### CT Findings
- CECT: +/- (Epi)dermoid, +/- ring-enhancement (abscess, arachnoiditis), or nerve root clumping [adhesive arachnoiditis; prior infection, (epi)dermoid rupture]
- Bone CT
  ○ Osseous findings range from normal → groove in lamina/spinous process → multilevel dysraphism

### MR Findings
- T1WI
  ○ Sinus tract hypointense to subcutaneous fat
    ▪ Curvilinear extraspinal tract passes inferiorly and ventrally to lumbodorsal fascia, turns upward to ascend within spinal canal
  ○ Dorsal dural tenting indicates → dural penetration
    ▪ Intradural sinus course nearly impossible to follow; indistinguishable from cauda equina, filum
  ○ +/- (Epi)dermoid cyst
    ▪ Dermoid: Hypo- → hyperintense (fat)

## DDx: Dorsal Dermal Sinus

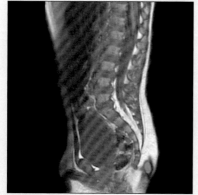

Coccygeal Dimple

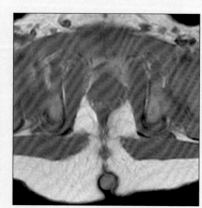

Coccygeal Dimple

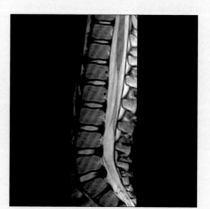

Epidermoid without DST

# DORSAL DERMAL SINUS

## Key Facts

### Terminology
- Dermal sinus tract (DST)

### Imaging Findings
- Best diagnostic clue: Hypointense curvilinear tract superimposed on hyperintense subcutaneous fat
- Osseous findings range from normal → groove in lamina/spinous process → multilevel dysraphism
- Dorsal dural tenting indicates → dural penetration
- Lumbosacral sinus ⇒ tethered cord, low-lying conus
- Thoracic, cervical sinuses ⇒ normal conus position

### Top Differential Diagnoses
- Low Sacrococcygeal Midline Dimple
- Pilonidal Sinus
- (Epi)dermoid Tumor without Dermal Sinus

### Pathology
- Focal incorporation of cutaneous ectoderm into neural ectoderm during disjunction at a circumscribed point only ⇒ focal segmental adhesion

### Clinical Issues
- Progressive neurological deterioration from cord tethering, (epi)dermoid enlargement, mass effect on spinal cord or cauda equina, sequelae of meningitis/abscess

### Diagnostic Checklist
- Dorsal dermal sinus must be differentiated from simple sacral dimple or pilonidal sinus
- Maintain a high index of suspicion for all dimples above intergluteal fold

---

- Epidermoid: Usually hypointense
- Extradural lesions may be subtle; look for nerve root or cord displacement
- Ruptured (epi)dermoid difficult to detect; look for nerve clumping, CSF "smudging"
  - +/- Tethered cord
    - Lumbosacral sinus ⇒ tethered cord, low-lying conus
    - Thoracic, cervical sinuses ⇒ normal conus position
- T2WI
  - May see hypointense tract in hyperintense CSF
  - +/- Hyperintense (epi)dermoid cyst
  - +/- Nerve root clumping (adhesive arachnoiditis)
- DWI: +/- Hyperintense epidermoid cyst
- T1 C+: +/- Intra/extramedullary abscess, infectious or chemical arachnoiditis

### Radiographic Findings
- Radiography: +/- Dysraphism, laminar defect

### Ultrasonographic Findings
- Grayscale Ultrasound
  - Shows entire length of tract from skin to spinal cord
    - Subcutaneous tract slightly hypoechoic, hard to detect
    - Echogenic subarachnoid tract clearly demonstrated within anechoic CSF
  - +/- Low-lying conus, thick filum, ↓ nerve mobility, intrathecal mass

### Non-Vascular Interventions
- Myelography: Dorsal dural tenting +/- (epi)dermoid, nerve root clumping

### Other Modality Findings
- Sagittal phase contrast cine MR
  - Loss of normal conus pulsation
  - Increased contrast between free-flowing CSF, solid epidermoid tumor

### Imaging Recommendations
- Best imaging tool: MR imaging
- Protocol advice

- Sagittal and axial T1WI, T2WI
  - Adjust window/level to best delineate subcutaneous tract
- Ultrasound supplements MR in infants < 1 year; use MR to confirm positive ultrasound study

## DIFFERENTIAL DIAGNOSIS

### Low Sacrococcygeal Midline Dimple
- 2-4% of infants
- Small (< 5 mm), low (< 2.5 cm from anus), extend inferiorly or horizontally toward coccyx
- Usually no associated masses, other cutaneous stigmata

### Pilonidal Sinus
- Common; nearly always incidental
- Low ostium, do not enter spinal canal

### (Epi)dermoid Tumor without Dermal Sinus
- No skin stigmata or sinus tract

## PATHOLOGY

### General Features
- General path comments
  - Three clinically important types of sinus tracts
    - Low sacral or coccygeal dermal sinuses form differently embryologically; always terminate in sacral or coccygeal fascia and never extend into subarachnoid space
    - Pilonidal sinus: Low ostium, do not enter spinal canal
    - Congenital dorsal dermal sinus + atypical dimple [large (> 5 mm), remote from anus (> 2.5 cm), combined with other lesions]
  - Midline dimple/pit is one of most common referrals to pediatric neurosurgeons
    - Regardless of depth, dimples below top of intergluteal crease end blindly and never extend intraspinally

# DORSAL DERMAL SINUS

- Sinus opening dermatomal level correlates with metameric cord level of attachment
- Etiology
  - Focal incorporation of cutaneous ectoderm into neural ectoderm during disjunction at a circumscribed point only ⇒ focal segmental adhesion
    - Spinal cord ascends relative to spinal canal, stretches adhesion into a long, tubular tract
- Epidemiology
  - Low sacrococcygeal dimple: 2-4% of all infants
  - Pilonidal sinus: Common
  - DST: Uncommon, midline > paramedian ostium
- Associated abnormalities
  - (Epi)dermoid tumor (30-50%)
    - Midline sinus ostia ⇒ usually dermoid
    - Paramedian ostia ⇒ epidermoid more common
    - May be multiple; most common at conus
  - Epidural/subdural abscess, meningitis, or intramedullary abscess 2° to bacteria ascending via tract
  - Lipoma (15-20%)
  - Cutaneous stigmata; angioma, pigment abnormalities, hypertrichosis, lipoma, skin tag, or (rarely) supranumerary sinus tracts

## Gross Pathologic & Surgical Features
- Sinus tract course varies short → long; may terminate extraspinal
- Intraspinal extension of sinus tract ≥ 50%
  - May terminate in subarachnoid space, conus medullaris, filum terminale, nerve root, fibrous nodule on cord surface, or (epi)dermoid cyst
- Palpable sinus tract
- (Epi)dermoid tumor
  - +/- Cheesy, oily material (dermoid) or discrete pearly white (epidermoid) tumor
  - Capsule often adherent to surrounding neural structures

## Microscopic Features
- Sinus tract lined by stratified squamous epithelium
- Epidermoid: Desquamated epithelium
- Dermoid: Skin adnexa

# CLINICAL ISSUES

## Presentation
- Most common signs/symptoms
  - Asymptomatic; incidentally noted skin dimple
  - Neurological deficits below level of tract secondary to tethering or cord compression
  - Other signs/symptoms
    - Meningitis, intraspinal abscess (retrograde passage of pathogens)
- Clinical Profile: Atypical sacral dimple with pinpoint ostium, cutaneous stigmata

## Demographics
- Age: Infancy through 3rd decade
- Gender: M = F

## Natural History & Prognosis
- Progressive neurological deterioration from cord tethering, (epi)dermoid enlargement, mass effect on spinal cord or cauda equina, sequelae of meningitis/abscess
  - Early surgical intervention ⇒ normal neurological development possible
- Most important factor influencing outcome is total excision of sinus before development of infection, neural compression

## Treatment
- Surgical excision of sinus tract, tethered cord release, and treatment of complications
- Long term antibiotics (if infected)

# DIAGNOSTIC CHECKLIST

## Consider
- Dorsal dermal sinus must be differentiated from simple sacral dimple or pilonidal sinus
- Regardless of depth, dimples below top of intergluteal crease end blindly and never extend intraspinally
- Maintain a high index of suspicion for all dimples above intergluteal fold

## Image Interpretation Pearls
- Critical to identify dermal sinus course and termination for surgical planning
- Up to 50% of dermal sinuses associated with (epi)dermoid tumor
- Dural "nipple" on sagittal image indicates dural penetration

# SELECTED REFERENCES

1. Gupta DK et al: An unusual presentation of lumbosacral dermal sinus with CSF leak and meningitis. A case report and review of the literature. Pediatr Neurosurg. 41(2):98-101, 2005
2. Tubbs RS et al: Isolated flat capillary midline lumbosacral hemangiomas as indicators of occult spinal dysraphism. J Neurosurg. 100(2):86-9, 2004
3. Ackerman LL et al: Spinal congenital dermal sinuses: a 30-year experience. Pediatrics. 112(3 Pt 1):641-7, 2003
4. Shah RK et al: Lower cervical dermal sinus tract and associated intraspinal abscess causing meningitis in a child. Emerg Radiol. 10(3):160-2, 2003
5. Ackerman LL et al: Cervical and thoracic dermal sinus tracts. A case series and review of the literature. Pediatr Neurosurg. 37(3):137-47, 2002
6. Lin KL et al: Sonography for detection of spinal dermal sinus tracts. J Ultrasound Med. 21(8):903-7, 2002
7. Aydin K et al: Thoracocervical dorsal dermal sinus associated with multiple vertebral body anomalies. Neuroradiology. 43(12):1084-6, 2001
8. Unsinn KM et al: US of the spinal cord in newborns: spectrum of normal findings, variants, congenital anomalies, and acquired diseases. Radiographics. 20(4):923-38, 2000
9. Weprin BE et al: Coccygeal pits. Pediatrics. 105(5):E69, 2000
10. Kanev PM et al: Dermoids and dermal sinus tracts of the spine. Neurosurg Clin N Am. 6(2):359-66, 1995

## IMAGE GALLERY

### Variant

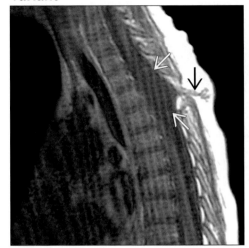 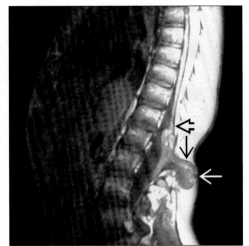

*(Left)* Sagittal T1WI MR demonstrates a thoracic dermal sinus tract ➡ with associated intradural (epi)dermoid tumor ➡. The dura tents outward at the point of sinus tract entry. *(Right)* Sagittal T1WI MR shows a large dermoid tumor ➡ within the spinal canal, backfilling the dermal sinus tract nearly to the cutaneous opening ➡ and tethering the low-lying conus ⇗.

### Variant

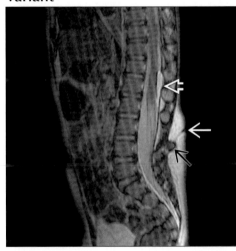 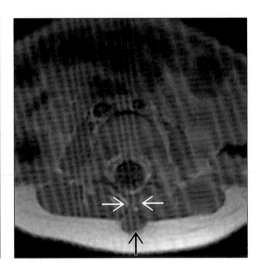

*(Left)* Sagittal T2WI MR demonstrates lumbar skin dimple ➡ with dermal sinus tract containing a small dermoid ➡. Low-lying spinal cord is affixed to dorsal lipoma ⇗. *(Right)* Axial T1 C+ MR confirms mild posterior dysraphism ➡ permitting the sinus tract access to thecal sac. The dermoid ➡ resides within the sinus tract, dorsal to the spinous process.

### Variant

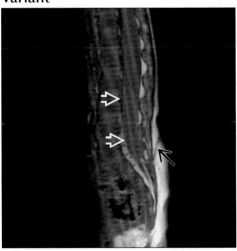 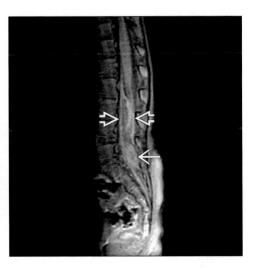

*(Left)* Sagittal T1WI MR in meningitis patient shows hypointense subcutaneous tract ➡ and abnormal intradural mass ⇗ (abscess, dermoid at surgery) filling the thecal sac. *(Right)* Sagittal T1 C+ MR confirms a mildly enhancing infected dermoid in the lower lumbar canal ➡ with peripherally enhancing intradural abscess collection rostrally ⇗.

# DERMOID AND EPIDERMOID TUMORS

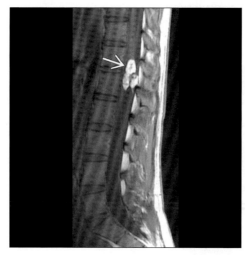

Sagittal T1WI MR shows a hyperintense mass ➡ in the region of the conus medullaris. The mass appears to be both intra- and extramedullary. T1 hyperintensity suggests dermoid.

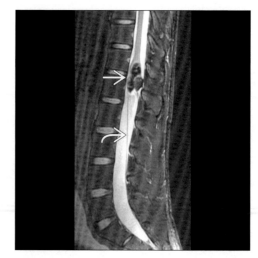

Sagittal T2WI MR using a fast steady state acquisition technique shows the mass ➡ to be markedly hypointense. Note the very straight, thick filum terminale ➡, which suggests tethering.

## TERMINOLOGY

### Abbreviations and Synonyms
- (Epi)dermoid, (epi)dermoid cyst

### Definitions
- Benign spinal tumor composed of cells that embryologically comprise skin and its appendages (hair follicles, sweat glands, and sebaceous glands)

## IMAGING FINDINGS

### General Features
- Best diagnostic clue: Lumbosacral or cauda equina CSF isointense/isodense mass
- Location
  - 40% intramedullary, 60% extramedullary; extradural rare
    - Dermoid: Lumbosacral (60%), cauda equina (20%), infrequent in the cervical and thoracic spine

- Epidermoid: Upper thoracic (17%), lower thoracic (26%), lumbosacral (22%), and cauda equina (35%)
  - Acquired epidermoids almost uniformly occur at cauda equina
- Size: Range: Tiny subpial masses → huge growths
- Morphology
  - Uni- or multilobular round/ovoid mass
  - Look for associated dermal sinus (in 15-20%)

### CT Findings
- CECT
  - Dermoid: Well-demarcated isodense mass ± regions of fat hypodensity, calcification
    - ± Minimal enhancement
  - Epidermoid: Well-circumscribed hypodense mass with attenuation similar to CSF ± calcification (rare)
    - Rarely hyperdense on nonenhanced images reflecting high protein content, hemorrhage, or cellular debris
    - Minimal to no enhancement unless infected
- Bone CT

---

## DDx: (Epi)dermoid Mimics

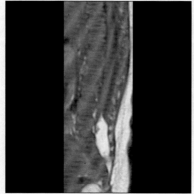

*Tethering Lipoma*

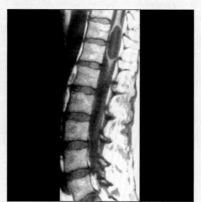

*Ventriculus Terminalis*

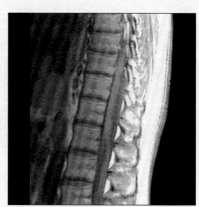

*Neurenteric Cyst*

# DERMOID AND EPIDERMOID TUMORS

## Key Facts

### Terminology
- (Epi)dermoid, (epi)dermoid cyst

### Imaging Findings
- 40% intramedullary, 60% extramedullary; extradural rare
- Dermoid: Well-demarcated isodense mass ± regions of fat hypodensity, calcification
- Epidermoid: Well-circumscribed hypodense mass with attenuation similar to CSF ± calcification (rare)
- Dermoid: T1 hypo- to hyperintense signal intensity mass
- Epidermoid: Usually T1 isointense to CSF, occasionally mildly hyperintense
- DWI: Distinguishes epidermoid (hyperintense) from arachnoid cyst (isointense to CSF)

### Top Differential Diagnoses
- Arachnoid Cyst
- Neurenteric Cyst

### Pathology
- Congenital (100% dermoid, 60% epidermoid)
- Acquired (40% epidermoid)

### Clinical Issues
- Slowly progressive compressive radiculopathy/myelopathy

### Diagnostic Checklist
- Diagnosis requires high index of suspicion; look for mass effect on regional structures
- FLAIR and DWI may distinguish epidermoid from CSF, arachnoid cyst

---

- Focal osseous erosion, spinal canal widening, flattening of pedicles and laminae at spinal level of mass

## MR Findings
- T1WI
  - Dermoid: T1 hypo- to hyperintense signal intensity mass
    - Hypointensity may reflect increased water content from sweat gland secretions
    - Fat hyperintensity is most specific for dermoid but least common appearance; intrinsic T1 shortening permits differentiation of dermoid from epidermoid
  - Epidermoid: Usually T1 isointense to CSF, occasionally mildly hyperintense
- T2WI
  - Typically, both show high T2 signal intensity
  - Dermoids may be very hypointense
- FLAIR: Mild hyperintensity to CSF may help detect occult epidermoid tumor, differentiate from arachnoid cyst
- DWI: Distinguishes epidermoid (hyperintense) from arachnoid cyst (isointense to CSF)
- T1 C+: ± Mild ring-enhancement; more avid contrast-enhancement if infected

## Radiographic Findings
- Radiography: Focal vertebral osseous erosion, spinal canal widening, and flattening of pedicles and laminae

## Ultrasonographic Findings
- Grayscale Ultrasound: Hypoechoic mass lesion with internal echoes, focal areas of hyperechogenicity (if fat present → dermoid)

## Non-Vascular Interventions
- Myelography
  - CSF or fat density mass adjacent to bright CSF; most useful in conjunction with CT
  - Frequently myelographic block if symptomatic
  - Largely replaced by FLAIR, DWI MR

## Imaging Recommendations
- Best imaging tool: MR; reserve CT myelography for patients with MR contraindications, inconclusive MR studies
- Protocol advice: Sagittal and axial T1WI and T2WI MR to include entire conus and cauda equina to coccyx

---

# DIFFERENTIAL DIAGNOSIS

## Arachnoid Cyst
- Follows CSF signal intensity/density on all sequences
- DWI MR useful to distinguish arachnoid cyst (isointense to CSF) from epidermoid (hyperintense)

## Neurenteric Cyst
- Intradural cyst; usually ventral to cord but may be dorsal or intramedullary
- ± Vertebral anomalies, hyperdense/hyperintense proteinaceous content
- Definitive diagnosis is pathological

---

# PATHOLOGY

## General Features
- General path comments: Benign tumor arising from cells that produce skin and its appendages (hair follicles, sweat glands, sebaceous glands)
- Etiology
  - Congenital (100% dermoid, 60% epidermoid)
    - Arise from dermal/epidermal rests or focal expansion of a dermal sinus
  - Acquired (40% epidermoid)
    - Iatrogenic lesion resulting from implantation of viable dermal and epidermal elements following lumbar puncture (non-trocar spinal needle) or following surgery (myelomeningocele closure)
    - Cells slowly grow until large enough to cause symptoms

# DERMOID AND EPIDERMOID TUMORS

- Link between lumbar puncture and subsequent epidermoid tumor is particularly strong in neonatal period
- Epidemiology
  - (Epi)dermoid comprise 1-2% of all spinal cord tumors, up to 10% of spinal cord tumors under age 15 years
  - Dermoid and epidermoid occur roughly equally in spine; ~ 40% single epidermoid, 35% single dermoid, and 5% multiple dermoid or epidermoid
- Associated abnormalities
  - Dermal sinus (15-20%)
  - Vertebral abnormalities (diastematomyelia, hemivertebra, scoliosis)
  - Closed dysraphism (anterior sacral meningocele, "spina bifida occulta") rare

## Gross Pathologic & Surgical Features

- Epidermoid
  - Striking white pearly sheen capsule; may be smooth, lobulated, or nodular
  - Cyst filled with creamy, waxy, pearly material
  - Either easy to shell out or firmly affixed to regional structures (result of local inflammation)
- Dermoid
  - Well-demarcated smooth mass; wall may be thickened by skin appendages or calcifications
  - Cyst filled with thick cheesy, buttery, yellowish material

## Microscopic Features

- Epidermoid
  - Outer connective tissue capsule lined with stratified squamous epithelium; calcification rare
  - Centrally contains desquamated epithelial keratin, cholesterol crystals; positive staining with antibodies to EMA and cytokeratin
- Dermoid
  - Uni- or multilocular; outer connective tissue capsule lined with stratified squamous epithelium containing hair follicles, sebaceous glands, and sweat glands
  - ± Inflammation (if ruptured)
  - Centrally contains desquamated epithelial keratin, lipid material

## CLINICAL ISSUES

### Presentation

- Most common signs/symptoms
  - Asymptomatic
  - Slowly progressive compressive radiculopathy/myelopathy
  - Other signs/symptoms
    - Cauda equina syndrome
    - Acute chemical meningitis secondary to rupture and discharge of inflammatory cholesterol crystals into CSF
    - Recurrent bacterial meningitis; most common in association with dermal sinus

### Demographics

- Age

---

- Dermoids usually cause symptoms during childhood
- Epidermoids are slower growing; symptoms usually arise in early adulthood
- Gender
  - Dermoids M = F
  - Epidermoids M > F

## Natural History & Prognosis

- Symptoms slowly progress if untreated
- Complete surgical resection offers best opportunity for good neurologic outcome
  - Incomplete resection frequently recurs; malignant transformation very rare

## Treatment

- Standard treatment is complete surgical excision
- Radiotherapy not established for the treatment of epidermoid cysts
  - May be an alternative to palliative operation or for patients who cannot undergo surgery

## DIAGNOSTIC CHECKLIST

### Consider

- Dermoid is a congenital lesion and presents during childhood/adolescence
- Epidermoid may be congenital or acquired, and usually arises in teens or adults
- Look for associated dermal sinus

### Image Interpretation Pearls

- Epidermoids/dermoids are frequently difficult to diagnosis on CT and MR
  - Diagnosis requires high index of suspicion; look for mass effect on regional structures
  - FLAIR and DWI may distinguish epidermoid from CSF, arachnoid cyst

## SELECTED REFERENCES

1. Chandra PS et al: Association of craniovertebral and upper cervical anomalies with dermoid and epidermoid cysts: report of four cases. Neurosurgery. 56(5):E1155; discussion E1155, 2005
2. Najjar MW et al: Dorsal intramedullary dermoids. Neurosurg Rev. 28(4):320-5, 2005
3. Ziv ET et al: Iatrogenic intraspinal epidermoid tumor: two cases and a review of the literature. Spine. 29(1):E15-8, 2004
4. Bretz A et al: Intraspinal epidermoid cyst successfully treated with radiotherapy: case report. Neurosurgery. 53(6):1429-31; discussion 1431-2, 2003
5. Amato VG et al: Intramedullary epidermoid cyst: preoperative diagnosis and surgical management after MRI introduction. Case report and updating of the literature. J Neurosurg Sci. 46(3-4):122-6, 2002
6. Graham D et al: Greenfield's Neuropathology. 7th ed. London, Arnold. 964-66, 2002
7. Kikuchi K et al: The utility of diffusion-weighted imaging with navigator-echo technique for the diagnosis of spinal epidermoid cysts. AJNR Am J Neuroradiol. 21(6):1164-6, 2000
8. Potgieter S et al: Epidermoid tumours associated with lumbar punctures performed in early neonatal life. Dev Med Child Neurol. 40(4):266-9, 1998

# DERMOID AND EPIDERMOID TUMORS

## IMAGE GALLERY

### Typical

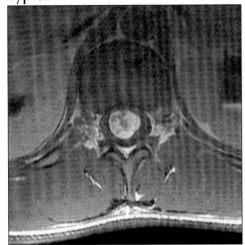 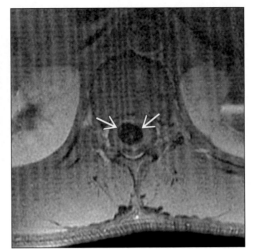

*(Left) Axial T1WI MR in the same patient as previous images shows the heterogeneous, hyperintense mass filling much of the spinal canal. (Right) Axial T1WI FS MR shows that the hyperintense signal completely disappears after ➡ application of the fat-suppression pulse, proving that the hyperintensity was due to fat in a dermoid.*

### Typical

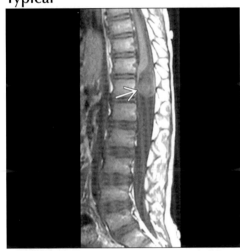 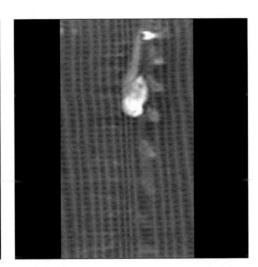

*(Left) Sagittal T1WI MR shows heterogeneous, mixed intensity mass ➡ in the region of the conus medullaris, displacing the cord tissue anteriorly. (Right) Sagittal DWI MR shows the mass to be hyperintense, indicating reduced diffusivity. This is a common finding in dermoid and epidermoid tumors.*

### Typical

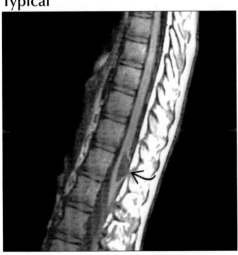 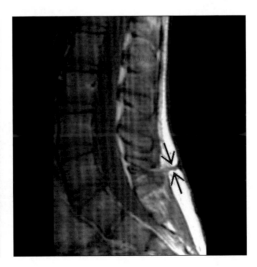

*(Left) Sagittal T1 C+ MR shows a hypointense intramedullary mass ➡ in the conus medullaris, expanding the cord at that location. No enhancement was seen after contrast administration. (Right) Axial T1WI MR shows defect ➡ in the subcutaneous fat at the lower lumbar level at the site of a cutaneous dimple; this was a dermal sinus. Conus lesion was a dermoid at the end of the sinus.*

# SEGMENTAL SPINAL DYSGENESIS

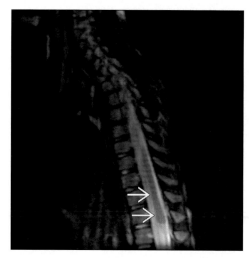

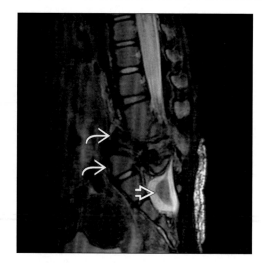

*Sagittal T2WI MR shows abnormally high termination of spinal cord* ➔ *within the thoracic region. Note abnormally shaped, blunted (instead of smoothly tapered) termination of spinal cord.*

*Sagittal T2WI MR (same patient as previous image) shows multiple dysplastic vertebrae* ➔ *in lumbar regions with severe kyphos and severe stenosis. Normal appearing distal cord* ➔ *is seen at level of sacrum.*

## TERMINOLOGY

### Abbreviations and Synonyms
- Segmental spinal dysgenesis (SSD), focal spinal hypoplasia

### Definitions
- Malformation characterized by region of dysmorphic, hypoplastic vertebrae and hypoplastic meninges and spinal cord between normal regions above and below

## IMAGING FINDINGS

### General Features
- Best diagnostic clue: Acute kyphosis with associated dysmorphic vertebrae and narrow canal
- Location: Lower thoracic and upper-mid lumbar spine

### CT Findings
- NECT
  - Region of several dysplastic vertebrae with acute, focal, severe kyphosis

- From rostral to caudal, vertebrae (bodies & posterior elements) become progressively more dysplastic & less completely segmented, then less dysplastic & better segmented
- Spinal canal narrows, then enlarges again
- Most common location: Caudal thoracic and lumbar regions
- CECT
  - CT myelography with intrathecal contrast
    - As vertebrae become dysplastic, thecal sac narrows, then nearly completely terminates
    - Spinal cord narrows and disappears rostral to sac
    - Below the dysplastic segment, thecal sac reappears
    - Spinal cord reappears caudal to reappearance of thecal sac

### MR Findings
- Dysplastic vertebrae are seen, similar to on CT
- Vertebrae, cord have normal signal intensity
- Spinal cord narrows, terminates at the upper level of dysplastic vertebrae
  - Termination of cord is blunted, often wedge-shaped
- Cord reappears below the dysplastic segments; has normal appearance

## DDx: Causes of Kyphosis

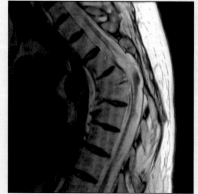

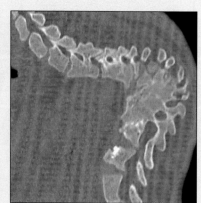

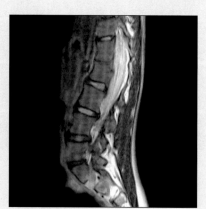

*Trauma*

*Post Infection*

*Segmentation Anomaly*

# SEGMENTAL SPINAL DYSGENESIS

## Key Facts

### Terminology
- Malformation characterized by region of dysmorphic, hypoplastic vertebrae and hypoplastic meninges and spinal cord between normal regions above and below

### Imaging Findings
- Location: Lower thoracic and upper-mid lumbar spine
- Region of small, dysplastic vertebrae, typically in lower thoracic or in lumbar spine

- Vertebrae, cord have normal signal intensity
- Spinal cord narrows, terminates at the upper level of dysplastic vertebrae
- Cord reappears below the dysplastic segments; has normal appearance

### Clinical Issues
- Progressive kyphosis as fetus or neonate
- Associated renal anomalies, neurogenic bladder
- Treat by bracing, then spinal fusion

---

- Termination of cord is often low (sacral levels)

## Radiographic Findings
- Radiography
  - Region of small, dysplastic vertebrae, typically in lower thoracic or in lumbar spine
  - Incomplete segmentation
  - Narrowing of spinal canal

## Imaging Recommendations
- Best imaging tool: MR
- Protocol advice: Thin-section sagittal, axial images

## DIFFERENTIAL DIAGNOSIS

### Osteomyelitis/Infection
- Severe kyphosis
- Normal thecal sac

### Post-Traumatic Myelomalacia
- Abnormal T2 hyperintensity ± hypointensity in narrowed cord

### Segmentation Anomaly
- Hemivertebrae, butterfly vertebrae

## PATHOLOGY

### General Features
- Etiology: Unknown: Probably malexpression of segmental genes

- Epidemiology: Very rare, occurs in neonates & infants

## Gross Pathologic & Surgical Features
- Dysplastic, incompletely segmented vertebrae
- Profoundly narrow spinal canal

## CLINICAL ISSUES

### Presentation
- Most common signs/symptoms
  - Progressive kyphosis as fetus or neonate
  - Variable lower extremity weakness, spasticity
- Other signs/symptoms
  - Associated renal anomalies, neurogenic bladder
  - May be associated with caudal regression

### Natural History & Prognosis
- Progressive deformity

### Treatment
- Treat by bracing, then spinal fusion

## SELECTED REFERENCES

1. Bristol RE et al: Segmental spinal dysgenesis: report of four cases and proposed management strategy. Childs Nerv Syst. 2006
2. Tortori-Donati P et al: Segmental spinal dysgenesis: neuroradiologic findings with clinical and embryologic correlation. AJNR Am J Neuroradiol. 20(3):445-56, 1999

III

6

19

## IMAGE GALLERY

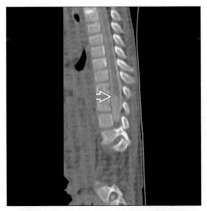 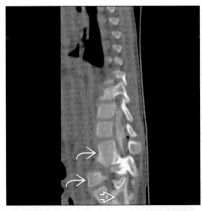 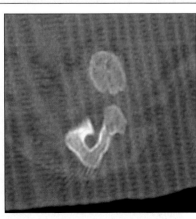

*(Left)* Sagittal CECT reformation with intrathecal contrast shows blunted cord termination ➾ above abrupt spinal curvature and apparent termination of thecal sac. *(Center)* Sagittal CECT reformation with intrathecal contrast (same patient as previous image) shows thecal sac terminating rostral to kyphosis & dysplastic vertebrae ➾. Normal thecal sac & cord ➾ appear below. *(Right)* Axial NECT shows very dysplastic vertebral body & posterior elements at site of the stenosis & kyphosis. Spinal canal is extremely small & thecal sac transiently terminates.

# CAUDAL REGRESSION SYNDROME

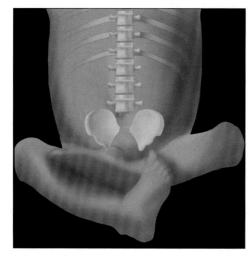

Coronal graphic of fetus demonstrates agenesis of the sacral vertebra, with medial displacement of the small iliac wings. The feet demonstrate talipes equinovarus (clubfoot) configuration.

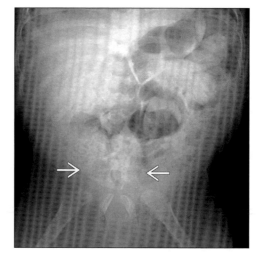

Anteroposterior radiograph demonstrates severe group 1 CRS, with the last intact vertebral body at approximately L3. Hypoplastic iliac wings ➔ are medially positioned.

## TERMINOLOGY

### Abbreviations and Synonyms
- Caudal regression syndrome (CRS), sacral agenesis, lumbosacral dysgenesis

### Definitions
- Constellation of caudal developmental growth abnormalities with associated regional soft tissue anomalies

## IMAGING FINDINGS

### General Features
- Best diagnostic clue: Dysgenetic lumbosacral vertebrae with abnormal distal spinal cord
- Location: Lumbosacral spine
- Size: Variable diminution of caudal spine
- Morphology
  - Spectrum ranging in severity from absent coccyx to complete lumbosacral agenesis
    - Partial or total unilateral dysgenesis with oblique lumbosacral joint

- Bilateral total lumbosacral agenesis; vertebral column terminates in thoracic spine
  - Caudal vertebral bodies often dysmorphic/fused
  - Severe canal narrowing rostral to last intact vertebra
    - Osseous vertebral excrescences, fibrous bands connecting bifid spinous processes, or severe distal dural tube stenosis

### CT Findings
- CECT: Lumbosacral dysgenesis with distal spinal stenosis

### MR Findings
- T1WI
  - Vertebral body dysgenesis/hypogenesis
  - Group 1: Distal spinal cord hypoplasia ("wedge-shaped" cord termination), severe sacral osseous anomalies
    - +/- Dilated central canal, conus cerebrospinal fluid (CSF) cyst
  - Group 2: Tapered, low-lying, distal cord elongation with tethering, less severe sacral anomalies
- T2WI: Same findings as T1WI; best for depicting dural stenosis

## DDx: Caudal Regression Syndrome

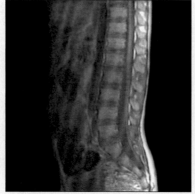

Tethered Spinal Cord

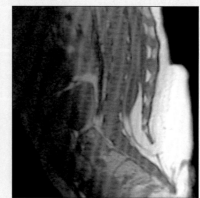

Lipomyelomeningocele

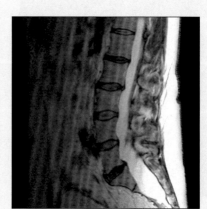

Intrasacral Meningocele

# CAUDAL REGRESSION SYNDROME

## Key Facts

### Terminology
- Caudal regression syndrome (CRS), sacral agenesis, lumbosacral dysgenesis

### Imaging Findings
- Best diagnostic clue: Dysgenetic lumbosacral vertebrae with abnormal distal spinal cord
- Spectrum ranging in severity from absent coccyx to complete lumbosacral agenesis
- Group 1: Blunt spinal cord termination above L1; central canal may be prominent
- Group 2: Elongated conus with thick filum +/- intraspinal lipoma

### Top Differential Diagnoses
- Tethered Spinal Cord
- Closed Spinal Dysraphism

- Occult Intrasacral Meningocele (OIM)

### Pathology
- Most severe cases ⇒ sirenomelia ("mermaid")
- Most cases sporadic
- 1/7,500 births (milder forms > severe forms)
- 15-20% are infants of diabetic mothers; 1% of offspring from diabetic mothers affected
- Genitourinary abnormalities (24%)

### Diagnostic Checklist
- MR imaging most useful imaging tool for characterizing abnormalities and surgical planning
- Caudal spine anomalies should be sought out in patients with genitourinary or anorectal anomalies and vice versa

---

- T1 C+: Hypertrophied dorsal root ganglia (DRG)/nerve roots may enhance

## Radiographic Findings
- Radiography: Dysgenetic/hypogenetic lumbosacral vertebrae

## Ultrasonographic Findings
- Grayscale Ultrasound
  - Group 1: Blunt spinal cord termination above L1; central canal may be prominent
  - Group 2: Elongated conus with thick filum +/- intraspinal lipoma

## Non-Vascular Interventions
- Myelography: Caudal hypogenesis +/- dural stenosis; most useful in conjunction with CT

## Imaging Recommendations
- Consider ultrasound for infant screening
- MR imaging to confirm ultrasound findings, treatment planning
  - Sagittal MR to demonstrate extent of lumbosacral deficiency, distal spinal cord morphology, and presence/absence of tethering
  - Axial MR to detect osseous spinal narrowing, hydromyelia, other associated lesions

## DIFFERENTIAL DIAGNOSIS

### Tethered Spinal Cord
- Low-lying spinal cord +/- thickened or fatty filum, no caudal dysgenesis
- Difficult to clinically discern from mild sacral dysgenesis
  - +/- Associated imaging abnormalities may help distinguish

### Closed Spinal Dysraphism
- Dorsal dysraphism without severe vertebral column agenesis

### Occult Intrasacral Meningocele (OIM)
- Sacrum thinned and remodeled, sometimes imitating caudal regression

## PATHOLOGY

### General Features
- General path comments
  - Sequela of caudal cell mass dysplasia with spectrum of severity
  - Lower extremity deformities, lumbosacral agenesis, anorectal abnormalities, renal/pulmonary hypoplasia characteristic
    - Most severe cases ⇒ sirenomelia ("mermaid")
    - 20% ⇒ tethering subcutaneous lesions (group 2)
- Genetics
  - Most cases sporadic
  - Dominantly inherited form recently described; defect in the HLBX9 homeobox gene (chromosome 7)
    - HLBX9 also expressed in pancreas ⇒ possible association between diabetic hyperglycemia and caudal regression
- Etiology
  - Normal caudal spine development ⇒ canalization and retrogressive differentiation
    - Anorectal and genitourinary structures form contemporaneously in close anatomic proximity
  - Disruption prior to 4th gestational week ⇒ caudal cell mass developmental abnormalities
    - Hyperglycemia, infectious, toxic, or ischemic insult postulated to impair spinal cord, vertebral formation
    - Signaling defects by retinoic acid and sonic hedgehog during blastogenesis and gastrulation
    - Abnormal neural tube, notochord development ⇒ impaired migration of neurons and mesodermal cells
- Epidemiology
  - 1/7,500 births (milder forms > severe forms)

# CAUDAL REGRESSION SYNDROME

- 15-20% are infants of diabetic mothers; 1% of offspring from diabetic mothers affected
- Association with VACTERL (10%), omphalocele, exstrophy bladder, imperforate anus, spinal anomalies (10%), and Currarino triad syndromic complexes
- Associated abnormalities
  - Tethered cord
    - ≈ 100% of CRS patients with conus terminating below L1
    - Thickened filum (65%) +/- dermoid or lipoma
  - Other spinal anomalies
    - Vertebral anomalies (22%), diastematomyelia, terminal hydromyelia (10%), myelomeningocele (35-50%), lipomyelomeningocele (10-20%), terminal myelocystocele (15%), anterior sacral meningocele
  - Congential cardiac defects (24%), pulmonary hypoplasia
  - Genitourinary abnormalities (24%)
    - Renal agenesis/ectopia, hydronephrosis, Müllerian duct malformations, urinary bladder malformation
  - Anorectal anomalies (particularly anal atresia)
    - Higher level of anal atresia ⇒ more severe lumbosacral dysgenesis, genitourinary anomalies
  - Orthopedic abnormalities; extreme cases ⇒ lower extremity fusion (sirenomelia)

## Gross Pathologic & Surgical Features
- Severity of vertebral dysgenesis, presence/absence of tethering, and osseous canal diameter impact surgical planning

## Microscopic Features
- Findings typical for tissue content

## Staging, Grading or Classification Criteria
- Group 1: More severe caudal dysgenesis with high-lying, club-shaped cord terminus (decreased number of anterior horn cells)
  - Distal cord hypoplasia with wedging seen in all with partial/complete dysgenesis and termination of spinal cord above L1
  - Termination of conus above L1 highly correlated with sacral malformations ending at S1 or above
- Group 2: Less severe dysgenesis with low-lying, tapered, distal cord tethered by tight filum, lipoma, lipomyelomeningocele, or terminal myelocystocele
  - Conus termination below L1 highly correlated with sacral malformations ending at S2 or below
  - Tethering is thus more common in milder sacral dysgenesis

# CLINICAL ISSUES

## Presentation
- Most common signs/symptoms
  - Neurogenic urinary bladder dysfunction (nearly all patients)
  - Sensorimotor paresis (group 2 > group 1)
    - Severity of motor deficit > sensory

- Sacral sensory sparing common, even in severe cases
  - Neurologically asymptomatic (group 1 > group 2)
- Clinical Profile
  - Broad clinical spectrum but always have narrow hips, hypoplastic gluteal muscles, shallow intergluteal cleft
  - Neurologic symptoms/signs range from mild foot disorders ⇒ complete lower extremity paralysis and distal leg atrophy
    - Motor level usually higher than sensory level
    - Level of vertebral aplasia correlates with motor but not sensory level

## Demographics
- Age
  - Severe cases identified in utero (obstetrical ultrasound) or at birth
  - Mild cases may not be identified until adulthood
- Gender: M = F

## Natural History & Prognosis
- Variable depending on severity

## Treatment
- Surgical untethering if clinically symptomatic
- Surgical release/duraplasty may improve neurological function in patients with distal spinal canal stenosis
- Orthopedic procedures to improve lower extremity functionality

# DIAGNOSTIC CHECKLIST

## Consider
- MR imaging most useful imaging tool for characterizing abnormalities and surgical planning

## Image Interpretation Pearls
- Caudal spine anomalies should be sought out in patients with genitourinary or anorectal anomalies and vice versa

# SELECTED REFERENCES

1. Merello E et al: HLXB9 homeobox gene and caudal regression syndrome. Birth Defects Res A Clin Mol Teratol. 76(3):205-9, 2006
2. Nievelstein RA et al: Magnetic resonance imaging in children with anorectal malformations: embryologic implications. J Pediatr Surg. 37(8):1138-45, 2002
3. Tortori-Donati P et al: Spinal dysraphism: a review of neuroradiological features with embryological correlations and proposal for a new classification. Neuroradiology. 42(7):471-91, 2000
4. Heij HA et al: Abnormal anatomy of the lumbosacral region imaged by magnetic resonance in children with anorectal malformations. Arch Dis Child. 74(5):441-4, 1996
5. Long FR et al: Tethered cord and associated vertebral anomalies in children and infants with imperforate anus: evaluation with MR imaging and plain radiography. Radiology. 200(2):377-82, 1996
6. Pang D: Sacral agenesis and caudal spinal cord malformations. Neurosurgery. 32(5): 755-78, discussion 778-9, 1993

# CAUDAL REGRESSION SYNDROME

## IMAGE GALLERY

### Typical

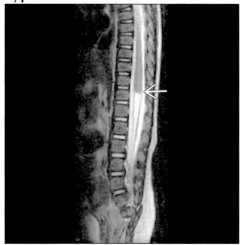
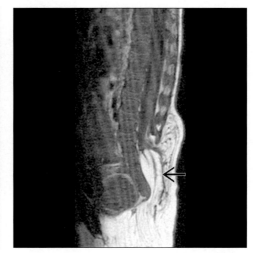

*(Left)* Sagittal T2WI MR (CRS group 1) demonstrates severe dysgenesis of the sacral vertebra and abrupt termination of the blunt "wedge-shaped" conus ➡ at T12. *(Right)* Sagittal T1WI MR (CRS group 2) reveals milder sacral dysgenesis and abnormal low-lying, tapered, tethered spinal cord terminating in a large terminal lipoma ➡.

### Typical

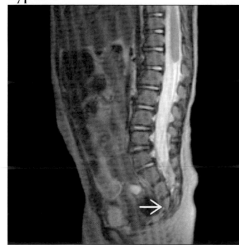
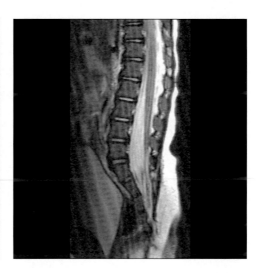

*(Left)* Sagittal T2WI MR (CRS group 1) shows a blunted spinal cord terminus ending at L1 vertebral level. The sacrum is hypoplastic, ending with a hypoplastic S4 vertebra ➡. S5 and coccyx are absent. *(Right)* Sagittal T2WI MR (CRS 2) demonstrates a mild variant of CRS, manifesting 4 sacral vertebrae with absence of S5 and the coccyx. The low-lying, tapered spinal cord is probably tethered.

### Variant

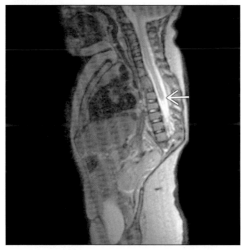
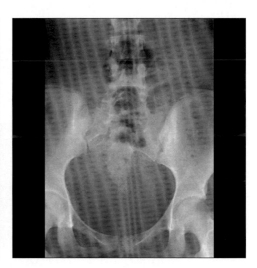

*(Left)* Sagittal T2WI MR (severe group 1 CRS) demonstrates high termination of "wedge-shaped" distal spinal cord ➡, lumbosacral agenesis, and multiple vertebral segmentation anomalies. *(Right)* Anteroposterior radiograph demonstrates partial absence of the left sacral alar wing (hemisacral agenesis).

# TETHERED SPINAL CORD

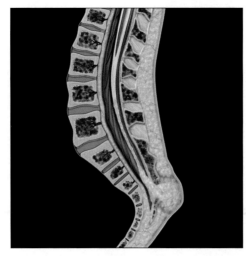

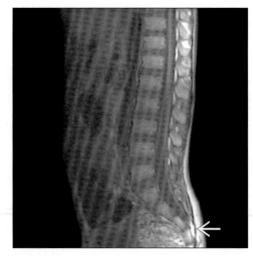

*Sagittal graphic shows a low-lying hydromyelic tethered cord with fibrolipoma inserting into a terminal lipoma. Lipoma is contiguous with subcutaneous fat through dorsal dysraphism.*

*Sagittal T1WI MR shows an elongated spinal cord extending to at least L5, subtly transitioning into a thickened filum terminale that terminates in a small terminal lipoma ➡.*

## TERMINOLOGY

### Abbreviations and Synonyms
- Tethered cord syndrome (TCS), tight filum terminale syndrome

### Definitions
- Symptoms and imaging findings referable to low-lying conus medullaris tethered by short, thick filum terminale

## IMAGING FINDINGS

### General Features
- Best diagnostic clue: Conus ends below L2 inferior endplate; tethered by thickened filum +/- fibrolipoma, terminal lipoma
- Location: Thoracolumbar junction → sacrum
- Size: Filum thickened (> 1 mm at L5-S1, axial MR)
- Morphology: Attenuated conus terminates lower than normal

### CT Findings
- NECT: Stretched, thinned cord with low-lying conus, thickened filum +/- fibrolipoma, dysraphism, vertebral segmentation and fusion anomalies

### MR Findings
- T1WI
  - Thickened filum +/- hyperintense lipoma
  - Filum thickness > 2 mm (L5-S1, axial MR)
  - +/- Low-lying conus; may be difficult to distinguish from thickened filum
  - Dorsal positioning of conus medullaris, filum terminale in thecal sac
    - Noted even in prone position; cord normally falls into anterior 2/3 of canal when prone
- T2WI
  - Findings similar to T1WI
  - +/- Hyperintense dilatation of conus central canal 2° to hydromyelia or myelomalacia (25%)
  - Fatty filum ⇒ chemical shift artifact
  - Dural sac widened; dorsal dura tense, tented posteriorly by thickened filum

## DDx: Tethered Cord Syndrome

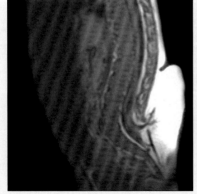

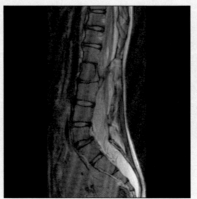

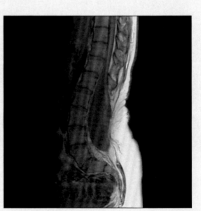

*Lipomyelomeningocele*

*Diastematomyelia*

*Post MMC Repair*

# TETHERED SPINAL CORD

## Key Facts

### Terminology
- Tethered cord syndrome (TCS), tight filum terminale syndrome
- Symptoms and imaging findings referable to low-lying conus medullaris tethered by short, thick filum terminale

### Imaging Findings
- Best diagnostic clue: Conus ends below L2 inferior endplate; tethered by thickened filum +/- fibrolipoma, terminal lipoma
- Size: Filum thickened (> 1 mm at L5-S1, axial MR)

### Top Differential Diagnoses
- Normal Variant Low-Lying Conus
- Open or Closed Spinal Dysraphism
- Post-Surgical Low-Lying Conus

### Pathology
- Widened dural sac; thickened filum closely applied to or indistinguishable from dural sac

### Clinical Issues
- Low back and leg pain; worst in morning, exacerbated by exertion
- Urinary bladder dysfunction

### Diagnostic Checklist
- Tethered cord syndrome is a clinical diagnosis; imaging role is detection of low-lying conus/thick filum, associated anatomic abnormalities for surgical decision making
- Measure filum thickness at L5/S1; stretching at more rostral levels may erroneously thin filum into "normal" size range

## Radiographic Findings
- Radiography
  - May be normal, but nearly always shows localized dysraphism or incomplete posterior fusion
  - +/- Scoliosis (20%)

## Ultrasonographic Findings
- Grayscale Ultrasound: +/- Low-lying conus, thickened filum terminale, reduced or absent spinal cord movement

## Other Modality Findings
- Phase contrast (PC) MR
  - ↓ Spinal cord motion
  - ≤ 1/3 show return of normal cord motion after untethering, even if symptoms resolve

## Imaging Recommendations
- Best imaging tool: Multiplanar MR
- Protocol advice
  - Ultrasound < 6 months old; confirm positive study with MR
  - Thin-section sagittal, axial T1WI and T2WI, phase contrast MR; extend axial slices to thecal sac termination

## DIFFERENTIAL DIAGNOSIS

### Normal Variant Low-Lying Conus
- Asymptomatic patient with normal filum thickness

### Open or Closed Spinal Dysraphism
- Spinal lipoma, myelomeningocele (MMC), meningocele, (epi)dermoid, diastematomyelia, dermal sinus tract

### Post-Surgical Low-Lying Conus
- Imaging shows low-lying conus irrespective of symptoms
  - Ultrasound, PC MR helpful to evaluate conus motion

  - Cannot exclude re-tethering by imaging alone; diagnosis must be made on clinical grounds

## PATHOLOGY

### General Features
- General path comments
  - Incomplete retrogressive differentiation with failure of terminal cord involution or failure of filum terminale to lengthen
  - Conus normally terminates at or above inferior L2 in ≥ 98% of normal population
    - Conus should be at normal position by birth → 2 months old
    - Conus terminating below L2/3 is always abnormal at any post-natal age
  - May not be distinct filum; spinal cord sometimes elongated, ends directly in small terminal lipoma
  - Significant number of patients presenting with typical clinical signs/symptoms of TCS show normal filum diameter, normal conus position
- Etiology: Tethering stretches nerve fibers, arterioles, and venules ⇒ impairs oxidative metabolism of conus and nerve roots ⇒ abnormal lumbosacral function
- Epidemiology: Prevalence unknown; probably more common than appreciated
- Associated abnormalities
  - Lumbosacral hypogenesis, VACTERL syndrome
  - Open or closed spinal dysraphism, incomplete posterior fusion (up to 100%)
    - Diastematomyelia, spinal lipoma, intrasacral or dorsal meningocele, lipomyelomeningocele, myelomeningocele
  - Cutaneous stigmata (50%)
  - Hydromyelia/myelomalacia (25%)
  - Scoliosis (functional adaption to ↓ length of spinal cord course, ↓ intramedullary tension)

### Gross Pathologic & Surgical Features
- Widened dural sac; thickened filum closely applied to or indistinguishable from dural sac

# TETHERED SPINAL CORD

- Thickened fibrotic filum (55%), small fibrolipoma within thickened filum (23%), or filar cyst (3%)
- Lack of viscoelasticity by filum stretch test during surgery

## Microscopic Features
- Tethered filum histologically abnormal, even if conus terminates at normal level
  - Normal filum ⇒ mainly collagen fibers
  - TCS filum ⇒ more connective tissue with dense collagen fibers, hyalinization and dilated capillaries, displacement of glial tissue

# CLINICAL ISSUES

## Presentation
- Most common signs/symptoms
  - Low back and leg pain; worst in morning, exacerbated by exertion
  - Gait spasticity, weakness, muscular atrophy
  - ↓ Sensation, abnormal lower extremity reflexes
  - Urinary bladder dysfunction
  - Orthopedic foot abnormalities (usually clubfoot)
  - Cutaneous stigmata (≤ 50%); simple dimple, hairy tuft, or hemangioma
- Clinical Profile
  - Adults and children present differently
    - Adults: Pain first (2° degenerative changes), followed later by weakness +/- incontinence
    - Children: Incontinence, scoliosis, weakness

## Demographics
- Age: Symptomatic presentation most common during rapid somatic growth (adolescent growth spurt, school age 4-8 years), or in elderly 2° kyphosis
- Gender: M = F

## Natural History & Prognosis
- Progressive, irreversible neurological impairment
  - Majority of patients show improvement or stabilization of neurological deficits following surgical untethering; motor weakness (12-60%), sensory dysfunction (40-60%), pain (50-88%), bladder dysfunction (19-67%)
  - Better outcome if symptom duration shorter or conus moves to more normal level following surgery
- Post-operative symptom recurrence rare; prompts consideration for re-tethering

## Treatment
- Symptomatic patients: Early prophylactic surgery
  - Resect tethering mass, release cord, and repair dura
- Asymptomatic patients with radiologic signs of tethering: Management controversial
  - Some advocate prophylactic surgery ⇒ low morbidity, prognosis for asymptomatic patients better than symptomatic
  - Others advocate prophylactic surgery only for asymptomatic adults who lead physically active lifestyles

# DIAGNOSTIC CHECKLIST

## Consider
- Clinical tethering may occur despite normal conus level, normal filum thickness
  - Tethered cord syndrome is a clinical diagnosis; imaging role is detection of low-lying conus/thick filum, associated anatomic abnormalities for surgical decision making
- Distinguish cord tethering 2° tight/thickened filum terminale from tethering due to other lesions: Lipoma, myelomeningocele, diastematomyelia

## Image Interpretation Pearls
- Measure filum thickness at L5/S1; stretching at more rostral levels may erroneously thin filum into "normal" size range
- Determine conus level using axial images; cauda equina may obscure conus tip on sagittal images ⇒ imitate elongated conus

# SELECTED REFERENCES

1. Bademci G et al: Prevalence of primary tethered cord syndrome associated with occult spinal dysraphism in primary school children in Turkey. Pediatr Neurosurg. 42(1):4-13, 2006
2. Rinaldi F et al: Tethered cord syndrome. J Neurosurg Sci. 49(4):131-5; discussion 135, 2005
3. Haro H et al: Long-term outcomes of surgical treatment for tethered cord syndrome. J Spinal Disord Tech. 17(1):16-20, 2004
4. Michelson DJ et al: Tethered cord syndrome in childhood: diagnostic features and relationship to congenital anomalies. Neurol Res. 26(7):745-53, 2004
5. Tubbs RS et al: Can the conus medullaris in normal position be tethered? Neurol Res. 26(7):727-31, 2004
6. Yamada S et al: Pathophysiology of tethered cord syndrome and other complex factors. Neurol Res. 26(7):722-6, 2004
7. Yamada S et al: Tethered cord syndrome: overview of diagnosis and treatment. Neurol Res. 26(7):719-21, 2004
8. Selcuki M et al: Is a filum terminale with a normal appearance really normal? Childs Nerv Syst. 19(1):3-10, 2003
9. Unsinn KM et al: US of the spinal cord in newborns: spectrum of normal findings, variants, congenital anomalies, and acquired diseases. Radiographics. 20(4):923-38, 2000
10. Iskandar BJ et al: Congenital tethered spinal cord syndrome in adults. J Neurosurg. 88(6):958-61, 1998
11. Selcuki M et al: Management of tight filum terminale syndrome with special emphasis on normal level conus medullaris (NLCM). Surg Neurol. 50(4):318-22; discussion 322, 1998
12. Sharif S et al: "Tethered cord syndrome"--recent clinical experience. Br J Neurosurg. 11(1):49-51, 1997
13. Yundt KD et al: Normal diameter of filum terminale in children: in vivo measurement. Pediatr Neurosurg. 27(5):257-9, 1997
14. Beek FJ et al: Sonographic determination of the position of the conus medullaris in premature and term infants. Neuroradiology. 38 Suppl 1:S174-7, 1996
15. Brunelle F et al: Lumbar spinal cord motion measurement with phase-contrast MR imaging in normal children and in children with spinal lipomas. Pediatr Radiol. 26(4):265-70, 1996

# TETHERED SPINAL CORD

## IMAGE GALLERY

### Typical

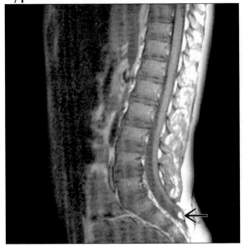
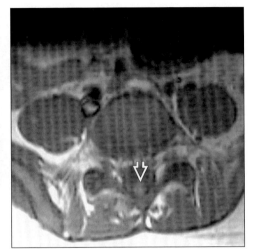

*(Left) Sagittal T1WI MR shows an elongated low-lying spinal cord extending to the S2 level, ending in a small terminal lipoma* →*. Focal sacral posterior dysraphism is also present. (Right) Axial T1WI MR confirms the presence of low-lying spinal cord* ⇒ *at the lumbosacral level.*

### Typical

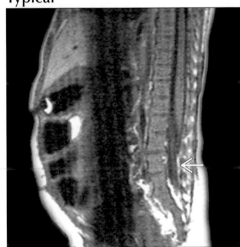
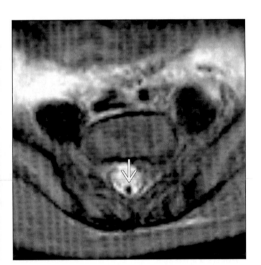

*(Left) Sagittal T1WI MR (VACTERL syndrome) shows an abnormally low-lying spinal cord, with the conus terminating at the inferior L3 vertebral level. The filum* → *contains fat. (Right) Axial T2WI FS MR (VACTERL syndrome) confirms fatty filum infiltration with marked signal loss on axial T2WI FS MR* →*.*

### Variant

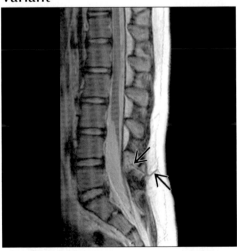
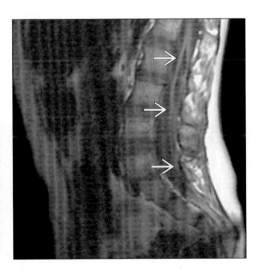

*(Left) Sagittal T2WI MR demonstrates a taut appearance of posteriorly positioned, low-lying conus with tip near L4. Further inspection of image reveals unsuspected dermal sinus tract* →*. (Right) Sagittal T1WI MR shows a low-lying hydromyelic spinal cord* ⇒ *inserting into the caudal thecal sac. This patient also had a horseshoe kidney (not shown).*

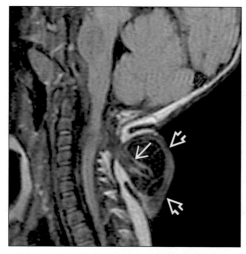

*Sagittal FLAIR MR shows small inner cyst ➡ extending into dorsal meningocele ➡ compatible with cervical myelocystocele. No hydromyelia was noted. (Courtesy C. Hoffman, MD).*

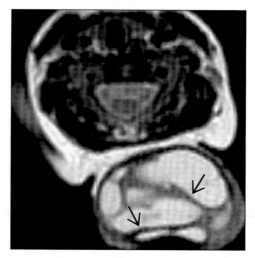

*Axial T2WI MR in same patient as previous image reveals the complex cystic mass. Note the low intensity of the tissue strands ➡ & absence of hydromyelia. (Courtesy C. Hoffman, MD).*

## TERMINOLOGY

### Abbreviations and Synonyms

- Cervical myelocystocele, thoracic myelocystocele

### Definitions

- Congenital skin covered malformation with dilated central spinal cord canal protruding dorsally through posterior dysraphic defect

## IMAGING FINDINGS

### General Features

- Best diagnostic clue: Enlarged central spinal cord canal protrudes through spina bifida defect into dorsal subcutaneous tissues
- Location: Cervical, cervicothoracic > thoracic
- Size: Small → large
- Morphology
  - Skin is normal to thick at base
    - Thin & discolored over dome
  - Pedunculated or sessile

### CT Findings

- NECT: Fluid density cyst protrudes through posterior osseous defect

### MR Findings

- T1WI
  - Hydromyelia (may be multiloculated)
  - Central spinal cord canal protrudes through dysraphic defect into dorsal subcutaneous tissues
- T2WI: Similar findings to T1WI

### Ultrasonographic Findings

- Grayscale Ultrasound
  - "Cyst within cyst"
  - Hydromyelic canal herniates into meninges to form inner cyst

### Non-Vascular Interventions

- Myelography
  - CT myelography may be useful to differentiate subarachnoid space from cyst
  - CT myelography may help identify fibroneurovascular stalks & median fibrous septa in cases with associated diastematomyelia

## DDx: Posterior Cervical & Thoracic Dysraphism

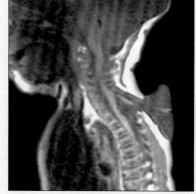

*Cervical Meningocele*

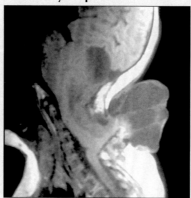

*Chiari III Malformation*

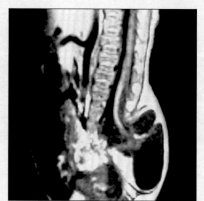

*Terminal Myelocystocele*

# NONTERMINAL MYELOCYSTOCELE

## Key Facts

### Terminology
- Cervical myelocystocele, thoracic myelocystocele

### Imaging Findings
- Best diagnostic clue: Enlarged central spinal cord canal protrudes through spina bifida defect into dorsal subcutaneous tissues
- Pedunculated or sessile
- Hydromyelia (may be multiloculated)
- "Cyst within cyst"

### Top Differential Diagnoses
- Cervical Meningocele/Myelomeningocele
- Chiari III Malformation
- Terminal Myelocystocele

### Pathology
- Unlike lumbar myelomeningoceles, cervical spinal dysraphisms covered by full thickness skin at base & thick opaque membrane at dome
- Hydromyelia cyst maintains continuity with distended central canal, herniates posteriorly into meningocele ("cyst within a cyst")

### Clinical Issues
- More favorable prognosis than myelomeningocele
- Motor deficit commonly develops; sensory & urologic deficits are uncommon

### Diagnostic Checklist
- Image entire spinal axis to exclude associated malformations

## Imaging Recommendations
- Best imaging tool
  - Multiplanar MR imaging
  - CT myelography may be a useful adjunct in complicated cases
- Protocol advice
  - Multiplanar T1WI and T2WI MR
  - Sagittal & axial planes most helpful

## DIFFERENTIAL DIAGNOSIS

### Cervical Meningocele/Myelomeningocele
- Failure of primary neurulation
- May be associated with Chiari II malformation
- Cervical meningocele
  - Single posterior cystic sac containing CSF, lined by arachnoid & dura
  - May have band of tissue tenting posterior aspect of cervical cord & extend into sac wall
  - Frequently contains neural tissue (neuroglial stalks, fibrovascular stalks); debated whether better described as meningocele or myelomeningocele
  - In contrast to cervical myelocystocele, meningocele patients generally do not have neurologic deficits but often develop mild orthopedic problems
  - Some authors propose that cervical meningocele & myelocystocele may be part of same spectrum, with diagnosis depending on presence or absence of associated hydromyelia
- Cervical myelomeningocele
  - Debated whether cervical myelomeningoceles really constitute a distinct pathologic entity or are better characterized as either meningocele or myelocystocele

### Chiari III Malformation
- Distinct pathological entity from nonterminal myelocystocele
- Ectopic cerebellar tissue herniates into sac

### Terminal Myelocystocele
- Abnormal secondary neurulation ⇒ inability of CSF to exit from early neural tube, terminal ventricle balloons into cyst disrupting overlying mesenchyme
- Association with omphalocele, bladder exstrophy, imperforate anus, caudal cell mass anomalies

## PATHOLOGY

### General Features
- General path comments
  - Cervical spinal dysraphism terminology in scientific literature is confusing and contradictory
  - Myelocystocele technically not cervical myelomeningocele because cord is fully neurulated at affected level
  - Nevertheless, some authors propose that cervical meningocele & myelocystocele are part of same spectrum
    - "Unifying hypothesis" of Steinbok & Cochrane
    - Presence or absence of associated hydromyelia helps distinguish cervical meningocele from myelocystocele
  - Unlike lumbar myelomeningoceles, cervical spinal dysraphisms covered by full thickness skin at base & thick opaque membrane at dome
    - Thick membrane rarely ruptures; CSF leak rare (unlike lumbar open dysraphism)
  - Hydromyelia cyst maintains continuity with distended central canal, herniates posteriorly into meningocele ("cyst within a cyst")
    - Outer cyst in continuity with subarachnoid space; skin covered wall composed of arachnoid & fibrous tissue
    - Inner cyst in continuity with distended central canal; wall contains neurons, glial tissue, & ependymal lining
- Etiology
  - May arise from partial limited closure of neural tube, failed disjunction of cutaneous ectoderm & hydromyelia

# NONTERMINAL MYELOCYSTOCELE

- Some authors propose that cervical meningocele & myelocystocele are spectrum of same underlying developmental abnormality
  - "Unifying hypothesis" of Steinbok & Cochrane
  - Eventual anomaly depends on presence or absence of associated hydromyelia
- Incomplete fusion of dorsal neural folds ⇒ failure of neural ectoderm to separate from cutaneous ectoderm
- Thin fibroneurovascular stalk containing neurons, glia, & peripheral nerves penetrates narrow dorsal dural opening
- Hydromyelic sac extends into subarachnoid space & posterior spinal cord wall becomes posterior sac wall
- Because myeloschisis extent is limited, superficial tissues achieve skin cover → skin covered malformation
- Epidemiology
  - Cervical dysraphism comprises 3-8% of all dysraphisms
  - Myelocystoceles very rare dysraphic malformation
- Associated abnormalities
  - Dermal sinus
  - Diastematomyelia
  - Vertebral segmentation anomalies
  - Chiari II malformation
  - Hydrocephalus
  - Cutaneous stigmata
  - Extraneural congenital malformations uncommon

## Gross Pathologic & Surgical Features
- Gross pathological findings
  - Most of cystic mass covered with full-thickness skin
  - Tough violaceous membrane covers cyst apex
  - Spinal cord & arachnoid herniate through posterior spina bifida
  - Localized expansion of subarachnoid space not necessary; uncommon in cervical myelocystoceles
  - Tethered spinal cord
- Surgical findings
  - Neuroglial stalk ⇒ meningocele
  - Fibrovascular stalk ⇒ meningocele
  - "Cyst within cyst" ⇒ true myelocystocele

## Microscopic Features
- Outer cyst composed of arachnoid & fibrous tissue
- Inner cyst lined by ependyma in contiguity with central spinal cord canal

# CLINICAL ISSUES

## Presentation
- Most common signs/symptoms
  - Neonate presents with dorsal midline skin covered cystic mass
    - Full thickness skin at base
    - Thick opaque membrane at dome
    - Typically normal neurological exam
- Other signs/symptoms
  - Occasionally infant presents with mild weakness or tone abnormality
  - Leakage of cerebrospinal fluid rare in cervical lesions

- Clinical Profile: Alpha fetoprotein (AFP) & acetylcholinesterase levels normal (skin covered)

## Natural History & Prognosis
- More favorable prognosis than myelomeningocele
- Motor deficit commonly develops; sensory & urologic deficits are uncommon
  - Patient usually neurologically normal at birth
  - Progressive neurological deficits develop during first year of life → extremity spasticity/weakness
  - Usually some motor deficit, orthopedic issues conspicuous by end of first decade

## Treatment
- Surgical resection of sac, intradural exploration, resection of tethering bands
- Orthopedic intervention for extremity motor deficits

# DIAGNOSTIC CHECKLIST

## Consider
- Image entire spinal axis to exclude associated malformations
- In complex cases, CT myelography may be a useful additional study

## Image Interpretation Pearls
- Myelocystocele characterized by "cyst within a cyst"

# SELECTED REFERENCES

1. Andronikou S et al: Cervical spina bifida cystica: MRI differentiation of the subtypes in children. Childs Nerv Syst. 22(4):379-384, 2006
2. Rossi A et al: Spectrum of nonterminal myelocystoceles. Neurosurgery. 58(3):509-15; discussion 509-15, 2006
3. Salomao JF et al: Cystic spinal dysraphism of the cervical and upper thoracic region. Childs Nerv Syst. 22(3):234-42, 2006
4. Salomao JF: Cervical meningocele in association with spinal abnormalities. Childs Nerv Syst. 21(1):4-5; author reply 6, 2005
5. Meyer-Heim AD et al: Cervical myelomeningocele--follow-up of five patients. Eur J Paediatr Neurol. 7(6):407-12, 2003
6. Nishio S et al: Cervical (myelo)meningocoele: report of 2 cases. J Clin Neurosci. 8(6):586-7, 2001
7. Perez LM et al: Urological outcome of patients with cervical and upper thoracic myelomeningocele. J Urol. 164(3 Pt 2):962-4, 2000
8. Sun JC et al: Cervical myelocystoceles and meningoceles: long-term follow-up. Pediatr Neurosurg. 33(3):118-22, 2000
9. Ankola PA et al: Picture of the month. Cervical myelomeningocele. Arch Pediatr Adolesc Med. 152(3):299-300, 1998
10. Nishino A et al: Cervical myelocystocele with Chiari II malformation: magnetic resonance imaging and surgical treatment. Surg Neurol. 49(3):269-73, 1998
11. Steinbok P et al: Cervical meningoceles and myelocystoceles: a unifying hypothesis. Pediatr Neurosurg. 23(6):317-22, 1995
12. Steinbok P: Dysraphic lesions of the cervical spinal cord. Neurosurg Clin N Am. 6(2):367-76, 1995
13. Pang D et al: Cervical myelomeningoceles. Neurosurgery. 33(3):363-72; discussion 372-3, 1993

# NONTERMINAL MYELOCYSTOCELE

## IMAGE GALLERY

### Typical

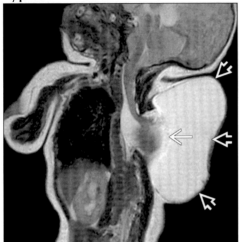
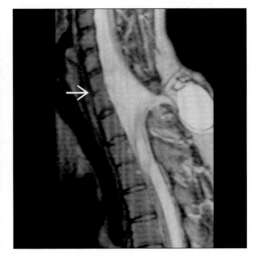

*(Left)* Sagittal T2WI MR shows thoracic myelocystocele with Chiari I malformation. Note signal dephasing within inner cyst ➡ residing in large outer cyst ➡. *(Right)* Sagittal T2WI MR shows hydromyelic spinal cord → "cyst within cyst". Dysplastic neural tissue & cysts protrude through narrow spinal dysraphism. Note vertebral segmentation failure ➡.

### Typical

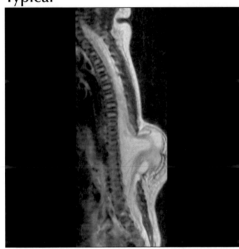
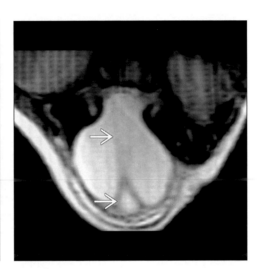

*(Left)* Sagittal T2WI MR demonstrates spinal cord extending through focal dysraphism into skin covered cystic mass. Note hydromyelia & characteristic "cyst within cyst". *(Right)* Axial T2WI MR (same patient as previous image) confirms "cyst within cyst" of thoracic myelocystocele. Note fibroneurovascular tissue ➡ tethering cord to dorsal sac.

III

6

31

### Typical

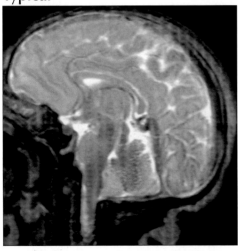
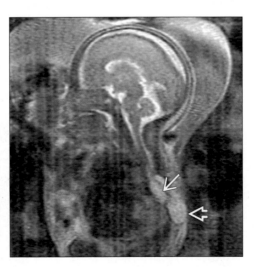

*(Left)* Sagittal T2WI FS MR in same patient as previous image shows mild Chiari I malformation with tonsillar ectopia. No stigmata of Chiari II malformation were detected. *(Right)* Sagittal T2WI MR of a fetus depicts a thoracic myelocystocele with dilated central spinal cord canal hydromyelic cyst ➡ within meningocele ➡. (Courtesy A. Kennedy, MD).

# TERMINAL MYELOCYSTOCELE

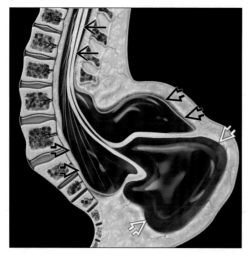

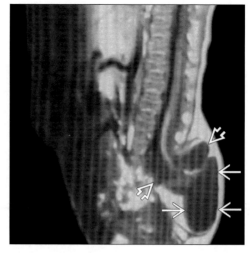

*Sagittal graphic displays a low-lying, hydromyelic spinal cord ➡️ piercing an expanded subarachnoid space (meningocele ⬛▷), to terminate in a terminal myelocystocele ⬛➡️.*

*Sagittal T1WI MR demonstrates a hypoplastic sacrum and low-lying tethered spinal cord with distal hydromyelia ➡️ traversing a meningocele ⬛➡️ produced by obstruction of subarachnoid space.*

## TERMINOLOGY

### Abbreviations and Synonyms
- Terminal syringocele

### Definitions
- Complex spinal malformation → hydromyelic low-lying tethered spinal cord traversing a meningocele to terminate in myelocystocele

## IMAGING FINDINGS

### General Features
- Best diagnostic clue: Hydromyelic tethered cord traversing dorsal meningocele to terminate in a dilated terminal ventricle
- Location: Sacrum/coccyx
- Size: Mass varies from small → huge (> 10 cm diameter)
- Morphology: Closed spinal dysraphism, large skin covered mass, terminal cord cyst traversing meningocele

### CT Findings
- NECT: Lumbosacral dysraphism

### MR Findings
- T1WI
  - Hypointense cephalic dorsal meningocele ⇒ back mass
  - Tethered distal cord shows "trumpet-like flaring" into hypointense caudal terminal cyst
  - +/- Lumbosacral hypogenesis
- T2WI
  - Hypointense dorsal fibrous band at cephalic margin of meningocele constrains cord
  - Fibrolipomatous tissue surrounds both sacs

### Radiographic Findings
- Radiography
  - Lumbosacral dysraphism/dysgenesis +/- soft tissue mass
  - +/- Pubic diastasis (usually + bladder exstrophy)

### Ultrasonographic Findings
- Grayscale Ultrasound

## DDx: Terminal Myelocystocele

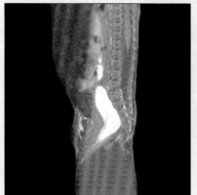

*Sacrococcygeal Teratoma*

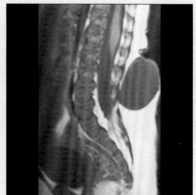

*Dorsal Meningocele*

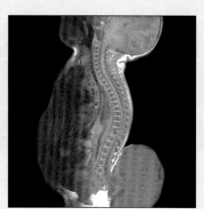

*Myelomeningocele*

# TERMINAL MYELOCYSTOCELE

## Key Facts

### Terminology
- Terminal syringocele
- Complex spinal malformation → hydromyelic low-lying tethered spinal cord traversing a meningocele to terminate in myelocystocele

### Imaging Findings
- Best diagnostic clue: Hydromyelic tethered cord traversing dorsal meningocele to terminate in a dilated terminal ventricle
- NECT: Lumbosacral dysraphism

### Top Differential Diagnoses
- Sacrococcygeal Teratoma (SGT)
- Simple Dorsal Meningocele
- Myelomeningocele
- Anterior Sacral Meningocele

### Pathology
- Skin covered lumbosacral dysraphism
- Arachnoid lined meningocele directly contiguous with spinal subarachnoid space
- Low-lying hydromyelic cord traverses meningocele, expands into large contiguous ependymal-lined terminal cyst

### Clinical Issues
- Presents at birth with large skin-covered back mass
- Majority neurologically intact at diagnosis

### Diagnostic Checklist
- Early diagnosis and surgery → best chance for normal neurological outcome
- Non-neurological prognosis largely linked to severity of associated anomalies

---

- Sagittal plane: Spinal cord passes through hypoechoic, dilated subarachnoid space (meningocele), terminates in cord cyst
- Axial plane: Bifid hydromyelic dorsal spinal cord within meningocele

### Non-Vascular Interventions
- Myelography
  - Hydromyelic cord passes through meningocele, terminates in separate sac caudal to contrast filled meningocele
  - Delayed imaging → +/- contrast imbibition into hydromyelic cord/terminal cyst

### Imaging Recommendations
- Best imaging tool: MR
- Protocol advice
  - Sagittal MR imaging for diagnosis and estimating length of hydromyelia, sizing cysts, and identifying associated abnormalities
  - Axial MR imaging to clarify extent of rachischisis, evaluate associated anomalies

## DIFFERENTIAL DIAGNOSIS

### Sacrococcygeal Teratoma (SGT)
- Similar clinical appearance of skin mass
- Distinguish by presence of solid tumor elements within cysts, calcifications

### Simple Dorsal Meningocele
- Dorsal meningocele protrudes thorough focal dysraphism
- Cord rarely tethered or hydromyelic

### Myelomeningocele
- Open spinal dysraphism; no skin covering, clinically obvious

### Anterior Sacral Meningocele
- Anterior meningocele protrudes thorough an enlarged sacral neural foramen into pelvis

## PATHOLOGY

### General Features
- General path comments
  - Classic pathological triad
    - Skin covered lumbosacral dysraphism
    - Arachnoid lined meningocele directly contiguous with spinal subarachnoid space
    - Low-lying hydromyelic cord traverses meningocele, expands into large contiguous ependymal-lined terminal cyst
  - Terminal cyst does not communicate directly with subarachnoid space
  - Some speculate → most severe manifestation of persistent terminal ventricle (ventriculus terminalis) spectrum
- Etiology
  - Postulated to result from deranged secondary neurulation of caudal cell mass; typically associated with other caudal tail-fold malformations
    - CSF unable to normally exit from early neural tube ⇒ terminal ventricle balloons into cyst ⇒ disrupts overlying dorsal mesenchyme but not superficial ectoderm
    - Posterior elements do not form normally ⇒ spina bifida with intact skin
    - Terminal ventricle dilatation ⇒ distends arachnoid cord lining ⇒ meningocele
    - Cyst bulk prevents cord ascent ⇒ tethered cord
    - After arachnoid formation, progressive distention of distal cord causes caudal bulge below end of meningocele into extra-arachnoid space and cephalically to expand distal cord, producing flaring of distal spinal cord
    - Disruption of caudal motor segments ⇒ progressive symptoms present at birth or that appear later
- Epidemiology
  - Rare: 1-5% of skin covered lumbosacral masses
    - Much more common in cloacal exstrophy patients
  - Sporadic; no familial incidence

# TERMINAL MYELOCYSTOCELE

- ○ Postulated associations with teratogens retinoic acid, hydantoin, ioperamid hydrochloride
- ○ No known association with diabetes mellitus (unlike caudal regression syndrome)
- • Associated abnormalities
  - ○ Cloacal exstrophy, imperforate anus, omphalocele, pelvic deformities, equinovarus, ambiguous hypoplastic genitalia, and renal abnormalities
  - ○ Syndromal associations
    - ▪ Caudal regression syndrome
    - ▪ OEIS syndrome constellation (omphalocele, exstrophy of the bladder, imperforate anus, and spinal anomalies)
  - ○ Chiari I and II malformations, hydrocephalus, and vertebral segmentation anomalies (rare)

## Gross Pathologic & Surgical Features
- • Lumbosacral dysraphism with hypoplastic, widely everted laminae
- • Proximal (smaller, rostral) sac resembles typical meningocele, with inner surface lined by arachnoid and thick fibrous layer
- • Distal spinal cord herniates under fibrous band between medial ends of most cephalic widely bifid lamina, traverses meningocele → terminal cyst (larger, caudal)
  - ○ Cord narrowed by fibrous band where it exits spinal canal, then widens distally due to concurrent hydromyelia
  - ○ Distal spinal nerve roots arise from ventral surface of intra-arachnoid segment of spinal cord, traverse meningocele, and re-enter spinal canal before exiting at their root sleeves or via bony clefts

## Microscopic Features
- • Meningocele lined by arachnoid, thick fibrous layer
- • Terminal cyst lined by ependyma, dysplastic glia; directly contiguous with central cord canal
- • Outer cord surface pia, arachnoid continuous with meningocele

# CLINICAL ISSUES

## Presentation
- • Most common signs/symptoms
  - ○ Presents at birth with large skin-covered back mass
    - ▪ Skin appears normal or exhibits hemangioma, nevus, or hypertrichosis
    - ▪ Rare patients without back mass present later with progressive neurological deficits
  - ○ Majority neurologically intact at diagnosis
  - ○ Later presentation or untreated lesion may develop progressive lower extremity paresis
- • Clinical Profile
  - ○ Usually neurologically intact at birth but may present with lower extremity sensorimotor deficits
  - ○ Large mass obliterates intergluteal cleft, extends upward from perineum for a variable distance
  - ○ +/- Concurrent midline cecal and paramedian bladder exstrophy, other visible anomalies

## Demographics
- • Age: Infancy

- • Gender: F > M

## Natural History & Prognosis
- • Normal intellectual potential
- • Mass size and deficits tend to progress with time, may be partially or totally reversible with prompt surgical repair
  - ○ Main goals of neurosurgical intervention are to reduce mass size and un-tether cord
  - ○ Operation soon after diagnosis is indicated to prevent progression of neurological abnormalities, cyst growth
  - ○ Persistent neurological deficits usually permanent
- • Overall prognosis is mainly related to other associated anomalies (OEIS constellation)
- • Patients with abdominal wall defects have ↑ incidence of neurological deficits

## Treatment
- • Early diagnosis and surgical repair maximizes probability of a normal neurological outcome
- • Delayed recognition and operation increase odds of onset or progression of lower extremity paresis

# DIAGNOSTIC CHECKLIST

## Consider
- • Early diagnosis and surgery → best chance for normal neurological outcome
- • Non-neurological prognosis largely linked to severity of associated anomalies

## Image Interpretation Pearls
- • Tethered hydromyelic cord traversing meningocele to terminate in a separate caudal cyst is unique imaging finding diagnostic of terminal myelocystocele

# SELECTED REFERENCES

1.  Gupta DK et al: Terminal myelocystoceles: a series of 17 cases. J Neurosurg. 103(4 Suppl):344-52, 2005
2.  James HE et al: Terminal myelocystocele. J Neurosurg. 103(5 Suppl):443-5, 2005
3.  Lemire RJ et al: Tumors and malformations of the caudal spinal axis. Pediatr Neurosurg. 38(4):174-80, 2003
4.  Kumar R et al: Terminal myelocystocele. Indian J Pediatr. 69(12):1083-6, 2002
5.  Midrio P et al: Prenatal diagnosis of terminal myelocystocele in the fetal surgery era: case report. Neurosurgery. 50(5):1152-4; discussion 1154-5, 2002
6.  Choi S et al: Long-term outcome of terminal myelocystocele patients. Pediatr Neurosurg. 32(2):86-91, 2000
7.  Tortori-Donati P et al: Spinal dysraphism: a review of neuroradiological features with embryological correlations and proposal for a new classification. Neuroradiology. 42(7):471-91, 2000
8.  Unsinn KM et al: US of the spinal cord in newborns: spectrum of normal findings, variants, congenital anomalies, and acquired diseases. Radiographics. 20(4):923-38, 2000
9.  Meyer SH et al: Terminal myelocystocele: important differential diagnosis in the prenatal assessment of spina bifida. J Ultrasound Med. 17(3):193-7, 1998
10. McLone DG et al: Terminal myelocystocele. Neurosurgery. 16(1):36-43, 1985

## IMAGE GALLERY

### Typical

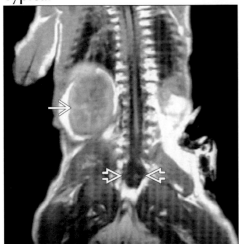
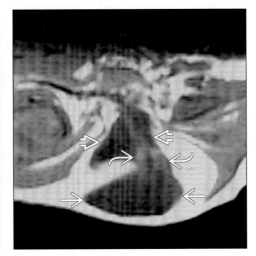

*(Left)* Coronal T1WI MR in the same patient as the first MR shows the meningocele ➡ as well as a single large right kidney ➡. Coronal MR is useful for detecting associated visceral anomalies. *(Right)* Axial T1WI MR depicts the low-lying distal spinal cord ➡ traversing the meningocele ➡ to end in a terminal hydromyelia sac ➡.

### Typical

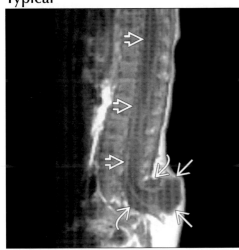
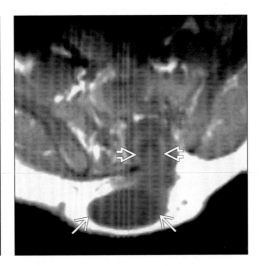

*(Left)* Sagittal T1WI MR demonstrates a low-lying hydromyelic spinal cord ➡ passing through the widened subarachnoid space meningocele ➡, flaring into a large subcutaneous terminal cyst ➡. *(Right)* Axial T1WI MR shows the hydromyelic spinal cord ➡ ending in a skin covered terminal cyst ➡ that classically defines terminal myelocystocele.

### Variant

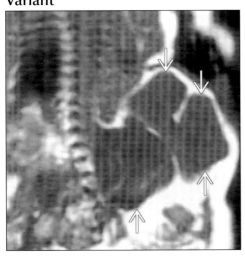
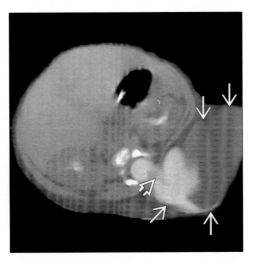

*(Left)* Coronal T1WI MR in a patient with caudal regression and cloacal exstrophy depicts the large, laterally directed CSF signal intensity meningocele ➡. *(Right)* Axial CECT following myelography shows spinal cord ➡ traversing a large meningocele sac ➡. The intrathecal contrast has incompletely filled the large, laterally directed meningocele.

# ANTERIOR SACRAL MENINGOCELE

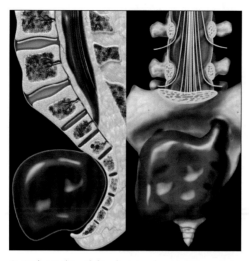
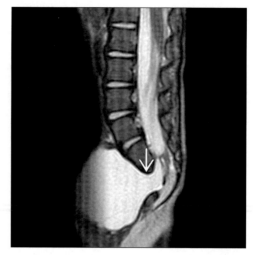

*Sagittal graphic (left) depicts characteristic anterior sacral "scimitar" remodeling by large anterior cyst. Coronal graphic (right) shows cyst origin through an enlarged neural foramen.*

*Sagittal T2WI MR demonstrates large presacral cyst contiguous with thecal sac through an enlarged sacral neural foramen ➡.*

## TERMINOLOGY

### Abbreviations and Synonyms
- Anterior sacral meningocele (ASM)

### Definitions
- Sacral meninges herniate anteriorly into the pelvis through focal erosion or hypogenesis of sacral +/- coccygeal vertebral segments

## IMAGING FINDINGS

### General Features
- Best diagnostic clue: Presacral cyst contiguous with thecal sac through an anterior sacral defect
- Location: Sacrum/coccyx
- Size: Variable
- Morphology
  - Uni- or multi-loculated cyst; usually devoid of neural tissue but may have traversing nerve roots
  - Sacral defect is 2° to neural foraminal widening
    - May be unilateral or bilateral, symmetrical or asymmetrical, and single or multiple level

### CT Findings
- CECT
  - Deficient sacrum with variably sized anterior cyst
    - +/- Nerve roots traversing sacral defect
  - +/- Lipoma/dermoid (hypodense)
  - Enhancement absent

### MR Findings
- T1WI
  - Deficient sacrum with variably sized presacral cyst
    - Sagittal images confirm cyst/thecal sac continuity
  - +/- Cord tethering
  - +/- Lipoma/dermoid (hyperintense)
- T2WI
  - Homogeneous hyperintense cerebrospinal fluid (CSF) signal intensity cyst (similar to thecal sac)
  - Best sequence to identify nerve roots traversing sacral defect
- T2* GRE
  - No hypointensity (calcification) within cyst wall
    - Distinguishes from sacrococcygeal teratoma
- DWI: Hypointense signal confirms CSF composition, excludes epidermoid cyst (hyperintense)
- T1 C+: No enhancement

## DDx: Anterior Sacral Meningocele

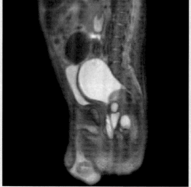
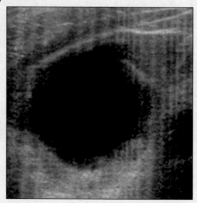
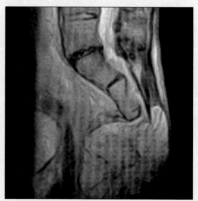

*Sacrococcygeal Teratoma*    *Ovarian Cyst*    *Chordoma*

# ANTERIOR SACRAL MENINGOCELE

## Key Facts

### Terminology
- Anterior sacral meningocele (ASM)
- Sacral meninges herniate anteriorly into the pelvis through focal erosion or hypogenesis of sacral +/- coccygeal vertebral segments

### Imaging Findings
- Best diagnostic clue: Presacral cyst contiguous with thecal sac through an anterior sacral defect
- Widened sacral canal and neural foramina
- Curved "scimitar" sacrum on lateral projection

### Top Differential Diagnoses
- Sacrococcygeal Teratoma (SCT)
- Ovarian Cyst
- Sacral Chordoma
- Neurenteric Cyst

- Cystic Neuroblastoma

### Pathology
- 5% of retrorectal tumors
- Associated abnormalities: Anorectal anomalies, epidermoid/dermoid tumor or other tethering lesion, Currarino triad

### Diagnostic Checklist
- MR imaging to identify and characterize cyst location and contents, confirm abnormal ultrasound findings
- Continuity of cyst with thecal sac necessary to ensure diagnosis
- Soft tissue mass or calcification implies tumor
- Presence/absence of neural tissue within cyst important for surgical planning

## Radiographic Findings
- Radiography
  - Widened sacral canal and neural foramina
  - Scalloping of anterior sacrum wall
    - Curved "scimitar" sacrum on lateral projection
  - +/- Scoliosis

## Ultrasonographic Findings
- Grayscale Ultrasound
  - Cystic hypoechoic pelvic mass anterior to sacrum
  - Complex internal echoes if prior/concurrent inflammation or infection

## Non-Vascular Interventions
- Myelography
  - Thecal sac continuity with cyst
    - Most useful in conjunction with NECT (CT myelography)
  - Rarely used unless MR contraindicated or non-diagnostic

## Imaging Recommendations
- Best imaging tool
  - MR imaging confirms cyst contiguity with thecal sac
    - T1WI also shows +/- epidermoid, lipoma/dermoid
    - T2WI demonstrates +/- entrapped neural tissue
  - CT imaging best depicts osseous defect, absence of calcification excludes teratoma
- Protocol advice
  - Ultrasound for initial screening during infancy
  - Sagittal and axial MR imaging to confirm positive ultrasound studies, pre-operative planning, and post-operative surveillance

## DIFFERENTIAL DIAGNOSIS

### Sacrococcygeal Teratoma (SCT)
- Cystic SCT may be difficult to distinguish from ASM
  - Look for soft tissue mass, enhancement, calcification

### Ovarian Cyst
- Ultrasound may reveal surrounding ovarian tissue that clinches diagnosis

### Sacral Chordoma
- Mixed solid/cystic destructive sacral mass
  - Bone CT shows destructive margins
  - Rare in children; peak incidence 5th → 6th decade

### Neurenteric Cyst
- Cyst usually within spinal canal +/- rachischisis, vertebral formation anomalies

### Cystic Neuroblastoma
- Search for calcifications, metastatic lesions

## PATHOLOGY

### General Features
- General path comments
  - 5% of retrorectal tumors
  - Osseous sacral remodeling in large meningoceles ⇒ classic "scimitar" shape
- Genetics
  - Sporadic (most patients)
  - Minority show inherited predisposition
    - Currarino triad: Autosomal dominant with variable penetration (HLXB 9 gene, chromosome 7q36)
    - Conditions where dural ectasia is prominent (NF1, Marfan, Homocystinuria)
- Etiology
  - Embryogenesis not definitively known; classified within caudal mass anomalies spectrum
    - Erosion or dysgenesis of sacral/coccygeal segments permits herniation of meningeal sac into anterior pelvis
  - Possible associations
    - Simple form: Marfan, NF1
    - Complicated form: Familial, partial sacral agenesis, imperforate anus or anal stenosis, and tethered cord

# ANTERIOR SACRAL MENINGOCELE

- Epidemiology: Rare; less common than dorsal meningoceles
- Associated abnormalities: Anorectal anomalies, epidermoid/dermoid tumor or other tethering lesion, Currarino triad

## Gross Pathologic & Surgical Features
- Widened sacral dural sac communicates with pelvic cyst through a narrow neck within sacral defect
- +/- Neural tissue within cyst sac

## Microscopic Features
- Characteristic features of dura; may reveal signs of prior inflammation

## CLINICAL ISSUES

### Presentation
- Most common signs/symptoms
  - Constipation, urinary frequency, incontinence, dysmenorrhea, dyspareunia, low back/pelvic pain
    - 2° to pressure on pelvic viscera
  - Other signs/symptoms
    - Sciatica, diminished rectal/detrusor tone, numbness/paresthesias in lower sacral dermatomes (nerve root pressure)
    - Intermittent positional high or low pressure headaches due to fluid shifts between ASM and spinal subarachnoid space
    - Superinfection +/- meningitis (uncommon)
- Clinical Profile
  - Most present with urinary or bowel complaints; ASM is discovered during imaging evaluation
  - Rare finding in headache patient
    - Classic: Low pressure headache on standing

### Demographics
- Age: Onset of symptoms in 2nd-3rd decade
- Gender
  - M = F (children)
  - M < F (adults)

### Natural History & Prognosis
- Good prognosis following successful repair

### Treatment
- Open posterior trans-sacral approach, patching of meningocele: Dural sac connection
  - Easier if cyst does not contain neural elements, permitting simple ligation of cyst neck
- Endoscopic approach ⇒ lower morbidity

## DIAGNOSTIC CHECKLIST

### Consider
- Ultrasound if mass identified in infant
- MR imaging to identify and characterize cyst location and contents, confirm abnormal ultrasound findings
- Bone CT to demonstrate characteristic osseous findings that permit a specific diagnosis

### Image Interpretation Pearls
- Continuity of cyst with thecal sac necessary to ensure diagnosis
- Soft tissue mass or calcification implies tumor
- Presence/absence of neural tissue within cyst important for surgical planning

## SELECTED REFERENCES

1.  Erdogmus B et al: Anterior sacral meningocele simulating ovarian cyst. J Clin Ultrasound. 2006
2.  Gardner PA et al: "Like mother, like son:" hereditary anterior sacral meningocele. Case report and review of the literature. J Neurosurg. 104(2 Suppl):138-42, 2006
3.  Marin-Sanabria EA et al: Presacral meningocele associated with hereditary sacral agenesis and treated surgically: evaluation in three members of the same family. Neurosurgery. 57(3):E597; discussion E597, 2005
4.  Bal S et al: A case with cauda equina syndrome due to bacterial meningitis of anterior sacral meningocele. Spine. 29(14):E298-9, 2004
5.  Morimoto K et al: Currarino triad as an anterior sacral meningocele. Pediatr Neurosurg. 40(2):97-8, 2004
6.  Rigante D et al: Anterior sacral meningocele in a patient with Marfan syndrome. Clin Neuropathol. 20(2):70-2, 2001
7.  Fitzpatrick MO et al: Anterior sacral meningocele associated with a rectal fistula. Case report and review of the literature. J Neurosurg (Spine). 91:124-7, 1999
8.  Shamoto H et al: Anterior sacral meningocele completely occupied by an epidermoid tumor. Childs Nerv Syst. 15(4):209-11, 1999
9.  Voyvodic F et al: Anterior sacral meningocele as a pelvic complication of Marfan syndrome. Aust N Z J Obstet Gynaecol. 39(2):262-5, 1999
10. Lee SC et al: Currarino triad: anorectal malformation, sacral bony abnormality, and presacral mass--a review of 11 cases. J Pediatr Surg. 32(1):58-61, 1997
11. Gaskill SJ et al: The Currarino triad: its importance in pediatric neurosurgery. Pediatr Neurosurg. 25(3):143-6, 1996
12. Kochling J et al: The Currarino syndrome--hereditary transmitted syndrome of anorectal, sacral and presacral anomalies. Case report and review of the literature. Eur J Pediatr Surg. 6(2):114-9, 1996
13. Funayama CA et al: Recurrent meningitis in a case of congenital anterior sacral meningocele and agenesis of sacral and coccygeal vertebrae. Arq Neuropsiquiatr. 53(4):799-801, 1995
14. Raftopoulos C et al: Anterior sacral meningocele and Marfan syndrome: a review. Acta Chir Belg. 93(1):1-7, 1993
15. Chamaa MT et al: Anterior-sacral meningocele; value of magnetic resonance imaging and abdominal sonography. A case report. Acta Neurochir (Wien). 109(3-4):154-7, 1991
16. McGuire RA Jr et al: Anterior sacral meningocele. Case report and review of the literature. Spine. 15(6):612-4, 1990
17. North RB et al: Occult, bilateral anterior sacral and intrasacral meningeal and perineurial cysts: case report and review of the literature. Neurosurgery. 27(6):981-6, 1990
18. Brem H et al: Neonatal diagnosis of a presacral mass in the presence of congenital anal stenosis and partial sacral agenesis. J Pediatr Surg. 24(10):1076-8, 1989
19. Lee KS et al: The role of MR imaging in the diagnosis and treatment of anterior sacral meningocele. Report of two cases. J Neurosurg. 69(4):628-31, 1988
20. Martin B et al: MR imaging of anterior sacral meningocele. J Comput Assist Tomogr. 12(1):166-7, 1988
21. Dyck P et al: Anterior sacral meningocele. Case report. J Neurosurg. 53(4):548-52, 1980

# ANTERIOR SACRAL MENINGOCELE

## IMAGE GALLERY

### Typical

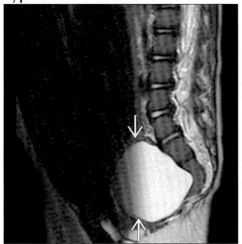

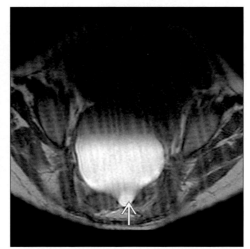

*(Left)* Sagittal T2WI MR shows characteristic "scimitar sacrum" with large presacral cyst ➡. Note remodeling of the sacrum that results in characteristic shape seen on plain radiographs. *(Right)* Axial T2WI MR confirms sacral neural foramen enlargement ➡, permitting ventral herniation and expansion of spinal meninges.

### Variant

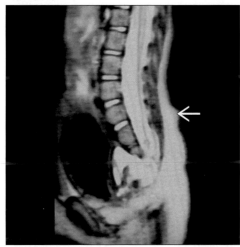

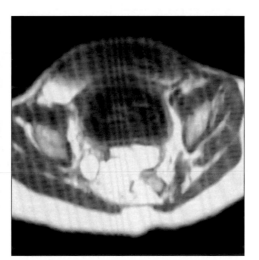

*(Left)* Sagittal T2WI MR reveals severe sacral dysplasia with low-lying tethered spinal cord, thickened filum terminale ➡ inserting into complex presacral mixed cystic and lipomatous mass. *(Right)* Axial T2WI MR confirms lipomatous cystic mass extending through the right neural foramen and remodeling the sacrum.

### Variant

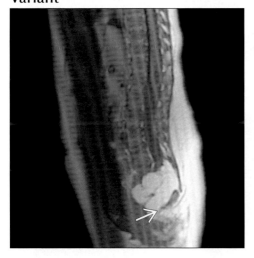

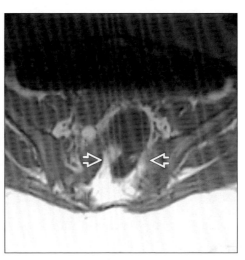

*(Left)* Sagittal T1WI MR reveals severe caudal regression and a complex fatty mass ➡ extending anteriorly through the sacrum into the pelvis. The conus demonstrates focal hydromyelia. *(Right)* Axial T1WI MR confirms complex cystic/fatty mass extending through an enlarged sacral foramen ➡ into the pelvis.

# DIASTEMATOMYELIA

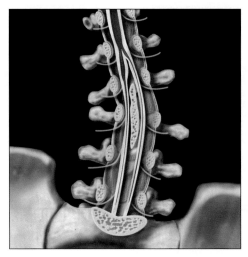

Coronal graphic demonstrates type I SCM with large osseous marrow-filled spur dividing syringomyelic tethered spinal cord into two hemicords contiguous with thoracic syrinx.

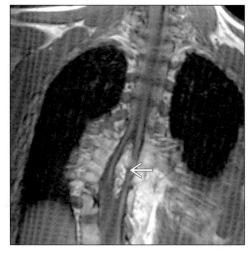

Coronal T1WI MR reveals multiple vertebral segmentation anomalies with bilateral posterior element and rib fusions. A large osseous midline spur ➡ splits the spinal cord (type I SCM).

## TERMINOLOGY

### Abbreviations and Synonyms
- Diastematomyelia (DSM), split cord malformation (SCM)

### Definitions
- Sagittal division of spinal cord into two hemicords, each with one central canal, dorsal horn, and ventral horn

## IMAGING FINDINGS

### General Features
- Best diagnostic clue
  - Fibrous or osseous spur splits spinal cord into two hemicords
  - Split cord and spur often occur in conjunction with intersegmental vertebral fusion
- Location: Thoracolumbar cleft (85% between T9 and S1) > > upper thoracic, cervical clefts
- Morphology
  - Hemicords usually (≈ 91%) reunite below cleft
    - +/- Spur (fibrous, osteocartilaginous, or osseous), thickened filum, cord tethering

### CT Findings
- Bone CT
  - Osseous spur often visible, fibrous spurs occult
  - Vertebral segmentation anomalies

### MR Findings
- T1WI
  - Two hemicords +/- syringohydromyelia (50%)
  - +/- Isointense (fibrous) or hyperintense (osseous: Contains marrow) spur
- T2WI
  - Two hemicords +/- syringohydromyelia (50%) in one or both cords, surrounded by bright cerebrospinal fluid (CSF)
  - Hypointense (fibrous or osseous) spur; fibrous spur best seen in axial or coronal plane
- T2* GRE: Myelographic effect produces bright CSF adjacent to dark bones, highlights hypointense spur

### Radiographic Findings
- Radiography

## DDx: More Examples of Diastematomyelia

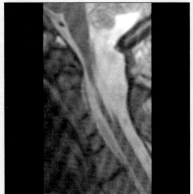

Type II, Klippel-Feil

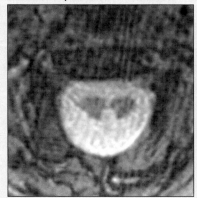

Type II, Klippel-Feil

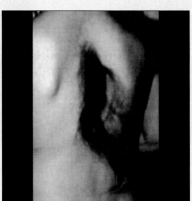

"Faun's Tail"

# DIASTEMATOMYELIA

## Key Facts

### Terminology
- Diastematomyelia (DSM), split cord malformation (SCM)
- Sagittal division of spinal cord into two hemicords, each with one central canal, dorsal horn, and ventral horn

### Imaging Findings
- Location: Thoracolumbar cleft (85% between T9 and S1) > > upper thoracic, cervical clefts
- Hemicords usually (≈ 91%) reunite below cleft
- Osseous spur often visible, fibrous spurs occult
- Vertebral segmentation anomalies
- Split cord; one or two dural tubes

### Top Differential Diagnoses
- Duplicated Spinal Cord (Diplomyelia)

### Pathology
- "Split notochord syndrome" spectrum
- Epidemiology: 5% of congenital scoliosis
- Congenital spinal deformities (85%)
- Nerve roots may become adherent to dura, tether cord ⇒ "meningocele manqué"

### Clinical Issues
- Cutaneous stigmata back indicates diastematomyelia level (> 50%); "faun's tail" hair patch most common

### Diagnostic Checklist
- Search for DSM in patients with cutaneous stigmata, intersegmental fusion of posterior elements, clinical tethered cord

---

- Quantify kyphoscoliosis, "count" level of vertebral segmentation anomalies
- Detects spur < 50% of cases

## Ultrasonographic Findings
- Grayscale Ultrasound
  - Obstetrical ultrasound → "extra" posterior echogenic focus, splaying of fetal posterior spinal elements
  - Post-natal imaging → spur, tethered cord

## Non-Vascular Interventions
- Myelography
  - Split cord; one or two dural tubes
  - Excellent delineation of spur location and meningocele manqué (if present); most useful in conjunction with CT

## Imaging Recommendations
- Best imaging tool: MR imaging
- Protocol advice
  - Consider ultrasound to screen infants with skin dimple or cutaneous marker
  - MR imaging most definitive
    - Coronal, axial images best demonstrate hemicords, spur
    - T1WI to evaluate for filum lesions (e.g., fibrolipoma), vertebral anomalies
    - T2WI to determine number of dural sacs, +/- syringohydromyelia
    - T2* GRE to detect spur
- Supplement with bone CT +/- myelography to optimally define spur anatomy for surgical planning
  - Sagittal, coronal reformats excellent for depicting osseous anatomy, extent of spur

## DIFFERENTIAL DIAGNOSIS

### Duplicated Spinal Cord (Diplomyelia)
- Two complete spinal cords, each with two anterior and two posterior horns and roots

- Exceedingly rare, seen only in presence of spinal canal duplication; many authors dispute its true existence, believe it represents a severe form of diastematomyelia

## PATHOLOGY

### General Features
- General path comments
  - Septum/filum fibrolipoma inhibits normal spinal cord movement during activity ⇒ symptoms
  - Spinal cord damage occurs via direct pressure and by traction ⇒ cord ischemia
  - Cleft focally splits cord, with single cord above and below split
    - Most (91%) hemicords reunite caudally to terminate in a single filum terminale
  - Roots may adhere to dura ⇒ "meningocele manqué"
- Genetics: Sporadic; rare familial cases described
- Etiology
  - "Split notochord syndrome" spectrum
    - Congenital splitting of notochord ⇒ "split notochord syndrome" spectrum; diastematomyelia, dorsal enteric fistula/sinus, and dorsal enteric cysts/diverticula
  - Notochord directly influences vertebral body formation ⇒ segmentation anomalies
    - Lateral notch produces hemivertebra
    - Cleft produces butterfly vertebra
- Epidemiology: 5% of congenital scoliosis
- Associated abnormalities
  - Other split notochord syndromes (20%)
  - Congenital spinal deformities (85%)
    - Segmentation and fusion anomalies (SFA)
    - Intersegmental laminar fusion (60%); virtually pathognomonic for diastematomyelia
    - Spinal dysraphism (myelocele/myelomeningocele 15-25%, hemimyelocele 15-20%)
    - Tethered spinal cord (75%); thickened filum terminale (40-90%)
    - Hydromyelia (50%) in one or both hemicords, usually above diastematomyelia

- Congenital scoliosis (79%)
- 15-20% of Chiari II malformations

## Gross Pathologic & Surgical Features

- Sagittal spinal cord split into symmetric or asymmetric hemicords, residing in either one or two dural tubes
  - Filum fibrolipoma common in all types
  - Symmetric: Each hemicord contains one central canal, dorsal horn/root, and ventral horn/root surrounded by pial layer
  - Asymmetric: Division of anterior or posterior hemicord: "Partial diastematomyelia"
- Two dural tubes, each with own pial, arachnoid, and dural sheaths for several spinal segments (50%)
  - Bony or cartilaginous spur at inferior cleft, originating from lamina or vertebral body
  - Vertebral anomalies more severe (block or butterfly vertebrae, hemivertebrae, and posterior spina bifida)
  - Hydromyelia common
- Single dural tube, subarachnoid space (50%)
  - No bony spur; nearly always have a fibrous band coursing thru inferior cleft inserting into dura → tethers cord
  - Vertebral anomalies less severe (usually butterfly vertebrae)
  - Nerve roots may become adherent to dura, tether cord ⇒ "meningocele manqué"

## Microscopic Features

- Single ependymal lined central canal, ventral horn/root, and dorsal horn/root per hemicord

## Staging, Grading or Classification Criteria

- Pang type I SCM
  - Separate dural sac, arachnoid space surrounds each hemicord
  - Osseous/fibrous spur
  - More commonly symptomatic than type II
- Pang type II SCM
  - Single dural sac, arachnoid space
  - No osseous spur; +/- adherent fibrous bands tether cord
  - Rarely symptomatic unless hydromyelia, tethering

# CLINICAL ISSUES

## Presentation

- Most common signs/symptoms
  - Clinically indistinguishable from other causes of tethered cord
  - Cutaneous stigmata back indicates diastematomyelia level (> 50%); "faun's tail" hair patch most common
  - Other signs/symptoms
    - Progressive kyphoscoliosis in older children, adults
    - Orthopedic foot problems (50%); especially clubfoot
    - Urologic dysfunction
- Clinical Profile
  - Mild cases normal +/- cutaneous stigmata
  - Severe cases → kyphoscoliosis, neurological and musculoskeletal abnormalities

## Demographics

- Age: Diagnosis in childhood; adult presentation uncommon
- Gender
  - Pediatric: F > > M (80-94%)
  - Adult: F > M (3.4:1)

## Natural History & Prognosis

- Stable or progressive disability if untreated
  - Late onset or previously stable patients may become symptomatic following relatively minor back injury or surgery requiring spinal manipulation
- ≥ 90% of patients stabilize or improve following surgery
  - Caveat: Scoliosis rarely affected by surgical untethering

## Treatment

- Surgical tethered cord release, spur resection, and dural repair for progressive symptoms, prophylactic precursor to scoliosis surgery

# DIAGNOSTIC CHECKLIST

## Consider

- Scrutinize images for presence of spur; type I SCM generally has more severe symptoms and anomalies, worse prognosis
- Search for DSM in patients with cutaneous stigmata, intersegmental fusion of posterior elements, clinical tethered cord

## Image Interpretation Pearls

- Segmentation anomalies + intersegmental laminar fusion virtually pathognomonic for diastematomyelia

# SELECTED REFERENCES

1. Rossi A et al: Spinal dysraphism: MR imaging rationale. J Neuroradiol. 31(1):3-24, 2004
2. Tubbs RS et al: Exclusive lower extremity mirror movements and diastematomyelia. Pediatr Neurosurg. 40(3):132-5, 2004
3. Balci S et al: Cervical diastematomyelia in cervico-oculo-acoustic (Wildervanck) syndrome: MRI findings. Clin Dysmorphol. 11(2):125-8, 2002
4. Tortori-Donati P et al: Magnetic resonance imaging of spinal dysraphism. Top Magn Reson Imaging. 12(6):375-409, 2001
5. Ersahin Y et al: Split spinal cord malformations in children. J Neurosurg. 88(1):57-65, 1998
6. Miller A et al: Evaluation and treatment of diastematomyelia. J Bone Joint Surg Am. 75(9):1308-17, 1993
7. Kaffenberger DA et al: Meningocele manque: radiologic findings with clinical correlation. AJNR Am J Neuroradiol. 13(4):1083-8, 1992
8. Pang D et al: Split cord malformation: Part I: A unified theory of embryogenesis for double spinal cord malformations. Neurosurgery. 31(3):451-80, 1992
9. Pang D et al: Split cord malformation: Part II: Clinical syndrome. Neurosurgery 31(3):481-500, 1992

# DIASTEMATOMYELIA

## IMAGE GALLERY

### Typical

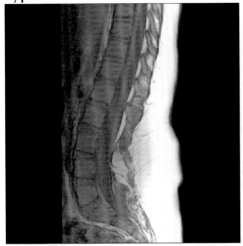

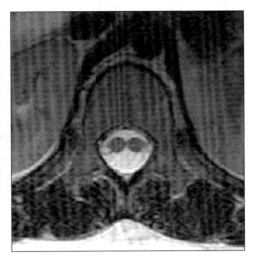

*(Left)* Sagittal T1WI MR demonstrates a low-lying spinal cord and lipomyelomeningocele with posterior dysraphism. Diastematomyelia (type II SCM) is occult on this midline sagittal image. *(Right)* Axial T2WI MR in same lipomyelomeningocele patient shows two separate hemicords residing within a single dural tube (type II SCM). No osseous or fibrous septum is identified.

### Variant

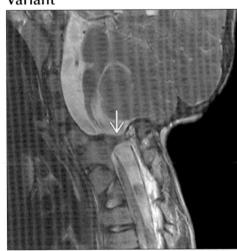

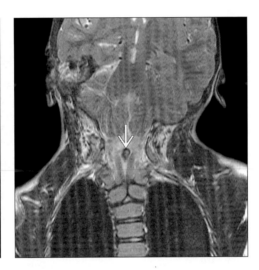

*(Left)* Sagittal T2WI MR depicts a large osseous spur ➡ arising from posterior vertebral body (type I SCM), piercing the spinal cord. Also present are multiple vertebral segmentation anomalies. *(Right)* Coronal T2WI MR reveals vertebral anomalies and osseous spur ➡ (type I SCM) that splits the high cervical spinal cord.

### Variant

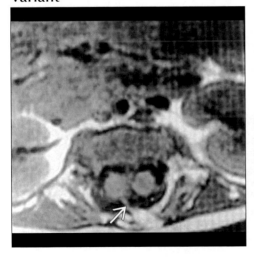

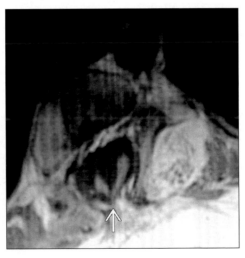

*(Left)* Axial T1WI MR shows a lumbar type II SCM. A fibrous band extending from right hemicord to dorsal dural sac ➡ tethers spinal cord (meningocele manqué). *(Right)* Axial T1WI MR demonstrates type II SCM with two hemicords in single dural tube. The hemicords are dorsally adherent to the dural sac ➡ (meningocele manqué).

# NEURENTERIC CYST, SPINAL

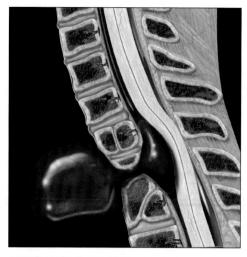

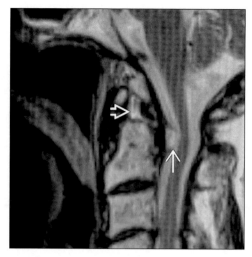

*Sagittal graphic demonstrates a large mediastinal enteric cyst extending into the ventral spinal canal through a patent canal of Kovalevsky, producing spinal cord compression.*

*Sagittal T2WI MR depicts a small extramedullary neurenteric cyst ➡ compressing the ventral spinal cord. There is a related C2 osseous defect ➡ and normal anterior C1 ring size.*

## TERMINOLOGY

### Abbreviations and Synonyms
- Spinal enterogenous cyst, spinal enteric cyst, spinal dorsal-enteric cyst

### Definitions
- Intraspinal cyst lined by enteric mucosa

## IMAGING FINDINGS

### General Features
- Best diagnostic clue: Intraspinal cyst + vertebral abnormalities (persistent canal of Kovalevsky, segmentation and fusion anomalies)
- Location: Thoracic (42%) > cervical (32%) > > lumbar spine, intracranial/basilar cisterns (rare)
- Size: Range small → large
- Morphology: Intraspinal or "dumbbell" shaped abdominal or mediastinal enteric/spinal cyst; ventral > dorsal, extramedullary (80-85%) > intramedullary (10-15%), midline > paramedian

### CT Findings
- CECT: Hypodense intraspinal cyst with minimal to no enhancement
- Bone CT
  - Focal osseous canal enlargement, widening of interpedicular distance
  - Vertebral anomalies (≤ 50%, usually pediatric patient); vertebral clefts, butterfly vertebra, segmentation anomalies

### MR Findings
- T1WI
  - Well-circumscribed fluid-intensity lesion +/- vertebral anomalies
    - Iso- → hyperintense (to CSF) depending on protein/mucin content
- T2WI
  - Well-circumscribed fluid-intensity cystic lesion
    - Hypo- → isointense (to CSF) depending on protein/mucin content
  - +/- Cord myeloschisis, focal cord atrophy
- T1 C+: Mild to no rim-enhancement

III

6

44

---

## DDx: Neurenteric Cyst

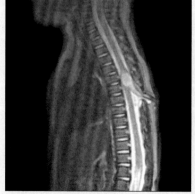

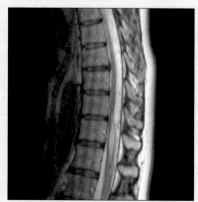

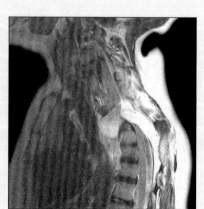

| *Epidermoid Tumor* | *Arachnoid Cyst* | *Anterior Meningocele* |

# NEURENTERIC CYST, SPINAL

## Key Facts

### Terminology
- Spinal enterogenous cyst, spinal enteric cyst, spinal dorsal-enteric cyst

### Imaging Findings
- Best diagnostic clue: Intraspinal cyst + vertebral abnormalities (persistent canal of Kovalevsky, segmentation and fusion anomalies)
- Location: Thoracic (42%) > cervical (32%) > > lumbar spine, intracranial/basilar cisterns (rare)
- Focal osseous canal enlargement, widening of interpedicular distance

### Top Differential Diagnoses
- (Epi)dermoid Cyst
- Arachnoid Cyst
- Anterior Thoracic Meningocele

### Pathology
- Single smooth unilocular (rarely multilocular) cyst containing clear or proteinaceous fluid (milky, cream-colored, yellowish, xanthochromic)
- Demonstrable cyst connection with spinal cord, vertebrae, or both; dorsal spinal-enteric tract traverses cartilage-lined canal of Kovalevsky through small dysplastic vertebra

### Clinical Issues
- Back/radicular pain
- Progressive paraparesis/paresthesias

### Diagnostic Checklist
- Degree of cord compression, size of cyst, and severity of associated anomalies determine disease course and prognosis

## Radiographic Findings
- Radiography
  - Enlarged spinal canal, widening of interpedicular distance
  - +/- Vertebral segmentation/fusion anomalies, midline circular vertebral defect (canal of Kovalevsky)

## Ultrasonographic Findings
- Grayscale Ultrasound: Hypoechoic intraspinal cyst

## Nuclear Medicine Findings
- Tc-99m cyst uptake (gastric mucosa) confirms diagnosis

## Non-Vascular Interventions
- Myelography
  - Focal spinal canal enlargement, contrast filling defect
    - Invaginating cyst mimics intramedullary lesion

## Imaging Recommendations
- Multiplanar T1WI, T2WI to assess for vertebral anomalies, cord compression, and cyst relationship to adjacent structures
- Bone CT/3D CT to characterize osseous anomalies, surgical planning

## DIFFERENTIAL DIAGNOSIS

### (Epi)dermoid Cyst
- Most common at conus/cauda equina level
- +/- Sinus tract, cord tethering, skin dimple

### Arachnoid Cyst
- CSF density/intensity on all pulse sequences
- Generally located within dorsal spinal canal
- Vertebral anomalies uncommon

### Anterior Thoracic Meningocele
- Anterior dumbbell shape, contiguous with dural sac

## PATHOLOGY

### General Features
- General path comments
  - Enteric cysts not limited to spinal column; may be found within brain, mediastinum, abdomen, pelvis, subcutaneous tissues
  - Neurenteric cyst is a subgroup of split notochord syndrome spectrum
    - Dorsal enteric diverticulum: Diverticulum from dorsal mesenteric border of bowel
    - Dorsal enteric enterogenous cyst: Prevertebral, intraspinal, postvertebral, mediastinal, or mesenteric location
    - Dorsal enteric sinus: Blind ending tract with opening on dorsal skin surface
    - Dorsal enteric fistula (most severe): Connects intestinal cavity with dorsal skin surface, traversing through soft tissues and spine
- Etiology
  - Putative derivation from abnormal connection between primitive endoderm and ectoderm during 3rd embryonic week
    - Notochord normally separates dorsal ectoderm (skin and spinal cord) and ventral endoderm (foregut)
    - Failure of separation ⇒ split notochord or notochord deviated to side of adhesion
    - Incomplete separation of notochord layer from the endoderm (primitive foregut) layer hinders development of mesoderm; a small piece of primitive gut becomes trapped in developing spinal canal
    - Embryo growth, adhesion may lengthen or partially obliterate; enteric and spinal structures connected through persistent canal of Kovalevsky in severe cases
- Epidemiology: Rare: 0.3-0.5% of spinal "tumors"
- Associated abnormalities

# NEURENTERIC CYST, SPINAL

○ Vertebral anomalies (≤ 50%): Anterior or posterior dysraphism, small dysplastic vertebral bodies, vertebral fusion, butterfly or hemivertebra, diastematomyelia (31%), lipoma (31%), dermal sinus tract, or tethered spinal cord (23%)
  ▪ Implies earlier developmental "error" than cases without vertebral anomalies
  ▪ More common if mediastinal or abdominal cysts
○ Klippel-Feil syndrome
○ Cutaneous stigmata
○ Alimentary duplication or fistulae, VACTERL syndrome

## Gross Pathologic & Surgical Features

• Single smooth unilocular (rarely multilocular) cyst containing clear or proteinaceous fluid (milky, cream-colored, yellowish, xanthochromic)
  ○ Demonstrable cyst connection with spinal cord, vertebrae, or both; dorsal spinal-enteric tract traverses cartilage-lined canal of Kovalevsky through small dysplastic vertebra

## Microscopic Features

• Thin-walled cyst lined by simple, pseudostratified, stratified cuboidal, or columnar epithelium +/- ciliated epithelium, goblet cells
• Ultrastructurally similar to brain Rathke cleft cyst, colloid cyst

## Staging, Grading or Classification Criteria

• World Health Organization (WHO) classification: "Other malformative tumors and tumor-like lesions"
• Three types based on histology (Wilkins and Odum)
  ○ Type A: Single layer or pseudostratified epithelium resembling respiratory (17%) or gastrointestinal (50%) epithelium, or both (33%)
  ○ Type B: Type A + mucous or serous glands, smooth muscle connective tissue, lymphoid tissue or nervous tissue
  ○ Type C: Type A + ependymal or other glial elements

# CLINICAL ISSUES

## Presentation

• Most common signs/symptoms
  ○ Back/radicular pain
  ○ Progressive paraparesis/paresthesias
  ○ Gait disturbance
  ○ Meningitis
    ▪ Mollaret → rupture into CSF
    ▪ Bacterial → seeding by enteric organisms
  ○ Other signs/symptoms
    ▪ Chronic fever and myelopathy 2° to secretion of TNF-α (usually infants)
    ▪ Congenital mirror movements of hands (very rare, seen in conjunction with diastematomyelia)
• Clinical Profile
  ○ Children present more commonly with cutaneous stigmata, spinal dysraphism symptoms
  ○ Adults present primarily with pain, myelopathy

## Demographics

• Age

○ 2nd → 4th decades (range 8 days → 72 years)
  ▪ Cysts with associated malformations present earlier than isolated cysts
• Gender: M:F = 3:2 to 2:1

## Natural History & Prognosis

• Some asymptomatic → diagnosis at autopsy
• Most show progressive neurological deterioration
• Significant symptomatic improvement following resection in many patients

## Treatment

• Primary treatment goal is complete surgical excision
  ○ Drainage, partial resection if complete excision not possible
  ○ Subtotal excision ⇒ recurrence

# DIAGNOSTIC CHECKLIST

## Consider

• Degree of cord compression, size of cyst, and severity of associated anomalies determine disease course and prognosis

## Image Interpretation Pearls

• Imaging appearance reflects cyst composition
• Look for associated mediastinal or abdominal cysts, connecting fistulae, or vertebral anomalies

# SELECTED REFERENCES

1. Setty H et al: Neurenteric cyst of the posterior mediastinum. Australas Radiol. 49(2):151-3, 2005
2. Hicdonmez T et al: Spontaneous hemorrhage into spinal neurenteric cyst. Childs Nerv Syst. 20(6):438-42, 2004
3. Shenoy SN et al: Spinal neurenteric cyst. Report of 4 cases and review of the literature. Pediatr Neurosurg. 40(6):284-92, 2004
4. Agrawal D et al: Intramedullary neurenteric cyst presenting as infantile paraplegia: a case and review. Pediatr Neurosy. 37(2):93-6, 2002
5. Graham D et al: Greenfield's Neuropathology. 7th ed. London, Arnold. 968-69, 2002
6. Kumar R et al: Intraspinal neurenteric cysts--report of three paediatric cases. Childs Nerv Syst. 17(10):584-8, 2001
7. Lippman CR et al: Intramedullary neurenteric cysts of the spine. Case report and review of the literature. J Neurosurg. 94(2 Suppl):305-9, 2001
8. Kadhim H et al: Spinal neurenteric cyst presenting in infancy with chronic fever and acute myelopathy. Neurology. 54(10):2011-5, 2000
9. Paleologos TS et al: Spinal neurenteric cysts without associated malformations. Are they the same as those presenting in spinal dysraphism? Br J Neurosurg. 14(3):185-94, 2000
10. Ellis AM et al: Intravertebral spinal neurenteric cysts: a unique radiographic sign--"the hole-in-one vertebra". J Pediatr Orthop. 17(6):766-8, 1997
11. Prasad VS et al: Cervico-thoracic neurenteric cyst: clinicoradiological correlation with embryogenesis. Childs Nerv Syst. 12(1):48-51, 1996
12. Gao PY et al: Neurenteric cysts: pathology, imaging spectrum, and differential diagnosis. International Journal of Neuroradiology. 1:17-27, 1995
13. Brooks BS et al: Neuroimaging features of neurenteric cysts: analysis of nine cases and review of the literature. AJNR Am J Neuroradiol. 14(3):735-46, 1993

# NEURENTERIC CYST, SPINAL

## IMAGE GALLERY

### Typical

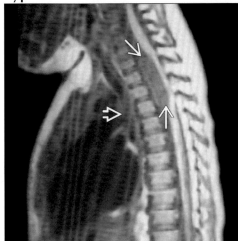
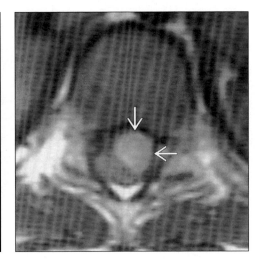

*(Left)* Sagittal T1WI MR reveals a large ventral cystic canal mass ➡ that compresses spinal cord. A prevertebral enteric cyst ➡ reveals similar signal characteristics. (Courtesy R. Boyer, MD). *(Right)* Axial T1WI MR shows a mildly hyperintense (proteinaceous) cyst ➡ within the ventrolateral spinal canal producing ventral spinal cord displacement and compression.

### Variant

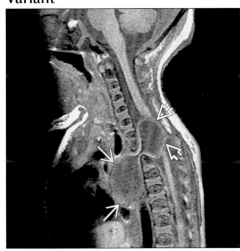
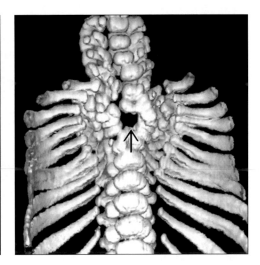

*(Left)* Sagittal T1WI MR shows a large dumbbell shaped neurenteric cyst ➡. The mediastinal enteric cyst ➡ extends into ventral spinal canal through a patent Canal of Kovalevsky. *(Right)* Coronal 3D bone CT shows a jumble of malformed vertebra and fused ribs with patent canal of Kovalevsky ➡, the portal between the mediastinum and spinal canal.

### Variant

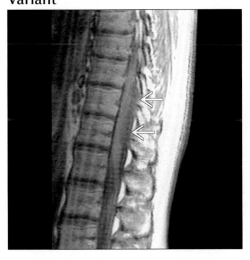
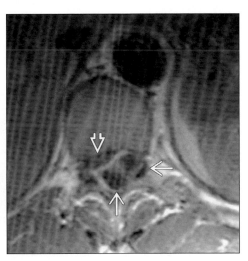

*(Left)* Sagittal T1WI MR demonstrates a complex dorsal multilocular extramedullary neurenteric cyst ➡. There is substantial spinal cord compression. *(Right)* Axial T1 C+ MR confirms extramedullary location of the multicystic rim enhancing mass ➡. There is severe spinal cord ➡ compression with ventral displacement.

# LATERAL MENINGOCELE

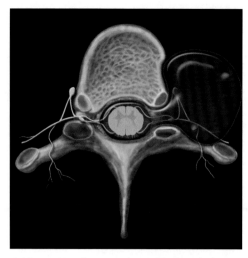

Axial graphic shows a large left lateral thoracic meningocele producing characteristic pedicular erosion, transverse process remodeling, and widening of the neural foramen.

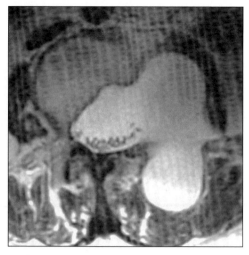

Axial T2WI MR NF1 demonstrates posterior vertebral remodeling and a large left lateral CSF-filled outpouching contiguous with thecal sac.

## TERMINOLOGY

### Definitions
- Meningeal dysplasia ⇒ CSF-filled dural/arachnoidal sac protrudes laterally through neural foramen

## IMAGING FINDINGS

### General Features
- Best diagnostic clue: CSF signal/density meningeal protrusion through neural foramen into adjacent intercostal/extrapleural space
- Location
  - Thoracic > lumbar spine
  - R > L; 10% bilateral
    - Bilateral meningoceles nearly always associated with neurofibromatosis type 1 (NF1), but may be seen in Marfan syndrome
- Size: Typical size 2-3 cm; range tiny ⇒ huge
- Morphology
  - CSF signal/density "cyst" adjacent to spine
    - Contiguous with neural foramen
    - +/- Sharply angled scoliosis at meningocele level

### CT Findings
- CTA: +/- Aortic aneurysm, dissection in context of systemic connective tissue disorder
- CECT
  - CSF density mass extends through enlarged neural foramen
  - No enhancement; useful to distinguish from nerve sheath tumor, nerve inflammation (CIDP)
- Bone CT
  - Wide neural foramen; +/- pedicular thinning, posterior vertebral scalloping (usually)
  - Reformatted images may show focal scoliosis (coronal plane) and dural ectasia (sagittal plane)

### MR Findings
- T1WI
  - CSF signal intensity (hypointense) mass in contiguity with thecal sac
  - Pedicular thinning, neural foraminal widening +/- posterior vertebral scalloping
- T2WI: CSF signal intensity (hyperintense) mass in contiguity with thecal sac; rarely see neural elements within meningocele

## DDx: Lateral Meningocele

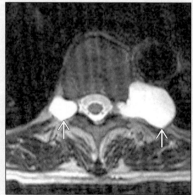

*Nerve Root Cysts*

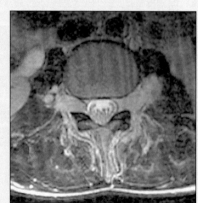

*CIDP*

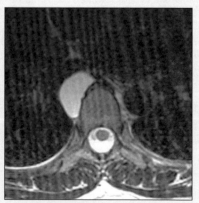

*Foregut Duplication Cyst*

# LATERAL MENINGOCELE

## Key Facts

### Imaging Findings
- Best diagnostic clue: CSF signal/density meningeal protrusion through neural foramen into adjacent intercostal/extrapleural space
- Thoracic > lumbar spine
- R > L; 10% bilateral
- Wide neural foramen; +/- pedicular thinning, posterior vertebral scalloping (usually)
- T1 C+: No enhancement; distinguishes from nerve sheath tumor or inflammation (CIDP)

### Top Differential Diagnoses
- Radicular (Meningeal) Cyst
- Chronic Inflammatory Demyelinating Polyneuropathy
- Foregut Duplication Cyst
- Nerve Sheath Tumor

### Pathology
- Strong association with NF1: 85%

### Clinical Issues
- Age: Most commonly present during 4th ⇒ 5th decades of life
- Gender: M = F
- Most remain asymptomatic unless very large or scoliosis causes symptoms

### Diagnostic Checklist
- Lateral meningocele prompts search for history/stigmata of NF1 or connective tissue disorder
- MR shows nonenhancing CSF signal intensity/density mass extending through an enlarged neural foramen

---

- T1 C+: No enhancement; distinguishes from nerve sheath tumor or inflammation (CIDP)

## Radiographic Findings
- Radiography
  - Pedicular erosion +/- neural foraminal enlargement
    - Often accompanied by scalloping of posterior vertebral bodies (dural ectasia)
    - +/- Sharply angled kyphosis/scoliosis (meningocele is near apex of deformity on convex side)

## Ultrasonographic Findings
- Grayscale Ultrasound
  - Posterior mediastinal or lumbar hypoechoic paraspinal cystic mass contiguous with an expanded spinal canal
    - Displaces and compresses adjacent spinal cord
  - Ultrasound is primary diagnostic tool in-utero, screening newborn infants
- Pulsed Doppler: No vascular flow pattern
- Color Doppler: Avascular hypoechoic mass

## Non-Vascular Interventions
- Myelography
  - Intrathecal contrast fills cyst from dural sac through an enlarged neural foramen
    - Confirms contiguity with thecal sac
    - Delayed imaging may be required
    - Consider placing patient with meningocele(s) dependently to improve contrast filling

## Imaging Recommendations
- Best imaging tool: MR imaging
- Protocol advice
  - Consider sonography for newborn screening; follow-up with MR to clarify positive ultrasound study
  - MR imaging for diagnosis, pre-operative planning
  - Bone CT to evaluate pedicles, vertebral bodies (particularly if surgery is contemplated)

## DIFFERENTIAL DIAGNOSIS

### Radicular (Meningeal) Cyst
- CSF signal intensity/density cyst within neural foramen
  - Cyst separate from dural sac, unlike meningocele
- Nerve root definable as discrete structure within or adjacent to cyst

### Chronic Inflammatory Demyelinating Polyneuropathy
- Solid fusiform nerve root enlargement, enhancement
- Clinical and laboratory findings characteristic

### Foregut Duplication Cyst
- Bronchogenic most common; may contain GI mucosa
  - Seldom contiguous with neural foramen
- Proximity to spinal canal +/- vertebral anomalies = neurenteric cyst

### Nerve Sheath Tumor
- Less hyperintense than CSF on T2WI, higher signal intensity than CSF on T1WI
- Contrast enhancement implies tumor
  - Caveats: Some schwannomas may appear cystic, and some neurofibromas minimally enhance

## PATHOLOGY

### General Features
- General path comments: Dural sac diverticulum, pedicular erosion, neural foraminal widening, and posterior vertebral scalloping
- Genetics
  - Strong association with NF1: 85%
    - Most common posterior mediastinal mass
  - Less common with Ehlers-Danlos, Marfan syndromes
- Etiology
  - Meningocele 2° to primary meningeal dysplasia

# LATERAL MENINGOCELE

- ▪ Meningeal weakness permits dural sac to focally stretch in response to repetitive CSF pulsation ⇒ enlarges neural foramina
  - ▪ Secondary osseous remodeling permits further herniation
  - ○ Posterior vertebral scalloping with dural dysplasia ⇒ same etiology
- Epidemiology: Uncommon in NF1 and inherited connective tissue disorders, but substantially more common than occurrence as an isolated lesion
- Associated abnormalities
  - ○ Occasionally isolated finding
  - ○ +/- Co-existent lumbar and thoracic lateral meningoceles
  - ○ +/- Findings specific to hereditary disorder
    - ▪ NF1: Dural ectasia, nerve sheath tumors, CNS neoplasms, pheochromocytomas, interstitial pulmonary fibrosis, skin and subcutaneous neurofibromas
    - ▪ Marfan syndrome: Dural ectasia, vascular dissection/aneurysm, lens dislocation, joint laxity

## Gross Pathologic & Surgical Features

- Scalloping of pedicles, laminae, and vertebral bodies adjacent to meningocele
- Enlarged central spinal canal, neural foramina
- Cord position variable; usually displaced away from meningocele
- Scoliosis convex toward meningocele

## Microscopic Features

- Dura/arachnoid lined outpouching of thecal sac

**6**

50

# CLINICAL ISSUES

## Presentation

- Most common signs/symptoms
  - ○ Asymptomatic (most common)
  - ○ Nonspecific motor or sensory symptoms referable to cord/nerve root compression
  - ○ Other signs/symptoms
    - ▪ Respiratory embarrassment (neonates); very large meningocele fills thoracic cavity
- Clinical Profile
  - ○ Asymptomatic patient (incidental discovery)
  - ○ +/- Scoliosis evaluation
  - ○ NF1: Cutaneous café-au-lait spots, cutaneous and subcutaneous neurofibromas, +/- kyphoscoliosis
  - ○ Connective tissue disorder: Frequently tall, joint hypermobility, lens dislocation, +/- normal intelligence, +/- scoliosis

## Demographics

- Age: Most commonly present during 4th ⇒ 5th decades of life
- Gender: M = F

## Natural History & Prognosis

- Most remain asymptomatic unless very large or scoliosis causes symptoms
- Most static in size; occasionally grow slowly
- May disappear after hydrocephalus shunting
- Excellent prognosis after surgical resection

## Treatment

- Options, risks, complications
  - ○ Surgical ligation of dural sac neck, resection of meningocele
  - ○ Correction/stabilization of scoliosis

# DIAGNOSTIC CHECKLIST

## Consider

- Lateral meningocele prompts search for history/stigmata of NF1 or connective tissue disorder

## Image Interpretation Pearls

- MR shows nonenhancing CSF signal intensity/density mass extending through an enlarged neural foramen

# SELECTED REFERENCES

1. Barkovich A: Pediatric Neuroimaging. 4th ed. Philadelphia, Lippincott Williams & Wilkins. 398, 667, 2005
2. Kubota M et al: Lateral thoracic meningocele presenting as a retromediastinal mass. Br J Neurosurg. 16(6):607-8, 2002
3. Baysefer A et al: Lateral intrathoracic meningocele associated with a spinal intradural arachnoid cyst. Pediatr Neurosurg. 35(2):107-10, 2001
4. Unsinn KM et al: US of the spinal cord in newborns: spectrum of normal findings, variants, congenital anomalies, and acquired diseases. Radiographics. 20(4):923-38, 2000
5. Zibis AH et al: Unusual causes of spinal foraminal widening. Eur Radiol. 10(1):144-8, 2000
6. Chen SS et al: Multiple bilateral thoracic meningoceles without neurofibromatosis: a case report. Zhonghua Yi Xue Za Zhi (Taipei). 61(12):736-40, 1998
7. Ball W: Pediatric Neuroradiology. Philadelphia, Lippincott-Raven. 727, 1997
8. Gripp KW et al: Lateral meningocele syndrome: three new patients and review of the literature. Am J Med Genet. 70(3):229-39, 1997
9. Strollo DC et al: Primary mediastinal tumors: part II. Tumors of the middle and posterior mediastinum. Chest. 112(5):1344-57, 1997
10. Gibbens DT et al: Chest case of the day. Lateral thoracic meningocele in a patient with neurofibromatosis. AJR Am J Roentgenol. 156(6):1299-300, 1991
11. Nakasu Y et al: Thoracic meningocele in neurofibromatosis: CT and MR findings. J Comput Assist Tomogr. 15(6):1062-4, 1991
12. Chee CP: Lateral thoracic meningocele associated with neurofibromatosis: total excision by posterolateral extradural approach. A case report. Spine. 14(1):129-31, 1989
13. Richaud J: Spinal meningeal malformations in children (without meningoceles or meningomyeloceles). Childs Nerv Syst. 4(2):79-87, 1988
14. Maiuri F et al: Lateral thoracic meningocele. Surg Neurol. 26(4):409-12, 1986
15. Weinreb JC et al: CT metrizamide myelography in multiple bilateral intrathoracic meningoceles. J Comput Assist Tomogr. 8(2):324-6, 1984
16. Erkulvrawatr S et al: Intrathoracic meningoceles and neurofibromatosis. Arch Neurol. 36(9):557-9, 1979
17. Booth AE: Lateral thoracic meningocele. J Neurol Neurosurg Psychiatry. 32(2):111-5, 1969
18. Bunner R: Lateral intrathoracic meningocele. Acta Radiol. 51(1):1-9, 1959

# LATERAL MENINGOCELE

## IMAGE GALLERY

### Typical

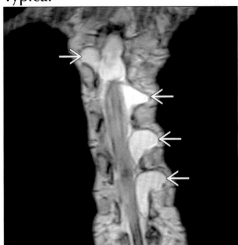

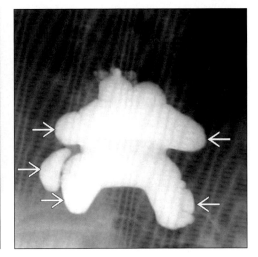

*(Left)* Coronal T2WI MR (Marfan syndrome) demonstrates bilateral small lateral meningoceles that erode the pedicles and project through the neural foramina ➡. *(Right)* Anteroposterior myelography NF1 shows bilateral lateral meningoceles ➡ extending through the neural foramina, in contiguity with the thecal sac.

### Typical

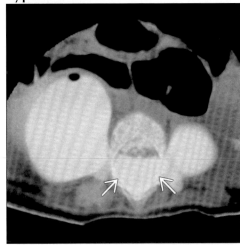

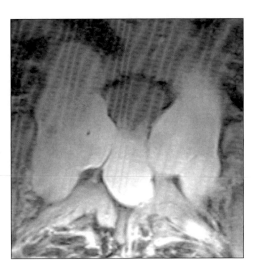

*(Left)* Axial bone CT following myelography reveals bilateral extension of large lateral meningoceles. The meningoceles remodel the central vertebral canal ➡, pushing the nerve roots anteriorly. *(Right)* Axial T2WI MR demonstrates extensive large bilateral lumbar lateral meningoceles that remodel the vertebral canal and neural foramina, and extend into the paraspinal tissues.

### Variant

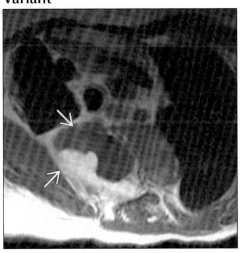

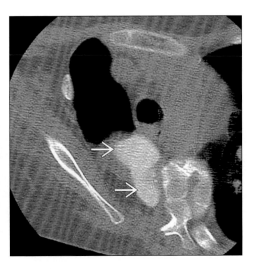

*(Left)* Axial T1WI MR depicts lateral extension of a complex meningocele ➡ into the right paraspinal tissues. Note scalloping of the posterior vertebral body and absence of the right pedicle. *(Right)* Axial bone CT following myelography displays intrathecal contrast within complex (fat containing) lateral meningocele ➡, confirming contiguity with thecal sac.

# DORSAL SPINAL MENINGOCELE

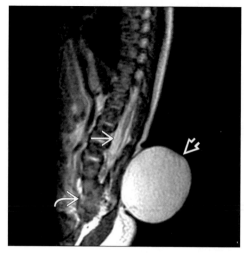

Sagittal T2WI MR shows large fluid-filled sacral dorsal sac → in an infant. No neural element is seen; conus → is low-lying and sacrum ↗ malformed. No fat covers over the sac.

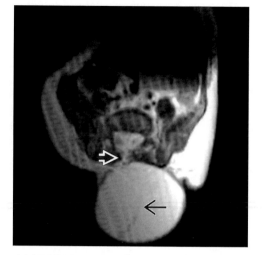

Axial T2WI MR in same infant as previous image shows connection → with spinal canal. Note absence of nervous tissue in sac. Curvilinear artifact → reflects pulsating CSF. Posterior fossa was normal.

## TERMINOLOGY

### Abbreviations and Synonyms
- Simple meningocele, simple spinal meningocele, posterior meningocele

### Definitions
- Dorsal meningeal herniation into subcutaneous tissue without neural malformation

## IMAGING FINDINGS

### General Features
- Best diagnostic clue: Skin-covered sac protruding though posterior bone defect
- Location: Anywhere along spine
- Size: Variable
- Morphology
  - Sessile or pedunculated
  - CSF filled sac with open neural arch(es)
  - Skin normal, fat usually absent
  - May (complex) or may not (simple) contain herniated neural tissue

### CT Findings
- NECT: Hypodense CSF dural sac
- Bone CT
  - Posterior dysraphism
    - Neural arch defect
    - Mild (localized) or severe (multisegmental)
    - ± Spinal canal widening, increased interpedicular distance

### MR Findings
- T1WI
  - Hypointense, CSF-intensity meningeal sac
  - Overlying skin intact (may be secondarily ulcerated) but fat usually missing
  - Nervous tissue
    - Conus medullaris typically normal position
    - Occasional herniation of filum or nerve roots into sac
    - Cord posteriorly displaced in cervical or thoracic meningoceles
- T2WI: Same, except CSF signal is hyperintense
- T2WI FS: Useful for bone morphology, segmentation (coronal)

---

## DDx: Other Posterior Neural Dysraphisms

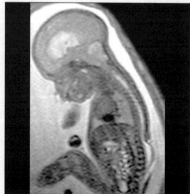
*Fetal Myelomeningocele*

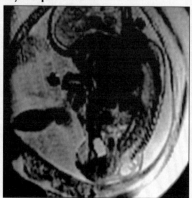
*Fetal Lipomyelomeningocele*

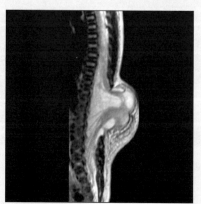
*Thoracic Myelocystocele*

# DORSAL SPINAL MENINGOCELE

## Key Facts

### Terminology
- Simple meningocele, simple spinal meningocele, posterior meningocele

### Imaging Findings
- Best diagnostic clue: Skin-covered sac protruding though posterior bone defect
- Best imaging tool: MR best to show dural sac, content & covering, cord
- Patient lying on side (not to compress the sac)
- Look for associations

### Top Differential Diagnoses
- Posterior Neural Dysraphisms
- Lateral Cystic Dilation of Root Sheaths
- Anterior Sacral Meningocele

### Pathology
- Nearly always contain ill-located nerve roots, ganglion cells, and/or glial nodules at surgery

### Clinical Issues
- Palpable skin-covered mass
- Patients usually neurologically normal
- Usually detected in fetus or neonate
- Associated cord/spine malformations may modify evolution
- Most patients require surgical resection, repair of dural defect

### Diagnostic Checklist
- "Simple" meningoceles are not free of complications

---

## Radiographic Findings
- Radiography: Cleft of neural arch(es); usually one or two vertebrae

## Ultrasonographic Findings
- Grayscale Ultrasound
  - Hypoechoic CSF-filled sac protrudes through posterior defect
    - ± Entrapped nervous tissue
  - Conus level and periodic motion
  - Primarily for fetal (delivery planning) or neonatal screening

## Non-Vascular Interventions
- Myelography
  - Conventional or with CT, when MR impossible/contraindicated
  - Neck of sac may appear occluded with fibrotic arachnoid

## Imaging Recommendations
- Best imaging tool: MR best to show dural sac, content & covering, cord
- Protocol advice
  - Patient lying on side (not to compress the sac)
  - Triplanar imaging for spine, cord, sac content and covering
  - T1, T2 & T2 FS, CISS/Fiesta
  - Look for possible causes for surgical difficulties
    - Entrapped roots attached to the sac
  - Look for associations
    - Neural abnormalities: Thick filum, low conus, split cord, hydromyelia, Chiari 1, epidermoid, lipoma
    - Vertebral abnormalities: Klippel-Feil, isolated hemivertebrae or other segmentation disorders

## DIFFERENTIAL DIAGNOSIS

### Posterior Neural Dysraphisms
- Terminology may be extremely confusing in the literature

- Myelomeningocele
  - Usually lumbosacral
  - Open dysraphism with exposed neural placode, midline skin defect
  - Chiari 2 features generally present (98%)
  - Rare cases located above lumbosacral segment sometimes referred to as "non-terminal myelocystoceles" in the literature
- Lipomyelomeningocele
  - Typically sacral
  - Lipoma continuous with subcutaneous fat through posterior bony defect, no skin defect
  - Cord tethered anterior to lipoma
  - Closed dysraphism, normal skin, no Chiari 2 features
- Myelocystocele
  - Most are sacral (terminal myelocystocele), but they may occur higher as well (true non-terminal myelocystocele)
  - Hydromyelic cyst protruding out of cord into meningocele
  - Closed dysraphism, fat present, no skin defect, no Chiari 2 spectrum features
  - Sometimes associated with cloacal extrophy

### Lateral Cystic Dilation of Root Sheaths
- Neurofibromatosis 1 (NF1): Multiple bilateral meningoceles through neural foramina
  - Part of spectrum of meningeal dysplasias in NF1
  - Usually thoracic
  - Syndrome of intracranial hypotension
- Tarlov cysts: Dilation of meningeal nerve sheaths at and lateral to neural foramina
  - Unknown mechanism
  - Low lumbar and sacral levels
  - Radicular pains

### Anterior Sacral Meningocele
- Anterior, pelvic
- May be simple, isolated, or associated with tethered cord, lipoma, dermoid/teratoma (e.g., Currarino triad)
- Sacral deformity ("scimitar")

# DORSAL SPINAL MENINGOCELE

## PATHOLOGY

### General Features
- General path comments
  - Always skin covered but skin may be dysplastic or ulcerated
  - Classically isolated but associated abnormalities possible
- Genetics: Unknown
- Etiology
  - Unknown
  - Classically: Assumed to be a posterior midline dehiscence of bony, fibrous tissues, with secondary meningeal sac herniation
  - But bony defect may occur without meningeal herniation
  - Herniation of neural tissue may develop secondarily
- Epidemiology: Rare: 1/10,000 live births
- Associated abnormalities
  - Hydrodynamic imbalance: Chiari I herniation possible, hydromyelia
  - Rarely developmental: Tethered cord, diastematomyelia, segmentation disorders

### Gross Pathologic & Surgical Features
- Nearly always contain ill-located nerve roots, ganglion cells, and/or glial nodules at surgery

### Microscopic Features
- Meningocele lined by arachnoid and thin-walled blood vessels; arachnoidal adhesions may obstruct neck of sac

## CLINICAL ISSUES

### Presentation
- Most common signs/symptoms
  - Palpable skin-covered mass
    - Typically diagnosed at birth, exceptionally incidental radiological discovery
  - Depressible, expands with Valsalva
- Other signs/symptoms
  - Back pain, headache, other manifestations of hydrodynamic imbalance
  - Radicular pain or deficits, sensory deficits, sphincters etc.
- Clinical Profile
  - Patients usually neurologically normal
    - Cervical, thoracic meningoceles more likely to be symptomatic than lumbar meningocele

### Demographics
- Age
  - In utero ⇒ adult life
    - Usually detected in fetus or neonate
- Gender: M = F

### Natural History & Prognosis
- Variable; depends on cyst size, contents & overlying skin
  - Skin ulceration
  - Function of entrapped roots may deteriorate

- Entrapment of nervous tissue may be progressive, secondary
- Associated cord/spine malformations may modify evolution

### Treatment
- Depends on size of sac
  - For cosmetic reasons mostly
  - Most patients require surgical resection, repair of dural defect
  - Often before release from nursery to home
  - Yet skin covering permits more "elective" surgical correction than for myelomeningocele
- Treatment of associated neurological/orthopedic disorders if needed

## DIAGNOSTIC CHECKLIST

### Consider
- "Simple" meningoceles are not free of complications

### Image Interpretation Pearls
- Simple meningocele may camouflage other malformations of spine and cord

## SELECTED REFERENCES

1. Arts MP et al: Thoracic meningocele, meningomyelocele or myelocystocele? Diagnostic difficulties, consequent implications and treatment. Pediatr Neurosurg. 40(2):75-9, 2004
2. Akay KM et al: The initial treatment of meningocele and myelomeningocele lesions in adulthood: experiences with seven patients. Neurosurg Rev. 26(3):162-7, 2003
3. Barazi SA et al: High and low pressure states associated with posterior sacral meningocele. Br J Neurosurg. 17(2):184-7, 2003
4. Bekavac I et al: Meningocele-induced positional syncope and retinal hemorrhage. AJNR Am J Neuroradiol. 24(5):838-9, 2003
5. Ersahin Y et al: Is meningocele really an isolated lesion? Childs Nerv Syst. 17(8):487-90, 2001
6. Unsinn KM et al: US of the spinal cord in newborns: spectrum of normal findings, variants, congenital anomalies, and acquired diseases. Radiographics. 20(4):923-38, 2000
7. Sattar TS et al: Pre-natal diagnosis of occult spinal dysraphism by ultrasonography and post-natal evaluation by MR scanning. Eur J Pediatr Surg. 8 Suppl 1:31-3, 1998
8. Steinbok P et al: Cervical meningoceles and myelocystoceles: a unifying hypothesis. Pediatr Neurosurg. 23(6):317-22, 1995
9. De La Paz RL: Congenital anomalies of the lumbosacral spine. Neuroimaging Clinics of North America. 3(3):429-31, 1993
10. Ebisu T et al: Neurenteric cysts with meningomyelocele or meningocele. Split notochord syndrome. Childs Nerv Syst. 6(8):465-7, 1990
11. Wolf YG et al: Thoraco-abdominal enteric duplication with meningocele, skeletal anomalies and dextrocardia. Eur J Pediatr. 149(11):786-8, 1990
12. Delashaw JB et al: Cervical meningocele and associated spinal anomalies. Childs Nerv Syst. 3(3):165-9, 1987
13. Erkulvrawatr S et al: Intrathoracic meningoceles and neurofibromatosis. Arch Neurol. 36(9):557-9, 1979

## IMAGE GALLERY

### Variant

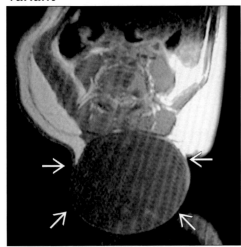

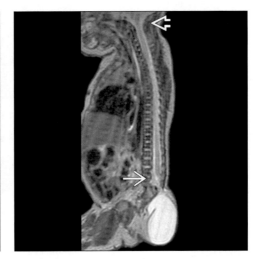

*(Left)* Axial T1WI MR in same infant as previous image shows fluid-filled sac with no nervous tissue within it. The skin covering is normal skin without subcutaneous fat ➡. *(Right)* Sagittal T2WI MR shows low sacral dorsal meningocele with low conus ➡ but no nervous tissue in the sac. Note normal cerebellum ⧩ without Chiari 2 features.

### Variant

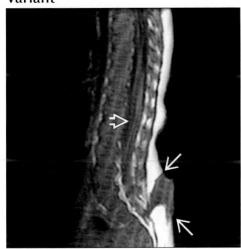

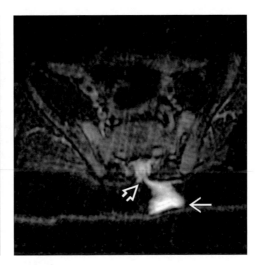

*(Left)* Sagittal T1WI MR shows posterior meningocele ➡ that is not elevated above skin level; conus ⧩ has a normal location. No other malformation was identified. *(Right)* Axial T2WI FS MR in same infant as previous image shows continuity between the sac and dural space ➡. Fat-saturation better depicts normal skin without any fat interposed between the sac and the skin ➡.

### Typical

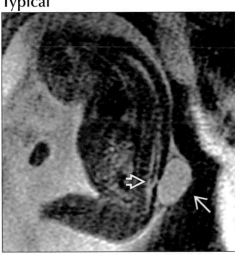

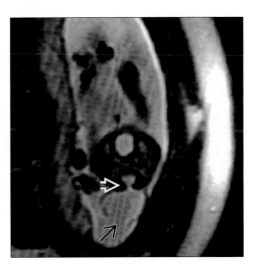

*(Left)* Sagittal T2WI MR in fetus shows large lumbar dorsal sac ➡, with no nervous tissue seen inside and no fat covering. Conus level ⧩ likely normal for gestational age. *(Right)* Axial T2WI MR in same fetus as previous image shows communication ⧩ between meningocele and spinal canal. The posterior discontinuity ➡ likely artifactual.

# NEUROFIBROMATOSIS TYPE 1, SPINE

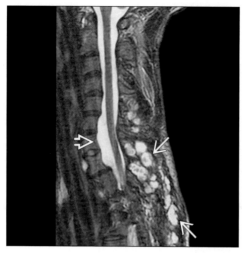

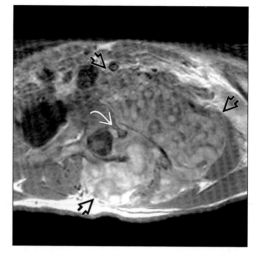

*Sagittal T2WI MR shows mild kyphotic angulation of the midcervical spine, lower cervical dural ectasia ⇨, and a PNF ➡ in the lower cervical/upper thoracic paraspinal soft tissues.*

*Axial T1 C+ MR (same patient as previous image) shows extensive PNF ⇨ in left paraspinal soft tissues. Pedicle ➡ is hypoplastic, and the neural foramen enlarged secondary to PNF & dural ectasia.*

## TERMINOLOGY

### Abbreviations and Synonyms
- Synonyms: NF1, von Recklinghausen disease, peripheral neurofibromatosis
- Abbreviations: Nerve root neurofibroma (NF), plexiform neurofibroma (PNF), malignant peripheral nerve sheath tumor (MPNST)

### Definitions
- Autosomal dominant mesodermal dysplasia characterized by plexiform and nerve root neurofibromas, spinal deformity, neoplastic and non-neoplastic brain lesions, and cutaneous stigmata

## IMAGING FINDINGS

### General Features
- Best diagnostic clue: Kyphoscoliosis ± multiple nerve root tumors, plexiform neurofibroma, dural ectasia/lateral meningocele
- Location: Entire craniospinal axis
- Size: Tumors range tiny → very large

- Morphology
  - Kyphosis/kyphoscoliosis often severe and bizarre
  - Neurogenic tumors localized to nerve roots as well as within plexiform nerve masses, cutaneous lesions

### CT Findings
- NECT
  - Hypodense fusiform or focal nerve root enlargement ± heterogeneous spinal cord expansion (glial tumor)
  - Dural ectasia ± CSF density lateral meningocele(s)
- CECT: Variable mild/moderate tumor enhancement
- Bone CT
  - Vertebral findings similar to radiography; canal, foraminal widening 2° dural ectasia ± spinal cord tumor

### MR Findings
- T1WI
  - Intramedullary glial cord tumors hypo → isointense to normal spinal cord
  - NF: Slight hyperintensity compared to muscle
- T2WI
  - Intramedullary tumors: Hyperintense to normal spinal cord

## DDx: Paraspinal Masses In Children

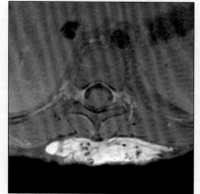

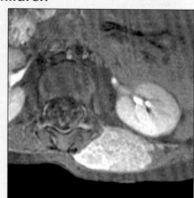

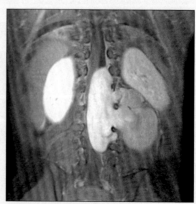

*Hemangioma*

*Leiomyosarcoma*

*Neuroblastoma*

# NEUROFIBROMATOSIS TYPE 1, SPINE

## Key Facts

### Terminology
- Synonyms: NF1, von Recklinghausen disease, peripheral neurofibromatosis

### Imaging Findings
- Best diagnostic clue: Kyphoscoliosis ± multiple nerve root tumors, plexiform neurofibroma, dural ectasia/lateral meningocele

### Top Differential Diagnoses
- Neurofibromatosis Type 2 (NF2, Central Neurofibromatosis)
- Chronic Inflammatory Demyelinating Polyneuropathy (CIDP)
- Congenital Hypertrophic Polyradiculoneuropathies
- Hemangioma, neuroblastoma, ganglioglioma, sarcoma, lymphoma, PNET

### Pathology
- Plexiform neurofibroma is the hallmark of NF1

### Clinical Issues
- Skeletal deformity common (25–40%)
- Palpable spinal or cutaneous mass
- Pigmentation anomalies (café-au-lait, axillary freckling, Lisch nodules) ≥ 90% NF1 patients

### Diagnostic Checklist
- Multiple nerve sheath tumors, ≥ 1 plexiform neurofibroma, bizarre kyphoscoliosis with deformed vertebra → consider NF1
- Absence of visible stigmata does not exclude NF1
- Characteristic PNF imaging appearance best displayed using fat-saturated T2WI or STIR MR imaging

---

- ○ NF: "Target sign" (hyperintense rim, low/intermediate signal intensity center) suggests neurogenic tumor; PNF > NF > MPNST
  - ■ Low T2 center corresponds to dense central core of collagen
- T1 C+
  - ○ Intramedullary tumors: Variable enhancement
  - ○ NF: Mild to moderate enhancement
    - ■ Target sign: Enhancing center, hypointense periphery
    - ■ Primary location → intraforaminal, paraspinal; intraspinal component less common

### Radiographic Findings
- Radiography: Kyphosis/scoliosis, scalloped vertebra, hypoplastic pedicles and posterior elements, ribbon ribs, enlarged neural foramen

### Nuclear Medicine Findings
- PET: FDG standard uptake value (SUV) MPNST > benign tumors

### Imaging Recommendations
- Best imaging tool: MR imaging
- Protocol advice
  - ○ Radiography to quantify and follow kyphosis, scoliosis
  - ○ Multiplanar enhanced MR (especially STIR, fat-saturated T2WI and T1 C+ MR) to evaluate cord, nerve pathology
  - ○ Bone CT to optimally define osseous anatomy for surgical planning

## DIFFERENTIAL DIAGNOSIS

### Neurofibromatosis Type 2 (NF2, Central Neurofibromatosis)
- Multiple intracranial schwannomas and meningiomas, spinal schwannomas and meningiomas
- Spinal deformity uncommon
- Pediatric presentation uncommon

### Chronic Inflammatory Demyelinating Polyneuropathy (CIDP)
- Repeated episodes of demyelination, remyelination ⇒ "onion skin" spinal, peripheral nerve enlargement
- Mimics PNF on imaging studies
- Occasional pediatric presentation (prevalence .5 per 100,000)

### Congenital Hypertrophic Polyradiculoneuropathies
- Charcot-Marie-Tooth, Dejerine-Sottas disease
- Nerve root enlargement mimics PNF on imaging studies
- No cutaneous stigmata of NF1

### Paraspinal Soft Tissue Tumors In Children
- Hemangioma, neuroblastoma, ganglioglioma, sarcoma, lymphoma, PNET

## PATHOLOGY

### General Features
- General path comments
  - ○ Plexiform neurofibroma is the hallmark of NF1
  - ○ Kyphoscoliosis is most common NF1 osseous abnormality; variable severity (usually mild; can be severe, progressive)
    - ■ Dystrophic scoliosis: Short-segment, sharply angulated, < 6 spinal segments, tendency → severe deformity
    - ■ Nondystrophic scoliosis: Similar to adolescent idiopathic curvature, usually 8-10 spinal segments, right convex
    - ■ Severe cervical kyphosis highly suggestive of NF1
  - ○ Dural ectasia: 1° meningeal/bone dysplasia, some cases 2° pressure erosion from intraspinal tumors
  - ○ "Ribbon" ribs 2° to bone dysplasia ± intercostal NF
- Genetics
  - ○ Autosomal dominant; chromosome 17q11.2, penetrance → 100%

- NF gene product (neurofibromin): Tumor suppressor; also involved in histogenesis of brain and nerves
  - Function of NF1 gene product in skeletal development/remodeling unknown
  - ~ 50% new mutations
- Etiology
  - Postulated that NF1 tumor suppression gene "switched off"
    - Leads to tissue proliferation, tumor development
- Epidemiology: Common (1:3,500 to 1:4,000)
- Associated abnormalities
  - Brain/skull abnormalities: Macrocephaly, focal areas of bright T2 signal abnormality, sphenoid wing dysplasia, glial tumors, hydrocephalus
  - ↑ Risk other neuroendocrine tumors (pheochromocytoma, carcinoid tumor), CML
  - Congenital bowing, pseudoarthrosis of tibia and forearm, massive extremity overgrowth
  - ↑ Fibromuscular dysplasia, vascular stenoses, intracranial aneurysms, moyamoya syndrome

## Gross Pathologic & Surgical Features
- Three types of spinal NF recognized in NF1
  - Localized NF (90% all NF)
    - Most common NF in both NF1, non-NF1 patients
    - Cutaneous and deep nerves, spinal nerve roots
    - NF1: Larger, multiple, more frequently involve large deep nerves (sciatic nerve, brachial plexus)
    - Malignant transformation rare
  - Diffuse NF
    - Infiltrating subcutaneous tumor; rarely affects spinal nerves; 90% **not** associated with NF1
  - Plexiform NF (pathognomonic for NF1)
    - Diffuse enlargement of major nerve trunks/branches ⇒ bulky rope-like ("bag of worms") nerve expansion with adjacent tissue distortion
    - Commonly large, bilateral, multilevel with predilection for sciatic nerve, brachial plexus
    - ~ 5% risk malignant degeneration → sarcoma

## Microscopic Features
- Neoplastic Schwann cells + perineural fibroblasts grow along nerve fascicles
  - Collagen fibers, mucoid/myxoid matrix, tumor, nerve fascicles intermixed
  - S-100 positive, mitotic figures rare unless malignant degeneration

## Staging, Grading or Classification Criteria
- Consensus Development Conference on Neurofibromatosis (NIH, 1987): 2 or more of the following criteria
  - > 6 café-au-lait spots measuring ≥ 15 mm in adults or 5 mm in children
  - ≥ 2 neurofibromas of any type or ≥ 1 plexiform neurofibroma
  - Axillary or inguinal freckling
  - Optic glioma
  - Two or more Lisch nodules (iris hamartomas)
  - Distinctive bony lesion (sphenoid wing dysplasia)
  - Thinning of long bone ± pseudoarthrosis
  - First-degree relative with NF1

# CLINICAL ISSUES

## Presentation
- Most common signs/symptoms
  - Skeletal deformity common (25-40%)
    - Focal or acute angle kyphoscoliosis ± myelopathy
    - Extremity bowing or overgrowth
  - Palpable spinal or cutaneous mass
    - With rapid growth or pain, suspect sarcomatous degeneration
  - Pigmentation anomalies (café-au-lait, axillary freckling, Lisch nodules) ≥ 90% NF1 patients

## Demographics
- Age: Childhood diagnosis; minimally affected patients may be diagnosed as adults
- Gender: M = F

## Natural History & Prognosis
- Kyphosis, scoliosis frequently progressive
- NF growth usually slow; rapid growth associated with pregnancy, puberty, or malignant transformation

## Treatment
- Conservative observation; intervention dictated by clinical symptomatology, appearance of neoplasm
- Surgical resection of symptomatic localized NF, spinal cord tumors
- PNF invasive, rarely resectable; observation ± biological or chemotherapeutic (thalidomide, antihistamines, maturation agents, antiangiogenic drugs) intervention
- Spinal fusion reserved for symptomatic or severe kyphoscoliosis

# DIAGNOSTIC CHECKLIST

## Consider
- Multiple nerve sheath tumors, ≥ 1 plexiform neurofibroma, bizarre kyphoscoliosis with deformed vertebra → consider NF1
- Absence of visible stigmata does not exclude NF1

## Image Interpretation Pearls
- Characteristic PNF imaging appearance best displayed using fat-saturated T2WI or STIR MR imaging

# SELECTED REFERENCES

1. Alwan S et al: Is osseous dysplasia a primary feature of neurofibromatosis 1 (NF1)? Clin Genet. 67(5):378-90, 2005
2. Khong PL et al: MR imaging of spinal tumors in children with neurofibromatosis 1. AJR Am J Roentgenol. 180(2):413-7, 2003
3. Packer RJ et al: Plexiform neurofibromas in NF1: toward biologic-based therapy. Neurology. 58(10):1461-70, 2002
4. Lin J et al: Cross-sectional imaging of peripheral nerve sheath tumors: characteristic signs on CT, MR imaging, and sonography. AJR Am J Roentgenol. 176(1):75-82, 2001
5. Murphey MD et al: From the archives of the AFIP. Imaging of musculoskeletal neurogenic tumors: radiologic-pathologic correlation. Radiographics. 19(5):1253-80, 1999

# NEUROFIBROMATOSIS TYPE 1, SPINE

## IMAGE GALLERY

### Typical

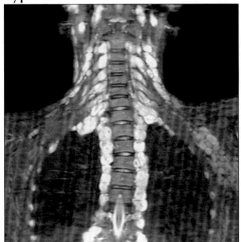
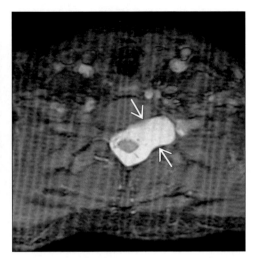

*(Left)* Coronal STIR MR of the cervical and thoracic spine shows bilateral neurofibromas at every spinal level, also in the brachial plexus, the soft tissues of the neck and the intercostal nerves. *(Right)* Axial STIR MR shows a left lateral meningocele ➡ at T1-T2 extending through a widened neural foramen. Lesion was isointense to CSF on T2 and T1 weighted images.

### Typical

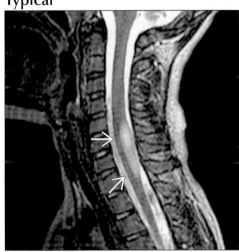
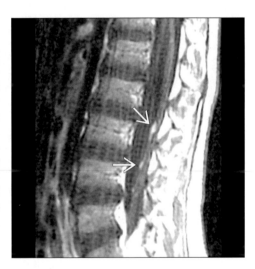

*(Left)* Sagittal T2WI MR in a 3 year old shows a well defined mass ➡ in the posterior cervicothoracic spinal cord. This low grade glioma was bright on T2 weighted images but did not enhance. *(Right)* Sagittal T1 C+ MR in the same patient as previous image shows multiple enhancing lesions ➡ in the lumbar spine. These intraspinal neurofibromas should not be mistaken for subarachnoid metastatic disease.

### Typical

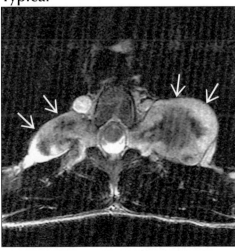
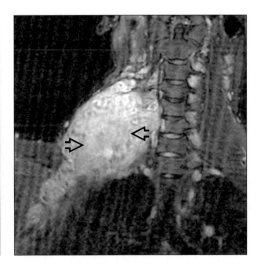

*(Left)* Axial T2WI MR shows bilateral large midthoracic neurofibromas ➡ foraminal and paravertebral in location. This was the only involved spinal level. *(Right)* Coronal STIR MR shows a large mass in the right brachial plexus. This mass had become painful, and the "target" appearance of PNF is not present in the deep portion ➡. Biopsy showed a MPNST.

# NEUROFIBROMATOSIS TYPE 2, SPINE

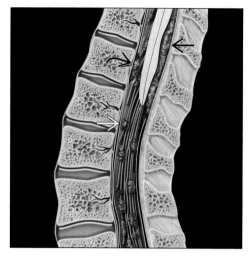

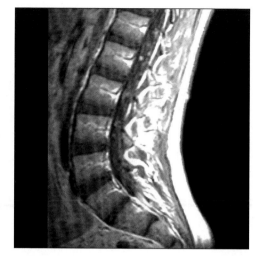

Sagittal graphic demonstrates numerous small schwannomas ➡ within cauda equina. Dorsal en plaque meningioma ⊡➜ indents conus, while ventral smaller meningioma ⊡➜ effaces subarachnoid space.

Sagittal T1 C+ MR reveals numerous enhancing nodules within cauda equina characteristic of schwannomas. Brain MR imaging (not shown) confirmed bilateral vestibular schwannomas.

## TERMINOLOGY

### Abbreviations and Synonyms
- NF2, nonsyndromic (NS)
- Bilateral acoustic neurofibromatosis, central neurofibromatosis (obsolete)

### Definitions
- Autosomal dominant from chromosomal 22 defect in which all patients develop CNS tumors
- Mnemonic for NF2 tumors = MISME (multiple inherited schwannomas, meningiomas, & ependymomas)

## IMAGING FINDINGS

### General Features
- Best diagnostic clue: Multiple spinal tumors of various histologic types
- Location
  - Schwannomas
    - Intradural, extramedullary; may occur anywhere in entire spine
    - Anatomic proximity to nerve root
    - May extend extradurally ("dumbbell")
  - Meningiomas: Intradural, extramedullary; typically thoracic spine, may occur anywhere
  - Ependymomas: Intramedullary; typically upper cervical cord or conus, may occur anywhere
- Size
  - Schwannomas: Tiny → several cms
  - Meningiomas: Vary; nodular studding → large
  - Ependymomas: Tiny → several cms
- Morphology
  - Schwannomas
    - Rounded, cystic when large
    - Dumbbell-shaped with extradural extension
  - Meningiomas: Flattened, dural attachment
  - Ependymomas: Elongated, heterogeneous

### CT Findings
- NECT: Similar appearance to nonsyndromic tumors

### MR Findings
- T1WI
  - Schwannomas
    - Intermediate signal intensity, ± hemorrhage or cystic degeneration

## DDx: Neurofibromatosis Type 2

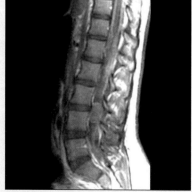

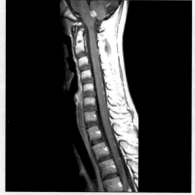

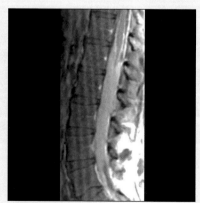

CSF Metastases     von Hippel Lindau     Lymphoma

# NEUROFIBROMATOSIS TYPE 2, SPINE

## Key Facts

### Terminology
- Mnemonic for NF2 tumors = MISME (multiple inherited schwannomas, meningiomas, & ependymomas)

### Imaging Findings
- Best diagnostic clue: Multiple spinal tumors of various histologic types
- Protocol advice: Contrast-enhanced MR best method for detecting lesions regardless of size

### Top Differential Diagnoses
- Metastasis
- Hemangioblastoma
- Non-Syndromic Schwannoma
- Non-Syndromic Meningioma
- Non-Syndromic Ependymoma

- Lymphoma

### Pathology
- Autosomal dominant
- 22q12 deletion → loss of NF2 gene product merlin (aka schwannomin)

### Clinical Issues
- Up to 50% present initially with hearing loss
- Up to 45% with extramedullary tumors exhibit signs/symptoms of cord compression
- Tumor resection is mainstay of NF2 treatment

### Diagnostic Checklist
- Multiple & different pathologic types of spinal tumors is highly suggestive of NF2
- Screen using MR C+ of brain & entire spine

---

- Meningiomas: Low → intermediate signal intensity
- Ependymomas
  - Iso- → mildly hyperintense signal intensity
- T2WI
  - Schwannomas
    - Hyperintense signal intensity, ± hemorrhage or cystic degeneration
  - Meningiomas
    - Variable, heterogeneous
  - Ependymomas: Usually well-defined, hyperintense signal intensity
  - Pitfall: Ill-defined hyperintense lesion → consider low grade astrocytoma
- T1 C+
  - Schwannomas: Avid enhancement; homogeneously when small, heterogeneously when large & cystic
  - Meningiomas: Avid homogeneous enhancement (often < schwannomas)
  - Ependymomas: Heterogeneous enhancement

### Imaging Recommendations
- Best imaging tool: Multiplanar C+ MR
- Protocol advice: Contrast-enhanced MR best method for detecting lesions regardless of size

## DIFFERENTIAL DIAGNOSIS

### Metastasis
- Originate from leptomeninges, eccentric

### Hemangioblastoma
- Associated with von-Hippel Lindau
- Originate from leptomeninges, may have associated cyst

### Non-Syndromic Schwannoma
- Imaging identical to syndromic tumors

### Non-Syndromic Meningioma
- Imaging identical to syndromic tumors

### Non-Syndromic Ependymoma
- Usually solitary, imaging identical to syndromic tumors

### Lymphoma
- Eccentric, may coat spinal cord pial surface

## PATHOLOGY

### General Features
- General path comments: Tumors of Schwann cells & meninges
- Genetics
  - Autosomal dominant
  - 22q12 deletion → loss of NF2 gene product merlin (aka schwannomin)
- Etiology
  - Chromosomal 22 deletion with eventual inactivation of merlin functionality
    - 1st event is chromosomal 22 loss
    - "Second hit theory": Remaining single NF2 copy is mutated (vast majority null mutations) → truncated, poorly or non-functional merlin protein
- Epidemiology
  - 1/50,000 live births worldwide
  - Intradural spinal tumors up to 65% patients on initial imaging
    - 84% have intramedullary tumors
    - 87% have intradural/extramedullary tumors

### Gross Pathologic & Surgical Features
- Multiple tumors of different histologic types

### Microscopic Features
- Merlin monoclonal antibody immunohistochemistry exhibits consistent Schwann cell immunostaining
- NF2 histopathology same as nonsyndromic tumors (with exception of multiplicity)

### Staging, Grading or Classification Criteria
- Definite NF2 diagnosis

# NEUROFIBROMATOSIS TYPE 2, SPINE

- Bilateral CN8 (vestibular) schwannomas
- 1st degree relative with NF2 & either unilateral early onset vestibular schwannoma (age < 30 years) or any 2 of meningioma, glioma, schwannoma, or juvenile posterior subcapsular lenticular opacity
- Presumptive NF2 diagnosis
  - Early onset unilateral CN8 schwannoma (age < 30 years) + one of meningioma, glioma, schwannoma, or juvenile posterior subcapsular lenticular opacity
  - Multiple meningiomas (> 2) + either unilateral vestibular schwannoma or one of glioma, schwannoma, or juvenile posterior subcapsular lenticular opacity
- Germline study findings support genotype-phenotype correlation of tumor grading
  - Nonsense & frameshift mutations
    - Usually severe disease phenotype; higher numbers of all spinal tumors, higher % of patients have intramedullary tumors, younger age at symptom onset or NF2 diagnosis
  - Missense mutations & large gene deletions
    - Usually mild disease phenotype
  - Splice-site mutations
    - Mild → severe phenotype depending on intron involved and effect on protein functionality

## CLINICAL ISSUES

### Presentation
- Most common signs/symptoms
  - Up to 50% present initially with hearing loss
  - Up to 45% with extramedullary tumors exhibit signs/symptoms of cord compression
    - Dependent on location
    - Weakness & sensory loss at or below level
    - Spasticity, pain, loss of bowel/bladder control
- Clinical Profile
  - Detection rates for genetic testing ~ 65%
  - Juvenile subcapsular lens opacities common
  - Retinal & choroidal hamartomas in 10-20%
  - Café-au-lait spots < 50%
  - Minimal to no cutaneous neurofibromas
  - Cutaneous schwannomas in 2/3

### Demographics
- Age: Genetic disease present at conception, become symptomatic 2nd-3rd decade
- Gender: M = F
- Ethnicity: No racial predilection

### Natural History & Prognosis
- Many have relatively normal lifespan
- Few patients require therapeutic intervention for intramedullary tumors (often remain quiescent)
- Intradural, extramedullary tumors frequently require surgical intervention
  - Percentage of patients with extramedullary tumors who undergo surgery 5x higher than percentage of patients with intramedullary tumors
  - Higher surgical rate is result of high number of tumors & frequent occurrence of cord compression

- Schwannomas present more often & in higher numbers than meningiomas → more surgical procedures overall
- Meningiomas account for a disproportionate number of symptomatic lesions
  - Meningiomas comprise ~ 12% of extramedullary tumors yet account for 37% of extramedullary tumors requiring excision

### Treatment
- Tumor resection is mainstay of NF2 treatment
- Intramedullary tumors: Monitor with regular imaging & appropriate clinical correlation
  - Relatively indolent course of most intramedullary tumors & anticipated burden from other spinal/intracranial tumors must be considered → standard aggressive management may not be warranted, even in symptomatic patient
- Intradural, extramedullary tumors: Early removal of rapidly growing or symptomatic tumors

## DIAGNOSTIC CHECKLIST

### Consider
- Multiple & different pathologic types of spinal tumors is highly suggestive of NF2

### Image Interpretation Pearls
- Screen using MR C+ of brain & entire spine
- Imaging follow-up of patients with spinal tumors based on knowledge of tumor location, number, & suspected histologic type

## SELECTED REFERENCES

1. Chen JC et al: Cervical dumbbell meningioma and thoracic dumbbell schwannoma in a patient with neurofibromatosis. Clin Neurol Neurosurg. 107(3):253-7, 2005
2. Cohen-Gadol AA et al: Spinal meningiomas in patients younger than 50 years of age: a 21-year experience. J Neurosurg. 98(3 Suppl):258-63, 2003
3. Patronas NJ et al: Intramedullary and spinal canal tumors in patients with neurofibromatosis 2: MR imaging findings and correlation with genotype. Radiology. 218(2):434-42, 2001
4. Evans DG et al: Neurofibromatosis type 2. J Med Genet. 37(12):897-904, 2000
5. den Bakker MA et al: Expression of the neurofibromatosis type 2 gene in human tissues. J Histochem Cytochem. 47(11):1471-80, 1999
6. Seppala MT et al: Multiple schwannomas: schwannomatosis or neurofibromatosis type 2? J Neurosurg. 89(1):36-41, 1998
7. Kluwe L et al: Identification of NF2 germ-line mutations and comparison with neurofibromatosis 2 phenotypes. Hum Genet. 98(5):534-8, 1996
8. Mautner VF et al: The neuroimaging and clinical spectrum of neurofibromatosis 2. Neurosurgery. 38(5):880-5; discussion 885-6, 1996
9. Mautner VF et al: Spinal tumors in patients with neurofibromatosis type 2: MR imaging study of frequency, multiplicity, and variety. AJR Am J Roentgenol. 165(4):951-5, 1995

# NEUROFIBROMATOSIS TYPE 2, SPINE

## IMAGE GALLERY

### Typical

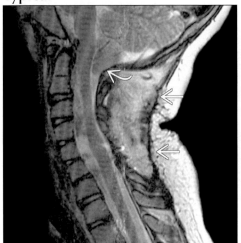
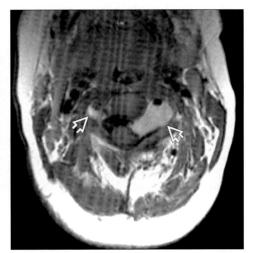

*(Left)* Sagittal T2WI MR demonstrates tumor remodeling of spinal canal and spinal cord deformity. Post-operative laminectomy changes ➡ and tonsillar herniation ➡ are apparent. *(Right)* Axial T1 C+ MR depicts bilateral nerve root schwannomas ➡. Left schwannoma shows characteristic "dumbbell" configuration reflecting concurrent intradural and extradural components.

### Variant

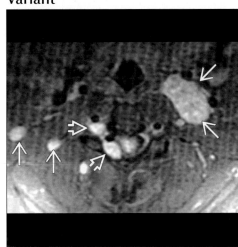
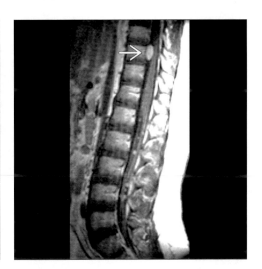

*(Left)* Axial T1 C+ FS MR shows enhancing spinal ➡ and extradural ➡ schwannomas. MR of brain showed unilateral vestibular schwannoma, bilateral trigeminal schwannomas. *(Right)* Sagittal T1 C+ MR shows many small cauda equina schwannomas and larger ventral schwannoma ➡ producing cord compression. Brain MR demonstrated bilateral vestibular schwannomas.

### Variant

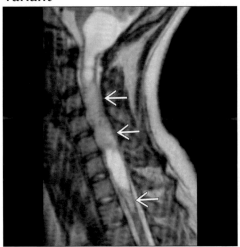
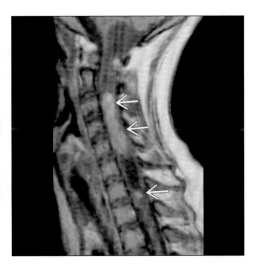

*(Left)* Sagittal T2WI MR demonstrates a large heterogeneous intramedullary mass ➡ with intermediate signal intensity solid tissue "capped" by cystic areas, characteristic of cellular ependymoma. *(Right)* Sagittal T1 C+ MR reveals expected heterogeneous enhancement ➡ of solid intramedullary tumor. Brain MR confirmed NF2 with bilateral enhancing vestibular and trigeminal schwannomas.

# DURAL DYSPLASIA

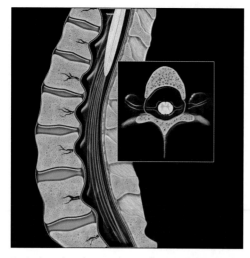

Sagittal graphic demonstrates scalloping of the posterior vertebral bodies with central canal enlargement. Also shown (inset) are bilateral lumbar lateral meningoceles.

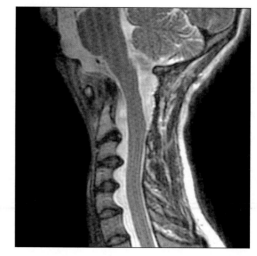

Sagittal T2WI MR (neurofibromatosis type 1) demonstrates striking posterior vertebral scalloping (C2 through C6) from dural dysplasia, producing widening of AP canal diameter.

## TERMINOLOGY

### Abbreviations and Synonyms
- Dural ectasia

### Definitions
- Patulous dural sac with posterior vertebral scalloping

## IMAGING FINDINGS

### General Features
- Best diagnostic clue: Smooth "C" shaped scalloping of posterior vertebral bodies with patulous dural sac
- Location
  - Lumbar > cervical, thoracic
    - Thoracic > lumbar in neurofibromatosis 1 (NF1)
- Size: Mild ⇒ extensive deformity
- Morphology: Expansile dural sac, spinal canal remodeling with posterior vertebral scalloping

### CT Findings
- CTA: +/- Arterial dissection or aneurysm (Marfan or Ehlers-Danlos syndrome)

- CECT
  - Posterior vertebral scalloping ⇒ spinal canal enlargement
    - Easiest to appreciate on sagittal images
  - Pedicular attenuation, widened interpediculate distance, erosion of anterior and posterior elements, patulous CSF density dural sac

### MR Findings
- T1WI
  - Posterior vertebral scalloping, expansion of osseous spinal canal, patulous dural sac, +/- kyphoscoliosis
  - +/- Pedicular thinning, lateral meningocele(s)
- T2WI
  - Similar findings to T1WI
  - Best evaluates position of neural elements relative to dural ectasia
- MRA: +/- Arterial dissection or aneurysm (Marfan, Ehlers-Danlos syndrome)

### Radiographic Findings
- Radiography
  - Smooth remodeling of posterior vertebral body, expansion of osseous spinal canal, +/- kyphoscoliosis
  - Osteopenia (homocystinuria)

## DDx: Dural Dysplasia

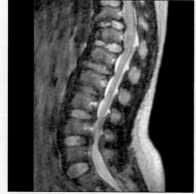

*Morquio (MPS IV)*

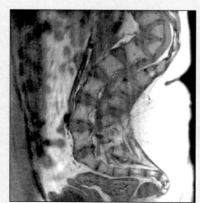

*Achondroplasia*

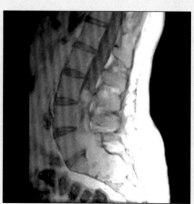

*Myxopapillary Ependymoma*

# DURAL DYSPLASIA

## Key Facts

### Terminology
- Dural ectasia
- Patulous dural sac with posterior vertebral scalloping

### Imaging Findings
- Best diagnostic clue: Smooth "C" shaped scalloping of posterior vertebral bodies with patulous dural sac
- Lumbar > cervical, thoracic
- Posterior vertebral scalloping, expansion of osseous spinal canal, patulous dural sac, +/- kyphoscoliosis
- +/- Pedicular thinning, lateral meningocele(s)

### Top Differential Diagnoses
- Congenital Vertebral Dysplasia
- Spinal Tumor or Syrinx
- Cauda Equina Syndrome of Ankylosing Spondylitis (AS)

### Pathology
- General path comments: Genetic predisposition ⇒ primary meningeal dysplasia ⇒ weakness in meninges ⇒ expansion, secondarily remodeling of posterior vertebral body and pedicular thinning ⇒ further dural sac expansion
- NF1: Autosomal dominant (chromosome 17q12)
- Marfan: Autosomal dominant (15q21.1)
- Homocystinuria: Autosomal recessive (21q22.3)
- Ehlers-Danlos: Autosomal dominant (many genes)

### Clinical Issues
- Moderate to severe back pain > 50% of Marfan patients; presence, degree of dural ectasia associated with back pain

## Ultrasonographic Findings
- Grayscale Ultrasound: Hypoechoic patulous dural sac, widening of spinal canal

## Angiographic Findings
- Conventional
  - Not useful for imaging spine deformity; primary utility is detecting associated vascular anomalies
  - Ascending aortic aneurysm ("tulip bulb configuration") suggests Marfan syndrome

## Non-Vascular Interventions
- Myelography: Posterior vertebral scalloping, contrast fills enlarged dural sac, +/- lateral meningocele(s)

## Imaging Recommendations
- MR shows osseous abnormalities well
- Additionally, MR is most useful modality to exclude syrinx or tumor as cause of canal enlargement before attributing to dural ectasia

# DIFFERENTIAL DIAGNOSIS

## Congenital Vertebral Dysplasia
- Achondroplasia, mucopolysaccharidosis, osteogenesis imperfecta (tarda)
- Search for appropriate family history, clinical stigmata

## Spinal Tumor or Syrinx
- Astrocytoma, ependymoma, nerve sheath tumor, syrinx
- Characteristic imaging findings lead to correct diagnosis

## Cauda Equina Syndrome of Ankylosing Spondylitis (AS)
- Irregular lumbar canal expansion
- Proposed etiology for dural ectasia; proliferative inflammatory synovium ⇒ cauda equina symptoms
- Imaging and clinical stigmata of AS typically present

# PATHOLOGY

## General Features
- General path comments: Genetic predisposition ⇒ primary meningeal dysplasia ⇒ weakness in meninges ⇒ expansion, secondarily remodeling of posterior vertebral body and pedicular thinning ⇒ further dural sac expansion
- Genetics
  - NF1: Autosomal dominant (chromosome 17q12)
  - Marfan: Autosomal dominant (15q21.1)
  - Homocystinuria: Autosomal recessive (21q22.3)
  - Ehlers-Danlos: Autosomal dominant (many genes)
- Etiology
  - NF1: Primary mesenchymal disorder
  - Marfan syndrome: Primary connective tissue defect unknown
  - Ehlers-Danlos: > 10 different types of collagen synthesis defects
  - Homocystinuria: Cystathionine beta-synthetase deficiency
- Epidemiology
  - NF1: 1/4,000, 50% new mutations; dural ectasia common
  - Marfan: 1/5,000 (United States); dural ectasia present > 60% patients
  - Homocystinuria: 1/344,000 worldwide; dural dysplasia less common than Marfan
  - Ehlers-Danlos: 1/400,000 worldwide; dural dysplasia less common than Marfan
- Associated abnormalities
  - Lateral thoracic or lumbar meningocele, anterior sacral meningocele
  - Kyphoscoliosis
  - Joint hypermobility, lens abnormalities, aneurysm, arterial dissection (connective tissue disorders)
  - Peripheral and central neoplasms (NF1)

## Gross Pathologic & Surgical Features
- Enlarged CSF thecal sac, remodeled posterior vertebral bodies
- Dura in ectatic areas is extremely thin, fragile

## Microscopic Features
- Dural thinning in ectatic areas

## CLINICAL ISSUES

### Presentation
- Most common signs/symptoms
  ○ Back pain +/- radiculopathy
    ■ Moderate to severe back pain > 50% of Marfan patients; presence, degree of dural ectasia associated with back pain
    ■ High prevalence of dural ectasia (41%) in Marfan patients without back pain however; mere presence of dural ectasia does not necessarily mean patient is symptomatic
  ○ Other signs/symptoms
    ■ Headache
    ■ Incontinence, pelvic symptoms
- Clinical Profile
  ○ NF1: Plexiform neurofibromas, kyphoscoliosis, optic nerve gliomas and other astrocytomas, café-au-lait spots, axillary freckling, extremity pseudoarthrosis
  ○ Marfan syndrome: Tall, joint hypermobility, arachnodactyly, kyphoscoliosis, joint and lens dislocations
  ○ Homocystinuria: Tall, arachnodactyly, scoliosis, mental retardation, seizures, lens dislocations
  ○ Ehlers-Danlos: +/- Tall, thin hyperelastic skin, hypermobile joints, fragile connective tissue

### Demographics
- Age: May present at any age depending on severity
- Gender: M = F
- Ethnicity
  ○ NF1: All ethnicities; higher in Arab-Israeli subpopulations
  ○ Marfan: All races, ethnicities
  ○ Homocystinuria: Northern European descent
  ○ Ehlers-Danlos: Caucasian, European descent

### Natural History & Prognosis
- Variable; dependent on underlying etiology
- Morbidity and mortality primarily related to vascular pathology
  ○ Vascular fragility ⇒ predisposition to arterial dissection or aneurysm ⇒ premature death

### Treatment
- Directed toward addressing underlying etiology
- Meningocele repair, scoliosis surgery for more severe cases

## DIAGNOSTIC CHECKLIST

### Consider
- Three disease categories produce posterior vertebral scalloping
  ○ Dural ectasia
  ○ Increased intraspinal pressure
  ○ Congenital vertebral dysplasia

- Important to determine underlying disorder for treatment planning, genetic counseling and determining prognosis

### Image Interpretation Pearls
- Recognition of specific imaging clues and integration of available clinical data permits a more specific diagnosis
- Look for imaging stigmata of etiological diseases
  ○ "Tulip bulb" aortic aneurysm ⇒ Marfan syndrome
  ○ Osteoporosis ⇒ homocystinuria
  ○ Pseudoarthrosis, CNS/PNS tumors ⇒ NF1

## SELECTED REFERENCES

1. Barkovich AJ: Pediatric Neuroimaging. 4th ed. Philadelphia, Lippincott Williams & Wilkins. 408, 2005
2. Nallamshetty L et al: Dural ectasia and back pain: review of the literature and case report. J Spinal Disord Tech. 15(4):326-9, 2002
3. Tubbs RS et al: Dural ectasia in neurofibromatosis. Pediatr Neurosurg. 37(6):331-2, 2002
4. Ahn NU et al: Dural ectasia and conventional radiography in the Marfan lumbosacral spine. Skeletal Radiol. 30(6):338-45, 2001
5. Oosterhof T et al: Quantitative assessment of dural ectasia as a marker for Marfan syndrome. Radiology. 220(2):514-8, 2001
6. Ahn NU et al: Dural ectasia in the Marfan syndrome: MR and CT findings and criteria. Genet Med. 2(3):173-9, 2000
7. Ahn NU et al: Dural ectasia is associated with back pain in Marfan syndrome. Spine. 25(12):1562-8, 2000
8. Rose PS et al: A comparison of the Berlin and Ghent nosologies and the influence of dural ectasia in the diagnosis of Marfan syndrome. Genet Med. 2(5):278-82, 2000
9. Schonauer C et al: Lumbosacral dural ectasia in type 1 neurofibromatosis. Report of two cases. J Neurosurg Sci. 44(3):165-8; discussion 169, 2000
10. Sponseller PD et al: Osseous anatomy of the lumbosacral spine in Marfan syndrome. Spine. 25(21):2797-802, 2000
11. De Paepe A: Dural ectasia and the diagnosis of Marfan's syndrome. Lancet. 354(9182):878-9, 1999
12. Fattori R et al: Importance of dural ectasia in phenotypic assessment of Marfan's syndrome. Lancet. 354(9182):910-3, 1999
13. Villeirs GM et al: Widening of the spinal canal and dural ectasia in Marfan's syndrome: assessment by CT. Neuroradiology. 41(11):850-4, 1999
14. Raff ML et al: Joint hypermobility syndromes. Curr Opin Rheumatol. 8(5):459-66, 1996
15. Helfen M et al: Intrathoracic dural ectasia mimicking neurofibroma and scoliosis. A case report. Int Orthop. 19(3):181-4, 1995
16. Bensaid AH et al: Neurofibromatosis with dural ectasia and bilateral symmetrical pedicular clefts: report of two cases. Neuroradiology. 34(2):107-9, 1992
17. Pyeritz RE et al: Dural ectasia is a common feature of the Marfan syndrome. Am J Hum Genet. 43(5):726-32, 1988
18. Stern WE: Dural ectasia and the Marfan syndrome. J Neurosurg. 69(2):221-7, 1988
19. Katz SG et al: Thoracic and lumbar dural ectasia in a two-year-old boy. Pediatr Radiol. 6(4):238-40, 1978

# DURAL DYSPLASIA

## IMAGE GALLERY

### Typical

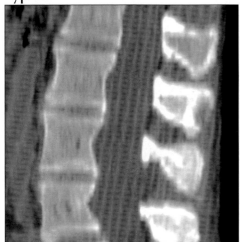
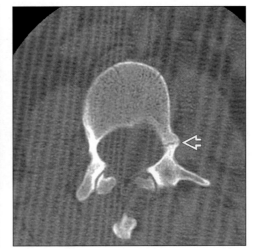

*(Left)* Sagittal bone CT shows curved posterior vertebral remodeling at multiple lumbar vertebral levels characteristic of dural dysplasia (neurofibromatosis type 1). *(Right)* Axial bone CT reveals vertebral remodeling and scalloping that enlarges anteroposterior canal diameter. There is also pseudoarthrosis from a non-healed fracture of a left pedicle ⇒.

### Variant

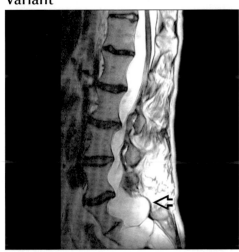
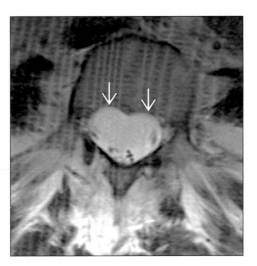

*(Left)* Sagittal T2WI MR reveals marked posterior vertebral scalloping. The sacral canal is markedly widened, with dural extension through the sacral foramina ⇒ from concurrent lateral meningocele. *(Right)* Axial T2WI MR shows widening of spinal canal with posterior vertebral scalloping ⇒. In dural dysplasia, the dural sac generally fills concavity produced in posterior vertebral body.

### Variant

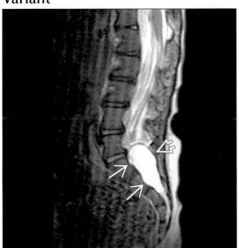
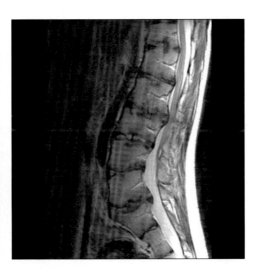

*(Left)* Sagittal T2WI MR (Marfan syndrome) demonstrates moderate posterior vertebral body scalloping ⇒, accompanied by a large intrasacral meningocele ⇒. *(Right)* Sagittal T2WI MR (Homocystinuria) reveals mild vertebral remodeling of dural dysplasia as well as marked degenerative intervertebral disc changes that result in severe spinal stenosis.

# LEUKEMIA, SPINE

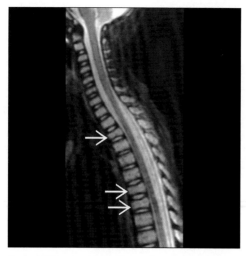

*Sagittal STIR MR demonstrates abnormal hyperintense marrow signal indicating leukemic marrow infiltration and multiple compression fractures ➡ precipitating initial leukemia presentation.*

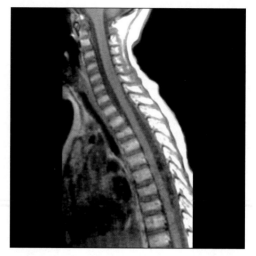

*Sagittal T1 C+ MR reveals diffuse abnormal marrow enhancement from leukemic marrow infiltration. Unlike this strong enhancement, normal red marrow will show minimal incremental enhancement.*

## TERMINOLOGY

### Abbreviations and Synonyms
- Acute lymphocytic leukemia (ALL), chronic lymphocytic leukemia (CLL), acute myelogenous leukemia (AML), chronic myelogenous leukemia (CML), granulocytic sarcoma, chloroma

### Definitions
- Acute or chronic myeloid or lymphoid white blood cell neoplasia with spinal involvement as component of systemic disease

## IMAGING FINDINGS

### General Features
- Best diagnostic clue: Diffuse osteopenia with multiple vertebral fractures +/- lytic spine lesions
- Location
  ○ Children: Multiple long bones and spine (14%)
  ○ Adults: Predominately axial skeleton

- Morphology: Osteopenia +/- moth eaten bone destruction of multiple vertebral bodies, leptomeningeal enhancement, focal mass ("chloroma")

### CT Findings
- NECT
  ○ Isodense soft tissue mass with adjacent bone destruction
  ○ Leptomeningeal disease: ↑ Density of lumbar theca, nerve root enlargement
- CECT: Variable enhancement
- Bone CT
  ○ Permeative bone destruction +/- focal lytic lesions, pathologic vertebral fractures

### MR Findings
- T1WI: Leukemic marrow, focal tumor masses relatively hypointense
- T2WI: Increased leukemic marrow signal intensity +/- focal vertebral mass, cord signal abnormality
- STIR: Hyperintense leukemic marrow
- T1 C+: Abnormal enhancement of marrow, focal lesion, or leptomeninges

---

## DDx: Spinal Leukemia

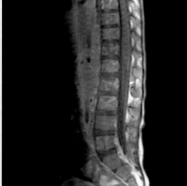

*Neuroblastoma*

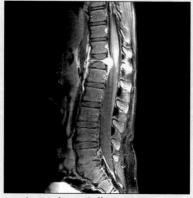

*Langerhans Cell Histiocytosis*

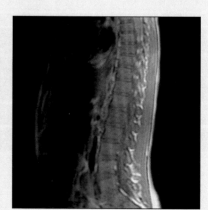

*Hodgkin Disease*

# LEUKEMIA, SPINE

## Key Facts

### Terminology
- Acute or chronic myeloid or lymphoid white blood cell neoplasia with spinal involvement as component of systemic disease

### Imaging Findings
- Best diagnostic clue: Diffuse osteopenia with multiple vertebral fractures +/- lytic spine lesions
- Radiographs may look normal, even if extensive disease
- Granulocytic sarcoma ⇒ focal lytic mass

### Top Differential Diagnoses
- Metastases
- Langerhans Cell Histiocytosis (LCH)
- Osteomyelitis
- Lymphoma

- Ewing Sarcoma

### Pathology
- Strong association with chromosomal abnormalities

### Clinical Issues
- Chronic leukemia may be asymptomatic
- Symptomatic patients present with fever, ↑ ESR, hepatosplenomegaly, lymphadenopathy, joint effusions, petechial and retinal hemorrhage, anemia, frequent infections

### Diagnostic Checklist
- MR sensitivity for leptomeningeal metastases < < laboratory CSF evaluation
- Consider leukemia in a patient with unexplained compression fractures

## Radiographic Findings
- Radiography
  - Diffuse vertebral, long bone osteopenia
    - Coarse cancellous trabeculation +/- pathologic vertebral compression fractures
    - Radiographs may look normal, even if extensive disease
  - +/- "Leukemic lines" (horizontal vertebral bands)
  - Granulocytic sarcoma ⇒ focal lytic mass

## Nuclear Medicine Findings
- Bone Scan: +/- ↑ Radiotracer uptake; often underestimates disease extent, especially in absence of significant cortical destruction

## Imaging Recommendations
- Best imaging tool: MR imaging
- Protocol advice
  - Multiplanar T1WI, T2WI (+ fat-saturation) or STIR, T1 C+ MR
  - Whole body STIR MRI (WBMR) proposed for staging, assessing lesion burden
  - Bone CT with multiplanar reformats to clarify osseous lesions, quantify compression fractures

## DIFFERENTIAL DIAGNOSIS

### Metastases
- Metastatic neuroblastoma or rhabdomyosarcoma in children, carcinomas in adults
- Multifocal bone involvement similar to leukemia

### Langerhans Cell Histiocytosis (LCH)
- Lytic lesion with periosteal reaction, endosteal scalloping, soft tissue mass
- May have systemic symptoms similar to leukemia

### Osteomyelitis
- Granulomatous or pyogenic; TB in particular may (relatively) spare disc spaces
- Periosteal reaction, soft tissue extension
- May have systemic symptoms similar to leukemia

### Lymphoma
- Older patient with large soft tissue mass; predilection for paraspinal, epidural locations
- Systemic lymphomatous metastasis or primary vertebral lesion

### Ewing Sarcoma
- Marked periosteal reaction + associated soft tissue mass
- No metaphyseal lucent lines
- May have systemic symptoms similar to leukemia

## PATHOLOGY

### General Features
- General path comments
  - Spinal leukemia may involve either single or multiple vertebral bodies
    - Most common spinal presentation is multiple compression fractures
  - Neuropathologic features include manifestations of primary disease, side effects of therapeutic procedures (radiation therapy, chemotherapy, BMT), and complications 2° to immunosuppression
    - Spinal manifestations of primary disease: Fractures, marrow or meningeal infiltration
    - Treatment effects: Secondary neoplasms (usually aggressive CNS tumors), hemorrhage, anterior lumbosacral radiculopathy (intrathecal methotrexate toxicity)
    - Immunosuppression complications: Fungal or other opportunistic infection
  - Granulocytic sarcoma (chloroma): Extramedullary neoplasm of immature granulocytic cells → focal lytic mass
    - Most common in AML (concurrent presentation ≤ 9.1% AML cases); rare aleukemic presentations reported
- Genetics
  - Strong association with chromosomal abnormalities
    - ALL: Trisomy 21, chromosomal translocations
    - CLL: Trisomy 12

- CML: 90% have Philadelphia chromosome t(9;22)
- Etiology
  - External factors: Alkylating drugs, ionizing radiation, chemicals (benzene)
  - Internal factors: Chromosomal abnormalities
  - Predisposing hematological disorders: Aplastic anemia, chronic myeloproliferative disorders
- Epidemiology
  - Most common malignancy of childhood (ALL: 75%, AML: 15-20%, CML: 5%)
  - 20th most common cause of cancer death (all age groups)
- Associated abnormalities
  - Long bone periostitis (12-25%), "leukemic" metaphyseal lines
  - Focal destruction of flat/tubular bones, pathologic fractures
  - Opportunistic infections, second malignancies
  - Chemotherapy-related complications

## Gross Pathologic & Surgical Features

- Hyperemic/hemorrhagic bone marrow with destruction of bony trabeculae, bone infarction

## Microscopic Features

- Diffuse bone marrow infiltration by poorly-differentiated hematologic cells
  - ALL: Infiltrates of small blue cells
  - AML: Auer rods (condensed lysosomal cytoplasmic rod shaped structures) diagnostic
  - CLL: Mature lymphocytes, < 55% atypical cells
  - CML: Leukocytosis with increase in basophils, eosinophils, neutrophils; Philadelphia chromosome t(9;22)

# CLINICAL ISSUES

## Presentation

- Most common signs/symptoms
  - Localized or diffuse bone pain
  - Recurrent para-articular arthralgias (75%)
- Clinical Profile
  - Chronic leukemia may be asymptomatic
  - Symptomatic patients present with fever, ↑ ESR, hepatosplenomegaly, lymphadenopathy, joint effusions, petechial and retinal hemorrhage, anemia, frequent infections

## Demographics

- Age
  - ALL: Peak 2-10 y
  - AML: Peak > 65 y
  - CML: Rare in childhood (< 5%), peak > 40 y
  - CLL: Peak 50-70 y
- Gender: M:F = 2:1

## Natural History & Prognosis

- 5 year survival (all leukemias): 25-30%
  - Children with ALL: 90% complete remission, 80% 5 year disease free survival
  - Adults with ALL: Remission in 60-80%, 20-30% 5 year disease free survival
  - AML: 45% 5 year survival

- CLL: 6 years median survival
- CML: 5 years median survival

## Treatment

- Chemotherapy
  - Induction phase, consolidation phase, maintenance therapy phase
  - Intrathecal chemotherapy for CNS involvement
- Radiation therapy
- Bone marrow transplant

# DIAGNOSTIC CHECKLIST

## Consider

- Marrow infiltration in child with osteoporosis raises suspicion for leukemia
- MR sensitivity for leptomeningeal metastases < < laboratory CSF evaluation

## Image Interpretation Pearls

- Consider leukemia in a patient with unexplained compression fractures

# SELECTED REFERENCES

1. Staebler M et al: Complications of lumbar puncture in a child treated for leukaemia. Pediatr Radiol. 35(11):1121-4, 2005
2. Kuhn J et al: Caffey's Pediatric Diagnostic Imaging. 10th ed. Philadelphia, Mosby. 710-11, 2004
3. Laffan EE et al: Whole-body magnetic resonance imaging: a useful additional sequence in paediatric imaging. Pediatr Radiol. 34(6):472-80, 2004
4. Porto L et al: Central nervous system imaging in childhood leukaemia. Eur J Cancer. 40(14):2082-90, 2004
5. Chang YW et al: Spinal MRI of vincristine neuropathy mimicking Guillain-Barre syndrome. Pediatr Radiol. 33(11):791-3, 2003
6. Sandoval C et al: Neurotoxicity of intrathecal methotrexate: MR imaging findings. AJNR Am J Neuroradiol. 24(9):1887-90, 2003
7. Anderson SC et al: Ventral polyradiculopathy with pediatric acute lymphocytic leukemia. Muscle Nerve. 25(1):106-10, 2002
8. Beckers R et al: Acute lymphoblastic leukaemia presenting with low back pain. Eur J Paediatr Neurol. 6(5):285-7, 2002
9. Vazquez E et al: Neuroimaging in pediatric leukemia and lymphoma: differential diagnosis. Radiographics. 22(6):1411-28, 2002
10. Buckland ME et al: Spinal chloroma presenting with triplegia in an aleukaemic patient. Pathology. 33(3):386-9, 2001
11. Carriere B et al: Vertebral fractures as initial signs for acute lymphoblastic leukemia. Pediatr Emerg Care. 17(4):258-61, 2001
12. Shalaby-Rana E et al: (99m)Tc-MDP scintigraphic findings in children with leukemia: value of early and delayed whole-body imaging. J Nucl Med. 42(6):878-83, 2001
13. Yavuz H et al: Transverse myelopathy: an initial presentation of acute leukemia. Pediatr Neurol. 24(5):382-4, 2001
14. Kim HJ et al: Spinal involvement of hematopoietic malignancies and metastasis: differentiation using MR imaging. Clin Imaging. 23(2):125-33, 1999
15. Sandhu GS et al: Granulocytic sarcoma presenting as cauda equina syndrome. Clin Neurol Neurosurg. 100(3):205-8, 1998

## IMAGE GALLERY

### Variant

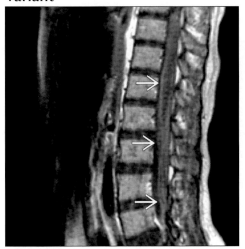
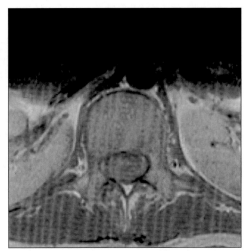

*(Left)* Sagittal T1 C+ MR demonstrates diffuse abnormal leptomeningeal and cauda equina enhancement ⇒ from disseminated intrathecal leukemic metastasis. *(Right)* Axial T1 C+ MR confirms diffuse leptomeningeal enhancement from disseminated intrathecal leukemic metastasis encircling the spinal cord and infiltrating the cauda equina.

### Variant

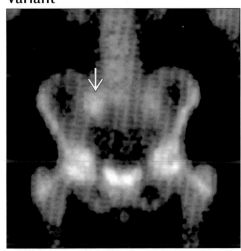
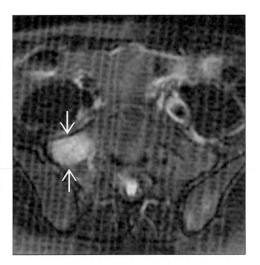

*(Left)* Coronal bone scan image of the pelvis reveals abnormal increased uptake within the right sacral ala ⇒, indicating a focal leukemic metastasis to the axial skeleton. *(Right)* Axial T2WI FS MR confirms abnormal T2 hyperintensity in the right sacral ala ⇒ from focal leukemic metastasis.

### Variant

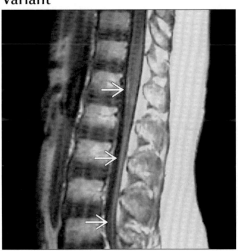
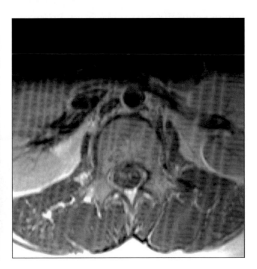

*(Left)* Sagittal T1 C+ MR demonstrate avid enhancement of anterior cord pia and ventral nerve roots ⇒ characteristic of chemotherapy-related anterior lumbar radiculopathy syndrome. *(Right)* Axial T1 C+ MR confirms that the avid enhancement of the anterior cord pia and ventral nerve roots is confined to the anterior roots only, and spares the dorsal roots.

# NEUROBLASTIC TUMOR

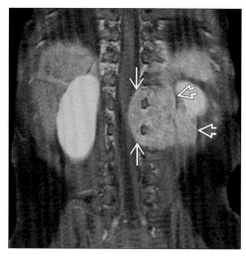 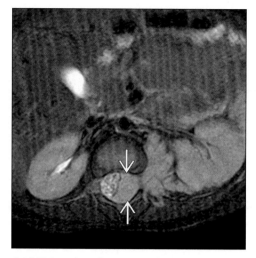

*Coronal T1 C+ FS MR shows transgression of a large paraspinal tumor ⇉ through the neural foramina into the spinal canal, producing an epidural mass ➡ and conus displacement.*

*Axial STIR MR best demonstrates the relationship of the primary paraspinal abdominal neuroblastoma and the local extension into the epidural space ⇉, compressing the thecal sac.*

## TERMINOLOGY

### Abbreviations and Synonyms
- Neuroblastic tumors (NT) = ganglioneuroma (GN), ganglioneuroblastoma (GNB), and neuroblastoma (NB)

### Definitions
- Embryonal tumors derived from neural crest cells

## IMAGING FINDINGS

### General Features
- Best diagnostic clue: Abdominal or thoracic paraspinal mass +/- intraspinal extension, calcification
- Location: Abdominal (40% adrenal, 25% paraspinal ganglia) > thoracic (15%) >, pelvic (5%) > cervical (3%); miscellaneous (12%)
- Size: Variable: 1-10 cm diameter
- Morphology: Marrow replacement, "dumbbell" paraspinal-intraspinal tumor

### CT Findings
- CECT: Enhancing paraspinal mass +/- epidural extension, finely stippled calcifications
- Bone CT
  - Widened neural foramina & intercostal spaces, pedicle erosion, adjacent rib splaying (GN, GNB) or destruction (NB)

### MR Findings
- T1WI
  - Hypointense → isointense paraspinal mass +/- epidural extension through neural foramina
  - +/- Hypointense marrow replacement
- T2WI: Hypointense → hyperintense paraspinal mass +/- epidural extension, spinal cord compression
- T1 C+: Variable enhancement +/- internal hemorrhage, necrosis

### Radiographic Findings
- Radiography
  - Widened paraspinal soft tissues +/- scoliosis
  - +/- Stippled abdominal or mediastinal calcifications

---

## DDx: Neuroblastic Tumors

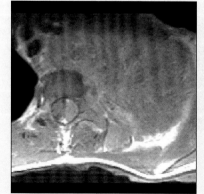 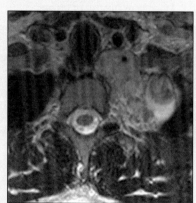 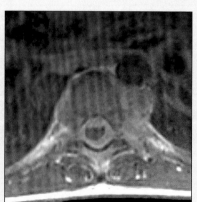

| *Ewing Sarcoma* | *Plexiform NF* | *Lymphoma* |

# NEUROBLASTIC TUMOR

## Key Facts

### Terminology
- Neuroblastic tumors (NT) = ganglioneuroma (GN), ganglioneuroblastoma (GNB), and neuroblastoma (NB)

### Imaging Findings
- Best diagnostic clue: Abdominal or thoracic paraspinal mass +/- intraspinal extension, calcification
- Location: Abdominal (40% adrenal, 25% paraspinal ganglia) > thoracic (15%) >, pelvic (5%) > cervical (3%); miscellaneous (12%)

### Top Differential Diagnoses
- Ewing Sarcoma
- Vertebral Metastasis
- Nerve Sheath Tumor

- Lymphoma
- Wilms Tumor

### Pathology
- Arise from primordial neural crest cell derivatives along sympathetic chain

### Clinical Issues
- Abdominal mass/pain, bone pain, fatigue, weight loss, blanching subcutaneous nodules
- Paraparesis/paraplegia (cord compression)

### Diagnostic Checklist
- Infants more often present with thoracic, cervical tumors; older children with abdominal tumors
- Critical to recognize epidural extension prior to surgery

## Ultrasonographic Findings
- Grayscale Ultrasound: Mixed echogenicity paraspinal mass; calcifications → posterior acoustic shadowing

## Nuclear Medicine Findings
- PET: Avid FDG uptake
- Bone Scan: Tc-99m MDP uptake in osseous metastatic lesions
- MIBG (metaiodobenzylguanidine)
  ○ Uptake by sympathetic catecholaminergic cells
    ▪ (123) I-MIBG for NB staging, post-therapy surveillance
    ▪ (131) I-MIBG shows early therapeutic promise for NB treatment

## Imaging Recommendations
- Best imaging tool
  ○ MR imaging for diagnosis, pre-surgical planning
  ○ MIBG for staging, post-treatment surveillance
- Protocol advice
  ○ Multiplanar enhanced MRI for tumor evaluation
  ○ Bone CT with multiplanar reformats to evaluate bone disease, detect calcifications
  ○ MIBG +/- bone scan for staging, surveillance

## DIFFERENTIAL DIAGNOSIS

### Ewing Sarcoma
- "Small round blue cell tumor"; relatively T2 hypointense
- Arises from adjacent flat bones (rib, chest wall, pelvis) → 2° vertebral invasion

### Vertebral Metastasis
- Variable signal intensity; imaging characteristics follow primary tumor
- Multifocal disease common

### Nerve Sheath Tumor
- Contiguous with neural foramen +/- "dumbbell" configuration

### Lymphoma
- Systemic metastasis or primary lesion; predilection for paraspinal, epidural locations

### Wilms Tumor
- Majority arise from renal parenchyma; distinctive histopathology, slightly older age facilitate distinction from NB

## PATHOLOGY

### General Features
- General path comments
  ○ Arise from primordial neural crest cell derivatives along sympathetic chain
    ▪ GN: Best differentiated, most benign, mature ganglion cells
    ▪ GNB: Intermediate malignant potential, varying proportions of neuroblastoma and mature ganglion cells
    ▪ NB: Poorly differentiated malignant "small round blue cell tumor"
- Genetics
  ○ Hereditary neuroblastoma predisposition ≤ 5% NB
  ○ 1p chromosomal deletion in 70-80% of NB patients
- Etiology: No specific environmental exposure or risk factors definitively identified
- Epidemiology: 7-10 new NB cases/1,000,000 children (US); true incidence of GNB, GN unknown because many asymptomatic
- Associated abnormalities: Orbit/skull/mandible osseous/dural metastases, "hair-on-end" periostitis, primary brain neuroblastoma (PNET)

### Gross Pathologic & Surgical Features
- GN, GNB: Firm gray-white nodules
- NB: Soft gray-tan nodules +/- hemorrhage, necrosis, calcification

### Microscopic Features
- GN: Mature ganglion cells, Schwann cells, neuritic processes

# NEUROBLASTIC TUMOR

- GNB: Internal spectrum ranging GN → NB
- NB: Undifferentiated neuroblasts, ganglion cells
  - Small uniform round blue cells containing dense hyperchromatic nuclei, scant cytoplasm
  - Homer-Wright pseudorosettes around central neuropil core (15-50%)

## Staging, Grading or Classification Criteria
- GN, GNB (intermixed-GNBi or nodular-GNBn), NB
- NB morphologic indicators: Undifferentiated (U), poorly differentiated (PD), differentiating (D)
- Evans anatomic staging for NB (prognosis: % survival)
  - Locoregional (combines stages 1-3)
    - 1: Confined to organ of interest (90%)
    - 2: Extension beyond organ but not crossing midline (75%)
    - 3: Extension crossing midline (include vertebral column) (30%)
  - Stage 4: Systemic, widespread distal metastases (10%)
  - Stage 4S: < 1 yr at diagnosis, metastatic disease confined to skin, liver, and bone marrow, may spontaneously regress (nearly 100% survival)

## CLINICAL ISSUES

### Presentation
- Most common signs/symptoms
  - Abdominal mass/pain, bone pain, fatigue, weight loss, blanching subcutaneous nodules
  - Paraparesis/paraplegia (cord compression)
  - Other signs/symptoms
    - Diarrhea (VIP syndrome)
    - Proptosis, periorbital/conjunctival ecchymoses ("raccoon eyes")
    - Opsoclonus-myoclonus-ataxia (OMA) paraneoplastic syndrome (2-3%)
    - Horner syndrome (cervical NB)
  - Laboratory findings
    - > 90% ↑ urine homovanillic acid (HVA) and/or vanillylmandelic acid (VMA)
    - ↑ Serum neuron-specific enolase (NSE), lactic dehydrogenase (LDH), ferritin
- Clinical Profile
  - Kerner-Morrison syndrome → intractable secretory diarrhea 2° VIP secretion (GN, GNB > NB)
  - Pepper syndrome: Infant with overwhelming liver metastatic NB → respiratory compromise
  - "Blueberry muffin baby": Infant with subcutaneous metastatic NB
  - Hutchinson syndrome: Widespread bone metastasis → bone pain, limping, pathologic fractures
  - NAT mimic: Metastatic retrobulbar neuroblastoma → rapidly progressive painless proptosis, periorbital ecchymosis

### Demographics
- Age: 40% < 1 yr, 35% 1-2 yr, and 25% > 2 yr at diagnosis; rare after age 10 yr
- Gender: M > F = 1.3:1

### Natural History & Prognosis
- GN prognosis excellent after surgical resection

- GNB prognosis dependent on proportion of GN, NB
- NB 5 year survival ≈ 83% for infants, 55% for children 1-5 years, and 40% for children > 5 years
  - Favorable prognostic indicators: Locoregional, stage 4s, ↓ n-myc amplification, hyperdiploid DNA
  - Unfavorable prognostic indicators: Stage 4 disease, ocular involvement, HER2/neu oncogene over-expression, ↑ NSE/LDH/serum ferritin, ↑ urine HVA/VMA, 1p chromosomal deletion

### Treatment
- Chemotherapy, surgery, radiation, steroids

## DIAGNOSTIC CHECKLIST

### Consider
- NB presentation depends on patient age, primary site, metastatic burden, metabolically active products
- Infants more often present with thoracic, cervical tumors; older children with abdominal tumors

### Image Interpretation Pearls
- Critical to recognize epidural extension prior to surgery

## SELECTED REFERENCES

1. Navarro S et al: Prognostic value of International Neuroblastoma Pathology Classification in localized resectable peripheral neuroblastic tumors: a histopathologic study of localized neuroblastoma European Study Group 94.01 Trial and Protocol. J Clin Oncol. 24(4):695-9, 2006
2. Bourdeaut F et al: Germline mutations of the paired-like homeobox 2B (PHOX2B) gene in neuroblastoma. Cancer Lett. 228(1-2):51-8, 2005
3. Gambini C et al: Neuroblastic tumors associated with opsoclonus-myoclonus syndrome: histological, immunohistochemical and molecular features of 15 Italian cases. Virchows Arch. 442(6):555-62, 2003
4. Peuchmaur M et al: Revision of the International Neuroblastoma Pathology Classification: confirmation of favorable and unfavorable prognostic subsets in ganglioneuroblastoma, nodular. Cancer. 98(10):2274-81, 2003
5. Pfluger T et al: Integrated imaging using MRI and 123I metaiodobenzylguanidine scintigraphy to improve sensitivity and specificity in the diagnosis of pediatric neuroblastoma. AJR Am J Roentgenol. 181(4):1115-24, 2003
6. Rha SE et al: Neurogenic tumors in the abdomen: tumor types and imaging characteristics. Radiographics. 23(1):29-43, 2003
7. Lonergan GJ et al: Neuroblastoma, ganglioneuroblastoma, and ganglioneuroma: radiologic-pathologic correlation. Radiographics. 22(4):911-34, 2002
8. Siegel MJ et al: Staging of neuroblastoma at imaging: report of the radiology diagnostic oncology group. Radiology. 223(1):168-75, 2002
9. Joshi VJ: Peripheral neuroblastic tumors: pathological classification based on recommendations of international neuroblastoma committee. Pediatr and Dev Path. 3:184-99, 2000
10. Schwab et al: Neuroblastic tumors of the adrenal gland and sympathetic nervous system, Kleihues and Cavenee (eds): pathology and Genetics of tumors of the nervous system. IARC press, Lyon. 153-161, 2000

# NEUROBLASTIC TUMOR

## IMAGE GALLERY

### Typical

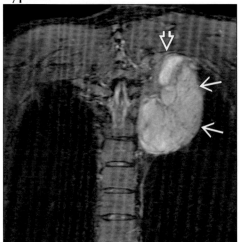

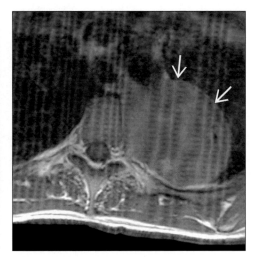

*(Left)* Coronal STIR MR depicts an intermediate signal intensity posterior mediastinal mass (ganglioneuroma ➡) that remodels an adjacent rib ➡ without marrow signal abnormality to suggest invasion. *(Right)* Axial T1 C+ MR (surgically proved ganglioneuroma) shows a left paraspinal mass ➡ with moderate heterogeneous enhancement and no adjacent rib invasion or neural foraminal encroachment.

### Typical

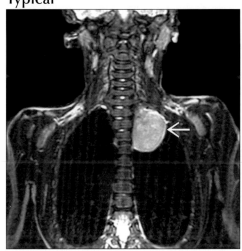

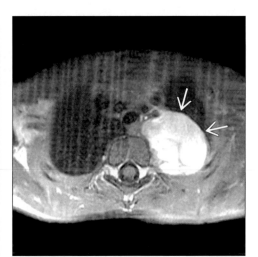

*(Left)* Coronal T2WI FS MR (ganglioneuroblastoma) depicts mildly hyperintense posterior mediastinal mass ➡ with no adjacent osseous marrow signal abnormality. *(Right)* Axial T1 C+ FS MR of posterior mediastinal ganglioneuroblastoma confirms that the well-circumscribed mass ➡ shows no gross invasion of neural foramen or spinal canal.

### Typical

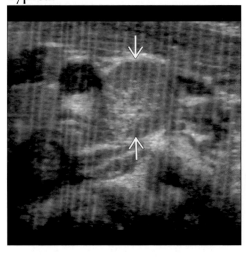

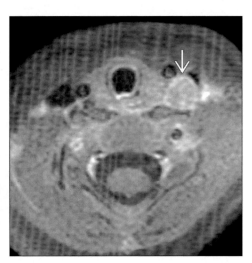

*(Left)* Axial ultrasound shows a well-circumscribed hyperechoic mass ➡ in the left carotid space. Color duplex ultrasound (not shown) confirmed prominent vascularity. *(Right)* Axial T1 C+ FS MR in same patient as previous image confirms a fusiform extradural mass in the left carotid space ➡. Surgical resection confirmed primary cervical neuroblastoma diagnosis.

# HARDWARE FAILURE

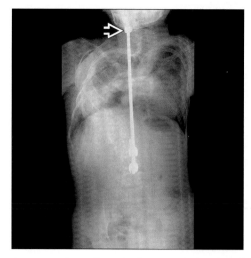 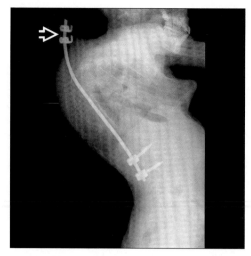

*Anteroposterior radiograph shows marked C-shaped scoliosis associated with neurofibromatosis type 1. The superior sublaminar hooks ▷ project to the right of the cervical spine.*

*Lateral radiograph demonstrates posterior displacement of the superior sublaminar hooks ▷, projecting through the skin. This was clinically obvious when the patient presented for follow-up.*

## TERMINOLOGY

### Abbreviations and Synonyms
- Spinal implant or metal failure

### Definitions
- Mechanical breakdown or hardware malfunction

## IMAGING FINDINGS

### General Features
- Best diagnostic clue: Fractured or malpositioned metallic implant
- Location: Any instrumented spinal segment

### CT Findings
- Bone CT
  - Peri-implant lucency (suggests loosening)
  - Cervical bicortical screws overextend beyond posterior vertebral cortex
  - Medial cortex penetration by suboptimally placed lumbar pedicle screw
  - Occult osseous fractures
  - Osseous nonunion, pseudoarthrosis

### MR Findings
- MR does not depict hardware location or integrity well
  - Extensive artifact from steel hardware
  - Titanium hardware produces less artifact
- MR most useful for demonstrating impact on surrounding soft tissue, cord morphology

### Radiographic Findings
- Radiography
  - Cervical spine
    - Loose cannulated screw bridging type II odontoid fracture
    - Broken or extruded screw
    - Fractured, ventrally displaced plate
    - Dislodged allograft
    - Broken or detached posterior cervical wire
  - Thoracolumbar and lumbosacral spine
    - Broken sublaminar or subpars wire
    - Bent, loose, or fractured pedicle screw
    - Disengaged hook
    - Broken or dislodged rod
    - Intervertebral cage/allograft migration
  - Pseudoarthrosis (any location)

---

## DDx: More Examples of Hardware Failure

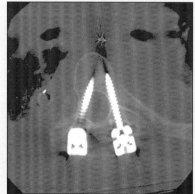 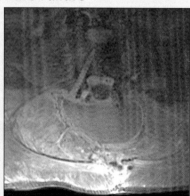 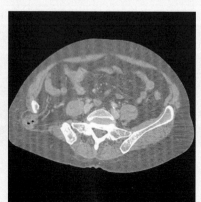

*Malpositioned Pedicle Screw* — *Post-Operative Infection* — *Hernia through Graft Harvest Site*

# HARDWARE FAILURE

## Key Facts

### Terminology
- Spinal implant or metal failure
- Mechanical breakdown or hardware malfunction

### Imaging Findings
- Best diagnostic clue: Fractured or malpositioned metallic implant
- Broken or extruded screw
- Fractured, ventrally displaced plate
- Bent, loose, or fractured pedicle screw
- Broken or dislodged rod
- Intervertebral cage/allograft migration
- Pseudoarthrosis on flexion/extension views
- 4 mm of translation or > 10° of angular motion between adjacent vertebrae
- Peri-implant lucency (suggests loosening)

- Plain films excellent for evaluating vertebral alignment, hardware integrity, fusion status
- CT evaluation if implant breakage suspected, but not definitive on radiography
- MR to identify soft tissue complications or spinal cord injury

### Pathology
- 2-45% re-operation rate for implant failure

### Clinical Issues
- Osseous fusion may occur even if hardware fails

### Diagnostic Checklist
- Important not only to evaluate hardware failure but also to look for complicating instability or osseous fracture

---

  - Lucency between bone graft and adjacent vertebra
  - Sclerosis, rounding of unfused bones
  - Development or progression of vertebral malalignment
  - Complication at graft harvest site

### Nuclear Medicine Findings
- Bone Scan
  - Increased uptake at fusion site suggests non-union
    - Nonspecific until one year after surgery

### Fluoroscopic Findings
- Pseudoarthrosis on flexion/extension views
  - 4 mm of translation or > 10° of angular motion between adjacent vertebrae
  - Up to 3 mm of translation within normal limits

### Other Modality Findings
- Anterior-posterior conventional tomogram
  - Lucency between sclerotic edges of bones suggests pseudoarthrosis

### Imaging Recommendations
- Best imaging tool
  - Plain films excellent for evaluating vertebral alignment, hardware integrity, fusion status
    - Cost-effective
    - Abnormalities frequently detected
    - Flexion extension views uncover motion when hardware failure present
  - CT evaluation if implant breakage suspected, but not definitive on radiography
    - Especially helpful with complex constructs and in osteopenic patients
    - Sagittal and coronal reformation necessary
  - MR to identify soft tissue complications or spinal cord injury
- Protocol advice
  - MR: Technique optimized to minimize susceptibility artifact
    - Low magnetic field strength
    - Fast spin echo technique, avoid gradient-echo sequences

- Higher receiver bandwidths
- Shorter TE
- Smaller voxel size
- Frequency encoding parallel to axis of hardware
  - CT: ↑ Kilovolt peaks/milliamperes to ↓ beam hardening

## DIFFERENTIAL DIAGNOSIS

None

## PATHOLOGY

### General Features
- General path comments
  - Hardware intended to stabilize fusion construct while awaiting successful osseous fusion
    - All hardware eventually fails if fusion does not occur in timely fashion
    - Fusion rate improved with direct current electrical stimulation
    - Fusion usually occurs after 6-9 months, up to 18 months
  - Fibrous union may provide satisfactory stability in absence of radiographic osseous fusion
    - Stability confirmed with dynamic flexion/extension views
- Genetics: No genetic predisposition
- Etiology
  - Excessive stress loading on implant
    - Implant malpositioning at surgery
    - Gross spinal instability
    - Failed fusion with pseudoarthrosis
  - Poor bone quality
    - Peri-implant bone resorption
    - Osteoporosis
    - Osteomyelitis
    - Residual or recurrent neoplasm
  - Multi-segmental construct
  - Unconstrained cervical fusion plates: Orozco, Casper
    - Screw not locked to plate

- ■ Risk of screw extrusion
- ○ Risks of pseudoarthrosis
  - ■ Smoking
  - ■ Obesity
  - ■ Diabetes
  - ■ Multiple spine surgeries
  - ■ Multilevel fusions
  - ■ ≥ Grade III anterolisthesis
- • Epidemiology
  - ○ 2-45% re-operation rate for implant failure
  - ○ Hardware failure in scoliosis surgery
    - ■ 31% with anterior approach
    - ■ 1% with posterior approach
  - ○ Unconstrained cervical fusion system
    - ■ 22-46% failure rate vs. 18% in constrained system
  - ○ Lumbar fusion with unconstrained pedicle screw system
    - ■ 22% failure rate
    - ■ 75% due to pseudoarthrosis
- • Associated abnormalities
  - ○ Pseudoarthrosis
  - ○ Spinal instability
  - ○ Osseous fractures
  - ○ Dural laceration
  - ○ Nerve injury

## CLINICAL ISSUES

### Presentation

- • Most common signs/symptoms
  - ○ May be incidental finding
  - ○ Other signs/symptoms
    - ■ Pain
    - ■ Tenderness
    - ■ Weakness
    - ■ Paresthesia
    - ■ Radiculopathy
- • Clinical Profile
  - ○ Hardware failure in early post-operative period
    - ■ Indication of continued gross spinal instability
  - ○ Development or progression of neurologic symptoms
    - ■ Osseous nonunion and/or hardware failure should be suspected

### Demographics

- • Gender: No sex predilection

### Natural History & Prognosis

- • Osseous fusion may occur even if hardware fails
  - ○ Broken hardware need not be removed if spine clinically & radiographically stable
- • Fibrous union without radiographic osseous fusion may be satisfactory
  - ○ Best demonstrated on dynamic flexion/extension views
- • Repeat surgical fusion may be necessary, especially if hardware failure occurs early

### Treatment

- • Conservative observation
- • Surgical revision to prevent nonunion & instability

## DIAGNOSTIC CHECKLIST

### Consider

- • Consult references describing expected hardware appearance

### Image Interpretation Pearls

- • Important not only to evaluate hardware failure but also to look for complicating instability or osseous fracture
- • Important to consider original indication for fusion in suspected implant failure
  - ○ Failed fusion for trauma may indicate unsuspected ligamentous injury
  - ○ Failed fusion for neoplasm may indicate tumor recurrence or progression

## SELECTED REFERENCES

1. Singh SK et al: Occipitocervical reconstruction with the Ohio Medical Instruments Loop: results of a multicenter evaluation in 30 cases. J Neurosurg. 98(3 Suppl):239-46, 2003
2. Bagchi K et al: Hardware complications in scoliosis surgery. Pediatr Radiol. 32(7):465-75, 2002
3. Smith JA et al: Does instrumented anterior scoliosis surgery lead to kyphosis, pseudarthrosis, or inadequate correction in adults? Spine. 27(5):529-34, 2002
4. Apfelbaum RI et al: Direct anterior screw fixation for recent and remote odontoid fractures. J Neurosurg. 93(2 Suppl):227-36, 2000
5. Deckey JE et al: Loss of sagittal plane correction after removal of spinal implants. Spine. 25(19):2453-60, 2000
6. Glassman SD et al: The durability of small-diameter rods in lumbar spinal fusion. J Spinal Disord. 13(2):165-7, 2000
7. Geiger F et al: Complications of scoliosis surgery in children with myelomeningocele. Eur Spine J. 8(1):22-6, 1999
8. Rodgers WB et al: Occipitocervical fusions in children. Retrospective analysis and technical considerations. Clin Orthop Relat Res. (364):125-33, 1999
9. Wetzel FT et al: Hardware failure in an unconstrained lumbar pedicle screw system. A 2-year follow-up study. Spine. 24(11):1138-43, 1999
10. Lowery GL et al: The significance of hardware failure in anterior cervical plate fixation. Patients with 2- to 7-year follow-up. Spine. 15;23(2):181-6; discussion 186-7, 1998
11. Wellman BJ et al: Complications of posterior articular mass plate fixation of the subaxial cervical spine in 43 consecutive patients. Spine. 23(2):193-200, 1998
12. Shapiro SA et al: Spinal instrumentation with a low complication rate. Surg Neurol. 48(6):566-74, 1997
13. Paramore CG et al: Radiographic and clinical follow-up review of Caspar plates in 49 patients. J Neurosurg. 84(6):957-61, 1996
14. Blumenthal S et al: Complications of the Wiltse Pedicle Screw Fixation System. Spine. 18(13):1867-71, 1993
15. McLain RF et al: Early failure of short-segment pedicle instrumentation for thoracolumbar fractures. A preliminary report. J Bone Joint Surg Am. 75(2):162-7, 1993
16. Slone RM et al: Spinal fixation. Part 3. Complications of spinal instrumentation. Radiographics. 13(4):797-816, 1993

## IMAGE GALLERY

### Typical

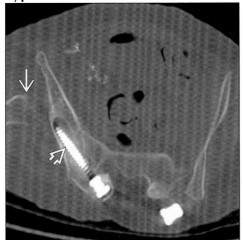
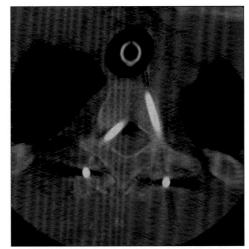

*(Left) Axial bone CT shows loosening of iliac wing screw ➡ following scoliosis hardware fixation. Note also dislocated right femoral head ➡ in myelomeningocele patient with neuromuscular scoliosis. (Right) Axial bone CT shows medial cortex penetration by suboptimally placed lumbar pedicle screw, missing the pedicle and crossing the right lateral central canal. (Courtesy S. Westra, MD).*

### Typical

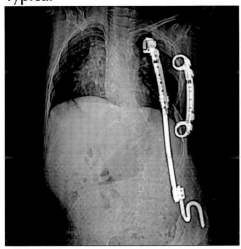
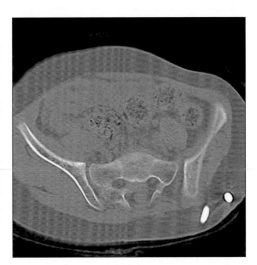

*(Left) Coronal radiograph shows two vertical expandable prosthetic titanium rib (VEPTR) devices for treatment of thoracic insufficiency. AP view fails to show posterior hardware displacement. (Right) Axial bone CT shows posterior displacement of the VEPTR device out of the iliac crest into the posterior soft tissues.*

### Typical

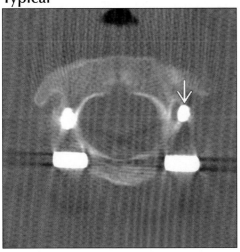
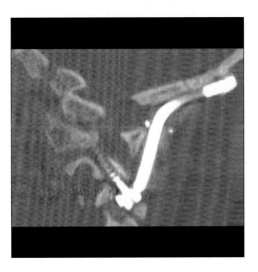

*(Left) Axial bone CT shows left C2 screw ➡ is loose, with surrounding lucency and lateral migration. (Right) Sagittal bone CT shows prominent lucency along C2 lateral mass screw placed for occipital to C2 fusion for craniovertebral junction instability.*

**III**

**6**

79

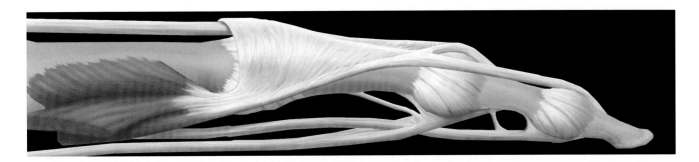

# INDEX

# INDEX

**i**

iii

# INDEX

# INDEX

# INDEX

# INDEX

i

# INDEX

# INDEX

i

# INDEX

# INDEX

# INDEX

Mitochondrial SURF1 mutations, maple syrup urine disease vs., **I:1–82i**, I:1–83

MLC. *See* Megaloencephalic leukoencephalopathy with subcortical cysts.

Molar tooth malformations, I:4–34 to I:4–37, **I:4–37i**
    Dandy Walker spectrum vs., I:4–23 to I:4–24
    differential diagnosis, **I:4–34i**, I:4–35

Morgagni syndrome of hyperostosis frontalis interna, fibrous dysplasia vs., I:6–57

Morning glory disc anomaly, coloboma vs., II:2–29

Morquio syndrome, dural dysplasia vs., **III:6–64i**

Moyamoya, I:7–30 to I:7–33, **I:7–33i**
    differential diagnosis, **I:7–30i**, I:7–31
    sickle cell disease of brain vs., I:1–145
    stroke vs., I:1–150

Mucocele, sinonasal, orbital dermoid and epidermoid cysts vs., **II:2–36i**, II:2–37

Mucolipidosis III, spinal mucopolysaccharidoses vs., III:2–43

Mucopolysaccharidoses, I:8–70 to I:8–73, **I:8–73i**
    Alexander disease vs., I:1–97
    cranial fossa "cyst-like" spaces with, glutaric aciduria type 1 vs., I:1–91
    craniovertebral junction variants vs., **III:1–12i**, III:1–13
    differential diagnosis, **I:8–70i**, I:8–71
    dural dysplasia vs., **III:6–64i**, III:6–65
    hypomyelination vs., I:1–45
    spinal, III:2–42 to III:2–45, **III:2–45i**
        congenital spinal stenosis vs., **III:2–18i**, III:2–19
        differential diagnosis, **III:2–42i**, III:2–43
        failure of vertebral formation vs., III:2–5
        kyphosis vs., **III:2–94i**
    thick skull vs., I:6–65

Multicystic encephalomalacia, porencephalic cyst vs., **I:1–192i**, I:1–193

Multifocal lesions
    hemorrhagic, diffuse axonal injury vs., **I:1–158i**, I:1–159
    nonhemorrhagic, diffuse axonal injury vs., I:1–159

Multiple sclerosis
    acute disseminated encephalomyelitis, vs., **I:1–124i**, I:1–125
    acute disseminated encephalomyelitis of spinal cord vs., **III:5–14i**, III:5–15
    idiopathic acute transverse myelitis vs., **III:5–18i**, III:5–19
    infectious, spinal cord astrocytoma vs., III:5–23
    leukodystrophies vs., I:1–50
    osmotic demyelination syndrome vs., **I:8–74i**
    pilocytic astrocytoma vs., I:4–8
    spinal cord ependymoma vs., III:5–27
    tumefactive, supratentorial PNET vs., I:1–181

Muscle-eye-brain disease, hemimegalencephaly vs., I:1–21

Muscular dystrophy, congenital, I:8–44 to I:8–47, **I:8–47i**

Muscular torticollis, fibromatosis colli vs., II:4–41

Mycobacterial adenitis, nontuberculous, first branchial apparatus anomalies vs., II:4–3

Myelin vacuolation syndromes, hypomyelination vs., **I:1–44i**, I:1–45

Myelination, normal, I:1–40 to I:1–43, **I:1–43i**. *See also* Hypomyelination.
    anatomy and imaging issues, I:1–40 to I:1–41
    and metabolic disease, I:1–40 to I:1–131

Myelitis
    autoimmune or inflammatory, spinal cord astrocytoma vs., III:5–23
    Guillain-Barré syndrome vs., III:5–11
    infectious, spinal cord astrocytoma vs., III:5–23
    transverse, idiopathic acute, III:5–18 to III:5–21, **III:5–21i**
        acute disseminated encephalomyelitis of spinal cord vs., **III:5–14i**, III:5–15
        differential diagnosis, **III:5–18i**, III:5–19
        spinal cord astrocytoma vs., **III:5–22i**, III:5–23
        spinal cord ependymoma vs., **III:5–26i**, III:5–27

Myelocele, lipomyelomeningocele vs., III:6–7

Myelocystocele
    dorsal spinal meningocele vs., **III:6–52i**, III:6–53
    nonterminal, III:6–28 to III:6–31, **III:6–31i**
    terminal, III:6–32 to III:6–35, **III:6–35i**
        differential diagnosis, **III:6–32i**, III:6–33
        nonterminal myelocystocele vs., **III:6–28i**, III:6–29

Myeloma, spinal extramedullary hematopoiesis vs., III:3–19

Myelomalacia
    post-traumatic, segmental spinal dysgenesis vs., **III:6–18i**, III:6–19
    syringomyelia vs., III:5–7
    ventriculus terminalis vs., III:5–3

Myelomeningocele, III:6–2 to III:6–5, **III:6–5i**
    cervical, nonterminal myelocystocele vs., **III:6–28i**, III:6–29
    differential diagnosis, **III:6–2i**, III:6–3
    dorsal spinal meningocele vs., **III:6–52i**, III:6–53
    lipomyelomeningocele vs., **III:6–6i**, III:6–7
    terminal myelocystocele vs., **III:6–32i**, III:6–33
    tethered spinal cord vs., **III:6–24i**, III:6–25

Myositis
    due to neck infection, fibromatosis colli vs., II:4–41
    orbital, orbital cellulitis vs., II:2–41

Myxoma, odontogenic, basal cell nevus syndrome vs., **I:8–22i**, I:8–23

i

xx

# INDEX

i

xxi

# INDEX

# INDEX

i

xxiv

# INDEX

# INDEX

# INDEX

# INDEX

i

# INDEX

**i**